IMMUNO BIOLOGY

the immune system in health and disease

6th EDITION

CD-ROM IN BACK
Poc

IMM
20

IMMUNO BIOLOGY
the immune system in health and disease
6th EDITION

Charles A. Janeway, Jr.
Yale University School of Medicine

Paul Travers
Anthony Nolan Research Institute, London

Mark Walport
Wellcome Trust, London

Mark J. Shlomchik
Yale University School of Medicine

Garland Science
Taylor & Francis Group
NEW YORK AND LONDON

CHURCHILL
LIVINGSTONE

Vice President:	Denise Schanck
Text Editor:	Eleanor Lawrence
Senior Publisher:	Jackie Harbor
Editorial Assistants:	Emma Catherall & Sbita Reandi
Production Editor:	Georgia Bushell
New Media Editor:	Michael Morales
Copyeditor:	Bruce Goatly
Indexer:	Merrall-Ross International Ltd
Illustration and Layout:	Matthew McClements, Blink Studio Ltd
Manufacturing:	Andrea Bosher & Georgia Bushell

Immunobiology Interactive:

Storyboards by:	Paul Travers
Narrated by:	Julie Theriot
Animations, Interface Design & Programming:	Matthew McClements & Tom McElderry, Blink Studio Ltd

Distributors:

Inside North America: Garland Science Publishing, 29 West 35th Street, New York, NY 10001-2299, USA.

Inside Japan: Nankodo Co. Ltd., 42-6, Hongo 3-Chrome, Bunkyo-ku, Tokyo, 113-8410, Japan.

Outside North America and Japan: Elsevier Ltd, Books Customer Services, Linacre House, Jordan Hill, Oxford, OX2 8DP, UK.

ISBN 0 8153 4101 6 (paperback) Garland Science Publishing
ISBN 0 4430 7310 4 (paperback) Churchill Livingstone
ISBN 0 4430 7309 0 (paperback) Churchill Livingstone International Student Edition

Library of Congress Cataloging-in-Publication Data
Immunobiology : the immune system in health and disease / Charles A. Janeway, Jr. .. [et al.].-- 6th ed.
    p. cm.
Includes bibliographical references and index.
 ISBN 0-8153-4101-6 (pbk.) -- ISBN 0-443-07310-4 (pbk.) -- ISBN 0-443-07309-0 (pbk.)
1. Immunology. 2. Immunity. I. Janeway, Charles.
QR181.I397 2005
616.07'9--dc22

2004007144

Published by Garland Science Publishing, a member of the Taylor & Francis Group, 29 West 35th Street, New York, NY 10001-2299, USA and 4 Park Square, Milton Park, Abingdon, Oxon, OX14 4RN, UK.

Printed in the United States of America.
15 14 13 12 11 10 9 8 7 6 5 4 3 2 1

In Memoriam
Charles Alderson Janeway Jr.
1943–2003

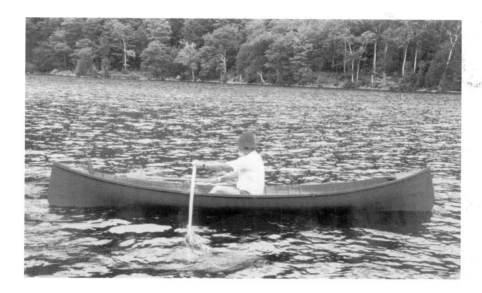

During the course of revising this edition of *Immunobiology*, to all our great sadness, Charlie Janeway died, having fought a long and hard battle against cancer. The photograph above he supplied for the launch of the first edition of *Immunobiology*, and shows him as he wanted to portray himself, doing one of the things he loved; visitors to his office in New Haven will all recognize the Adirondack guide boat whose plans had a prominent place on his wall. In this, as in so many ways, Charlie was a larger than life figure, from his ubiquitous red hat, to his big voice, to his even bigger intellect, and we will all miss him greatly.

Charlie was the origin of this textbook, the raw material for which was a collection of his lecture notes, and a continual inspiration for it. Charlie's vision was comprehensive. The key chapter for him—Chapter 10 in this edition—he would always refer to as "Space, Time and Architecture", in which the individual components of recognition and effector functions are brought together in a grand synthesis to show the integrated development of the immune response from the initial contact of pathogens with the innate immune system through to the generation of adaptive immune memory. The recognition of the importance of the spatial and temporal context in which immune responses develop, together with the understanding of the key role of innate immunity in initiating and orchestrating the adaptive response, marked an evolutionary step in the current understanding of the immune system. His personal style and clarity of thought about immunobiology is imprinted throughout this book, and in future editions we know we will still be working with Charlie. We dedicate this edition to him.

Paul Travers
Mark Walport
Mark Shlomchik

Preface to the sixth edition

This book is intended as an introductory text for use in immunology courses for medical students, advanced undergraduate biology students, graduate students, and scientists in other fields who want to know more about the immune system. It attempts to present the field of immunology from a consistent viewpoint, that of the host's interaction with an environment containing many species of potentially harmful microbes. The justification for this approach is that the absence of one or more components of the immune system is virtually always made clear by an increased susceptibility to one or more specific infections. Thus, first and foremost, the immune system exists to protect the host from infection, and its evolutionary history must have been shaped largely by this challenge. Other aspects of immunology, such as allergy, autoimmunity, graft rejection, and immunity to tumors, are treated as variations on this basic protective function. In these cases the nature of the antigen is the major variable.

In this, the sixth edition of this book, the chapter plan remains essentially the same as in the previous edition, although the order of the topics within some of the chapters has been altered to place related material together. Each chapter has been updated to incorporate new observations that extend our knowledge and understanding of the immune system. Moreover, each chapter now ends with a number of discussion questions relating to the topics described within the chapter. These questions can be used for review or as the basis for discussion, either in class or in informal study groups. The accompanying CD-ROM, *Immunobiology Interactive*, has been expanded and enhanced.

The mechanisms of innate immunity are treated early in the book, in Chapter 2, as an important protective system in its own right and a necessary precursor to the adaptive immune response. The coverage of Toll receptors has been extended and updated to reflect the rapid progress in this field in the past three years, and the description of the different families of activating and inhibitory NK receptors has been extended to reflect the growing understanding of these. After a discussion of innate immunity the emphasis shifts to adaptive immunity, because we know far more about this subject thanks to the efforts of the vast majority of immunologists. The central theme of the subsequent text is clonal selection of lymphocytes.

As in the fifth edition we consider the two lymphoid lineages, B lymphocytes and T lymphocytes, together rather than separately, because it seems to us that common mechanisms work in both cell types. Treating them together facilitates comparison and eliminates redundancies. The first instance of common mechanisms is lymphocyte recognition of antigen by means of receptors that result from RAG-dependent rearrangement of gene segments. The second shared theme is the similar course of development of B cells and T cells from a common precursor cell, B cells in the bone marrow, and T cells in the thymus, both of which are dependent on similar stromal cells. The third parallel is the promotion of the survival of T cells by self-MHC:self-peptide ligands and of B cells by environmental and possibly self ligands. We also treat activation and signaling through B-cell and T-cell receptors together, because their similarities again outweigh their differences, and in our detailed description of signaling pathways we now include information on the interaction of the signaling pathways with the cytoskeleton that allows signals through cell surface receptors to change the shape and behaviour of immune cells. We also describe the organization of the signaling molecules within cell membranes, with new material describing lipid rafts in signaling and describing in more detail the immunological synapse—the interface between a lymphocyte and an antigen-presenting cell.

We have kept discussions of T-cell and B-cell activation and their effector functions separate, because completely different mechanisms are involved: B cells act by secreting their antigen-specific receptors in the form of antibodies, whereas T cells work by direct interaction with infected cells and by releasing cytokines that have profound effects on other cells of the immune system. Another distinction between activated B and T cells is the somatic genetic changes—somatic hypermutation and isotype switching—that B cells alone undergo.

We synthesize all of this information in Chapter 10, where we treat the immune system, including the mucosal immune system, as a single, integrated system. In this chapter, speaking in general and specific terms, we ask, "How does the immune system in healthy individuals protect its host from an infection?" This chapter pulls together much of the information learned in the individual chapters and synthesizes it into our view of the whole. In this edition we include recent advances in our understanding of the nature of immunological memory and of the signals that are required to maintain antigen-specific lymphocytes in the repertoire.

The subsequent three chapters deal mainly with how diseases such as HIV/AIDS, autoimmunity, or allergy can be caused by inherited or acquired immunodeficiencies or by failures or malfunction of immunological mechanisms. As our understanding of the causes of disease grows, so these chapters have been extended with descriptions of syndromes for which underlying gene defects have newly been identified. In particular, the chapter in which we describe autoimmunity and transplantation has been extensively revised to reflect our new understanding of the mechanisms by which self-tolerance is maintained. These chapters, which describe the failures of the immune system to maintain health, are followed by a chapter on how the immune response can be manipulated by vaccination and other means in attempts to combat not only infectious diseases, but transplant rejection and cancer as well.

The book ends with an extensively revised chapter, now Chapter 15, on the evolution of the immune system. This reflects new information that is starting to come out of genome sequencing projects, especially for those organisms that may hold clues to the origins of the vertebrate adaptive immune system.

Diseases and immunological deficiencies are cross-referenced to the fourth edition of the clinical companion text *Case Studies in Immunology* by Fred Rosen and Raif Geha (ISBN: 0815341024). This text presents major topics in

Case Studies in Immunology

immunology as background to a selection of real clinical cases that serve to reinforce and extend the basic science. A marginal icon in *Immunobiology* provides the reader with a link to the relevant Case Study, where the science is applied in a clinical setting. There are seven new cases in the fourth edition, bringing the total number to 42.

The sixth edition of *Immunobiology* includes a CD-ROM with original immunological animations based on figures in the book and videos selected from visually compelling experiments. All the animations and videos are accompanied by a voice-over narration read by Julie Theriot, Stanford University School of Medicine. The CD also contains an archive of all the figures in the book, loaded into PowerPoint® presentations. There is one presentation for each chapter of the book, and the figures follow the order of the chapter. Instructors who adopt *Immunobiology* for their course will also have access to Garland Science Classwire™*. The Classwire course management system allows instructors to build websites for their courses easily. It also serves as an online archive for instructors' resources. After registering for Classwire, instructors will be able to download all of the figures from *Immunobiology*, which are available in JPEG and PowerPoint formats, and all of the videos and animations on the CD. Additional videos and animations, not found on the CD, will be available on the book's website and on the Classwire system. Additionally, instructors may download resources from other Garland Science textbooks. Please visit the Garland Science Publishing website at www.garlandscience.com or e-mail science@garland.com for additional information on Classwire.

This book would not exist without the able efforts of the 'Garland Crew'. Emma Catherall, Georgia Bushell, Michael Morales, Sbita Reandi, and Denise Schanck have been extremely helpful to all of us and kept the book running. Many others have contributed to getting the book out. Eleanor Lawrence is our invaluable editor and substitute conscience, always wanting to get the book not just to read well, but to read correctly. The illustrations, although sketched mainly by the authors, are largely the work of Matthew McClements. The CD-ROM storyboards were created by Paul Travers and animated by Matthew McClements and Tom McElderry. Finally, we would like to acknowledge the efforts of Adam Sendroff, who markets the book in North America. All of these individuals have helped to make the book work, and we are truly grateful to them.

Paul Travers would like to thank Rose Zamoyska for her infinite patience and support over the many editions of the text. Mark Walport would like to thank his wife, Julia, and children, Louise, Robert, Emily and Fiona, for their patience and support while he was occupied by matters immunological. Mark Shlomchik would like to thank his wife, Ann Haberman, for her constant support, patience, understanding and immunological advice and his daughter, Mariel, for all of the same (save the immunological advice!). Finally, Charles Janeway's wife, Kim Bottomly, and daughters, Katherine, Hannah, and Megan, were a source of inspiration to him. We are grateful to them as well.

We would like to give great thanks to all those people who read parts or all of the chapters of the fifth edition, as well as drafts of the sixth edition, and advised us on how to make them better. They are listed by chapter on page xi. We would also like to absolve them of any responsibility for errors that are still in the text; we take full responsibility for all of them.

Charles A. Janeway, Jr
Paul Travers
Mark Walport
Mark J. Shlomchik

(*Classwire is a trademark of Chalkfree, Inc.)

Immunobiology Interactive

The *Immunobiology Interactive* CD-ROM contains figures from the book loaded into PowerPoint® presentations, one presentation for each chapter of the book. The videos and animations, which run in a self-contained interface on the CD, cover material from Chapters 4 through 11 as follows. Videos are indicated with a (V).

Section II
4.1   Somatic Recombination
5.1   MHC Class I Processing
5.2   Intracellular *Listeria* Infection (V)
5.3   MHC Class II Processing

Section III
6.1   Lipid Rafts
6.2   TCR Signaling
6.3   Activated T cell (V)
6.4   MAP Kinase
6.5   Cytokine Signaling
6.6   Chemokine Signaling
6.7   Induction of Apoptosis
6.8   Apoptosis (V)
7.1   T-Cell Development
7.2   Lymph Node Development

Section IV
8.1   T-Cell Killing
8.2   Dendritic Cell Migration
8.3   TCR–APC Interaction
8.4   Immunological Synapse (V)
8.5   T-Cell Granule Release
9.1   Phagocytosis
9.2   Complement System
10.1   The Immune Response
10.2   Rolling Adhesion
10.3   Leukocytes Rolling (V)
10.4   Leukocyte Extravasation
10.5   Chemotaxis (V)
10.6   Lymphocyte Trafficking
10.7   Lymphocyte Homing (V)
10.8   Germinal Centers

Section V
11.1   Antigenic Drift
11.2   Antigenic Shift

The videos and animations are rendered in QuickTime format and can be extracted from the CD for presentation purposes. Please see the 'Read Me' file on the CD for details.

Acknowledgments

We would like to thank the following experts who read parts or the whole of the fifth edition chapters indicated and provided us with invaluable advice in developing this sixth edition.

Chapter 1: Jonathan Howard, Institute for Genetics, University of Cologne; William E. Paul, National Institute of Allergies and Infectious Diseases.

Chapter 2: Bruce Beutler, Scripps Research Institute; Christine Biron, Brown University, Providence; Mike Carroll, Harvard University Medical School, Jason Cyster, University of California at San Francisco, Craig Gerard, Children's Hospital, Harvard Medical School; Siamon Gordon, Sir William Dunn School of Pathology, University of Oxford; Lewis Lanier, University of California at San Francisco; Robert Lehrer, University of California, Los Angeles; Jerry McGhee, University of Alabama; Ruslan Medzhitov, Howard Hughes Medical Institute, Yale University School of Medicine; Tim Springer, Harvard University Medical School; Wayne Yokoyama, Washington University in St Louis.

Chapter 3: Nicholas Gascoigne, Scripps Research Institute; Sherie Morrison, University of California at Los Angeles; Ian Wilson, Scripps Research Institute.

Chapter 4: Michael P. Cancro, University of Pennsylvania; David Schatz, Yale University School of Medicine.

Chapter 5: Pamela Bjorkman, California Institute of Technology; Peter Cresswell, Yale University School of Medicine.

Chapter 6: Michael Dustin, New York University School of Medicine; Michael Reth, Albert Ludwigs University and Max Planck Institute of Immunobiology; Arthur Weiss, Howard Hughes Medical Institute, University of California, San Francisco.

Chapter 7: Harald von Boehmer, Dana-Farber Cancer Institute, Harvard Medical School; Paul Kincade, Oklahoma Medical Research Foundation; David Nemazee, Scripps Research Institute; John Owen, Birmingham Medical School; David Schatz, Yale University School of Medicine.

Chapter 8: Tim Mosmann, University of Rochester Medical Center; Alan Sher, Laboratory of Parasitic Diseases, NIAID, NIH; Miguel J. Stadecker, Tufts Medical School, Boston; Jurg Tschopp, University of Lausanne.

Chapter 9: Pamela Bjorkman, California Institute of Technology; John Cambier, National Jewish Center for Medical Research; David Gray, Edinburgh University; Garnett Kelsoe, Duke University Medical Center, Durham; Ian MacLennan, University of Birmingham Medical School; Jeff Ravetch, The Rockefeller University, New York.

Chapter 10: Martin Bachmann, Cytos Biotechnology, Zurich; Arturo Casadevall, Albert Einstein College of Medicine, Yeshiva University; Peter Doherty, St Judes Children's Residential Hospital, Memphis; Hans Hengartner, Institute for Experimental Immunology, University of Zurich; Jerry McGhee, University of Alabama; Michael Potter, National Cancer Institute, NIH.

Chapter 11: Arturo Casadevall, Albert Einstein College of Medicine, Yeshiva University; Max Cooper, Comprehensive Cancer Center, University of Alambama; Alain Fischer, Group Hospitalier Necker-Enfants Malades, Paris; Fred Rosen, Center for Blood Research, Harvard University Medical School; Bruce Walker, Partners AIDS Research Center, Massachusetts General Hospital; Robin Weiss, Windeyer Institute of Medical Sciences, London.

Chapter 12: Bob Coffman, DNAX Research Institute of Molecular and Cellular Biology, California; Stephen J. Galli, Stanford University; Raif S. Geha, Children's Hospital, Harvard Medical School; Barry Kay, National Heart and Lung Institute, Imperial College of Science, Technology and Medicine.

Chapter 13: J. Alastair Gracie, University of Glasgow; Brian Kotzin, University of Colorado Health Sciences Center; Fadi Lakkis, Yale University; Ann Marshak Rothstein, Boston University; Herman Waldmann, University of Oxford.

Chapter 14: Erol Fikrig, Yale University School of Medicine; Richard Insel, University of Rochester Medical Center; Ashley Knights, University of Tubingen; Elias Lolis, Yale University School of Medicine; Graham Pawelec, University of Tubingen; Ellen Vitetta, University of Texas Southwestern Medical Center at Dallas.

Chapter 15
We would like to thank the following experts who helped to develop this concluding chapter: Martin Flajnik, University of Maryland, Baltimore; Gary Litman, Children's Research Institute, University of South Florida College of Medicine; Ferenc Livak, University of Maryland, Baltimore; Ruslan Medzhitov, Howard Hughes Medical Institute, Yale University School of Medicine; L. Courtney Smith, George Washington University.

Appendix III: Anne Cooke, University of Cambridge.

Appendix IV: Jason Cyster, University of California at San Francisco; Barrett Rollins, Dana Farber Cancer Institute.

Photographs

Chapter 1

Fig. 1.1 reproduced courtesy of Yale University, Harvey/John Hay Whitney Medical Library.

Fig. 1.10 center and right photographs from Clark, M. et al.: **Inoculum composition and Salmonella pathogenicity island 1 regulate M-cell invasion and epithelial destruction by Salmonella typhimurium.** *Infect. Immun.* 1998, **66**:724–731 © 1998 American Society for Microbiology.

Fig. 1.26 photographs from *PNAS* 1988, **85**:5210–5214.

Chapter 2

Fig. 2.13 photograph from Galan, J., and Zhou, D.: **Striking a balance: Modulation of the actin cytoskeleton by Salmonella.** *PNAS* 2000, **97**:8754–8761 © 2000 National Academy of Sciences, U.S.A.

Fig. 2.21 photograph from Thiel, S., and Reid, K.B.M.: **Structures and functions associated with the group of mammalian lectins containing collagen-like sequences.** *FEBS Lett.* 1989, **250**:78–84 © 1989 with permission from Elsevier.

Fig. 2.24 photograph from Lu, J.H. et al.: **Binding of the pentamer/hexamer forms of mannan-binding protein to zymosan activates the proenzyme C1r2C1s complex, of the classical pathway of complement, without involvement of C1q.** *J. Immunol.* 1990, **144**:2287–2294 © 1990 The American Association of Immunologists, Inc.

Fig. 2.35 photographs from Bhakdi, S. et al.: **Functions and relevance of the terminal complement sequence.** *Blut* 1990, **60**:309–318 © 1990 Springer-Verlag.

Fig. 2.47 model structure from Emsley, J. et al.: **Structure of pentameric human serum amyloid P component.** *Nature* 1994, 367:338–345 © 1994 Macmillan Magazines Limited.

Chapter 3

Fig. 3.1 panel a from Harris, L. et al.: **The three-dimensional structure of an impact monoclonal antibody for canine lymphoma.** *Nature* 1992, **360**:369–372 © 1992 Macmillan Magazines Limited.

Fig. 3.4 photograph from Green, N.M.: **Electron microscopy of the immunoglobulins.** *Adv. Immunol.* 1969, **11**:1–30 © 1969 with permission from Elsevier.

Fig. 3.10 from Amit, A.C. et al.: **3-Dimensional structure of an antigen-antibody complex at 2.8A resolution.** *Science* 1986, **233**:747–753 © 1986 AAAS.

Fig. 3.13 model structures from Garcia, K.C. et al.: **T cell receptor binding MHC:peptide complex.** *Science* 1996, **274**:209–219 © 1996 AAAS.

Fig. 3.18 from Jones, Y.: **CD8 and TCR binding to MHC class I.** *Nature* 1997, **387**:630–634 © 1997 Macmillan Magazines Limited.

Fig. 3.27 from Garcia, K.C. et al.: **T cell receptor binding MHC:peptide complex.** *Science* 1996, **274**:209–219 © 1996 AAAS.

Fig. 3.28 from Reinherz, E.L. et al.: **The crystal structure of a T cell receptor in complex with peptide and MHC class II.** *Science* 1999, **286**:1913–1921 © 1999 AAAS.

Chapter 4

Fig. 4.23 photographs from Davies, A.C. et al.: **On the structure of polymeric IgM.** *Eur. J. Immunol.* 1988, **18**:1001–1008 © 1988 Wiley-VCH.

Chapter 5

Fig. 5.3 bottom panel from Velarde, G. et al.: **Three dimensional structure of Transporter Associated with Antigen Processing (TAP) obtained by single particle image analysis.** *J. Biochem.* 2002, **276**:46054–46063 © 2002 American Society for Biochemistry and Molecular Biology.

Fig. 5.4 from Lowe, J. et al.: **Crystal structure of a proteosome.** *Science* 1995, **268**:533–539 © 1995 AAAS.

Fig. 5.5 from Whitby, F.G. et al.: **Structural basis for the activation of 20S proteosomes by 11s regulators.** *Nature* 2000, **408**:115–120 © 2000 Nature Publishing Group.

Fig. 5.8 model structure reprinted from Cresswell, P.: **Invariant chain structure and MHC Class II function.** *Cell* 1996, **84**:505–507 © 1996 with permission from Elsevier.

Fig. 5.19 molecular model from Fields, B. et al.: **Crystal structure of a T-cell receptor β-chain complexed with a superantigen.** *Nature* 1996, **384**:188–192 © 1996 Macmillan Magazines Limited.

Chapter 7

Fig. 7.4 photograph b from Witte, P.L.: **Relationships between B-lineage lymphocytes and stromal cells in long-term bone marrow cultures.** *Eur. J. Immunol.* 1987, **17**:1473–1484 © 1987 Wiley-VCH.

Fig. 7.11 photographs from Surh, C.D., and Sprent, J.: **T-cell apoptosis detected in situ during positive and negative selection in the thymus.** *Nature* 1994, **372**:100–103 © 1994 Macmillan Magazines Limited.

Fig. 7.34 photographs from Wack, A., and Kioussis, D.: **Direct visualization of thymocyte apoptosis in neglect, acute and steady-state negative selection.** *Int. Immunol.* 1996, **8**:1537–1548 © 1996 Oxford University Press.

Chapter 8

Fig. 8.2 fluorescent micrographs from Pierre, P., and Turley, S. et al.: **Immunofluorescence of dendritic cell migration and maturation.** *Nature* 1997, **388**:787–792 © 1997 Macmillan Magazines Limited.

Fig. 8.29 panel c from Henkart, P.A., and Martx, E. (eds): *Second International Workshop on Cell Mediated Cytotoxicity* © 1985 Kluwer/Plenum Publishers.

Fig. 8.36 panels a and b from Henkart, P.A., and Martx, E. (eds): *Second International Workshop on Cell Mediated Cytotoxicity* © 1985 Kluwer/Plenum Publishers.

Fig. 8.36 panel c from Podack, E.: **The molecular mechanism of lymphocyte-mediated tumor cell lysis.** *Immunol. Today* 1985, **6**:21–27 © 1985 with permission from Elsevier.

Chapter 9

Fig. 9.15 left panel from Szakal, A.K. et al.: **Isolated follicular dendritic cells: cytochemical antigen localization, Nomarski, SEM, and TEM morphology.** *J. Immunol.* 1985, **134**:1349–1359 © 1985 The American Association of Immunologists, Inc.

Fig. 9.15 center and right panels from Szakal, A.K. et al.: **Microanatomy of lymphoid tissue during humoral immune responses: structure function relationships.** *Ann. Rev. Immunol.* 1989, **7**:91–109 © 1989 Annual Reviews www.annualreviews.org.

Fig. 9.27 from Davis, A.C. et al.: **On the structure of polymeric IgM.** *Eur. J. Immunol.* 1988, **18**:1001–1008 © 1988 Wiley-VCH.

Chapter 11

Fig. 11.6 photographs reprinted from Kaplan, G., and Cohn, Z.A.: **The immunobiology of leprosy.** *Int. Rev. Exp. Pathol.* 1986, **28**:45–78 © 1986 with permission from Elsevier.

Fig. 11.26 data from Wei, X. et al.: **Viral dynamics in human immunodefiency virus type 1 infection.** *Nature* 1995, **373**:117–122.

Fig. 11.28 based on data from Palella, F.J. et al.: **Declining morbidity and morality among patients with advanced human immunodefiency virus infection. HIV Outpatient Study Investigators.** *N. Engl. J. Med.* 1998, **338**:853–860.

Chapter 12

Fig. 12.4 photograph from Roitt, I. et al.: *Immunology, 5th edn.* © 1998 with permission from Elsevier.

Fig. 12.20 photographs from Finotto, S. et al.: **Development of spontaneous airway changes consistent with human asthma in mice lacking T-bet.** *Science* 2002, **295**:336–338 © 2002 AAAS.

Chapter 13

Fig. 13.3 photograph from Wraith, D. et al.: **Antigen recognition in autoimmune encephalomyelitis and the potential for peptide-mediated immunotherapy.** *Cell* 1989, **59**:247–255 © 1989 with permission from Elsevier.

Chapter 14

Fig. 14.8 data from Miller, D.H. et al.: **A controlled trial of natalizumab for relapsing multiple sclerosis.** *N. Engl. J. Med.* 2003, **348**:15–23.

Fig. 14.16 photographs reprinted from Herberman, R., and Callewaert, D.: *Mechanisms of Cytotoxicity by Natural Killer Cells* © 1985 with permission from Elsevier.

Appendix 1

Fig. A.32 data from Aubert, G. et al.: **Cytomegalovirus-specific cellular immune responses and viremia in recipients of allogenic stem cell transplants.** *J. Infect. Dis.* 2001, **184**:955–963 © 2001 University of Chicago Press.

Fig. A.39 from Alizadeh, A.A. et al.: **Distinct types of diffuse large B-cell lymphoma identified by gene expression profiling.** *Nature* 2000, **403**:503–511 © 2000 Nature Publishing Group.

Contents

Detailed Contents

Part II THE RECOGNITION OF ANTIGEN

Chapter 3 Antigen Recognition by B-cell and T-cell Receptors

Chapter 4 The Generation of Lymphocyte Antigen Receptors

Part IV   THE ADAPTIVE IMMUNE RESPONSE

Chapter 8   T Cell-Mediated Immunity   319

Chapter 9   The Humoral Immune Response   367

Part V · THE IMMUNE SYSTEM IN HEALTH AND DISEASE

Chapter 11 Failures of Host Defense Mechanisms 461

Chapter 12 Allergy and Hypersensitivity 517

PART I

AN INTRODUCTION TO IMMUNOBIOLOGY AND INNATE IMMUNITY

Basic Concepts in Immunology

1

Immunology is a relatively new science. Its origin is usually attributed to **Edward Jenner** (Fig. 1.1), who discovered in 1796 that cowpox, or vaccinia, induced protection against human smallpox, an often fatal disease. Jenner called his procedure vaccination, and this term is still used to describe the inoculation of healthy individuals with weakened or attenuated strains of disease-causing agents to provide protection from disease. Although Jenner's bold experiment was successful, it took almost two centuries for smallpox vaccination to become universal, an advance that enabled the World Health Organization to announce in 1979 that smallpox had been eradicated (Fig. 1.2), arguably the greatest triumph of modern medicine.

When Jenner introduced vaccination he knew nothing of the infectious agents that cause disease: it was not until late in the 19th century that **Robert Koch** proved that infectious diseases are caused by **microorganisms**, each one responsible for a particular disease, or **pathology**. We now recognize four broad categories of disease-causing microorganisms, or **pathogens**: these are **viruses**, **bacteria**, pathogenic **fungi**, and other relatively large and complex eukaryotic organisms collectively termed **parasites**.

The discoveries of Koch and other great 19th-century microbiologists stimulated the extension of Jenner's strategy of vaccination to other diseases. In the 1880s, **Louis Pasteur** devised a vaccine against cholera in chickens, and developed a rabies vaccine that proved a spectacular success upon its first trial in a boy bitten by a rabid dog. These practical triumphs led to a search for the mechanism of protection and to the development of the science of immunology. In the early 1890s, **Emil von Behring** and **Shibasaburo Kitasato** discovered that the serum of animals immune to diphtheria or tetanus contained a specific "antitoxic activity"—later called **antibodies**—that could confer short-lived immunity on unimmunized individuals.

A specific **immune response**, such as the production of antibodies against a particular pathogen, is known as an **adaptive immune response**, because it occurs during the lifetime of an individual as an adaptation to infection with that pathogen. In many cases, an adaptive immune response confers lifelong **protective immunity** to reinfection with the same pathogen. This distinguishes such responses from **innate immunity**, which, at the time that von Behring and Kitasato were developing serum therapy, was known chiefly

Fig. 1.1 Edward Jenner. Portrait by John Raphael Smith. Reproduced courtesy of Yale University, Harvey Cushing/John Hay Whitney Medical Library.

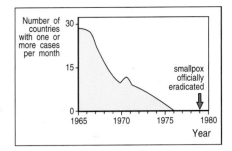

Fig. 1.2 The eradication of smallpox by vaccination. After a period of 3 years in which no cases of smallpox were recorded, the World Health Organization was able to announce in 1979 that smallpox had been eradicated, and vaccination stopped. Unfortunately, a few laboratory stocks were retained, and there are fears that the virus might have fallen into the hands of terrorists.

through the work of the great Russian immunologist **Elie Metchnikoff**. Metchnikoff discovered that many microorganisms could be engulfed and digested by **phagocytic cells**, which he called **macrophages**. These cells are immediately available to combat a wide range of pathogens without requiring prior exposure and are a key component of the innate immune system. Antibodies, by contrast, are produced only after infection, and such antibodies are specific for the infecting pathogen. The antibodies present in a given person therefore directly reflect the infections to which he or she has been exposed.

Indeed, it quickly became clear that specific antibodies can be induced against a vast range of substances. Such substances are known as **antigens** because they can stimulate *anti*body *gen*eration. We shall see, however, that not all adaptive immune responses entail the production of antibodies, and the term antigen is now used in a broader sense to describe any substance that can be recognized by the adaptive immune system.

Both innate immunity and adaptive immune responses depend upon the activities of white blood cells, or **leukocytes**. Innate immunity largely involves **granulocytes** and macrophages. Granulocytes, also called **polymorphonuclear leukocytes**, are a diverse collection of white blood cells whose prominent granules give them their characteristic staining patterns; they include the **neutrophils**, which are phagocytic. The macrophages of humans and other vertebrates are presumed to be the direct evolutionary descendants of the phagocytic cells present in simpler animals, such as those that Metchnikoff observed in sea stars. Adaptive immune responses depend upon **lymphocytes**, which provide the lifelong immunity that can follow exposure to disease or vaccination. The innate and adaptive immune systems together provide a remarkably effective defense system. It ensures that, although we spend our lives surrounded by potentially pathogenic microorganisms, we become ill only relatively rarely. Many infections are handled successfully by the innate immune system and cause no disease; others that cannot be resolved by innate immunity trigger an adaptive immune response and are then overcome successfully, followed by lasting immunological memory.

The main focus of this book will be on the diverse mechanisms of adaptive immunity, whereby specialized classes of lymphocytes recognize and target pathogenic microorganisms or the cells infected with them. We shall see, however, that the actions of the innate immune system are a prerequisite for the development of adaptive immunity and that cells involved in innate immune responses also participate in adaptive immune responses. Indeed, most of the effector actions that the adaptive immune system uses to destroy invading microorganisms depend upon linking antigen-specific recognition to the activation of effector mechanisms that are also used in innate host defense.

In this chapter, we first introduce the cells of the immune system, and the tissues in which they develop and through which they circulate or migrate. In later sections, we outline the specialized functions of the different types of cells and the mechanisms by which they eliminate infection.

The components of the immune system.

The cells of the immune system originate in the **bone marrow**, where many of them also mature. They then migrate to guard the peripheral tissues, circulating in the blood and in a specialized system of vessels called the **lymphatic system**. During this recirculation, they receive so-called 'tonic signals' via their receptors that contribute to their survival.

1-1   The white blood cells of the immune system derive from precursors in the bone marrow.

All the cellular elements of blood, including the red blood cells that transport oxygen, the platelets that trigger blood clotting in damaged tissues, and the white blood cells of the immune system, derive ultimately from the same cells—the **hematopoietic stem cells** in the bone marrow. As these stem cells can give rise to all the different types of blood cells, they are often known as pluripotent hematopoietic stem cells. Initially, they give rise to stem cells of more limited potential, which are the immediate progenitors of red blood cells, platelets, and the two main categories of white blood cells. The different types of blood cell and their lineage relationships are summarized in Fig. 1.3. We shall be concerned here with all the cells derived from the common lymphoid progenitor and the myeloid progenitor, apart from the megakaryocytes and red blood cells.

The **myeloid progenitor** is the precursor of the granulocytes, macrophages, dendritic cells, and mast cells of the innate immune system. Macrophages are one of the three types of phagocyte in the immune system and are distributed widely in the body tissues, where they play a critical part in innate immunity. They are the mature form of **monocytes**, which circulate in the blood and differentiate continuously into macrophages upon migration into the tissues. **Dendritic cells** are specialized to take up antigen, process it, and display it for recognition by T lymphocytes. Immature dendritic cells migrate from the blood to reside in the tissues and are both phagocytic and **macropinocytic**, ingesting large amounts of the surrounding extracellular fluid. They continuously migrate from the tissues bearing self antigens and induce tolerance as they lack the necessary co-stimulatory molecules. Upon encountering a pathogen, they rapidly mature, express co-stimulatory molecules, and migrate to lymph nodes.

Mast cells, whose blood-borne precursors are not well defined, also differentiate in the tissues. They mainly reside near small blood vessels and, when activated, release substances that affect vascular permeability. Although best known for their role in orchestrating allergic responses, they are believed to play a part in protecting mucosal surfaces against pathogens.

The granulocytes are so called because they have densely staining granules in their cytoplasm; they are also sometimes called polymorphonuclear leukocytes because of their oddly shaped nuclei. There are three types of granulocyte, all of which are relatively short lived, and they are produced in increased numbers during immune responses, when they leave the blood to migrate to sites of infection or inflammation. Neutrophils, which are the third phagocytic cell of the immune system, are the most numerous and most important cellular component of the innate immune response: hereditary deficiencies in neutrophil function lead to overwhelming bacterial infection, which is fatal if untreated. **Eosinophils** are thought to be important chiefly in defense against parasitic infections, because their numbers increase when the body has a parasitic infection. The function of **basophils** is probably similar and complementary to that of mast cells; we shall discuss the functions of these cells in Chapter 9 and their role in allergic inflammation in Chapter 12. The cells of the myeloid lineage are shown in Fig. 1.4.

The **common lymphoid progenitor** gives rise to the lymphocytes, with which most of this book will be concerned, and to the natural killer cells (NK cells) of innate immunity. In addition, it is also able to give rise to dendritic cells that appear indistinguishable from those derived from the common myeloid progenitor. However, as there are more common myeloid progenitors than there are common lymphoid progenitors, the majority of the dendritic cells in the body develop from common myeloid progenitors.

Fig. 1.3. All the cellular elements of the blood, including the cells of the immune system, arise from pluripotent hematopoietic stem cells in the bone marrow. These pluripotent cells divide to produce two types of stem cells—a common lymphoid progenitor that gives rise to natural killer (NK) cells and T and B lymphocytes, and a common myeloid progenitor that gives rise to different types of leukocytes (white blood cells), erythrocytes (red blood cells), and the megakaryocytes that produce platelets important in blood clotting. T and B lymphocytes are distinguished by their sites of differentiation—the thymus and bone marrow, respectively—and by the possession of antigen receptors. Mature T and B lymphocytes circulate between the blood and peripheral

lymphoid tissues. After encounter with antigen, B cells differentiate into antibody-secreting plasma cells, while T cells differentiate into effector T cells with a variety of functions. Unlike T and B cells, NK cells lack antigen specificity. The leukocytes are the monocytes, the myeloid dendritic cells, and neutrophils, eosinophils and basophils. The latter three are either termed granulocytes, because of the cytoplasmic granules whose staining gives these cells a distinctive appearance in blood smears, or polymorphonuclear leukocytes, because of their irregularly shaped nuclei. They circulate in the blood and enter tissues only at sites of infection or inflammation, to which neutrophils are recruited to phagocytose bacteria. Eosinophils and basophils are recruited to sites of allergic inflammation, and appear to be involved in defense against parasites. Immature dendritic cells travel through the blood to enter peripheral tissues. When they encounter a potential pathogen, they mature and migrate to lymphoid tissues, where they activate antigen-specific T lymphocytes. The common lymphoid progenitor also gives rise to some dendritic cells; as these are a minor subpopulation, for clarity this developmental pathway has not been illustrated. Monocytes also enter tissues, where they differentiate into phagocytic macrophages. Mast cells also complete their maturation in tissues; they are mainly important in allergic responses.

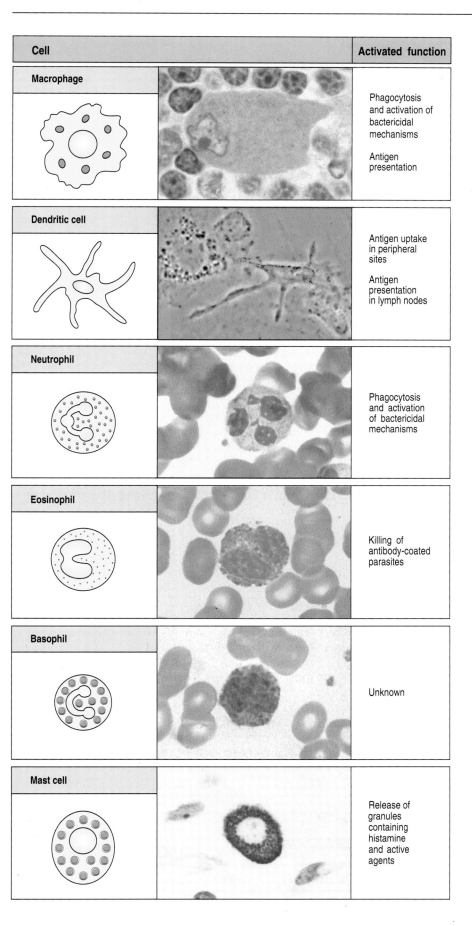

Cell		Activated function
Macrophage		Phagocytosis and activation of bactericidal mechanisms Antigen presentation
Dendritic cell		Antigen uptake in peripheral sites Antigen presentation in lymph nodes
Neutrophil		Phagocytosis and activation of bactericidal mechanisms
Eosinophil		Killing of antibody-coated parasites
Basophil		Unknown
Mast cell		Release of granules containing histamine and active agents

Fig. 1.4 Myeloid cells in innate and adaptive immunity. Cells of the myeloid lineage perform various important functions in the immune response. The cells are shown schematically on the left in the form in which they will be represented throughout the rest of the book. A photomicrograph of each cell type is shown in the center panels. Macrophages and neutrophils are primarily phagocytic cells that engulf pathogens and destroy them in intracellular vesicles, a function they perform in both innate and adaptive immune responses. Dendritic cells are phagocytic when they are immature and can take up pathogens; after maturing, they act as antigen-presenting cells to T cells, initiating adaptive immune responses. Macrophages can also present antigens to T cells and can activate them. The other myeloid cells are primarily secretory cells that release the contents of their prominent granules upon activation via antibody during an adaptive immune response. Eosinophils are thought to be involved in attacking large antibody-coated parasites such as worms, whereas the function of basophils is less clear. Mast cells are tissue cells that trigger a local inflammatory response to antigen by releasing substances that act on local blood vessels. Photographs courtesy of N. Rooney, R. Steinman, and D. Friend.

Fig. 1.5 Lymphocytes are mostly small and inactive cells. The left panel shows a light micrograph of a small lymphocyte surrounded by red blood cells. Note the condensed chromatin of the nucleus, indicating little transcriptional activity, the relative absence of cytoplasm, and the small size. The right panel shows a transmission electron micrograph of a small lymphocyte. Again, note the condensed chromatin, the scanty cytoplasm, the absence of rough endoplasmic reticulum, and other evidence of functional inactivity. Photographs courtesy of N. Rooney.

There are two major types of lymphocyte: **B lymphocytes** or **B cells**, which when activated differentiate into **plasma cells** that secrete antibodies; and **T lymphocytes** or **T cells**, of which there are two main classes. One class differentiates on activation into **cytotoxic T cells**, which kill cells infected with viruses, whereas the second class of T cells differentiates into cells that activate other cells such as B cells and macrophages.

 Most lymphocytes are small, featureless cells with few cytoplasmic organelles and much of the nuclear chromatin inactive, as shown by its condensed state (Fig. 1.5). This appearance is typical of inactive cells, and it is not surprising that, as recently as the early 1960s, textbooks could describe these cells, now the central focus of immunology, as having no known function. Indeed, these small lymphocytes have no functional activity until they encounter antigen as well as molecules induced by innate immunity known as **co-stimulatory molecules**, which provide signals necessary to trigger their proliferation and the differentiation of their specialized functional characteristics.

Lymphocytes are remarkable in being able to mount a specific immune response against virtually any foreign antigen. This is possible because each individual lymphocyte matures bearing a unique variant of a prototype antigen receptor, so that the population of T and B lymphocytes collectively bears a huge repertoire of receptors that are highly diverse in their antigen-binding sites. The **B-cell antigen receptor**, or **B-cell receptor** (**BCR**), is a membrane-bound form of the antibody that the B cell will secrete after activation and differentiation to plasma cells. Antibody molecules as a class are known as **immunoglobulins**, often shortened to **Ig**, and the antigen receptor of B lymphocytes is therefore also known as **membrane immunoglobulin** (**mIg**). The **T-cell antigen receptor**, usually simply called the **T-cell receptor** (**TCR**), is related to immunoglobulin but is quite distinct from it, as it is specially adapted to detect antigens derived from foreign proteins or pathogens that have entered into host cells. We shall describe the structures of these lymphocyte antigen receptors in detail in Chapters 3 and 4, and the way in which their diversity of binding sites is created as lymphocytes develop in Chapter 7.

Natural killer (NK) cell
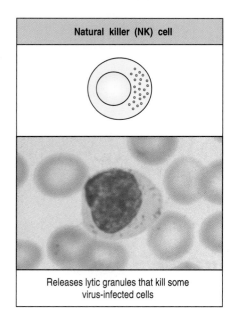
Releases lytic granules that kill some virus-infected cells

Fig. 1.6 Natural killer (NK) cells. These are large granular lymphoid-like cells with important functions in innate immunity. Although lacking antigen-specific receptors, they can detect and attack herpes virus-infected cells. Photograph courtesy of B. Smith.

A third lineage of lymphoid cells, the NK cells, lack antigen-specific receptors and are part of the innate immune system. These cells circulate in the blood as large lymphocytes with distinctive granules (Fig. 1.6). They are able to recognize and kill some abnormal cells, for example some tumor cells and cells infected with herpes viruses.

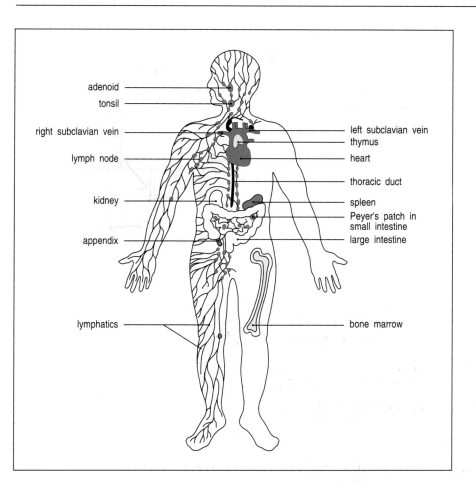

Fig. 1.7 The distribution of lymphoid tissues in the body. Lymphocytes arise from stem cells in bone marrow, and differentiate in the central lymphoid organs (yellow), B cells in bone marrow and T cells in the thymus. They migrate from these tissues and are carried in the bloodstream to the peripheral or secondary lymphoid organs (blue), the lymph nodes, spleen, and lymphoid tissues associated with mucosa, like the gut-associated tonsils, Peyer's patches, and appendix. The peripheral lymphoid organs are the sites of lymphocyte activation by antigen, and lymphocytes recirculate between the blood and these organs until they encounter their specific antigen. T cells receive survival signals from dendritic cells (DCs) in the periphery, whereas the source of the survival signals for B cells is thought to be in the lymphoid follicles. Lymphatics drain extracellular fluid from the peripheral tissues, through the lymph nodes and into the thoracic duct, which empties into the left subclavian vein. This fluid, known as lymph, carries antigen taken up by DCs and macrophages to the lymph nodes and recirculating lymphocytes from the lymph nodes back into the blood. Lymphoid tissue is also associated with other mucosa such as the bronchial linings (not shown).

1-2   Lymphocytes mature in the bone marrow or the thymus.

The **lymphoid organs** are organized tissues containing large numbers of lymphocytes in a framework of nonlymphoid cells. In these organs, the interactions lymphocytes make with nonlymphoid cells are important either to lymphocyte development, to the initiation of adaptive immune responses, or to their survival and maintenance. Lymphoid organs can be divided broadly into **central** or **primary lymphoid organs**, where lymphocytes are generated, and **peripheral** or **secondary lymphoid organs**, where adaptive immune responses are initiated and where lymphocytes are maintained. The central lymphoid organs are the bone marrow and the **thymus**, an organ in the upper chest; the location of the thymus, and of the other lymphoid organs, is shown schematically in Fig. 1.7.

Both B and T lymphocytes originate in the bone marrow, but only the B lymphocytes mature there; the precursor T lymphocytes migrate to the thymus to undergo their maturation. Thus B lymphocytes are so-called because they are bone-marrow derived, and T lymphocytes because they are thymus derived. Once they have completed their maturation, both types of lymphocyte enter the bloodstream, from which they migrate to the peripheral lymphoid organs.

1-3 The peripheral lymphoid organs are specialized to trap antigen-bearing dendritic cells, to allow initiation of adaptive immune responses, and to provide signals that sustain recirculating lymphocytes.

Pathogens can enter the body by many routes and set up an infection anywhere, but antigen and lymphocytes will eventually encounter each other in the peripheral lymphoid organs—the lymph nodes, spleen, and the mucosal lymphoid tissues (see Fig. 1.7). Lymphocytes are continually recirculating through these tissues, to which antigen is also carried from sites of infection, primarily within macrophages and dendritic cells. Within the lymphoid organs, specialized cells such as mature dendritic cells display the antigen to lymphocytes.

The **lymph nodes** are highly organized lymphoid structures located at the points of convergence of vessels of the lymphatic system, which is an extensive system that collects extracellular fluid from the tissues and returns it to the blood. This extracellular fluid is produced continuously by filtration from the blood and is called **lymph**. The vessels are **lymphatic vessels** or **lymphatics** (see Fig. 1.7). **Afferent lymphatic vessels** drain fluid from the tissues and also carry antigen-bearing cells from infected tissues to the lymph nodes, where they are trapped. In the lymph nodes, B lymphocytes are localized in **follicles**, with T cells more diffusely distributed in surrounding **paracortical areas**, also referred to as **T-cell zones**. Some of the B-cell follicles include **germinal centers**, where B cells are undergoing intense proliferation after encountering their specific antigen and their cooperating T cells (Fig. 1.8). B and T lymphocytes are segregated in a similar fashion in the other peripheral lymphoid tissues, and we shall see that this organization promotes the crucial interactions that occur between antigen-presenting cells and T cells, and between activated antigen-specific T cells and B cells upon encountering antigen.

Fig. 1.8 Organization of a lymph node. As shown in the diagram on the left, a lymph node consists of an outermost cortex and an inner medulla. The cortex is composed of an outer cortex of B cells organized into lymphoid follicles, and deep, or paracortical, areas made up mainly of T cells and dendritic cells. When an immune response is underway, some of the follicles contain central areas of intense B-cell proliferation called germinal centers and are known as secondary lymphoid follicles. These reactions are very dramatic, but eventually die out as senescent germinal centers. Lymph draining from the extracellular spaces of the body carries antigens in phagocytic dendritic cells and phagocytic macrophages from the tissues to the lymph node via the afferent lymphatics. Lymph leaves by the efferent lymphatics in the medulla. The medulla consists of strings of macrophages and antibody-secreting plasma cells known as the medullary cords. Naive lymphocytes enter the node from the bloodstream through specialized postcapillary venules (not shown) and leave with the lymph through the efferent lymphatic. The light micrograph shows a section through a lymph node, with prominent follicles containing germinal centers. Magnification × 7. Photograph courtesy of N. Rooney.

The **spleen** is a fist-sized organ just behind the stomach (see Fig. 1.7) that collects antigen from the blood. It also collects and disposes of senescent red blood cells. Its organization is shown schematically in Fig. 1.9. The bulk of the spleen is composed of **red pulp**, which is the site of red blood cell disposal. The

Fig. 1.9 Organization of the lymphoid tissues of the spleen. The schematic at top right shows that the spleen consists of red pulp (pink areas in the top panel), which is a site of red blood cell destruction, interspersed with the lymphoid white pulp. An enlargement of a small section of a mouse spleen (center) shows the arrangement of discrete areas of white pulp (yellow and blue) around central arterioles. Lymphocytes and antigen-loaded dendritic cells come together in the periarteriolar lymphoid sheath. Most of the white pulp is shown in transverse section, with two portions in longitudinal section. The bottom two schematics show enlargements of a transverse section (lower left) and longitudinal section (lower right) of white pulp. In each area of white pulp, blood carrying lymphocytes and antigen flows from a trabecular artery into a central arteriole. Cells and antigen then pass into a marginal sinus and drain into a trabecular vein. The marginal sinus is surrounded by a marginal zone of lymphocytes. Within the marginal sinus and surrounding the central arteriole is the periarteriolar lymphoid sheath (PALS), made up of T cells. The follicles consist mainly of B cells; in secondary follicles a germinal center is surrounded by a B-cell corona. Although the organization of the spleen is similar to that of a lymph node, antigen enters the spleen from the blood rather than from the lymph. The light micrograph at bottom left shows a transverse section of white pulp of human spleen immunostained for mature B cells. The main structural differences between human and mouse spleen are that there is no marginal sinus between the follicular B-cell corona (Co) and the marginal zone (MZ), the marginal zone surrounds the lymphoid follicle only, not the periarteriolar lymphocyte sheath (PALS), and both follicle and PALS are surrounded by a perifollicular zone (PFZ). The follicular arteriole emerges in the PALS (arrowhead at bottom) traverses the follicle, goes through the marginal zone and opens into the perifollicular zone (upper arrowheads). GC, germinal center; RP, red pulp; arrowheads, central arteriole. Photograph courtesy of N.M. Milicevic.

Fig. 1.10 Organization of typical gut-associated lymphoid tissue. As the diagram on the left shows, the bulk of the tissue is B cells, organized in a large and highly active domed follicle. T cells occupy the areas between follicles. The antigen enters across a specialized epithelium made up of so-called M cells. Although this tissue looks very different from other lymphoid organs, the basic divisions are maintained. The light micrograph in the center shows a section through the gut wall. The dome of gut-associated lymphoid tissue can be seen lying beneath the epithelial tissues. The micrograph at the upper right shows the surface of the gut epithelium overlaying a dome of gut-associated lymphoid tissue. A roughly circular patch of specialized epithelial cells called follicle-associated epithelium can be distinguished, which at higher magnification, as shown in the lower right hand micrograph, contain the M cells through which antigens can pass into the gut-associated lymphoid tissues. The M cells have either a microvillus morphology (shown labeled M) or can produce membrane ruffles, as in the M cell indicated by the arrow. Center photograph courtesy of N. Rooney. Magnification × 16. Right photographs courtesy of B.H. Hirst.

lymphocytes surround the arterioles entering the organ, forming areas of **white pulp**, the inner region of which is divided into a **periarteriolar lymphoid sheath** (**PALS**), containing mainly T cells, and a flanking **B-cell corona**.

The **gut-associated lymphoid tissues** (**GALT**), which include the **tonsils**, **adenoids**, **appendix**, and specialized structures called **Peyer's patches** in the small intestine, collect antigen from the epithelial surfaces of the gastrointestinal tract. In Peyer's patches, which are the most important and highly organized of these tissues, the antigen is collected by specialized epithelial cells called **multi-fenestrated** or **M cells** (Fig. 1.10). The lymphocytes form a follicle consisting of a large central dome of B lymphocytes surrounded by smaller numbers of T lymphocytes. Similar but more diffuse aggregates of lymphocytes protect the respiratory epithelium, where they are known as **bronchial-associated lymphoid tissue** (**BALT**), and other mucosa, where they are known simply as **mucosal-associated lymphoid tissue** (**MALT**). Collectively, the mucosal immune system is estimated to contain as many lymphocytes as all the rest of the body, and they form a specialized set of cells obeying somewhat different rules than those in the peripheral lymphoid organs.

Although very different in appearance, the lymph nodes, spleen, and mucosal-associated lymphoid tissues all share the same basic architecture. Each of these tissues operates on the same principle, trapping antigen ingested by dendritic cells or macrophages from sites of infection and presenting it to migratory small lymphocytes, thus inducing adaptive immune responses. The peripheral lymphoid tissues also provide sustaining signals to the lymphocytes that do not encounter their specific antigen, so that they continue to survive and recirculate until they do encounter their specific antigen or undergo apoptosis. This is important in maintaining the correct numbers of circulating T and B lymphocytes, and ensures that only those lymphocytes with the potential to respond to foreign antigen are sustained.

1-4   Lymphocytes circulate between blood and lymph.

Small B and T lymphocytes that have matured in the bone marrow and thymus but have not yet encountered their specific antigen are referred to as **naive lymphocytes**. These cells circulate continually from the blood into the peripheral lymphoid tissues, which they enter by squeezing between the specialized endothelial cells that appear to be larger than those found elsewhere in the body and are called **high endothelial venules (HEV)**. They are then returned to the blood via the lymphatic vessels (Fig. 1.11) or, in the case of the spleen, return directly to the blood. In the event of an infection, lymphocytes that recognize the infectious agent are arrested in the lymphoid tissue, where they proliferate and differentiate into **effector cells** capable of combating the infection.

When an infection occurs in the periphery, for example, large amounts of antigen are taken up by dendritic cells and macrophages which then travel from the site of infection through the afferent lymphatic vessels into the **draining lymph nodes** (see Fig. 1.11). In the lymph nodes, these cells display the antigen to recirculating T lymphocytes, where they also help to activate antigen-specific T cells. B cells that encounter antigen as they migrate through the lymph node are also arrested and activated, with the help of some of the activated T cells. Once the antigen-specific lymphocytes have undergone a period of proliferation and differentiation, they leave the lymph nodes as effector cells through the **efferent lymphatic vessel** (see Fig. 1.8).

Because they are involved in initiating adaptive immune responses, the peripheral lymphoid tissues are not static structures but vary quite dramatically depending upon whether or not infection is present. The diffuse mucosal lymphoid tissues may appear in response to infection and then disappear, whereas the architecture of the organized tissues changes in a more defined way during an infection. For example, the B-cell follicles of the lymph nodes expand as B lymphocytes proliferate to form germinal centers (see Fig. 1.8), and the entire lymph node enlarges, a phenomenon familiarly known as swollen glands.

Summary.

Immune responses are mediated by leukocytes, which derive from precursors in the bone marrow. A pluripotent hematopoietic stem cell gives rise to the lymphocytes responsible for adaptive immunity, and also to myeloid lineages that participate in both innate and adaptive immunity. Neutrophils, eosinophils, and basophils are collectively known as granulocytes; they circulate in the blood unless recruited to act as effector cells at sites of infection and inflammation. Macrophages and mast cells complete their differentiation in the tissues where they act as effector cells in the front line of host defense and initiate inflammation. Macrophages phagocytose bacteria and recruit other phagocytic cells, the neutrophils, from the blood. Mast cells are exocytic and are thought to orchestrate the defense against parasites as well as triggering allergic inflammation; they recruit eosinophils and basophils, which are also exocytic. Dendritic cells enter the tissues as immature phagocytes where they specialize in ingesting antigens. These antigen-presenting cells subsequently migrate into lymphoid tissue. These cells collectively are key players in innate immunity.

There are two major types of lymphocyte: B lymphocytes, which mature in the bone marrow, and T lymphocytes, which mature in the thymus. The bone marrow and thymus are thus known as the central or primary lymphoid organs. Mature lymphocytes bearing antigen-specific receptors recirculate continually from the bloodstream through the peripheral or secondary lymphoid organs, returning to the bloodstream through the lymphatic vessels. Most adaptive immune responses are triggered when a recirculating T cell recognizes its specific antigen on the surface of an activated dendritic cell. The three major types of peripheral lymphoid tissue are the spleen, which collects antigens from the blood; the lymph nodes, which collect antigen

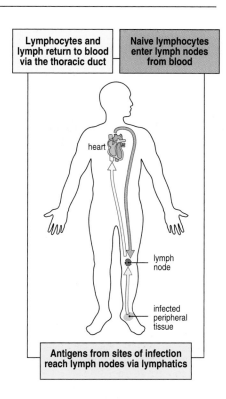

Lymphocytes and lymph return to blood via the thoracic duct

Naive lymphocytes enter lymph nodes from blood

heart

lymph node

infected peripheral tissue

Antigens from sites of infection reach lymph nodes via lymphatics

Fig. 1.11 Circulating lymphocytes encounter antigen in peripheral lymphoid organs. Naive lymphocytes recirculate constantly through peripheral lymphoid tissue, here illustrated as a lymph node behind the knee or a popliteal lymph node. Here, they may encounter their specific antigen, draining from an infected site in the foot. These so-called draining lymph nodes are the sites at which lymphocytes may become activated by encountering their specific ligand.

from sites of infection in the tissues; and the mucosal-associated lymphoid tissues, which collect antigens from the epithelial surfaces of the body. Adaptive immune responses are initiated in these peripheral lymphoid tissues: T cells that encounter antigen proliferate and differentiate into antigen-specific effector cells, while B cells, with the active help of T cells, proliferate and differentiate into antibody-secreting cells.

Principles of innate and adaptive immunity.

The macrophages and neutrophils of the innate immune system provide a first line of defense against many common microorganisms and are essential for the control of common infections. However, they cannot always eliminate infectious microorganisms. The lymphocytes of the adaptive immune system have evolved to provide a more versatile means of defense, which, in addition, provides increased protection against subsequent reinfection with the same pathogen. The cells of the innate immune system, however, play a crucial part in the initiation and subsequent direction of adaptive immune responses, as well as participating in the removal of pathogens that have been targeted by an adaptive immune response. Moreover, because there is a delay of 4–7 days before the initial adaptive immune response takes effect, the innate immune response plays a critical role in controlling infections during this period.

1-5   Most infectious agents induce inflammatory responses by activating innate immunity.

Microorganisms such as bacteria that penetrate the epithelial surfaces of the body for the first time are met immediately by cells and molecules that can mount an innate immune response. Phagocytic macrophages conduct the defense against bacteria by means of surface receptors that are able to recognize and bind common constituents of many bacterial surfaces. The same is true for viral infections, fungal infections, and infections with parasites. The cell walls of bacteria, for example, bind to these receptors and trigger the macrophage to engulf the bacterium and also induce the secretion of biologically active molecules. Activated macrophages secrete **cytokines**, which are defined as proteins released by cells that affect the behavior of other cells that bear receptors for them. They also release proteins known as **chemokines** that attract cells with specific **chemokine receptors** such as neutrophils and monocytes from the bloodstream (Fig. 1.12). The cytokines and chemokines released by macrophages in response to bacterial, viral, or fungal pathogen constituents initiate the process known as **inflammation**. Local inflammation and the phagocytosis of invading bacteria may also be triggered as a result of the activation of **complement** on the bacterial cell surface. Complement is a system of plasma proteins that activates a cascade of proteolytic reactions on microbial surfaces but not on host cells, coating these surfaces with fragments that are recognized and bound by phagocytic receptors on macrophages. This cascade of reactions also releases small peptides that contribute to inflammation.

Inflammation is traditionally defined by the four Latin words *calor*, *dolor*, *rubor*, and *tumor*, meaning heat, pain, redness, and swelling, all of which reflect the effects of cytokines and other inflammatory mediators on the local blood vessels. Dilation and increased permeability of the blood vessels during inflammation lead to increased local blood flow and the leakage of fluid, and account for the heat, redness, and swelling. Cytokines and complement

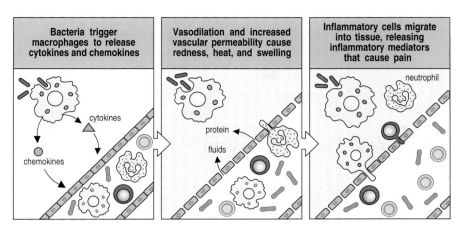

Bacteria trigger macrophages to release cytokines and chemokines	Vasodilation and increased vascular permeability cause redness, heat, and swelling	Inflammatory cells migrate into tissue, releasing inflammatory mediators that cause pain

Fig. 1.12 Infection triggers an inflammatory response. Macrophages encountering bacteria or other classes of microbes in tissues are triggered to release cytokines that increase the permeability of blood vessels, allowing fluid and proteins to pass into the tissues. They also produce chemokines, which direct the migration of neutrophils to the site of infection. The stickiness of the endothelial cells of the blood vessel wall is also changed, so that cells adhere to the wall and are able to crawl through it; first neutrophils and then monocytes are shown entering the tissue from a blood vessel. The accumulation of fluid and cells at the site of infection causes the redness, swelling, heat, and pain known collectively as inflammation. Neutrophils and macrophages are the principal inflammatory cells. Later in an immune response, activated lymphocytes can also contribute to inflammation.

fragments also have important effects on the adhesive properties of the endothelium, causing circulating leukocytes to stick to the endothelial cells of the blood vessel wall and migrate between them to the site of infection, to which they are attracted by chemokines. The migration of cells into the tissue and their local actions account for the pain. The main cell types seen in an inflammatory response in its initial phases are neutrophils, which are recruited into the inflamed, infected tissue in large numbers. Like macrophages, they have surface receptors for common bacterial constituents and for complement, and they are the principal cells that engulf and destroy the invading microorganisms. The influx of neutrophils is followed a short time later by monocytes that rapidly differentiate into macrophages. Macrophages and neutrophils are thus also known as **inflammatory cells**. Inflammatory responses later in an infection also involve lymphocytes, which have meanwhile been activated by microbial antigens that are generated in dendritic cells that have drained from the site of the infection to local lymph nodes via the afferent lymphatics.

The innate immune response makes a crucial contribution to the activation of adaptive immunity. The inflammatory response increases the flow of lymph, containing antigen in antigen-bearing cells, into lymphoid tissue, while complement fragments on microbial surfaces and induced changes in cells that have taken up microorganisms provide signals that synergize in activating lymphocytes whose receptors bind to specific microbial antigens. Macrophages that have phagocytosed bacteria and subsequently become activated can also activate T lymphocytes. However, the cells that specialize in presenting antigen to T lymphocytes and initiating adaptive immunity are the dendritic cells.

1-6   Activation of specialized antigen-presenting cells is a necessary first step for induction of adaptive immunity.

The induction of an adaptive immune response begins when a pathogen is ingested by an **immature dendritic cell** in the infected tissue. These specialized phagocytic cells are resident in most tissues and are long-lived compared to other white blood cells such as neutrophils, which live for only a few days. Most of these derive from the same myeloid precursors as macrophages, and migrate from the bone marrow to their peripheral stations, where their role is to survey the local environment for pathogens. Eventually, these tissue-resident dendritic cells migrate through the lymph to the regional lymph nodes where they interact with recirculating naive lymphocytes.

Fig. 1.13 Dendritic cells initiate adaptive immune responses. Immature dendritic cells resident in a tissue take up pathogens and their antigens by macropinocytosis and by receptor-mediated endocytosis. They are stimulated by recognition of the presence of pathogens to migrate through the lymphatics to regional lymph nodes, where they arrive as fully mature nonphagocytic dendritic cells that express both antigen and the necessary surface molecules to stimulate clonal expansion. In the lymph node, the mature dendritic cell encounters and activates antigen-specific naive T lymphocytes, which enter the node from the blood through a specialized blood vessel known from its cuboidal endothelial cells as a high endothelial venule (HEV).

| Immature dendritic cells reside in peripheral tissues | Dendritic cells migrate via afferent lymphatics to regional lymph nodes | Mature dendritic cell in the deep cortex |

The immature dendritic cell carries receptors on its surface that recognize common features of many pathogens, such as bacterial cell wall peptido-glycans. As with macrophages and neutrophils, binding of a bacterium to these receptors stimulates the dendritic cell to engulf the pathogen and degrade it intracellularly. Immature dendritic cells are also continually taking up extracellular material, including any virus particles or bacteria that may be present, by the receptor-independent mechanism of **macropinocytosis**. The function of dendritic cells, however, is not primarily to destroy pathogens but to carry pathogen antigens to peripheral lymphoid organs and there present them to T lymphocytes. When a dendritic cell takes up a pathogen in infected tissue, it becomes activated and travels to a nearby lymph node. On activation, the dendritic cell matures into a highly effective **antigen-presenting cell** (**APC**) and undergoes changes that enable it to activate pathogen-specific lymphocytes that it encounters in the lymph node (Fig. 1.13). Activated dendritic cells secrete cytokines that influence both innate and adaptive immune responses, making these cells essential gatekeepers that determine whether and how the immune system responds to the presence of infectious agents. We shall consider the maturation of dendritic cells and their central role in presenting antigens to T lymphocytes in Chapter 8.

1-7 The innate immune system provides an initial discrimination between self and nonself.

As we have described in the previous section, the activation of dendritic cells to become antigen-presenting cells is a crucial step in the activation of lymphocytes to produce an adaptive immune response. Dendritic cells, whether of the myeloid or lymphoid lineage, form part of the innate immune system and share with other cells of innate immunity families of receptors that recognize simple molecules and molecular patterns expressed by bacterial and fungal pathogens and which stimulate phagocytosis by the immature dendritic cell. Signaling through these innate immune receptors activates the dendritic cell, enabling it, in turn, to activate the naive T lymphocytes of the adaptive immune system. Thus, the adaptive immune response is essentially initiated by an explicit recognition of nonself by the innate immune system. This requirement was recognized experimentally long before the discovery of dendritic cells and their activation and signaling properties. It was found that in order to obtain adaptive immune responses to purified antigens, it was essential to add killed bacteria or bacterial extracts to the pure antigen. This additional material was termed an **adjuvant**, as it helped the response to the immunizing antigen (*adjuvare* is Latin for 'to help'). Finding suitable adjuvants is still an important part of vaccine preparation; we describe modern adjuvant formulations in Appendix I.

1-8 Lymphocytes activated by antigen give rise to clones of antigen-specific cells that mediate adaptive immunity.

The defense systems of innate immunity are effective in combating many pathogens. They are constrained, however, by relying on germline-encoded receptors to recognize microorganisms that can evolve more rapidly than the hosts they infect. This may explain why the cells and molecules of the innate immune system can only recognize microorganisms that bear surface molecules or internal structures, such as unmethylated CpG DNA, that are common to many pathogens and that have been conserved over the course of evolution. Not surprisingly, many pathogenic bacteria have evolved a protective capsule that enables them to conceal their surface molecules and thereby avoid being recognized and phagocytosed. Viruses almost always go through a phase in their life cycles where their genome is expressed as double-stranded RNA, which is recognized by a different inherited receptor. Viruses and encapsulated bacteria can, however, still be taken up by dendritic cells through the nonreceptor-dependent process of macropinocytosis. Molecules that reveal their infectious nature can then be unmasked, and the dendritic cell activated to present their antigens to lymphocytes. The recognition mechanism used by the lymphocytes of the adaptive immune response has evolved to overcome any constraints faced by the innate immune system, and this enables recognition of an almost infinite diversity of antigens, so that each different pathogen can be targeted specifically.

Instead of bearing several different receptors, each recognizing a different feature shared by many pathogens, each naive lymphocyte entering the bloodstream bears antigen receptors of a single specificity. The specificity of these receptors is determined by a unique genetic mechanism that operates during lymphocyte development in the bone marrow and the thymus to generate millions of different variants of the genes encoding the receptor molecules. Thus, although an individual lymphocyte carries receptors of only one specificity, the specificity of each lymphocyte is different. This ensures that the billions of lymphocytes in the body collectively carry millions of different antigen receptor specificities—the **lymphocyte receptor repertoire** of the individual. During a person's lifetime these lymphocytes undergo a process akin to natural selection; only those lymphocytes that encounter an antigen to which their receptor binds will be activated to proliferate and differentiate into effector cells.

This selective mechanism was first proposed in the 1950s by **Macfarlane Burnet** to explain why antibodies, which can be induced in response to virtually any antigen, are produced in each individual only to those antigens to which he or she is exposed. He postulated the pre-existence in the body of many different potential antibody-producing cells, each having the ability to make antibody of a different specificity and displaying on its surface a membrane-bound version of the antibody that served as a receptor for that antigen. On binding antigen, the cell is activated to divide and to produce many identical progeny, which are collectively known as a **clone**; these cells can now secrete **clonotypic** antibodies with a specificity identical to that of the surface receptor that first triggered activation and clonal expansion (Fig. 1.14). Burnet called this the **clonal selection theory** of antibody production.

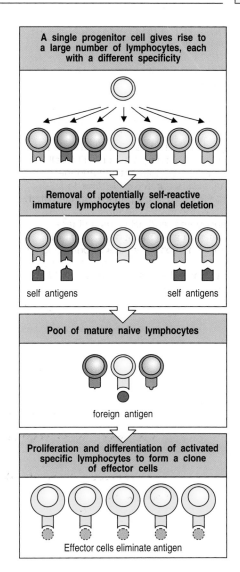

Fig. 1.14 Clonal selection. Each lymphoid progenitor gives rise to a large number of lymphocytes, each bearing a distinct antigen receptor. Lymphocytes with receptors that bind ubiquitous self antigens are eliminated before they become fully mature, ensuring tolerance to such self antigens. When a foreign antigen interacts with the receptor on a mature naive lymphocyte, that cell is activated and starts to divide. It gives rise to a clone of identical progeny, all of whose receptors bind the same antigen. Antigen specificity is thus maintained as the progeny proliferate and differentiate into effector cells. Once antigen has been eliminated by these effector cells, the immune response ceases, although some lymphocytes are retained to mediate immunological memory.

(Figure labels:)
A single progenitor cell gives rise to a large number of lymphocytes, each with a different specificity

Removal of potentially self-reactive immature lymphocytes by clonal deletion

self antigens   self antigens

Pool of mature naive lymphocytes

foreign antigen

Proliferation and differentiation of activated specific lymphocytes to form a clone of effector cells

Effector cells eliminate antigen

Fig. 1.15 The four basic principles of clonal selection.

Postulates of the clonal selection hypothesis
Each lymphocyte bears a single type of receptor with a unique specificity
Interaction between a foreign molecule and a lymphocyte receptor capable of binding that molecule with high affinity leads to lymphocyte activation
The differentiated effector cells derived from an activated lymphocyte will bear receptors of identical specificity to those of the parental cell from which that lymphocyte was derived
Lymphocytes bearing receptors specific for ubiquitous self molecules are deleted at an early stage in lymphoid cell development and are therefore absent from the repertoire of mature lymphocytes

1-9   Clonal selection of lymphocytes is the central principle of adaptive immunity.

Remarkably, at the time that Burnet formulated his theory, nothing was known of the antigen receptors of lymphocytes; indeed the function of lymphocytes themselves was still obscure. Lymphocytes did not take center stage until the early 1960s, when **James Gowans** discovered that removal of the small lymphocytes from rats resulted in the loss of all known adaptive immune responses. These immune responses were restored when the small lymphocytes were replaced. This led to the realization that lymphocytes must be the units of clonal selection, and their biology became the focus of the new field of **cellular immunology**.

Clonal selection of lymphocytes with diverse receptors elegantly explained adaptive immunity but it raised one significant conceptual problem. If the antigen receptors of lymphocytes are generated randomly during the lifetime of an individual, how are lymphocytes prevented from recognizing antigens on the tissues of the body and attacking them? **Ray Owen** had shown in the late 1940s that genetically different twin calves with a common placenta, and thus a shared placental blood circulation, were immunologically **tolerant** of one another's tissues. That is why they did not make an immune response against each other. **Peter Medawar** then showed in 1953 that exposure to foreign tissues during embryonic development caused mice to become immunologically unresponsive, or tolerant, to these tissues. Burnet proposed that developing lymphocytes that are potentially self-reactive are removed before they can mature, a process known as **clonal deletion**. He has since been proved right in this too, although the mechanisms of tolerance are still being worked out, as we shall see when we discuss the development of lymphocytes in Chapter 7.

Clonal selection of lymphocytes is the single most important principle in adaptive immunity. Its four basic postulates are listed in Fig. 1.15. The last of the problems posed by the clonal selection theory—how the diversity of lymphocyte antigen receptors is generated—was solved in the 1970s when advances in molecular biology made it possible to clone the genes encoding antibody molecules.

1-10 The structure of the antibody molecule illustrates the central puzzle of adaptive immunity.

Antibodies, as discussed above, are the secreted form of the B-cell receptor. Because they are produced in very large quantities in response to antigen, they can be studied by traditional biochemical techniques; indeed, their structure was understood long before recombinant DNA technology made it possible to study the membrane-bound antigen receptors of B lymphocytes. The startling feature that emerged from the biochemical studies was that an antibody molecule is composed of two distinct regions. One is a **constant region** that can take one of only four or five biochemically distinguishable forms; the other is a **variable region** that can be composed of an apparently infinite variety of different sequences, forming subtly different structures that allow it to bind specifically to an equally vast variety of antigens.

This division is illustrated in the simple schematic diagram in Fig. 1.16, where the antibody is depicted as a Y-shaped molecule, with the constant region shown in blue and the variable region in red. The two variable regions, which are identical in any one antibody molecule, determine the antigen-binding specificity of the antibody; the constant region determines how the antibody disposes of the pathogen once it is bound.

Each antibody molecule has a two-fold axis of symmetry and is composed of two identical heavy chains and two identical light chains (Fig. 1.17). Heavy and light chains both have variable and constant regions; the variable regions of a heavy and a light chain combine to form an antigen-binding site, so that both chains contribute to the antigen-binding specificity of the antibody molecule. The structure of antibody molecules will be described in detail in Chapter 3, and the functional properties of antibodies conferred by their constant regions will be considered in Chapters 4 and 9. For the time being, we are concerned only with the properties of antibody molecules as antigen receptors, and how the diversity of the variable regions is generated.

1-11 Each developing lymphocyte generates a unique antigen receptor by rearranging its receptor gene segments.

How are antigen receptors with an almost infinite range of specificities encoded by a finite number of genes? This question was answered in 1976, when **Susumu Tonegawa** discovered that the genes for immunoglobulin variable regions are inherited as sets of **gene segments**, each encoding a part of the variable region of one of the immunoglobulin polypeptide chains (Fig. 1.18). During B-cell development in the bone marrow, these gene segments are irreversibly joined by DNA recombination to form a stretch of DNA encoding a complete variable region. Because there are many different gene segments in each set, and different gene segments are joined together in different cells, each cell generates unique genes for the variable regions of the heavy and light chains of the immunoglobulin molecule. Once these recombination events have succeeded in producing a functional receptor, further rearrangement is prohibited. Thus each lymphocyte expresses only one receptor specificity.

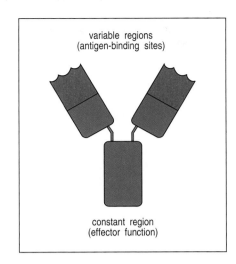

Fig. 1.16 Schematic structure of an antibody molecule. The two arms of the Y-shaped antibody molecule contain the variable regions that form the two identical antigen-binding sites. The stem can take one of only a limited number of forms and is known as the constant region. This region engages effector mechanisms that are activated by antigens to eliminate pathogens.

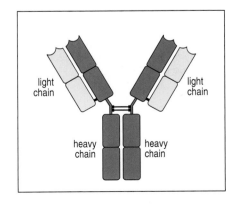

Fig. 1.17 Antibodies are made up of four protein chains. There are two types of chain in an antibody molecule: a larger chain called the heavy chain (green), and a smaller one called the light chain (yellow). Each chain has both a variable and a constant region, and there are two identical light chains and two identical heavy chains in each antibody molecule.

Inherited gene segments

Unique combination of segments becomes joined by somatic gene rearrangement

Chains pair to give a unique receptor for each lymphocyte

Fig. 1.18 The diversity of lymphocyte antigen receptors is generated by somatic gene-segment rearrangements. Different parts of the variable regions of antigen receptors are encoded by sets of gene segments. During a lymphocyte's development, one member of each set of gene segments is joined randomly to the others by an irreversible process of DNA recombination. The juxtaposed gene segments make up a complete gene that encodes the variable part of one chain of the receptor, and is unique to that cell. This random rearrangement is repeated for the set of gene segments encoding the other chain. The rearranged genes are expressed to produce the two types of polypeptide chain. These come together to form a unique antigen receptor on the lymphocyte surface. Each lymphocyte bears many copies of its unique receptor.

This mechanism has three important consequences. First, it enables a limited number of gene segments to generate a vast number of different proteins. Second, because each cell assembles a different set of gene segments, each cell expresses a unique receptor specificity. Third, because gene segment rearrangement involves an irreversible change in a cell's DNA, all the progeny of that cell will inherit genes encoding the same receptor specificity. This general scheme was later also confirmed for the genes encoding the antigen receptor on T lymphocytes. The main distinctions between B- and T-lymphocyte receptors are that the immunoglobulin that serves as the B-cell antigen receptor has two identical antigen-recognition sites and can also be secreted, whereas the T-cell antigen receptor has a single antigen-recognition site and is always a cell-surface molecule. We shall see later that these receptors also recognize antigen in very different ways.

The potential diversity of lymphocyte receptors generated in this way is enormous. Just a few hundred different gene segments can combine in different ways to generate thousands of different receptor chains. The diversity of lymphocyte receptors is further amplified by junctional diversity, created by adding or subtracting nucleotides in the process of joining the gene segments, and by the fact that each receptor is made by pairing two different variable chains, each encoded in distinct sets of gene segments. A thousand different chains of each type could thus generate 10^6 distinct antigen receptors through this **combinatorial diversity**. Thus, a small amount of genetic material can encode a truly staggering diversity of receptors. Only a subset of these randomly generated receptor specificities survive the selective processes that shape the peripheral lymphocyte repertoire; nevertheless, there are lymphocytes of at least 10^8 different specificities in an individual human at any one time. These provide the raw material on which clonal selection acts.

1-12 Development and survival of lymphocytes are determined by signals received through their antigen receptors.

Equally amazing as the generation of millions of specificities of lymphocyte antigen receptors is the shaping of this repertoire during lymphocyte development and the homeostatic maintenance of such an extensive repertoire in the periphery. How are the most useful receptor specificities selected, and how are the numbers of peripheral lymphocytes, and the percentages of B cells and T cells, kept relatively constant? The answer seems to be that lymphocyte maturation and survival are regulated by signals received through their antigen receptors. Strong signals received through the antigen receptor by an immature lymphocyte cause it to die or undergo further receptor rearrangement, and in these ways, self-reactive receptor specificities are deleted from the repertoire. However, a complete absence of signals from the antigen receptor can also lead to cell death. It seems that in order to survive, lymphocytes must periodically receive survival signals from their environment via their antigen receptors. In this way, the body can ensure that each receptor is functional, and the environment can thus regulate the number and type of lymphocytes in the population at any given time. These survival signals appear to be delivered by other cells in the lymphoid organs and must derive, at least in part, from the body's own molecules, the **self antigens**, as altering the self environment alters the life-span of lymphocytes in that environment. Developing B cells in the bone marrow interact with stromal cells, while their final maturation and continued recirculation appears to depend on survival signals received from the B-cell follicles of peripheral lymphoid tissue. T lymphocytes receive survival signals from self molecules on specialized epithelial cells in the thymus during development, and from the same or similar molecules expressed by dendritic cells in the lymphoid tissues in the periphery. The self ligands that interact with the T-cell receptor to deliver these signals are partially defined, being composed of known cell-surface molecules complexed with undefined peptides from other self proteins in the cell. These same cell-surface molecules function to present foreign antigens to T cells, as we shall explain in Section 1-17, and in Chapter 5. They select only a subset of T-cell receptors for survival, but these are the receptors most likely to be useful in responding to foreign antigens, as we shall see in Chapter 7.

Lymphocytes that fail to receive survival signals, and those that are clonally deleted because they are self-reactive, undergo a form of cell suicide called **apoptosis** or **programmed cell death**. Apoptosis, derived from a Greek word meaning the falling of leaves from the trees, occurs in all tissues, at a relatively constant rate in each tissue, and is a means of regulating the number of cells in the body. It is responsible, for example, for the death and shedding of skin cells, the turnover of liver cells, and the death of the oldest intestinal epithelial cells at the tips of the villi, that are constantly replaced by new cells formed at the base of the crypts. Thus, it should come as no surprise that immune system cells are regulated through the same mechanism. Each day the bone marrow produces many millions of new neutrophils, monocytes, red blood cells, and lymphocytes, and this production must be balanced by an equal loss of these cells. Regulated loss of all these blood cells occurs by apoptosis, and the dying cells are finally phagocytosed by specialized macrophages in the liver and spleen. Lymphocytes are a special case, because the loss of an individual naive lymphocyte means the loss of a receptor specificity from the repertoire, while each newly matured cell that survives will contribute a different specificity. The survival signals received through the antigen receptors appear to regulate this process by inhibiting the apoptosis of individual lymphocytes, thus regulating the maintenance and composition of the lymphocyte repertoire. We shall return to the question of which ligands deliver these signals, and how they contribute to shaping and maintaining the receptor repertoire, in Chapter 7.

1-13 Lymphocytes proliferate in response to antigen in peripheral lymphoid organs, generating effector cells and immunological memory.

The large diversity of lymphocyte receptors means that there will usually be at least a few that can bind to any given foreign antigen. However, because each lymphocyte has a different receptor, the numbers of lymphocytes that can bind and respond to any given antigen is very small. To generate sufficient antigen-specific effector lymphocytes to fight an infection, a lymphocyte with an appropriate receptor specificity must be activated to proliferate before its progeny finally differentiate into effector cells. This **clonal expansion** is a feature common to all adaptive immune responses. As we have seen, lymphocyte activation and proliferation is initiated in the draining lymphoid tissues, where naive lymphocytes and activated antigen-presenting cells can come together. Antigens are thus presented to the naive recirculating lymphocytes as they migrate through the lymphoid tissue before returning to the bloodstream via the efferent lymph. On recognizing its specific antigen on an activated antigen-presenting cell, a small lymphocyte stops migrating and enlarges. The chromatin in its nucleus becomes less dense, nucleoli appear, the volume of both the nucleus and the cytoplasm increases, and new mRNAs and new proteins are synthesized. Within a few hours, the cell looks completely different and is known as a **lymphoblast** (Fig. 1.19).

The lymphoblasts now begin to divide, normally duplicating themselves two to four times every 24 hours for 3 to 5 days, so that one naive lymphocyte gives rise to a clone of around 1000 daughter cells of identical specificity. These then differentiate into effector cells (see Fig. 1.19). In the case of B cells,

Fig. 1.19 Transmission electron micrographs of lymphocytes at various stages of activation to effector function. Small resting lymphocytes (top panel) have not yet encountered antigen. Note the scanty cytoplasm, the absence of rough endoplasmic reticulum, and the condensed chromatin, all indicative of an inactive cell. This could be either a T cell or a B cell. Small circulating lymphocytes are trapped in lymph nodes when their receptors encounter antigen on antigen-presenting cells. Stimulation by antigen induces the lymphocyte to become an active lymphoblast (center panel). Note the large size, the nucleoli, the enlarged nucleus with diffuse chromatin, and the active cytoplasm; again, T and B lymphoblasts are similar in appearance. This cell undergoes repeated division, which is followed by differentiation to effector function. The bottom panels show effector T and B lymphocytes. Note the large amount of cytoplasm with prominent nucleoli, abundant mitochondria, and the presence of rough endoplasmic reticulum, all hallmarks of active cells. The rough endoplasmic reticulum is especially prominent in plasma cells (effector B cells), which are synthesizing and secreting very large amounts of protein in the form of antibody. Photographs courtesy of N. Rooney.

the differentiated effector cells are the plasma cells which secrete antibody; in the case of T cells, the effector cells are able to destroy infected cells or activate other cells of the immune system. These changes also affect the recirculation of antigen-specific lymphocytes. Changes in the cell-adhesion molecules they express on their surface allow effector lymphocytes to migrate into sites of infection or stay in the lymphoid organs to activate B cells.

After a naive lymphocyte has been activated, it takes 4 to 5 days before clonal expansion is complete and the lymphocytes have differentiated into effector cells. That is why adaptive immune responses occur only after a delay of several days. Effector cells have only a limited life-span and most of the antigen-specific cells generated by the clonal expansion of small lymphocytes eventually undergo apoptosis. However, a significant number persist after antigen has been eliminated. These cells are known as **memory cells** and form the basis of **immunological memory**, which ensures a more rapid and effective response on a second encounter with a pathogen and thereby usually provides lasting protective immunity.

The characteristics of immunological memory are readily observed by comparing the antibody response of an individual to a first or **primary immunization** with the same response elicited in the same individual by a **secondary** or **booster immunization** with the same antigen. As shown in Fig. 1.20, the **secondary antibody response** occurs after a shorter lag phase, achieves a markedly higher level, and produces antibodies of higher **affinity**, or strength of binding, for the antigen. We shall describe the mechanisms of these remarkable changes in Chapters 9 and 10. The cellular basis of immunological memory is the clonal expansion and clonal differentiation of cells specific for the eliciting antigen, and it is therefore entirely antigen specific.

It is immunological memory that enables successful vaccination and prevents reinfection with pathogens that have been repelled successfully by an adaptive immune response. Immunological memory is the most important biological consequence of the development of adaptive immunity, although its cellular and molecular basis is still not fully understood, as we shall see in Chapter 10.

1-14   Interaction with other cells as well as with antigen is necessary for lymphocyte activation.

Peripheral lymphoid tissues are specialized not only to trap phagocytic cells that have ingested antigen (see Sections 1-3 and 1-6) but also to promote their interactions with lymphocytes that are needed to initiate an adaptive immune response. The spleen and lymph nodes, in particular, are highly organized for the latter function.

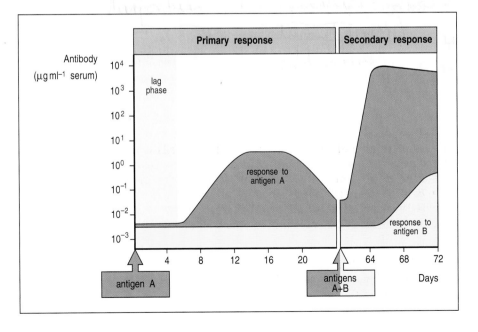

Fig. 1.20 The course of a typical antibody response. The first encounter with an antigen produces a primary response. Antigen A introduced at time zero encounters little specific antibody in the serum. After a lag phase, antibody against antigen A (blue) appears; its concentration rises to a plateau, and then gradually declines. This is typical of a primary response. When the serum is tested for antibody against another antigen, B (yellow), there is little present, demonstrating the specificity of the antibody response. When the animal is later challenged with a mixture of antigens A and B, a very rapid and intense secondary response to A occurs. This illustrates immunological memory, the ability of the immune system to make a second response to the same antigen more efficiently and effectively, providing the host with a specific defense against infection. This is the main reason for giving booster injections after an initial vaccination. Note that the response to B resembles the initial or primary response to A, as this is the first encounter of the host with antigen B.

Fig. 1.21 Two signals are required for lymphocyte activation. As well as receiving a signal through their antigen receptor, mature naive lymphocytes must also receive a second signal to become activated. For T cells (left panel), this second signal is delivered by an antigen-presenting cell such as the dendritic cell shown here. For B cells (right panel), the second signal is usually delivered by an activated T cell.

All lymphocyte responses to antigen require not only the signal that results from antigen binding to lymphocyte receptors, but also a second signal, which is delivered by another cell by means of cell-surface molecules known generally as co-stimulatory molecules. Naive T cells are usually stimulated by activated dendritic cells (Fig. 1.21, left panel) but for naive B cells (Fig. 1.21, right panel), the second signal is delivered by an activated effector T cell. Because of their ability to deliver activating signals to naive T lymphocytes, activated dendritic cells are known as antigen-presenting cells. Macrophages and B cells presenting foreign antigen on their surface can also be induced to express co-stimulatory molecules and thus can activate naive T cells. These three specialized antigen-presenting cells of the immune system are illustrated in Fig. 1.22. Dendritic cells are the most important of the three in this respect, with a central role in the initiation of adaptive immune responses (see Section 1-6). Macrophages can also mediate innate immune responses directly and make a crucial contribution to the effector phase of the adaptive immune response.

Thus, we need to add a final postulate to the clonal selection theory. A naive lymphocyte can only be activated by cells that not only bear specific antigen but also co-stimulatory molecules, whose expression is regulated by innate immunity. Contact with antigen-presenting cells that have not been induced to express these co-stimulatory molecules leads to inactivation of lymphocytes, or clonal anergy. This, in turn, helps to explain the need for microbial constituents in all effective adjuvants. We shall return to these topics in Chapter 2.

Summary.

The early innate systems of defense, which depend on invariant receptors recognizing common features of pathogens, are crucially important, but they can be overcome by many pathogens, and they do not lead to immunological memory. The abilities to recognize all pathogens specifically and to provide enhanced protection against reinfection are the unique features of adaptive immunity, which is based on clonal selection of lymphocytes bearing antigen-specific receptors. The clonal selection of lymphocytes provides a theoretical framework for understanding all the key features of an adaptive immune response. Each lymphocyte carries cell-surface receptors of a single specificity, generated by the random recombination of variable receptor gene segments and the pairing of distinct variable chains: immunoglobulin heavy and light chains, or the two chains of T-cell receptors. This process

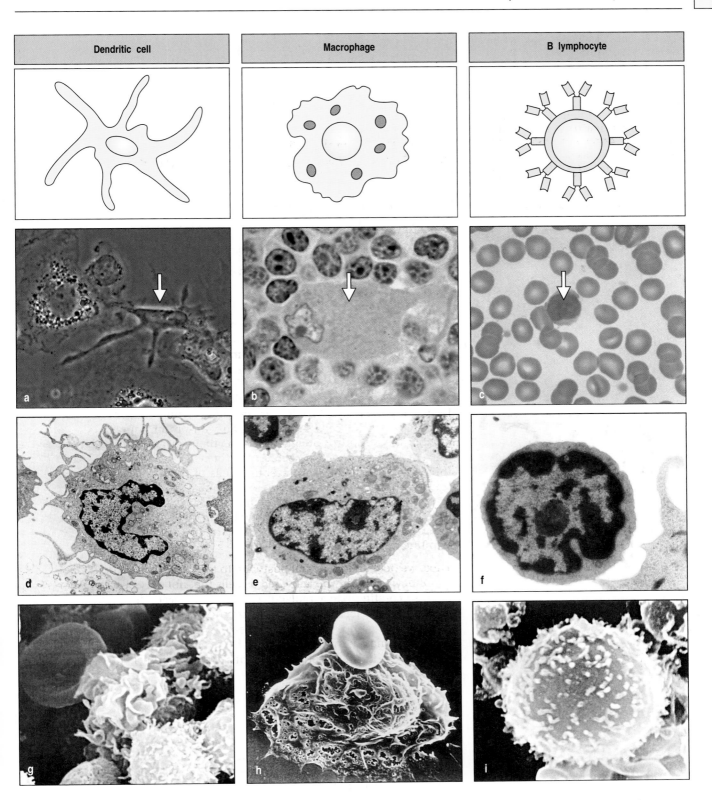

Fig. 1.22 The antigen-presenting cells. The three types of antigen-presenting cell are shown in the form in which they will be depicted throughout this book (top row), as they appear in the light microscope (second row; the relevant cell is indicated by an arrow), by transmission electron microscopy (third row) and by scanning electron microscopy (bottom row). Mature dendritic cells are found in lymphoid tissues and are derived from immature tissue dendritic cells that interact with many distinct types of pathogen. Macrophages are specialized to internalize extracellular pathogens, especially after they have been coated with antibody, and to present their antigens. B cells have antigen-specific receptors that enable them to internalize large amounts of specific antigen, process it, and present it. Photographs courtesy of R.M. Steinman (a); N. Rooney (b, c, e, f); S. Knight (d, g); and P.F. Heap (h, i).

produces lymphocytes each bearing a distinct receptor so that the total repertoire of receptors can recognize virtually any antigen. If the receptor on a lymphocyte is specific for a ubiquitous self antigen, the cell is eliminated by encountering the antigen early in its development, while survival signals received through the antigen receptor select and maintain a functional lymphocyte receptor repertoire. Adaptive immunity is initiated when an innate immune response fails to eliminate a new infection, and activated antigen-presenting cells bearing this antigen are delivered to the draining lymphoid tissues. When a recirculating lymphocyte encounters its specific foreign antigen in peripheral lymphoid tissues, it is induced to proliferate and its progeny then differentiate into effector cells that can eliminate the infectious agent. A subset of these proliferating lymphocytes differentiates into memory cells, ready to respond rapidly to the same pathogen if it is encountered again. The details of these processes of recognition, development, and differentiation form the main material of the central three parts of this book.

The recognition and effector mechanisms of adaptive immunity.

Clonal selection describes the basic operating principle of the adaptive immune response but not how it defends the body against infection. In the last part of this chapter, we outline the mechanisms by which pathogens are detected by lymphocytes and are eventually destroyed in a successful adaptive immune response. The distinct lifestyles of different pathogens require different response mechanisms, not only to ensure their destruction but also for their detection and recognition (Fig. 1.23). We have already seen that there are two different kinds of antigen receptor: the surface immunoglobulin of B cells, and the smaller antigen receptor of T cells. These surface receptors are adapted to recognize antigen in two different ways: B cells recognize antigen that is present outside the cells of the body, where, for example, most bacteria are found. T cells, by contrast, can detect antigens generated inside infected cells, for example those due to viruses.

The immune system protects against four classes of pathogen		
Type of pathogen	**Examples**	**Diseases**
Extracellular bacteria, parasites, fungi	*Streptococcus pneumoniae* *Clostridium tetani* *Trypanosoma brucei* *Pneumocystis carinii*	Pneumonia Tetanus Sleeping sickness *Pneumocystis* pneumonia
Intracellular bacteria, parasites	*Mycobacterium leprae* *Leishmania donovani* *Plasmodium falciparum*	Leprosy Leishmaniasis Malaria
Viruses (intracellular)	Variola Influenza Varicella	Smallpox Flu Chickenpox
Parasitic worms (extracellular)	*Ascaris* *Schistosoma*	Ascariasis Schistosomiasis

Fig. 1.23 The major types of pathogen confronting the immune system and some of the diseases they cause.

The **effector mechanisms** that operate to eliminate pathogens in an adaptive immune response are essentially identical to those of innate immunity. Indeed, it seems likely that specific recognition by clonally distributed receptors evolved as a late addition to existing innate effector mechanisms to produce the present-day adaptive immune response. We begin by outlining the effector actions of antibodies, which depend almost entirely on recruiting cells and molecules of the innate immune system.

1-15   Antibodies deal with extracellular forms of pathogens and their toxic products.

Antibodies, which were the first specific product of the adaptive immune response to be identified, are found in the fluid component of blood, or **plasma**, and in extracellular fluids. Because body fluids were once known as humors, immunity mediated by antibodies is known as **humoral immunity**.

As we have seen in Fig. 1.16, antibodies are Y-shaped molecules whose arms form two identical antigen-binding sites. These are highly variable from one molecule to another, providing the diversity required for specific antigen recognition. The stem of the Y, which defines the **class** of the antibody and determines its functional properties, takes one of only five major forms, or **isotypes**. Each of the five antibody classes engages a distinct set of effector mechanisms for disposing of antigen once it is recognized. We shall describe the isotypes and their actions in detail in Chapters 4 and 9.

The simplest and most direct way in which antibodies can protect from pathogens or their toxic products is by binding to them and thereby blocking their access to cells that they might infect or destroy (Fig. 1.24, left panels). This is known as **neutralization** and is important for protection against bacterial toxins and against pathogens such as viruses, which can thus be prevented from entering cells and replicating.

Binding by antibodies, however, is not sufficient on its own to arrest the replication of bacteria that multiply outside cells. In this case, one role of antibody is to enable a phagocytic cell to ingest and destroy the bacterium. This is important for the many bacteria that are resistant to direct recognition by phagocytes; instead, the phagocytes recognize the constant region of the antibodies coating the bacterium (see Fig. 1.24, middle panels). The coating of pathogens and foreign particles in this way is known as **opsonization**.

The third function of antibodies is to activate a system of plasma proteins known as **complement**. The complement system, which we shall discuss in detail in Chapter 2, can also be activated without the help of antibodies on many microbial surfaces, and therefore contributes to innate as well as adaptive immunity. The pores formed by activated complement components can directly destroy certain bacteria, and this is important in a few bacterial infections (see Fig. 1.24, right panels). However, the main function of complement, like that of the antibodies themselves, is to coat the surface of pathogens and enable phagocytes to engulf and destroy bacteria that they would otherwise not recognize. Complement also enhances the bactericidal actions of phagocytes; indeed it is so-called because it 'complements' the activities of antibodies.

Antibodies of different isotypes are found in different compartments of the body and differ in the effector mechanisms that they recruit, but all pathogens and particles bound by antibody are eventually delivered to phagocytes for ingestion, degradation, and removal from the body (see Fig. 1.24, bottom panels). The complement system and the phagocytes that antibodies recruit are not themselves antigen-specific; they depend upon antibody molecules to

Fig. 1.24 Antibodies can participate in host defense in three main ways. The left panels show antibodies binding to and neutralizing a bacterial toxin, thus preventing it from interacting with host cells and causing pathology. Unbound toxin can react with receptors on the host cell, whereas the toxin:antibody complex cannot. Antibodies also neutralize complete virus particles and bacterial cells by binding and inactivating them. The antigen:antibody complex is eventually scavenged and degraded by macrophages. Antibodies coating an antigen render it recognizable as foreign by phagocytes (macrophages and neutrophils), which then ingest and destroy it; this is called opsonization. The middle panels show opsonization and phagocytosis of a bacterial cell. The right panels show activation of the complement system by antibodies coating a bacterial cell. Bound antibodies form a receptor for the first protein of the complement system, which eventually forms a protein complex on the surface of the bacterium that, in some cases, can kill the bacterium directly. More generally, complement coating favors taking up and destroying of the bacterium by phagocytes. Thus, antibodies target pathogens and their toxic products for disposal by phagocytes.

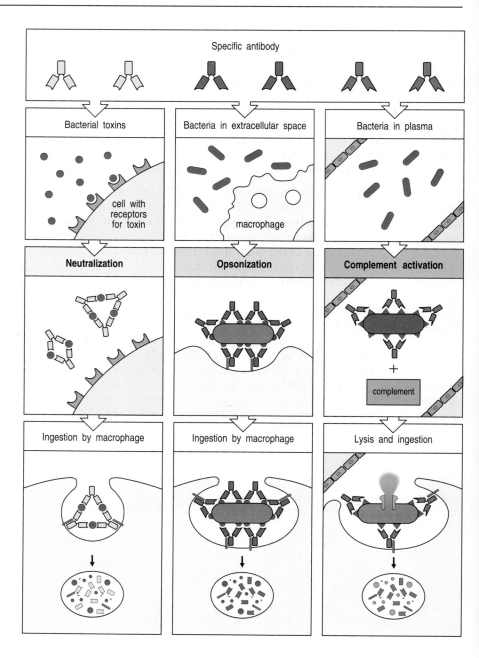

mark the particles as foreign. Producing antibodies is the sole effector function of B cells. T cells, by contrast, have a variety of effector actions.

1-16   T cells are needed to control intracellular pathogens and to activate B-cell responses to most antigens.

Pathogens are accessible to antibodies only in the blood and the extracellular spaces. However, some bacterial pathogens and parasites, and all viruses, replicate inside cells where they cannot be detected by antibodies. The destruction of these invaders is the function of the T lymphocytes, or T cells, which are responsible for the **cell-mediated immune responses** of adaptive immunity.

Cell-mediated reactions depend on direct interactions between T lymphocytes and cells bearing the antigen that the T cells recognize. The actions of cytotoxic T cells are the most direct. These recognize any of the body's cells that are infected with viruses, which replicate inside cells, using the biosynthetic machinery of the cell itself. The replicating virus eventually kills the cell, releasing new virus particles. Antigens derived from the replicating virus are, however, displayed on the surface of infected cells, where they are recognized by cytotoxic T cells. These cells can then control the infection by killing the infected cell before viral replication is complete (Fig. 1.25). Cytotoxic T cells typically express the molecule CD8 on their cell surfaces.

T lymphocytes that activate the cells they recognize are marked by the expression of the cell-surface molecule CD4 instead of CD8. CD4 T lymphocytes can be divided into two subsets, which carry out different functions in defending the body, in particular from bacterial infections. One subset of CD4 T lymphocytes is important in the control of intracellular bacterial infections. Some bacteria grow only in the intracellular membrane-bounded vesicles of macrophages; important examples are *Mycobacterium tuberculosis* and *M. leprae*, the pathogens that cause tuberculosis and leprosy. Bacteria phagocytosed by macrophages are usually destroyed in the lysosomes, which contain a variety of enzymes and antimicrobial substances. Intracellular bacteria survive because the vesicles they occupy do not fuse with the lysosomes. These infections can be controlled by a subset of CD4 T cells, known as **T$_H$1 cells**, which activate macrophages, inducing the fusion of their lysosomes with the vesicles containing the bacteria and at the same time stimulating other antibacterial mechanisms of the phagocyte (Fig. 1.26). T$_H$1 cells also release cytokines and chemokines that attract macrophages to the site of infection.

Fig. 1.25 Mechanism of host defense against intracellular infection by viruses. Cells infected by viruses are recognized by specialized T cells called cytotoxic T cells, which kill the infected cells directly. The killing mechanism involves the activation of enzymes known as caspases, which contain cysteine in their active site and cleave after aspartic acid. These in turn activate a cytosolic nuclease in the infected cell, which cleaves host and viral DNA. Panel a is a transmission electron micrograph showing the plasma membrane of a cultured CHO cell (the Chinese hamster ovary cell line) infected with influenza virus. Many virus particles can be seen budding from the cell surface. Some of these have been labeled with a monoclonal antibody that is specific for a viral protein and is coupled to gold particles, which appear as the solid black dots in the micrograph. Panel b is a transmission electron micrograph of a virus-infected cell (V) surrounded by cytotoxic T lymphocytes. Note the close apposition of the membranes of the virus-infected cell and the T cell (T) in the upper left corner of the micrograph, and the clustering of the cytoplasmic organelles in the T cell between its nucleus and the point of contact with the infected cell. Panel a courtesy of M. Bui and A. Helenius; panel b courtesy of N. Rooney.

Fig. 1.26 Mechanism of host defense against intracellular infection by mycobacteria. Mycobacteria are engulfed by macrophages but resist being destroyed by preventing fusion with lysosomes of the intracellular vesicles in which they reside, thus protecting them from being killed. However, when the phagocyte is recognized and activated by a T_H1 cell, this causes fusion of the phagocytic vesicle with lysosomes containing bactericidal agents. In resting macrophages, the mycobacteria persist and replicate in these vesicles. Macrophage activation is controlled by T_H1 cells, both to avoid tissue damage and to save energy. The light micrographs (bottom row) show resting (left) and activated (right) macrophages infected with mycobacteria. The cells have been stained with an acid-fast red dye to reveal mycobacteria. These are prominent as red-staining rods in the resting macrophages but have been eliminated from the activated macrophages. Photographs courtesy of G. Kaplan.

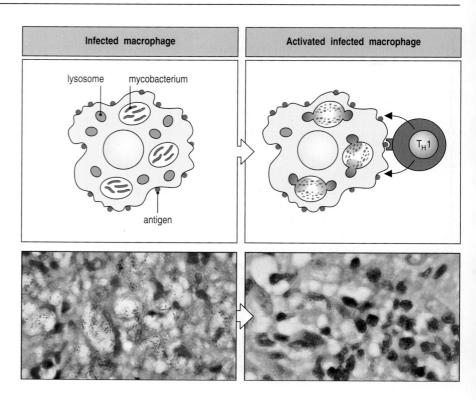

T cells carrying CD4 destroy intracellular pathogens by killing infected cells and by activating macrophages but they also have a central role in the destruction of extracellular pathogens by activating B cells. A second subset of CD4 T cells, called **T_H2 cells**, is specialized for this task. T_H2 cells are, for example, involved in stimulating B cells to produce certain classes of antibodies. We shall see in Chapter 9, when we discuss the humoral immune response in detail, that only a few antigens with special properties can activate naive B lymphocytes on their own. Most antigens require an accompanying signal from T cells before they can stimulate B cells to proliferate and differentiate into cells secreting antibody (see Fig. 1.21).

The ability of T cells to activate B cells was discovered long before it was recognized that a functionally distinct class of T cells activates macrophages, and the term 'helper T cell,' or T_H, was originally coined to describe T cells that 'help' B cells produce antibody. The designation 'helper' was later extended to all CD4 T cells, including those that activate macrophages (hence the H in T_H1). We consider this usage confusing and throughout this book we will only use the term 'helper T cell' in connection with the activation of B cells for antibody production, whether by T_H1 or T_H2 cells.

1-17   T cells are specialized to recognize foreign antigens as peptide fragments bound to proteins of the major histocompatibility complex.

All the effects of T lymphocytes depend on interactions with target cells containing foreign proteins. Cytotoxic CD8 T cells and primed T_H1 cells interact with antigens produced by pathogens that have infected the target cell or that have been ingested by it. Helper T cells, in contrast, recognize and interact with B cells that have bound and internalized foreign antigen by means of their surface immunoglobulin. In all cases, T cells recognize their targets by detecting peptide fragments derived from the foreign proteins, after these peptides have been captured by specialized molecules in the host cell and displayed by them at the cell surface. The molecules that display peptide antigen to T cells are membrane glycoproteins encoded in a cluster of genes bearing the cumbersome name **major histocompatibility complex**, which is usually abbreviated to **MHC**.

The MHC was originally identified in mice as a genetic locus controlling the acceptance or rejection of transplanted tumors, later being shown to control the acceptance or rejection of transplanted tissues in general. The human **MHC molecules** were first discovered as the result of attempts to use skin grafts from donors to repair badly burned pilots and bomb victims during World War II. The patients rejected the grafts, which were recognized as being 'foreign.' It was soon appreciated from studies in mice that this rejection was due to an immune response, and eventually genetic experiments using in-bred strains of mice showed that rapid rejection of skin grafts is caused by differences in a single genetic region. Because they control the compatibility of tissue grafts, these genes became known as 'histocompatibility genes.' Later, it was found that several closely linked and highly **polymorphic** genes specify histocompatibility, which led to the term major histocompatibility complex. The central role of the MHC in antigen recognition by T cells, which we shall discuss in Chapter 5, was discovered later still, revealing the true physiological function of the proteins encoded by the MHC. This, in turn, led to an explanation for the major effect on tissue compatibility for which they were named. We shall discuss these diverse functions of MHC molecules in Chapters 3, 5, 7, 8, and 13.

1-18   Two major types of T cell recognize peptides bound to proteins of two different classes of MHC molecule.

There are two types of MHC molecule, called MHC class I molecules and MHC class II molecules. These differ in several subtle ways but share most of their major structural features. The most important of these is formed by the two outer extracellular domains of these molecules, which combine to create a long cleft in which a single peptide fragment is trapped during the synthesis and assembly of the MHC molecule inside the cell. The MHC molecule bearing its cargo of peptide is then transported to the cell surface, where it displays the peptide to T cells (Fig. 1.27). The antigen receptors of T lymphocytes are specialized to recognize a foreign antigenic peptide bound to an MHC molecule. A T cell with a receptor specific for the complex formed between that particular foreign peptide and an MHC molecule can then recognize and respond to the antigen-presenting cell.

The most important differences between the two classes of MHC molecule lie not in their structure but in the source of the peptides that they trap and carry to the cell surface. **MHC class I molecules** collect peptides derived from proteins synthesized in the cytosol and are thus able to display fragments of viral proteins on the cell surface (Fig. 1.28). **MHC class II molecules** bind peptides derived from proteins in intracellular vesicles, and thus display

Fig. 1.27 Major histocompatibility complex (MHC) molecules on the cell surface display peptide fragments of antigens. MHC molecules are membrane proteins whose outer extracellular domains form a cleft in which a peptide fragment is bound. These fragments are derived from proteins degraded inside the cell, including both self and foreign protein antigens. The peptides are bound by the newly synthesized MHC molecule before it reaches the cell surface. There are two kinds of MHC molecule—MHC class I and MHC class II—with related but distinct structures and functions. Both MHC class I and MHC class II molecules are trimers of two protein chains and the bound self or nonself peptide.

Fig. 1.28 MHC class I molecules present antigen derived from proteins in the cytosol. In cells infected with viruses, viral proteins are synthesized in the cytosol. Peptide fragments of viral proteins are transported into the endoplasmic reticulum (ER) where they are bound by MHC class I molecules, which then deliver the peptides to the cell surface.

peptides derived from pathogens living in macrophage vesicles or internalized by phagocytic cells and B cells (Fig. 1.29). We shall see in Chapter 5 exactly how peptides from these different sources are made accessible to the two types of MHC molecule.

Having reached the cell surface with their peptide cargo, the two classes of MHC molecule are recognized by different functional classes of T cell. MHC class I molecules bearing viral peptides are recognized by CD8-bearing cytotoxic T cells, which then kill the infected cell (Fig. 1.30); MHC class II molecules bearing peptides derived from pathogens taken up into vesicles are recognized by CD4-bearing T_H1 or T_H2 cells (Fig. 1.31).

The antigen-specific activation of these effector T cells is aided by co-receptors on the T-cell surface that distinguish between the two classes of MHC molecule; cytotoxic cells express the CD8 co-receptor, which binds MHC class I molecules, whereas MHC class II specific T cells express the CD4 co-receptor, which has specificity for MHC class II molecules. However, even before T cells have encountered the specific foreign antigen that activates them to differentiate into effector cells, they express the appropriate co-receptor to match the specificity of their receptor for MHC class I or MHC class II molecules. The

Fig. 1.29 MHC class II molecules present antigen originating in intracellular vesicles. Some bacteria infect cells and grow in intracellular vesicles. Peptides derived from such bacteria are bound by MHC class II molecules and transported to the cell surface (top row). MHC class II molecules also bind and transport peptides derived from antigen that has been bound and internalized by B-cell antigen receptor-mediated uptake into intracellular vesicles (bottom row).

maturation of T cells into either CD8 or CD4 T cells reflects the testing of T-cell receptor specificity that occurs during development, and the selection of T cells that can receive survival signals from self MHC molecules in the periphery. Exactly how this selective process works, and how it maximizes the usefulness of the T-cell repertoire is a central question in immunology, and is a major topic of Chapter 7.

On recognizing their targets, the three types of T cell are stimulated to release different sets of effector molecules. These can directly affect their target cells or help to recruit other effector cells in ways we shall discuss in Chapter 8. These effector molecules include many cytokines, which have a crucial role in the clonal expansion of lymphocytes as well as in innate immune responses and in the effector actions of most cells of the immune system. Thus, understanding the actions of cytokines is central to understanding the various behaviors of the immune system. The actions of all the known cytokines are summarized in Appendix III, and of the T-cell-derived cytokines in Chapter 8.

1-19   Defects in the immune system result in increased susceptibility to infection.

We tend to take for granted the ability of our immune systems to free our bodies of infection and prevent its recurrence. In some people, however, parts of the immune system fail. In the most severe of these **immunodeficiency diseases**, adaptive immunity is completely absent, and death occurs in infancy from overwhelming infection unless heroic measures are taken. Other less catastrophic failures lead to recurrent infections with particular types of pathogen, depending on the particular deficiency. Much has been learned about the functions of the different components of the human immune system through the study of these immunodeficiencies.

More than 25 years ago, a devastating form of immunodeficiency appeared, the **acquired immune deficiency syndrome**, or **AIDS**, which is itself caused by an infectious agent. This disease destroys T cells, dendritic cells, and macrophages bearing the CD4 co-receptor, leading to infections caused by intracellular bacteria and other pathogens normally controlled by such cells. These infections are the major cause of death from this increasingly prevalent immunodeficiency disease, which is discussed fully in Chapter 11 together with inherited immunodeficiencies.

AIDS is caused by a virus, the **human immunodeficiency virus-1**, or **HIV-1**, that has evolved several strategies by which it not only evades but also subverts the protective mechanisms of the adaptive immune response. Such strategies are typical of many successful pathogens and we shall examine a

Fig. 1.30 Cytotoxic CD8 T cells recognize antigen presented by MHC class I molecules and kill the cell. The peptide:MHC class I complex on virus-infected cells is detected by antigen-specific cytotoxic T cells. Cytotoxic T cells are preprogrammed to kill the cells they recognize.

Fig. 1.31 CD4 T cells recognize antigen presented by MHC class II molecules. On recognition of their specific antigen on infected macrophages, T_H1 cells activate the macrophage, leading to the destruction of the intracellular bacteria (left panel). When T_H2 or T_H1 helper T cells recognize antigen on B cells, they activate these cells to proliferate and differentiate into antibody-producing plasma cells (right panel).

variety of them in Chapter 11. The conquest of many of the world's leading diseases, including malaria and diarrheal diseases (the leading killers of children) as well as the more recent threat from AIDS, depends upon a better understanding of the pathogens that cause them and their interactions with the cells of the immune system.

1-20   Understanding adaptive immune responses is important for the control of allergies, autoimmune disease, and organ graft rejection.

The main function of our immune system is to protect the human host from infectious agents. However, many medically important diseases are associated with a normal immune response directed against an inappropriate antigen, often in the absence of infectious disease. Immune responses directed at noninfectious antigens occur in **allergy**, where the antigen is an innocuous foreign substance, in **autoimmune disease**, where the response is to a self antigen, and in **graft rejection**, where the antigen is borne by a transplanted foreign cell. What we call a successful immune response or a failure, and whether the response is considered harmful or beneficial to the host, depends not on the response itself but rather on the nature of the antigen (Fig. 1.32).

Allergic diseases, which include asthma, are an increasingly common cause of disability in the developed world, and many other important diseases are now recognized as autoimmune. An autoimmune response directed against pancreatic β cells is the leading cause of diabetes in the young. In allergies and autoimmune diseases, the powerful protective mechanisms of the adaptive immune response cause serious damage to the patient.

Immune responses to harmless antigens, to body tissues, or to organ grafts are, like all other immune responses, highly specific. At present, the usual way to treat these responses is with **immunosuppressive drugs**, which inhibit all immune responses, desirable and undesirable. If it were possible to suppress only those lymphocyte clones responsible for the unwanted response, the disease could be cured or the grafted organ protected without impeding protective immune responses. There is hope that this dream of antigen-specific **immunoregulation** to control unwanted immune responses could become a reality, as antigen-specific suppression of immune responses can

Fig. 1.32 Immune responses can be beneficial or harmful depending on the nature of the antigen. Beneficial responses are shown in white, harmful responses in red shaded boxes. Where the response is beneficial, its absence is harmful.

Antigen	Effect of response to antigen	
	Normal response	Deficient response
Infectious agent	Protective immunity	Recurrent infection
Innocuous substance	Allergy	No response
Grafted organ	Rejection	Acceptance
Self organ	Autoimmunity	Self tolerance
Tumor	Tumor immunity	Cancer

be induced experimentally, although the molecular basis of this suppression is not fully understood. We shall see in Chapter 10 how the mechanisms of immune regulation are beginning to emerge from a better understanding of the functional subsets of lymphocytes and the cytokines that control them, and we shall discuss the present state of understanding of allergies, autoimmune disease, graft rejection, and immunosuppressive drugs in Chapters 12–14.

1-21   Vaccination is the most effective means of controlling infectious diseases.

Although the specific suppression of immune responses must await advances in basic research on immune regulation and its application, the deliberate stimulation of an immune response by immunization, or vaccination, has achieved many successes in the two centuries since Jenner's pioneering experiment.

Mass immunization programs have led to the virtual eradication of several diseases that used to be associated with significant morbidity (illness) and mortality (Fig. 1.33). Immunization is considered so safe and so important that most states in the United States require children to be immunized against up to seven common childhood diseases. Impressive as these accomplishments are, there are still many diseases for which we lack effective vaccines. And even where vaccines for diseases such as measles or polio can be used effectively in developed countries, technical and economic problems can prevent their widespread use in developing countries, where mortality from these diseases is still high. The tools of modern immunology and molecular biology are being applied to develop new vaccines and improve old ones, and we shall discuss these advances in Chapter 14. The prospect of controlling these important diseases is tremendously exciting. The guarantee of good health is a critical step toward population control and economic development. At a cost of pennies per person, great hardship and suffering can be alleviated.

Summary.

Lymphocytes have two distinct recognition systems specialized for detection of extracellular and intracellular pathogens. B cells have cell-surface immunoglobulin molecules as receptors for antigen and, upon activation, secrete the immunoglobulin as soluble antibody that provides defense against pathogens in the extracellular spaces of the body. T cells have receptors that recognize peptide fragments of intracellular pathogens transported to the cell surface by the glycoproteins of the MHC. Two classes of MHC molecule transport peptides from different intracellular compartments to present them to distinct types of effector T cell: cytotoxic CD8 T cells that kill infected target cells, and CD4 T cells that mainly activate macrophages and B cells. Thus, T cells are crucially important for both the humoral and cell-mediated responses of adaptive immunity. The adaptive immune response seems to have engrafted specific antigen recognition by highly diversified receptors onto innate defense systems, which have a central role in the effector actions of both B and T lymphocytes. The vital role of adaptive immunity in fighting infection is illustrated by the immunodeficiency diseases and the problems caused by pathogens that succeed in evading or subverting an adaptive immune response. The antigen-specific suppression of adaptive immune responses is the goal of treatment for important human diseases involving inappropriate activation of lymphocytes, whereas the specific stimulation of an adaptive immune response is the basis of successful vaccination.

Fig. 1.33 Successful vaccination campaigns. Diphtheria, polio, and measles and its consequences have been virtually eliminated in the United States, as shown in these three graphs. SSPE stands for subacute sclerosing panencephalitis, a brain disease that is a late consequence of measles infection in a few patients. When measles was prevented, SSPE disappeared 15–20 years later. However, as these diseases have not been eradicated worldwide, immunization must be maintained in a very high percentage of the population to prevent their reappearance.

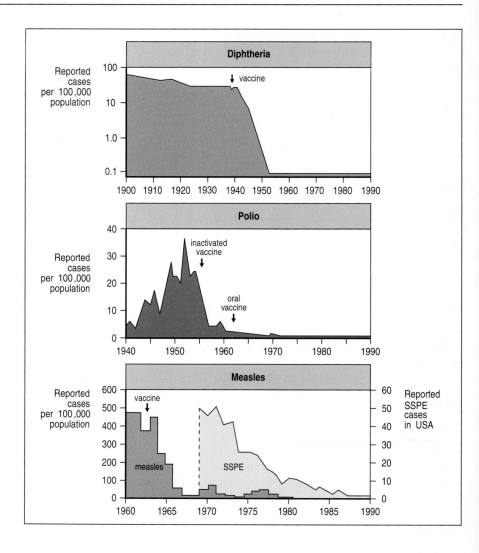

Summary to Chapter 1.

The immune system defends the host against infection. Innate immunity serves as a first line of defense but lacks the ability to recognize certain pathogens and to provide the specific protective immunity that prevents re-infection. Adaptive immunity is based on clonal selection from a repertoire of lymphocytes bearing highly diverse antigen-specific receptors that enable the immune system to recognize any foreign antigen. In the adaptive immune response, antigen-specific lymphocytes proliferate and differentiate into effector cells that eliminate pathogens. Host defense requires different recognition systems and a wide variety of effector mechanisms to seek out and destroy the wide variety of pathogens in their various habitats within the body and at its external and internal surfaces. Not only can the adaptive immune response eliminate a pathogen but, in the process, it also generates increased numbers of differentiated memory lymphocytes through clonal selection, and this allows a more rapid and effective response upon reinfection. The regulation of immune responses, whether to suppress them when unwanted or to stimulate them in the prevention of infectious disease, is the major medical goal of research in immunology.

General references.

Historical background

Burnet, F.M.: *The Clonal Selection Theory of Acquired Immunity.* London, Cambridge University Press, 1959.

Gowans, J.L.: **The Lymphocyte—a disgraceful gap in medical knowledge.** *Immunol. Today* 1996, **17**:288–291.

Landsteiner, K.: *The Specificity of Serological Reactions,* 3rd edn. Boston, Harvard University Press, 1964.

Metchnikoff, E.: *Immunity in the Infectious Diseases,* 1st edn. New York, Macmillan Press, 1905.

Silverstein, A.M.: *History of Immunology,* 1st edn. London, Academic Press, 1989.

Biological background

Alberts, B., Bray, D., Lewis, J., Raff, M., Roberts, K., and Watson, J.D.: *Molecular Biology of the Cell,* 3rd edn. New York, Garland Publishing, 1994.

Lodish, H., Berk, A., Zipursky, S.L., Matsudaira, P., Baltimore, D., and Darnell, J.: *Molecular Cell Biology,* 4th edn. New York, W.H. Freeman and Company, 2000.

Mims, C., Nash, A., and Stephen, J. *Mims' Pathogenesis of Infectious Disease.* 5th edn. London, Academic Press, 2001.

Ryan, K.J. (ed): *Medical Microbiology,* 3rd edn. East Norwalk, CT, Appleton-Lange, 1994.

Stryer, L.: *Biochemistry,* 4th edn. New York, Freeman, 1995.

Primary journals devoted solely or primarily to immunology

Autoimmunity
Clinical and Experimental Immunology
Comparative and Developmental Immunology
European Journal of Immunology
Immunity
Immunogenetics
Immunology
Infection and Immunity
International Immunology
Journal of Autoimmunity
Journal of Experimental Medicine
Journal of Immunology
Nature Immunology
Regional Immunology
Thymus

Primary journals with frequent papers in immunology

Cell
Current Biology
EMBO Journal
Journal of Biological Chemistry
Journal of Cell Biology
Journal of Clinical Investigation
Molecular Cell Biology
Nature
Nature Cell Biology
Proceedings of the National Academy of Sciences, USA
Science

Review journals in immunology

Annual Reviews in Immunology
Contemporary Topics in Microbiology and Immunology
Current Opinion in Immunology
Immunogenetics Reviews
Immunological Reviews
Immunology Today
Proceedings of the International Congress of Immunology, **1–10**, *1971–1992, 1998.*
Research in Immunology
Seminars in Immunology
The Immunologist
The Immunologist, **3**: *Proceedings Issue, 9th International Congress of Immunology.*

Advanced textbooks in immunology, compendia, etc.

Lachmann, P.J., Peters, D.K., Rosen, F.S., and Walport, M.J. (eds): *Clinical Aspects of Immunology,* 5th edn. Oxford, Blackwell Scientific Publications, 1993.

Mak, T.W. and Simard, J.J.L.: *Handbook of Immune Response Genes.* New York, Plenum Press, 1998.

Paul, W.E. (ed): *Fundamental Immunology,* 4th edn. New York, Lippincott-Raven, 1998.

Roitt, I.M., and Delves, P.J. (eds): *Encyclopedia of Immunology,* 3rd edn. London/San Diego, Academic Press, 1992.

Rosen, F.S., and Geha, R.S.: *Case Studies in Immunology: A Clinical Companion,* 3rd edn. New York, Garland Publishing, 2001.

Innate Immunity

2

Throughout this book we will examine the individual mechanisms by which the adaptive immune response acts to protect the host from pathogenic infectious agents. In this chapter, however, we will examine the role of those innate, nonadaptive defenses that form early barriers to the establishment of infection. The microorganisms that are encountered daily in the life of a normal healthy individual only occasionally cause perceptible disease. Most are detected and destroyed within minutes or hours by defense mechanisms that do not require a prolonged period of induction because they do not rely on the clonal expansion of antigen-specific lymphocytes: these are the mechanisms of **innate immunity**.

The time course and different phases of an encounter with a new pathogen are summarized in Fig. 2.1. The innate immune mechanisms act immediately, and are followed by **early induced responses**, which can be activated by infection but do not generate **immunological memory**. Only if an infectious organism can breach these early lines of defense will an **adaptive immune response** ensue, with the generation of antigen-specific effector cells that target the specific pathogen, and memory cells that can prevent reinfection with the same microorganism. The power of adaptive immune responses is due to their antigen specificity, which we will be studying in the following chapters. However, they harness, and also depend upon, many of the effector mechanisms used by the innate immune system, which we will describe in this chapter.

Fig. 2.1 The response to an initial infection occurs in three phases. The effector mechanisms that remove the infectious agent (for example, phagocytes and complement) are similar or identical in each phase, but the first two phases rely on the recognition of pathogens by germline-encoded receptors of the innate immune system, whereas adaptive immunity uses variable antigen-specific receptors that are produced as a result of gene segment rearrangements. Adaptive immunity occurs late, because the rare B and T cells specific for the invading pathogen must first undergo clonal expansion before they differentiate into effector cells that can clear the infection.

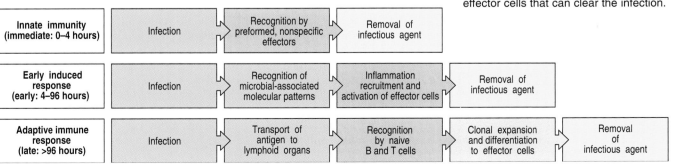

Whereas the adaptive immune system uses a large repertoire of receptors encoded by rearranging gene segments to recognize a huge variety of antigens (see Section 1-10), innate immunity depends upon germline-encoded receptors to recognize features that are common to many pathogens. In fact, as we will see, the mechanisms of innate immunity discriminate very effectively between host cells and pathogens, and this ability to discriminate between self and nonself, and to recognize broad classes of pathogens, contributes to the induction of an appropriate adaptive immune response.

In the first part of the chapter we will consider the fixed defenses of the body: the epithelia that line the internal and external surfaces of the body, and the phagocytes that lie beneath all epithelial surfaces and that can engulf and digest invading microorganisms. As well as killing microorganisms directly, the activities of these phagocytes induce the next phase of the innate immune response. In this phase an inflammatory response recruits new phagocytic cells to the site of infection as well as humoral effector molecules that cooperate with the phagocytes in the engulfment of the pathogens. In addition, the initiating steps of the adaptive immune response take place, so that if the infection is not cleared by these innate responses, an adaptive immune response will ensue; this involves specific recognition of the pathogen and, ultimately, produces antigen-specific immunological memory that, in most cases, ensures long-lasting immunity to the pathogen.

Second, we will take a closer look at the ancient system of pattern-recognition receptors used by the innate immune system to identify pathogens and discriminate them from self antigens. As well as directing the immediate destruction of pathogens, we shall see how stimulation of some of these receptors on macrophages and dendritic cells leads to their becoming cells that can effectively present antigen to T lymphocytes, thus initiating an adaptive immune response. The third part of the chapter is devoted to a system of plasma proteins known as the complement system. This important element of humoral innate immunity interacts with microorganisms to promote their removal by phagocytic cells. In the last part of the chapter we shall describe how the cytokines and chemokines produced by activated phagocytes and dendritic cells induce the later phases of the innate immune response, such as the acute-phase response. We shall also encounter another cell of the innate immune system, the natural killer or NK cell, which contributes to innate host defense against viruses and other intracellular pathogens.

The front line of host defense.

Microorganisms that cause pathology in humans and animals enter the body at different sites and produce disease by a variety of mechanisms. Many different infectious agents can cause pathology, and those that do are referred to as **pathogenic microorganisms** or **pathogens**. Invasions by microorganisms are initially countered, in all vertebrates, by innate defense mechanisms that preexist in all individuals and begin to act within minutes of the encounter of the host with the infectious agent. Only when the innate host defenses are bypassed, evaded, or overwhelmed is an adaptive immune response required. In the first part of this chapter we will describe briefly the infectious strategies used by microbes to evade recognition by the innate immune system before examining the innate host defenses that, in most cases, prevent infection from becoming established. We will examine the defense functions of the epithelial surfaces of the body, the role of antimicrobial peptides and proteins, and the defense of body tissues by macrophages and neutrophils, which bind to and ingest invading microorganisms in a process known as **phagocytosis**.

Routes of infection for pathogens			
Route of entry	**Mode of transmission**	**Pathogen**	**Disease**
Mucosal surfaces			
Airway	Inhaled droplet	Influenza virus	Influenza
	Spores	*Neisseria meningitidis*	Meningococcal meningitis
		Bacillus anthracis	Inhalation anthrax
Gastrointestinal tract	Contaminated water or food	*Salmonella typhi*	Typhoid fever
		Rotavirus	Diarrhea
Reproductive tract	Physical contact	*Treponema pallidum*	Syphilis
		HIV	AIDS
External epithelia			
External surface	Physical contact	*Trichophyton*	Athlete's foot
Wounds and abrasions	Minor skin abrasions	*Bacillus anthracis*	Cutaneous anthrax
	Puncture wounds	*Clostridium tetani*	Tetanus
	Handling infected animals	*Francisella tularensis*	Tularemia
Insect bites	Mosquito bites (*Aedes aegypti*)	Flavivirus	Yellow fever
	Deer tick bites	*Borrelia burgdorferi*	Lyme disease
	Mosquito bites (*Anopheles*)	*Plasmodium* spp.	Malaria

Fig. 2.2 Pathogens infect the body through a variety of routes.

2-1   Infectious agents must overcome innate host defenses to establish a focus of infection.

Our bodies are constantly exposed to microorganisms present in our environment, including infectious agents that have been shed from other infected individuals. Contact with these microorganisms may occur through external or internal epithelial surfaces: the respiratory tract mucosa provides a route of entry for airborne microorganisms, the gastrointestinal mucosa for microorganisms in food and water, insect bites and wounds allow microorganisms to penetrate the skin, and direct contact between individuals offers opportunities for infection of the skin, the gut, and the mucosa of the reproductive tract (Fig. 2.2).

In spite of this exposure, infectious disease is fortunately quite infrequent. The epithelial surfaces of the body serve as an effective barrier against most microorganisms, and they are rapidly repaired if wounded. Furthermore, most of the microorganisms that do succeed in crossing an epithelial surface are efficiently removed by innate immune mechanisms that function in the underlying tissues. Thus, in most cases these defenses, which we will examine in more detail in subsequent sections, prevent a site of infection from becoming established. It is difficult to know how many infections are repelled in this way, because there are no symptoms of such infections and no measurable response to them. It is clear, however, that the microorganisms that a normal human being inhales or ingests, or that enter through minor wounds, are mostly held at bay or eliminated, because they seldom cause clinical disease.

Infectious disease occurs when a microorganism succeeds in evading or overwhelming innate host defenses to establish a local site of infection, and replicates there to allow its further transmission within our bodies. In some cases, such as athlete's foot, the initial infection remains local and does not cause significant pathology. In other cases the infectious agent causes significant pathology as it spreads through the lymphatics or the bloodstream, or as a result of secreting toxins.

Pathogen spread is often countered by an inflammatory response that recruits more effector cells and molecules of the innate immune system from local blood vessels (Fig. 2.3), while inducing clotting further downstream so that pathogens cannot spread through the blood. The induced responses of innate immunity act over several days while an adaptive immune response gets underway in response to pathogen molecules delivered to local lymphoid tissue by dendritic cells. An adaptive immune response differs from innate immunity in its ability to target specific features of the pathogen. This response will usually clear the infection, and protect the host against reinfection with the same pathogen, by producing effector cells and antibodies against the pathogen, and immunological memory of that pathogen.

2-2 The epithelial surfaces of the body make up the first lines of defense against infection.

Fig. 2.3 An infection and the response to it can be divided into a series of stages. These are illustrated here for an infectious microorganism entering through a wound in the skin. The infectious agent must first adhere to the epithelial cells and then cross the epithelium. A local immune response may prevent the infection from becoming established. If not, it helps to contain the infection and also delivers the infectious agent, carried in lymph and inside dendritic cells, to local lymph nodes. This initiates the adaptive immune response and eventual clearance of the infection. The role of γ:δ T cells is uncertain, as we shall see in Section 2-29, and this is indicated by the question mark.

Our body surfaces are defended by epithelia, which provide a physical barrier between the internal milieu and the external world that contains pathogens (Fig. 2.4). Epithelial cells are held together by tight junctions, which effectively form a seal against the external environment. Epithelia comprise the skin and the linings of the body's tubular structures—the gastrointestinal, respiratory, and urogenital tracts. Infections occur only when the pathogen can colonize or cross through these barriers, and because the dry, protective layers of the skin present a more formidable barrier, pathogen entry most often occurs through the internal epithelial surfaces, which represent the vast majority of epithelial surfaces of our bodies. The importance of epithelia in protection against infection is obvious when the barrier is breached, as in wounds, burns, and loss of the integrity of the body's internal epithelia, where infection is a major cause of mortality and morbidity. In the absence of wounding or disruption, pathogens

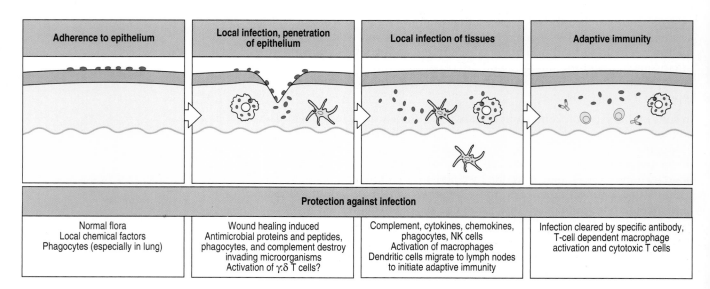

Adherence to epithelium	Local infection, penetration of epithelium	Local infection of tissues	Adaptive immunity
Protection against infection			
Normal flora Local chemical factors Phagocytes (especially in lung)	Wound healing induced Antimicrobial proteins and peptides, phagocytes, and complement destroy invading microorganisms Activation of γ:δ T cells?	Complement, cytokines, chemokines, phagocytes, NK cells Activation of macrophages Dendritic cells migrate to lymph nodes to initiate adaptive immunity	Infection cleared by specific antibody, T-cell dependent macrophage activation and cytotoxic T cells

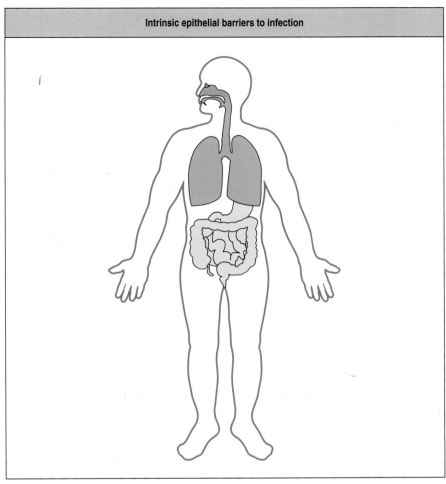

Intrinsic epithelial barriers to infection

Fig. 2.4 Many barriers prevent pathogens from crossing epithelia and colonizing tissues. Surface epithelia provide mechanical, chemical, and microbiological barriers to infection.

	Skin	Gut	Lungs	Eyes/nose
Mechanical	Epithelial cells joined by tight junctions			
	Longitudinal flow of air or fluid		Movement of mucus by cilia	
Chemical	Fatty acids	Low pH		Salivary enzymes (lysozyme)
		Enzymes (pepsin)		
	Antibacterial peptides			
Microbiological	Normal flora			

normally cross epithelial barriers by binding to molecules on the epithelial surfaces of our internal organs, or establish an infection by adhering to and colonizing these surfaces. This specific attachment allows the pathogen to infect the epithelial cell, to damage the epithelium so it can be crossed, or, in the case of colonizing pathogens, to avoid being dislodged by the flow of air or fluid across the epithelial surface.

The internal epithelia are known as **mucosal epithelia** because they secrete a viscous fluid called mucus, which contains many glycoproteins called mucins. Microorganisms coated in mucus may be prevented from adhering to the epithelium, and in mucosal epithelia such as that of the respiratory tract, microorganisms can be expelled in the flow of mucus driven by the beating of epithelial cilia. The efficacy of mucus flow in clearing infection is illustrated by people with defective mucus secretion or inhibition of ciliary movement, as occurs in the inherited disease **cystic fibrosis**. Such individuals frequently develop lung infections caused by bacteria that colonize the epithelial surface but do not cross it. In the gut, peristalsis is an important mechanism for keeping both food and infectious agents moving through the body. Failure of peristalsis is typically accompanied by the overgrowth of pathogenic bacteria within the intestinal lumen.

Our surface epithelia are more than mere physical barriers to infection; they also produce chemical substances that are microbicidal or that inhibit microbial growth. For example, the antibacterial enzymes lysozyme and phospholipase A are secreted in tears and saliva, and saliva contains several histatins—histidine-rich peptides with antimicrobial properties. The acid pH of the stomach and the digestive enzymes, bile salts, fatty acids, and lysolipids found in the upper gastrointestinal tract create a substantial chemical barrier to infection. Further down the intestinal tract, antibacterial and antifungal peptides called cryptdins or α-defensins are made by Paneth cells, which are resident in the base of the crypts in the small intestine beneath the epithelial stem cells. Related antimicrobial peptides, the β-defensins, are made by other epithelia, primarily in the respiratory and urogenital tracts, skin, and tongue. Such antimicrobial peptides have a role in the immune defense of many organisms, including humans and other vertebrates that also can make an adaptive immune response. Even more striking is resistance to infection in insects and other invertebrates and even plants, in which innate immunity comprises the only system of host defense. All these organisms produce antimicrobial peptides. These are cationic peptides that are thought to kill bacteria by damaging the bacterial cell membrane.

Another type of antimicrobial protein is secreted into the fluid that bathes the epithelial surfaces of the lung. This fluid contains two proteins—surfactant proteins A and D, usually abbreviated as SP-A and SP-D—that bind to and coat the surfaces of pathogens so that they are more easily phagocytosed by macrophages that have left the subepithelial tissues to enter the alveoli of the lung. These proteins are members of the collectin family, so called because they contain both collagen-like and lectin (sugar-binding) domains. Coating of a particle with proteins that facilitate its phagocytosis is known as **opsonization**, and we will meet several other examples of this defense strategy in this and later chapters.

In addition to these defenses, most epithelial surfaces are associated with a normal flora of nonpathogenic bacteria that compete with pathogenic microorganisms for nutrients and for attachment sites on epithelial cells. The normal flora can also produce antimicrobial substances, such as the lactic acid produced by vaginal lactobacilli, some strains of which also produce antimicrobial peptides (bacteriocins). When the nonpathogenic bacteria are killed by antibiotic treatment, pathogenic microorganisms frequently replace them and cause disease.

2-3   After entering tissues, many pathogens are recognized, ingested, and killed by phagocytes.

If a microorganism crosses an epithelial barrier and begins to replicate in the tissues of the host, in most cases it is immediately recognized by the mononuclear phagocytes, or **macrophages**, that reside in these tissues. Macrophages mature continuously from monocytes that leave the circulation to migrate into tissues throughout the body. They are found in especially large numbers in connective tissue, in the submucosal layer of the gastrointestinal tract, in the lung (where they are also found in both the interstitium and the alveoli), along certain blood vessels in the liver (where they are known as **Kupffer cells**), and throughout the spleen, where they remove senescent blood cells. The second major family of phagocytes—the **neutrophils**, or **polymorphonuclear neutrophilic leukocytes** (**PMNs** or polys)—are short-lived cells that are abundant in the blood, but they are not present in normal, healthy tissues. Both of these phagocytic cells have a key role in innate immunity because they can recognize, ingest, and destroy many pathogens without the aid of an adaptive immune response.

Macrophages, located in the submucosal tissues, are the first cells to encounter pathogens, but they are soon reinforced by the recruitment of large numbers of neutrophils to sites of infection. Macrophages and neutrophils recognize pathogens by means of their cell-surface receptors that can discriminate between the surface molecules displayed by pathogens and those of the host. These receptors, which we will examine in more detail later in this chapter, include the macrophage mannose receptor, which is found on macrophages but not on monocytes or neutrophils, scavenger receptors, which bind many negatively charged ligands such as lipoteichoic acids, which are cell-wall components of Gram-positive bacteria, and CD14, a receptor for bacterial lipopolysaccharide (LPS), found predominantly on monocytes and macrophages (Fig. 2.5). Ligation of many of these cell-surface receptors by pathogens leads to phagocytosis of the pathogen, followed by its death inside the phagocyte. Phagocytosis is an active process, in which the bound pathogen is first surrounded by the phagocyte membrane and then internalized in a membrane-bounded vesicle known as a **phagosome** or endocytic vacuole. The phagosome then becomes acidified, killing most pathogens. In addition to being phagocytic, macrophages and neutrophils have membrane-bounded granules, called **lysosomes**, that contain enzymes, proteins, and peptides that can mediate an intracellular antimicrobial response. The phagosome fuses with one or more lysosomes to generate a **phagolysosome** in which the lysosomal contents are released to destroy the pathogen (see Fig. 2.5).

Upon phagocytosis, macrophages and neutrophils also produce a variety of other toxic products that help kill the engulfed microorganism (Fig. 2.6). The most important of these are nitric oxide (NO), the superoxide anion (O_2^-), and hydrogen peroxide (H_2O_2), which are directly toxic to bacteria. Nitric oxide is produced by a high-output form of nitric oxide synthase, iNOS2. Superoxide is generated by a multicomponent, membrane-associated NADPH oxidase in a process known as the **respiratory burst** because it is

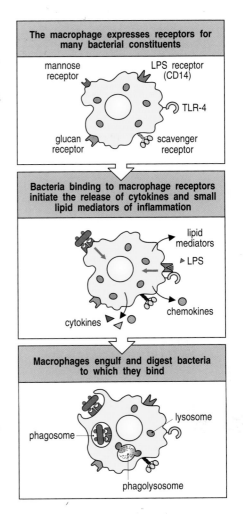

The macrophage expresses receptors for many bacterial constituents

mannose receptor

LPS receptor (CD14)

TLR-4

glucan receptor

scavenger receptor

Bacteria binding to macrophage receptors initiate the release of cytokines and small lipid mediators of inflammation

lipid mediators

LPS

chemokines

cytokines

Macrophages engulf and digest bacteria to which they bind

phagosome

lysosome

phagolysosome

Fig. 2.5 Macrophages are activated by pathogens and both engulf them and initiate inflammatory responses. Macrophages derive from circulating monocytes. They have many of the same characteristics but they acquire new functions and new receptors when they become resting cells in the connective tissues throughout the body. Macrophages express receptors for many bacterial components, including receptors for bacterial carbohydrates (mannose and glucan receptors), lipids (LPS receptor) and other pathogen-derived components (Toll-like receptors (TLRs) and scavenger receptor). Binding of bacteria to macrophage receptors stimulates the phagocytosis and uptake of pathogens into intracellular vesicles, where they are destroyed. Signaling through some receptors, such as the Toll receptors, in response to bacterial components causes the secretion of 'pro-inflammatory cytokines' such as interleukin-1β (IL-1β), IL-6, and tumor necrosis factor-α (TNF-α).

Fig. 2.6 Bactericidal agents produced or released by phagocytes on the ingestion of microorganisms. Most of these agents are made by both macrophages and neutrophils. Some of them are toxic; others, such as lactoferrin, work by binding essential nutrients and preventing their uptake by the bacteria. The same substances can be released by phagocytes interacting with large antibody-coated surfaces such as parasitic worms or host tissues. As these agents are also toxic to host cells, phagocyte activation can cause extensive tissue damage during an infection.

Class of mechanism	Specific products
Acidification	pH=~3.5–4.0, bacteriostatic or bactericidal
Toxic oxygen-derived products	Superoxide O_2^-, hydrogen peroxide H_2O_2, singlet oxygen $^1O_2^{\bullet}$, hydroxyl radical $OH^{\bullet}$, hypohalite OCl^-
Toxic nitrogen oxides	Nitric oxide NO
Antimicrobial peptides	Defensins and cationic proteins
Enzymes	Lysozyme—dissolves cell walls of some Gram-positive bacteria. Acid hydrolases—further digest bacteria
Competitors	Lactoferrin (binds Fe) and vitamin B_{12}-binding protein

accompanied by a transient increase in oxygen consumption and is converted by the enzyme superoxide dismutase into H_2O_2 (Fig. 2.7); further chemical and enzymatic reactions produce a range of toxic chemicals from hydrogen peroxide, including the hydroxyl radical ($OH^{\bullet}$) and the hypochlorite (OCl^-) and hypobromite (OBr^-) ions. Neutrophils are short-lived cells, dying soon after they have accomplished a round of phagocytosis. Dead and dying neutrophils are a major component of the **pus** that forms in some infections; bacteria that give rise to such infections are thus known as **pyogenic** or **pus-forming bacteria**. Macrophages, in contrast, are long-lived and continue to generate new lysosomes. Patients with chronic granulomatous disease have a genetic deficiency of NADPH oxidase, which means that their phagocytes do not produce the toxic oxygen derivatives characteristic of the respiratory burst, and so are less able to kill ingested microorganisms and clear an infection. People with this defect are unusually susceptible to bacterial and fungal infections, especially in infancy.

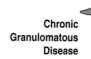

Chronic Granulomatous Disease

Macrophages can phagocytose pathogens and produce the respiratory burst immediately on encountering an infecting microorganism, and this can be sufficient to prevent an infection from becoming established. In the 19th century the cellular immunologist **Elie Metchnikoff** believed that the innate response of macrophages encompassed all host defense and, indeed, it is now clear that invertebrates, such as the sea star that he was studying, rely entirely on innate immunity for their defense against infection. Although this is not the case in humans and other vertebrates, the innate response of macrophages still provides an important front line of host defense that must be overcome if a microorganism is to establish an infection that can be passed on to a new host.

A key feature that distinguishes pathogenic from nonpathogenic microorganisms is their ability to overcome innate immune defenses. Pathogens have developed a variety of strategies to avoid immediate destruction by macrophages. Many extracellular pathogenic bacteria coat themselves with a thick polysaccharide capsule that is not recognized by any phagocyte receptor. Other pathogens, for example mycobacteria, have evolved ways to grow inside macrophage phagosomes by inhibiting their acidification and fusion with lysosomes. Without such devices, a microorganism must enter the body in sufficient numbers to simply overwhelm the immediate innate host defenses and to establish a focus of infection.

A second important effect of the interaction between pathogens and tissue macrophages is the activation of macrophages to release **cytokines**, **chemokines** (chemoattractant cytokines), and other mediators that set up a state of inflammation in the tissue and bring neutrophils and plasma proteins to the site of an infection. It is thought that the pathogen induces cytokine and chemokine secretion by signals delivered through some of the receptors to which it binds, and we will see later how this occurs in response to LPS. Receptors that signal the presence of pathogens and induce cytokines also have another important role. This is to induce the expression of so-called co-stimulatory molecules on macrophages and on **dendritic cells**, another type of phagocytic cell present in tissues, thus enabling these antigen-presenting cells to initiate an adaptive immune response (see Section 1-6).

The cytokines released by macrophages make an important contribution both to local inflammation and to other induced but nonadaptive responses that occur in the first few days of a new infection. We will be describing the role of individual cytokines in these induced responses in the last part of this chapter. However, because an inflammatory response is usually initiated within hours of infection or wounding, we will outline here how it occurs and how it contributes to host defense.

2-4 Pathogen recognition and tissue damage initiate an inflammatory response.

Inflammation plays three essential roles in combating infection. The first is to deliver additional effector molecules and cells to sites of infection, to augment the killing of invading microorganisms by the front-line macrophages. The second is to provide a physical barrier in the form of microvascular co-agulation to prevent the spread of the infection in the bloodstream. The third is to promote the repair of injured tissue, a nonimmunological role that we will not discuss further. Inflammation at the site of infection is initiated by the response of macrophages to pathogens.

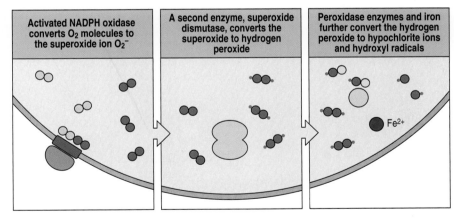

Fig. 2.7 The respiratory burst in macrophages and neutrophils is caused by a transient increase in oxygen consumption during the production of microbicidal oxygen metabolites. Ingestion of microorganisms activates the phagocyte to assemble the multi-subunit enzyme NADPH oxidase from its components. The active enzyme converts molecular oxygen to the superoxide ion O_2^-, and other oxygen free radicals. Superoxide ion is then converted by the enzyme superoxide dismutase to hydrogen peroxide, which can kill microorganisms and is also converted by other enzymes and by chemical reactions with ferrous (Fe^{2+}) ions to microbicidal hypochlorite and hydroxyl radicals.

Inflammatory responses are operationally characterized by pain, redness, heat, and swelling at the site of an infection, reflecting four types of change in the local blood vessels, as shown in Fig. 2.8. The first is an increase in vascular diameter, leading to increased local blood flow—hence the heat and redness—and a reduction in the velocity of blood flow, especially along the inner walls of small blood vessels. The second change is that the endothelial cells lining the blood vessel are activated to express **adhesion molecules** that promote the binding of circulating leukocytes. The combination of slowed blood flow and adhesion molecules allows leukocytes to attach to the endothelium and migrate into the tissues, a process known as **extravasation**, which we will describe in detail later. All these changes are initiated by the cytokines and chemokines produced by activated macrophages. Once inflammation has begun, the first white blood cells attracted to the site of infection are neutrophils. These are followed by monocytes, which differentiate into additional tissue macrophages (Fig. 2.9). Macrophages in different tissues were originally given different names—microglial cells in neural tissue, or Kupffer cells in the liver; generically these cells are sometimes referred to as mononuclear phagocytes. In the later stages of inflammation, other leukocytes such as eosinophils and lymphocytes also enter the infected site. The third major change in the local blood vessels is an increase in vascular permeability. Thus, instead of being tightly joined together, the endothelial cells lining the blood vessel walls become separated, leading to an exit of fluid and proteins from the blood and their local accumulation in the tissue. This accounts for the swelling, or **edema**, and pain—as well as the accumulation of plasma proteins that aid in host defense. The fourth change, clotting in microvessels in the site of infection, also contributes to host defense by preventing the spread of the pathogen via the blood.

These changes are induced by a variety of inflammatory mediators released as a consequence of the recognition of pathogens by macrophages. These include the lipid mediators of inflammation—**prostaglandins**, **leukotrienes**, and **platelet-activating factor** (**PAF**)—which are rapidly produced by macrophages through enzymatic pathways that degrade membrane phospholipids. Their actions are followed by those of the chemokines and cytokines that are synthesized and secreted by macrophages in response to

| Cytokines produced by macrophages cause dilation of local small blood vessels | Leukocytes move to periphery of blood vessel as a result of increased expression of adhesion molecules | Leukocytes extravasate at site of infection | Blood clotting occurs in the microvessels |

Fig. 2.8 Infection stimulates macrophages to release cytokines and chemokines that initiate an inflammatory response. Cytokines produced by tissue macrophages at the site of infection cause dilation of local small blood vessels and changes in the endothelial cells of their walls. These changes lead to the movement of leukocytes, such as neutrophils and monocytes, out of the blood vessel (extravasation) and into the infected tissue, guided by chemokines produced by the activated macrophages. The blood vessels also become more permeable, allowing plasma proteins and fluid to leak into the tissues. Together, these changes cause the characteristic inflammatory signs of heat, pain, redness, and swelling at the site of infection.

Monocyte binds adhesion molecules on vascular endothelium near sites of infection and gets chemokine signal	The monocyte migrates into the surrounding tissue	Monocyte differentiates into a macrophage and migrates to the site of infection

Fig. 2.9 Monocytes circulating in the blood recognize blood vessel walls near sites of inflammation and leave the bloodstream, to migrate into the tissue toward the site of infection and inflammation. The initial interactions are mediated by adhesion molecules that first capture the monocyte from the bloodstream and cause it to adhere to the vascular endothelium. Chemokines bound to the vascular endothelium then signal the monocyte to migrate across the endothelium into the underlying tissue. The monocyte, now differentiating into a macrophage, continues to migrate, under the influence of chemokines released during inflammatory responses, toward the site of infection.

pathogens. The cytokine **tumor necrosis factor-α (TNF-α)**, for example, is a potent activator of endothelial cells.

As we will see in the third part of this chapter, another way in which pathogen recognition rapidly triggers an inflammatory response is through activation of the complement cascade. One of the cleavage products of the complement reaction is a peptide called C5a. C5a is a potent mediator of inflammation, with several different activities. In addition to increasing vascular permeability and inducing the expression of some adhesion molecules, it acts as a powerful chemoattractant for neutrophils and monocytes. C5a also activates phagocytes and local **mast cells**, which are in turn stimulated to release their granules containing the small inflammatory molecule histamine and the cytokine TNF-α.

If wounding has occurred, the injury to blood vessels immediately triggers two other protective enzyme cascades. The **kinin system** is an enzymatic cascade of plasma pro-enzymes that is triggered by tissue damage to produce several inflammatory mediators, including the vasoactive peptide **bradykinin**. This causes an increase in vascular permeability that promotes the influx of plasma proteins to the site of tissue injury. It also causes pain, which, although unpleasant to the victim, draws attention to the problem and leads to immobilization of the affected part of the body, which helps to limit the spread of the infection.

The **coagulation system** is another enzymatic cascade of **pro-enzymes** or **zymogens** that is triggered after damage to blood vessels. This leads to the formation of a fibrin clot, whose normal role is to prevent blood loss. However, in innate immunity, its role prevents any of the infectious microorganisms from entering the bloodstream. Both these cascades have an important role in the inflammatory response to pathogens even if wounding or gross tissue injury has not occurred, because they are also triggered by endothelial cell activation. Thus, within minutes of the penetration of tissues by a pathogen, the inflammatory response causes an influx of proteins and cells that may control the infection. It also forms a physical barrier in the form of blood clots to limit the spread of infection and makes the host fully aware of the local infection.

Summary.

The mammalian body is susceptible to infection by many pathogens, which must first make contact with the host and then establish a focus of infection in order to cause disease. These pathogens differ greatly in their lifestyles, the structures of their surfaces, and their mechanisms of pathogenesis, so an equally diverse set of defensive responses from the host immune system is required. The first phase of host defense consists of those mechanisms that are present and ready to resist an invader at any time. The epithelial surfaces of the body keep pathogens out and protect against colonization and against viruses and bacteria that enter the body through specialized cell-surface interactions. This happens by preventing pathogen adherence and by secreting antimicrobial enzymes and peptides. Bacteria, viruses, and parasites that overcome this barrier are faced immediately by tissue macrophages equipped with surface receptors that can bind and phagocytose many different types of pathogen. This, in turn, leads to an inflammatory response, which causes the accumulation of phagocytic neutrophils and macrophages at the site of infection. In addition to the cellular innate immune response described here, plasma proteins accumulate at the site of infection, including the complement components that provide circulating or humoral innate immunity, as will be described in the third part of this chapter. Innate immunity provides a front line of host defense through effector mechanisms that engage the pathogen directly, act immediately on contact with it, and are unaltered in their ability to resist a subsequent challenge with either the same or a different pathogen. These mechanisms often succeed in preventing an infection from becoming established. If not, they are reinforced through the recruitment and increased production of further effector cells and molecules in a series of induced responses that we will consider in the last part of this chapter. These induced innate responses often fail to clear the infection. In that case, dendritic cells, macrophages, and other cells activated in the early innate immune response help to initiate the development of an adaptive immune response.

Pattern recognition in the innate immune system.

Although the innate immune system lacks the fine specificity of adaptive immunity that is necessary to produce immunological memory, it can distinguish self from nonself. We have already seen how this occurs in the response of macrophages to pathogenic microbes. In this part of the chapter we will look more closely at the receptors that activate the innate immune response, including those that recognize pathogens directly and signal for a cellular innate immune response. Proteins that recognize features common to many pathogens occur as receptors on macrophages, neutrophils and dendritic cells, and also as secreted molecules. Their general characteristics are contrasted with the antigen-specific receptors of adaptive immunity in Fig. 2.10. Unlike the receptors that mediate adaptive immunity, the receptors of the innate immune system are not clonally distributed; a given set of receptors will be present on all cells of the same cell type. The binding of specific components of pathogens by these receptors gives rise to very rapid responses, which are put into effect without the delay imposed by the clonal expansion of lymphocytes needed in the adaptive immune response.

Receptors of the innate immune system mediate several different functions. Many are phagocytic receptors that stimulate ingestion of the pathogens they recognize. Some are chemotactic receptors, such as the fMet-Leu-Phe receptor that binds the N-formylated peptides produced by bacteria. This

Receptor characteristic	Innate immunity	Adaptive immunity
Specificity inherited in the genome	Yes	No
Expressed by all cells of a particular type (eg, macrophages)	Yes	No
Triggers immediate response	Yes	No
Recognizes broad classes of pathogen	Yes	No
Interacts with a range of molecular structures of a given type	Yes	No
Encoded in multiple gene segments	No	Yes
Requires gene rearrangement	No	Yes
Clonal distribution	No	Yes
Able to discriminate between even closely related molecular structures	No	Yes

Fig. 2.10 Comparison of the characteristics of recognition molecules of the innate and adaptive immune systems. The innate immune system uses receptors that are encoded by complete genes inherited through the germline, whereas the adaptive immune system uses antigen receptors encoded in gene segments that are assembled into complete T-cell and B-cell receptor genes during lymphocyte development, a process that leads to each individual cell expressing a receptor of unique specificity. As a result, receptors of the innate immune system are deployed nonclonally (that is, by all the cells of a given cell type), whereas the antigen receptors of the adaptive immune system are clonally distributed on individual lymphocytes.

receptor guides neutrophils to sites of infection. A third function, which may be mediated by some of the phagocytic receptors as well as by specialized signaling receptors, is to induce effector molecules that contribute to the induced responses of innate immunity and molecules that influence the initiation and nature of any subsequent adaptive immune response. In this part of the chapter we will first examine the recognition properties of the receptors that bind pathogens directly. We will then focus on an evolutionarily primitive recognition and signaling system, originally discovered on account of its role in embryonic development in the fruitfly *Drosophila melanogaster*. It is now known to have a key role in defense against infection in plants, adult insects, and vertebrates, including mammals. The receptor mediating these functions in *Drosophila* is known as Toll. The homologous proteins in mammals have been named the **Toll-like receptors** (**TLRs**). The role of TLRs is to activate phagocytes and tissue dendritic cells to respond to pathogens by secreting chemokines and cytokines, and to express the co-stimulatory molecules needed to activate adaptive immunity.

2-5 Receptors with specificity for pathogen molecules recognize patterns of repeating structural motifs.

The surfaces of microorganisms typically bear repeating patterns of molecular structure, as do their nucleic acids. Bacterial DNA, for example, contains unmethylated repeats of the dinucleotide CpG. Viruses almost invariably express double-stranded RNA as part of their life cycles. The innate immune system recognizes such pathogens by means of receptors that bind to features of these regular patterns; these receptors are sometimes known as **pattern-recognition receptors**.

The **mannose-binding lectin** (**MBL**) is one such receptor, which is present as a free protein in blood plasma. As we shall see in the next part of this chapter, it can initiate the MB-lectin pathway of complement activation. As illustrated in Fig. 2.11, pathogen recognition and discrimination from self by MBL is due to recognition of a particular orientation of certain sugar residues, as well as

Fig. 2.11 Mannose-binding lectin recognizes bacterial surfaces by their particular spacing of carbohydrate residues. Mannose-binding lectin (MBL) is a plasma protein that is part of the pathogen-recognition system of innate immunity. It binds to certain bacterial surfaces that display a particular spatial arrangement of mannose or fucose residues. Note that the presence of these residues is not enough to ensure binding; the orientation of the binding sites in the MBL is fixed, and only if the mannose and fucose residues have the correct spacing will the MBL be able to bind. Once coated with MBL, the bacteria are more susceptible to phagocytosis.

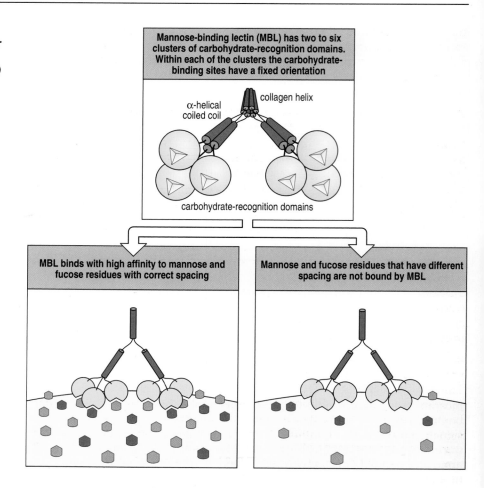

their spacing, which is found only on microbes and not on host cells. We have already met two other members of this family of proteins, the collectins, in Section 2-2—SP-A and SP-D—which are part of the innate immune defenses at mucosal surfaces. Collectins are made in the liver as part of the acute-phase response and can opsonize bacteria, as described in the last part of the chapter. The interaction of these soluble receptors with pathogens leads in turn to binding of the receptor–pathogen complex by phagocytes, either through interactions with the pathogen-bound receptor or through phagocyte receptors for complement, which also becomes bound to the pathogen. The outcome is the phagocytosis and killing of the bound pathogen (see Section 2-3) and the induction of other cellular responses.

Phagocytes are also equipped with several cell-surface receptors that recognize pathogen surfaces directly. Among these are the **macrophage mannose receptor** (see Fig. 2.5). This receptor is a cell-bound C-type (calcium-dependent) lectin that binds certain sugar molecules found on the surface of many bacteria and some viruses, including the human immunodeficiency virus (HIV). Its recognition properties are very similar to those of mannose-binding lectin (see Fig. 2.11) and, like mannose-binding lectin, it is a multipronged molecule with several carbohydrate-recognition domains. Because it is a transmembrane cell-surface receptor, however, it can function directly as a phagocytic receptor.

A second set of phagocytic receptors, called **scavenger receptors**, recognize various anionic polymers and acetylated low-density lipoproteins. These receptors are a structurally heterogeneous set of molecules, existing in at least six distinct molecular forms. Some scavenger receptors recognize structures that are shielded by sialic acid on normal host cells. These receptors are also involved in the removal of senescent red blood cells that have lost their sialic acid, as well as in the recognition and removal of pathogens. There are other recognition targets, many of which still need to be characterized.

2-6   Receptors on phagocytes can signal the presence of pathogens.

In addition to triggering phagocytosis, binding of pathogens to some of the receptors on the macrophage cell surface can also trigger the induced responses of innate immunity, as we will see later in this chapter. Stimulation of certain receptors by pathogen products also leads macrophages and dendritic cells to produce the cell-surface display of co-stimulatory molecules, that eventually leads to the induction of adaptive immunity. The best-defined activation pathway of this type is triggered through a family of evolutionarily conserved transmembrane receptors that seem to function exclusively as signaling receptors. These receptors, known as the **Toll-like receptors** (TLRs), were first described in the fruitfly. In the fly they recognize a cleaved protein product called spaetzle: in the fly embryo this recognition triggers formation of the dorso-ventral axis, whereas in the adult fly it triggers an intracellular cascade that leads to the formation of antimicrobial peptides in response to infections.

In mammals, Toll-like receptor 4, or **TLR-4** on macrophages, signals the presence of LPS by associating with CD14, the macrophage receptor for LPS. TLR-4 is also involved in the immune response to at least one virus, the respiratory syncytial virus, although in this case the exact nature of the stimulating ligand is not yet known. Another mammalian Toll-like receptor, TLR-2, signals the presence of a different set of microbial constituents, which include the peptidoglycans of Gram-positive bacteria, although how it recognizes these is not known. TLR-4 and TLR-2 induce similar but distinct signals, as shown by the distinct responses resulting from LPS signaling through TLR-4 and peptidoglycan signaling through TLR-2. There are now 10 distinct proteins in the Toll-like receptor family of proteins in mammals, and further functions of Toll-like receptors may soon be revealed as mice lacking one or other of these proteins are produced and their phenotypes are analyzed.

2-7   Each of the 10 Toll-like receptors in humans recognizes a particular molecular structure that is present in many pathogens.

There are 10 expressed *TLR* genes in mice and humans, and each is devoted to recognizing a distinct set of molecular patterns that are not found in normal vertebrates. These patterns are characteristic of components of pathogenic microorganisms at one or other stage of infection. Although certain Toll-like receptor proteins can form heterodimers, this is not the rule; TLR-4, for instance, can only form homodimers. Because there are only 10 functional *TLR* genes, the Toll-like receptors have limited specificity compared with the antigen receptors of the adaptive immune system and have evolved to recognize certain microbe-associated molecular patterns. But although the diversity of the Toll-like receptors is limited, they still recognize a broad range of pathogenic microorganisms. The 10 known TLRs can recognize elements of most microbes, as illustrated in Fig. 2.12.

Innate immune recognition by Toll-like receptors	
Toll-like receptor	**Ligand**
TLR-1 dimer	Peptidoglycan Lipoproteins Lipoarabinomannan (mycobacteria) GPI (*T. cruzi*) Zymosan (yeast)
TLR-2/TLR-6 dimer	
TLR-3	dsRNA
TLR-4 dimer (plus CD14)	LPS (Gram-negative bacteria)
TLR-5	Flagellin
TLR-9	Unmethylated CpG DNA

Fig. 2.12 Innate immune recognition by Toll-like receptors. Each of the known TLRs recognizes one or more microbial molecular patterns, generally by direct interaction with molecules on the pathogen surface. GPI, glycosylphosphatidylinositol; *T. cruzi*, the protozoan parasite *Trypanosoma cruzi*; dsRNA, double-stranded RNA.

Fig. 2.13 Certain pathogens can invade directly through the intestinal or other internal epithelia. In the case of *Salmonella typhi*, which causes typhoid fever, shown here in the process of migrating through the intestinal epithelium, the long flagella are recognized by Toll-like receptors on macrophages and dendritic cells in the underlying tissues and provoke an innate response that helps to control the infection. Photograph courtesy of J. Galan.

2-8 The effects of bacterial lipopolysaccharide on macrophages are mediated by CD14 binding to TLR-4.

Bacterial LPS is a cell-wall component of Gram-negative bacteria, such as *Salmonella*, which has long been known to induce a reaction in the infected host. The systemic injection of LPS causes a collapse of the circulatory and respiratory systems, a condition known as **shock**. These dramatic effects of LPS are seen in humans as **septic shock** and are caused by the overwhelming secretion of cytokines, particularly of TNF-α, as a result of an uncontrolled systemic bacterial infection. We will discuss the pathogenesis of septic shock later in this chapter and shall see that it is an undesirable consequence of the same effector actions of TNF-α that are important in containing local infections. LPS acts through TLR-4, and the benefits of TLR-4 signaling are clearly illustrated by mutant mice that lack TLR-4 function: although resistant to septic shock, they are highly sensitive to LPS-bearing pathogens such as *Salmonella typhimurium*, a natural pathogen of mice. The same principles are seen in humans infected with *Salmonella typhi*, the cause of typhoid fever. This bacterium invades across the mucosal membranes (Fig. 2.13) but can be recognized by macrophages and other innate phagocytic cells because it expresses both LPS and flagellin, which allows it to activate two TLRs—TLR-4 and TLR-5 (see Fig. 2.12). The consequence of this is the activation of the NFκB signaling pathway in the cell and the subsequent stimulation of TNF-α production by macrophages. Thus, systemic infection with *S. typhi* is capable of causing systemic shock in humans by the same mechanism provoked by *S. typhimurium* in mice, by inducing a systemic production of TNF-α. *S. typhi*, in common with many pathogenic bacteria, expresses what is called a type III secretion system, a microhomolog of a syringe, allowing the bacterium to secrete molecules directly across the cell membrane of mammalian cells and into the cytosol. Using its type III secretion system, *S. typhi* is able to transfer into the cytosol of macrophages protease molecules that inhibit both the NFκB signaling pathway and the production of TNF-α, perhaps as an escape mechanism to allow the bacterium to evade the innate immune response.

When TLR-4 interacts with LPS bound to CD14, this sends a signal to the cell nucleus that activates the transcription factor NFκB (Fig. 2.14). We will describe the signaling pathway used by all TLRs in detail in Chapter 6. This signaling pathway was first discovered as the pathway used by the Toll receptor to determine dorso-ventral body pattern during embryogenesis in the fruitfly *Drosophila*, and we will therefore call it the **Toll pathway**. The pathway is

LPS in body fluids is bound by an acute-phase protein, LPS-binding protein (LBP)

LPS   LBP   CD14

The LPS:LBP complex transfers LPS to CD14 on the surface of phagocytes

TLR-4

Having bound LPS, CD14 interacts with Toll-like receptor 4 (TLR-4) resulting in activation of NFκB in the nucleus

Fig. 2.14 Bacterial lipopolysaccharide signals through the Toll-like receptor TLR-4 to activate the transcription factor NFκB. TLR-4 on macrophages is activated by the binding of bacterial lipopolysaccharide (LPS) through two other proteins. In the plasma, LPS is bound by the soluble LPS-binding protein, which then loads its bound LPS onto the glycosylphosphatidylinositol (GPI)-tethered peripheral membrane protein CD14. This LPS:CD14 complex then triggers the membrane protein TLR-4 to signal to the nucleus, activating the transcription factor NFκB, which in turn activates genes encoding proteins involved in defense against infection.

Cytokines secreted by macrophages and dendritic cells			
Cytokine	Main producer	Acts upon	Effect
IL-1	Macrophages Keratinocytes	Lymphocytes	Enhances responses
		Liver	Induces acute-phase protein secretion
IL-6	Macrophages Dendritic cells	Lymphocytes	Enhances responses
		Liver	Induces acute-phase protein secretion
CXCL8 (IL-8)	Macrophages Dendritic cells	Phagocytes	Chemoattractant for neutrophils
IL-12	Macrophages Dendritic cells	Naive T cells	Diverts immune response to type 1, proinflammatory, cytokine secretion
TNF-α	Macrophages Dendritic cells	Vascular endothelium	Induces changes in vascular endothelium (expression of cell-adhesion molecules (E- and P-selectin), changes in cell–cell junctions with increased fluid loss, local blood clotting)

Fig. 2.15 Important cytokines secreted by macrophages in response to bacterial products include IL-1β, IL-6, CXCL8, IL-12, and TNF-α. TNF-α is an inducer of a local inflammatory response that helps to contain infections; it also has systemic effects, many of which are harmful (see Section 2-24). The chemokine CXCL8 is also involved in the local inflammatory response, helping to attract neutrophils into the site of infection. IL-1β, IL-6, and TNF-α have a crucial role in inducing the acute-phase response in the liver (see Section 2-25) and induce fever, which favors effective host defense in several ways. IL-12 activates the natural killer (NK) cells of the innate immune response, and favors the differentiation of CD4 T cells into the T_H1 subset during an adaptive immune response.

also known to participate in defense against infection in adult flies and in the induction of innate immune responses in vertebrates. A similar pathway is used by plants in their defense against viruses and other plant pathogens. Thus, the Toll pathway is an ancient signaling pathway that seems to be used in innate immune defense in most or all multicellular organisms. In the next section we will use the Toll-like receptors to illustrate the typical innate immune responses provoked by pathogen components.

2-9 Activation of Toll-like receptors triggers the production of pro-inflammatory cytokines and chemokines, and the expression of co-stimulatory molecules.

The Toll signaling pathway in adult flies results in the production of several antimicrobial peptides that contribute to the fly's defense against infection. In humans and all other vertebrates examined, activation of NFκB by the Toll pathway leads to the production of several important mediators of innate immunity, such as cytokines (Fig. 2.15) and chemokines (see Fig. 2.40) (Appendices III and IV provide a detailed listing of these important mediators.) The Toll pathway also leads to the surface expression of **co-stimulatory molecules** that are essential for the induction of adaptive immune responses. These molecules, called **B7.1** (**CD80**) and **B7.2** (**CD86**), are cell-surface proteins that are expressed by both macrophages and tissue dendritic cells in response to LPS signaling through TLR-4 (Fig. 2.16). It is these molecules, along with the antigenic microbial peptides presented by MHC class II proteins on dendritic cells and macrophages (see Section 1-18), which activate naive CD4 T cells (Fig. 2.17). These cells, in turn, are needed to initiate most adaptive immune responses. To encounter a naive CD4 T cell, the antigen-presenting dendritic cell must also migrate to a nearby lymph node through which circulating naive T cells pass, and this migration is stimulated by cytokines such as TNF-α, which are also induced through signaling by TLR-4. Thus, the activation of adaptive immunity depends on molecules induced as a consequence of innate immune recognition and signaling.

Fig. 2.16 Bacterial LPS induces changes in Langerhans' cells, stimulating them to migrate and initiate adaptive immunity to infection by activating CD4 T cells. Langerhans' cells are immature dendritic cells resident in the skin. During a bacterial infection they are activated by LPS through the Toll signaling pathway. This induces two types of change in the Langerhans' cells. The first is a change in behavior and location. From being resting cells in the skin they become activated migrating cells in the afferent lymphatics, and eventually fully mature dendritic cells in the regional lymph nodes. The second is a drastic alteration in their cell-surface molecules. Resting Langerhans' cells in the skin are highly phagocytic and macropinocytic, but lack the ability to activate T lymphocytes. Mature dendritic cells in the lymph nodes have lost the ability to ingest antigen but have gained the ability to stimulate T cells. This is due to an increase in the number of MHC molecules on their surface and the expression of the co-stimulatory molecules CD80 (B7.1) and CD86 (B7.2).

Substances such as LPS that induce co-stimulatory activity have been used for years in mixtures that are co-injected with protein antigens to enhance their immunogenicity. These substances are known as **adjuvants** (see Appendix I, Section A-4), and it was found empirically that the best adjuvants contained microbial components. A range of microbial components (see Fig. 2.12) can induce macrophages and tissue dendritic cells to express co-stimulatory molecules and cytokines. The exact profile of cytokines produced by the macrophage or dendritic cell varies according to the receptors stimulated and, as we shall see in Chapters 8 and 10, the cytokines secreted will in turn influence the functional character of the adaptive immune response that develops. In this way the ability of the innate immune system to discriminate between different types of pathogen is used to ensure an appropriate type of adaptive immune response.

Summary.

The innate immune system uses several different receptors to recognize and respond to pathogens. Those that recognize pathogen surfaces directly often bind to repeating patterns, for example of carbohydrate or lipid moieties, that are characteristic of microbial surfaces but are not found on host cells. Some of these receptors, such as the macrophage mannose receptor, directly stimulate phagocytosis, whereas others are produced as secreted molecules that promote the phagocytosis of pathogens by opsonization or by the activation of complement, as we shall see in the next part of this chapter. The innate immune system receptors that recognize pathogens also have an important role in signaling for the induced innate responses that are responsible for local inflammation, the recruitment of new effector cells, the containment of local infection, and the initiation of an adaptive immune response. Such signals can be transmitted through a family of signaling receptors, known as the Toll-like receptors (TLRs), that have been highly conserved across evolutionary time and serve to activate host defense through a signaling pathway that operates in most multicellular organisms. In vertebrates, TLRs also have a key role in enabling the initiation of adaptive immunity. TLR-4 detects the presence of Gram-negative bacteria through its association with the peripheral membrane protein CD14, which is a receptor for bacterial LPS. Other TLRs respond to other molecular patterns found on or in pathogens. TLRs activate the transcription factor NFκB, which then induces the transcription of a variety of genes, including those for the cytokines, chemokines, and co-stimulatory molecules that have essential roles in directing the course of the adaptive immune response later in infection.

Fig. 2.17 For naive T cells to be activated by antigen, the antigen must be presented to them by an activated antigen-presenting cell that also expresses co-stimulatory molecules. Antigen is recognized by the T-cell receptor in the form of a peptide bound to an MHC molecule on an antigen-presenting cell (APC), such as a macrophage or dendritic cell. However, the T cell will be activated only if the antigen-presenting cell also expresses the co-stimulatory molecules CD80 or CD86.

The complement system and innate immunity.

Complement was discovered by **Jules Bordet** many years ago as a heat-labile component of normal plasma that augments the opsonization and killing of bacteria by antibodies. This activity was said to 'complement' the antibacterial·activity of antibody; hence the name. Although first discovered as an effector arm of the antibody response, complement can also be activated early in infection in the absence of antibodies. Indeed, it now seems clear that complement first evolved as part of the innate immune system, where it still has an important role.

The **complement system** is made up of many distinct plasma proteins that react with one another to opsonize pathogens and induce a series of inflammatory responses that help to fight infection. Several complement proteins are proteases that are themselves activated by proteolytic cleavage. Such enzymes are called zymogens and were first found in the gut. The digestive enzyme pepsin, for example, is stored inside cells and secreted as an inactive precursor enzyme, pepsinogen, which is only cleaved to pepsin in the acid environment of the stomach. The advantage to the host of not being auto-digested is obvious.

In the complement system, the precursor zymogens are widely distributed throughout body fluids and tissues without adverse effect. At sites of infection, however, they are activated locally and trigger a series of potent inflammatory events. The complement system activates through a triggered-enzyme cascade. In such a cascade, an active complement enzyme generated by cleavage of its zymogen precursor then cleaves its substrate, another complement zymogen, to its active enzymatic form. This in turn cleaves and activates the next zymogen in the complement pathway. In this way, the activation of a small number of complement proteins at the start of the pathway is hugely amplified by each successive enzymatic reaction, resulting in the rapid generation of a disproportionately large complement response. As might be expected, there are many regulatory mechanisms to prevent uncontrolled complement activation. The blood coagulation system is another example of a triggered-enzyme cascade. In this case, a small injury to a blood vessel wall can lead to the development of a large thrombus.

Fig. 2.18 Schematic overview of the complement cascade. There are three pathways of complement activation: the classical pathway, which is triggered by the binding of complement component C1q to antibody complexed with antigen by the direct binding of C1q to the pathogen surface, or by the binding of C1q to C-reactive protein bound to the pathogen; the MB-lectin pathway, which is triggered by mannose-binding lectin, a normal serum constituent that binds some encapsulated bacteria; and the alternative pathway, which is triggered directly on pathogen surfaces. All of these pathways generate a crucial enzymatic activity that, in turn, generates the effector molecules of complement. The three main consequences of complement activation are opsonization of pathogens, the recruitment of inflammatory cells, and the direct killing of pathogens.

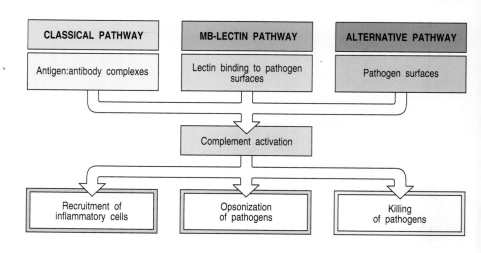

There are three distinct pathways through which complement can be activated on pathogen surfaces. These pathways depend on different molecules for their initiation, but they converge to generate the same set of effector molecules (Fig. 2.18). There are also three ways in which the complement system protects against infection. First, it generates large numbers of activated complement proteins that bind covalently to pathogens, opsonizing them for engulfment by phagocytes bearing receptors for complement. Second, the small fragments of some complement proteins act as chemoattractants to recruit more phagocytes to the site of complement activation, and also to activate these phagocytes. Third, the terminal complement components damage certain bacteria by creating pores in the bacterial membrane.

2-10 Complement is a system of plasma proteins that interacts with pathogens to mark them for destruction by phagocytes.

In the early phases of an infection, the complement cascade can be activated on the surface of a pathogen through one or more of the three pathways shown in Fig. 2.19. **The classical pathway** is initiated by the binding of C1q, the first protein in the complement cascade, to the pathogen surface. C1q can bind to the surface of pathogens in one of three ways. It can bind directly to surface components of some bacteria, including certain proteins of bacterial cell walls and polyanionic surface structures, such as lipoteichoic acid on Gram-positive bacteria. Second, C1q binds to C-reactive protein, an acute-phase protein of human plasma that binds to phosphocholine residues in bacterial polysaccharides, such as pneumococcal C polysaccharide; hence the name C-reactive protein. Third, C1q is a key link between the effector mechanisms of innate and adaptive immunity by binding to antibody:-antigen complexes. The **mannose-binding lectin pathway** (**MB-lectin pathway**) is initiated by binding of the mannose-binding lectin (MBL), a serum protein whose level increases during the acute-phase response, to mannose-containing carbohydrates on bacteria or viruses. Finally, the **alternative pathway** can be initiated by the binding of spontaneously activated C3 in plasma to the surface of a pathogen.

Each pathway follows a sequence of reactions to generate a protease called a **C3 convertase**. These reactions are known as the 'early' events of complement activation, and consist of triggered-enzyme cascades in which inactive complement zymogens are successively cleaved to yield two fragments, the larger of which is an active serine protease. The active protease is retained at the pathogen surface, and this ensures that the next complement zymogen in the pathway is also cleaved and activated at the pathogen surface. By contrast, the small peptide fragment is released from the site of the reaction and can act as a soluble mediator.

The C3 convertases formed by these early events of complement activation are bound covalently to the pathogen surface. Here they cleave C3 to generate large amounts of **C3b**, the main effector molecule of the complement system, and C3a, a weak peptide mediator of inflammation. The C3b molecules act as opsonins; they bind covalently to the pathogen and thereby target it for destruction by phagocytes equipped with receptors for C3b. C3b also binds to the C3 convertase to form a **C5 convertase** that produces the most important small peptide mediator of inflammation, **C5a**, as well as a large active fragment, **C5b**, that initiates the 'late' events of complement activation. These comprise a sequence of polymerization reactions in which the terminal complement components interact to form a **membrane-attack complex**, which creates a pore in the cell membranes of certain pathogens that can lead to their death.

The nomenclature of complement proteins is often a significant obstacle to understanding this system, and before discussing the complement cascade in more detail we will explain the naming of the complement proteins. All components of the classical complement pathway and the membrane-attack complex are designated by the letter C followed by a number. The native components have a simple number designation, for example, C1 and C2, but unfortunately the components were numbered in the order of their discovery rather than the sequence of reactions. The reaction sequence is C1, C4,

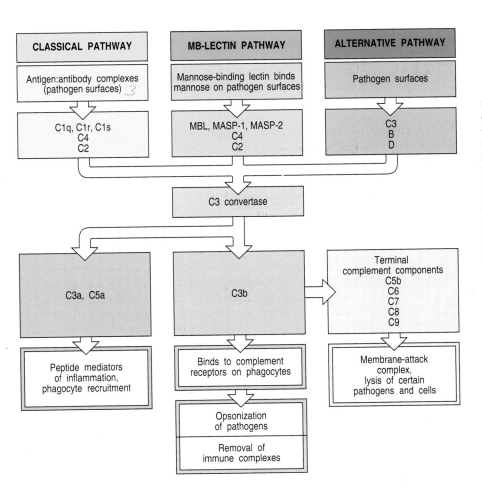

Fig. 2.19 Overview of the main components and effector actions of complement. The early events of all three pathways of complement activation involve a series of cleavage reactions that culminate in the formation of an enzymatic activity called a C3 convertase, which cleaves complement component C3 into C3b and C3a. The production of the C3 convertase is the point at which the three pathways converge and the main effector functions of complement are generated. C3b binds covalently to the bacterial cell membrane and opsonizes the bacteria, enabling phagocytes to internalize them. C3a is a peptide mediator of local inflammation. C5a and C5b are generated by the cleavage of C5b by a C5 convertase formed by C3b bound to the C3 convertase (not shown in this simplified diagram). C5a is also a powerful peptide mediator of inflammation. C5b triggers the late events in which the terminal components of complement assemble into a membrane-attack complex that can damage the membrane of certain pathogens.

Functional protein classes in the complement system	
Binding to antigen:antibody complexes and pathogen surfaces	C1q
Binding to mannose on bacteria	MBL
Activating enzymes	C1r C1s C2b Bb D MASP-1 MASP-2
Membrane-binding proteins and opsonins	C4b C3b
Peptide mediators of inflammation	C5a C3a C4a
Membrane-attack proteins	C5b C6 C7 C8 C9
Complement receptors	CR1 CR2 CR3 CR4 C1qR
Complement-regulatory proteins	C1INH C4bp CR1 MCP DAF H I P CD59

Fig. 2.20 Functional protein classes in the complement system.

C2, C3, C5, C6, C7, C8, and C9. The products of the cleavage reactions are designated by added lower-case letters, the larger fragment being designated b and the smaller a; thus, for example, C4 is cleaved to C4b, the large fragment of C4 that binds covalently to the surface of the pathogen, and C4a, a small fragment with weak pro-inflammatory properties. The components of the alternative pathway, instead of being numbered, are designated by different capital letters, for example factor B and factor D. As with the classical pathway, their cleavage products are designated by the addition of lower-case a and b: thus, the large fragment of B is called Bb and the small fragment Ba. Finally, in the mannose-binding lectin pathway, the first enzymes to be activated are known as the *m*annose-binding-lectin-*a*ssociated *s*erine *p*roteases, MASP-1 and MASP-2, after which the pathway is essentially the same as the classical pathway. Activated complement components are often designated by a horizontal line, for example, $\overline{C2b}$; however, we will not use this convention. It is also useful to be aware that the large active fragment of C2 was originally designated C2a, and is still called that in some texts and research papers. Here, for consistency, we will call all large fragments of complement b, so the large active fragment of C2 will be designated C2b; this can be remembered by the mnemonic 'b' stands for 'big.'

The formation of C3 convertase activity is pivotal in complement activation, leading to the production of the principal effector molecules, and initiating the late events. In the classical and MB-lectin pathways the C3 convertase is formed from membrane-bound C4b complexed with C2b, designated C4b2b. In the alternative pathway, a homologous C3 convertase is formed from membrane-bound C3b complexed with Bb, C3bBb. The alternative pathway can act as an amplification loop for all three pathways, because it is initiated by the binding of C3b.

It is clear that a pathway leading to such potent inflammatory and destructive effects, and which, moreover, has a series of built-in amplification steps, is potentially dangerous and must be subject to tight regulation. One important safeguard is that key activated complement components are rapidly inactivated unless they bind to the pathogen surface on which their activation was initiated. There are also several points in the pathway at which regulatory proteins act on complement components to prevent the inadvertent activation of complement on host cell surfaces, thereby protecting them from accidental damage. We will return to these regulatory mechanisms later.

We have now introduced all the relevant components of complement and are ready for a more detailed account of their functions. To help in distinguishing the different components according to their functions, we will use a color code in the figures in this part of the chapter. This is introduced in Fig. 2.20, where all the components of complement are grouped by function.

2-11   The classical pathway is initiated by activation of the C1 complex.

The classical pathway has a role in both innate and adaptive immunity. As we will see in Chapter 9, the first component of this pathway, C1q, links the adaptive humoral immune response to the complement system by binding to antibodies complexed with antigens. C1q can, however, also bind directly to the surface of certain pathogens and thus trigger complement activation in the absence of antibody. It can also bind to C-reactive protein bound to phosphocholine on bacteria. Therefore the complement proteins can act in the absence of adaptive immunity, and represent the humoral arm of innate immunity.

C1q is part of the C1 complex, which comprises a single C1q molecule bound to two molecules each of the zymogens C1r and C1s. C1q has six globular heads, linked together by a collagen-like tail, which surround the $(C1r:C1s)_2$

Fig. 2.21 The first protein in the classical pathway of complement activation is C1, which is a complex of C1q, C1r, and C1s. C1q is composed of six identical subunits with globular heads and long collagen-like tails. The tails combine to bind to two molecules each of C1r and C1s, forming the C1 complex C1q:C1r$_2$:C1s$_2$. The heads can bind to the constant regions of immunoglobulin molecules or directly to the pathogen surface, causing a conformational change in C1r, which then cleaves and activates the C1s zymogen. Photograph ($\times$ 500,000) courtesy of K.B.M. Reid.

complex (Fig. 2.21). Binding of more than one of the C1q heads to a pathogen surface or to the Fc portions of antibodies in an immune complex causes a conformational change in the (C1r:C1s)$_2$ complex, which leads to the activation of an autocatalytic enzymatic activity in C1r; the active form of C1r then cleaves its associated C1s to generate an active serine protease.

Once activated, the C1s enzyme acts on the next two components of the classical pathway, cleaving C4 and then C2 to generate two large fragments, C4b and C2b, which together form the C3 convertase of the classical pathway. In the first step, C1s cleaves C4 to produce C4b, which may bind covalently to the surface of the pathogen. The covalently attached C4b then binds one molecule of C2, making it susceptible, in turn, to cleavage by C1s. C1s cleaves C2 to produce the large fragment C2b, which is itself a serine protease. C4b2b, the complex of C4b with the active serine protease C2b, remains covalently linked to the surface of the pathogen as the C3 convertase of the classical pathway. Its most important activity is to cleave large numbers of C3 molecules to produce C3b molecules that coat the pathogen surface. At the same time, the other cleavage product, C3a, initiates a local inflammatory response. These reactions, which comprise the classical pathway of complement activation, are shown in schematic form in Fig. 2.22; the proteins involved, and their active forms, are listed in Fig. 2.23.

Fig. 2.22 The classical pathway of complement activation generates a C3 convertase that deposits large numbers of C3b molecules on the pathogen surface. The steps in the reaction are outlined here and detailed in the text. The cleavage of C4 by C1s exposes a reactive group on C4b that allows it to bind covalently to the pathogen surface. C4b then binds C2, making it susceptible to cleavage by C1s. The larger C2b fragment is the active protease component of the C3 convertase. It cleaves many molecules of C3 to produce C3b, which binds to the pathogen surface, and C3a, an inflammatory mediator.

Fig. 2.23 The proteins of the classical pathway of complement activation.

Proteins of the classical pathway of complement activation		
Native component	**Active form**	**Function of the active form**
C1 (C1q: C1r$_2$:C1s$_2$)	C1q	Binds directly to pathogen surfaces or indirectly to antibody bound to pathogens, thus allowing autoactivation of C1r
	C1r	Cleaves C1s to active protease
	C1s	Cleaves C4 and C2
C4	C4b	Covalently binds to pathogen and opsonizes it. Binds C2 for cleavage by C1s
	C4a	Peptide mediator of inflammation (weak activity)
C2	C2b	Active enzyme of classical pathway C3/C5 convertase: cleaves C3 and C5
	C2a	Precursor of vasoactive C2 kinin
C3	C3b	Many molecules of C3b bind to pathogen surface and act as opsonins. Initiates amplification via the alternative pathway. Binds C5 for cleavage by C2b
	C3a	Peptide mediator of inflammation (intermediate activity)

2-12 The mannose-binding lectin pathway is homologous to the classical pathway.

The MB-lectin pathway uses a protein very similar to C1q to trigger the complement cascade. This protein, called **mannose-binding lectin** (**MBL**), introduced earlier in Fig. 2.11, is a member of the collectin family of proteins, of which SP-A and SP-D are also members (see Section 2-2). Mannose-binding lectin binds specifically to mannose residues, and to certain other sugars, which are accessible and arranged in a pattern that allows binding on many pathogens, as shown schematically in Fig. 2.11. On vertebrate cells, however, these are covered by other sugar groups, especially by sialic acid. Thus, MBL is able to initiate complement activation by binding to pathogen surfaces while avoiding activation on host cell surfaces. It is present at low concentrations in normal plasma of most individuals, and, as we will see in the last part of this chapter, its production by the liver is increased during the acute-phase reaction driven by the innate immune response.

Mannose-binding lectin, like C1q, is a two- to six-headed molecule that forms a complex with two protease zymogens, which in the case of the MBL complex are **MASP-1** and **MASP-2** (Fig. 2.24). MASP-2 is closely homologous to C1r and C1s, and MASP-1 is a slightly more distantly related cousin; all four enzymes are likely to have evolved from gene duplication of a common precursor. When the MBL complex binds to a pathogen surface, MASP-2 is activated to cleave C4 and C2. The role, if any, of MASP-1 in complement activation is uncertain. Thus the MB-lectin pathway initiates complement activation in a closely similar way to the classical pathway, forming a C3 convertase from C2b bound to C4b. People deficient in MBL experience a substantial increase in infections during early childhood, indicating the importance of the MB-lectin pathway for host defense. The age window of susceptibility to infections associated with MBL deficiency illustrates the particular importance of innate host defense mechanisms in early child-hood, which is a time before the child's adaptive immune responses are fully matured and after maternal antibodies transferred across the placenta and in colostrum have been lost.

2-13 Complement activation is largely confined to the surface on which it is initiated.

We have seen that the classical and MB-lectin pathways of complement activation are initiated by proteins that bind to pathogen surfaces. During the triggered-enzyme cascade that follows, it is important that activating events are confined to this same site, so that C3 activation also occurs on the surface of the pathogen, and not in the plasma or on host cell surfaces. This is achieved principally by the covalent binding of C4b to the pathogen surface. Cleavage of C4 exposes a highly reactive thioester bond on the C4b molecule that allows it to bind covalently to molecules in the immediate vicinity of its site of activation. In innate immunity, C4 cleavage is catalyzed by a C1 or MBL complex bound to the pathogen surface, and C4b can bind adjacent proteins or carbohydrates on the pathogen surface. If C4b does not rapidly form this bond, the thioester bond is cleaved by reaction with water and this hydrolysis reaction irreversibly inactivates C4b (Fig. 2.25). This helps to prevent C4b from diffusing from its site of activation on the microbial surface and becoming coupled to host cells.

C2 becomes susceptible to cleavage by C1s only when it is bound by C4b, and the C2b serine protease is thereby also confined to the pathogen surface, where it remains associated with C4b, forming the C3 convertase C4b2b. The activation of C3 molecules thus also occurs at the surface of the pathogen. Furthermore, the C3b cleavage product is also rapidly inactivated unless it binds covalently by the same mechanism as C4b, and it therefore opsonizes only the surface on which complement activation has taken place.

2-14 Hydrolysis of C3 causes initiation of the alternative pathway of complement.

The alternative pathway is so named because it was discovered as a second, or 'alternative,' pathway for complement activation after the classical pathway had been defined. This pathway can proceed on many microbial surfaces in the absence of specific antibody, and it leads to the generation of a distinct C3 convertase designated C3bBb. In contrast to the classical and MB-lectin pathways of complement activation, the alternative pathway does not depend on a pathogen-binding protein for its initiation; instead it is initiated through the spontaneous hydrolysis of C3, as shown in the top three panels of Fig. 2.26. The distinctive components of the pathway are listed in Fig. 2.27. Several mechanisms ensure that the activation pathway will only proceed on the surface of a pathogen.

C3 is abundant in plasma, and C3b is produced at a significant rate by spontaneous cleavage (also known as 'tickover'). This occurs through the spontaneous hydrolysis of the thioester bond in C3 to form $C3(H_2O)$, which has an altered conformation, allowing binding of the plasma protein **factor B**. The binding of B by $C3(H_2O)$ then allows a plasma protease called **factor D** to cleave factor B to Ba and Bb, the latter remaining associated with $C3(H_2O)$ to form the $C3(H_2O)Bb$ complex. This complex is a fluid-phase C3 convertase, and although it is only formed in small amounts it can cleave many molecules of C3 to C3a and C3b. Much of this C3b is inactivated by hydrolysis, but some attaches covalently, through its reactive thioester group, to the surfaces of pathogens or of host cells. C3b bound in this way is able to bind factor B,

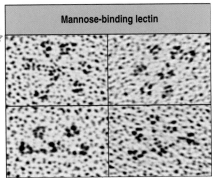

Fig. 2.24 Mannose-binding lectin forms a complex with serine proteases that resembles the complement C1 complex. Mannose-binding lectin (MBL) forms clusters of two to six carbohydrate-binding heads around a central collagen-like stalk. This structure, easily discernible under the electron microscope (lower panels), has been described as looking like 'a bunch of tulips.' Associated with this complex are two serine proteases, MBL-associated serine protease 1 (MASP-1) and 2 (MASP-2). The structural disposition of the MASP proteins in the complex is not yet determined. On binding of MBL to bacterial surfaces, these serine proteases become activated and can then activate the complement system by cleaving and activating C4 and C2. Photograph courtesy of K.B.M. Reid.

Fig. 2.25 Cleavage of C4 exposes an active thioester bond that causes the large fragment, C4b, to bind covalently to nearby molecules on the bacterial cell surface. Intact C4 consists of an α, a β, and a γ chain with a shielded thioester bond on the α chain. This is exposed when the α chain is cleaved by C1s to produce C4b. The thioester bond (marked by an arrow in the third panel) is rapidly hydrolyzed (that is, cleaved by water), inactivating C4b unless it reacts with hydroxyl or amino groups to form a covalent linkage with molecules on the pathogen surface. The homologous protein C3 has an identical reactive thioester bond that is also exposed on the C3b fragment when C3 is cleaved by C2b. The covalent attachment of C3b and C4b enables these molecules to act as opsonins and is important in confining complement activation to the pathogen surface.

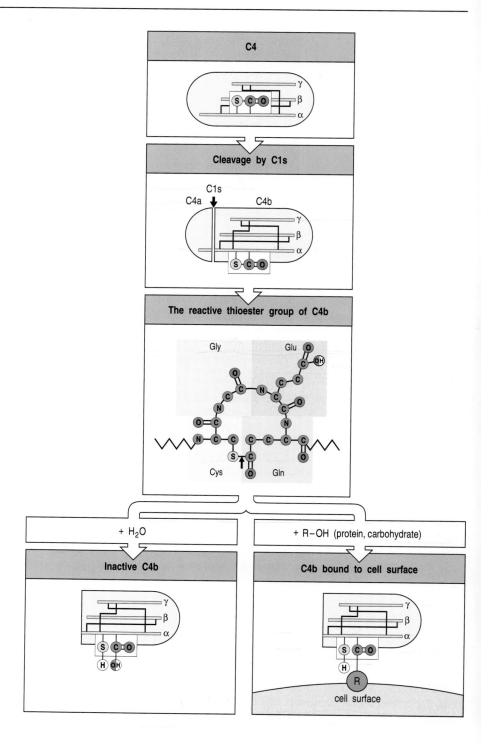

allowing its cleavage by factor D to yield the small fragment Ba and the active protease Bb. This results in formation of the alternative pathway C3 convertase, C3bBb (Fig. 2.28).

When C3b binds to host cells, several complement-regulatory proteins, present in the plasma and on host cell membranes, combine to prevent complement activation from proceeding. These proteins interact with C3b and either prevent the convertase from forming or promote its rapid dissociation. Thus, the complement receptor 1 (CR1) and a membrane-attached protein known as **decay-accelerating factor** (**DAF** or **CD55**) compete with factor B for

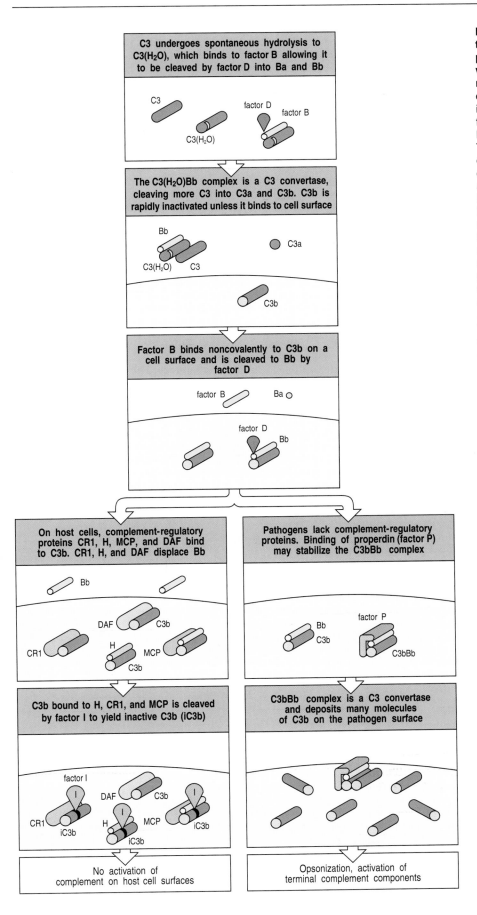

Fig. 2.26 Complement activated by the alternative pathway attacks pathogens while sparing host cells, which are protected by complement regulatory proteins. The complement component C3 is cleaved spontaneously in plasma to give $C3(H_2O)$, which binds factor B and enables the bound factor B to be cleaved by factor D (top panel). The resulting soluble C3 convertase cleaves C3 to give C3a and C3b, which can attach to host cells or pathogen surfaces (second panel). Covalently bound C3b binds factor B, which in turn is rapidly cleaved by factor D to Bb, which remains bound to C3b to form a C3 convertase, and Ba, which is released (third panel). If C3bBb forms on the surface of host cells (bottom left panels), it is rapidly inactivated by complement-regulatory proteins expressed by the host cell: complement receptor 1 (CR1), decay-accelerating factor (DAF), and membrane cofactor of proteolysis (MCP). Host cell surfaces also favor the binding of factor H from plasma. CR1, DAF, and factor H displace Bb from C3b, and CR1, MCP, and factor H catalyze the cleavage of bound C3b by the plasma protease factor I to produce inactive C3b (known as iC3b). Bacterial surfaces (bottom right panels) do not express complement-regulatory proteins and favor the binding of properdin (factor P), which stabilizes the C3bBb convertase activity. This convertase is the equivalent of C4b2b of the classical pathway (see Fig. 2.22).

Fig. 2.27 The proteins of the alternative pathway of complement activation.

Proteins of the alternative pathway of complement activation		
Native component	Active fragments	Function
C3	C3b	Binds to pathogen surface, binds B for cleavage by D, C3bBb is C3 convertase and C3b₂Bb is C5 convertase
Factor B (B)	Ba	Small fragment of B, unknown function
	Bb	Bb is active enzyme of the C3 convertase C3bBb and C5 convertase C3b₂Bb
Factor D (D)	D	Plasma serine protease, cleaves B when it is bound to C3b to Ba and Bb
Properdin (P)	P	Plasma protein with affinity for the C3bBb convertase on bacterial cells

Factor I
Deficiency

binding to C3b on the cell surface, and can displace Bb from a convertase that has already formed. Convertase formation can also be prevented by cleaving C3b to its inactive derivative iC3b. This is achieved by a plasma protease, **factor I** in conjunction with C3b-binding proteins that can act as cofactors, such as CR1 and **membrane cofactor of proteolysis** (**MCP** or **CD46**), another host cell membrane protein. **Factor H** is yet another complement-regulatory protein in plasma that binds C3b and, like CR1, it is able to compete with factor B to displace Bb from the convertase in addition to acting as a cofactor for factor I. Factor H binds preferentially to C3b bound to vertebrate cells because it has an affinity for the sialic acid residues present on these cells.

By contrast, because pathogen surfaces lack these regulatory proteins and sialic acid residues, the C3bBb convertase can form and persist. Indeed, this process may be favored by a positive regulatory factor, known as **properdin** or **factor P**, which binds to many microbial surfaces and stabilizes the convertase. Deficiencies in factor P are associated with a heightened susceptibility to infection with *Neisseria* species.

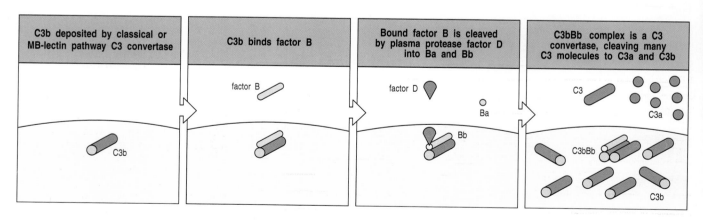

Fig. 2.28 The alternative pathway of complement activation can amplify the classical or the MB-lectin pathway by forming an alternative C3 convertase and depositing more C3b molecules on the pathogen. C3b deposited by the classical or MB-lectin pathway can bind factor B, making it susceptible to

cleavage by factor D. The C3bBb complex is the C3 convertase of the alternative pathway of complement activation and its action, like that of C4b2b, results in the deposition of many molecules of C3b on the pathogen surface.

Once formed, the C3bBb convertase rapidly cleaves yet more C3 to C3b, which can bind to the pathogen and either act as an opsonin or reinitiate the pathway to form another molecule of C3bBb convertase. Thus, the alternative pathway activates through an amplification loop that can proceed on the surface of a pathogen but not on a host cell. This same amplification loop enables the alternative pathway to contribute to complement activation initially triggered through the classical or MB-lectin pathways (see Fig. 2.19).

Deficiency of the C8 Complement Component

The C3 convertases resulting from activation of the classical and MB-lectin pathways (C4b2b) and from the alternative pathway (C3bBb) are apparently distinct. However, understanding of the complement system is simplified somewhat by recognition of the close evolutionary relationships between the different complement proteins (Fig. 2.29). Thus the complement zymogens, factor B and C2, are closely related proteins encoded by homologous genes located in tandem within the major histocompatibility complex (MHC) on human chromosome 6. Furthermore, their respective binding partners, C3 and C4, both contain thioester bonds that provide the means of covalently attaching the C3 convertases to a pathogen surface. Only one component of the alternative pathway seems entirely unrelated to its functional equivalents in the classical and MB-lectin pathways: the initiating serine protease, factor D. Factor D can also be singled out as the only activating protease of the complement system to circulate as an active enzyme rather than a zymogen. This is both necessary for the initiation of the alternative pathway through spontaneous C3 cleavage, and safe for the host because factor D has no other substrate than factor B when bound to C3b. This means that factor D finds its substrate only at a very low level in plasma, and at pathogen surfaces where the alternative pathway of complement activation is allowed to proceed.

Comparison of the different pathways of complement activation illustrates the general principle that most of the immune effector mechanisms that can be activated in a nonclonal fashion as part of the early nonadaptive host response against infection have been harnessed during evolution to be used as

Fig. 2.29 There is a close relationship between the factors of the alternative, MB-lectin, and classical pathways of complement activation. Most of the factors are either identical or the products of genes that have duplicated and then diverged in sequence. The proteins C4 and C3 are homologous and contain the unstable thioester bond by which their large fragments, C4b and C3b, bind covalently to membranes. The genes encoding proteins C2 and B are adjacent in the class III region of the MHC and arose by gene duplication. Factor H, CR1, and C4BP regulatory proteins share a repeat sequence common to many complement-regulatory proteins. The greatest divergence between the pathways is in their initiation: in the classical pathway the C1 complex binds either to certain pathogens or to bound antibody and in the latter it serves to convert antibody binding into enzyme activity on a specific surface; in the MB-lectin pathway, mannose-binding lectin (MBL) associates with a serine protease, activating MBL-associated serine protease (MASP), to serve the same function as C1r:C1s; in the alternative pathway this enzyme activity is provided by factor D.

Step in pathway	Protein serving function in pathway			Relationship
	Alternative (innate)	MB-lectin	Classical	
Initiating serine protease	D	MASP	C1s	Homologous (C1s and MASP)
Covalent binding to cell surface	C3b	C4b		Homologous
C3/C5 convertase	Bb	C2b		Homologous
Control of activation	CR1 H	CR1 C4BP		Identical Homologous
Opsonization	C3b			Identical
Initiation of effector pathway	C5b			Identical
Local inflammation	C5a, C3a			Identical
Stabilization	P	None		Unique

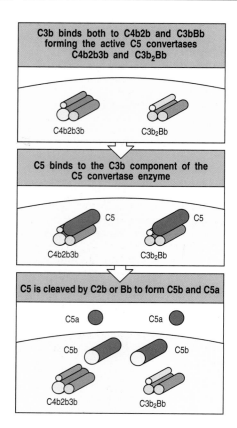

Fig. 2.30 Complement component C5 is cleaved when captured by a C3b molecule that is part of a C5 convertase complex. As shown in the top panel, C5 convertases are formed when C3b binds either the classical or MB-lectin pathway C3 convertase C4b2b to form C4b2b3b, or the alternative pathway C3 convertase C3bBb to form C3b₂Bb. C5 binds to C3b in these complexes (center panel). The bottom panel shows how C5 is cleaved by the active enzyme C2b or Bb to form C5b and the inflammatory mediator C5a. Unlike C3b and C4b, C5b is not covalently bound to the cell surface. The production of C5b initiates the assembly of the terminal complement components.

effector mechanisms of adaptive immunity. It is almost certain that the adaptive response evolved by adding specific recognition to the original non-adaptive system. This is illustrated particularly clearly in the complement system, because here the components are defined and the functional homologs can be seen to be evolutionarily related.

2-15 Surface-bound C3 convertase deposits large numbers of C3b fragments on pathogen surfaces and generates C5 convertase activity.

The formation of C3 convertases is the point at which the three pathways of complement activation converge, because both the classical pathway and MB-lectin pathway convertase C4b2b and the alternative pathway convertase C3bBb have the same activity, and they initiate the same subsequent events. They both cleave C3 to C3b and C3a. C3b binds covalently through its thioester bond to adjacent molecules on the pathogen surface; otherwise it is inactivated by hydrolysis. C3 is the most abundant complement protein in plasma, occurring at a concentration of 1.2 mg ml⁻¹, and up to 1000 molecules of C3b can bind in the vicinity of a single active C3 convertase (see Fig. 2.28). Thus, the main effect of complement activation is to deposit large quantities of C3b on the surface of the infecting pathogen, where it forms a covalently bonded coat that, as we will see, can signal the ultimate destruction of the pathogen by phagocytes.

The next step in the cascade is the generation of the C5 convertases. In the classical and the MB-lectin pathways, a C5 convertase is formed by the binding of C3b to C4b2b to yield C4b2b3b. By the same token, the C5 convertase of the alternative pathway is formed by the binding of C3b to the C3 convertase to form C3b₂Bb. C5 is captured by these C5 convertase complexes through binding to an acceptor site on C3b, and is then rendered susceptible to cleavage by the serine protease activity of C2b or Bb. This reaction, which generates C5b and C5a, is much more limited than cleavage of C3, as C5 can be cleaved only when it binds to C3b that is part of the C5 convertase complex. Thus, complement activated by all three pathways leads to the binding of large numbers of C3b molecules on the surface of the pathogen, the generation of a more limited number of C5b molecules, and the release of C3a and C5a (Fig. 2.30).

2-16 Ingestion of complement-tagged pathogens by phagocytes is mediated by receptors for the bound complement proteins.

The most important action of complement is to facilitate the uptake and destruction of pathogens by phagocytic cells. This occurs by the specific recognition of bound complement components by **complement receptors (CRs)** on phagocytes. These complement receptors bind pathogens opsonized with complement components: opsonization of pathogens is a major function of C3b and its proteolytic derivatives. C4b also acts as an opsonin but has a relatively minor role, largely because so much more C3b than C4b is generated.

The six known types of receptor for bound complement components are listed, with their functions and distributions, in Fig. 2.31. The best characterized is the C3b receptor **CR1 (CD35)**, which is expressed on both macrophages and polymorphonuclear leukocytes. Binding of C3b to CR1 cannot by itself stimulate phagocytosis, but it can lead to phagocytosis in the presence of other immune mediators that activate macrophages. For example, the small complement fragment C5a can activate macrophages to ingest bacteria bound to their CR1 receptors (Fig. 2.32). C5a binds to another receptor expressed by macrophages, the **C5a receptor**, which has seven membrane-spanning domains. Receptors

Receptor	Specificity	Functions	Cell types
CR1 (CD35)	C3b, C4b iC3b	Promotes C3b and C4b decay Stimulates phagocytosis Erythrocyte transport of immune complexes	Erythrocytes, macrophages, monocytes, polymorphonuclear leukocytes, B cells, FDC
CR2 (CD21)	C3d, iC3b, C3dg Epstein–Barr virus	Part of B-cell co-receptor Epstein–Barr virus receptor	B cells, FDC
CR3 (Mac-1) (CD11b/ CD18)	iC3b	Stimulates phagocytosis	Macrophages, monocytes, polymorphonuclear leukocytes, FDC
CR4 (gp150, 95) (CD11c/ CD18)	iC3b	Stimulates phagocytosis	Macrophages, monocytes, polymorphonuclear leukocytes, dendritic cells
C5a receptor	C5a	Binding of C5a activates G protein	Endothelial cells, mast cells, phagocytes
C3a receptor	C3a	Binding of C3a activates G protein	Endothelial cells, mast cells, phagocytes

Fig. 2.31 Distribution and function of receptors for complement proteins on the surfaces of cells. There are several different receptors specific for different bound complement components and their fragments. CR1 and CR3 are especially important in inducing phagocytosis of bacteria with complement components on their surface. CR2 is found mainly on B cells, where it is also part of the B-cell co-receptor complex and the receptor by which the Epstein–Barr virus selectively infects B cells, causing infectious mononucleosis. CR1 and CR2 share structural features with the complement-regulatory proteins that bind C3b and C4b. CR3 and CR4 are integrins; CR3 is known to be important for leukocyte adhesion and migration, whereas CR4 is only known to function in phagocytic responses. The C5a and C3a receptors are seven-span G-protein-coupled receptors. FDC, follicular dendritic cells; these are not involved in innate immunity and are discussed in later chapters.

of this type couple with intracellular guanine-nucleotide-binding proteins called G proteins, and the C5a receptor signals in this way. Proteins associated with the extracellular matrix, such as fibronectin, can also contribute to phagocyte activation; these are encountered when phagocytes are recruited to connective tissue and activated there. C3a, which has inflammatory activities similar to those of C5a, although it is a less potent chemoattractant, binds to its own specific receptor, the C3a receptor, which is homologous in structure to the C5a receptor.

Three other complement receptors—**CR2** (also known as **CD21**), **CR3** (**CD11b:CD18**), and **CR4** (**CD11c:CD18**)—bind to inactivated forms of C3b that remain attached to the pathogen surface. Like several other key components of complement, C3b is subject to regulatory mechanisms and can be cleaved into derivatives that cannot form an active convertase. One of the inactive derivatives of C3b, known as iC3b (see Section 2-14) acts as an opsonin in its own right when bound by the complement receptors CR2 or CR3. Unlike the binding of iC3b to CR1, the binding of iC3b to CR3 is sufficient on its own to stimulate phagocytosis. A second breakdown product of C3b, called **C3dg**, binds only to CR2. CR2 is found on B cells as part of a co-receptor complex that can augment the signal received through the antigen-specific immunoglobulin receptor. Thus a B cell whose antigen receptor is specific for a given pathogen will receive a strongly augmented signal on binding this pathogen if it is also coated with C3dg. The activation of complement can therefore contribute to producing a strong antibody response (see Chapters 6 and 9). This example of how an innate humoral immune response can contribute to activating adaptive humoral immunity parallels the contribution made by the innate cellular response of macrophages and dendritic cells to the initiation of a T-cell response, which we will discuss later in this chapter.

Fig. 2.32 The anaphylatoxin C5a can enhance the phagocytosis of opsonized microorganisms. Activation of complement, either by the alternative or by the MB-lectin pathway, leads to the deposition of C3b on the surface of the microorganism (left panel). C3b can be bound by the complement receptor CR1 on the surface of phagocytes, but this on its own is insufficient to induce phagocytosis (center panel). Phagocytes also express receptors for the anaphylatoxin C5a, and binding of C5a will now activate the cell to phagocytose microorganisms bound through CR1 (right panel).

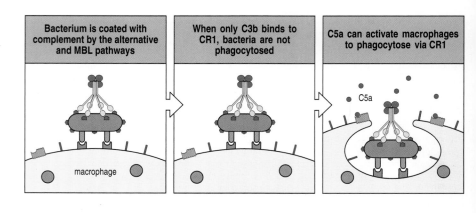

| Bacterium is coated with complement by the alternative and MBL pathways | When only C3b binds to CR1, bacteria are not phagocytosed | C5a can activate macrophages to phagocytose via CR1 |

The central role of opsonization by C3b and its inactive fragments in the destruction of extracellular pathogens can be seen in the effects of various complement deficiency diseases. Whereas individuals deficient in any of the late components of complement are relatively unaffected, individuals deficient in C3 or in molecules that catalyze C3b deposition show increased susceptibility to infection by a wide range of extracellular bacteria, as we will see in Chapter 11.

2-17   Small fragments of some complement proteins can initiate a local inflammatory response.

The small complement fragments C3a, C4a, and C5a act on specific receptors (see Fig. 2.31) to produce local inflammatory responses. When produced in large amounts or injected systemically, they induce a generalized circulatory collapse, producing a shock-like syndrome similar to that seen in a systemic allergic reaction involving IgE antibodies (see Chapter 12). Such a reaction is termed **anaphylactic shock** and these small fragments of complement are therefore often referred to as **anaphylatoxins**. Of the three, C5a has the highest specific biological activity. All three induce smooth muscle contraction and increase vascular permeability, but C5a and C3a also act on the endothelial cells lining blood vessels to induce adhesion molecules. In addition, C3a and C5a can activate the mast cells that populate submucosal tissues to release mediators such as histamine and TNF-α that cause similar effects. The changes induced by C5a and C3a recruit antibody, complement, and phagocytic cells to the site of an infection (Fig. 2.33), and the increased fluid in the tissues hastens the movement of pathogen-bearing antigen-presenting cells to the local lymph nodes, contributing to the prompt initiation of the adaptive immune response.

C5a also acts directly on neutrophils and monocytes to increase their adherence to vessel walls, their migration toward sites of antigen deposition, and their ability to ingest particles. C5a also increases the expression of CR1 and CR3 on the surfaces of these cells. In this way, C5a, and to a smaller extent C3a and C4a, act in concert with other complement components to hasten the destruction of pathogens by phagocytes. C5a and C3a signal through transmembrane receptors that activate G proteins; thus the action of C5a in attracting neutrophils and monocytes is analogous to that of chemokines, which also act via G proteins to control cell migration.

2-18 The terminal complement proteins polymerize to form pores in membranes that can kill certain pathogens.

One of the important effects of complement activation is the assembly of the terminal components of complement (Fig. 2.34) to form a membrane-attack complex. The reactions leading to the formation of this complex are shown schematically and microscopically in Fig. 2.35. The end result is a pore in the lipid bilayer membrane that destroys membrane integrity. This is thought to kill the pathogen by destroying the proton gradient across the pathogen's cell membrane.

The first step in the formation of the membrane-attack complex is the cleavage of C5 by a C5 convertase to release C5b (see Fig. 2.30). In the next stages, shown in Fig. 2.35, C5b initiates the assembly of the later complement components and their insertion into the cell membrane. First, one molecule of C5b binds one molecule of C6, and the C5b6 complex then binds one molecule of C7. This reaction leads to a conformational change in the constituent molecules, with the exposure of a hydrophobic site on C7, which inserts into the lipid bilayer. Similar hydrophobic sites are exposed on the later components C8 and C9 when they are bound to the complex, allowing these proteins also to insert into the lipid bilayer. C8 is a complex of two proteins, C8β and C8α-γ. The C8β protein binds to C5b, and the binding of C8β to the membrane-associated C5b67 complex allows the hydrophobic domain of C8α-γ to insert into the lipid bilayer. Finally, C8α-γ induces the polymerization of 10 to 16 molecules of C9

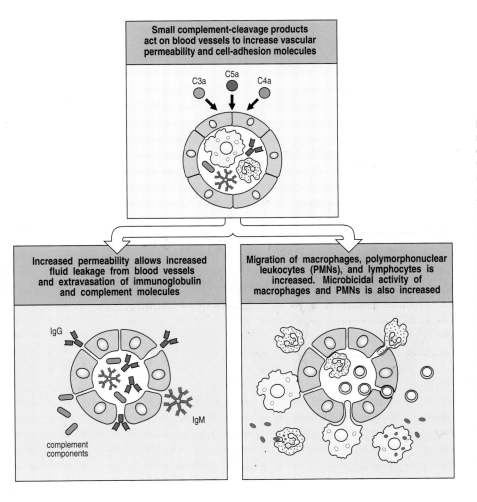

Fig. 2.33 Local inflammatory responses can be induced by small complement fragments, especially C5a. The small complement fragments are differentially active: C5a is more active than C3a, which is more active than C4a. They cause local inflammatory responses by acting directly on local blood vessels, stimulating an increase in blood flow, increased vascular permeability, and increased binding of phagocytes to endothelial cells. C5a also activates mast cells (not shown) to release mediators, such as histamine and TNF-α, that contribute to the inflammatory response. The increase in vessel diameter and permeability leads to the accumulation of fluid and protein. Fluid accumulation increases lymphatic drainage, bringing pathogens and their antigenic components to nearby lymph nodes. The antibodies, complement, and cells thus recruited participate in pathogen clearance by enhancing phagocytosis. The small complement fragments can also directly increase the activity of the phagocytes.

Fig. 2.34 The terminal complement components assemble to form the membrane-attack complex.

The terminal complement components that form the membrane-attack complex		
Native protein	**Active component**	**Function**
C5	C5a	Small peptide mediator of inflammation (high activity)
	C5b	Initiates assembly of the membrane-attack system
C6	C6	Binds C5b; forms acceptor for C7
C7	C7	Binds C5b6; amphiphilic complex inserts in lipid bilayer
C8	C8	Binds C5b67; initiates C9 polymerization
C9	$C9_n$	Polymerizes to C5b678 to form a membrane-spanning channel, lysing cell

into a pore-forming structure called the membrane-attack complex. The membrane-attack complex, shown schematically and by electron microscopy in Fig. 2.35, has a hydrophobic external face, allowing it to associate with the lipid bilayer, but a hydrophilic internal channel. The diameter of this channel is about 100 Å, allowing the free passage of solutes and water across the lipid bilayer. The disruption of the lipid bilayer leads to the loss of cellular homeostasis, the disruption of the proton gradient across the membrane, the penetration of enzymes such as lysozyme into the cell, and the eventual destruction of the pathogen.

Although the effect of the membrane-attack complex is very dramatic, particularly in experimental demonstrations in which antibodies against red blood cell membranes are used to trigger the complement cascade, the significance of these components in host defense seems to be quite limited. So far, deficiencies in complement components C5–C9 have been associated with susceptibility only to *Neisseria* species, the bacteria that cause the sexually transmitted disease gonorrhea and a common form of bacterial meningitis. Thus, the opsonizing and inflammatory actions of the earlier components of the complement cascade are clearly more important for host defense against infection. Formation of the membrane-attack complex seems to be important only for the killing of a few pathogens, although, as we will see in Chapter 13, it might well have a major role in immunopathology.

2-19   Complement control proteins regulate all three pathways of complement activation and protect the host from its destructive effects.

Given the destructive effects of complement, and the way in which its activation is rapidly amplified through a triggered-enzyme cascade, it is not surprising that there are several mechanisms to prevent its uncontrolled activation. As we have seen, the effector molecules of complement are generated through the sequential activation of zymogens, which are present in plasma in an inactive form. The activation of these zymogens usually occurs on a pathogen surface, and the activated complement fragments produced in the ensuing cascade of reactions usually bind nearby or are rapidly inactivated by hydrolysis. These two features of complement activation act as safeguards against uncontrolled activation. Even so, all complement components

Fig. 2.35 Assembly of the membrane-attack complex generates a pore in the lipid bilayer membrane. The sequence of steps and their approximate appearance are shown here in schematic form. C5b triggers the assembly of a complex of one molecule each of C6, C7, and C8, in that order. C7 and C8 undergo conformational changes that expose hydrophobic domains that insert into the membrane. This complex causes moderate membrane damage in its own right, and also serves to induce the polymerization of C9, again with the exposure of a hydrophobic site. Up to 16 molecules of C9 are then added to the assembly to generate a channel 100 Å in diameter in the membrane. This channel disrupts the bacterial cell membrane, killing the bacterium. The electron micrographs show erythrocyte membranes with membrane-attack complexes in two orientations, end on and side on. Photographs courtesy of S. Bhakdi and J. Tranum-Jensen.

are activated spontaneously at a low rate in plasma, and activated complement components will sometimes bind proteins on host cells. The potentially damaging consequences are prevented by a series of complement control proteins, summarized in Fig. 2.36, which regulate the complement cascade at different points. As we saw in discussing the alternative pathway of complement activation (see Section 2-14), many of these control proteins specifically protect host cells while allowing complement activation to proceed on pathogen surfaces. The complement control proteins therefore allow complement to distinguish self from nonself.

The reactions that regulate the complement cascade are shown in Fig. 2.37. The top two panels show how the activation of C1 is controlled by a plasma serine protease inhibitor or **serpin**, the C1 inhibitor (C1INH). C1INH binds the active enzymes C1r:C1s and causes them to dissociate from C1q, which remains bound to the pathogen. In this way, C1INH limits the time during which active C1s is able to cleave C4 and C2. By the same means, C1INH limits the spontaneous activation of C1 in plasma. Its importance can be seen in the C1INH deficiency disease **hereditary angioneurotic edema**, in which chronic spontaneous complement activation leads to the production of excess cleaved fragments of C4 and C2. The small fragment of C2, C2a, is further

Hereditary Angioneurotic Edema

Fig. 2.36 The proteins that regulate the activity of complement.

Regulatory proteins of the classical and alternative pathways	
Name (symbol)	**Role in the regulation of complement activation**
C1 inhibitor (C1INH)	Binds to activated C1r, C1s, removing them from C1q
C4-binding protein (C4BP)	Binds C4b, displacing C2b; cofactor for C4b cleavage by I
Complement receptor 1 (CR1)	Binds C4b, displacing C2b, or C3b displacing Bb; cofactor for I
Factor H (H)	Binds C3b, displacing Bb; cofactor for I
Factor I (I)	Serine protease that cleaves C3b and C4b; aided by H, MCP, C4BP, or CR1
Decay-accelerating factor (DAF)	Membrane protein that displaces Bb from C3b and C2b from C4b
Membrane cofactor protein (MCP)	Membrane protein that promotes C3b and C4b inactivation by I
CD59 (protectin)	Prevents formation of membrane-attack complex on autologous or allogenic cells. Widely expressed on membranes

cleaved into a peptide, the C2 kinin, which causes extensive swelling—the most dangerous being local swelling in the trachea, which can lead to suffocation. Bradykinin, which has similar actions to C2 kinin, is also produced in an uncontrolled fashion in this disease, as a result of the lack of inhibition of another plasma protease, kallikrein, which is activated by tissue damage and also regulated by C1INH. This disease is fully corrected by replacing C1INH. The large activated fragments of C4 and C2, which normally combine to form the C3 convertase, do not damage host cells in such patients because C4b is rapidly inactivated in plasma (see Fig. 2.25) and the convertase does not form. Furthermore, any convertase that accidentally forms on a host cell is inactivated by the mechanisms described below.

The thioester bond of activated C3 and C4 is extremely reactive and has no mechanism for distinguishing an acceptor hydroxyl or amine group on a host cell from a similar group on the surface of a pathogen. A series of protective mechanisms, mediated by other proteins, has evolved to ensure that the binding of a small number of C3 or C4 molecules to host cell membranes results in minimal formation of C3 convertase and little amplification of complement activation. We have already encountered most of these mechanisms in the description of the alternative pathway (see Fig. 2.26), but we will consider them again here, because they are important regulators of the classical pathway convertase as well (see Fig. 2.37, second and third rows). The mechanisms can be divided into three categories. The first catalyze the cleavage of any C3b or C4b that does bind to host cells into inactive products. The complement-regulatory enzyme responsible is the plasma serine protease factor I; it circulates in active form but can cleave C3b and C4b only when they are bound to a membrane cofactor protein. In these circumstances, factor I cleaves C3b, first into iC3b and then further to C3dg, thus permanently inactivating it. C4b is similarly inactivated by cleavage into C4c and C4d. There are two cell-membrane proteins that bind C3b and C4b and possess cofactor activity for factor I; these are CR1 and MCP (see Section 2-14). Microbial cell walls lack these protective proteins and cannot promote the breakdown of

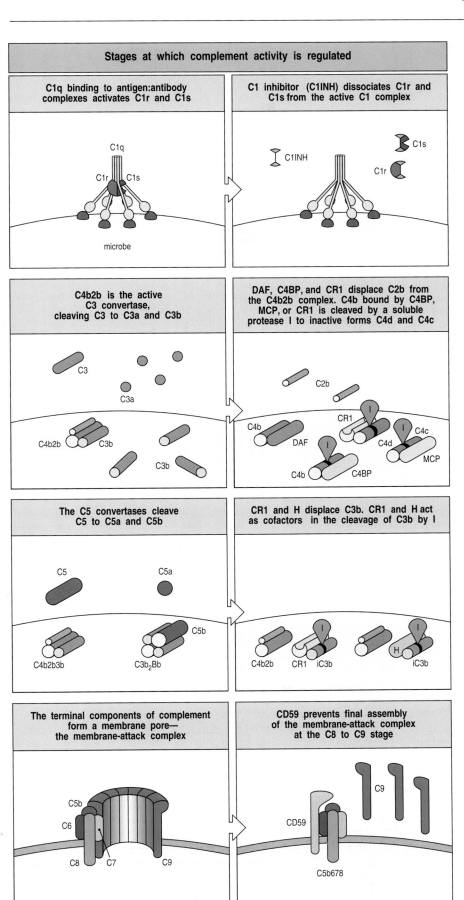

Stages at which complement activity is regulated

C1q binding to antigen:antibody complexes activates C1r and C1s

C1q
C1r C1s
microbe

C1 inhibitor (C1INH) dissociates C1r and C1s from the active C1 complex

C1INH
C1s
C1r

C4b2b is the active C3 convertase, cleaving C3 to C3a and C3b

C3
C3a
C4b2b   C3b
C3b

DAF, C4BP, and CR1 displace C2b from the C4b2b complex. C4b bound by C4BP, MCP, or CR1 is cleaved by a soluble protease I to inactive forms C4d and C4c

C2b
CR1
C4b
DAF
C4c
C4d
MCP
C4b   C4BP

The C5 convertases cleave C5 to C5a and C5b

C5
C5a
C5b
C4b2b3b   C3b₂Bb

CR1 and H displace C3b. CR1 and H act as cofactors in the cleavage of C3b by I

C4b2b   CR1   iC3b
H   iC3b

The terminal components of complement form a membrane pore— the membrane-attack complex

C5b
C6
C8   C7   C9

CD59 prevents final assembly of the membrane-attack complex at the C8 to C9 stage

C9
CD59
C5b678

Fig. 2.37 Complement activation is regulated by a series of proteins that serve to protect host cells from accidental damage. These act on different stages of the complement cascade, dissociating complexes or catalyzing the enzymatic degradation of covalently bound complement proteins. Stages in the complement cascade are shown schematically down the left side of the figure, with the control reactions on the right. The alternative pathway C3 convertase is similarly regulated by DAF, CR1, MCP, and factor H.

Factor I
Deficiency

C3b and C4b. Instead, these proteins act as binding sites for factor B and C2, promoting complement activation. The importance of factor I can be seen in people with genetic factor I deficiency. Because of uncontrolled complement activation, complement proteins rapidly become depleted and such people suffer repeated bacterial infections, especially with ubiquitous pyogenic bacteria.

There are also plasma proteins with cofactor activity for factor I. C4b is bound by a cofactor known as **C4b-binding protein** (**C4BP**), which mainly acts as a regulator of the classical pathway in the fluid phase. C3b is bound in both the fluid phase and at cell membranes by a cofactor protein called factor H (see Section 2-14). Factor H is an important complement regulator at cell membranes, and at first sight it is not obvious how factor H can distinguish between C3b bound to host cells and that bound to a pathogen. However, the carbohydrate content of the cell membranes of bacterial pathogens differs from that of their hosts and this is the basis for the protective effect of factor H. Factor H has affinity for the terminal sialic acids of host cell membrane glycoproteins and this increases the binding of factor H to any C3b deposited on host cells. In contrast, factor H has a much lower affinity for C3b deposited on the cell walls of many bacteria, and factor B binds in preference, resulting in the amplification of complement activation on bacterial cell surfaces. In effect, factor H and factor B compete for binding to C3b bound to cells. If factor B 'wins,' as typically happens on a pathogen surface, then more C3bBb C3 convertase forms and complement activation is amplified. If factor H 'wins,' as occurs on cells of the host, then the bound C3b is catabolized by factor I to iC3b and C3dg and complement activation is inhibited.

The competition between factor H and factor B for binding to surface-bound C3b is an example of the second mechanism for inhibiting complement activation on host cell membranes. Several proteins competitively inhibit the binding of C2 to cell-bound C4b and of factor B to cell-bound C3b, thereby inhibiting convertase formation. These proteins bind to C3b and C4b on the cell surface, and also mediate protection against complement through the third mechanism, which is to augment the dissociation of C4b2b and C3bBb convertases that have already formed. Host cell membrane molecules that regulate complement through both these mechanisms include DAF and CR1, which promote the dissociation of convertase in addition to their cofactor activity. All the proteins that bind the homologous C4b and C3b molecules share one or more copies of a structural element called the short consensus repeat (SCR), complement control protein (CCP) repeat, or (especially in Japan) the sushi domain.

In addition to the mechanisms for preventing C3 convertase formation and C4 and C3 deposition on cell membranes, there are also inhibitory mechanisms that prevent the inappropriate insertion of the membrane-attack complex into membranes. We saw in Section 2-18 that the membrane-attack complex polymerizes onto C5b molecules created by the action of C5 convertase. This complex mainly inserts into cell membranes adjacent to the site of the C5 convertase; that is, close to the site of complement activation on a pathogen. However, some newly formed membrane-attack complexes may diffuse from the site of complement activation and insert into adjacent host cell membranes. Several plasma proteins bind to the C5b67 complex and thereby inhibit its random insertion into cell membranes. The most important is probably C8β itself, when it binds to C5b67 in the fluid phase. Host cell membranes also contain an intrinsic protein, **CD59** or **protectin**, which inhibits the binding of C9 to the C5b678 complex (see Fig. 2.37, bottom row). CD59 and DAF are both linked to the cell surface by a glycosylphosphatidylinositol (GPI) tail, like many other peripheral membrane proteins. One of the enzymes involved in the synthesis of GPI tails is encoded on the X chromosome. In people with a somatic mutation in this gene in a clone of hematopoietic cells, both CD59 and DAF fail to function. This causes the disease **paroxysmal nocturnal hemoglobinuria**, which is characterized by episodes of intravascular red blood cell lysis by complement. Red blood cells that lack CD59 only are also susceptible to destruction as a result of spontaneous activation of the complement cascade.

Summary.

The complement system is one of the major mechanisms by which pathogen recognition is converted into an effective host defense against initial infection. Complement is a system of plasma proteins that can be activated directly by pathogens or indirectly by pathogen-bound antibody, leading to a cascade of reactions that occurs on the surface of pathogens and generates active components with various effector functions. There are three pathways of complement activation: the classical pathway, which is triggered directly by pathogen or indirectly by antibody binding to the pathogen surface; the MB-lectin pathway; and the alternative pathway, which also provides an amplification loop for the other two pathways. All three pathways can be initiated independently of antibody as part of innate immunity. The early events in all pathways consist of a sequence of cleavage reactions in which the larger cleavage product binds covalently to the pathogen surface and contributes to the activation of the next component. The pathways converge with the formation of a C3 convertase enzyme, which cleaves C3 to produce the active complement component C3b. The binding of large numbers of C3b molecules to the pathogen is the central event in complement activation. Bound complement components, especially bound C3b and its inactive fragments, are recognized by specific complement receptors on phagocytic cells, which engulf pathogens opsonized by C3b and its inactive fragments. The small cleavage fragments of C3, C4, and especially C5 recruit phagocytes to sites of infection and activate them by binding to specific trimeric G-protein-coupled receptors. Together, these activities promote the uptake and destruction of pathogens by phagocytes. The molecules of C3b that bind the C3 convertase itself initiate the late events, binding C5 to make it susceptible to cleavage by C2b or Bb. The larger C5b fragment triggers the assembly of a membrane-attack complex, which can result in the lysis of certain pathogens. The activity of complement components is modulated by a system of regulatory proteins that prevent tissue damage as a result of inadvertent binding of activated complement components to host cells or of spontaneous activation of complement components in plasma.

Induced innate responses to infection.

In the final part of this chapter we will look at the induced responses of innate immunity. These depend on the cytokines and chemokines that are produced in response to pathogen recognition, and we will introduce these first. The chemokines are a large family of chemoattractant molecules with a central role in leukocyte migration, and because adhesion molecules also have a central role in this process we will also consider them briefly. This will be followed by a description of how macrophage-derived chemokines and cytokines promote the phagocytic response through the recruitment and production of fresh phagocytes and opsonizing molecules, while containing the spread of infection to the bloodstream through the activation of clotting mechanisms. We will also look at the role of the cytokines known as **interferons**, which are induced by viral infection, and at a class of lymphoid cells, known as **natural killer (NK) cells**, that are activated by interferons to contribute to innate host defense against viruses and other intracellular pathogens. We will also discuss the **innate-like lymphocytes (ILLs)**, which contribute to rapid responses to infection by acting early but use a limited set of antigen-receptor gene segments (see Section 1-11) to make immunoglobulins and T-cell receptors. These cells have a role in host defense, but only if the proteins that promote antigen-receptor gene rearrangement, RAG-1 and RAG-2, are present. (We will describe these proteins and their role in adaptive immune lymphocytes in detail in Chapter 4.) ILLs are therefore, by definition, members of the adaptive immune system, but they behave more like a part of the innate immune system.

The induced innate responses can either succeed in clearing the infection or contain it while an adaptive response develops. Adaptive immunity harnesses many of the same effector mechanisms that are used by the innate immune system, but adaptive immunity is able to target them with much greater precision. Thus antigen-specific T cells activate the microbicidal and cytokine-secreting properties of macrophages harboring pathogens, while antibodies activate complement, act as direct opsonins for phagocytes, and stimulate NK cells to kill infected cells. In addition, the adaptive immune response uses cytokines and chemokines, in a manner similar to that of innate immunity, to induce inflammatory responses that promote the influx of antibodies and effector lymphocytes to sites of infection. The effector mechanisms described here therefore serve as a primer for the later chapters that focus on adaptive immunity.

2-20   Activated macrophages secrete a range of cytokines that have a variety of local and distant effects.

Cytokines (see Appendix III) are small proteins (approximately 25 kDa) that are released by various cells in the body, usually in response to an activating stimulus, and they induce responses through binding to specific receptors. They can act in an autocrine manner, affecting the behavior of the cell that releases the cytokine, in a paracrine manner, affecting the behavior of adjacent cells, and some cytokines are stable enough to act in an endocrine manner, affecting the behavior of distant cells, although this depends on their ability to enter the circulation and on their half-life in the blood.

The cytokines secreted by macrophages in response to pathogens are a structurally diverse group of molecules that include interleukin-1β (IL-1β), IL-6, IL-12, TNF-α, and the chemokine IL-8 (now known as CXCL8). The name **interleukin (IL)** followed by a number (for example IL-1, IL-2, and so on) was coined in an attempt to develop a standardized nomenclature for molecules secreted by, and acting on, leukocytes. However, this became confusing when an ever-increasing number of cytokines with diverse origins, structures, and effects were discovered, and although the IL designation is still used, it is hoped that eventually a nomenclature based on cytokine structure will be developed (Fig. 2.38). The cytokines and their receptors are grouped according to their structure in the appendices at the end of this book (Appendix III). There are two major structural families of cytokines: the hematopoietin family, which includes growth hormones and also many interleukins with roles in both adaptive and innate immunity, and the TNF family, which again functions in both innate and adaptive immunity and includes many members that are membrane-bound. Of the macrophage-derived interleukins shown in Fig. 2.39, IL-6 belongs to the large family of hematopoietins, TNF-α is obviously part of the TNF family, and IL-1 and IL-12 are structurally distinct. All have important local and systemic effects that contribute to both innate and adaptive immunity, and these are summarized in Fig. 2.39.

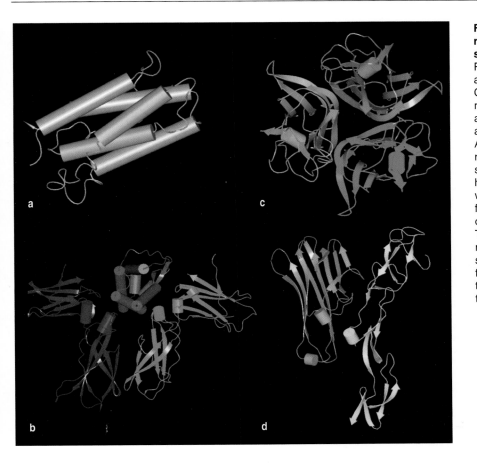

Fig. 2.38 Cytokines and their receptors can be grouped into a small number of structural families. Representatives of the hematopoietin and TNF families are shown here. Cytokines are in the top row with their receptors below. The hematopoietins are represented by IL-4 (panel a). They are small single-chain proteins. A hypothetical model of the dimeric IL-4 receptor structure (based on the known structure of the related human growth hormone receptor) is shown in panel b, with bound IL-4 in red. Tumor necrosis factor (TNF) and its related molecules occur as trimers, as shown in panel c. The structure of one subunit of a TNF receptor binding a monomeric TNF is shown in panel d. The other structural families of immunological interest are the interferons and their receptors and the chemokines and their receptors.

The recognition of different classes of pathogen may involve signaling through distinct receptors and result in some variation in the cytokines induced. The study of this is still in its infancy, but it is thought to be a way in which appropriate responses can be selectively activated as the released cytokines orchestrate the next phase of host defense. We will see how TNF-α, which is elicited by LPS-bearing pathogens, is particularly important in containing infection by these pathogens, and how the release of different chemokines can recruit and activate different types of effector cell.

2-21 Chemokines released by phagocytes and dendritic cells recruit cells to sites of infection.

Among the cytokines released by tissues in the earliest phases of infection are members of a family of chemoattractant cytokines known as **chemokines**. These small proteins induce directed chemotaxis in nearby responsive cells and were discovered only relatively recently. Because they were first detected in cytokine assays, they were initially named interleukins: interleukin-8 (now known as CXCL8) was the first chemokine to be cloned and characterized, and it remains typical of this family. All the chemokines are related in amino acid sequence, and their receptors are all integral membrane proteins containing seven membrane-spanning helices. This structure is characteristic of receptors such as rhodopsin (Fig. 2.40) and the muscarinic acetylcholine receptor, which are coupled to G proteins; the chemokine receptors also signal through coupled G proteins. Chemokines function mainly as chemoattractants for leukocytes, recruiting monocytes, neutrophils, and other effector cells from the blood to sites of infection. They can be released by many different types of cell and they serve to guide cells involved in innate immunity

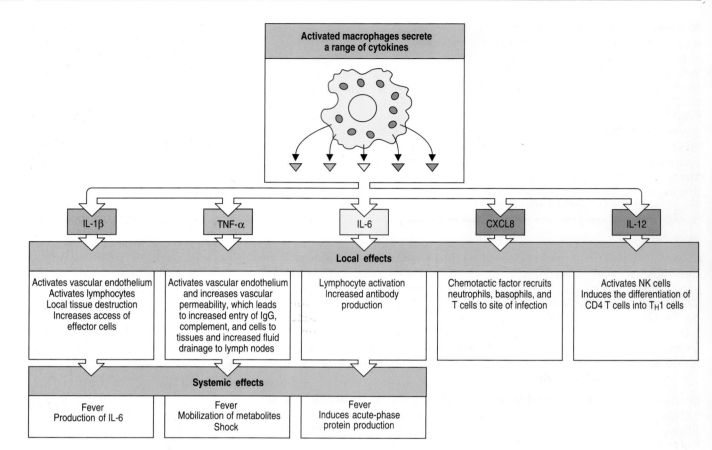

Fig. 2.39 Important cytokines secreted by macrophages in response to bacterial products include IL-1, IL-6, CXCL8, IL-12, and TNF-α. TNF-α is an inducer of a local inflammatory response that helps to contain infections. It also has systemic effects, many of which are harmful (see Section 2-24). The chemokine CXCL8 is also involved in the local inflammatory response, helping to attract neutrophils to the site of infection. IL-1, IL-6, and TNF-α have a critical role in inducing the acute-phase response in the liver (see Section 2-25) and induce fever, which favors effective host defense in various ways. IL-12 activates natural killer (NK) cells and favors the differentiation of CD4 T cells into the T$_H$1 subset in adaptive immunity.

to sites of infection. They also guide the lymphocytes in adaptive immunity, as we will learn in Chapters 8–10. Some chemokines also function in lymphocyte development and migration, and in angiogenesis (the growth of new blood vessels). The properties of a variety of chemokines are listed in Fig. 2.41 (see also Appendix IV). Quite why there are so many chemokines is not yet known, but it may reflect their importance in delivering cells to their correct location, as seems to be the case for lymphocytes.

Members of the chemokine family fall mostly into two broad groups—CC chemokines with two adjacent cysteines near the amino terminus, and CXC chemokines, in which the equivalent two cysteine residues are separated by a single amino acid. The two groups of chemokines act on different sets of receptors. CC chemokines bind to CC chemokine receptors, of which there are nine, designated CCR1–9. CXC chemokines bind to CXC receptors; there are six of these, CXCR1–6. These receptors are expressed on different cell types, which are consequently attracted by different chemokines. In general, CXC chemokines with a Glu-Leu-Arg tripeptide motif immediately before the first cysteine promote the migration of neutrophils. CXCL8 is an example of this type of chemokine. Other CXC chemokines that lack this motif, such as the B-lymphocyte chemokine (CXCL13), guide lymphocytes to their proper destination in the B-cell areas of the spleen, lymph nodes, and gut. The CC chemokines promote the migration of monocytes, lymphocytes, or other cell types. An example is macrophage chemoattractant protein-1 (CCL2). CXCL8 and CCL2 have similar, although complementary, functions: CXCL8 induces neutrophils to leave the bloodstream and migrate into the surrounding tissues; CCL2, by contrast, acts on monocytes, inducing their migration from the bloodstream to become tissue macrophages. Other CC chemokines such as CCL5 may promote the infiltration into tissues of a range of leukocytes, including effector T cells (see Section 10-8), with individual chemokines acting on different subsets of cells. The only known chemokine with only one cysteine (XCL1) was originally called lymphotactin; it is thought to attract T-cell precursors to the thymus by binding to XCR1. The chemokine fractalkine is unusual in several ways: it has three amino acid residues between the two cysteines, making it a CX_3CL chemokine. Most unusually, it exists in two forms, one tethered to the membrane of the endothelial and epithelial cells that express it, where it serves as an adhesion protein, and a soluble form released from the cell surface, which acts, like other chemokines, as a chemoattractant. We will return to the chemokines in Chapter 10.

The role of chemokines such as CXCL8 and CCL2 in cell recruitment is twofold. First, they act on the leukocyte as it rolls along endothelial cells at sites of inflammation, converting this rolling into stable binding by triggering a change of conformation in the adhesion molecules known as leukocyte integrins. This allows the leukocyte to cross the blood vessel wall by squeezing between the endothelial cells, as we will see when we describe the process of extravasation. Second, the chemokine directs the migration of the leukocyte along a gradient of chemokine molecules bound to the extracellular matrix and the surfaces of endothelial cells. This gradient increases in concentration toward the site of infection.

Chemokines can be produced by a wide variety of cell types in response to bacterial products, viruses, and agents that cause physical damage, such as silica, alum, or the urate crystals that occur in gout. Thus, infection or physical damage to tissues sets in motion the production of chemokine gradients that can direct phagocytes to the sites where they are needed. In addition, peptides that act as chemoattractants for neutrophils are made by bacteria themselves. All bacteria produce proteins with an amino-terminal N-formylated methionine, and, as discovered many years ago, the fMet-Leu-Phe (fMLP) peptide is a potent chemotactic factor for inflammatory cells, especially neutrophils. The fMLP receptor is also a G-protein-coupled receptor, like the receptors for chemokines and for the complement fragments C5a, C3a, and C4a. Thus, there is a common mechanism for attracting neutrophils, whether by complement fragments, chemokines, or bacterial peptides. Neutrophils are the first cells to arrive in large numbers at a site of infection, with monocytes and immature dendritic cells being recruited later.

The complement peptide C5a and the chemokines CXCL8 and CCL2 also activate their respective target cells, so that not only are neutrophils and macrophages brought to potential sites of infection but, in the process, they are armed to deal with any pathogens they may encounter there. In particular, neutrophils exposed to CXCL8 and the cytokine TNF-α are activated to produce the respiratory burst that generates oxygen radicals and nitric oxide, and to release their stored lysosomal contents, thus contributing both to host defense and to the tissue destruction and pus formation seen in local sites, especially those infected with pyogenic bacteria.

Chemokines do not act alone in cell recruitment. They also require the action of vasoactive mediators to bring leukocytes close to the blood vessel endothelium (see Section 2-4) and cytokines such as TNF-α to induce the necessary adhesion molecules on the endothelial cells. We will now turn to the molecules that mediate leukocyte adherence to the endothelium, and then describe the process of leukocyte extravasation step-by-step as it has been shown for both neutrophils and monocytes.

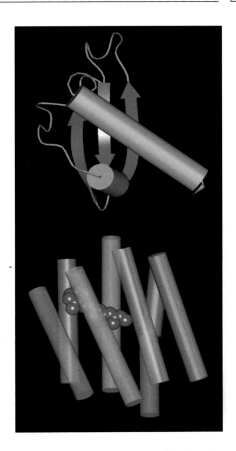

Fig. 2.40 Chemokines are a family of proteins of similar structure that bind to chemokine receptors, themselves part of a large family of G-protein-coupled receptors. The chemokines are represented here by CXCL8 (upper structure). The receptors for the chemokines are members of the family of seven-span receptors, which also includes the photoreceptor protein rhodopsin and many other receptors. They have seven transmembrane helices, and all the family interact with G proteins. The first solved structure of a seven-span membrane protein was of the bacterial protein bacteriorhodopsin; it is depicted here (lower structure), showing the orientation of the seven transmembrane helices (blue) with the bound ligand (in this case retinal) in red. Essentially all of this structure would be embedded within the cell membrane. Cylinders represent α helices and arrows β strands.

Fig. 2.41 Properties of selected chemokines. Chemokines fall mainly into two related but distinct groups. The CXC chemokines, the genes for which in humans are mainly found in a cluster on chromosome 17, have an amino-acid residue (X) between two invariant cysteines (C) in the amino-terminal region. CC chemokines, which in humans are mostly encoded in one region of chromosome 4, have these two invariant cysteines adjacent. These classes can be divided further by the presence or absence of an amino-acid triplet (ELR: glutamic acid-leucine-arginine) preceding the first of these invariant cysteines. All the chemokines that attract neutrophils have this motif, whereas most of the other CXC chemokines, including those that interact with receptors CXCR3, 4, and 5, lack it. A C chemokine with only one cysteine at this location, and fractalkine, a CX₃C chemokine, are encoded elsewhere in the genome. Each chemokine interacts with one or more receptors, and affects one or more types of cell. A comprehensive list of chemokines and their receptors is given in Appendix IV.

Class	Chemokine	Produced by	Receptors	Cells attracted	Major effects
CXC	CXCL8 (IL-8)	Monocytes Macrophages Fibroblasts Keratinocytes Endothelial cells	CXCR1 CXCR2	Neutrophils Naive T cells	Mobilizes, activates and degranulates neutrophils Angiogenesis
	CXCL7 (PBP, β-TG NAP-2)	Platelets	CXCR2	Neutrophils	Activates neutrophils Clot resorption Angiogenesis
	CXCL1 (GROα) CXCL2 (GROβ) CXCL3 (GROγ)	Monocytes Fibroblasts Endothelium	CXCR2	Neutrophils Naive T cells Fibroblasts	Activates neutrophils Fibroplasia Angiogenesis
	CXCL10 (IP-10)	Keratinocytes Monocytes T cells Fibroblasts Endothelium	CXCR3	Resting T cells NK cells Monocytes	Immunostimulant Antiangiogenic Promotes T$_H$1 immunity
	CXCL12 (SDF-1)	Stromal cells	CXCR4	Naive T cells Progenitor (CD34⁺) B cells	B-cell development Lymphocyte homing Competes with HIV-1
	CXCL13 (BLC)	Stromal cells	CXCR5	B cells	Lymphocyte homing
CC	CCL3 (MIP-1α)	Monocytes T cells Mast cells Fibroblasts	CCR1, 3, 5	Monocytes NK and T cells Basophils Dendritic cells	Competes with HIV-1 Antiviral defense Promotes T$_H$1 immunity
	CCL4 (MIP-1β)	Monocytes Macrophages Neutrophils Endothelium	CCR1, 3, 5	Monocytes NK and T cells Dendritic cells	Competes with HIV-1
	CCL2 (MCP-1)	Monocytes Macrophages Fibroblasts Keratinocytes	CCR2B	Monocytes NK and T cells Basophils Dendritic cells	Activates macrophages Basophil histamine release Promotes T$_H$2 immunity
	CCL5 (RANTES)	T cells Endothelium Platelets	CCR1, 3, 5	Monocytes NK and T cells Basophils Eosinophils Dendritic cells	Degranulates basophils Activates T cells Chronic inflammation
	CCL11 (Eotaxin)	Endothelium Monocytes Epithelium T cells	CCR3	Eosinophils Monocytes T cells	Role in allergy
	CCL18 (DC-CK)	Dendritic cells	?	Naive T cells	Role in activating naive T cells
C	XCL1 (Lymphotactin)	CD8>CD4 T cells	CXCR1	Thymocytes Dendritic cells NK cells	Lymphocyte trafficking and development
CXXXC (CX₃C)	CX3CL1 (Fractalkine)	Monocytes Endothelium Microglial cells	CX₃CR1	Monocytes T cells	Leukocyte–endothelial adhesion Brain inflammation

2-22 Cell-adhesion molecules control interactions between leukocytes and endothelial cells during an inflammatory response.

The recruitment of activated phagocytes to sites of infection is one of the most important functions of innate immunity. Recruitment occurs as part of the inflammatory response and is mediated by cell-adhesion molecules that are induced on the surface of the local blood vessel endothelium. Before we consider the process of inflammatory cell recruitment, we will first describe some of the cell-adhesion molecules involved.

A significant barrier to understanding cell-adhesion molecules is their nomenclature. Most cell-adhesion molecules, especially those on leukocytes, which are relatively easy to analyze functionally, were named after the effects of specific monoclonal antibodies directed against them; only later were these characterized by gene cloning. Their names therefore bear no relation to their structure. For instance, the **leukocyte functional antigens LFA-1**, **LFA-2**, and **LFA-3**, are actually members of two different protein families. In Fig. 2.42, the adhesion molecules are grouped according to their molecular structure, which is shown in schematic form, alongside their different names, sites of expression, and ligands. Three families of adhesion molecules are important for leukocyte recruitment. The **selectins** are membrane glycoproteins with a distal lectin-like domain that binds specific carbohydrate groups. Members of this family are induced on activated endothelium and initiate endothelium–leukocyte interactions by binding to fucosylated oligosaccharide ligands on passing leukocytes (see Fig. 2.42).

The next step in leukocyte recruitment depends on tighter adhesion, which is due to the binding of **intercellular adhesion molecules (ICAMs)** on the endothelium to heterodimeric proteins of the **integrin** family on leukocytes. The leukocyte integrins important for extravasation are **LFA-1** ($\alpha_L{:}\beta_2$, also known as CD11a/CD18) and **CR3** ($\alpha_M{:}\beta_2$, complement receptor type 3, also known as CD11b/CD18 or Mac-1; we met CR3 in Section 2-16 as a receptor for iC3b, but this is just one of the ligands for this integrin) and they both bind to **ICAM-1** and to **ICAM-2** (Fig. 2.43). Strong adhesion between

	Name	Tissue distribution	Ligand
Selectins Bind carbohydrates. Initiate leukocyte–endothelial interaction *P-selectin*	P-selectin (PADGEM, CD62P)	Activated endothelium and platelets	PSGL-1, sialyl-Lewis^x
	E-selectin (ELAM-1, CD62E)	Activated endothelium	Sialyl-Lewis^x
Integrins Bind to cell-adhesion molecules and extracellular matrix. Strong adhesion *LFA-1*	$\alpha_L{:}\beta_2$ (LFA-1, CD11a/CD18)	Monocytes, T cells, macrophages, neutrophils, dendritic cells	ICAMs
	$\alpha_M{:}\beta_2$ (CR3, Mac-1, CD11b/CD18)	Neutrophils, monocytes, macrophages	ICAM-1, iC3b, fibrinogen
	$\alpha_x{:}\beta_2$ (CR4, p150.95, CD11c/CD18)	Dendritic cells, macrophages, neutrophils	iC3b
	$\alpha_5{:}\beta_1$ (VLA-5, CD49d/CD29)	Monocytes, macrophages	Fibronectin
Immunoglobulin superfamily Various roles in cell adhesion. Ligand for integrins *ICAM-1*	ICAM-1 (CD54)	Activated endothelium	LFA-1, Mac1
	ICAM-2 (CD102)	Resting endothelium, dendritic cells	LFA-1
	VCAM-1 (CD106)	Activated endothelium	VLA-4
	PECAM (CD31)	Activated leukocytes, endothelial cell–cell junctions	CD31

Fig. 2.42 Adhesion molecules involved in leukocyte interactions. Several structural families of adhesion molecules have a role in leukocyte migration, homing, and cell–cell interactions: the selectins, the integrins, and proteins of the immunoglobulin superfamily. The figure shows schematic representations of an example from each family, a list of other family members that participate in leukocyte interactions, their cellular distribution, and their ligand in adhesive interactions. The family members shown here are limited to those that participate in inflammation and other innate immune mechanisms. The same molecules and others participate in adaptive immunity and will be considered in Chapters 8 and 10. The nomenclature of the different molecules in these families is confusing because it often reflects the way in which the molecules were first identified rather than their related structural characteristics. Alternative names for each of the adhesion molecules are given in parentheses. Sulfated sialyl-Lewis^x, which is recognized by P- and E-selectin, is an oligosaccharide present on the cell-surface glycoproteins of circulating leukocytes. Sulfation can occur at either the sixth carbon atom of the galactose or the *N*-acetyl-glucosamine, but not both.

Leukocyte
Adhesion Deficiency

[handwritten notes: cytokines of TNF α → selectins on endothelium interact w/ neutrophils; integrin bind ICAM on endothelium; ICAM endo → integrin neutrophil or monocytes]

leukocytes and endothelial cells is promoted by the induction of ICAM-1 on inflamed endothelium and the activation of a **conformational change** in LFA-1 and CR3 that occurs in the response to chemokines. The importance of the leukocyte integrins in inflammatory cell recruitment is illustrated by the disease **leukocyte adhesion deficiency**, which stems from a defect in the β_2 chain common to both LFA-1 and CR3. People with this disease suffer from recurrent bacterial infections and impaired healing of wounds.

The activation of endothelium is driven by interactions with macrophage cytokines, particularly TNF-α, which induce the rapid externalization of granules called **Weibel–Palade bodies** in the endothelial cells. These granules contain preformed **P-selectin**, which is thus expressed within minutes on the surface of local endothelial cells after the production of TNF-α by macrophages. Shortly after the appearance of P-selectin on the cell surface, mRNA encoding **E-selectin** is synthesized, and within 2 hours, the endothelial cells are expressing mainly E-selectin. Both these proteins interact with the sulfated-sialyl-Lewis^x that is present on the surface of neutrophils.

Resting endothelium carries low levels of ICAM-2, apparently in all vascular beds. This may be used by circulating monocytes to navigate out of the vessels and into their tissue sites. This monocyte migration happens continuously and essentially ubiquitously. However, upon exposure to TNF-α, local expression of ICAM-1 is strongly induced on the endothelium of small vessels near or within the infectious focus. ICAM-1 in turn binds to LFA-1 or CR3 on circulating monocytes and polymorphonuclear leukocytes, in particular neutrophils, as shown in Fig. 2.43. Cell-adhesion molecules have many other roles in the body, directing many aspects of tissue and organ development. In this brief description we have considered only those that participate in the recruitment of inflammatory cells in the hours to days after the establishment of an infection.

2-23 Neutrophils make up the first wave of cells that cross the blood vessel wall to enter inflammatory sites.

The physical changes that accompany the initiation of the inflammatory response have been described in Section 2-4; here we give a step-by-step account of how the required effector cells are recruited into sites of infection. Under normal conditions, leukocytes flow in the center of small blood vessels, where blood flow is fastest. In inflammatory sites, the vessels are dilated and the slower blood flow allows the leukocytes to move out of the center of the blood vessel and interact with the vascular endothelium. Even in the absence of infection, monocytes migrate continuously into the tissues, where they differentiate into macrophages. During an inflammatory response, the induction of adhesion molecules on the endothelial cells by the infection focus, as well as induced changes in the adhesion molecules expressed on leukocytes, recruit large numbers of circulating leukocytes, initially neutrophils and later monocytes, into the site of an infection. The migration of leukocytes out of blood vessels, a process known as **extravasation**, is thought to occur in four steps. We will describe this process as it is known to occur for monocytes and neutrophils (Fig. 2.44).

The first step involves selectins. P-selectin appears on endothelial cell surfaces within a few minutes of exposure to leukotriene B4, the complement fragment C5a, or histamine, which is released from mast cells in response to C5a. The appearance of P-selectin can also be induced by exposure to TNF-α or LPS, and both of these have the additional effect of inducing the synthesis of a second selectin, E-selectin, which appears on the endothelial cell surface a few hours later. These selectins recognize the sulfated-sialyl-Lewis^x moiety of certain leukocyte glycoproteins that are exposed on the tips of leukocyte

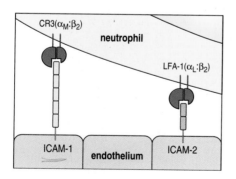

Fig. 2.43 Phagocyte adhesion to vascular endothelium is mediated by integrins. Vascular endothelium, when it is activated by inflammatory mediators, expresses two adhesion molecules—ICAM-1 and ICAM-2. These are ligands for integrins expressed by phagocytes—α_L:β_2 (also called LFA-1 or CD11a:CD18) and α_M:β_2 (also called CR3, Mac-1, or CD11b:CD18).

Selectin-mediated adhesion to leukocyte sialyl-Lewis^x is weak, and allows leukocytes to roll along the vascular endothelial surface

s-Le^x

Blood flow →

E-selectin

basement membrane

Rolling adhesion	Tight binding	Diapedesis	Migration

CXCL8R (IL-8 receptor)

LFA-1(α_L:β_2)

s-Le^x

ICAM-1

E-selectin

CD31

chemokine CXCL8 (IL-8)

Fig. 2.44 Neutrophils leave the blood and migrate to sites of infection in a multistep process mediated through adhesive interactions that are regulated by macrophage-derived cytokines and chemokines. The first step (top panel) involves the reversible binding of leukocytes to vascular endothelium through interactions between selectins induced on the endothelium and their carbohydrate ligands on the leukocyte, shown here for E-selectin and its ligand the sialyl-Lewis^x moiety (s-Le^x). This interaction cannot anchor the cells against the shearing force of the flow of blood, and instead they roll along the endothelium, continually making and breaking contact. The binding does, however, allow stronger interactions, which occur as a result of the induction of ICAM-1 on the endothelium and the activation of its receptors LFA-1 and CR3 (Mac-1) (not shown) on the leukocyte by contact with a chemokine such as CXCL8. Tight binding between these molecules arrests the rolling and allows the leukocyte to squeeze between the

endothelial cells forming the wall of the blood vessel (to extravasate). The leukocyte integrins LFA-1 and CR3 are required for extravasation, and for migration toward chemoattractants. Adhesion between molecules of CD31, expressed on both the leukocyte and the junction of the endothelial cells, is also thought to contribute to extravasation. The leukocyte also needs to traverse the basement membrane; it penetrates this with the aid of a matrix metalloproteinase enzyme that it expresses at the cell surface. Finally, the leukocyte migrates along a concentration gradient of chemokines (here shown as CXCL8) secreted by cells at the site of infection. The electron micrograph shows a neutrophil extravasating between endothelial cells. The blue arrow indicates the pseudopod that the neutrophil is inserting between the endothelial cells. Photograph ($\times$ 5500) courtesy of I. Bird and J. Spragg.

microvilli. The interaction of P-selectin and E-selectin with these glyco-proteins allows monocytes and neutrophils to adhere reversibly to the vessel wall, so that circulating leukocytes can be seen to 'roll' along endothelium that has been treated with inflammatory cytokines (Fig. 2.44, top panel). This adhesive interaction permits the stronger interactions of the next step in leukocyte migration.

This second step depends on interactions between the leukocyte integrins LFA-1 and CR3 with molecules on endothelium such as ICAM-1, which can also be induced on endothelial cells by TNF-α, and ICAM-2 (Fig. 2.44, bottom panel). LFA-1 and CR3 normally adhere only weakly, but CXCL8 or other chemokines, bound to proteoglycans on the surface of endothelial cells, trigger a conformational change in LFA-1 and CR3 on the rolling leukocyte, which greatly increases the adhesive properties of the neutrophil. In consequence, the leukocyte attaches firmly to the endothelium and its rolling is arrested.

In the third step the leukocyte extravasates, or crosses the endothelial wall. This step also involves LFA-1 and CR3, as well as a further adhesive interaction involving an immunoglobulin-related molecule called **PECAM** or **CD31**, which is expressed both on the leukocyte and at the intercellular junctions of endothelial cells. These interactions enable the phagocyte to squeeze between the endothelial cells. It then penetrates the basement membrane with the aid of enzymes that break down the extracellular matrix proteins of the basement membrane. The movement through the basement membrane is known as **diapedesis**, and it enables phagocytes to enter the subendothelial tissues.

The fourth and final step in extravasation is the migration of leukocytes through the tissues under the influence of chemokines. Chemokines such as CXCL8 and CCL2 (see Section 2-21) are produced at the site of infection and bind to proteoglycans in the extracellular matrix and on similar molecules on endothelial cell surfaces. This forms a matrix-associated concentration gradient of chemokine on a solid surface along which the leukocyte can migrate to the focus of infection (see Fig. 2.44). CXCL8 is released by the macrophages that first encounter pathogens and recruits neutrophils, which enter the infected tissue in large numbers in the early part of the induced response. Their influx usually peaks within the first 6 hours of an inflammatory response, whereas monocytes can be recruited later, through the action of chemokines such as CCL2. Once in an inflammatory site, neutrophils are able to eliminate many pathogens by phagocytosis. They act as phagocytic effectors in an innate immune response through receptors that opsonize or capture infectious agents and their derived components through innate immune recognition as well as by recognizing pathogens directly. In addition, as we will see in Chapter 9, they act as phagocytic effectors in humoral adaptive immunity. The importance of neutrophils is dramatically illustrated by diseases or treatments that severely reduce neutrophil numbers. Such patients are said to have **neutropenia**, and they are very susceptible to infection with a wide range of pathogens and commensal organisms. Restoring neutrophil levels in such patients by transfusion of neutrophil-rich blood fractions or by stimulating their production with specific growth factors largely corrects this susceptibility.

2-24 Tumor necrosis factor-α is an important cytokine that triggers local containment of infection but induces shock when released systemically.

Inflammatory mediators also stimulate endothelial cells to express proteins that trigger blood clotting in the local small vessels, occluding them and thus cutting off blood flow. This can be important in preventing the pathogen from entering the bloodstream and spreading through the blood to organs all over the body. Instead, the fluid that has leaked into the tissue in the early phases of an infection carries the pathogen, usually enclosed in dendritic cells, via the lymph to the regional lymph nodes, where an adaptive immune response can be initiated. The importance of TNF-α in the containment of local infection is illustrated by experiments in which rabbits were infected locally with a bacterium. Normally, the infection would be contained at the site of the inoculation; if, however, an injection of anti-TNF-α antibody was also given to block the action of TNF-α, the infection spread via the blood to other organs.

Once an infection spreads to the bloodstream, however, the same mechanisms by which TNF-α so effectively contains local infection instead become catastrophic (Fig. 2.45). The presence of infection in the bloodstream, known as **sepsis**, is accompanied by the release of TNF-α by macrophages in the liver, spleen, and other systemic sites. The systemic release of TNF-α causes vasodilation, which leads to a loss of blood pressure, increased vascular permeability, leading to a loss of plasma volume, and eventually to shock. In septic shock, disseminated intravascular coagulation (blood clotting) is also triggered by TNF-α, leading to the generation of clots in many small vessels and the massive consumption of clotting proteins, thus causing the patient's ability to clot blood appropriately to be lost. This condition frequently leads to the failure of vital organs such as the kidneys, liver, heart, and lungs, which are quickly compromised by the failure of normal perfusion; consequently, septic shock has a very high mortality rate.

Mice with a mutant TNF-α receptor gene are resistant to septic shock; however, such mice are also unable to control local infection. The features of TNF-α that make it so valuable in containing local infection are precisely those that give it a central role in the pathogenesis of septic shock. It is clear from the evolutionary conservation of TNF-α that its benefits in the former area far outweigh the devastating consequences of its systemic release.

2-25   Cytokines released by phagocytes activate the acute-phase response.

As well as their important local effects, the cytokines produced by macrophages have long-range effects that contribute to host defense. One of these is the elevation of body temperature, which is caused mainly by TNF-α, IL-1β, and IL-6. These are termed **endogenous pyrogens** because they cause fever and derive from an endogenous source rather than from bacterial components such as LPS, which is an exogenous pyrogen. Fever is generally beneficial to host defense; most pathogens grow better at lower temperatures and adaptive immune responses are more intense at elevated temperatures. Host cells are also protected from the deleterious effects of TNF-α at raised temperatures.

The effects of TNF-α, IL-1, and IL-6 are summarized in Fig. 2.46. One of the most important of these is the initiation of a response known as the **acute-phase response** (Fig. 2.47). This involves a shift in the proteins synthesized and secreted by the liver into the plasma and results from the action of IL-1, IL-6, and TNF-α on hepatocytes. In the acute-phase response, levels of some plasma proteins go down, while levels of others increase markedly. The proteins whose synthesis is induced by TNF-α, IL-1, and IL-6 are called **acute-phase proteins**. Several of these are of particular interest because they mimic the action of antibodies, but, unlike antibodies, these proteins have broad specificity for pathogen-associated molecular patterns and depend only on the presence of cytokines for their production.

One of these proteins, the **C-reactive protein**, is a member of the **pentraxin** protein family, so called because they are formed from five identical subunits. C-reactive protein is another example of a multipronged pathogen-recognition molecule, and binds to the phosphocholine portion of certain bacterial and fungal cell-wall lipopolysaccharides. Phosphocholine is also found in mammalian cell membrane phospholipids, but it cannot be bound by C-reactive protein. When C-reactive protein binds to a bacterium, it is not only able to opsonize it but can also activate the complement cascade by binding to C1q, the first component of the classical pathway of complement

Fig. 2.45 The release of TNF-α by macrophages induces local protective effects, but TNF-α can have damaging effects when released systemically. The panels on the left show the causes and consequences of local release of TNF-α, and the panels on the right show the causes and consequences of systemic release. Both left and right central panels illustrate the common effects of TNF-α, and acts on blood vessels, especially venules, to increase blood flow, to increase vascular permeability to fluid, proteins, and cells, and to increase endothelial adhesiveness for leukocytes and platelets. Local release thus allows an influx into the infected tissue of fluid, cells, and proteins that participate in host defense. Later, blood clots form in the small vessels, preventing spread of the infection via the blood, and the accumulated fluid and cells drain to regional lymph nodes, where the adaptive immune response is initiated. When there is a systemic infection, or sepsis, with bacteria that elicit TNF-α production, then TNF-α is released into the blood by macrophages in the liver and spleen and acts in a similar way on all small blood vessels. The result is shock, disseminated intravascular coagulation with depletion of clotting factors and consequent bleeding, multiple organ failure, and frequently death. These effects require the presence of the Toll-like receptor TLR-4 on macrophages, which provides the initial signal in response to LPS.

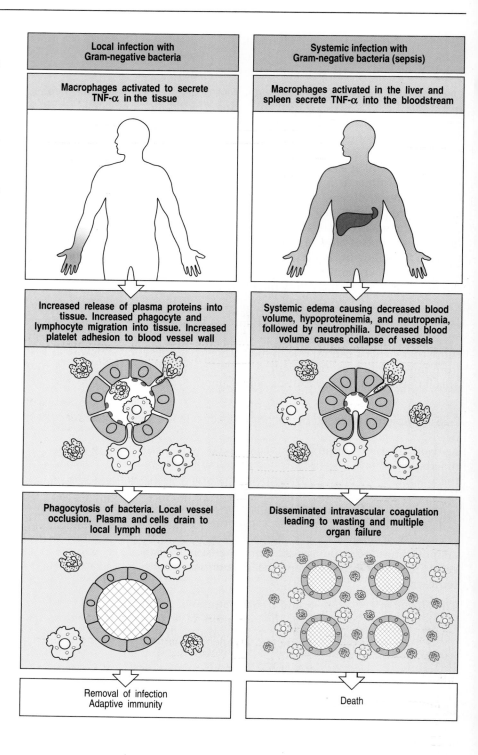

activation, as we learnt in Section 2-10. The interaction with C1q involves the collagen-like parts of C1q rather than the globular heads contacted by pathogen surfaces, but the same cascade of reactions is initiated.

The second acute-phase protein of interest is the mannose-binding lectin, which we have already met as a pathogen-binding molecule (see Fig. 2.11) and as a trigger for the complement cascade (see Section 2-10). Mannose-binding lectin is found in normal serum at low levels but is produced in increased amounts during the acute-phase response. It acts as an opsonin for monocytes, which, unlike tissue macrophages, do not express the

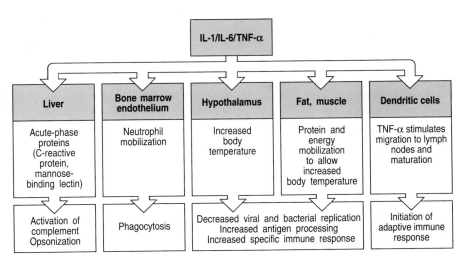

Fig. 2.46 The cytokines TNF-α, IL-1, and IL-6 have a wide spectrum of biological activities that help to coordinate the body's responses to infection. IL-1, IL-6, and TNF-α activate hepatocytes to synthesize acute-phase proteins, and bone marrow endothelium to release neutrophils. The acute-phase proteins act as opsonins, whereas the disposal of opsonized pathogens is augmented by the enhanced recruitment of neutrophils from the bone marrow. IL-1, IL-6, and TNF-α are also endogenous pyrogens, raising body temperature, which is believed to help in eliminating infections. A major effect of these cytokines is to act on the hypothalamus, altering the body's temperature regulation, and on muscle and fat cells, altering energy mobilization to increase the body temperature. At elevated temperatures, bacterial and viral replication are decreased, whereas the adaptive immune response operates more efficiently.

macrophage mannose receptor. Two other proteins with opsonizing properties that are produced by the liver in increased quantities during the acute-phase response are the pulmonary surfactant proteins SP-A and SP-D. Like mannose-binding lectin, these are members of the collectin family, binding to pathogen surfaces through globular lectin-domains attached to a collagen-like stalk. SP-A and SP-D are found along with macrophages in the alveolar fluid of the lung and are important in promoting the phagocytosis of respiratory pathogens such as *Pneumocystis carinii*, one of the main causes of pneumonia in patients with AIDS.

Thus, within a day or two, the acute-phase response provides the host with several proteins with the functional properties of antibodies but able to bind a broad range of pathogens. However, unlike the antibodies we shall learn about in Chapters 3 and 9 they have no structural diversity and are made in response to any stimulus that triggers the release of TNF-α, IL-1, and IL-6. Therefore, unlike antibodies, their synthesis is not specifically induced and targeted.

A final distant effect of the cytokines produced by phagocytes is to induce a **leukocytosis**, an increase in circulating neutrophils. The neutrophils come from two sources: the bone marrow, from which mature leukocytes are released in increased numbers; and sites in blood vessels where they are attached loosely to endothelial cells. Thus, the effects of these cytokines contribute to the control of infection while the adaptive immune response is being developed. As shown in Fig. 2.46, TNF-α also has a role in stimulating the migration of dendritic cells from their sites in peripheral tissues to the lymph node and in their maturation into nonphagocytic but highly co-stimulatory antigen-presenting cells.

2-26 Interferons induced by viral infection make several contributions to host defense.

Infection of cells with viruses induces the production of proteins that are known as **interferons**, because they were found to interfere with viral replication in previously uninfected tissue culture cells. They are believed to have a similar role *in vivo*, blocking the spread of viruses to uninfected cells. These antiviral effector molecules, called **interferon-α (IFN-α)** and **interferon-β (IFN-β)**, are quite distinct from **interferon-γ (IFN-γ)**. This cytokine is not directly induced by viral infection but is produced later and does have an important role in the adaptive immune response to intracellular pathogens,

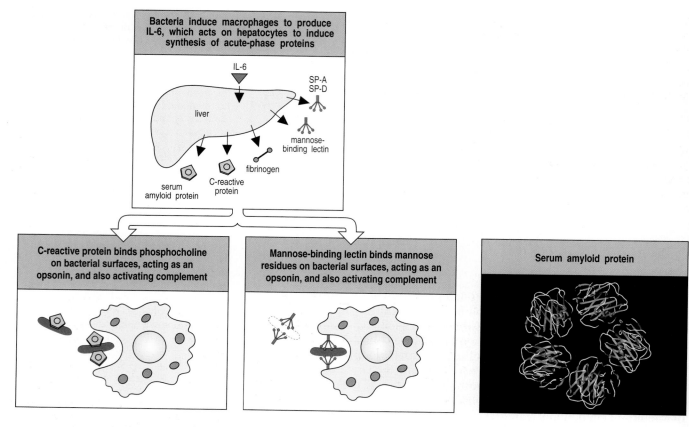

Fig. 2.47 The acute-phase response produces molecules that bind pathogens but not host cells. Acute-phase proteins are produced by liver cells in response to cytokines released by macrophages in the presence of bacteria. They include serum amyloid protein (SAP) (in mice but not humans), C-reactive protein (CRP), fibrinogen, and mannose-binding lectin (MBL). SAP and CRP are homologous in structure; both are pentraxins, forming five-membered discs, as shown for SAP (photograph on the right). CRP binds phosphocholine on certain bacterial and fungal surfaces but does not recognize it in the form in which it is found in host cell membranes. It both acts as an opsonin in its own right and activates the classical complement pathway by binding C1q to augment opsonization. MBL is a member of the collectin family, which includes the lung surfactant proteins SP-A and SP-D. It also resembles C1q in its structure. Like CRP, MBL can act as an opsonin in its own right, as can SP-A and SP-D. Model structure courtesy of J. Emsley.

as we will see below. IFN-α, actually a family of several closely related proteins, and IFN-β, the product of a single gene, are synthesized by many cell types after their infection by diverse viruses. Interferon synthesis is thought to occur in response to the presence of double-stranded RNA, because synthetic double-stranded RNA is a potent inducer of interferons α and β. Double-stranded RNA, which is not found in mammalian cells, forms the genome of some viruses and might be made as part of the infectious cycle of all viruses. Therefore, double-stranded RNA might be the common element in interferon induction. It is recognized as a distinct pattern by the Toll-like receptor **TLR-3**.

Interferons make several contributions to defense against viral infection (Fig. 2.48). An obvious and important effect is the induction of a state of resistance to viral replication in all cells. IFN-α and IFN-β secreted by the infected cell bind to a common cell-surface receptor, known as the **interferon receptor**, on both the infected cell and nearby uninfected cells. The interferon receptor, like many other cytokine receptors, is coupled to a **Janus-family tyrosine kinase**, through which it signals. This signaling pathway, which we will describe in detail in Chapter 6, rapidly induces new gene transcription as the

Janus-family kinases directly phosphorylate signal-transducing activators of transcription known as **STAT proteins**. The STAT proteins undergo dimerization when they are phosphorylated, which allows them to translocate to the nucleus where they activate the transcription of several different genes. In this way, interferons α and β induce the synthesis of several host-cell proteins that contribute to the inhibition of viral replication.

One of these is the enzyme oligoadenylate synthetase, which polymerizes ATP into a series of 2′–5′-linked oligomers (nucleotides in nucleic acids are normally linked 3′–5′). These activate an endoribonuclease that then degrades viral RNA. A second protein activated by IFN-α and IFN-β is a serine–threonine kinase called **PKR kinase**. This enzyme phosphorylates the eukaryotic protein synthesis initiation factor eIF-2, inhibiting translation and thus further contributing to the inhibition of viral replication.

Another interferon-inducible protein called **Mx** is known to be required for cellular resistance to influenza virus replication. Mice that lack the gene for Mx are highly susceptible to infection with the influenza virus, whereas mice that can make Mx are not susceptible to influenza.

Another way in which interferons protect the host against viruses is by increasing the cellular immune response to these pathogens. The adaptive immune response to viruses depends on their effective presentation to T cells as viral peptide fragments complexed with MHC class I molecules at the cell surface. Interferons promote this by inducing an increased synthesis and expression of MHC class I molecules. Interferons also activate NK cells to kill virus-infected cells and to release cytokines. Although of lymphoid origin, NK cells do not have antigen-specific receptors and are therefore part of the innate immune system, as we shall see in the next section. It is not entirely clear what allows them to discriminate between infected and uninfected cells.

NK cells possess both activating and inhibitory receptors. The former, as the name suggests, activate the NK cells, causing the release of cytokines such as interferon-γ and the directed killing of the stimulating cell through the release of cytotoxic granules containing granzymes and perforin. This killing mechanism is the same as that used by cytotoxic T cells and will be described in detail when we describe the functions of that effector T-cell population (Chapter 8). The immunoglobulin receptor of NK cells is also capable of activating NK cells to release their cytotoxic granules, allowing NK cells to mediate what is called **antibody-dependent cellular cytotoxicity**, or **ADCC**.

The inhibitory receptors balance the signals transduced by the activating receptors, and can inhibit killing when bound to their ligands, which are in most cases normal MHC class I molecules. This means that the higher the expression of MHC class I on a cell surface, the more protected it is against destruction by NK cells. Therefore, interferons protect uninfected host cells from NK cells by inducing the expression of MHC class I molecules, while activating the NK cells to kill infected cells. Interferons also promote the release of effector cytokines by NK cells.

2-27 NK cells are activated by interferons and macrophage-derived cytokines to serve as an early defense against certain intracellular infections.

Natural killer cells (**NK cells**) develop in the bone marrow from the common lymphoid progenitor cell and circulate in the blood. They are larger than T and B lymphocytes, have distinctive cytoplasmic granules, and are functionally identified by their ability to kill certain lymphoid tumor cell lines *in vitro* without the need for prior immunization or activation. The mechanism of NK cell killing is the same as that used by the cytotoxic T cells generated in

Fig. 2.48 Interferons are antiviral proteins produced by cells in response to viral infection. The interferons (IFN)-α and -β have three major functions. First, they induce resistance to viral replication in uninfected cells by activating genes that cause the destruction of mRNA and inhibit the translation of viral and some host proteins. Second, they can induce MHC class I expression in most cell types in the body, thus enhancing their resistance to NK cells; they may also induce increased synthesis of MHC class I molecules in cells that are newly infected by virus, thus making them more susceptible to killing by CD8 cytotoxic T cells (see Chapter 8). Third, they activate NK cells, which then kill virus-infected cells selectively.

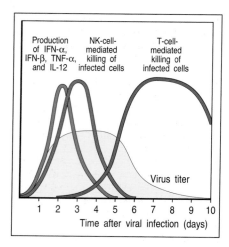

Fig. 2.49 Natural killer cells (NK cells) are an early component of the host response to virus infection.
Experiments in mice have shown that IFN-α, IFN-β, and the cytokines TNF-α and IL-12 appear first, followed by a wave of NK cells, which together control virus replication but do not eliminate the virus. Virus elimination is accomplished when virus-specific CD8 T cells are produced. Without NK cells, the levels of some viruses are much higher in the early days of the infection, and can be lethal unless treated vigorously with antiviral compounds.

an adaptive immune response; cytotoxic granules are released onto the surface of the bound target cell, and the effector proteins they contain penetrate the cell membrane and induce programmed cell death. However, NK cell killing is triggered by invariant receptors that recognize components of infected cell surfaces, and their known function in host defense is in the early phases of infection with several intracellular pathogens, particularly herpes viruses, the protozoan parasite *Leishmania*, and the bacterium *Listeria monocytogenes*.

NK cells are activated in response to interferons or macrophage-derived cytokines. Although NK cells that can kill sensitive targets can be isolated from uninfected individuals, this activity is increased by 20–100 times when NK cells are exposed to IFN-α and IFN-β or to the NK-cell-activating factor IL-12, which is one of the cytokines produced early in many infections. Activated NK cells serve to contain virus infections while the adaptive immune response is generating antigen-specific cytotoxic T cells that can clear the infection (Fig. 2.49).

At present the only clue to the physiological function of NK cells in humans comes from rare patients deficient in NK cells. Such patients prove to be highly susceptible to early phases of herpes virus infection. A similar finding has recently been made in mice infected with another herpes virus, murine cytomegalovirus.

IL-12, in synergy with TNF-α, can also elicit the production of large amounts of IFN-γ by NK cells, and this secreted IFN-γ is crucial in controlling some infections before CD8 T cells have been activated to produce IFN-γ. One example is the response to *Listeria monocytogenes*. Mice that lack T and B lymphocytes are initially quite resistant to this pathogen; however, antibody-mediated depletion of NK cells or neutralization of TNF-α or IFN-γ or their receptors renders these mice highly susceptible, so that they die a few days after infection, before an adaptive immune response can be mounted.

2-28 NK cells possess receptors for self molecules that prevent their activation by uninfected cells.

If NK cells are to defend the body against infection with viruses and other pathogens, they must have some mechanism for distinguishing infected from uninfected cells. Exactly how this is achieved has not yet been worked out, but recognition of 'altered self' is thought to be involved. NK cells have two types of surface receptor that control their cytotoxic activity. One type is an 'activating receptor' that triggers killing by the NK cell. Several types of receptor provide this activation signal, including members of the C-type lectins.

A second set of receptors inhibit this activation and prevent NK cells from killing normal host cells. These 'inhibitory receptors' are specific for MHC class I alleles, which helps to explain why NK cells selectively kill target cells bearing low levels of MHC class I molecules. Altered expression of MHC class I molecules may be a common feature of cells infected by intracellular pathogens, because many of these pathogens have developed strategies to interfere with the ability of MHC class I molecules to capture and display peptides to T cells. Thus, one possible mechanism by which NK cells distinguish infected from uninfected cells is by recognizing alterations in MHC class I expression (Fig. 2.50). Another is that they recognize changes in cell-surface glycoproteins induced by viral or bacterial infection.

The receptors that regulate the activity of NK cells fall into two families (see Fig. 2.51). One is composed of receptors homologous to C-type lectins and is called the NK receptor complex, or NKC. The other is composed of receptors

MHC class I on normal cells is recognized by killer cell immunoglobulin-like receptors (KIRs) or by lectin-like CD94:NKG2 heterodimers on NK cells, which inhibit signals from activating receptors

KIR 3D

NK cell

KIR 2D

CD94:NKG2

MHC class I

NK cell activating ligand

NK cell does not kill the normal cell

'Altered' or absent MHC class I cannot stimulate a negative signal. The NK cell is triggered by signals from activating receptors

Activated NK cell releases granule contents, inducing apoptosis in target cell

Fig. 2.50 Possible mechanisms by which NK cells distinguish infected from uninfected cells. A proposed mechanism of recognition is shown. NK cells can use several different receptors that signal them to kill, including lectin-like activating receptors, or 'killer receptors,' that recognize carbohydrate on self cells. However, another set of receptors—called Ly49 in the mouse, and killer immunoglobulin-like receptors (KIRs) in humans—recognize MHC class I molecules and inhibit killing by NK cells by overruling the actions of the killer receptors. This inhibitory signal is lost when the target cells do not express MHC class I and perhaps also in cells infected with virus, which might inhibit MHC class I expression or alter its conformation. Another possibility is that normal uninfected cells respond to IFN-α and IFN-β by increasing expression of MHC class I molecules, making them resistant to killing by activated NK cells. In contrast, infected cells can fail to increase MHC class I expression, making them targets for activated NK cells. Ly49 and KIR belong to different protein families—the C-type lectins for Ly49 and the immunoglobulin superfamily for KIRs. The KIRs are made in two forms, p58 (KIR2D) and p70 (KIR3D), which differ by the presence of one immunoglobulin domain (3D and 2D).

with immunoglobulin-like domains; hence their name, *K*iller cell *I*mmunoglobulin-like *R*eceptors, or KIRs. The KIR genes form part of a larger cluster of immunoglobulin-like receptors known as the leukocyte receptor complex, or LRC. Both the NKC and LRC clusters are present in mice and in humans, but mice lack the KIR genes and therefore rely on the C-type lectin-like receptors of the NKC to control their NK-cell activity.

One complication in understanding the regulation of NK cell activity is that the same structural families of NK receptors contain both activating and inhibitory receptors. In human and mouse, NK cells express a heterodimer of two C-type lectins, called CD94 and NKG2, which interacts with nonpolymorphic MHC class I-like molecules, including HLA-E in humans and Qa-1 in mice, that bind the leader peptides of other MHC class I molecules. Thus, this receptor could be sensitive to the presence of several different MHC class I alleles. In humans, the NKG2 family has six members, NKG2A, B, C, D, E, and F. Of these, for example, NKG2A and B are inhibitory, whereas NKG2C and D are activating. In mice, Ly49H, a member of the Ly49 C-type lectin family, seems to be distinct, because binding of this molecule is an activating event that triggers a cytotoxic response, whereas binding to the other Ly49 members is inhibitory.

Fig. 2.51 The genes that encode NK receptors fall into two families. The first, the leukocyte receptor complex (LRC), comprises a large cluster of genes encoding a family of proteins composed of immunoglobulin-like domains. These include the killer immunoglobulin-like receptors (KIRs) expressed by NK cells, the leukocyte immunoglobulin-like receptor (LILR) and the leukocyte-associated immunoglobulin-like receptor (LAIR) gene families. The signaling lectins (SIGLECs), and members of the CD66 family are located nearby. In humans, this complex is located on chromosome 19. The second gene cluster is called the natural killer complex (NKC), and encodes a receptor family that includes the NKG2 proteins as well as CD94, with which an NKG2 molecule pairs to form a functional receptor. This complex is located on human chromosome 12. Figure based on data courtesy of J. Trowsdale, University of Cambridge.

The KIR gene products come in either a low-molecular-weight form, called KIR-2D, or a higher-molecular-weight form called KIR-3D, depending on whether they have two or three immunoglobulin-like domains. In this family, too, some members are activating while others are inhibitory. It even seems that for one KIR gene there are two alleles, of which one is activating and the other is inhibitory. Other inhibitory NK receptors specific for the products of the MHC class I loci are rapidly being defined, and all are members of either the immunoglobulin-like KIR family or the Ly49-like C-type lectins. We will discuss the motifs on the cytoplasmic portions of the receptors that lead to activation or inhibition in Chapter 6. Clearly, the regulation of NK-cell activity is complex and whether any individual NK cell is activated by another cell will depend on the overall balance of activating and inhibitory receptors

Signaling by the inhibitory NK receptors suppresses the killing activity of NK cells. This means that NK cells will not kill healthy, genetically identical cells with normal expression of MHC class I molecules, such as the other cells of the body. Virus-infected cells, however, can become susceptible to killing by NK cells by a variety of mechanisms. First, some viruses inhibit all protein synthesis in their host cells, so synthesis of MHC class I proteins would be blocked in infected cells, even while being augmented by the secretion of interferon in uninfected cells. The reduced level of MHC class I expression in infected cells would make them correspondingly less able to inhibit NK cells through their MHC-specific receptors, and therefore more susceptible to killing. Second, some viruses can selectively prevent the export of MHC class I molecules, which might allow the infected cell to evade recognition by the cytotoxic T cells of the adaptive immune response but would make them susceptible to killing by NK cells. Virus infection alters the glycosylation of cellular proteins, perhaps allowing recognition by allowing NK-activating receptors to dominate, or by removing the normal ligand for the inhibitory receptors. Such a mechanism could allow infected cells to be detected even when the level of MHC class I expression had not been altered.

Clearly, much remains to be learned about this innate mechanism of cytotoxic attack and its physiological relevance. The role of MHC molecules in allowing NK cells to detect intracellular infections is of particular interest because these same molecules govern the response of T cells to intracellular pathogens. It is possible that NK cells, which use a diverse set of nonclonal receptors to detect altered MHC, represent the modern remnants of the evolutionary forebears of T cells, which evolved rearranging genes that encode a vast repertoire of antigen-specific receptors geared to recognizing altered MHC.

2-29 Several lymphocyte subpopulations behave as innate-like lymphocytes.

Receptor gene rearrangements are a defining characteristic of the lymphocytes of the adaptive immune system, and they allow the generation of an infinite variety of receptors, each expressed by a different individual T cell or B cell (see Section 1-11). However, there are several minor lymphocyte subsets that express only a very limited diversity of receptors, encoded by a few common gene segment rearrangements. Because their receptors are relatively invariant and because they occur only in specific locations within the body, these lymphocytes do not need to undergo clonal expansion before responding effectively to the antigens they recognize; they are therefore known as **innate-like lymphocytes** (**ILLs**) (Fig. 2.52).

One type of ILL is the intraepithelial subset of **γ:δ T cells**. The γ:δ T cells are themselves a minor subset of the T cells introduced in Chapter 1. However, their antigen receptors are composed of a γ chain and a δ chain rather than the α and β chains that make up the antigen receptors on the majority subset of T cells involved in adaptive immunity. γ:δ T cells were discovered purely as a consequence of their having immunoglobulin-like receptors encoded by rearranged genes, and their function is still being clarified.

One of their most striking features is their division into two highly distinct sets of cells. One set of γ:δ T cells is found in the lymphoid tissue of all vertebrates and, like B cells and the α:β T cells, they have highly diversified T-cell receptors. By contrast, intraepithelial γ:δ T cells occur variably in different vertebrates, and commonly display receptors of very limited diversity, particularly in the skin and the female reproductive tract of mice, where the γ:δ T cells are essentially homogeneous in any one site. On the basis of this limited diversity and lack of recirculation, it has been proposed that intraepithelial γ:δ T cells may recognize ligands that are derived from the epithelium in which they reside, but which are expressed only when a cell has become infected. Candidate ligands are heat-shock proteins, MHC class IB molecules, and unorthodox nucleotides and phospholipids; there is evidence of recognition of all these ligands by γ:δ T cells.

Unlike α:β T cells, γ:δ T cells do not generally recognize antigen as peptides presented by MHC molecules; instead, they seem to recognize their target antigens directly, and thus could recognize and respond rapidly to molecules expressed by many different cell types. Recognition of molecules expressed as a consequence of infection, rather than of pathogen-specific antigens themselves, would distinguish intraepithelial γ:δ T cells from other lymphocytes and would place them in the innate-like class.

Innate-like lymphocytes		
B-1 cells	**Epithelial γ:δ cells**	**NK T cells**
Make natural antibody, protect against infection with *Streptococcus pneumoniae*	Produce cytokines rapidly	Produce cytokines rapidly
Ligands not MHC associated	Ligands are MHC class IB associated	Ligands are lipids bound to CD1d
Cannot be boosted	Cannot be boosted	Cannot be boosted

Fig. 2.52 The three main classes of innate-like lymphocytes and their properties.

B-1 cell binds bacterial capsular polysaccharide or cell-wall components and receives a signal (IL-5) from accessory cells

IL-5

B-1 cell

B-1 cell secretes IgM anti-polysaccharide antibody

IgM

IgM binds polysaccharide capsule

Activation of complement and removal of bacteria

Fig. 2.53 B-1 cells might be important in the response to carbohydrate antigens such as bacterial polysaccharides. These T-cell-independent responses occur rapidly, with antibody appearing within 48 hours after infection, presumably because there is a high frequency of precursors of the responding lymphocytes so that little clonal expansion is required. In the absence of antigen-specific T-cell help, only IgM is made and, in mice, these responses therefore work mainly through the activation of complement, which is most efficient when the antibody is of the IgM isotype.

Another subset of lymphocytes with antigen receptors of limited diversity is the B-1 subset of B cells. B-1 cells are distinguished from other B cells by the cell-surface protein CD5 and have properties quite distinct from those of the conventional B cells that mediate adaptive humoral immunity. B-1 cells are in many ways analogous to intraepithelial γ:δ T cells: they arise early in ontogeny, they use a distinctive and limited set of gene rearrangements to make their receptors, they are self-renewing in the periphery, and they are the predominant lymphocyte in a distinctive microenvironment—the peritoneal and pleural cavities. B-1 cells seem to make antibody responses mainly to polysaccharide antigens and can produce antibodies of the IgM class without needing help from T cells (Fig. 2.53). Although these responses can be augmented by T cells, they first appear within 48 hours of exposure to antigen, and so T cells cannot be involved. Thus, B-1 cells are not active in an antigen-specific adaptive immune response. The lack of an antigen-specific interaction with helper T cells might explain why immunological memory is not generated as a result of B-1 cell responses: repeated exposures to the same antigen elicit similar, or decreased, responses with each exposure. These responses, although generated by lymphocytes with rearranging receptors, therefore resemble innate rather than adaptive immune responses.

As with γ:δ T cells, the precise role of B-1 cells in host defense is uncertain. Mice that are deficient in B-1 cells are more susceptible to infection with *Streptococcus pneumoniae* because they fail to produce an antibody against the phospholipid headgroup phosphocholine that effectively protects against this organism. A significant fraction of the B-1 cells can make antibodies of this specificity, and because no antigen-specific T-cell help is required, a potent response can be produced early in infection with this pathogen. Whether human B-1 cells have the same role is not certain.

A third subset of ILLs, known as NK T cells, exists both in the thymus and in peripheral lymphoid organs. These cells express an invariant T-cell receptor α chain, paired with one of three different β chains, and are able to recognize glycolipid antigens. The main response of NK T cells seems to be the rapid secretion of cytokines, including IL-4, IL-10, and IFN-γ, and it is thought that these cells may have a primarily regulatory function. We shall encounter these unusual cells again in Chapter 10.

From an evolutionary perspective, it is interesting to note that γ:δ T cells seem to defend the body surfaces, whereas B-1 cells defend the body cavity. Both cell types are relatively limited in their range of specificities and in the efficiency of their responses. It is possible that these two cell types represent a transitional phase in the evolution of the adaptive immune response, guarding the two main compartments of primitive organisms—the epithelial surfaces and the body cavity. It is not yet clear whether they are still critical to host defense or whether they represent an evolutionary relic. Nevertheless, because each cell type is prominent in certain sites in the body and contributes to responses against certain pathogens, they must be incorporated into our thinking about host defense.

A final component of the body's innate immune defenses are antibodies that are known as 'natural antibodies'. This 'natural IgM' is encoded by rearranged antibody genes that have not undergone further diversification by somatic hypermutation. It makes up a considerable amount of the IgM circulating in humans and does not seem to be the consequence of an antigen-specific adaptive immune response to infection. It has a low affinity for many microbial pathogens and is highly cross-reactive, even binding to some self molecules. Furthermore, it is not known whether it is produced in response to the normal flora of the epithelial surfaces of the body or in response to self. However, it can have a role in host defense against *Streptococcus pneumoniae* by binding to phosphocholine in the bacterial cell envelope, leading to clearance of the bacteria before they become dangerous.

Summary.

Innate immunity uses a variety of induced effector mechanisms to clear an infection or, failing that, to hold it in check until the pathogen can be recognized by the adaptive immune system. These effector mechanisms are all regulated by germline-encoded receptor systems that are able to discriminate between normal self molecules on uninfected cells and infectious nonself ligands. Thus the phagocyte's ability to discriminate between self and pathogen controls its release of pro-inflammatory chemokines and cytokines that act together to recruit more phagocytic cells to the site of infection. Especially prominent is the early recruitment of neutrophils that can recognize pathogens directly. Furthermore, cytokines released by tissue phagocytic cells induce fever, the production of acute-phase response proteins, including the pathogen-binding mannose-binding lectin and C-reactive protein, and the mobilization of antigen-presenting cells that induce the adaptive immune response. Viral pathogens are recognized by the cells in which they replicate, leading to the production of interferons that serve to inhibit viral replication and to activate NK cells, which in turn can distinguish infected from uninfected cells. As we will see later in this book, cytokines, chemokines, phagocytic cells, and NK cells are all effector mechanisms that are also employed in the adaptive immune response, which uses variable receptors to target specific pathogen antigens.

Summary to Chapter 2.

The innate system of host defense against infection is made up of several distinct components. The first of these are the barrier functions of the body's epithelia, which can simply prevent an infection from becoming established. Next, there are cells and molecules available to control or destroy the pathogen once it has breached the epithelial defenses. The most important of these are the tissue macrophages, which mediate cellular defense of the borders. The understanding of how the innate immune system recognizes pathogens is rapidly growing, and structural studies, such as those of mannose-binding lectin, have begun to reveal in detail how innate immune receptors can distinguish pathogen surfaces from those of host cells. Furthermore, the identification of the receptor for bacterial LPS and its link to human TLR-4 has opened a window onto innate immune recognition of microbe-associated molecular patterns. Recognition by the innate immune system leads to the elimination of invading pathogens through various effector mechanisms. Most of these have been known for a long time; indeed, the elimination of microorganisms by phagocytosis was the first immune response to be observed. However, more is being learned all the time; the chemokines, for example, have only been known of for about 15 years, and over 50 chemokine proteins have now been discovered. The complement system of proteins mediates humoral innate immunity of the tissue spaces and the blood. The induction of powerful effector mechanisms on the basis of innate immune recognition through germline-encoded receptors clearly has some dangers. Indeed, the double-edged sword embodied by the effects of the cytokine TNF-α—beneficial when it is released locally but disastrous when it is released systemically—illustrates the evolutionary knife-edge down which all innate mechanisms of host defense travel. The innate immune system can be viewed as a defense system that mainly frustrates the establishment of a focus of infection; however, even when it is inadequate to this function, it can still set the scene for the adaptive immune response, which forms an essential part of host defense in humans. Thus, having introduced the study of immunology with a consideration of innate immune function, we will now turn our attention to the adaptive immune response. This has been the focus of nearly all studies in immunology, because it is much easier to follow and experiment by using reagents and responses that are specific for defined antigens.

Chapter 2 questions.

2.1   The innate immune system uses two different strategies to identify pathogens: recognition of nonself and recognition of self. (a) Give examples of each and discuss how each example contributes to the ability of the organism to protect itself from infection. (b) What are the disadvantages of these different strategies?

2.2   The complement system gives rise to inflammatory signals, opsonins and molecules that lyse bacteria directly. (a) Describe the general properties of each class and discuss their utility in host defense. (b) Say which you think is most important in host defense, and why.

2.3   "The Toll receptors represent the most ancient pathways of host defense." Is this statement justified? Give an explanation for your answer.

2.4   Elie Metchnikoff discovered the protective role of macrophages by observing what happened in a starfish injured by a sea urchin spine. Describe the sequence of events that would follow were you to be speared by a sea urchin spine.

2.5   The complement system is a cascade of enzymes capable of producing powerful deleterious effects. (a) How is complement harnessed to protect us rather than creating harm? (b) What happens when things go wrong?

2.6   During their development and in order to perform their various functions efficiently, cells of the immune system must find their way to the correct part of the body. How do they manage to do this?

General references.

Ezekowitz, R.A.B., and Hoffman, J.: **Innate immunity.** *Curr. Opin. Immunol.* 1998, **10**:9–53.

Fearon, D.T., and Locksley, R.M.: **The instructive role of innate immunity in the acquired immune response.** *Science* 1996, **272**:50–53.

Gallin, J.I., Goldstein, I.M., and Snyderman, R. (eds): *Inflammation—Basic Principles and Clinical Correlates*, 3rd edn. New York, Raven Press, 1999.

Janeway, C.A., Jr, and Medzhitov, R.: **Innate immune recognition.** *Annu. Rev. Immunol.* 2002, **20**:197–216.

Mandell, G.L., Bennett, J.E., and Dolin, R. (eds): *Principles and Practice of Infectious Diseases*, 4th edn. New York, Churchill Livingstone, 1995.

Salyers, A.A., and Whitt, D.D.: *Bacterial Pathogenesis, A Molecular Approach.* Washington, DC, ASM Press, 1994.

Section references.

2-1 Infectious agents must overcome innate host defenses to establish a focus of infection.

Gibbons, R.J.: How microorganisms cause disease, in Gorbach, S.L., Bartlett, J.G., and Blacklow, N.R. (eds): *Infectious Diseases.* Philadelphia, W.B. Saunders Co., 1992.

Hornef, M.W., Wick, M.J., Rhen, M., and Normark, S.: **Bacterial strategies for overcoming host innate and adaptive immune responses.** *Nat. Immunol.* 2002, **3**:1033–1040.

2-2 The epithelial surfaces of the body make up the first lines of defense against infection.

Gallo, R.L., Murakami, M., Ohtake, T., and Zaiou, M.: **Biology and clinical relevance of naturally occurring antimicrobial peptides.** *J. Allergy Clin. Immunol.* 2002, **110**:823–831.

Gudmundsson, G.H., and Agerberth, B.: **Neutrophil antibacterial peptides, multifunctional effector molecules in the mammalian immune system.** *J. Immunol. Methods* 1999, **232**:45–54.

Koczulla, A.R., and Bals, R.: **Antimicrobial peptides: current status and therapeutic potential.** *Drugs* 2003, **63**:389–406.

Risso, A.: **Leukocyte antimicrobial peptides: multifunctional effector molecules of innate immunity.** *J. Leukoc. Biol.* 2000, **68**:785–792.

Zaiou, M., and Gallo, R.L.: **Cathelicidins, essential gene-encoded mammalian antibiotics.** *J. Mol. Med.* 2002, **80**:549–561.

2-3 After entering tissues, many pathogens are recognized, ingested, and killed by phagocytes.

Aderem, A., and Underhill, D.M.: **Mechanisms of phagocytosis in macrophages.** *Annu. Rev. Immunol.* 1999, **17**:593–623.

Beutler, B., and Rietschel, E.T.: **Innate immune sensing and its roots: the story of endotoxin.** *Nat. Rev. Immunol.* 2003, **3**:169–176.

Bogdan, C., Rollinghoff, M., and Diefenbach, A.: **Reactive oxygen and reactive nitrogen intermediates in innate and specific immunity.** *Curr. Opin. Immunol.* 2000, **12**:64–76.

Dahlgren, C., and Karlsson, A.: **Respiratory burst in human neutrophils.** *J. Immunol. Methods* 1999, **232**:3–14.

Harrison, R.E., and Grinstein, S.: **Phagocytosis and the microtubule cytoskeleton.** *Biochem. Cell Biol.* 2002, **80**:509–515.

2-4 Pathogen recognition and tissue damage initiate an inflammatory response.

Chertov, O., Yang, D., Howard, O.M., and Oppenheim, J.J.: **Leukocyte granule proteins mobilize innate host defenses and adaptive immune responses.** *Immunol. Rev.* 2000, **177**:68–78.

Kohl, J.: **Anaphylatoxins and infectious and noninfectious inflammatory diseases.** *Mol. Immunol.* 2001, **38**:175–187.

Mekori, Y.A., and Metcalfe, D.D.: **Mast cells in innate immunity.** *Immunol. Rev.* 2000, **173**:131–140.

Svanborg, C., Godaly, G., and Hedlund, M.: **Cytokine responses during mucosal infections: role in disease pathogenesis and host defence.** *Curr. Opin. Microbiol.* 1999, **2**:99–105.

van der Poll, T.: **Coagulation and inflammation.** *J. Endotoxin Res.* 2001, **7**:301–304.

2-5 Receptors with specificity for pathogen molecules recognize patterns of repeating structural motifs.

Apostolopoulos, V., and McKenzie, I.F.: **Role of the mannose receptor in the immune response.** *Curr. Mol. Med.* 2001, **1**:469–474.

Feizi, T.: **Carbohydrate-mediated recognition systems in innate immunity.** *Immunol. Rev.* 2000, **173**:79–88.

Gough, P.J., and Gordon, S.: **The role of scavenger receptors in the innate immune system.** *Microbes Infect.* 2000, **2**:305–311.

Heine, H., and Lien, E.: **Toll-like receptors and their function in innate and adaptive immunity.** *Int. Arch. Allergy Immunol.* 2003, **130**:180–192.

Kaisho, T., and Akira, S.: **Critical roles of toll-like receptors in host defense.** *Crit. Rev. Immunol.* 2000, **20**:393–405.

Linehan, S.A., Martinez-Pomares, L., and Gordon, S.: **Macrophage lectins in host defence.** *Microbes Infect.* 2000, **2**:279–288.

Podrez, E.A., Poliakov, E., Shen, Z., Zhang, R., Deng, Y., Sun, M., Finton, P.J., Shan, L., Gugiu, B., Fox, P.L., et al.: **Identification of a novel family of oxidized phospholipids that serve as ligands for the macrophage scavenger receptor CD36.** *J. Biol. Chem.* 2002, **277**:38503–38516.

Turner, M.W., and Hamvas, R.M.: **Mannose-binding lectin: structure, function, genetics and disease associations.** *Rev. Immunogenet.* 2000, **2**:305–322.

2-6 Receptors on phagocytes can signal the presence of pathogens.

Kopp, E.B., and Medzhitov, R.: **The Toll-receptor family and control of innate immunity.** *Curr. Opin. Immunol.* 1999, **11**:13–18.

Medzhitov, R., and Janeway, C.A., Jr: **How does the immune system distinguish self from nonself?** *Semin. Immunol.* 2000, **12**:185–188; discussion 257–344.

Medzhitov, R., and Janeway, C.A., Jr: **The toll receptor family and microbial recognition.** *Trends Microbiol.* 2000, **8**:452–456.

Peiser, L., De Winther, M.P., Makepeace, K., Hollinshead, M., Coull, P., Plested, J., Kodama, T., Moxon, E.R., and Gordon, S.: **The class A macrophage scavenger receptor is a major pattern recognition receptor for Neisseria meningitidis which is independent of lipopolysaccharide and not required for secretory responses.** *Infect. Immun.* 2002, **70**:5346–5354.

2-7 Each of the 10 Toll-like receptors in humans recognizes a particular molecular structure that is present in many pathogens.

Barton, G.M., and Medzhitov, R.: **Toll-like receptors and their ligands.** *Curr. Top. Microbiol. Immunol.* 2002, **270**:81–92.

2-8 The effects of bacterial lipopolysaccharide on macrophages are mediated by CD14 binding to TLR-4.

Beutler, B.: **Endotoxin, toll-like receptor 4, and the afferent limb of innate immunity.** *Curr. Opin. Microbiol.* 2000, **3**:23–28.

Beutler, B., and Rietschel, E.T.: **Innate immune sensing and its roots: the story of endotoxin.** *Nat. Rev. Immunol.* 2003, **3**:169–176.

2-9 Activation of Toll-like receptors triggers the production of pro-inflammatory cytokines and chemokines, and the expression of co-stimulatory molecules.

Bowie, A., and O'Neill, L.A.: **The interleukin-1 receptor/Toll-like receptor superfamily: signal generators for pro-inflammatory interleukins and microbial products.** *J. Leukoc. Biol.* 2000, **67**:508–514.

Brightbill, H.D., Libraty, D.H., Krutzik, S.R., Yang, R.B., Belisle, J.T., Bleharski, J.R., Maitland, M., Norgard, M.V., Plevy, S.E., Smale, S.T., et al.: **Host defense mechanisms triggered by microbial lipoproteins through toll-like receptors.** *Science* 1999, **285**:732–736.

Dalpke, A., and Heeg, K.: **Signal integration following Toll-like receptor triggering.** *Crit. Rev. Immunol.* 2002, **22**:217–250.

Heine, H., and Lien, E.: **Toll-like receptors and their function in innate and adaptive immunity.** *Int. Arch. Allergy Immunol.* 2003, **130**:180–192.

2-10   Complement is a system of plasma proteins that interacts with pathogens to mark them for destruction by phagocytes.

Frank, M.M.: **Complement deficiencies.** *Pediatr. Clin. North Am.* 2000, **47**:1339–1354.

Frank, M.M., and Fries, L.F.: **The role of complement in inflammation and phagocytosis.** *Immunol. Today* 1991, **12**:322–326.

Tomlinson, S.: **Complement defense mechanisms.** *Curr. Opin. Immunol.* 1993, **5**:83–89.

2-11   The classical pathway is initiated by activation of the C1 complex.

Arlaud, G.J., Gaboriaud, C., Thielens, N.M., Budayova-Spano, M., Rossi, V., and Fontecilla-Camps, J.C.: **Structural biology of the C1 complex of complement unveils the mechanisms of its activation and proteolytic activity.** *Mol. Immunol.* 2002, **39**:383–394.

Cooper, N.R.: **The classical complement pathway. Activation and regulation of the first complement component.** *Adv. Immunol.* 1985, **37**:151–216.

2-12   The mannose-binding lectin pathway is homologous to the classical pathway.

Dodds, A.W.: **Which came first, the lectin/classical pathway or the alternative pathway of complement?** *Immunobiology* 2002, **205**:340–354.

Gal, P., and Ambrus, G.: **Structure and function of complement activating enzyme complexes: C1 and MBL-MASPs.** *Curr. Protein Pept. Sci.* 2001, **2**:43–59.

Jack, D.L., Klein, N.J., and Turner, M.W.: **Mannose-binding lectin: targeting the microbial world for complement attack and opsonophagocytosis.** *Immunol. Rev.* 2001, **180**:86–99.

Lu, J., Teh, C., Kishore, U., and Reid, K.B.: **Collectins and ficolins: sugar pattern recognition molecules of the mammalian innate immune system.** *Biochim. Biophys. Acta* 2002, **1572**:387–400.

Rabinovich, G.A., Rubinstein, N., and Toscano, M.A.: **Role of galectins in inflammatory and immunomodulatory processes.** *Biochim. Biophys. Acta* 2002, **1572**:274–284.

Schwaeble, W., Dahl, M.R., Thiel, S., Stover, C., and Jensenius, J.C.: **The mannan-binding lectin-associated serine proteases (MASPs) and MAp19: four components of the lectin pathway activation complex encoded by two genes.** *Immunobiology* 2002, **205**:455–466.

2-13   Complement activation is largely confined to the surface on which it is initiated.

Cicardi, M., Bergamaschini, L., Cugno, M., Beretta, A., Zingale, L.C., Colombo, M., and Agostoni, A.: **Pathogenetic and clinical aspects of C1 inhibitor deficiency.** *Immunobiology* 1998, **199**:366–376.

2-14   Hydrolysis of C3 causes initiation of the alternative pathway of complement.

Fijen, C.A., van den Bogaard, R., Schipper, M., Mannens, M., Schlesinger, M., Nordin, F.G., Dankert, J., Daha, M.R., Sjoholm, A.G., Truedsson, L., and Kuijper, E.J.:

Properdin deficiency: molecular basis and disease association. *Mol. Immunol.* 1999, **36**:863–867.

Xu, Y., Narayana, S.V., and Volanakis, J.E.: **Structural biology of the alternative pathway convertase.** *Immunol. Rev.* 2001, **180**:123–135.

2-15   Surface-bound C3 convertase deposits large numbers of C3b fragments on pathogen surfaces and generates C5 convertase activity.

Rawal, N., and Pangburn, M.K.: **Structure/function of C5 convertases of complement.** *Int. Immunopharmacol.* 2001, **1**:415–422.

2-16   Ingestion of complement-tagged pathogens by phagocytes is mediated by receptors for the bound complement proteins.

Ehlers, M.R.: **CR3: a general purpose adhesion-recognition receptor essential for innate immunity.** *Microbes Infect.* 2000, **2**:289–294.

Fijen, C.A., Bredius, R.G., Kuijper, E.J., Out, T.A., De Haas, M., De Wit, A.P., Daha, M.R., and De Winkel, J.G.: **The role of Fcg receptor polymorphisms and C3 in the immune defence against *Neisseria meningitidis* in complement-deficient individuals.** *Clin. Exp. Immunol.* 2000, **120**:338–345.

Linehan, S.A., Martinez-Pomares, L., and Gordon, S.: **Macrophage lectins in host defence.** *Microbes Infect.* 2000, **2**:279–288.

Ravetch, J.V.: **A full complement of receptors in immune complex diseases.** *J. Clin. Invest.* 2002, **110**:1759–1761.

Ross, G.D.: **Regulation of the adhesion versus cytotoxic functions of the Mac-1/CR3alphaMbeta2-integrin glycoprotein.** *Crit. Rev. Immunol.* 2000, **20**:197–222.

2-17   Small fragments of some complement proteins can initiate a local inflammatory response.

Kohl, J.: **Anaphylatoxins and infectious and noninfectious inflammatory diseases.** *Mol. Immunol.* 2001, **38**:175–187.

Kildsgaard, J., Hollmann, T.J., Matthews, K.W., Bian, K., Murad, F., and Wetsel, R.A.: **Cutting edge: targeted disruption of the C3a receptor gene demonstrates a novel protective anti-inflammatory role for C3a in endotoxin-shock.** *J. Immunol.* 2000, **165**:5406–5409.

Monsinjon, T., Gasque, P., Ischenko, A., and Fontaine, M.: **C3A binds to the seven transmembrane anaphylatoxin receptor expressed by epithelial cells and triggers the production of IL-8.** *FEBS Lett.* 2001, **487**:339–346.

Schraufstatter, I.U., Trieu, K., Sikora, L., Sriramarao, P., and DiScipio, R.: **Complement c3a and c5a induce different signal transduction cascades in endothelial cells.** *J. Immunol.* 2002, **169**:2102–2110.

2-18   The terminal complement proteins polymerize to form pores in membranes that can kill certain pathogens.

Bhakdi, S., and Tranum-Jensen, J.: **Complement lysis: a hole is a hole.** *Immunol. Today* 1991, **12**:318–320.

Parker, C.L., and Sodetz, J.M.: **Role of the human C8 subunits in complement-mediated bacterial killing: evidence that C8 gamma is not essential.** *Mol. Immunol.* 2002, **39**:453–458.

Scibek, J.J., Plumb, M.E., and Sodetz, J.M.: **Binding of human complement C8 to C9: role of the N-terminal modules in the C8 alpha subunit.** *Biochemistry* 2002, **41**:14546–14551.

Wang, Y., Bjes, E.S., and Esser, A.F.: **Molecular aspects of complement-mediated bacterial killing. Periplasmic conversion of C9 from a protoxin to a toxin.** *J. Biol. Chem.* 2000, **275**:4687–4692.

2-19   Complement control proteins regulate all three pathways of complement activation and protect the host from its destructive effects.

Blom, A.M., Rytkonen, A., Vasquez, P., Lindahl, G., Dahlback, B., and Jonsson, A.B.: **A novel interaction between type IV pili of *Neisseria gonorrhoeae* and the** human complement regulator C4B-binding protein. *J. Immunol.* 2001, **166**:6764–6770.

Jiang, H., Wagner, E., Zhang, H., and Frank, M.M.: **Complement 1 inhibitor is a regulator of the alternative complement pathway.** *J. Exp. Med.* 2001, **194**:1609–1616.

Kirschfink, M.: **Controlling the complement system in inflammation.** *Immunopharmacology* 1997, **38**:51–62.

Kirschfink, M.: **C1-inhibitor and transplantation.** *Immunobiology* 2002, **205**:534–541.

Liszewski, M.K., Farries, T.C., Lublin, D.M., Rooney, I.A., and Atkinson, J.P.: **Control of the complement system.** *Adv. Immunol.* 1996, **61**:201–283.

Miwa, T., Zhou, L., Hilliard, B., Molina, H., and Song, W.C.: **Crry, but not CD59 and DAF, is indispensable for murine erythrocyte protection in vivo from spontaneous complement attack.** *Blood* 2002, **99**:3707–3716.

Pangburn, M.K.: **Host recognition and target differentiation by factor H, a regulator of the alternative pathway of complement.** *Immunopharmacology* 2000, **49**:149–157.

Singhrao, S.K., Neal, J.W., Rushmere, N.K., Morgan, B.P., and Gasque, P.: **Spontaneous classical pathway activation and deficiency of membrane regulators render human neurons susceptible to complement lysis.** *Am. J. Pathol.* 2000, **157**:905–918.

Smith, G.P., and Smith, R.A.: **Membrane-targeted complement inhibitors.** *Mol. Immunol.* 2001, **38**:249–255.

Suankratay, C., Mold, C., Zhang, Y., Lint, T.F., and Gewurz, H.: **Mechanism of complement-dependent haemolysis via the lectin pathway: role of the complement regulatory proteins.** *Clin. Exp. Immunol.* 1999, **117**:442–448.

Suankratay, C., Mold, C., Zhang, Y., Potempa, L.A., Lint, T.F., and Gewurz, H.: **Complement regulation in innate immunity and the acute-phase response: inhibition of mannan-binding lectin-initiated complement cytolysis by C-reactive protein (CRP).** *Clin. Exp. Immunol.* 1998, **113**:353–359.

Zipfel, P.F., Jokiranta, T.S., Hellwage, J., Koistinen, V., and Meri, S.: **The factor H protein family.** *Immunopharmacology* 1999, **42**:53–60.

2-20 Activated macrophages secrete a range of cytokines that have a variety of local and distant effects.

Larsson, B.M., Larsson, K., Malmberg, P., and Palmberg, L.: **Gram positive bacteria induce IL-6 and IL-8 production in human alveolar macrophages and epithelial cells.** *Inflammation* 1999, **23**:217–230.

Ozato, K., Tsujimura, H., and Tamura, T.: **Toll-like receptor signaling and regulation of cytokine gene expression in the immune system.** *Biotechniques* 2002, Suppl:66–69,70,72 *C₃a, C5a.*

Svanborg, C., Godaly, G., and Hedlund, M.: **Cytokine responses during mucosal infections: role in disease pathogenesis and host defence.** *Curr. Opin. Microbiol.* 1999, **2**:99–105.

2-21 Chemokines released by phagocytes and dendritic cells recruit cells to sites of infection.

Kunkel, E.J., and Butcher, E.C.: **Chemokines and the tissue-specific migration of lymphocytes.** *Immunity* 2002, **16**:1–4.

Luster, A.D.: **The role of chemokines in linking innate and adaptive immunity.** *Curr. Opin. Immunol.* 2002, **14**:129–135.

Matsukawa, A., Hogaboam, C.M., Lukacs, N.W., and Kunkel, S.L.: **Chemokines and innate immunity.** *Rev. Immunogenet.* 2000, **2**:339–358.

Ono, S.J., Nakamura, T., Miyazaki, D., Ohbayashi, M., Dawson, M., and Toda, M.: **Chemokines: roles in leukocyte development, trafficking, and effector function.** *J. Allergy Clin. Immunol.* 2003, **111**:1185–1199.

Scapini, P., Lapinet-Vera, J.A., Gasperini, S., Calzetti, F., Bazzoni, F., and Cassatella, M.A.: **The neutrophil as a cellular source of chemokines.** *Immunol. Rev.* 2000, **177**:195–203.

Yoshie, O.: **Role of chemokines in trafficking of lymphocytes and dendritic cells.** *Int. J. Hematol.* 2000, **72**:399–407.

2-22 Cell-adhesion molecules control interactions between leukocytes and endothelial cells during an inflammatory response.

Alon, R., and Feigelson, S.: **From rolling to arrest on blood vessels: leukocyte tap dancing on endothelial integrin ligands and chemokines at sub-second contacts.** *Semin. Immunol.* 2002, **14**:93–104.

Bunting, M., Harris, E.S., McIntyre, T.M., Prescott, S.M., and Zimmerman, G.A.: **Leukocyte adhesion deficiency syndromes: adhesion and tethering defects involving beta 2 integrins and selectin ligands.** *Curr. Opin. Hematol.* 2002, **9**:30–35.

D'Ambrosio, D., Albanesi, C., Lang, R., Girolomoni, G., Sinigaglia, F., and Laudanna, C.: **Quantitative differences in chemokine receptor engagement generate diversity in integrin-dependent lymphocyte adhesion.** *J. Immunol.* 2002, **169**:2303–2312.

Johnston, B., and Butcher, E.C.: **Chemokines in rapid leukocyte adhesion triggering and migration.** *Semin. Immunol.* 2002, **14**:83–92.

Ley, K.: **Integration of inflammatory signals by rolling neutrophils.** *Immunol. Rev.* 2002, **186**:8–18.

Shahabuddin, S., Ponath, P., and Schleimer, R.P.: **Migration of eosinophils across endothelial cell monolayers: interactions among IL-5, endothelial-activating cytokines, and C-C chemokines.** *J. Immunol.* 2000, **164**:3847–3854.

Vestweber, D.: **Lymphocyte trafficking through blood and lymphatic vessels: more than just selectins, chemokines and integrins.** *Eur. J. Immunol.* 2003, **33**:1361–1364.

2-23 Neutrophils make up the first wave of cells that cross the blood vessel wall to enter inflammatory sites.

Bochenska-Marciniak, M., Kupczyk, M., Gorski, P., and Kuna, P.: **The effect of recombinant interleukin-8 on eosinophils' and neutrophils' migration in vivo and in vitro.** *Allergy* 2003, **58**:795–801.

Godaly, G., Bergsten, G., Hang, L., Fischer, H., Frendeus, B., Lundstedt, A.C., Samuelsson, M., Samuelsson, P., and Svanborg, C.: **Neutrophil recruitment, chemokine receptors, and resistance to mucosal infection.** *J. Leukoc. Biol.* 2001, **69**:899–906.

Gompertz, S., and Stockley, R.A.: **Inflammation—role of the neutrophil and the eosinophil.** *Semin. Respir. Infect.* 2000, **15**:14–23.

Lee, S.C., Brummet, M.E., Shahabuddin, S., Woodworth, T.G., Georas, S.N., Leiferman, K.M., Gilman, S.C., Stellato, C., Gladue, R.P., Schleimer, R.P., and Beck, L.A.: **Cutaneous injection of human subjects with macrophage inflammatory protein-1 alpha induces significant recruitment of neutrophils and monocytes.** *J. Immunol.* 2000, **164**:3392–3401.

Worthylake, R.A., and Burridge, K.: **Leukocyte transendothelial migration: orchestrating the underlying molecular machinery.** *Curr. Opin. Cell Biol.* 2001, **13**:569–577.

2-24 Tumor necrosis factor-α is an important cytokine that triggers local containment of infection but induces shock when released systemically.

Cairns, C.B., Panacek, E.A., Harken, A.H., and Banerjee, A.: **Bench to bedside: tumor necrosis factor-alpha: from inflammation to resuscitation.** *Acad. Emerg. Med.* 2000, **7**:930–941.

Dellinger, R.P.: **Inflammation and coagulation: implications for the septic patient.** *Clin. Infect. Dis.* 2003, **36**:1259–1265.

Pfeffer, K.: **Biological functions of tumor necrosis factor cytokines and their receptors.** *Cytokine Growth Factor Rev.* 2003, **14**:185–191.

Sriskandan, S., and Cohen, J.: **Gram-positive sepsis. Mechanisms and differences from gram-negative sepsis.** *Infect. Dis. Clin. North Am.* 1999, **13**:397–412.

2-25 Cytokines released by phagocytes activate the acute-phase response.

Bopst, M., Haas, C., Car, B., and Eugster, H.P.: **The combined inactivation of tumor necrosis factor and interleukin-6 prevents induction of the major acute phase proteins by endotoxin.** *Eur. J. Immunol.* 1998, **28**:4130–4137.

Ceciliani, F., Giordano, A., and Spagnolo, V.: **The systemic reaction during inflammation: the acute-phase proteins.** *Protein Pept. Lett.* 2002, **9**:211–223.

He, R., Sang, H., and Ye, R.D.: **Serum amyloid A induces IL-8 secretion through a G protein-coupled receptor, FPRL1/LXA4R.** *Blood* 2003, **101**:1572–1581.

Horn, F., Henze, C., and Heidrich, K.: **Interleukin-6 signal transduction and lymphocyte function.** *Immunobiology* 2000, **202**:151–167.

Mold, C., Rodriguez, W., Rodic-Polic, B., and Du Clos, T.W.: **C-reactive protein mediates protection from lipopolysaccharide through interactions with Fc gamma R.** *J. Immunol.* 2002, **169**:7019–7025.

Sheth, K., and Bankey, P.: **The liver as an immune organ.** *Curr. Opin. Crit. Care* 2001, **7**:99–104.

Volanakis, J.E.: **Human C-reactive protein: expression, structure, and function.** *Mol. Immunol.* 2001, **38**:189–197.

2-26 Interferons induced by viral infection make several contributions to host defense.

Balachandran, S., Roberts, P.C., Brown, L.E., Truong, H., Pattnaik, A.K., Archer, D.R., and Barber, G.N.: **Essential role for the dsRNA-dependent protein kinase PKR in innate immunity to viral infection.** *Immunity* 2000, **13**:129–141.

Barber, G.N.: **Host defense, viruses and apoptosis.** *Cell Death Differ.* 2001, **8**:113–126.

Barnes, B., Lubyova, B., and Pitha, P.M.: **On the role of IRF in host defense.** *J. Interferon Cytokine Res.* 2002, **22**:59–71.

Bogdan, C.: **The function of type I interferons in antimicrobial immunity.** *Curr. Opin. Immunol.* 2000, **12**:419–424.

Brierley, M.M., and Fish, E.N.: **Review: IFN-alpha/beta receptor interactions to biologic outcomes: understanding the circuitry.** *J. Interferon Cytokine Res.* 2002, **22**:835–845.

Durbin, J.E., Fernandez-Sesma, A., Lee, C.K., Rao, T.D., Frey, A.B., Moran, T.M., Vukmanovic, S., Garcia-Sastre, A., and Levy, D.E.: **Type I IFN modulates innate and specific antiviral immunity.** *J. Immunol.* 2000, **164**:4220–4228.

Kadowaki, N., Antonenko, S., Lau, J.Y., and Liu, Y.J.: **Natural interferon alpha/beta-producing cells link innate and adaptive immunity.** *J. Exp. Med.* 2000, **192**:219–226.

Levy, D.E., and Garcia-Sastre, A.: **The virus battles: IFN induction of the antiviral state and mechanisms of viral evasion.** *Cytokine Growth Factor Rev.* 2001, **12**:143–156.

Shtrichman, R., and Samuel, C.E.: **The role of gamma interferon in antimicrobial immunity.** *Curr. Opin. Microbiol.* 2001, **4**:251–259.

2-27 NK cells are activated by interferons and macrophage-derived cytokines to serve as an early defense against certain intracellular infections.

Biron, C.A., Nguyen, K.B., Pien, G.C., Cousens, L.P., and Salazar-Mather, T.P.: **Natural killer cells in antiviral defense: function and regulation by innate cytokines.** *Annu. Rev. Immunol.* 1999, **17**:189–220.

Carnaud, C., Lee, D., Donnars, O., Park, S.H., Beavis, A., Koezuka, Y., and Bendelac, A.: **Cutting edge: Cross-talk between cells of the innate immune system: NKT cells rapidly activate NK cells.** *J. Immunol.* 1999, **163**:4647–4650.

Dascher, C.C., and Brenner, M.B.: **CD1 antigen presentation and infectious disease.** *Contrib. Microbiol.* 2003, **10**:164–182.

Godshall, C.J., Scott, M.J., Burch, P.T., Peyton, J.C., and Cheadle, W.G.: **Natural killer cells participate in bacterial clearance during septic peritonitis through in-**

teractions with macrophages. *Shock* 2003, **19**:144–149.

Orange, J.S., Fassett, M.S., Koopman, L.A., Boyson, J.E., and Stromigner, J.L.: **Viral evasion of natural killer cells.** *Nat. Immunol.* 2002, **3**:1006–1012.

Salazar-Mather, T.P., Hamilton, T.A., and Biron, C.A.: **A chemokine-to-cytokine-to-chemokine cascade critical in antiviral defense.** *J. Clin. Invest.* 2000, **105**:985–993.

Seki, S., Habu, Y., Kawamura, T., Takeda, K., Dobashi, H., Ohkawa, T., and Hiraide, H.: **The liver as a crucial organ in the first line of host defense: the roles of Kupffer cells, natural killer (NK) cells and NK1.1 Ag+ T cells in T helper 1 immune responses.** *Immunol. Rev.* 2000, **174**:35–46.

2-28 NK cells possess receptors for self molecules that prevent their activation by uninfected cells.

Borrego, F., Kabat, J., Kim, D.K., Lieto, L., Maasho, K., Pena, J., Solana, R., and Coligan, J.E.: **Structure and function of major histocompatibility complex (MHC) class I specific receptors expressed on human natural killer (NK) cells.** *Mol. Immunol.* 2002, **38**:637–660.

Boyington, J.C., and Sun, P.D.: **A structural perspective on MHC class I recognition by killer cell immunoglobulin-like receptors.** *Mol. Immunol.* 2002, **38**:1007–1021.

Brown, M.G., Dokun, A.O., Heusel, J.W., Smith, H.R., Beckman, D.L., Blattenberger, E.A., Dubbelde, C.E., Stone, L.R., Scalzo, A.A., and Yokoyama, W.M.: **Vital involvement of a natural killer cell activation receptor in resistance to viral infection.** *Science* 2001, **292**:934–937.

Robbins, S.H., and Brossay, L.: **NK cell receptors: emerging roles in host defense against infectious agents.** *Microbes Infect.* 2002, **4**:1523–1530.

Trowsdale, J.: **Genetic and functional relationships between MHC and NK receptor genes.** *Immunity* 2001, **15**:363–374.

Vilches, C., and Parham, P.: **KIR: diverse, rapidly evolving receptors of innate and adaptive immunity.** *Annu. Rev. Immunol.* 2002, **20**:217–251.

2-29 Several lymphocyte subpopulations behave as innate-like lymphocytes.

Bos, N.A., Cebra, J.J., and Kroese, F.G.: **B-1 cells and the intestinal microflora.** *Curr. Top. Microbiol. Immunol.* 2000, **252**:211–220.

Chan, W.L., Pejnovic, N., Liew, T.V., Lee, C.A., Groves, R., and Hamilton, H.: **NKT cell subsets in infection and inflammation.** *Immunol. Lett.* 2003, **85**:159–163.

Chatenoud, L.: **Do NKT cells control autoimmunity?** *J. Clin. Invest.* 2002, **110**:747–748.

Galli, G., Nuti, S., Tavarini, S., Galli-Stampino, L., De Lalla, C., Casorati, G., Dellabona, P., and Abrignani, S.: **CD1d-restricted help to B cells by human invariant natural killer T lymphocytes.** *J. Exp. Med.* 2003, **197**:1051–1057.

Kronenberg, M., and Gapin, L.: **The unconventional lifestyle of NKT cells.** *Nat. Rev. Immunol.* 2002, **2**:557–568.

Reid, R.R., Woodcock, S., Prodeus, A.P., Austen, J., Kobzik, L., Hechtman, H., Moore, F.D., Jr, and Carroll, M.C.: **The role of complement receptors CD21/CD35 in positive selection of B-1 cells.** *Curr. Top. Microbiol. Immunol.* 2000, **252**:57–65.

Sharif, S., Arreaza, G.A., Zucker, P., Mi, Q.S., and Delovitch, T.L.: **Regulation of autoimmune disease by natural killer T cells.** *J. Mol. Med.* 2002, **80**:290–300.

Stober, D., Jomantaite, I., Schirmbeck, R., and Reimann, J.: **NKT cells provide help for dendritic cell-dependent priming of MHC class I-restricted CD8+ T cells in vivo.** *J. Immunol.* 2003, **170**:2540–2548.

Zinkernagel, R.M.: **A primitive T cell-independent mechanism of intestinal mucosal IgA responses to commensal bacteria.** *Science* 2000, **288**:2222–2226.

PART I

THE RECOGNITION OF ANTIGEN

Antigen Recognition by B-cell and T-cell Receptors

3

We have learned in Chapter 2 that the body is defended by innate immune responses, but these only work to control pathogens that have certain molecular patterns or that induce interferons and other secreted yet nonspecific defenses. Most crucially, they do not allow memory to form because they operate through receptors that are coded in the genome. Thus, innate immunity is good for preventing pathogens from growing freely in the body, but it does not lead to the most important feature of adaptive immunity, which is long-lasting memory of a specific pathogen.

To fight the wide range of pathogens an individual will encounter, the lymphocytes of the adaptive immune system have evolved to recognize a great variety of different antigens from bacteria, viruses, and other disease-causing organisms. The antigen-recognition molecules of B cells are the **immunoglobulins**, or **Ig**. These proteins are produced by B cells in a vast range of antigen specificities, each B cell producing immunoglobulin of a single specificity (see Sections 1-8 to 1-10). Membrane-bound immunoglobulin on the B-cell surface serves as the cell's receptor for antigen, and is known as the **B-cell receptor** (**BCR**). Immunoglobulin of the same antigen specificity is secreted as **antibody** by terminally differentiated B cells—the plasma cells. The secretion of antibodies, which bind pathogens or their toxic products in the extracellular spaces of the body, is the main effector function of B cells in adaptive immunity.

Antibodies were the first molecules involved in specific immune recognition to be characterized, and are still the best understood. The antibody molecule has two separate functions: one is to bind specifically to molecules from the pathogen that elicited the immune response; the other is to recruit other cells and molecules to destroy the pathogen once the antibody is bound to it. For example, binding by antibody neutralizes viruses and marks pathogens for destruction by phagocytes and complement, as described in Section 1-15. These functions are structurally separated in the antibody molecule, one part of which specifically recognizes and binds to the pathogen or antigen whereas the other engages different effector mechanisms. The antigen-binding region varies extensively between antibody molecules and is thus known as the **variable region** or **V region**. The variability of antibody molecules allows each antibody to bind a different specific antigen, and the total repertoire of antibodies made by a single individual is large enough to ensure that virtually any structure can be recognized. The region of the antibody molecule that engages the effector functions of the immune system does not vary in the same way and is thus known as the **constant region** or **C region**. It comes in five main forms, which are each specialized for activating different effector mechanisms. The membrane-bound B-cell receptor does not have these effector functions, because the C region remains inserted in the membrane of the

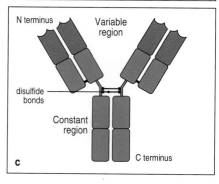

Fig. 3.1 Structure of an antibody molecule. Panel a illustrates a ribbon diagram based on the X-ray crystallographic structure of an IgG antibody, showing the course of the backbones of the polypeptide chains. Three globular regions form a Y shape. The two antigen-binding sites are at the tips of the arms, which are tethered to the trunk of the Y by a flexible hinge region. A schematic representation of the structure in a is given in panel b, illustrating the four-chain composition and the separate domains comprising each chain. Panel c shows a simplified schematic representation of an antibody molecule that will be used throughout this book. C terminus, carboxy terminus; N terminus, amino terminus. Panel a courtesy of A. McPherson and L. Harris.

B cell. Its function is as a receptor that recognizes and binds antigen by the V regions exposed on the surface of the cell, thus transmitting a signal that causes B-cell activation, leading to clonal expansion and specific antibody production.

The antigen-recognition molecules of T cells are made solely as membrane-bound proteins and function only to signal T cells for activation. These **T-cell receptors** (**TCRs**) are related to immunoglobulins both in their protein structure—having both V and C regions—and in the genetic mechanism that produces their great variability (see Section 1-11 and Chapter 4). However, the T-cell receptor differs from the B-cell receptor in an important way: it does not recognize and bind antigen directly, but instead recognizes short peptide fragments of pathogens' protein antigens, which are bound to **MHC molecules** on the surfaces of other cells.

The MHC molecules are glycoproteins encoded in the large cluster of genes known as the **major histocompatibility complex** (**MHC**) (see Sections 1-17 and 1-18). Their most striking structural feature is a cleft running across their outermost surface, in which a variety of peptides can be bound. As we shall discuss further in Chapter 5, MHC molecules show great genetic variation in the population. Most people are heterozygous for the MHC molecules: they express two allelic forms of each MHC locus, which increases the range of pathogen-derived peptides that can be bound. T-cell receptors recognize features of both the peptide antigen and the MHC molecule to which it is bound. This introduces an extra dimension to antigen recognition by T cells, known as **MHC restriction**, because any given T-cell receptor is specific not simply for a foreign peptide antigen but for a unique combination of a peptide and a particular MHC molecule. The ability of T-cell receptors to recognize MHC molecules, and their selection during T-cell development for the ability to recognize the particular MHC molecules expressed by an individual, are topics we shall return to in Chapters 5 and 7.

In this chapter we focus on the structure and antigen-binding properties of immunoglobulins and T-cell receptors. Although B cells and T cells recognize foreign molecules in two distinct fashions, the receptor molecules they use for this task are very similar in structure. We will see how this basic structure can accommodate great variability in antigen specificity, and how it enables immunoglobulins and T-cell receptors to perform their functions as the antigen-recognition molecules of the adaptive immune response.

The structure of a typical antibody molecule.

Antibodies are the secreted form of the B-cell receptor. An antibody is identical to the B-cell receptor of the cell that secretes it except for a small portion of the carboxy terminus of the heavy-chain C region. In the case of the B-cell receptor the carboxy terminus is a hydrophobic membrane-anchoring sequence, and in the case of antibody it is a hydrophilic sequence that allows secretion. As they are soluble, and secreted in large quantities, antibodies are easily obtainable and easily studied. For this reason, most of what we know about the B-cell receptor comes from the study of antibodies.

Antibody molecules are roughly Y-shaped molecules consisting of three equal-sized portions, connected by a flexible tether. Three schematic representations of antibody structure, which has been determined by X-ray crystallography, are shown in Fig. 3.1. The aim of this part of the chapter is to explain how this structure is formed and how it allows antibody molecules to perform their dual tasks—binding on the one hand to a wide variety of antigens, and on the other hand to a limited number of effector molecules and cells. As we will see, each of these tasks is performed by separable parts of the molecule. The two arms of the Y end in regions that vary between different antibody molecules—the V regions. These are involved in antigen binding, whereas the stem of the Y, or the C region, is far less variable and is the part that interacts with effector cells and molecules.

All antibodies are constructed in the same way from paired heavy and light polypeptide chains, and the generic term immunoglobulin is used for all such proteins. Within this general category, however, five different classes of immunoglobulins—IgM, IgD, IgG, IgA, and IgE—can be distinguished by their C regions, which will be described more fully in Chapter 4. More subtle differences confined to the V region account for the specificity of antigen binding. We will use the IgG antibody molecule as an example to describe the general structural features of immunoglobulins.

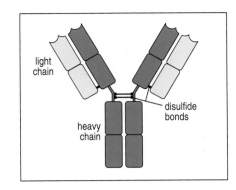

Fig. 3.2 Immunoglobulin molecules are composed of two types of protein chain: heavy chains and light chains. Each immunoglobulin molecule is made up of two heavy chains (green) and two light chains (yellow) joined by disulfide bonds so that each heavy chain is linked to a light chain and the two heavy chains are linked together.

3-1   IgG antibodies consist of four polypeptide chains.

IgG antibodies are large molecules with a molecular weight of approximately 150 kDa and are composed of two different kinds of polypeptide chain. One, of approximately 50 kDa, is termed the **heavy** or **H chain**, and the other, of 25 kDa, is termed the **light** or **L chain** (Fig. 3.2). Each IgG molecule consists of two heavy chains and two light chains. The two heavy chains are linked to each other by disulfide bonds and each heavy chain is linked to a light chain by a disulfide bond. In any given immunoglobulin molecule, the two heavy chains and the two light chains are identical, giving an antibody molecule two identical antigen-binding sites (see Fig. 3.1), and thus the ability to bind simultaneously to two identical structures.

Two types of light chain, termed **lambda (λ)** and **kappa (κ)**, are found in antibodies. A given immunoglobulin has either κ chains or λ chains, never one of each. No functional difference has been found between antibodies having λ or κ light chains, and either type of light chain can be found in antibodies of any of the five major classes. The ratio of the two types of light chain varies from species to species. In mice, the average κ to λ ratio is 20:1, whereas in humans it is 2:1 and in cattle it is 1:20. The reason for this variation is unknown. Distortions of this ratio can sometimes be used to detect the abnormal proliferation of a clone of B cells. These would all express the identical light chain, and thus an excess of λ light chains in a person might indicate the presence of a B-cell tumor producing λ chains.

By contrast, the class, and thus the effector function, of an antibody is defined by the structure of its heavy chain. There are five main **heavy-chain classes** or **isotypes**, some of which have several subtypes, and these determine the functional activity of an antibody molecule. The five major classes of immunoglobulin are **immunoglobulin M (IgM)**, **immunoglobulin D (IgD)**, **immunoglobulin G (IgG)**, **immunoglobulin A (IgA)**, and **immunoglobulin E (IgE)**. Their heavy chains are denoted by the corresponding lower-case Greek letter (μ, δ, γ, α, and ε, respectively). IgG is by far the most abundant immunoglobulin and has several subclasses (IgG1, 2, 3, and 4 in humans). Their distinctive functional properties are conferred by the carboxy-terminal part of the heavy chain, where it is not associated with the light chain. We will describe the structure and functions of the different heavy-chain isotypes in Chapter 4. The general structural features of all the isotypes are similar, and we will consider IgG, the most abundant isotype in plasma, as a typical antibody molecule.

3-2   Immunoglobulin heavy and light chains are composed of constant and variable regions.

The amino acid sequences of many immunoglobulin heavy and light chains have been determined and reveal two important features of antibody molecules. First, each chain consists of a series of similar, although not identical, sequences, each about 110 amino acids long. Each of these repeats corresponds to a discrete, compactly folded region of protein structure known as a protein domain. The light chain is made up of two such **immunoglobulin domains**, whereas the heavy chain of the IgG antibody contains four (see Fig. 3.1a). This suggests that the immunoglobulin chains have evolved by repeated duplication of an ancestral gene corresponding to a single domain.

The second important feature revealed by comparisons of amino acid sequences is that the amino-terminal sequences of both the heavy and light chains vary greatly between different antibodies. The variability in sequence is limited to approximately the first 110 amino acids, corresponding to the first domain, whereas the remaining domains are constant between immunoglobulin chains of the same isotype. The amino-terminal **variable domains (V domains)** of the heavy and light chains (V_H and V_L, respectively) together make up the V region of the antibody and confer on it the ability to bind specific antigen, whereas the **constant domains (C domains)** of the heavy and light chains (C_H and C_L, respectively) make up the C region (see Fig. 3.1b, c). The multiple heavy-chain C domains are numbered from the amino-terminal end to the carboxy terminus, for example C_H1, C_H2, and so on.

3-3   The antibody molecule can readily be cleaved into functionally distinct fragments.

The protein domains described above associate to form larger globular domains. Thus, when fully folded and assembled, an antibody molecule comprises three equal-sized globular portions joined by a flexible stretch of polypeptide chain known as the **hinge region** (see Fig. 3.1b). Each arm of this Y-shaped structure is formed by the association of a light chain with the amino-terminal half of a heavy chain, whereas the trunk of the Y is formed by the pairing of the carboxy-terminal halves of the two heavy chains. The association of the heavy and light chains is such that the V_H and V_L domains are paired, as are the C_H1 and C_L domains. The C_H3 domains pair with each other but the C_H2 domains do not interact; carbohydrate side chains attached to the C_H2 domains lie between the two heavy chains. The two antigen-binding sites are formed by the paired V_H and V_L domains at the ends of the two arms of the Y (see Fig. 3.1b).

Proteolytic enzymes (proteases) that cleave polypeptide sequences have been used to dissect the structure of antibody molecules and to determine which parts of the molecule are responsible for its various functions. Limited digestion with the protease papain cleaves antibody molecules into three fragments (Fig. 3.3). Two fragments are identical and contain the antigen-binding activity. These are termed the **Fab fragments**, for Fragment antigen binding. The Fab fragments correspond to the two identical arms of the antibody molecule, each of which consists of a complete light chain paired with the V_H and C_H1 domains of a heavy chain. The other fragment contains no antigen-binding activity but was originally observed to crystallize readily, and for this reason was named the **Fc fragment**, for Fragment crystallizable. This fragment corresponds to the paired C_H2 and C_H3 domains and is the part of the antibody molecule that interacts with effector molecules and cells. The functional differences between heavy-chain isotypes lie mainly in the Fc fragment.

Fig. 3.3 The Y-shaped immunoglobulin molecule can be dissected by partial digestion with proteases. Upper panels: papain cleaves the immunoglobulin molecule into three pieces, two Fab fragments and one Fc fragment. The Fab fragment contains the V regions and binds antigen. The Fc fragment is crystallizable and contains C regions. Lower panels: pepsin cleaves immunoglobulin to yield one $F(ab0_2$ fragment and many small pieces of the Fc fragment, the largest of which is called the pFc0fragment. $F(ab0_2$ is written with a prime because it contains a few more amino acids than Fab, including the cysteines that form the disulfide bonds.

The protein fragments obtained after proteolysis are determined by where the protease cuts the antibody molecule in relation to the disulfide bonds that link the two heavy chains. These lie in the hinge region between the C_H1 and C_H2 domains and, as illustrated in Fig. 3.3, papain cleaves the antibody molecule on the amino-terminal side of the disulfide bonds. This releases the two arms of the antibody as separate Fab fragments, whereas in the Fc fragment the carboxy-terminal halves of the heavy chains remain linked.

Another protease, pepsin, cuts in the same general region of the antibody molecule as papain but on the carboxy-terminal side of the disulfide bonds (see Fig. 3.3). This produces a fragment, the **F(ab')$_2$ fragment**, in which the two antigen-binding arms of the antibody molecule remain linked. In this case the remaining part of the heavy chain is cut into several small fragments. The F(ab')$_2$ fragment has exactly the same antigen-binding characteristics as the original antibody but is unable to interact with any effector molecule. It is thus of potential value in therapeutic applications of antibodies as well as in research into the functional role of the Fc portion.

Genetic engineering techniques also now permit the construction of many different antibody-related molecules. One important type is a truncated Fab comprising only the V domain of a heavy chain linked by a stretch of synthetic peptide to a V domain of a light chain. This is called **single-chain Fv**, named from **F**ragment **v**ariable. Fv molecules may become valuable therapeutic agents because of their small size, which allows them to penetrate tissues readily. They can be coupled to protein toxins to yield immunotoxins with potential application, for example, in tumor therapy in the case of a Fv specific for a tumor antigen (see Chapter 14).

3-4   The immunoglobulin molecule is flexible, especially at the hinge region.

The hinge region that links the Fc and Fab portions of the antibody molecule is in reality a flexible tether, allowing independent movement of the two Fab arms, rather than a rigid hinge. This has been demonstrated by electron microscopy of antibodies bound to **haptens**. These are small molecules of various sorts, typically about the size of a tyrosine side chain. They can be recognized by antibody but are able to stimulate the production of anti-hapten antibodies only when linked to a larger protein **carrier** (see Appendix I, Section A-1). An antigen made of two identical hapten molecules joined by a short flexible region can link two or more anti-hapten antibodies, forming dimers, trimers, tetramers, and so on, which can be seen by electron microscopy (Fig. 3.4). The shapes formed by these complexes demonstrate that antibody molecules are flexible at the hinge region. Some flexibility is also found at the junction between the V and C domains, allowing bending and rotation of the V domain relative to the C domain. For example, in the antibody molecule shown in Fig. 3.1a, not only are the two hinge regions clearly bent differently, but the angle between the V and C domains in each of the two Fab arms is also different. This range of motion has led to the junction between the V and C domains being referred to as a 'molecular ball-and-socket joint.' Flexibility at both the hinge and the V–C junction enables the binding of both arms of an antibody molecule to sites that are various distances apart, for example, sites on bacterial cell-wall polysaccharides. Flexibility at the hinge also enables the antibodies to interact with the antibody-binding proteins that mediate immune effector mechanisms.

Fig. 3.4 Antibody arms are joined by a flexible hinge. An antigen consisting of two hapten molecules (red balls in diagrams) that can cross-link two antigen-binding sites is used to create antigen:antibody complexes, which can be seen in the electron micrograph. Linear, triangular, and square forms are seen, with short projections or spikes. Limited pepsin digestion removes these spikes (not shown in the figure), which therefore correspond to the Fc portion of the antibody; the F(ab′)₂ pieces remain cross-linked by antigen. The interpretation of the complexes is shown in the diagrams. The angle between the arms of the antibody molecules varies, from 0° in the antibody dimers, through 60° in the triangular forms, to 90° in the square forms, showing that the connections between the arms are flexible. Photograph (× 300,000) courtesy of N.M. Green.

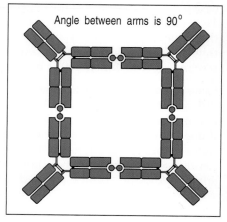

3-5   The domains of an immunoglobulin molecule have similar structures.

As we saw in Section 3-2, immunoglobulin heavy and light chains are composed of a series of discrete protein domains, all of which have a similar folded structure. Within this basic three-dimensional structure there are distinct differences between V and C domains. The structural similarities and differences can be seen in the diagram of a light chain in Fig. 3.5. Each domain is constructed from two **β sheets**, which are elements of protein structure made up of strands of the polypeptide chain (β strands) packed together; the sheets are linked by a disulfide bridge and together form a roughly barrel-shaped structure, known as a **β barrel**. The distinctive folded structure of the immunoglobulin protein domain is known as the **immunoglobulin fold**.

Both the essential similarity of V and C domains and the critical difference between them are most clearly seen in the bottom panels of Fig. 3.5, where the cylindrical domains are opened out to reveal how the polypeptide chain folds to create each of the β sheets and how it forms flexible loops as it changes direction. The main difference between the V and C domains is that the V domain is larger, with an extra loop. We will see in Section 3-6 that the flexible loops of the V domains form the antigen-binding site of the immunoglobulin molecule.

Fig. 3.5 The structure of immunoglobulin constant and variable domains. The upper panels show schematically the folding pattern of the constant (C) and variable (V) domains of an immunoglobulin light chain. Each domain is a barrel-shaped structure in which strands of polypeptide chain (β strands) running in opposite directions (antiparallel) pack together to form two β sheets (shown in yellow and green in the diagram of the C domain), which are held together by a disulfide bond. The way the polypeptide chain folds to give the final structure can be seen more clearly when the sheets are opened out, as shown in the lower panels. The β strands are lettered sequentially with respect to the order of their occurrence in the amino acid sequence of the domains; the order in each β sheet is characteristic of immunoglobulin domains. The β strands C′ and C″ that are found in the V domains but not in the C domains are indicated by a blue shaded background. The characteristic four-strand plus three-strand (C-region type domain) or four-strand plus five-strand (V-region type domain) arrangements are typical immunoglobulin superfamily domain building blocks, found in a whole range of other proteins as well as antibodies and T-cell receptors.

Many of the amino acids that are common to C and V domains of immunoglobulin chains lie in the core of the immunoglobulin fold and are essential for its stability. For that reason, other proteins having sequences similar to those of immunoglobulins are believed to form domains of similar structure, and in many cases this has been demonstrated by crystallography. These **immunoglobulin-like domains** are present in many other proteins of the immune system, and in proteins involved in cell–cell recognition in the nervous system and other tissues. Together with the immunoglobulins and the T-cell receptors, they make up the extensive **immunoglobulin superfamily**.

Summary.

The IgG antibody molecule is made up of four polypeptide chains, comprising two identical light chains and two identical heavy chains, and can be thought of as forming a flexible Y-shaped structure. Each of the four chains has a variable (V) region at its amino terminus, which contributes to the antigen-binding site, and a constant (C) region, which determines the isotype. The isotype of the heavy chain determines the functional properties of the antibody. The light chains are bound to the heavy chains by many noncovalent interactions and by disulfide bonds, and the V regions of the heavy and light chains pair in each arm of the Y to generate two identical antigen-binding sites, which lie at the tips of the arms of the Y. The possession of two antigen-binding sites allows antibody molecules to cross-link antigens and to bind them much more stably. The trunk of the Y, called the Fc fragment, is composed of the carboxy-terminal domains of the heavy chains. Joining the arms of the Y to the trunk are the flexible hinge regions. The Fc fragment and hinge regions differ in antibodies of different isotypes, thus determining their functional properties. However, the overall organization of the domains is similar in all isotypes.

The interaction of the antibody molecule with specific antigen.

We have described the structure of the antibody molecule and how the V regions of the heavy and light chains fold and pair to form the antigen-binding site. In this part of the chapter we look at the antigen-binding site in more detail. We discuss the different ways in which antigens can bind to antibody and address the question of how variation in the sequences of the antibody V domains determines the specificity for antigen.

3-6 Localized regions of hypervariable sequence form the antigen-binding site.

The V regions of any given antibody molecule differ from those of every other. Sequence variability is not, however, distributed evenly throughout the V region but is concentrated in certain segments. The distribution of variable amino acids can be seen clearly in what is termed a **variability plot** (Fig. 3.6), in which the amino acid sequences of many different antibody V regions are compared. Three particularly variable segments can be identified in both the V_H and V_L domains. They are designated **hypervariable regions** and are denoted HV1, HV2, and HV3. In the heavy chains these are

Fig. 3.6 There are discrete regions of hypervariability in V domains. A variability plot derived from comparison of the amino acid sequences of several dozen heavy-chain and light-chain V domains. At each amino acid position the degree of variability is the ratio of the number of different amino acids seen in all of the sequences together to the frequency of the most common amino acid. Three hypervariable regions (HV1, HV2, and HV3) are indicated in red and are also known as the complementarity-determining regions, CDR1, CDR2, and CDR3. They are flanked by less variable framework regions (FR1, FR2, FR3, and FR4, shown in blue or yellow).

roughly from residues 30 to 36, from 49 to 65, and from 95 to 103, respectively, while in the light chains they are roughly from residues 28 to 35, from 49 to 59, and from 92 to 103, respectively. The most variable part of the domain is in the HV3 region. The regions between the hypervariable regions, which comprise the rest of the V domain, show less variability and are termed the **framework regions**. There are four such regions in each V domain, designated FR1, FR2, FR3, and FR4.

The framework regions form the β sheets that provide the structural framework of the domain, whereas the hypervariable sequences correspond to three loops at the outer edge of the β barrel, which are juxtaposed in the folded domain (Fig. 3.7). Thus, not only is sequence diversity concentrated in particular parts of the V domain, but it is localized to a particular region on the surface of the molecule. When the V_H and V_L domains are paired in the antibody molecule, the hypervariable loops from each domain are brought together, creating a single hypervariable site at the tip of each arm of the molecule. This is the binding site for antigen, the **antigen-binding site** or **antibody combining site**. The six hypervariable loops determine antigen specificity by forming a surface complementary to the antigen, and are more commonly termed the **complementarity-determining regions**, or **CDRs** (there are three CDRs from each of the heavy and light chains, namely **CDR1**, **CDR2**, and **CDR3**). Because CDRs from both V_H and V_L domains contribute to the antigen-binding site, it is the combination of the heavy and the light chain, and not either alone, that determines the final antigen specificity. Thus, one way in which the immune system is able to generate antibodies of different specificities is by generating different combinations of heavy- and light-chain V regions. This means of producing variability is known as **combinatorial diversity**; we will encounter a

Fig. 3.7 The hypervariable regions lie in discrete loops of the folded structure. When the hypervariable regions (CDRs) are positioned on the structure of a V domain it can be seen that they lie in loops that are brought together in the folded structure. In the antibody molecule, the pairing of a heavy and a light chain brings together the hypervariable loops from each chain to create a single hypervariable surface, which forms the antigen-binding site at the tip of each arm.

second form of combinatorial diversity when we consider in Chapter 4 how the genes encoding the heavy- and light-chain V regions are created from smaller segments of DNA.

3-7   Antibodies bind antigens via contacts with amino acids in CDRs, but the details of binding depend upon the size and shape of the antigen.

In early investigations of antigen binding to antibodies, the only available sources of large quantities of a single type of antibody molecule were tumors of antibody-secreting cells. The antigen specificities of the tumor-derived antibodies were unknown, so that many compounds had to be screened to identify ligands that could be used to study antigen binding. In general, the substances found to bind to these antibodies were haptens (see Section 3-4) such as phosphorylcholine or vitamin K_1. Structural analysis of complexes of antibodies with their hapten ligands provided the first direct evidence that the hypervariable regions form the antigen-binding site, and demonstrated the structural basis of specificity for the hapten. Subsequently, with the discovery of methods of generating monoclonal antibodies (see Appendix I, Section A-12), it became possible to make large amounts of pure antibodies specific for many different antigens. This has provided a more general picture of how antibodies interact with their antigens, confirming and extending the view of antibody–antigen interactions derived from the study of haptens.

The surface of the antibody molecule formed by the juxtaposition of the CDRs of the heavy and light chains creates the site to which an antigen binds. Clearly, as the amino acid sequences of the CDRs are different in different antibodies, so are the shapes of the surfaces created by these CDRs. As a general principle, antibodies bind ligands whose surfaces are complementary to that of the antibody. A small antigen, such as a hapten or a short peptide, generally binds in a pocket or groove lying between the heavy- and light-chain V domains (Fig. 3.8a and b). Other antigens, such as a protein molecule, can be of the same size as, or larger than, the antibody molecule itself, and cannot fit into a groove or pocket. In these cases, the interface between the two molecules is often an extended surface that involves all of the CDRs and, in some cases, part of the framework region of the antibody (Fig. 3.8c). This surface need not be concave but can be flat, undulating, or even convex. In some cases, antibody molecules with elongated CDR3 loops can protrude a 'finger' into recesses in the surface of the antigen, as is shown in Fig. 3.8d, where an antibody binding to the HIV gp120 antigen projects a long loop against its target.

3-8   Antibodies bind to conformational shapes on the surfaces of antigens.

The biological function of antibodies is to bind to pathogens and their products, and to facilitate their removal from the body. An antibody generally recognizes only a small region on the surface of a large molecule such as a polysaccharide or protein. The structure recognized by an antibody is called an **antigenic determinant** or **epitope**. Some of the most important pathogens have polysaccharide coats, and antibodies that recognize epitopes formed by

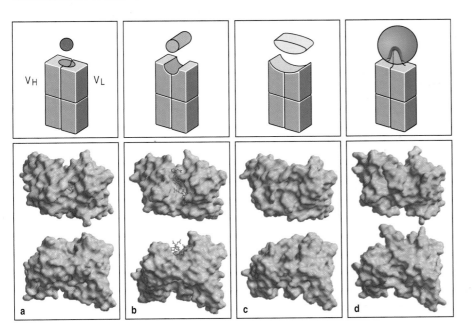

Fig. 3.8 Antigens can bind in pockets, or grooves, or on extended surfaces in the binding sites of antibodies. The panels in the top row show schematic representations of the different types of binding site in a Fab fragment of an antibody: first panel, pocket; second panel, groove; third panel, extended surface; and fourth panel, protruding surface. Below are examples of each type. Panel a: the top image shows the molecular surface of the interaction of a small hapten with the complementarity-determining regions (CDRs) of a Fab fragment as viewed looking into the antigen-binding site. The ferrocene hapten, shown in green, is bound into the antigen-binding pocket (yellow). In the bottom image (and in those of panels b, c, and d) the molecule has been rotated by about 90° to give a side-on view of the binding site. Panel b: in a complex of an antibody with a peptide from the human immunodeficiency virus (HIV), the peptide (green) binds along a groove (yellow) formed between the heavy- and light-chain V domains. Panel c: complex between hen egg-white lysozyme and the Fab fragment of its corresponding antibody (HyHel5). The surface on the antibody that comes into contact with the lysozyme is colored yellow. All six CDRs of the antigen-binding site are involved in the binding. Panel d: an antibody molecule against the HIV gp120 antigen has elongated CDR3 loops that protrude into a recess in the surface of the antigen. The structure of the complex between this antibody and gp120 has not been solved, and so the yellow area on the images in the lower panels represents the extent of the CDR regions rather than the actual region of contact between antibody and antigen. Photographs courtesy of I.A. Wilson and R.L. Stanfield.

the sugar subunits of these molecules are essential in providing immune protection from such pathogens. In many cases, however, the antigens that provoke an immune response are proteins. For example, protective antibodies against viruses recognize viral coat proteins. In such cases, the structures recognized by the antibody are located on the surface of the protein. Such sites are likely to be composed of amino acids from different parts of the polypeptide chain that have been brought together by protein folding. Antigenic determinants of this kind are known as **conformational** or **discontinuous epitopes** because the structure recognized is composed of segments of the protein that are discontinuous in the amino acid sequence of the antigen but are brought together in the three-dimensional structure. In contrast, an epitope composed of a single segment of polypeptide chain is termed a **continuous** or **linear epitope**. Although most antibodies raised against intact, fully folded proteins recognize discontinuous epitopes, some will bind peptide fragments of the protein. Conversely, antibodies raised against peptides of a protein or against synthetic peptides corresponding to part of its sequence are occasionally found to bind to the natural folded protein. This makes it possible, in some cases, to use synthetic peptides in vaccines that aim at raising antibodies against a pathogen protein.

3-9 Antigen–antibody interactions involve a variety of forces.

The interaction between an antibody and its antigen can be disrupted by high salt concentrations, by extremes of pH, by detergents, and sometimes by competition with high concentrations of the pure epitope itself. The binding is therefore a reversible noncovalent interaction. The forces, or bonds, involved in these noncovalent interactions are outlined in Fig. 3.9.

Electrostatic interactions occur between charged amino acid side chains, as in salt bridges. Interactions also occur between electric dipoles, as in hydrogen bonds, or can involve short-range van der Waals forces. High salt concentrations and extremes of pH disrupt antigen–antibody binding by weakening electrostatic interactions and/or hydrogen bonds. This principle

Fig. 3.9 The noncovalent forces that hold together the antigen:antibody complex. Partial charges found in electric dipoles are shown as δ⁺ or δ⁻. Electrostatic forces diminish as the inverse square of the distance separating the charges, whereas van der Waals forces, which are more numerous in most antigen–antibody contacts, fall off as the sixth power of the separation and therefore operate only over very short ranges. Covalent bonds never occur between antigens and naturally produced antibodies.

Noncovalent forces	Origin	
Electrostatic forces	Attraction between opposite charges	$-NH_3^{\oplus}$ $\overset{\ominus}{OOC}-$
Hydrogen bonds	Hydrogen shared between electronegative atoms (N,O)	$\underset{\delta^-}{N}-\underset{\delta^+}{H}--\underset{\delta^-}{O}=C$
Van der Waals forces	Fluctuations in electron clouds around molecules oppositely polarize neighboring atoms	$\delta^+ \rightleftharpoons \delta^-$ $\delta^- \rightleftharpoons \delta^+$
Hydrophobic forces	Hydrophobic groups interact unfavorably with water and tend to pack together to exclude water molecules. The attraction also involves van der Waals forces	

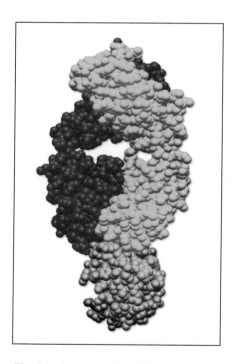

Fig. 3.10 The complex of lysozyme with the antibody D1.3. The interaction of the Fab fragment of D1.3 with hen egg-white lysozyme is shown, with the lysozyme in blue, the heavy chain in purple and the light chain in yellow. A glutamine residue of lysozyme, shown in red, protrudes between the two V domains of the antigen-binding site and makes hydrogen bonds that are important to the antigen–antibody binding. Courtesy of R.J. Poljak.

is employed in the purification of antigens with the use of affinity columns of immobilized antibodies, and vice versa for antibody purification (see Appendix I, Section A-5). Hydrophobic interactions occur when two hydrophobic surfaces come together to exclude water. The strength of a hydrophobic interaction is proportional to the surface area that is hidden from water. For some antigens, hydrophobic interactions probably account for most of the binding energy. In some cases, water molecules are trapped in pockets in the interface between antigen and antibody. These trapped water molecules, especially those between polar amino acid residues, may also contribute to binding and hence to the specificity of the antibody.

The contribution of each of these forces to the overall interaction depends on the particular antibody and antigen involved. A striking difference between antibody interactions with protein antigens and most other natural protein–protein interactions is that antibodies often possess many aromatic amino acids in their antigen-binding sites. These amino acids participate mainly in van der Waals and hydrophobic interactions, and sometimes in hydrogen bonds. In general, the hydrophobic and van der Waals forces operate over very short ranges and serve to pull together two surfaces that are complementary in shape: hills on one surface must fit into valleys on the other for good binding to occur. In contrast, electrostatic interactions between charged side chains, and hydrogen bonds bridging oxygen and/or nitrogen atoms, accommodate specific features or reactive groups while strengthening the interaction overall.

For example, in the complex of hen egg-white lysozyme with the antibody D1.3 (Fig. 3.10), strong hydrogen bonds are formed between the antibody and a particular glutamine in the lysozyme molecule that protrudes between the V_H and V_L domains. Lysozymes from partridge and turkey have another amino acid in place of the glutamine and do not bind to the antibody. In the high-affinity complex of hen egg-white lysozyme with another antibody, HyHel5 (see Fig. 3.8c), two salt bridges between two basic arginines on the surface of the lysozyme interact with two glutamic acids, one each from the V_H CDR1 and CDR2 loops. Again, lysozymes that lack one of the two arginine residues show a 1000-fold decrease in affinity. Although overall surface complementarity must have an important role in antigen–antibody interactions, in most antibodies that have been studied at this level of detail only a few residues make a major contribution to the binding energy and hence to the final specificity of the antibody. Although many antibodies naturally bind their ligands with high affinity, genetic engineering by site-directed mutagenesis can further tailor an antibody's binding to its complementary epitope.

Summary.

X-ray crystallographic analysis of antigen:antibody complexes has demonstrated that the hypervariable loops (complementarity-determining regions) of immunoglobulin V regions determine the specificity of antibodies. With protein antigens, the antibody molecule contacts the antigen over a broad area of its surface that is complementary to the surface recognized on the antigen. Electrostatic interactions, hydrogen bonds, van der Waals forces, and hydrophobic interactions can all contribute to binding. Depending on the size of the antigen, amino acid side chains in most or all of the hypervariable loops make contact with antigen and determine both the specificity and the affinity of the interaction. Other parts of the V region play little part in the direct contact with the antigen but provide a stable structural framework for the hypervariable loops and help to determine their position and conformation. Antibodies raised against intact proteins usually bind to the surface of the protein and make contact with residues that are discontinuous in the primary structure of the molecule; they may, however, occasionally bind peptide fragments of the protein, and antibodies raised against peptides derived from a protein can sometimes be used to detect the native protein molecule. Peptides binding to antibodies usually bind in the cleft between the V regions of the heavy and light chains, where they make specific contact with some, but not necessarily all, of the hypervariable loops. This is also the usual mode of binding for carbohydrate antigens and small molecules such as haptens.

Antigen recognition by T cells.

In contrast to the immunoglobulins, which interact with pathogens and their toxic products in the extracellular spaces of the body, T cells only recognize foreign antigens that are displayed on the surfaces of the body's own cells. These antigens can derive from pathogens such as viruses or intracellular bacteria, which replicate within cells, or from pathogens or their products that cells have internalized by endocytosis from the extracellular fluid.

T cells can detect the presence of an intracellular pathogen because infected cells display, on their surface, peptide fragments derived from the pathogen's proteins. These foreign peptides are delivered to the cell surface by specialized host-cell glycoproteins. These are encoded in a large cluster of genes that were first identified by their powerful effects on the immune response to transplanted tissues. For that reason, the gene complex was called the **major histocompatibility complex** (**MHC**), and the peptide-binding glycoproteins are still known as MHC molecules. The recognition of antigen as a small peptide fragment bound to an MHC molecule and displayed at the cell surface is one of the most distinctive features of T cells, and will be the focus of this part of the chapter. How peptide fragments of antigen become complexed with MHC molecules will be considered in Chapter 5.

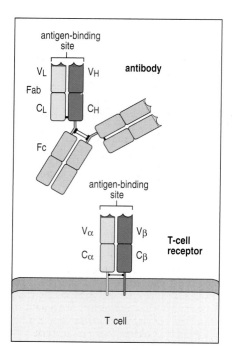

Fig. 3.11 The T-cell receptor resembles a membrane-bound Fab fragment. The Fab fragment of an antibody molecule is a disulfide-linked heterodimer, each chain of which contains one immunoglobulin C domain and one V domain; the juxtaposition of the V domains forms the antigen-binding site (see Section 3-6). The T-cell receptor is also a disulfide-linked heterodimer, with each chain containing an immunoglobulin C-like domain and an immunoglobulin V-like domain. As in the Fab fragment, the juxtaposition of the V domains forms the site for antigen recognition.

In this part of the chapter we describe the structure and properties of the T-cell antigen receptor, the T-cell receptor (or TCR for short). As might be expected from their function as highly variable antigen-recognition structures, T-cell receptors are closely related to antibody molecules in the structure of their genes. There are, however, important differences between T-cell receptors and immunoglobulins that reflect the special features of antigen recognition by the T-cell receptor, and its lack of effector functions.

3-10 The antigen receptor on T cells is very similar to a Fab fragment of immunoglobulin.

T-cell receptors were first identified by using monoclonal antibodies that bound only one cloned T-cell line but not others and that could specifically inhibit antigen recognition by that clone of T cells, or specifically activate them (see Appendix I, Section A-19). These **clonotypic** antibodies were then used to show that each T cell bears about 30,000 identical antigen-receptor molecules on its surface, each receptor consisting of two different polypeptide chains, termed the **T-cell receptor α (TCRα) and β (TCRβ) chains**, linked by a disulfide bond. These α:β heterodimers are very similar in structure to the Fab fragment of an immunoglobulin molecule (Fig. 3.11), and they account for antigen recognition by most T cells. A minority of T cells bear an alternative, but structurally similar, receptor made up of a different pair of polypeptide chains designated γ and δ. The **γ:δ T-cell receptors** seem to have different antigen-recognition properties from the **α:β T-cell receptors**, and the function of γ:δ T cells in immune responses is not yet entirely clear. In the rest of this chapter we shall use the term T-cell receptor to mean the α:β receptor, except where specified otherwise. Both types of T-cell receptor differ from the membrane-bound immunoglobulin that serves as the B-cell receptor: a T-cell receptor has only one antigen-binding site, whereas a B-cell receptor has two; and T-cell receptors are never secreted, whereas immunoglobulin can be secreted as antibody.

Our initial insights into the structure and function of the α:β T-cell receptor came from studies of cloned cDNA encoding the receptor chains. The amino acid sequences predicted from T-cell receptor cDNAs show clearly that both chains of the T-cell receptor have an amino-terminal variable (V) region with homology to an immunoglobulin V domain, a constant (C) region with homology to an immunoglobulin C domain, and a short hinge region containing a cysteine residue that forms the interchain disulfide bond (Fig. 3.12). Each chain spans the lipid bilayer by a hydrophobic transmembrane domain, and ends in a short cytoplasmic tail. These close similarities of T-cell receptor chains to the heavy and light immunoglobulin chains first enabled prediction of the structural resemblance of the T-cell receptor heterodimer to a Fab fragment of immunoglobulin.

The three-dimensional structure of the T-cell receptor has been determined by X-ray crystallography; the structure is indeed similar to that of a Fab fragment,

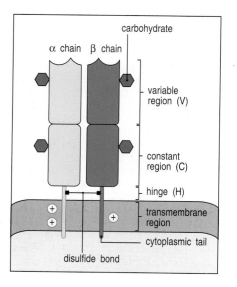

Fig. 3.12 Structure of the T-cell receptor. The T-cell receptor heterodimer is composed of two transmembrane glycoprotein chains, α and β. The extracellular portion of each chain consists of two domains, resembling immunoglobulin V and C domains, respectively. Both chains have carbohydrate side chains attached to each domain. A short segment, analogous to an immunoglobulin hinge region, connects the immunoglobulin-like domains to the membrane and contains the cysteine residue that forms the interchain disulfide bond. The transmembrane helices of both chains are unusual in containing positively charged (basic) residues within the hydrophobic transmembrane segment. The α chain carries two such residues; the β chain has one.

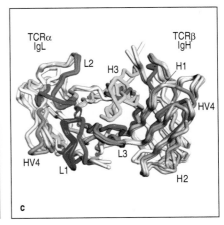

Fig. 3.13 The crystal structure of an α:β T-cell receptor resolved at 2.5 Å. In panels a and b the α chain is shown in pink and the β chain in blue. Disulfide bonds are shown in green. In panel a, the T-cell receptor is viewed from the side as it would sit on a cell surface, with the CDR loops that form the antigen-binding site (labeled 1, 2, and 3) arrayed across its relatively flat top. In panel b, the $C_α$ and $C_β$ domains are shown. The $C_α$ domain does not fold into a typical immunoglobulin-like domain; the face of the domain away from the $C_β$ domain is mainly composed of irregular strands of polypeptide rather than β sheet. The intramolecular disulfide bond joins a β strand to this segment of α helix. The interaction between the $C_α$ and $C_β$ domains is assisted by carbohydrate (colored gray and labeled on the figure), with a sugar group from the $C_α$ domain making hydrogen bonds to the $C_β$ domain. In panel c, the T-cell receptor is shown aligned with the antigen-binding sites from three different antibodies. This view is looking down into the binding site. The $V_α$ domain of the T-cell receptor is aligned with the V_L domains of the antigen-binding sites of the antibodies, and the $V_β$ domain is aligned with the V_H domains. The CDRs of the T-cell receptor and immunoglobulin molecules are colored, with CDRs 1, 2, and 3 of the TCR shown in red and the HV4 loop in orange. For the immunoglobulin V domains, the CDR1 loops of the heavy chain (H1) and light chain (L1) are shown in light and dark blue, respectively, and the CDR2 loops (H2, L2) in light and dark purple, respectively. The heavy-chain CDR3 loops (H3) are in yellow; the light-chain CDR3s (L3) are in bright green. The HV4 loops of the TCR (orange) have no hypervariable counterparts in immunoglobulins. Model structures courtesy of I.A. Wilson.

as was suspected from earlier studies of the genes that encoded it. The T-cell receptor chains fold in much the same way as those of a Fab fragment (Fig. 3.13a), although the final structure appears a little shorter and wider. There are, however, some distinct differences between T-cell receptors and Fab fragments. The most striking difference is in the $C_α$ domain, where the fold is unlike that of any other immunoglobulin-like domain. The half of the domain that is juxtaposed with the $C_β$ domain forms a β sheet similar to that found in other immunoglobulin-like domains, but the other half of the domain is formed of loosely packed strands and a short segment of α helix (Fig. 3.13b). The intramolecular disulfide bond, which in immunoglobulin-like domains normally joins two β strands, in a $C_α$ domain joins a β strand to this segment of α helix.

There are also differences in the way in which the domains interact. The interface between the V and C domains of both T-cell receptor chains is more extensive than in antibodies, which may make the hinge joint between the domains less flexible. The interaction between the $C_α$ and $C_β$ domains is distinctive as it might be assisted by carbohydrate, with a sugar group from the $C_α$ domain making a number of hydrogen bonds to the $C_β$ domain (see Fig. 3.13b). Finally, a comparison of the variable binding sites shows that, although the CDR loops align fairly closely with those of antibody molecules, there is some relative displacement (Fig. 3.13c). This is particularly marked in the $V_α$ CDR2 loop, which is oriented at roughly right angles to the equivalent loop in antibody V domains, as a result of a shift in the β strand that anchors one end of the loop from one face of the domain to the other. A strand displacement also causes a change in the orientation of the $V_β$ CDR2 loop in two of the seven $V_β$ domains whose structures are known. As yet, the crystallographic structures of only seven T-cell receptors have been solved to this level of resolution, so it remains to be seen to what degree all T-cell receptors share these features, and whether there is more variability to be discovered.

3-11   A T-cell receptor recognizes antigen in the form of a complex of a foreign peptide bound to an MHC molecule.

Antigen recognition by T-cell receptors clearly differs from recognition by B-cell receptors and antibodies. Antigen recognition by B cells involves direct binding of immunoglobulin to the intact antigen and, as discussed in Section 3-8, antibodies typically bind to the surface of protein antigens, contacting amino acids that are discontinuous in the primary structure but are brought together in the folded protein. T cells, in contrast, were found to respond to short contiguous amino acid sequences in proteins. These sequences were often buried within the native structure of the protein and thus could not be

Fig. 3.14 Differences in the recognition of hen egg-white lysozyme by immunoglobulins and T-cell receptors. Antibodies can be shown by X-ray crystallography to bind epitopes on the surface of proteins, as shown in panel a, where the epitopes for three antibodies are shown on the surface of hen egg-white lysozyme (see also Fig. 3.10). In contrast, the epitopes recognized by T-cell receptors need not lie on the surface of the molecule, because the T-cell receptor recognizes not the antigenic protein itself but a peptide fragment of the protein. The peptides corresponding to two T-cell epitopes of lysozyme are shown in panel b. One epitope, shown in blue, lies on the surface of the protein but a second, shown in red, lies mostly within the core and is inaccessible in the folded protein. For this residue to be accessible to the T-cell receptor, the protein must be unfolded and processed. Panel a courtesy of S. Sheriff.

recognized directly by T-cell receptors unless some unfolding of the protein antigen and its 'processing' into peptide fragments had occurred (Fig. 3.14).

The nature of the antigen recognized by T cells became clear with the realization that the peptides that stimulate T cells are recognized only when bound to an MHC molecule. These cell-surface glycoproteins are encoded by genes within the major histocompatibility complex (MHC). The ligand recognized by the T cell is thus a complex of peptide and MHC molecule. The evidence for involvement of the MHC in T-cell recognition of antigen was at first indirect, but it has recently been proved conclusively by stimulating T cells with purified peptide:MHC complexes. The T-cell receptor interacts with this ligand by making contacts with both the MHC molecule and the antigen peptide.

3-12   T cells with different functions are distinguished by CD4 and CD8 cell-surface proteins and recognize peptides bound to different classes of MHC molecule.

T cells fall into two major classes that have different effector functions. The two classes are distinguished by the expression of the cell-surface proteins **CD4** and **CD8**. These two types of T cell differ in the class of MHC molecule

Fig. 3.15 The structures of the CD4 and CD8 co-receptor molecules. The CD4 molecule contains four immunoglobulin-like domains, as shown in diagrammatic form in panel a, and as a ribbon diagram of the crystal structure in panel b. The amino-terminal domain, D_1, is similar in structure to an immunoglobulin V domain. The second domain, D_2, although clearly related to an immunoglobulin domain, is different from both V and C domains and has been termed a C2 domain. The first two domains of CD4 form a rigid rodlike structure that is linked to the two carboxy-terminal domains by a flexible link. The binding site for MHC class II molecules is thought to involve both the D_1 and D_2 domains. The CD8 molecule is a heterodimer of an α and a β chain covalently linked by a disulfide bond; an alternative form of CD8 exists as a homodimer of α chains. The heterodimer is depicted in panel a, whereas the ribbon diagram in panel b is of the homodimer. CD8α and CD8β chains have very similar structures, each having a single domain resembling an immunoglobulin V domain and a stretch of polypeptide chain, believed to be in a relatively extended conformation, that anchors the V-like domain to the cell membrane.

Fig. 3.16 The binding sites for CD4 and CD8 on MHC class II and class I molecules lie in the immunoglobulin-like domains. The binding sites for CD4 and CD8 on the MHC class II and class I molecules, respectively, lie in the immunoglobulin-like domains nearest to the membrane and distant from the peptide-binding cleft. In panel a, the binding of CD4 to an MHC class II molecule is shown. The α chain of the MHC class II molecule is shown in pink, and the β chain in white, while CD4 is shown in gold. Only the first two domains of the CD4 molecule are shown. The binding site for CD4 lies at the base of the β_2 domain of an MHC class II molecule and does not seem to involve interactions with the base of the α_1 and β_1 domains. In panel b, the binding of CD8 to an MHC class I molecule is shown. The class I heavy chain and β_2-microglobulin are shown in white and pink, respectively, and the two chains of the CD8 dimer are shown in light and dark purple. The structure is actually of the binding of the CD8α homodimer, but the CD8α:β heterodimer is believed to bind in the same way. The orientation of the MHC class I molecule in this figure matches that of the MHC class II molecule in panel a, and you can see that the binding site for CD8 on the MHC class I molecule lies in a similar position to that of CD4 in the MHC class II molecule. However, although the binding site for CD8 lies at the base of the α_3 domain of the MHC class I molecule it also involves the base of the α_1 and α_2 domains, and thus the binding of CD8 to MHC class I is not completely equivalent to the binding of CD4 to MHC class II.

that they recognize. There are two classes of MHC molecule—**MHC class I** and **MHC class II**—which differ in their structure and expression pattern on tissues of the body (see Section 3-13). CD4 and CD8 were known as markers for different functional sets of T cells for some time before it became clear that they have an important role in the direct recognition of MHC class II and MHC class I molecules, respectively. CD4 binds to the MHC class II molecule and CD8 to the MHC class I molecule. During antigen recognition, depending on the type of T cell, CD4 or CD8 molecules associate on the T-cell surface with the T-cell receptor and bind to invariant sites on the MHC portion of the composite MHC:peptide ligand. This binding is required for the T cell to make an effective response, and so CD4 and CD8 are called **co-receptors**.

CD4 is a single-chain molecule composed of four immunoglobulin-like domains (Fig. 3.15). The first two domains (D_1 and D_2) of the CD4 molecule are packed tightly together to form a rigid rod about 60 Å long, which is joined by a flexible hinge to a similar rod formed by the third and fourth domains (D_3 and D_4). CD4 binds MHC class II molecules through a region that is located mainly on a lateral face of the first domain, D_1. Because CD4 binds to a site on the β_2 domain of the MHC class II molecule that is well away from the site where the T-cell receptor binds (Fig. 3.16a), the CD4 molecule and the T-cell receptor can bind the same peptide:MHC class II complex. CD4 interacts strongly with a cytoplasmic tyrosine kinase called **Lck**, and can deliver this tyrosine kinase into close proximity to the signaling components of the T-cell receptor complex. This results in enhancement of the signal that is generated when the T-cell receptor binds its peptide:MHC class II ligand, as we will discuss further in Chapter 6. When CD4 and the T-cell receptor can simultaneously bind to the same MHC class II:peptide complex, the sensitivity of a T cell to antigen presented by MHC class II molecules is markedly increased; the T cell in this case requires 100-fold less antigen for activation.

CD4 binding to an MHC class II molecule on its own is weak, and it is not clear whether such binding would be able to transmit a signal to the interior of the T cell. As shown in Fig. 3.17, CD4 can form homodimers through a site in the D_4 domain, which leaves the MHC-binding site free to interact with an MHC class II molecule. Thus, the CD4 dimer could cross-link two MHC class II molecules and therefore the two T-cell receptors bound to them. Whether the dimerization of CD4 is important in its co-receptor function is not known at present.

Fig. 3.17 CD4 can form dimers. The structure of the extracellular domains of the CD4 molecule has been determined by X-ray crystallography. Two molecules of CD4 (blue and green) can interact with each other through their D_4 domains, forming homodimers. The site that binds MHC class II molecules remains available in such dimers.

Fig. 3.18 CD8 binds to a site on MHC class I molecules distant from that to which the T-cell receptor binds. The relative positions of the T-cell receptor and CD8 molecules bound to the same MHC class I molecule can be seen in this hypothetical reconstruction of the interaction of an MHC class I molecule (the α chain is shown in green; β$_2$-microglobulin (dull yellow) can be seen faintly in the background) with a T-cell receptor and CD8. The α and β chains of the T-cell receptor are shown in pink and purple, respectively. The CD8 structure is that of a CD8α homodimer, but is colored to represent the likely orientation of the subunits in the heterodimer, with the CD8α subunit in red and the CD8β subunit in blue. Courtesy of G. Gao.

Although CD4 and CD8 both function as co-receptors, their structures are quite distinct. The CD8 molecule is a disulfide-linked heterodimer consisting of an α and a β chain, each containing a single immunoglobulin-like domain linked to the membrane by a segment of extended polypeptide chain (see Fig. 3.15). This segment is extensively glycosylated, which is thought to be important in maintaining this polypeptide in an extended conformation and protecting it from cleavage by proteases. CD8α chains can also form homodimers, although these are not found when the CD8β chains are present. The CD8α homodimer may have a specific function in recognizing a specialized subset of non-classical MHC class I molecules that we will describe in Chapter 5.

CD8 binds weakly to an invariant site in the α$_3$ domain of an MHC class I molecule (see Fig. 3.16b), which is equivalent to the site in MHC class II molecules to which CD4 binds. Although so far only the interaction of the CD8α homodimer with MHC class I is known in detail, it is clear from this that the MHC class I binding site of the CD8 α:β heterodimer is formed by the interaction of the CD8α and β chains. In addition, CD8 (most probably through the α chain) interacts with residues in the base of the α$_2$ domain of the MHC class I molecule. The strength of binding of CD8 to the MHC class I molecule can be influenced by the glycosylation of the CD8 molecule; increased numbers of sialic acid residues added to the CD8 carbohydrate structures decrease the strength of the interaction. The pattern of sialylation of CD8 changes during the maturation of T cells and also on activation, and although this might have a role in modulating recognition by CD8 T cells, the significance of these changes is not yet known.

By binding to the membrane-proximal domains of the MHC class I and class II molecules, the co-receptors leave the upper surface of the MHC molecule exposed and free to interact simultaneously with a T-cell receptor, as shown for CD8 in Fig. 3.18. Both CD4 and CD8 bind Lck—in the case of the CD8α:β heterodimer through the cytoplasmic tail of the α chain—and bring it into close proximity to the T-cell receptor. And as with CD4, the presence of CD8 increases the sensitivity of T cells to antigen presented by MHC class I molecules about 100-fold. Thus, CD4 and CD8 have similar functions and bind to the same approximate location in MHC class I and MHC class II molecules even though the structures of the two co-receptor proteins are only distantly related.

3-13 The two classes of MHC molecule are expressed differentially on cells.

MHC class I and MHC class II molecules have distinct distributions among cells that reflect the different effector functions of the T cells that recognize them (Fig. 3.19). MHC class I molecules present peptides from pathogens, commonly viruses, to CD8 cytotoxic T cells, which are specialized to kill any cell that they specifically recognize. Because viruses can infect any nucleated cell, almost all such cells express MHC class I molecules, although the level of constitutive expression varies from one cell type to the next. For example, cells of the immune system express abundant MHC class I on their surface, whereas liver cells (hepatocytes) express relatively low levels (see Fig. 3.19). Non-nucleated cells, such as mammalian red blood cells, express little or no MHC class I, and thus the interior of red blood cells is a site in which an infection can go undetected by cytotoxic T cells. Because red blood cells cannot support viral replication, this is of no great consequence for viral infection, but it might be the absence of MHC class I that allows the *Plasmodium* species that cause malaria to live in this privileged site.

In contrast, the main function of the CD4 T cells that recognize MHC class II molecules is to activate other effector cells of the immune system. Thus MHC class II molecules are normally found on B lymphocytes, dendritic cells, and macrophages—cells that participate in immune responses—but not on

Tissue	MHC class I	MHC class II
Lymphoid tissues		
T cells	+++	+*
B cells	+++	+++
Macrophages	+++	++
Other antigen-presenting cells (eg Langerhans' cells)	+++	+++
Epithelial cells of the thymus	+	+++
Other nucleated cells		
Neutrophils	+++	–
Hepatocytes	+	–
Kidney	+	–
Brain	+	–†
Non-nucleated cells		
Red blood cells	–	–

Fig. 3.19 The expression of MHC molecules differs between tissues. MHC class I molecules are expressed on all nucleated cells, although they are most highly expressed in hematopoietic cells. MHC class II molecules are normally expressed only by a subset of hematopoietic cells and by thymic stromal cells, although they may be expressed by other cell types on exposure to the inflammatory cytokine interferon-γ. *In humans, activated T cells express MHC class II molecules, whereas in mice all T cells are MHC class II-negative. †In the brain, most cell types are MHC class II-negative, but microglia, which are related to macrophages, are MHC class II-positive.

other tissue cells (see Fig. 3.19). When CD4 T cells recognize peptides bound to MHC class II molecules on B cells, they stimulate the B cells to produce antibody. Similarly, CD4 T cells recognizing peptides bound to MHC class II molecules on macrophages activate these cells to destroy the pathogens in their vesicles. We shall see in Chapter 8 that MHC class II molecules are also expressed on specialized antigen-presenting cells in lymphoid tissues where naive T cells encounter antigen and are first activated. The expression of both MHC class I and MHC class II molecules is regulated by cytokines, in particular interferons, released in the course of immune responses. Interferon-γ (IFN-γ), for example, increases the expression of MHC class I and MHC class II molecules, and can induce the expression of MHC class II molecules on certain cell types that do not normally express them. Interferons also enhance the antigen-presenting function of MHC class I molecules by inducing the expression of key components of the intracellular machinery that enables peptides to be loaded onto the MHC molecules.

3-14 The two classes of MHC molecule have distinct subunit structures but similar three-dimensional structures.

The two classes of MHC molecule differ from each other in their structure and also have different distributions on the cells of the body. Their different structures enable the two classes of MHC molecules to serve distinct functions in antigen presentation, binding peptides from different intracellular

Fig. 3.20 The structure of an MHC class I molecule determined by X-ray crystallography. Panel a shows a computer graphic representation of a human MHC class I molecule, HLA-A2, which has been cleaved from the cell surface by the enzyme papain. The surface of the molecule is shown, colored according to the domains shown in panels b–d and described below. Panels b and c show a ribbon diagram of that structure. Shown schematically in panel d, the MHC class I molecule is a heterodimer of a membrane-spanning α chain (molecular weight 43 kDa) bound noncovalently to β2-microglobulin (12 kDa), which does not span the membrane. The α chain folds into three domains: α1, α2, and α3. The α3 domain and β2-microglobulin show similarities in amino acid sequence to immunoglobulin C domains and have similar folded structures, whereas the α1 and α2 domains fold together into a single structure consisting of two segmented α helices lying on a sheet of eight antiparallel β strands. The folding of the α1 and α2 domains creates a long cleft or groove, which is the site at which peptide antigens bind to the MHC molecules. The transmembrane region and the short stretch of peptide that connects the external domains to the cell surface are not seen in panels a and b because they have been removed by the digestion with papain. As can be seen in panel c, looking down on the molecule from above, the sides of the cleft are formed from the inner faces of the two α helices; the β-pleated sheet formed by the pairing of the α1 and α2 domains creates the floor of the cleft. We shall use the schematic representation in panel d throughout this text.

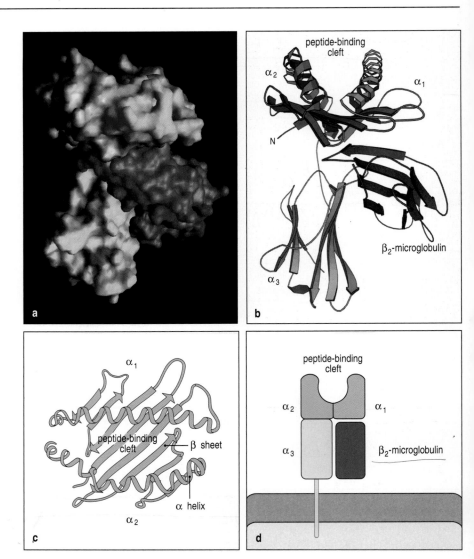

sites and activating different subsets of T cells, as we will see in Chapter 5. Despite their differences in subunit structure, however, MHC class I and MHC class II molecules are closely related in overall structure. In both classes, the two paired protein domains nearest to the membrane resemble immunoglobulin domains, whereas the two domains furthest away from the membrane fold together to create a long cleft, or groove, which is the site at which a peptide binds. Purified peptide:MHC class I and peptide:MHC class II complexes have been characterized structurally, allowing us to describe in detail both the MHC molecules themselves and the way in which they bind peptides.

MHC class I structure is outlined in Fig. 3.20. MHC class I molecules consist of two polypeptide chains, a larger α chain encoded in the MHC genetic locus, and a smaller noncovalently associated chain, **β2-microglobulin**, which is not polymorphic and is not encoded in the MHC locus, instead being encoded on a separate chromosome, chromosome 15 in humans. Only the class I α chain spans the membrane. The complete molecule has four domains, three formed from the MHC-encoded α chain, and one contributed by β2-microglobulin. The α3 domain and β2-microglobulin have a folded structure that closely resembles that of an immunoglobulin domain. The most remarkable feature of MHC class I molecules is the structure of the

Fig. 3.21 MHC class II molecules resemble MHC class I molecules in overall structure. The MHC class II molecule is composed of two transmembrane glycoprotein chains, α (34 kDa) and β (29 kDa), as shown schematically in panel d. Each chain has two domains, and the two chains together form a compact four-domain structure similar to that of the MHC class I molecule (compare with panel d of Fig. 3.20). Panel a shows a computer graphic representation of the surface of the MHC class II molecule, in this case the human protein HLA-DR1, and panel b shows the equivalent ribbon diagram. The α_2 and β_2 domains, like the α_3 and β_2-microglobulin domains of the MHC class I molecule, have amino acid sequence and structural similarities to immunoglobulin C domains; in the MHC class II molecule the two domains forming the peptide-binding cleft are contributed by different chains and are therefore not joined by a covalent bond (see panels c and d). Another important difference, not apparent in this diagram, is that the peptide-binding groove of the MHC class II molecule is open at both ends.

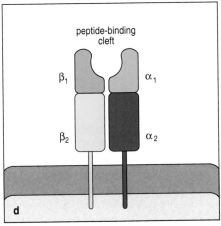

folded α_1 and α_2 domains. These two domains form the walls of a cleft on the surface of the molecule; this is the site of peptide binding. They are also sites of polymorphisms that determine T-cell antigen recognition (see Chapter 5).

An MHC class II molecule consists of a noncovalent complex of two chains, α and β, both of which span the membrane (Fig. 3.21). The MHC class II α and β chains are both encoded within the MHC. The crystallographic structure of the MHC class II molecule shows that it is folded very much like the MHC class I molecule. The major differences lie at the ends of the peptide-binding cleft, which are more open in MHC class II molecules than in MHC class I molecules. The main consequence of this is that the ends of a peptide bound to an MHC class I molecule are substantially buried within the molecule, whereas the ends of peptides bound to MHC class II molecules are not. Again, the sites of major polymorphism are located in the peptide-binding cleft (see Chapter 5); in an MHC class II molecule these are formed by the α_1 and β_1 domains.

In both MHC class I and class II molecules, bound peptides are sandwiched between the two α-helical segments of the MHC molecule (Fig. 3.22). The T-cell receptor interacts with this compound ligand, making contacts both with the MHC molecule and with the peptide antigen fragment.

Fig. 3.22 MHC molecules bind peptides tightly within the cleft. When MHC molecules are crystallized with a single synthetic peptide antigen, the details of peptide binding are revealed. In MHC class I molecules (panels a and c) the peptide is bound in an elongated conformation with both ends tightly bound at either end of the cleft. In MHC class II molecules (panels b and d) the peptide is also bound in an elongated conformation but the ends of the peptide are not tightly bound and the peptide extends beyond the cleft. The upper surface of the peptide:MHC complex is recognized by T cells, and is composed of residues of the MHC molecule and the peptide. In representations c and d, the electrostatic potential of the MHC molecule surface is shown, with blue areas indicating a positive potential and red a negative potential.

3-15   Peptides are stably bound to MHC molecules, and also serve to stabilize the MHC molecule on the cell surface.

An individual can be infected by a wide variety of different pathogens, the proteins of which will not generally have peptide sequences in common. If T cells are to be alerted to all possible infections, the MHC molecules on each cell (both class I and class II) must be able to bind stably to many different peptides. This behavior is quite distinct from that of other peptide-binding receptors, such as those for peptide hormones, which usually bind only a single type of peptide. The crystal structures of peptide:MHC complexes have helped to show how a single binding site can bind peptides with high affinity while retaining the ability to bind a wide variety of different peptides.

An important feature of the binding of peptides to MHC molecules is that the peptide is bound as an integral part of the MHC molecule's structure, and MHC molecules are unstable when peptides are not bound. The stability of peptide binding is important because, otherwise, peptide exchanges occurring at the cell surface would prevent peptide:MHC complexes from being reliable indicators of infection or of uptake of a specific antigen. As a result of this stability, when MHC molecules are purified from cells, their bound peptides co-purify with them, and this has enabled the peptides bound by specific MHC molecules to be analyzed. The peptides are released from the MHC molecules by denaturing the complex in acid; they can then be purified and sequenced. Pure synthetic peptides can also be incorporated into previously empty MHC molecules and the structure of the complex determined, revealing details of the contacts between the MHC molecule and the peptide. From the sequences of peptides bound to specific MHC molecules, combined with structural analysis of the peptide:MHC complex, a detailed picture of the binding interactions has been built up. We first discuss the peptide-binding properties of MHC class I molecules.

3-16   MHC class I molecules bind short peptides of 8–10 amino acids by both ends.

The binding of a peptide in the peptide-binding cleft of an MHC class I molecule is stabilized at both ends by contacts between atoms in the free amino and carboxy termini of the peptide and invariant sites that are found at each end of the cleft of all MHC class I molecules (Fig. 3.23). These contacts are thought to be the main stabilizing contacts for peptide:MHC class I complexes because synthetic peptide analogs lacking terminal amino and carboxyl groups fail to bind stably to MHC class I molecules. Other residues in the peptide serve as additional anchors. Peptides that bind to MHC class I molecules are usually 8–10 amino acids long. Peptides longer than this are thought to be able to bind to MHC class I molecules, particularly if they can bind at their carboxy-terminal end, but are subsequently cleaved by exopeptidases present in the endoplasmic reticulum. The peptide lies in an elongated conformation along the groove; variations in peptide length seem to be accommodated, in most cases, by a kinking in the peptide backbone. However, two examples of MHC class I molecules in which the peptide is able to extend out of the groove at the carboxy terminus suggest that some length variation can also be accommodated in this way.

These interactions give all MHC class I molecules their broad peptide-binding specificity. In addition, MHC molecules are highly polymorphic. There are hundreds of different versions, or alleles, of the MHC class I genes in the human population as a whole, and each individual carries only a small selection of them. The main differences between the allelic MHC variants are found at certain sites in the peptide-binding cleft, resulting in different amino acids in key peptide-interaction sites in the different MHC variants. The consequence of this is that the different MHC variants preferentially bind different peptides. The peptides that can bind to a given MHC variant have the same or very similar amino acid residues at two or three particular positions

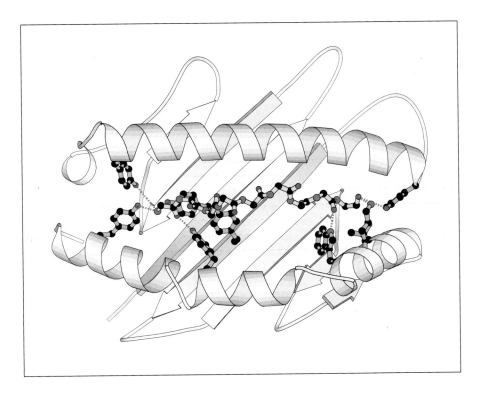

Fig. 3.23 Peptides are bound to MHC class I molecules by their ends. MHC class I molecules interact with the backbone of a bound peptide (shown in yellow) through a series of hydrogen bonds and ionic interactions (shown as dotted blue lines) at each end of the peptide. The amino terminus of the peptide is to the left, the carboxy terminus to the right. Black circles are carbon atoms; red are oxygen; blue are nitrogen. The amino acid residues in the MHC molecule that form these bonds are common to all MHC class I molecules and their side chains are shown in full (in gray) on a ribbon diagram of the MHC class I groove. A cluster of tyrosine residues common to all MHC class I molecules forms hydrogen bonds to the amino terminus of the bound peptide, while a second cluster of residues forms hydrogen bonds and ionic interactions with the peptide backbone at the carboxy terminus and with the carboxy terminus itself.

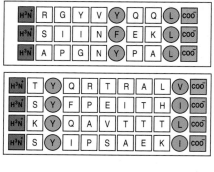

Fig. 3.24 Peptides bind to MHC molecules through structurally related anchor residues. Peptides eluted from two different MHC class I molecules are shown in the upper and lower panels, respectively. The anchor residues (green) differ for peptides that bind different alleles of MHC class I molecules but are similar for all peptides that bind to the same MHC molecule. The anchor residues that bind a particular MHC molecule need not be identical, but are always related (for example, phenylalanine (F) and tyrosine (Y) are both aromatic amino acids, whereas valine (V), leucine (L), and isoleucine (I) are all large hydrophobic amino acids). Peptides also bind to MHC class I molecules through their amino (blue) and carboxy (red) termini.

along the peptide sequence. The amino acid side chains at these positions insert into pockets in the MHC molecule that are lined by the polymorphic amino acids. Because the binding of these side chains anchors the peptide to the MHC molecule, the peptide residues involved have been called **anchor residues**. Both the position and identity of these anchor residues can vary, depending on the particular MHC class I variant that is binding the peptide. However, most peptides that bind to MHC class I molecules have a hydrophobic (or sometimes basic) anchor residue at the carboxy terminus (Fig. 3.24). Whereas changing an anchor residue will in most cases prevent the peptide from binding, not every synthetic peptide of suitable length that contains these anchor residues will bind the appropriate MHC class I molecule, and so the overall binding must also depend on the nature of the amino acids at other positions in the peptide. In some cases, particular amino acids are preferred in certain positions, whereas in others the presence of particular amino acids prevents binding. These additional amino acid positions are called 'secondary anchors'. These features of peptide binding enable an individual MHC class I molecule to bind a wide variety of different peptides, yet allow different MHC class I allelic variants to bind different sets of peptides.

3-17   The length of the peptides bound by MHC class II molecules is not constrained.

Peptide binding to MHC class II molecules has also been analyzed by elution of bound peptides and by X-ray crystallography, and differs in several ways from peptide binding to MHC class I molecules. Peptides that bind to MHC class II molecules are at least 13 amino acids long and can be much longer. The clusters of conserved residues that bind the two ends of a peptide in MHC class I molecules are not found in MHC class II molecules, and the ends of the peptide are not bound. Instead, the peptide lies in an extended conformation along the MHC class II peptide-binding groove. It is held in this groove both by peptide side chains that protrude into shallow and deep pockets lined by polymorphic residues, and by interactions between the peptide backbone and side chains of conserved amino acids that line the peptide-binding cleft in all MHC class II molecules (Fig. 3.25). Although there are fewer crystal structures of MHC class II-bound peptides than of peptides bound to MHC class I, the available data show that amino acid side chains at residues 1, 4, 6, and 9 of an MHC class II-bound peptide can be held in these binding pockets.

The binding pockets of MHC class II molecules are more permissive in their accommodation of different amino acid side chains than are those of the MHC class I molecule, making it more difficult to define anchor residues and to predict which peptides will be able to bind particular MHC class II molecules (Fig. 3.26). Nevertheless, by comparing the sequences of known binding peptides it is usually possible to detect a pattern of permissive amino acids for each of the different alleles of MHC class II molecules, and to model how the amino acids of this peptide sequence motif will interact with the amino acids that make up the peptide-binding cleft in the MHC class II molecule. Because the peptide is bound by its backbone and allowed to emerge from both ends of the binding groove, there is, in principle, no upper limit to the length of peptides that could bind to MHC class II molecules. However, it seems that longer peptides bound to MHC class II molecules are trimmed by peptidases to a length of 13–17 amino acids in most cases. Like MHC class I molecules, MHC class II molecules that lack bound peptide are unstable, but the critical stabilizing interactions that the peptide makes with the MHC class II molecule are not yet known.

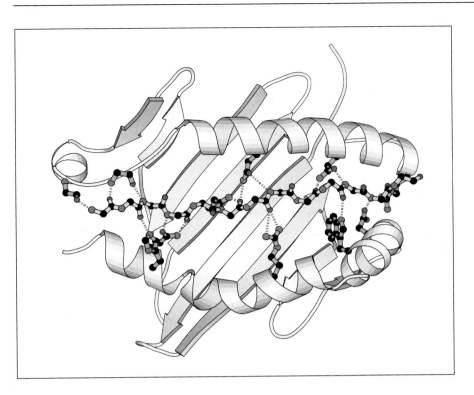

Fig. 3.25 Peptides bind to MHC class II molecules by interactions along the length of the binding groove. A peptide (yellow; shown as the peptide backbone only, with the amino terminus to the left and the carboxy terminus to the right) is bound by an MHC class II molecule through a series of hydrogen bonds (dotted blue lines) that are distributed along the length of the peptide. The hydrogen bonds toward the amino terminus of the peptide are made with the backbone of the MHC class II polypeptide chain, whereas throughout the peptide's length bonds are made with residues that are highly conserved in MHC class II molecules. The side chains of these residues are shown in gray upon the ribbon diagram of the MHC class II groove.

Fig. 3.26 Peptides that bind MHC class II molecules are variable in length and their anchor residues lie at various distances from the ends of the peptide. The sequences of a set of peptides that bind to the mouse MHC class II A^k allele are shown in the upper panel. All contain the same core sequence (shaded) but differ in length. In the lower panel, different peptides binding to the human MHC class II allele HLA-DR3 are shown. Anchor residues are shown as green circles. The lengths of these peptides can vary, and so by convention the first anchor residue is denoted as residue 1. Note that all of the peptides share a hydrophobic residue in position 1, a negatively charged residue (aspartic acid (D) or glutamic acid (E)) in position 4, and a tendency to have a basic residue (lysine (K), arginine (R), histidine (H), glutamine (Q), or asparagine (N)) in position 6 and a hydrophobic residue (for example, tyrosine (Y), leucine (L), phenylalanine (F)) in position 9.

3-18   The crystal structures of several MHC:peptide:T-cell receptor complexes all show the same T-cell receptor orientation over the MHC:peptide complex.

At the time that the first X-ray crystallographic structure of a T-cell receptor was published, a structure of the same T-cell receptor bound to a peptide:MHC class I ligand was also produced. This structure (Fig. 3.27), which had been forecast by site-directed mutagenesis of the MHC class I molecule, showed the T-cell receptor aligned diagonally over the peptide and the peptide-binding groove, with the TCRα chain lying over the α$_2$ domain and the amino-terminal end of the bound peptide, the TCRβ chain lying over the α$_1$ domain and the carboxy-terminal end of the peptide, and the CDR3 loops of both TCRα and TCRβ chains meeting over the central amino acids of the peptide. The T-cell receptor is threaded through a valley between the two high points on the two surrounding α helices that form the walls of the peptide-binding cleft.

Analysis of other MHC class I:peptide:T-cell receptor complexes and of MHC class II:peptide:T-cell receptor complexes (Fig. 3.28) shows that all of them have a very similar orientation, particularly for the V$_α$ domain, although some variability does occur in the location and orientation of the V$_β$ domain. In this orientation, the V$_α$ domain makes contact primarily with the amino terminus of the bound peptide, whereas the V$_β$ domain contacts primarily the carboxy terminus of the bound peptide. Both chains also interact with the α helices of the MHC class I molecule (see Fig. 3.27). The T-cell receptor contacts are not symmetrically distributed over the MHC molecule, so whereas the V$_α$ CDR1 and CDR2 loops are in close contact with the helices of the MHC:peptide complex around the amino terminus of the bound peptide, the β-chain CDR1 and CDR2 loops, which interact with the complex at the carboxy terminus of the bound peptide, have variable contributions to the binding. This suggests that the V$_α$ contacts are responsible for the conserved orientation of the T-cell receptor on the MHC:peptide complex.

Comparison of the three-dimensional structure of the T-cell receptor with that of the same T-cell receptor complexed to its MHC:peptide ligand could address the question of whether the T-cell receptor, like some other receptors, undergoes a conformational change, or 'induced fit,' in its three-dimensional structure when it binds its specific ligand. So far there is no certain answer, owing to the limitations of the available structures. For one thing, all the T-cell receptors analyzed so far are either bound to ligands that do not produce activation, or bound to ligands that can activate them, but comparable

Fig. 3.27 The T-cell receptor binds to the MHC:peptide complex. Panel a: the T-cell receptor binds to the top of the MHC:peptide complex, straddling, in the case of the MHC class I molecule shown here, both the α$_1$ and α$_2$ domain helices. The CDRs of the T-cell receptor are indicated in color: the CDR1 and CDR2 loops of the β chain in light and dark blue, respectively; and the CDR1 and CDR2 loops of the α chain in light and dark purple, respectively. The α chain CDR3 loop is in yellow, and the β chain CDR3 loop is in green. The β chain HV4 loop is red. The thick yellow line P1–P8 is the bound peptide. Panel b: the outline of the T-cell receptor antigen-binding site (thick black line) is superimposed on the top surface of the MHC:peptide complex (the peptide is shaded dull yellow). The T-cell receptor lies diagonally across the MHC:peptide complex, with the α and β CDR3 loops of the T-cell receptor (3α, 3β, yellow and green, respectively) contacting the center of the peptide. The α chain CDR1 and CDR2 loops (1α, 2α, light and dark purple, respectively) contact the MHC helices at the amino terminus of the bound peptide, whereas the β chain CDR1 and CDR2 loops (1β, 2β, light and dark blue, respectively) make contact with the helices at the carboxy terminus of the bound peptide. Courtesy of I.A. Wilson.

unliganded receptor structures are not available. Moreover, none of the structures contains the CD3 subunits of the T-cell receptor, which are actually responsible for the signaling properties of the receptor. Subtly different peptides can have strikingly different effects when the same T cell recognizes the peptides complexed with MHC. This could be due to differences in how T-cell receptor conformation is altered by binding related, yet different, ligands.

From an examination of these structures it is hard to predict whether the main binding energy is contributed by T-cell receptor contacts with the bound peptide, or by T-cell receptor contacts with the MHC molecule. Measurements of the kinetics of T-cell receptor binding to MHC:peptide ligands suggest that the interactions between the T-cell receptor and the MHC molecule might predominate at the start of the contact, guiding the receptor into the correct position where a second, more detailed, interaction with the peptide as well as the MHC molecule dictates the final outcome of the interaction—binding or dissociation. As with antibody–antigen interactions, only a few amino acids at the interface may provide the essential contacts that determine the specificity and strength of binding. It is known that alterations as simple as changing a leucine to isoleucine in the peptide are sufficient to alter the T-cell response from strong killing to absolutely no response at all. Studies show that mutations of single residues in the presenting MHC molecules can have the same effect. Thus, the specificity of T-cell recognition involves both the peptide and its presenting MHC molecule. This dual specificity underlies the MHC restriction of T-cell responses, a phenomenon that was observed long before the peptide-binding properties of MHC molecules were known. We will recount the story of how MHC restriction was discovered when we return to the issue of how MHC polymorphism affects antigen recognition by T cells in Chapter 5. Another consequence of this dual specificity is a need for T-cell receptors to be able to interact appropriately with the antigen-presenting surface of MHC molecules. It seems that there is some inherent specificity for MHC molecules encoded in the T-cell receptor genes, as well as selection during T-cell development for a repertoire of receptors able to interact appropriately with the particular MHC molecules present in that individual. We will discuss the evidence for this in Chapter 7.

3-19   A distinct subset of T cells bears an alternative receptor made up of γ and δ chains.

During the search for the gene for the TCRα chain, another T-cell receptor-like gene was unexpectedly discovered. This gene was named TCRγ, and its discovery led to a search for further T-cell receptor genes. Another receptor chain was identified by using antibody against the predicted sequence of the γ chain and was called the δ chain. It was soon discovered that a minority population of T cells bore a distinct type of T-cell receptor made up of γ:δ heterodimers rather than α:β heterodimers. The development of these cells is described in Sections 7-13 and 7-14.

The crystallographic structure of a γ:δ T-cell receptor reveals that, as expected, it is similar in shape to α:β T-cell receptors (Fig. 3.29). γ:δ T-cell receptors may be specialized to bind certain kinds of ligands, including heat-shock proteins and nonpeptide ligands such as phosphorylated ligands or mycobacterial lipid antigens. It seems likely that γ:δ T-cell receptors are not restricted by the 'classical' MHC class I and class II molecules. They may bind the free antigen, much as immunoglobulins do, and/or they may bind to peptides or other antigens presented by nonclassical MHC-like molecules. These are proteins that resemble MHC class I molecules but are relatively nonpolymorphic. We still know little about how γ:δ T-cell receptors bind antigen and thus how these cells function, and what

Fig. 3.28 The T-cell receptor interacts with MHC class I and MHC class II molecules in a similar fashion. The structure of a T-cell receptor binding to an MHC class II molecule has been determined, and shows the T-cell receptor binding to an equivalent site, and in an equivalent orientation, to the way in which T-cell receptors bind to MHC class I molecules (see Fig. 3.27). The structure of the molecules is shown in a cartoon form, with the MHC class II α and β chains shown in light green and orange respectively. Only the Vα and Vβ domains of the T-cell receptor are shown, colored in blue. The peptide is colored red, and carbohydrate residues are indicated in gray. The T-cell receptor sits in a shallow saddle formed between the MHC class II α and β chain α-helical regions, at roughly 90° to the long axis of the MHC class II molecule and the bound peptide. Courtesy of E.L. Reinherz.

α:β T-cell receptor

a

γ:δ T-cell receptor

b

Fig. 3.29 Structures of α:β and γ:δ T-cell receptors. The structures of the α:β and the γ:δ T-cell receptors have both been determined by X-ray crystallography, and are shown here in cartoon form. The α:β T-cell receptor is shown in panel a, with the α chain colored red and the β chain blue. Panel b shows the γ:δ receptor, with the γ chain colored gray and the δ chain pink. Both receptors have very similar structures, somewhat resembling that of a Fab fragment of an immunoglobulin molecule.

their role is in immune responses. The structure and rearrangement of the genes for γ:δ T-cell receptors is covered in Sections 4-19 and 7-13 and the functions of γ:δ T cells are considered in Chapter 10.

Summary.

The receptor for antigen on most T cells, the α:β T-cell receptor, is composed of two protein chains, TCRα and TCRβ, and resembles in many respects a single Fab fragment of immunoglobulin. T-cell receptors are always membrane-bound. α:β T-cell receptors do not recognize antigen in its native state, as do the immunoglobulin receptors of B cells, but recognize a composite ligand of a peptide antigen bound to an MHC molecule. MHC molecules are highly polymorphic glycoproteins encoded by genes in the major histocompatibility complex (MHC). Each MHC molecule binds a wide variety of different peptides, but the different variants each preferentially recognize sets of peptides with particular sequence and physical features. The peptide antigen is generated intracellularly, and bound stably in a peptide-binding cleft on the surface of the MHC molecule. There are two classes of MHC molecule, and these are bound in their nonpolymorphic domains by CD8 and CD4 molecules that distinguish two different functional classes of α:β T cells. CD8 binds MHC class I molecules and can bind simultaneously to the same class I MHC:peptide complex being recognized by a T-cell receptor, thus acting as a co-receptor and enhancing the T-cell response; CD4 binds MHC class II molecules and acts as a co-receptor for T-cell receptors that recognize class II MHC:peptide ligands. A T-cell receptor interacts directly both with the antigenic peptide and with polymorphic features of the MHC molecule that displays it, and this dual specificity underlies the MHC restriction of T-cell responses. A second type of T-cell receptor, composed of a γ and a δ chain, is structurally similar to the α:β T-cell receptor but seems to bind different ligands, including nonpeptide ligands. It is thought not to be MHC restricted. It is found on a minority population of T cells, the γ:δ T cells, whose biological function is still not clear.

Summary to Chapter 3.

B cells and T cells use different, but structurally similar, molecules to recognize antigen. The antigen-recognition molecules of B cells are immunoglobulins, and are made both as a membrane-bound receptor for antigen, the B-cell receptor, and as secreted antibodies that bind antigens and elicit humoral effector functions. The antigen-recognition molecules of T cells, in contrast, are made only as cell-surface receptors. Immunoglobulins and T-cell receptors are highly variable molecules, with the variability concentrated in that part of the molecule, the variable (V) region, that binds to antigen. Immunoglobulins bind a wide variety of chemically different antigens, whereas the major α:β type of T-cell receptor predominantly recognizes peptide fragments of foreign proteins bound to the MHC molecules that are ubiquitous on cell surfaces.

Binding of antigen by immunoglobulins has chiefly been studied by using antibodies. The binding of antibody to its corresponding antigen is highly specific, and this specificity is determined by the shape and physicochemical properties of the antigen-binding site. The part of the antibody that elicits effector functions, once the variable part has bound an antigen, is located at the other end of the molecule from the antigen-binding sites, and is termed the constant region. There are five main functional classes of antibody, each encoded by a different type of constant region. As we will see in Chapter 9, these interact with different components of the immune system to incite an inflammatory response and eliminate the antigen.

T-cell receptors differ in several respects from the B-cell immunoglobulins. Among the most important of these differences is the absence of a secreted form of the receptor. This reflects the functional differences between T cells and B cells. B cells deal with pathogens and their protein products circulating within the body; secretion of a soluble antigen-recognition molecule by the activated B cell after antigen has been encountered enables them to mop up antigen effectively throughout the extracellular spaces of the body. T cells, in contrast, are specialized for cell–cell interactions. They either kill cells that are infected with intracellular pathogens and that bear foreign antigenic peptides on their surface, or interact with cells of the immune system that have taken up foreign antigen and are displaying it on the cell surface. They thus have no requirement for a soluble, secreted receptor.

An additional distinctive feature of the T-cell receptor compared with immunoglobulins is that it recognizes a composite ligand made up of the foreign peptide bound to a self MHC molecule. This forces T cells to interact with infected body cells to become activated. Each T-cell receptor is specific for a particular combination of peptide and a self MHC molecule.

MHC molecules are encoded by a family of highly polymorphic genes; although each individual expresses several, this represents only a small selection of all possible variants. During T-cell development, the T-cell receptor repertoire is selected so that the T cells of each individual recognize antigen only in conjunction with their own MHC molecules. Expression of multiple variant MHC molecules, each with a different peptide-binding repertoire, helps to ensure that T cells from an individual will be able to recognize at least some peptides generated from nearly every pathogen.

Chapter 3 questions.

3.1 The immunoglobulin superfamily is one of the most abundant families of protein domain structures. (a) What are the characteristics of an immunoglobulin domain and how do the subtypes of these domains differ? (b) Give examples of immunoglobulin superfamily domains in proteins of different function.

3.2 How do antibodies, which all have the same basic shape, recognize antigens of a wide variety of different shapes?

3.3 T cells must deliver effector functions appropriate for the cellular localization of pathogens, whereas B cells are not so constrained. How does this account for the different recognition properties of B- and T-cell antigen receptors?

3.4 Describe the similarities and the differences between B- and T-cell antigen receptors.

3.5 What role do MHC molecules have in the activation of antigen-specific T cells?

General references.

Ager, A., Callard, R., Ezine, S., Gerard, C., and Lopez-Botet, M.: **Immune receptor Supplement.** *Immunol. Today* 1996, **17**.

Davies, D.R., and Chacko, S.: **Antibody structure.** *Acc. Chem. Res.* 1993, **26**:421–427.

Frazer, K., and Capra, J.D.: Immunoglobulins: structure and function, in Paul W.E. (ed): *Fundamental Immunology*, 4th edn. New York, Raven Press, 1998.

Garcia, K.C., Teyton, L., and Wilson, I.A.: **Structural basis of T cell recognition.** *Annu. Rev. Immunol.* 1999, **17**:369–397.

Germain, R.N.: **MHC-dependent antigen processing and peptide presentation: providing ligands for T lymphocyte activation.** *Cell* 1994, **76**:287–299.

Honjo, T., and Alt, F.W. (eds): *Immunoglobulin Genes*, 2nd edn. London, Academic Press, 1996.

Moller, G. (ed): **Origin of major histocompatibility complex diversity.** *Immunol. Rev.* 1995, **143**:5–292.

Poljak, R.J.: **Structure of antibodies and their complexes with antigens.** *Mol. Immunol.* 1991, **28**:1341–1345.

Section references.

3-1   IgG antibodies consist of four polypeptide chains.

Edelman, G.M.: **Antibody structure and molecular immunology.** *Scand. J. Immunol.* 1991, **34**:4–22.

Faber, C., Shan, L., Fan, Z., Guddat, L.W., Furebring, C., Ohlin, M., Borrebaeck, C.A.K., and Edmundson, A.B.: **Three-dimensional structure of a human Fab with high affinity for tetanus toxoid.** *Immunotechnology* 1998, **3**:253–270.

Harris, L.J., Larson, S.B., Hasel, K.W., Day, J., Greenwood, A., and McPherson, A.: **The 3-dimensional structure of an intact monoclonal antibody for canine lymphoma.** *Nature* 1992, **360**:369–372.

3-2   Immunoglobulin heavy and light chains are composed of constant and variable regions.

Han, W.H., Mou, J.X., Sheng, J., Yang, J., and Shao, Z.F.: **Cryo-atomic force microscopy—a new approach for biological imaging at high resolution.** *Biochemistry* 1995, **34**:8215–8220.

3-3   The antibody molecule can readily be cleaved into functionally distinct fragments.

Porter, R.R.: **Structural studies of immunoglobulins.** *Scand. J. Immunol.* 1991, **34**:382–389.

Yamaguchi, Y., Kim, H., Kato, K., Masuda, K., Shimada, I., and Arata, Y.: **Proteolytic fragmentation with high specificity of mouse IgG—mapping of proteolytic cleavage sites in the hinge region.** *J. Immunol. Meth.* 1995, **181**:259–267.

3-4   The immunoglobulin molecule is flexible, especially at the hinge region.

Gerstein, M., Lesk, A.M., and Chothia, C.: **Structural mechanisms for domain movements in proteins.** *Biochemistry* 1994, **33**:6739–6749.

Jimenez, R., Salazar, G., Baldridge, K.K., and Romesberg, F.E.: **Flexibility and molecular recognition in the immune system.** *Proc. Natl Acad. Sci. USA* 2003, **100**:92–97.

Saphire, E.O., Stanfield, R.L., Crispin, M.D., Parren, P.W., Rudd, P.M., Dwek, R.A., Burton, D.R., and Wilson, I.A.: **Contrasting IgG structures reveal extreme asymmetry and flexibility.** *J. Mol. Biol.* 2002, **319**:9–18.

3-5   The domains of an immunoglobulin molecule have similar structures.

Barclay, A.N., Brown, M.H., Law, S.K., McKnight, A.J., Tomlinson, M.G., and van der Merwe, P.A. (eds): *The Leukocyte Antigen Factsbook*, 2nd edn. London, Academic Press, 1997.

Brummendorf, T., and Lemmon, V.: **Immunoglobulin superfamily receptors: cis-interactions, intracellular adapters and alternative splicing regulate adhesion.** *Curr. Opin. Cell Biol.* 2001, **13**:611–618.

Marchalonis, J.J., Jensen, I., and Schluter, S.F.: **Structural, antigenic and evolutionary analyses of immunoglobulins and T cell receptors.** *J. Mol. Recog.* 2002, **15**:260–271.

Ramsland, P.A., and Farrugia, W.: **Crystal structures of human antibodies: a detailed and unfinished tapestry of immunoglobulin gene products.** *J. Mol. Recog.* 2002, **15**:248–259.

3-6   Localized regions of hypervariable sequence form the antigen-binding site.

Chitarra, V., Alzari, P.M., Bentley, G.A., Bhat, T.N., Eisele, J.L., Houdusse, A., Lescar, J., Souchon, H., and Poljak, R.J.: **Three-dimensional structure of a heteroclitic antigen–antibody cross-reaction complex.** *Proc. Natl Acad. Sci. USA* 1993, **90**:7711–7715.

Decanniere, K., Muyldermans, S., and Wyns, L.: **Canonical antigen-binding loop structures in immunoglobulins: more structures, more canonical classes?** *J. Mol. Biol.* 2000, **300**:83–91.

Gilliland, L.K., Norris, N.A., Marquardt, H., Tsu, T.T., Hayden, M.S., Neubauer, M.G., Yelton, D.E., Mittler, R.S., and Ledbetter, J.A.: **Rapid and reliable cloning of antibody variable regions and generation of recombinant single-chain antibody fragments.** *Tissue Antigens* 1996, **47**:1–20.

Johnson, G., and Wu, T.T.: **Kabat Database and its applications: 30 years after the first variability plot.** *Nucleic Acids Res.* 2000, **28**:214–218.

Wu, T.T., and Kabat, E.A.: **An analysis of the sequences of the variable regions of Bence Jones proteins and myeloma light chains and their implications for antibody complementarity.** *J. Exp. Med.* 1970, **132**:211–250.

Xu, J., Deng, Q., Chen, J., Houk, K.N., Bartek, J., Hilvert, D., and Wilson, I.A.: **Evolution of shape complementarity and catalytic efficiency from a primordial antibody template.** *Science* 1999, **286**:2345–2348.

3-7   Antibodies bind antigens via contacts with amino acids in CDRs, but the details of binding depend upon the size and shape of the antigen.

&

3-8   Antibodies bind to conformational shapes on the surfaces of antigens.

Ban, N., Day, J., Wang, X., Ferrone, S., and McPherson, A.: **Crystal structure of an anti-anti-idiotype shows it to be self-complementary.** *J. Mol. Biol.* 1996, **255**:617–627.

Davies, D.R., and Cohen, G.H.: **Interactions of protein antigens with antibodies.** *Proc. Natl Acad. Sci. USA* 1996, **93**:7–12.

Decanniere, K., Desmyter, A., Lauwereys, M., Ghahroudi, M.A., Muyldermans, S., and Wyns, L.: **A single-domain antibody fragment in complex with RNase A: non-canonical loop structures and nanomolar affinity using two CDR loops.** *Structure Fold Des* 1999, **7**:361–370.

Padlan, E.A.: **Anatomy of the antibody molecule.** *Mol. Immunol.* 1994, **31**:169–217.

Saphire, E.O., Parren, P.W., Pantophlet, R., Zwick, M.B., Morris, G.M., Rudd, P.M., Dwek, R.A., Stanfield, R.L., Burton, D.R., and Wilson, I.A.: **Crystal structure of a neutralizing human IGG against HIV-1: a template for vaccine design.** *Science* 2001, **293**:1155–1159.

Stanfield, R.L., and Wilson, I.A.: **Protein–peptide interactions.** *Curr. Opin. Struct. Biol.* 1995, **5**:103–113.

Tanner, J.J., Komissarov, A.A., and Deutscher, S.L.: **Crystal structure of an antigen-binding fragment bound to single-stranded DNA.** *J. Mol. Biol.* 2001, **314**:807–822.

Wilson, I.A., and Stanfield, R.L.: **Antibody-antigen interactions: new structures and new conformational changes.** *Curr. Opin. Struct. Biol.* 1994, **4**:857–867.

3-9   Antigen–antibody interactions involve a variety of forces.

Braden, B.C., and Poljak, R.J.: **Structural features of the reactions between antibodies and protein antigens.** *FASEB J.* 1995, **9**:9–16.

Braden, B.C., Goldman, E.R., Mariuzza, R.A., and Poljak, R.J.: **Anatomy of an antibody molecule: structure, kinetics, thermodynamics and mutational studies of the antilysozyme antibody D1.3.** *Immunol. Rev.* 1998, **163**:45–57.

Ros, R., Schwesinger, F., Anselmetti, D., Kubon, M., Schäfer, R., Plückthun, A., and Tiefenauer, L.: **Antigen binding forces of individually addressed single-chain Fv antibody molecules.** *Proc. Natl Acad. Sci. USA* 1998, **95**:7402–7405.

3-10   The antigen receptor on T cells is very similar to a Fab fragment of immunoglobulin.

Al-Lazikani, B., Lesk, A.M., and Chothia, C.: **Canonical structures for the hypervariable regions of T cell αβ receptors.** *J. Mol. Biol.* 2000, **295**:979–995.

Kjer-Nielsen, L., Clements, C.S., Brooks, A.G., Purcell, A.W., McCluskey, J., and Rossjohn, J.: **The 1.5 Å crystal structure of a highly selected antiviral T cell receptor provides evidence for a structural basis of immunodominance.** *Structure (Camb.)* 2002, **10**:1521–1532.

Machius, M., Cianga, P., Deisenhofer, J., and Ward, E.S.: **Crystal structure of a T cell receptor Vα₁₁ (AV11S5) domain: new canonical forms for the first and second complementarity determining regions.** *J. Mol. Biol.* 2001, **310**:689–698.

3-11   A T-cell receptor recognizes antigen in the form of a complex of a foreign peptide bound to an MHC molecule.

Baker, B.M., Gagnon, S.J., Biddison, W.E., and Wiley, D.C.: **Conversion of a T cell antagonist into an agonist by repairing a defect in the TCR/peptide/MHC interface: implications for TCR signaling.** *Immunity* 2000, **13**:475–484.

Davis, M.M., Boniface, J.J., Reich, Z., Lyons, D., Hampl, J., Arden, B., and Chien, Y.: **Ligand recognition by αβ T cell receptors.** *Annu. Rev. Immunol.* 1998, **16**:523–544.

Hennecke, J., and Wiley, D.C.: **Structure of a complex of the human αβ T cell receptor (TCR) HA1.7, influenza hemagglutinin peptide, and major histocompatibility complex class II molecule, HLA-DR4 (DRA*0101 and DRB1*0401): insight into TCR cross-restriction and alloreactivity.** *J. Exp. Med.* 2002, **195**:571–581.

Hennecke, J., Carfi, A., and Wiley, D.C.: **Structure of a covalently stabilized complex of a human αβ T-cell receptor, influenza HA peptide and MHC class II molecule, HLA-DR1.** *EMBO J.* 2000, **19**:5611–5624.

Luz, J.G., Huang, M., Garcia, K.C., Rudolph, M.G., Apostolopoulos, V., Teyton, L., and Wilson, I.A.: **Structural comparison of allogeneic and syngeneic T cell receptor-peptide-major histocompatibility complex complexes: a buried alloreactive mutation subtly alters peptide presentation substantially increasing Vβ interactions.** *J. Exp. Med.* 2002, **195**:1175–1186.

3-12   T cells with different functions are distinguished by CD4 and CD8 cell-surface proteins and recognize peptides bound to different classes of MHC molecule.

Gao, G.F., Tormo, J., Gerth, U.C., Wyer, J.R., McMichael, A.J., Stuart, D.I., Bell, J.I., Jones, E.Y., and Jakobsen, B.Y.: **Crystal structure of the complex between human CD8αα and HLA-A2.** *Nature* 1997, **387**:630–634.

Gaspar, R., Jr., Bagossi, P., Bene, L., Matko, J., Szollosi, J., Tozser, J., Fesus, L., Waldmann, T.A., and Damjanovich, S.: **Clustering of class I HLA oligomers with CD8 and TCR: three-dimensional models based on fluorescence resonance energy transfer and crystallographic data.** *J. Immunol.* 2001, **166**:5078–5086.

Kim, P.W., Sun, Z.Y., Blacklow, S.C., Wagner, G., and Eck, M.J.: **A zinc clasp structure tethers Lck to T cell coreceptors CD4 and CD8.** *Science* 2003, **301**:1725–1728.

Moldovan, M.C., Yachou, A., Levesque, K., Wu, H., Hendrickson, W.A., Cohen, E.A., and Sekaly, R.P.: **CD4 dimers constitute the functional component required for T cell activation.** *J. Immunol.* 2002, **169**:6261–6268.

Wang, J.H., and Reinherz, E.L.: **Structural basis of T cell recognition of peptides bound to MHC molecules.** *Mol. Immunol.* 2002, **38**:1039–1049.

Wu, H., Kwong, P.D., and Hendrickson, W.A.: **Dimeric association and segmental variability in the structure of human CD4.** *Nature* 1997, **387**:527–530.

Zamoyska, R.: **CD4 and CD8: modulators of T cell receptor recognition of antigen and of immune responses?** *Curr. Opin. Immunol.* 1998, **10**:82–86.

3-13   The two classes of MHC molecule are expressed differentially on cells.

Steimle, V., Siegrist, C.A., Mottet, A., Lisowska-Grospierre, B., and Mach, B.: **Regulation of MHC class II expression by interferon-γ mediated by the transactivator gene CIITA.** *Science* 1994, **265**:106–109.

3-14   The two classes of MHC molecule have distinct subunit structures but similar three-dimensional structures.

&

3-15   Peptides are stably bound to MHC molecules, and also serve to stabilize the MHC molecule on the cell surface.

Bouvier, M.: **Accessory proteins and the assembly of human class I MHC molecules: a molecular and structural perspective.** *Mol. Immunol.* 2003, **39**:697–706.

Dessen, A., Lawrence, C.M., Cupo, S., Zaller, D.M., and Wiley, D.C.: **X-ray crystal structure of HLA-DR4 (DRA*0101, DRB1*0401) complexed with a peptide from human collagen II.** *Immunity* 1997, **7**:473–481.

Fremont, D.H., Hendrickson, W.A., Marrack, P., and Kappler, J.: **Structures of an MHC class II molecule with covalently bound single peptides.** *Science* 1996, **272**:1001–1004.

Fremont, D.H., Matsumura, M., Stura, E.A., Peterson, P.A. and Wilson, I.A.: **Crystal structures of two viral peptides in complex with murine MHC class 1 H-2Kb.** *Science* 1992, **257**:919–927.

Fremont, D.H., Monnaie, D., Nelson, C.A., Hendrickson, W.A., and Unanue, E.R.: **Crystal structure of I-Ak in complex with a dominant epitope of lysozyme.** *Immunity* 1998, **8**:305–317.

Macdonald, W.A., Purcell, A.W., Mifsud, N.A., Ely, L.K., Williams, D.S., Chang, L., Gorman, J.J., Clements, C.S., Kjer-Nielsen, L., Koelle, D.M., Burrows, S.R., Tait, B.D., Holdsworth, R., Brooks, A.G., Lovrecz, G.O., Lu, L., Rossjohn, J., and McCluskey, J.: **A naturally selected dimorphism within the HLA-B44 supertype alters class I structure, peptide repertoire, and T cell recognition.** *J. Exp. Med.* 2003, **198**:679–691.

Zhu, Y., Rudensky, A.Y., Corper, A.L., Teyton, L., and Wilson, I.A.: **Crystal structure of MHC class II I-Ab in complex with a human CLIP peptide: prediction of an I-Ab peptide-binding motif.** *J. Mol. Biol.* 2003, **326**:1157–1174.

3-16   MHC class I molecules bind short peptides of 8–10 amino acids by both ends.

Bouvier, M., and Wiley, D.C.: **Importance of peptide amino and carboxyl termini to the stability of MHC class I molecules.** *Science* 1994, **265**:398–402.

Govindarajan, K.R., Kangueane, P., Tan, T.W., and Ranganathan, S.: **MPID: MHC-Peptide Interaction Database for sequence-structure-function information on peptides binding to MHC molecules.** *Bioinformatics* 2003, **19**:309–310.

Saveanu, L., Fruci, D., and van Endert, P.: **Beyond the proteasome: trimming, degradation and generation of MHC class I ligands by auxiliary proteases.** *Mol. Immunol.* 2002, **39**:203–215.

Weiss, G.A., Collins, E.J., Garboczi, D.N., Wiley, D.C., and Schreiber, S.L.: **A tricyclic ring system replaces the variable regions of peptides presented by three alleles of human MHC class I molecules.** *Chem. Biol.* 1995, **2**:401–407.

3-17 The length of the peptides bound by MHC class II molecules is not constrained.

Conant, S.B., and Swanborg, R.H.: **MHC class II peptide flanking residues of exogenous antigens influence recognition by autoreactive T cells.** *Autoimmun. Rev.* 2003, **2**:8–12.

Guan, P., Doytchinova, I.A., Zygouri, C., and Flower, D.R.: **MHCPred: a server for quantitative prediction of peptide-MHC binding.** *Nucleic Acids Res.* 2003, **31**:3621–3624.

Lippolis, J.D., White, F.M., Marto, J.A., Luckey, C.J., Bullock, T.N., Shabanowitz, J., Hunt, D.F., and Engelhard, V.H.: **Analysis of MHC class II antigen processing by quantitation of peptides that constitute nested sets.** *J. Immunol.* 2002, **169**:5089–5097.

Park, J.H., Lee, Y.J., Kim, K.L., and Cho, E.W.: **Selective isolation and identification of HLA-DR-associated naturally processed and presented epitope peptides.** *Immunol. Invest.* 2003, **32**:155–169.

Rammensee, H.G.: **Chemistry of peptides associated with MHC class I and class II molecules.** *Curr. Opin. Immunol.* 1995, **7**:85–96.

Rudensky, A.Y., Preston-Hurlburt, P., Hong, S.C., Barlow, A., and Janeway, C.A., Jr.: **Sequence analysis of peptides bound to MHC class II molecules.** *Nature* 1991, **353**:622.

Sercarz, E.E., and Maverakis, E.: **MHC-guided processing: binding of large antigen fragments.** *Nat. Rev. Immunol.* 2003, **3**:621–629.

Sinnathamby, G., and Eisenlohr, L.C.: **Presentation by recycling MHC class II molecules of an influenza hemagglutinin-derived epitope that is revealed in the early endosome by acidification.** *J. Immunol.* 2003, **170**:3504–3513.

3-18 The crystal structures of several MHC:peptide:T-cell receptor complexes all show the same T-cell receptor orientation over the MHC:peptide complex.

Buslepp, J., Wang, H., Biddison, W.E., Appella, E., and Collins, E.J.: **A correlation between TCR Vα docking on MHC and CD8 dependence: implications for T cell selection.** *Immunity* 2003, **19**:595–606.

Ding, Y.H., Smith, K.J., Garboczi, D.N., Utz, U., Biddison, W.E., and Wiley, D.C.: **Two human T cell receptors bind in a similar diagonal mode to the HLA-A2/Tax peptide complex using different TCR amino acids.** *Immunity* 1998, **8**:403–411.

Garcia, K.C., Degano, M., Pease, L.R., Huang, M., Peterson, P.A., Leyton, L., and Wilson, I.A.: **Structural basis of plasticity in T cell receptor recognition of a self peptide-MHC antigen.** *Science* 1998, **279**:1166–1172.

Sant'Angelo, D.B., Waterbury, G., Preston-Hurlburt, P., Yoon, S.T., Medzhitov, R., Hong, S.C., and Janeway, C.A., Jr.: **The specificity and orientation of a TCR to its peptide-MHC class II ligands.** *Immunity* 1996, **4**:367–376.

Teng, M.K., Smolyar, A., Tse, A.G.D., Liu, J.H., Liu, J., Hussey, R.E., Nathenson, S.G., Chang, H.C., Reinherz, E.L., and Wang, J.H.: **Identification of a common docking topology with substantial variation among different TCR-MHC-peptide complexes.** *Curr. Biol.* 1998, **8**:409–412.

3-19 A distinct subset of T cells bears an alternative receptor made up of γ and δ chains.

Allison, T.J., and Garboczi, D.N.: **Structure of γδ T cell receptors and their recognition of non-peptide antigens.** *Mol. Immunol.* 2002, **38**:1051–1061.

Allison, T.J., Winter, C.C., Fournie, J.J., Bonneville, M., and Garboczi, D.N.: **Structure of a human γδ T-cell antigen receptor.** *Nature* 2001, **411**:820–824.

Carding, S.R., and Egan, P.J.: **γδ T cells: functional plasticity and heterogeneity.** *Nature Rev. Immunol.* 2002, **2**:336–345.

Das, H., Wang, L., Kamath, A., and Bukowski, J.F.: **Vγ2Vδ2 T-cell receptor-mediated recognition of aminobisphosphonates.** *Blood* 2001, **98**:1616–1618.

Wilson, I.A., and Stanfield, R.L.: **Unraveling the mysteries of γδ T cell recognition.** *Nature Immunol.* 2001, **2**:579–581.

Wu, J., Groh, V., and Spies, T.: **T cell antigen receptor engagement and specificity in the recognition of stress-inducible MHC class I-related chains by human epithelial γδ T cells.** *J. Immunol.* 2002, **169**:1236–1240.

The Generation of Lymphocyte Antigen Receptors

Lymphocyte antigen receptors, in the form of immunoglobulins on B cells and T-cell receptors on T cells, are the means by which lymphocytes sense the presence of antigens in their environment. Individual lymphocytes bear numerous copies of a single antigen receptor with a unique antigen-binding site, which determines the antigens that that lymphocyte can bind. Because each person possesses billions of lymphocytes, these cells collectively enable a response to a great variety of antigens. The wide range of antigen specificities in the antigen-receptor repertoire is due to variation in the amino-acid sequence at the antigen-binding site, which is made up from the variable (V) regions of the receptor protein chains. In each chain the V region is linked to an invariant constant (C) region, which provides effector or signaling functions.

Given the importance of a diverse repertoire of lymphocyte receptors in the defense against infection, it is not surprising that a complex and elegant genetic mechanism has evolved for generating these highly variable proteins. Each receptor-chain variant cannot be encoded in full in the genome, as this would require more genes for antigen receptors than there are genes in the entire genome. Instead, we will see that the V regions of the receptor chains are encoded in several pieces—so-called gene segments. These are assembled in the developing lymphocyte by somatic DNA recombination to form a complete V-region sequence, a mechanism known generally as **gene rearrangement**. The fully assembled V-region sequence comprises two or three types of V gene segment. Each type of gene segment is present in multiple copies in the germline genome. The selection of a gene segment of each type during gene rearrangement occurs at random, and the large number of possible different combinations accounts for much of the diversity of the receptor repertoire.

In the first two parts of this chapter we will describe the gene rearrangement mechanism that generates the V regions of immunoglobulin and T-cell receptor genes. The basic mechanism is common to both B cells and T cells, and involves the same enzymes. We will describe the details of the enzymology of this recombination process, the evolution of which was probably critical to the evolution of the vertebrate adaptive immune system.

In B cells, but not T cells, the rearranged V region undergoes modification, known as **somatic hypermutation**. This does not occur until after B cells encounter and become activated by antigen. In these cells, the V regions of the assembled immunoglobulin genes undergo a high rate of point mutation that creates additional diversity within the expanding clone of B cells responding to antigen.

In the third part of the chapter we consider the limited, but functionally important, diversity of immunoglobulin C regions. The C regions of T-cell receptors do not show such diversity because they function only as part of a membrane-bound antigen receptor. Their role is to anchor and support the

V regions at the cell surface as well as linking the binding of antigen by the V regions to the receptor-associated intracellular signaling complex. The C regions of immunoglobulins also serve these functions but in addition the C regions of the heavy chain are responsible for the effector functions of the secreted immunoglobulins, or antibodies, made by activated B cells. These C_H regions come in several different versions, or isotypes, each of which has a different effector function. In B cells that have become activated by antigen, the heavy-chain V region can become associated with a different C_H region by a further somatic recombination event, in the process known as **isotype switching**. This enables the different heavy-chain C regions, each with a different function, to be represented among antibodies of the same antigen specificity.

The generation of diversity in immunoglobulins.

Virtually any substance can be the target of an antibody response. Furthermore, the response even to a simple antigen bearing a single antigenic determinant is diverse, comprising many different antibody molecules, each with a subtly different specificity for the antigen and a unique affinity, or binding strength. The total number of antibody specificities available to an individual is known as the **antibody repertoire**, or **immunoglobulin repertoire**, and in humans is at least 10^{11}. The number of antibody specificities present at any one time is, however, limited by the total number of B cells in an individual, as well as by each individual's encounters with antigens.

Before it was possible to examine the immunoglobulin genes directly, there were two main hypotheses for the origin of this diversity. The **germline theory** held that there is a separate gene for each different immunoglobulin chain and that the antibody repertoire is largely inherited. By contrast, **somatic diversification theories** proposed that the observed repertoire is generated from a limited number of inherited V-region sequences that undergo alteration within B cells during the individual's lifetime. Cloning of the immunoglobulin genes revealed that elements of both theories were correct and that the DNA sequence encoding each V region is generated by rearrangements of a relatively small group of inherited gene segments. Diversity is further enhanced by the process of somatic hypermutation in mature activated B cells. Thus the somatic diversification theory was essentially correct, although the concept of multiple germline genes embodied in the germline theory also proved true.

4-1   Immunoglobulin genes are rearranged in antibody-producing cells.

In nonlymphoid cells, the gene segments encoding the greater part of the V region of an immunoglobulin chain are some considerable distance away from the sequence encoding the C region. In mature B lymphocytes, however, the assembled V-region sequence lies much nearer the C region, as a consequence of gene rearrangement. Rearrangement within the immunoglobulin genes was originally discovered over 25 years ago, when the techniques of restriction enzyme analysis and Southern blotting first made it possible to study the organization of the immunoglobulin genes in both B cells and nonlymphoid cells. In these procedures, chromosomal DNA is first cut with a restriction enzyme, and the DNA fragments containing particular V- and C-region sequences are identified by hybridization with radiolabeled DNA probes specific for the relevant DNA sequences. In germline DNA, from nonlymphoid

Fig. 4.1 Immunoglobulin genes are rearranged in B cells. The two photographs on the left (germline DNA) show a Southern blot of a restriction enzyme digest of DNA from nonlymphoid cells from a normal person. The locations of immunoglobulin DNA sequences are identified by hybridization with V- and C-region probes. The V and C regions are found in distinct DNA fragments in the nonlymphoid DNA. The two photographs on the right (B-cell DNA) are of the same restriction digest of DNA from peripheral blood lymphocytes from a patient with chronic lymphocytic leukemia (see Chapter 7), in which a single clone of B cells is greatly expanded. The malignant B cells express the V region from which the V-region probe was obtained and, owing to their predominance in the cell population, this unique rearrangement can be detected. In this DNA, the V and C regions are found in the same fragment, which is a different size from either the C- or the V-region germline fragments. Although not shown in this figure, a population of normal B lymphocytes has many different rearranged genes, so they yield a smear of DNA fragment sizes, which are not visible as a crisp band. Photographs courtesy of S. Wagner and L. Luzzatto.

Germline DNA		B-cell DNA	
C-region fragment	V-region fragment	C-region fragment	V-region fragment

cells, the V- and C-region sequences identified by the probes are on separate DNA fragments. However, in DNA from an antibody-producing B cell these V- and C-region sequences are on the same DNA fragment, showing that a rearrangement of the DNA has occurred. A typical experiment using human DNA is shown in Fig. 4.1.

This simple experiment showed that segments of genomic DNA within the immunoglobulin genes are rearranged in cells of the B-lymphocyte lineage, but not in other cells. This process of rearrangement is known as **somatic recombination**, to distinguish it from the meiotic recombination that takes place during the production of gametes.

4-2   Complete genes that encode a V region are generated by the somatic recombination of separate gene segments.

The V region, or V domain, of an immunoglobulin heavy or light chain is encoded by more than one gene segment. For the light chain, the V domain is encoded by two separate DNA segments. The first segment encodes the first 95–101 amino acids of the light chain and is termed a **V gene segment** because it encodes most of the V domain. The second segment encodes the remainder of the V domain (up to 13 amino acids) and is termed a **joining** or **J gene segment**.

The rearrangements that lead to the production of a complete immunoglobulin light-chain gene are shown in Fig. 4.2 (center panel). The joining of a V and a J gene segment creates a continuous exon that encodes the whole of the light-chain V region. In the unrearranged DNA, the V gene segments are located relatively far away from the C region. The J gene segments are located close to the C region, however, and the joining of a V gene segment to a J gene segment also brings the V gene segment close to a C-region sequence. The J gene segment of the rearranged V region is separated from a C-region sequence only by a short intron. In the experiment shown in Fig. 4.1, the germline DNA fragment identified by the 'V-region probe' contains the V gene segment, and that identified by the 'C-region probe' actually contains both the J gene segment and the C-region sequence. To make a complete immunoglobulin light-chain messenger RNA, the V-region exon is joined to the C-region sequence by RNA splicing after transcription (see Fig. 4.2).

A heavy-chain V region is encoded in three gene segments. In addition to the V and J gene segments (denoted V_H and J_H to distinguish them from the light-chain V_L and J_L), there is a third gene segment called the **diversity** or D_H **gene segment**, which lies between the V_H and J_H gene segments. The process of recombination that generates a complete heavy-chain V region is shown in

Light chain	Heavy chain

Fig. 4.2 V-region genes are constructed from gene segments. Light-chain V-region genes are constructed from two segments (center panel). A variable (V) and a joining (J) gene segment in the genomic DNA are joined to form a complete light-chain V-region exon. Immunoglobulin chains are extracellular proteins and the V gene segment is preceded by an exon encoding a leader peptide (L), which directs the protein into the cell's secretory pathways and is then cleaved. The light-chain C region is encoded in a separate exon and is joined to the V-region exon by splicing of the light-chain RNA to remove the L-to-V and the J-to-C introns. Heavy-chain V regions are constructed from three gene segments (right panel). First, the diversity (D) and J gene segments join, then the V gene segment joins to the combined DJ sequence, forming a complete V_H exon. A heavy-chain C-region gene is encoded by several exons. The C-region exons, together with the leader sequence, are spliced to the V-domain sequence during processing of the heavy-chain RNA transcript. The leader sequence is removed after translation and the disulfide bonds that link the polypeptide chains are formed. The hinge region is shown in purple.

Fig. 4.2 (right panel), and occurs in two separate stages. In the first, a D_H gene segment is joined to a J_H gene segment; then a V_H gene segment rearranges to DJ_H to make a complete V_H-region exon. As with the light-chain genes, RNA splicing joins the assembled V-region sequence to the neighboring C-region gene.

4-3 For each immunoglobulin chain, multiple contiguous V-region gene segments are present on a stretch of chromosome.

For simplicity, we have so far discussed the formation of a complete immunoglobulin V-region sequence as though there were only a single copy of each gene segment. In fact, there are multiple copies of all the gene segments in germline DNA. It is the random selection of just one gene segment of each type to assemble a V region that makes possible the great diversity of

V regions among immunoglobulins. The numbers of functional gene segments of each type in the human genome, as determined by gene cloning and sequencing, are shown in Fig. 4.3. Not all the gene segments discovered are functional, as a proportion have accumulated mutations that prevent them from encoding a functional protein. These are termed 'pseudogenes.' Because there are many V, D, and J gene segments in germline DNA, no single one is essential. This reduces the evolutionary pressure on each gene segment to remain intact, and has resulted in a relatively large number of pseudogenes. Since some of these pseudogenes can undergo rearrangement just like a normal functional gene segment, a significant proportion of rearrangements will incorporate a pseudogene and thus be nonfunctional.

We saw in Section 3-1 that there are three sets of immunoglobulin chains, the heavy chains and two equivalent types of light chain, the κ and λ chains. The immunoglobulin gene segments forming each of these chains are organized into three clusters or genetic loci—the κ, λ, and heavy-chain loci—each of which can assemble a complete V-region sequence. These are on different chromosomes and each is organized slightly differently, as shown for humans in Fig. 4.4. At the λ light-chain locus, located on chromosome 22, a cluster of V_λ gene segments is followed by four sets of J_λ gene segments each linked to a single C_λ gene. In the κ light-chain locus, on chromosome 2, the cluster of V_κ gene segments is followed by a cluster of J_κ gene segments, and then by a single C_κ gene. The organization of the heavy-chain locus, on chromosome 14, resembles that of the κ locus, with separate clusters of V_H, D_H, and J_H gene segments and of C_H genes. The heavy-chain locus differs in one important way: instead of a single C region, it contains a series of C regions arrayed one after the other, each of which corresponds to a different isotype. B cells initially express IgM and IgD, which is accomplished by alternative mRNA splicing (see Section 4-17). The expression of other isotypes, such as IgG, subsequently occurs through DNA rearrangements referred to as isotype switching, which will be described in Section 4-18.

Number of functional gene segments in human immunoglobulin loci		
Segment	**Light chains**	**Heavy chain**
	κ	λ	H
Variable (V)	40	30	40
Diversity (D)	0	0	25
Joining (J)	5	4	6

Fig. 4.3 The numbers of functional gene segments for the V regions of human heavy and light chains. These numbers are derived from exhaustive cloning and sequencing of DNA from one individual and exclude all pseudogenes (mutated and nonfunctional versions of a gene sequence). Owing to genetic polymorphism, the numbers will not be the same for all people.

Fig. 4.4 The germline organization of the immunoglobulin heavy- and light-chain loci in the human genome. The genetic locus for the λ light chain (chromosome 22) has about 30 functional V_λ gene segments and four pairs of functional J_λ gene segments and C_λ genes. The κ locus (chromosome 2) is organized in a similar way, with about 40 functional V_κ gene segments accompanied by a cluster of five J_κ gene segments but with a single C_κ gene. In approximately 50% of individuals, the entire cluster of V_κ gene segments has undergone an increase by duplication (not shown for simplicity). The heavy-chain locus (chromosome 14) has about 40 functional V_H gene segments and a cluster of around 25 D_H segments lying between these V_H gene segments and six J_H gene segments. The heavy-chain locus also contains a large cluster of C_H genes that are described in Fig. 4.19. For simplicity we have shown only a single C_H gene in this diagram without illustrating its separate exons, have omitted pseudogenes, and have shown all V gene segments in the same orientation. L, leader sequence. This diagram is not to scale: the total length of the heavy-chain locus is over 2 megabases (2 million bases), whereas some of the D segments are only six bases long.

The human V gene segments can be grouped into families in which each member shares at least 80% DNA sequence identity with all others in the family. Both the heavy-chain and κ-chain V gene segments can be subdivided into seven such families, whereas there are eight families of V_λ gene segments. The families can be grouped into clans, made up of families that are more similar to each other than to families in other clans. Human V_H gene segments fall into three such clans. All the V_H gene segments identified from amphibians, reptiles, and mammals also fall into the same three clans, suggesting that these clans existed in a common ancestor of these modern animal groups. Thus, the V gene segments that we see today have arisen by a series of gene duplications and diversification through evolutionary time.

4-4 Rearrangement of V, D, and J gene segments is guided by flanking DNA sequences.

For a proper immunoglobulin or T-cell receptor chain to be expressed, DNA rearrangements must take place at the correct locations relative to the V, D, or J gene segment coding regions. In addition, joins must be regulated such that a V gene segment joins to a D or J and not to another V. DNA rearrangements are guided by conserved noncoding DNA sequences that are found adjacent to the points at which recombination takes place. These sequences consist of a conserved block of seven nucleotides—the **heptamer** 5′CACAGTG3′—which is always contiguous with the coding sequence, followed by a nonconserved region known as the **spacer**, which is either 12 or 23 nucleotides long, followed by a second conserved block of nine nucleotides—the **nonamer** 5′ACAAAAACC3′ (Fig. 4.5). The spacer varies in sequence but its conserved length corresponds to one or two turns of the DNA double helix. This brings the heptamer and nonamer sequences to the same side of the DNA helix, where they can be bound by the complex of proteins that catalyzes recombination. The heptamer–spacer–nonamer sequence motif is called a **recombination signal sequence (RSS)** and is always found directly adjacent to the coding sequence of V, D, or J gene segments.

Recombination normally occurs between gene segments located on the same chromosome. A gene segment flanked by an RSS with a 12-base-pair (bp) spacer typically can be joined only to one flanked by a 23-bp spacer RSS. This is known as the **12/23 rule**. Thus, for the heavy chain, a D_H gene segment can be joined to a J_H gene segment and a V_H gene segment to a D_H gene segment, but V_H gene segments cannot be joined to J_H gene segments directly, as both V_H and J_H gene segments are flanked by 23-bp spacers and the D_H gene segments have 12-bp spacers on both sides (see Fig. 4.5).

It is now apparent, however, that, even though it violates the 12/23 rule, direct joining of one D gene segment to another can occur in most species, albeit infrequently. In humans, D–D fusion is found in approximately 5% of

Fig. 4.5 Conserved heptamer and nonamer sequences flank the gene segments encoding the V regions of heavy (H) and light (λ and κ) chains. The spacer between the heptamer (pink) and nonamer (blue) sequences is always either approximately 12 bp (orange) or approximately 23 bp (purple), and joining almost always involves a 12-bp and a 23-bp recombination signal sequence.

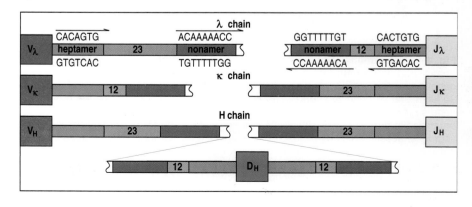

antibodies and is the major mechanism accounting for the unusually long CDR3 loops found in some heavy chains. By creating extra-long CDR3s and unusual amino-acid combinations, these D–D fusions add further to the diversity of the antibody repertoire.

The mechanism of DNA rearrangement is similar for the heavy- and light-chain loci, although only one joining event is needed to generate a light-chain gene whereas two are needed to generate a complete heavy-chain gene. When the coding sequences of the two gene segments are in the same orientation in the DNA, rearrangement (Fig. 4.6, left panels) involves the looping-out and deletion of the DNA between two gene segments. A second mode of recombination can occur between two gene segments that have opposite transcriptional orientations. The mechanism of recombination is essentially the same, but the DNA that lies between the two gene segments meets a different fate (Fig. 4.6, right panels). When the RSSs in such cases are brought together and recombination takes place, the intervening DNA is not lost from the chromosome but is retained in an inverted orientation. This mode of recombination is less common, although such rearrangements account for about half of all V_κ to J_κ joins; because the transcriptional orientation of half of the human V_κ gene segments is opposite to that of the J_κ gene segments.

Fig. 4.6 V-region gene segments are joined by recombination. In every V-region recombination event, the recombination signal sequences (RSSs) flanking the gene segments are brought together to allow recombination to take place. For simplicity, the recombination of a light-chain gene is illustrated; for the heavy-chain gene, two separate recombination events are required to generate a functional V region. In some cases, as shown in the left panels, the V and J gene segments have the same transcriptional orientation. Juxtaposition of the RSSs results in the looping out of the intervening DNA. The 12-bp-spaced RSSs are shown in orange, the 23-bp-spaced RSSs in purple. Recombination occurs at the ends of the heptamer sequences in the RSSs, creating a signal joint and releasing the intervening DNA in the form of a closed circle. Subsequently, the joining of the V and J gene segments creates the coding joint. In other cases, illustrated in the right panels, the V and J gene segments are initially oriented in opposite transcriptional directions. Bringing together the RSSs in this case requires a more complex looping of the DNA. Joining the ends of the two heptamer sequences now results in the inversion and integration of the intervening DNA. Again, the joining of the V and J segments creates a functional V-region exon.

RAG protein complexes bind to 12 and 23 bp spaced recombination signal sequences (RSSs)

The protein complexes bind to each other, bringing together the segments to be joined

The DNA is cleaved to create hairpin structures at the ends of the immunoglobulin gene segments

Other proteins (Ku70:Ku80, and DNA-dependent protein kinases) bind to the hairpins and the cleaved RSS ends

The DNA hairpins are cleaved at random. Additional bases may be added by terminal deoxynucleotidyl transferase (TdT) or subtracted by exonuclease to generate imprecise ends

DNA ligase IV, along with XRCC4, joins the ends of the gene segments to form the coding joint and the RSS ends to form the signal joint

coding joint

signal joint

4-5   The reaction that recombines V, D, and J gene segments involves both lymphocyte-specific and ubiquitous DNA-modifying enzymes.

The molecular mechanism of V-region DNA rearrangement, or **V(D)J recombination**, is illustrated in Fig. 4.7. The two RSSs are brought together by interactions between proteins that specifically recognize the length of spacer and thus enforce the 12/23 rule for recombination. The DNA molecule is then broken in two places and rejoined in a different configuration. The ends of the heptamer sequences are joined precisely in a head-to-head fashion to form a **signal joint**; when the joining segments are in direct orientation, the signal joint is in a circular piece of extrachromosomal DNA (see Fig. 4.6, left panels), which is lost from the genome when the cell divides. The V and J gene segments, which remain on the chromosome, join to form what is called the **coding joint**. As we shall discuss, this junction is imprecise, and consequently generates much additional variability in the V-region sequence.

The complex of enzymes that act in concert to carry out somatic V(D)J recombination is termed the **V(D)J recombinase**. The products of the two genes *RAG-1* and *RAG-2* (**recombination-activating genes**) comprise the lymphoid-specific components of the recombinase. This pair of genes is expressed in developing lymphocytes only while they are engaged in assembling their antigen receptors, as described in more detail in Chapter 7. They are essential for V(D)J recombination. Indeed, these genes, when expressed together, are sufficient to confer on nonlymphoid cells such as fibroblasts the capacity to rearrange exogenous segments of DNA that contain appropriate RSSs; this is how *RAG-1* and *RAG-2* were initially discovered.

Although the RAG proteins are required for V(D)J recombination, they are not the only enzymes in the recombinase. The remaining enzymes are ubiquitously expressed DNA-modifying proteins that are involved in double-stranded DNA repair, DNA bending, or the modification of the ends of the broken DNA strands. They include the enzyme DNA ligase IV, the enzyme DNA-dependent protein kinase (DNA-PK), Ku, a well-known autoantigen, which is a heterodimer (Ku70:Ku80) that associates tightly with DNA-PK, and Artemis, a protein involved in the opening of covalently closed DNA 'hairpin' structures.

Fig. 4.7 Enzymatic steps in the rearrangement of immunoglobulin gene segments. Rearrangement begins with the binding of RAG-1, RAG-2, and high-mobility group (HMG) proteins (not shown). These RAG-1:RAG-2 complexes (domes, colored light orange or light purple for clarity although they are identical at each recombination site) recognize the recombination signal sequences (arrows) flanking the coding sequences to be joined (red and yellow rectangles). These are then brought together (second panel), following which the RAG complex is activated to cut one strand of the double-stranded DNA precisely at the end of the heptamer sequences (third panel). The 30hydroxyl group of the cut end of this DNA strand then reacts with the complementary uncut strand, forming a hairpin on the coding end and leaving a double-stranded break at the end of the heptamer sequence. Subsequently, through the action of additional essential proteins such as Ku70:Ku80 (indicated in blue) that join the complex (fourth panel) along with the RAG proteins, the DNA hairpin is cleaved at a random site to yield either a flush or single-strand extended DNA end (depending on the exact site of hairpin cleavage). This end is then modified by the action of TdT and exonuclease (indicated in pink, fifth panel), which randomly creates diverse, imprecise ends. Finally (sixth panel) the two heptamer sequences, which are not modified, are ligated to form the precise signal joint, while the coding joint is also ligated, both by the action of DNA ligase IV.

V(D)J recombination is a multistep enzymatic process in which the first re-action is an endonucleolytic cleavage requiring the coordinated activity of both RAG proteins. Initially, two RAG protein complexes, each containing RAG-1, RAG-2, and high-mobility group proteins, recognize and align the two RSSs that target the cleavage reaction (see Fig. 4.7). RAG-1 is thought to specifically recognize the nonamer of the RSS. At this stage, the 12/23 rule is established through mechanisms that are still poorly understood. The endonuclease activity of the RAG protein complexes then makes two sin-gle-strand DNA breaks at sites just 5′ of each bound RSS, leaving a free 3′-OH group at the end of each coding segment. This 3′-OH group then attacks the phosphodiester bond on the other strand, creating a DNA 'hair-pin' at the end of the gene segment coding region. This process simultane-ously creates a flush double-stranded break at the ends of the two heptamer signal sequences. The DNA ends do not float apart, however, but are held tightly in a complex by the RAG proteins and other associated DNA repair enzymes until the join is completed. The two RSSs are precisely joined to form the signal joint. Coding joint formation is more complex. First, the DNA hairpin is nicked open by a single-stranded break. It is not clear whether this step is accomplished by the RAG proteins or by Artemis. The nicking can happen at various points along the hairpin, which leads to sequence variability in the eventual joint. The DNA repair enzymes in the complex then modify the opened hairpins by removing nucleotides by ex-onuclease activity and by randomly adding nucleotides, using the enzyme **terminal deoxynucleotidyl transferase, TdT**. It is not known whether addi-tion and deletion of nucleotides at the ends of coding regions occur simul-taneously or in a defined order. Finally, DNA ligase IV joins the processed ends together, thus reconstituting a chromosome that includes the re-arranged gene. This enzymatic process creates diversity in the joint be-tween gene segments (see Section 4-8), while ensuring that the RSS ends are ligated without modification and that unintended genetic damage such as a chromosomal break is avoided.

The recombination mechanism controlled by the RAG proteins shares many interesting features with the mechanism by which retroviral integrases cat-alyze the insertion of retroviral DNA into the genome, and also with the transposition mechanism used by transposons (mobile genetic elements that encode their own transposase, allowing them to excise and reinsert themselves in the genome). Even the structure of the *RAG* genes themselves, which lie close together in the chromosome and lack the usual mammalian introns, is reminiscent of a transposon. Indeed, it has recently been shown that the RAG complex can act as a transposase *in vitro*. These features have provoked speculation that the RAG complex originated as a transposase whose function was adapted by vertebrates to allow V gene segment recom-bination, thus leading to the advent of the vertebrate adaptive immune sys-tem. Consistent with this idea, no genes homologous to the *RAG* genes have been found in nonvertebrates.

The *in vivo* roles of the enzymes involved in V(D)J recombination have been established through natural or artificially induced mutations. Mice in which either of the *RAG* genes is knocked out suffer a complete block in lymphocyte development at the gene-rearrangement stage. Mice lacking TdT do not add extra nucleotides to the joints between gene segments. A mutation that was discovered some time ago results in mice that make only trivial numbers of B and T cells. Such mice suffer from a **s**evere **c**ombined **i**mmune **d**eficiency— hence the name *scid* for this mutation. These mice have subsequently been found to have a mutation in the enzyme DNA-PK that prevents the efficient rejoining of DNA at gene segment junctions. Mutations of other proteins that are involved in DNA joining also give the *scid* phenotype.

4-6 The diversity of the immunoglobulin repertoire is generated by four main processes.

The gene rearrangement that combines two or three gene segments to form a complete V-region exon generates diversity in two ways. First, there are multiple different copies of each type of gene segment, and different combinations of gene segments can be used in different rearrangement events. This **combinatorial diversity** is responsible for a substantial part of the diversity of the heavy- and light-chain V regions. Second, **junctional diversity** is introduced at the joints between the different gene segments as a result of addition and subtraction of nucleotides by the recombination process. A third source of diversity is also combinatorial, arising from the many possible different combinations of heavy- and light-chain V regions that pair to form the antigen-binding site in the immunoglobulin molecule. The two means of generating combinatorial diversity alone could give rise, in theory, to approximately 1.9×10^6 different antibody molecules (see Section 4-7). Coupled with junctional diversity, it is estimated that as many as 10^{11} different receptors could make up the repertoire of receptors expressed by naive B cells. Finally, somatic hypermutation introduces point mutations into the rearranged V-region genes of activated B cells, creating further diversity that can be selected for enhanced binding to antigen. We will discuss these mechanisms at greater length in the following sections.

4-7 The multiple inherited gene segments are used in different combinations.

There are multiple copies of the V, D, and J gene segments, each of which is capable of contributing to an immunoglobulin V region. Many different V regions can therefore be made by selecting different combinations of these segments. For human κ light chains, there are approximately 40 functional V_κ gene segments and five J_κ gene segments, and thus potentially 200 different V_κ regions. For λ light chains there are approximately 30 functional V_λ gene segments and four J_λ gene segments, yielding 120 possible V_λ regions. So, in all, 320 different light chains can be made as a result of combining different light-chain gene segments. For the heavy chains of humans, there are 40 functional V_H gene segments, approximately 25 D_H gene segments, and six J_H gene segments, and thus around 6000 different possible V_H regions ($40 \times 25 \times 6 \approx 6000$). During B-cell development, rearrangement at the heavy-chain gene locus to produce any one of the possible heavy chains is followed by several rounds of cell division before light-chain gene rearrangement takes place. The particular combination of gene segments used to produce a heavy chain does not seem to restrict substantially the choice of gene segments that can be recombined to assemble a light-chain variable region. Because both the heavy- and the light-chain V regions contribute to antibody specificity, each of the 320 different light chains could be combined with each of the approximately 6000 heavy chains to give around 1.9×10^6 different antibody specificities. This theoretical estimate of combinatorial diversity is based on the number of germline V gene segments contributing to functional antibodies (see Fig. 4.3); the total number of V gene segments is larger, but the additional gene segments are pseudogenes and do not appear in expressed immunoglobulin molecules.

In practice, combinatorial diversity is likely to be less than one might expect from the theoretical calculations above. One reason for this is that not all V gene segments are used at the same frequency; some are common in antibodies, while others are found only rarely. Also, not every heavy chain can pair with every light chain: certain combinations of V_H and V_L regions result in failure to assemble a stable immunoglobulin molecule. Cells that have heavy and light chains that cannot pair may continue to undergo light-chain gene rearrangement until a suitable light chain is produced, or may be eliminated, but in both cases a heavy- and light-chain combination that does not pair is lost from the repertoire. Nevertheless, it is thought that most heavy and light chains can pair with each other, and that this type of combinatorial diversity has a major role in the formation of an immunoglobulin repertoire with a wide range of specificities.

4-8 Variable addition and subtraction of nucleotides at the junctions between gene segments contributes to the diversity of the third hypervariable region.

Of the three hypervariable loops in the protein chains of immunoglobulins, two are encoded within the V gene segment DNA. The third (HV3 or CDR3, see Fig. 3.6) falls at the joint between the V gene segment and the J gene segment, and in the heavy chain is partly encoded by the D gene segment. In both heavy and light chains, the diversity of CDR3 is significantly increased by the addition and deletion of nucleotides at two steps in the formation of the junctions between gene segments. The added nucleotides are known as **P-nucleotides** and **N-nucleotides** and their addition is illustrated in Fig. 4.8.

P-nucleotides are so called because they make up palindromic sequences added to the ends of the gene segments. After the formation of the DNA hairpins as described in Section 4-5, the recombinase protein complex, possibly through the action of the Artemis protein, catalyzes a single-stranded cleavage at a random point within the coding sequence but near the original point at which the hairpin was first formed. When this cleavage occurs at a different point from the initial break, a single-stranded tail is formed from a few nucleotides of the coding sequence plus the complementary nucleotides from the other DNA strand (see Fig. 4.8). In most light-chain gene rearrangements, DNA repair enzymes then fill in complementary nucleotides on the single-stranded tails, which would leave short palindromic sequences at the joint if the ends were rejoined without any further exonuclease activity (see below). In heavy-chain gene rearrangements and in some human light-chain genes, however, N-nucleotides are first added by a quite different mechanism.

Fig. 4.8 The introduction of P- and N-nucleotides at the joints between gene segments during immunoglobulin gene rearrangement. The process is illustrated for a D_H to J_H rearrangement; however, the same steps occur in V_H to D_H and in V_L to J_L rearrangements. After formation of the DNA hairpins (first and second panels), the two heptamer sequences are ligated to form the signal joint (not shown here), while RAG proteins cleave the DNA hairpin at a random site to yield a single-stranded DNA end (third panel). Depending on the site of cleavage, this single-stranded DNA may contain nucleotides that were originally complementary in the double-stranded DNA and which therefore form short DNA palindromes, as indicated by the blue-shaded box. Such stretches of nucleotides that originate from the complementary strand are known as P-nucleotides. For example, the sequence GA at the end of the D segment shown is complementary to the preceding sequence TC. Where the enzyme terminal deoxynucleotidyl transferase (TdT) is present, nucleotides are added at random to the ends of the single-stranded segments (fourth panel), indicated by the shaded box surrounding these nontemplated, or N, nucleotides. The two single-stranded ends then pair (fifth panel). Exonuclease trimming of unpaired nucleotides (sixth panel) and repair of the coding joint by DNA synthesis and ligation (bottom panel) leaves both the P- and N-nucleotides present in the final coding joint (indicated by shading in the bottom panel). The randomness of insertion of P- and N-nucleotides makes an individual P-N region a valuable marker for following an individual B-cell clone as it develops, for instance in studies of somatic hypermutation (see Fig. 4.9).

N-nucleotides are so called because they are nontemplate-encoded. They are added by the enzyme TdT to single-stranded ends of the coding DNA after hairpin cleavage. After the addition of up to 20 nucleotides by this enzyme, the two single-stranded stretches at the ends of the gene segments form base pairs over a short region. Repair enzymes then trim off any nonmatching bases, synthesize complementary bases to fill in the remaining single-stranded DNA, and ligate it to the P-nucleotides (see Fig. 4.8). N-nucleotides are found especially in the V–D and D–J junctions of the assembled heavy-chain gene; they are less common in light-chain genes because TdT is maximally expressed during the period in B-cell development when the assembly of the heavy-chain gene takes place (see Chapter 7), which occurs before light-chain gene segment rearrangement.

Nucleotides can also be deleted at gene segment junctions. This is accomplished by as-yet-unidentified exonucleases. Thus, the length of heavy-chain CDR3 can be even shorter than the smallest D segment. In some instances it is difficult, if not impossible, to recognize the D segment that contributed to CDR3 formation because of the excision of most of its nucleotides. Deletions may also erase the traces of P-nucleotide palindromes introduced at the time of hairpin opening. For this reason, many completed V(D)J joins do not show obvious evidence of P-nucleotides.

As the total number of nucleotides added by these processes is random, the added nucleotides often disrupt the reading frame of the coding sequence beyond the joint. Such frameshifts will lead to a nonfunctional protein, and DNA rearrangements leading to such disruptions are known as **nonproductive rearrangements**. As roughly two in every three rearrangements will be nonproductive, many B-cell progenitors never succeed in producing functional immunoglobulin molecules and therefore never become mature B cells. Thus, junctional diversity is achieved only at the expense of considerable wastage. We will discuss this further in Chapter 7.

4-9   Rearranged V genes are further diversified by somatic hypermutation.

The mechanisms for generating diversity described so far all take place during the rearrangement of gene segments in the initial development of B cells in the central lymphoid organs. There is an additional mechanism that generates diversity throughout the V region and that operates on B cells in peripheral lymphoid organs after functional immunoglobulin genes have been assembled. This process, known as **somatic hypermutation**, introduces point mutations into the V regions of the rearranged heavy- and light-chain genes at a very high rate, giving rise to mutant B-cell receptors on the surface of the B cells (Fig. 4.9).

In mice and humans, somatic hypermutation occurs only when B cells respond to antigen along with signals from activated T cells. The immunoglobulin C-region gene, and other genes expressed in the B cell, are not affected, whereas the rearranged V_H and V_L genes are mutated even if they are nonproductive rearrangements and are not expressed. The pattern of nucleotide base changes in nonproductive V-region genes illustrates the result of somatic hypermutation without selection for enhanced binding to antigen. The base changes are distributed throughout the V region, but not completely randomly: there are certain 'hotspots' of mutation that indicate a preference for characteristic short motifs of four or five nucleotides, and perhaps also certain ill-defined secondary structural features. The pattern of base changes in the V regions of expressed immunoglobulin genes is different. Mutations that alter amino-acid sequences in the conserved framework regions will tend to disrupt basic antibody structure and are selected against. Some of the mutant immunoglobulin molecules bind antigen better than the original B-cell

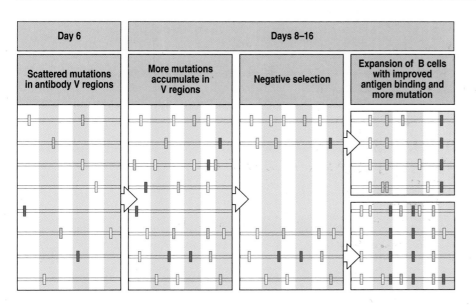

Day 6	Days 8–16		
Scattered mutations in antibody V regions	More mutations accumulate in V regions	Negative selection	Expansion of B cells with improved antigen binding and more mutation

Fig. 4.9 Somatic hypermutation introduces variation into the rearranged immunoglobulin variable region that is subject to negative and positive selection to yield improved antigen binding. In some circumstances it is possible to follow the process of somatic hypermutation by sequencing immunoglobulin variable regions at different time points after immunization. The result of one such experiment is depicted here. Within a few days of immunization, it is found that the variable regions within a particular clone of responding B cells have begun to acquire mutations (first panel). Each variable region is represented by a horizontal line, on which the positions of the mutations are represented by vertical bars. These may be silent (yellow bars), neutral (pink bars), deleterious (red bars), or positive (blue bars). Over the course of the next week, more mutations accumulate (second panel). Those B cells whose variable regions have accumulated deleterious mutations and can no longer bind antigen die, a process of negative selection (third panel). Those B cells whose variable regions have acquired mutations that result in improved antigen binding are able to compete effectively for binding to the antigen, and receive signals that drive their proliferation and expansion, along with continued mutation (fourth panel). This process of mutation and selection can actually go through multiple cycles (not shown for simplicity) during the second and third weeks of the germinal center reaction. In this way, over time, the antigen-binding efficiency of the antibody response is improved.

receptors, and B cells expressing them are preferentially selected to mature into antibody-secreting cells. This gives rise to a phenomenon called **affinity maturation** of the antibody population, which we will discuss in more detail in Chapters 9 and 10. The result of selection for enhanced binding to antigen is that base changes that alter amino-acid sequences, and thus protein structure, tend to be clustered in the CDRs, whereas silent mutations that preserve amino-acid sequence and do not alter protein structure are scattered throughout the V region.

The mechanism of somatic hypermutation is poorly defined, but several recent discoveries shed some light. It is known that mutation requires the presence of **enhancers**, DNA sequences that enhance the transcription of immunoglobulin genes in B cells, as well as a transcriptional promoter. The promoter, and the sequences that are the target of mutation, need not derive from immunoglobulin V genes, however. It has been shown experimentally that hypermutation can occur in any sequence as long as there is an active promoter and an immunoglobulin enhancer. Thus, specific sequences that target a gene for mutation must lie within the immunoglobulin enhancer, and the identity of these is currently being defined. In addition, it has recently been discovered that deficiency of an enzyme called **activation-induced cytidine deaminase (AID)** blocks the accumulation of somatic hypermutations. The mechanism by which this enzyme contributes to hypermutation is rapidly being clarified. Although it was originally thought to be an RNA-editing enzyme (on the basis of homology with other known RNA-editing enzymes), it turns out that AID can deaminate DNA directly at cytosine. Depending on how this DNA lesion is repaired, it can lead to a permanent base change at the deaminated site. This mechanism explains some of the known biases of somatic hypermutation such as transition-type mutations from C to T or G to A. More difficult to explain is how DNA deamination at C residues explains mutations at A–T base pairs, also common in somatic hypermutation. It is possible that when repair mechanisms are triggered by the initial base-pair mismatch at a deaminated C residue, nicks in DNA are created and there is error-prone repair leading to mutation at adjacent A–T base pairs. The relationship between these mechanisms and double-stranded DNA breaks, which are also associated with mutating V regions, is unknown. Interestingly, a deficiency of AID enzyme also abrogates the rearrangement of C-region genes that underlies the immunoglobulin class switching seen in activated B cells (see Section 4-18).

Activation-induced Cytidine Deaminase (AID) Deficiency

Fig. 4.10 The diversification of chicken immunoglobulins occurs through gene conversion. In chickens, all B cells express the same surface immunoglobulin (sIg) initially; there is only one active V, D, and J gene segment for the chicken heavy-chain gene and one active V and J gene segment for each of the light-chain genes (top left panel). Gene rearrangement can thus produce only a single receptor specificity. Immature B cells expressing this receptor migrate to the bursa of Fabricius, where the expression of sIg induces cell proliferation (center panels). Gene conversion events introduce sequences from adjacent V pseudogenes into the expressed gene, creating diversity in the receptors (bottom panels). Some of these gene conversions will inactivate the previously expressed gene (not shown). If a B cell can no longer express sIg after such a gene conversion, it is eliminated.

4-10   In some species, most immunoglobulin gene diversification occurs after gene rearrangement.

In birds, rabbits, cows, pigs, sheep, and horses there is little or no germline diversity in the V, D, and J gene segments that are rearranged to form the genes for the initial B-cell receptors, and the rearranged V-region sequences are identical or similar in most immature B cells. These B cells then migrate to specialized microenvironments, the best known of which is the bursa of Fabricius in chickens. Here, B cells proliferate rapidly, and their rearranged immunoglobulin genes undergo further diversification. In birds and rabbits this occurs by a process that includes **gene conversion**, in which an upstream V segment pseudogene exchanges short sequences with the expressed rearranged V-region gene (Fig. 4.10). It seems that gene conversion is related to somatic hypermutation in its mechanism, because gene conversion in a chicken B-cell line has been shown to require AID. In sheep and cows, diversification is the result of somatic hypermutation, which occurs in an organ known as the ileal Peyer's patch. Somatic hypermutation, independent of T cells and a particular driving antigen, also contributes to immunoglobulin diversification in birds, sheep, and rabbits.

Summary.

The extraordinary diversity of the immunoglobulin repertoire is achieved in several ways. Perhaps the most important factor that enables this diversity is that V regions are encoded by separate gene segments, which are brought together by somatic recombination to make a complete V-region gene. Many different V-region gene segments are present in the genome of an individual, and provide a heritable source of diversity. The RAG proteins are the unique lymphocyte-specific factors that are absolutely required to catalyze this rearrangement process. The evolution of RAG proteins, which coincided with the appearance of the modern vertebrate adaptive immune system, enabled this strategy—combinatorial diversity—in which the random recombination of separate V, D, and J gene segments forms a complete V-region exon. A substantial fraction of the functional diversity of immunoglobulins comes from the joining process itself. Variability at the joints between segments is generated by the insertion of random numbers of P- and N-nucleotides and by variable deletion of nucleotides at the ends of some coding sequences. The association of different light- and heavy-chain V regions to form the antigen-binding site of an immunoglobulin molecule contributes further diversity. Finally, after an immunoglobulin has been expressed, the coding sequences for its V regions are modified by somatic hypermutation upon stimulation of the B cell by antigen and in some species via mutation that occurs before antigen stimulation. The combination of all these sources of diversity generates a vast repertoire of antibody specificities from a relatively limited number of genes.

T-cell receptor gene rearrangement.

The mechanism by which B-cell antigen receptors are generated is such a powerful means of creating diversity that it is not surprising that the antigen receptors of T cells bear structural resemblances to immunoglobulins and are generated by the same mechanism. In this part of the chapter we describe the organization of the T-cell receptor loci and the generation of the genes for the individual T-cell receptor chains.

4-11   The T-cell receptor gene segments are arranged in a similar pattern to immunoglobulin gene segments and are rearranged by the same enzymes.

Like immunoglobulin light and heavy chains, T-cell receptor α and β chains each consist of a variable (V) amino-terminal region and a constant (C) region (see Section 3-10). The organization of the TCRα and TCRβ loci is shown in Fig. 4.11. The organization of the gene segments is broadly homologous to

Fig. 4.11 The germline organization of the human T-cell receptor α and β loci. The arrangement of the gene segments resembles that at the immunoglobulin loci, with separate variable (V), diversity (D), joining (J) gene segments, and constant (C) genes. The TCRα locus (chromosome 14) consists of 70–80 V_α gene segments, each preceded by an exon encoding the leader sequence (L). How many of these V_α gene segments are functional is not known exactly. A cluster of 61 J_α gene segments is located a considerable distance from the V_α gene segments. The J_α gene segments are followed by a single C gene, which contains separate exons for the constant and hinge domains and a single exon encoding the transmembrane and cytoplasmic regions (not shown). The TCRβ locus (chromosome 7) has a different organization, with a cluster of 52 functional V_β gene segments located distantly from two separate clusters each containing a single D gene segment together with six or seven J gene segments and a single C gene. Each TCRβ C gene has separate exons encoding the constant domain, the hinge, the transmembrane region, and the cytoplasmic region (not shown). The TCRα locus is interrupted between the J and V gene segments by another T-cell receptor locus—the TCRδ locus (not shown here; see Fig. 4.15).

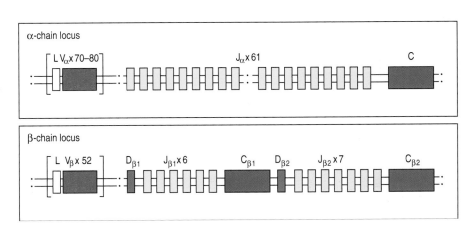

that of the immunoglobulin gene segments (see Sections 4-2 and 4-3). The TCRα locus, like those for the immunoglobulin light chains, contains V and J gene segments (V_α and J_α). The TCRβ locus, like that for the immunoglobulin heavy chain, contains D gene segments in addition to V_β and J_β gene segments.

The T-cell receptor gene segments rearrange during T-cell development to form complete V-domain exons (Fig. 4.12). T-cell receptor gene rearrangement takes place in the thymus; the order and regulation of the rearrangements will be dealt with in detail in Chapter 7. Essentially, however, the mechanics of gene rearrangement are similar for B and T cells. The T-cell receptor gene segments are flanked by heptamer and nonamer recombination signal sequences (RSSs) that are homologous to those flanking immunoglobulin gene segments (see Section 4-4 and Fig. 4.5) and are recognized by the same enzymes. The DNA circles resulting from gene rearrangement (see Fig. 4.6) are known as T-cell receptor rearrangement circles (TRECs) and are used as markers for T cells of thymic origin. All known defects in genes that control V(D)J recombination affect T cells and B cells equally, and animals with these genetic defects lack functional lymphocytes altogether (see Section 4-5). A further shared feature of immunoglobulin and T-cell receptor gene rearrangement is the presence of P- and N-nucleotides in the junctions between the V, D, and J gene segments of the rearranged TCRβ gene. In T cells, P- and N-nucleotides are also added between the V and J gene segments of all rearranged TCRα genes, whereas only about half the V–J joints in immunoglobulin light-chain genes are modified by N-nucleotide addition and these are often left without any P-nucleotides as well (Fig. 4.13, and see Section 4-8).

The main differences between the immunoglobulin genes and those encoding T-cell receptors reflect the fact that all the effector functions of B cells depend upon secreted antibodies whose different heavy-chain C-region isotypes trigger distinct effector mechanisms. The effector functions of T cells, in contrast, depend upon cell–cell contact and are not mediated directly by

Fig. 4.12 T-cell receptor α- and β-chain gene rearrangement and expression. The TCRα- and β-chain genes are composed of discrete segments that are joined by somatic recombination during development of the T cell. Functional α- and β-chain genes are generated in the same way that complete immunoglobulin genes are created. For the α chain (upper part of figure), a V_α gene segment rearranges to a J_α gene segment to create a functional V-region exon. Transcription and splicing of the VJ_α exon to C_α generates the mRNA that is translated to yield the T-cell receptor α-chain protein. For the β chain (lower part of figure), like the immunoglobulin heavy chain, the variable domain is encoded in three gene segments, V_β, D_β, and J_β. Rearrangement of these gene segments generates a functional VDJ_β V-region exon that is transcribed and spliced to join to C_β; the resulting mRNA is translated to yield the T-cell receptor β chain. The α and β chains pair soon after their synthesis to yield the α:β T-cell receptor heterodimer. Not all J gene segments are shown, and the leader sequences preceding each V gene segment are omitted for simplicity.

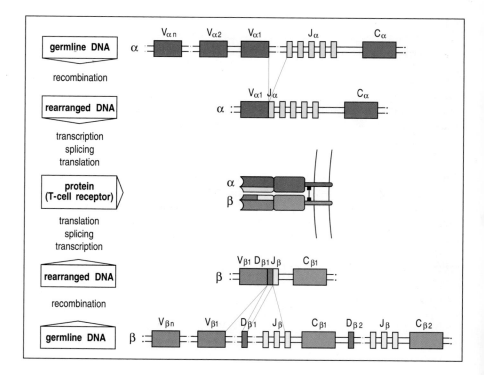

Element	Immunoglobulin		α:β T-cell receptors	
	H	κ+λ	β	α
Variable segments (V)	40	70	52	~70
Diversity segments (D)	25	0	2	0
D segments read in three frames	rarely	–	often	–
Joining segments (J)	6	5(κ) 4(λ)	13	61
Joints with N- and P-nucleotides	2	50% of joints	2	1
Number of V gene pairs	1.9×10^6		5.8×10^6	
Junctional diversity	$\sim 3 \times 10^7$		$\sim 2 \times 10^{11}$	
Total diversity	$\sim 5 \times 10^{13}$		$\sim 10^{18}$	

Fig. 4.13 The numbers of human T-cell receptor gene segments and the sources of T-cell receptor diversity compared with those of immunoglobulins. Note that only about half of human κ chains contain N-nucleotides. Somatic hypermutation as a source of diversity in immunoglobulins is not included in this figure.

the T-cell receptor, which serves only for antigen recognition. Thus, the C regions of the TCRα and TCRβ loci are much simpler than those of the immunoglobulin heavy-chain locus. There is only one C_α gene and, although there are two C_β genes, they are very closely homologous and there is no known functional distinction between their products. The T-cell receptor C-region genes encode only transmembrane polypeptides.

4-12   T-cell receptors concentrate diversity in the third hypervariable region.

The three-dimensional structure of the antigen-recognition site of a T-cell receptor looks much like that of an antibody molecule (see Sections 3-11 and 3-7, respectively). In an antibody, the center of the antigen-binding site is formed by the CDR3s of the heavy and light chains. The structurally equivalent third hypervariable loops (CDR3s) of the T-cell receptor α and β chains, to which the D and J gene segments contribute, also form the center of the antigen-binding site of a T-cell receptor; the periphery of the site consists of the CDR1 and CDR2 loops, which are encoded within the germline V gene segments for the α and β chains.

The extent and pattern of variability in T-cell receptors and immunoglobulins reflect the distinct nature of their ligands. Whereas the antigen-binding sites of immunoglobulins must conform to the surfaces of an almost infinite variety of different antigens, and thus come in a wide variety of shapes and chemical properties, the ligand for the major class of human T-cell receptor (α:β) is always a peptide bound to an MHC molecule. As a group, the antigen-recognition sites of T-cell receptors would therefore be predicted to have a less variable shape, with most of the variability focused on the bound antigenic peptide occupying the center of the surface in contact with the receptor. Indeed, the less variable CDR1 and CDR2 loops of a T-cell receptor will mainly contact the relatively less variable MHC component of the ligand, whereas the highly variable CDR3 regions will mainly contact the unique peptide component (Fig. 4.14).

Fig. 4.14 The most variable parts of the T-cell receptor interact with the peptide bound to an MHC molecule. The positions of the CDR loops of a T-cell receptor are shown as colored tubes, which in this figure are superimposed onto the MHC:peptide complex (gray). The CDR1 loops of the α and β chains of the TCR are shown in turquoise and dark blue respectively, the CDR2 loops in fawn and yellow respectively, and the CDR3 loops in magenta and red. The CDR3 loops lie in the center of the interface between the TCR and the MHC:peptide complex, and make direct contacts with the antigenic peptide.

The structural diversity of T-cell receptors is attributable mainly to combinatorial and junctional diversity generated during the process of gene rearrangement. It can be seen from Fig. 4.13 that the variability in T-cell receptor chains is focused on the junctional region encoded by V, D, and J gene segments and modified by P- and N-nucleotides. The TCRα locus contains many more J gene segments than either of the immunoglobulin light-chain loci: in humans, 61 J_α gene segments are distributed over about 80 kb of DNA, whereas immunoglobulin light-chain loci have only five J gene segments at most (see Fig. 4.13). Because the TCRα locus has so many J gene segments, the variability generated in this region is even greater for T-cell receptors than for immunoglobulins. Thus, most of the diversity resides in the CDR3 loops that form the center of the antigen-binding site.

4-13   γ:δ T-cell receptors are also generated by gene rearrangement.

A minority of T cells bear T-cell receptors composed of γ and δ chains (see Section 3-19). The organization of the TCRγ and TCRδ loci (Fig. 4.15) resembles that of the TCRα and TCRβ loci, although there are important differences. The cluster of gene segments encoding the δ chain is found entirely within the TCRα locus, between the V_α and the J_α gene segments. Because all V_α gene segments are oriented such that rearrangement will delete the intervening DNA, any rearrangement at the α locus results in the loss of the δ locus. There are substantially fewer V gene segments at the TCRγ and TCRδ loci than at either the TCRα or TCRβ loci or any of the immunoglobulin loci. Increased junctional variability in the δ chains may compensate for the small number of V gene segments and has the effect of focusing almost all the variability in the γ:δ receptor in the junctional region. As we have seen, the amino acids encoded by the junctional regions lie at the center of the T-cell receptor binding site.

T cells bearing γ:δ receptors are a distinct lineage of T cells whose functions are at present unclear. The ligands for these receptors are also largely unknown (see Section 3-19). Some γ:δ T-cell receptors seem to be able to recognize

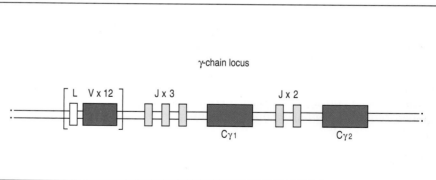

Fig. 4.15 The organization of the T-cell receptor γ- and δ-chain loci in humans. The TCRγ and TCRδ loci, like the TCRα and TCRβ loci, have discrete V, D, and J gene segments, and C genes. Uniquely, the locus encoding the δ chain is located entirely within the α-chain locus. The three D_δ gene segments, three J_δ gene segments, and the single δ C gene lie between the cluster of V_α gene segments and the cluster of J_α gene segments. There are two V_δ gene segments located near the δ C gene, one just upstream of the D regions and one in inverted orientation just downstream of the C gene (not shown). In addition, there are 6 V_δ gene segments interspersed among the V_α gene segments. Five are shared with V_α and can be used by either locus and one which is unique to the δ locus. The human TCRγ locus resembles the TCRβ locus in having two C genes each with its own set of J gene segments. The mouse γ locus (not shown) has a more complex organization and there are three functional clusters of γ gene segments, each containing V and J gene segments and a C gene. Rearrangement at the γ and δ loci proceeds as for the other T-cell receptor loci, with the exception that during TCRδ rearrangement both D segments can be used in the same gene. The use of two D segments greatly increases the variability of the δ chain, mainly because extra N-region nucleotides can be added at the junction between the two D gene segments as well as at the V–D and D–J junctions.

antigen directly, much as antibodies do, without the requirement for presentation by an MHC molecule or processing of the antigen. Detailed analysis of the rearranged V regions of γ:δ T-cell receptors shows that they resemble the V regions of antibody molecules more than they resemble the V regions of α:β T-cell receptors.

4-14 Somatic hypermutation does not generate diversity in T-cell receptors.

When we discussed the generation of antibody diversity in Section 4-9, we saw that somatic hypermutation increases the diversity of all three complementarity-determining regions of both immunoglobulin chains. Somatic hypermutation does not occur in T-cell receptor genes, so that variability of the CDR1 and CDR2 regions is limited to that of the germline V gene segments. All the diversity in T-cell receptors is generated during rearrangement and is consequently focused on the CDR3 regions.

Why T-cell and B-cell receptors differ in their abilities to undergo somatic hypermutation is not clear, but several explanations can be suggested on the basis of the functional differences between T and B cells. Because the central role of T cells is to stimulate both humoral and cellular immune responses, it is crucially important that T cells do not react with self proteins. T cells that recognize self antigens are rigorously purged during development (see Chapter 7) and the absence of somatic hypermutation helps to ensure that somatic mutants recognizing self proteins do not arise later in the course of immune responses. This constraint does not apply with the same force to B-cell receptors, as B cells usually require T-cell help to secrete antibodies. A B cell whose receptor mutates to become self-reactive would, under normal circumstances, fail to make antibody for lack of self-reactive T cells to provide this help (see Chapter 9).

A further argument is that T cells already interact with a self component, namely the MHC molecule that makes up the major part of the ligand for the receptor, and thus might be unusually prone to developing self-recognition capability through somatic hypermutation. In this case, the converse argument can also be made: because T-cell receptors must be able to recognize self-MHC molecules as part of their ligand, it is important to avoid somatic mutation that might result in the loss of recognition and the consequent loss of any ability to respond. However, the strongest argument for this difference between immunoglobulins and T-cell receptors is the simple one that somatic hypermutation is an adaptive specialization for B cells alone, because they must make very high-affinity antibodies to carry out effector functions in the extracellular fluids. We will see in Chapter 9 that they do this through somatic hypermutation followed by selection for antigen binding.

Summary.

T-cell receptors are structurally similar to immunoglobulins and are encoded by homologous genes. T-cell receptor genes are assembled by somatic recombination from sets of gene segments in the same way that the immunoglobulin genes are. Diversity is distributed differently in immunoglobulins and T-cell receptors: the T-cell receptor loci have roughly the same number of V gene segments but more J gene segments, and there is greater diversification of the junctions between gene segments during gene rearrangement. Moreover, functional T-cell receptors are not known to diversify their V genes after rearrangement through somatic hypermutation. This leads to a T-cell receptor in which the highest diversity is in the central part of the receptor, which in the case of α:β T-cell receptors contacts the bound peptide fragment of the ligand. Most of the diversity among γ:δ T-cell receptors is also in CDR3, but how this affects ligand binding is less clear because γ:δ T cells directly recognize poorly characterized ligands which in some cases are independent of MHC molecules.

Structural variation in immunoglobulin constant regions.

So far we have focused on the structural variation inherent in the assembly of the V regions of the antibody molecule and T-cell receptor. We have seen how this variation creates a diverse repertoire of antigen specificities, and we have also considered how these variable regions are attached to constant regions in the monovalent heterodimeric T-cell receptor, and the Y-shaped four-chain structure of the divalent immunoglobulin molecule. We have, however, discussed only the general structural features of the immunoglobulin C region as illustrated by IgG, the most abundant type of antibody in plasma (see Section 3-1). Immunoglobulins can be made in several different classes, or isotypes, and we next consider how this structural variation is generated by linking different heavy-chain C regions to the same variable region. The heavy-chain C regions (C_H), which determine the class or isotype of the antibody and thus its effector functions, are encoded in separate genes located downstream of the V genes at the heavy-chain locus. Initially, only the first two of these, the C_μ and C_δ genes, are expressed in conjunction with an assembled V gene. Thus naive B cells have both IgM and IgD on their surface. During the course of an antibody response, activated B cells can switch to the expression of individual downstream C_H genes by a process of somatic recombination known as isotype switching. In this part of the chapter we consider the structural features that distinguish the C_H regions of antibodies of the five major isotypes and confer on them their specialized functional properties as well as the means of isotype switching.

Unlike a T-cell receptor gene, an immunoglobulin gene can produce both a transmembrane protein product that acts as the B-cell receptor and a secreted product that acts as an antibody. We shall discuss how alternative RNA splicing allows the production of a membrane-bound and a secreted immunoglobulin with the same antigen specificity.

4-15   Transmembrane and secreted forms of immunoglobulin are generated from alternative heavy-chain transcripts.

Immunoglobulins of all heavy-chain isotypes can be produced either in secreted form or as a membrane-bound receptor. All B cells initially express the transmembrane form of IgM; after stimulation by antigen, some of their progeny differentiate into plasma cells producing the secreted form of IgM, whereas others undergo isotype switching to express transmembrane immunoglobulins of a different isotype followed by the production of secreted antibody of the new isotype.

The membrane forms of all isotypes are monomers comprising two heavy and two light chains: IgM and IgA polymerize only when they are secreted (see Section 4-20). In its membrane-bound form, the immunoglobulin heavy chain has a hydrophobic transmembrane domain of about 25 amino-acid residues at the carboxy terminus, which anchors it to the surface of the B lymphocyte. This transmembrane domain is absent from the secreted form, whose carboxy terminus is a hydrophilic secretory tail. The two different carboxy termini of the transmembrane and secreted forms of immunoglobulin heavy chains are encoded in separate exons, and production of the two forms is achieved by alternative RNA processing (Fig. 4.16). The last two exons of each C_H gene contain the sequences encoding the secreted

Fig. 4.16 Transmembrane and secreted forms of immunoglobulins are derived from the same heavy-chain sequence by alternative RNA processing. Each heavy-chain C gene has two exons (membrane-coding (MC) yellow) that encode the transmembrane region and cytoplasmic tail of the transmembrane form, and a secretion-coding (SC) sequence (orange) that encodes the carboxy terminus of the secreted form. In the case of IgD, the SC sequence is present on a separate exon, but for the other isotypes, including IgM as shown here, the SC sequence is contiguous with the last C-domain exon. The events that dictate whether a heavy-chain RNA will result in a secreted or transmembrane immunoglobulin occur during processing of the initial transcript. Each heavy-chain C gene has two potential polyadenylation sites (shown as pA_s and pA_m). In the upper panel, the transcript is cleaved and polyadenylated (AAA) at the second site (pA_m). Splicing between a site located between the $C_\mu 4$ exon and the SC sequence, and a second site at the 5' end of the MC exons, results in removal of the SC sequence and joining of the MC exons to the $C_\mu 4$ exon. This generates the transmembrane form of the heavy chain. In the lower panel, the primary transcript is cleaved and polyadenylated at the first site (pA_s), eliminating the MC exons and giving rise to the secreted form of the heavy chain. Note that the SC portion of the mRNA becomes part of the intron when splicing generates the membrane form, while it is part of the $C_\mu 4$ exon and is not spliced out when the secreted form is made.

and the transmembrane regions respectively; if the primary transcript is cleaved and polyadenylated at a site downstream of these exons, the sequence encoding the carboxy terminus of the secreted form is removed by splicing, and the cell-surface form of immunoglobulin is produced. Alternatively, if the primary transcript is cleaved at the polyadenylation site located before the last two exons, only the secreted molecule can be produced. This differential RNA processing is illustrated for C_μ in Fig. 4.16, but it occurs in the same way for all isotypes.

In activated B cells that differentiate to become antibody-secreting plasma cells, most of the transcripts are spliced to the secreted rather than the transmembrane form of whichever isotype the B cell happens to express.

4-16 The immunoglobulin heavy-chain isotypes are distinguished by the structure of their constant regions.

The five main isotypes of immunoglobulin are IgM, IgD, IgG, IgE, and IgA. In humans, IgG antibodies can be further subdivided into four subclasses (IgG1, IgG2, IgG3, and IgG4), whereas IgA antibodies are found as two subclasses (IgA1 and IgA2). The IgG isotypes in humans are named in order of their abundance in serum, with IgG1 being the most abundant. The heavy chains that define these isotypes are designated by the lower-case Greek letters μ, δ, γ, ε, and α, as shown in Fig. 4.17, which also lists the major physical properties of the different human isotypes. IgM forms pentamers in serum, which accounts for its high molecular weight. Secreted IgA can occur as either a monomer or a dimer.

Fig. 4.17 The properties of the human immunoglobulin isotypes. IgM is so called because of its size: although monomeric IgM is only 190 kDa, it normally forms pentamers, known as macroglobulin (hence the M), of very large molecular weight (see Fig. 4.18). IgA dimerizes to give a molecular weight of around 390 kDa in secretions. IgE antibody is associated with immediate-type hypersensitivity. When fixed to tissue mast cells, IgE has a much longer half-life than its half-life in plasma shown here. The activation of the alternative pathway of complement by IgA1 is caused not by its Fc portion but by its Fab portion. A subset of human V_H regions (clan 3, see Section 4-3) also binds staphylococcal Protein A through the Fab portion.

	Immunoglobulin								
	IgG1	IgG2	IgG3	IgG4	IgM	IgA1	IgA2	IgD	IgE
Heavy chain	γ_1	γ_2	γ_3	γ_4	μ	α_1	α_2	δ	ε
Molecular weight (kDa)	146	146	165	146	970	160	160	184	188
Serum level (mean adult mg ml⁻¹)	9	3	1	0.5	1.5	3.0	0.5	0.03	5×10^{-5}
Half-life in serum (days)	21	20	7	21	10	6	6	3	2
Classical pathway of complement activation	++	+	+++	−	+++	−	−	−	−
Alternative pathway of complement activation	−	−	−	−	−	+	−	−	−
Placental transfer	+++	+	++	−/+	−	−	−	−	−
Binding to macrophage and phagocyte Fc receptors	+	−	+	−/+	−	+	+	−	+
High-affinity binding to mast cells and basophils	−	−	−	−	−	−	−	−	+++
Reactivity with staphylococcal Protein A	+	+	−/+	+	−	−	−	−	−

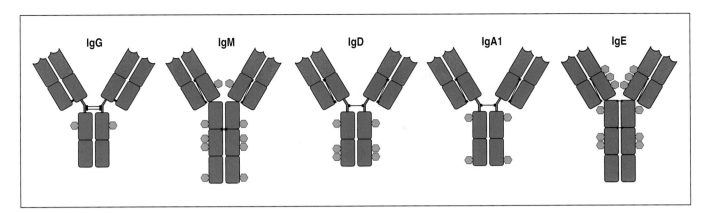

Sequence differences between immunoglobulin heavy chains cause the various isotypes to differ in several characteristic respects. These include the number and location of interchain disulfide bonds, the number of attached oligosaccharide moieties, the number of C domains (see Section 3-2), and the length of the hinge region (Fig. 4.18). IgM and IgE heavy chains contain an extra C domain that replaces the hinge region found in γ, δ, and α chains. The absence of the hinge region does not imply that IgM and IgE molecules lack flexibility; electron micrographs of IgM molecules binding to ligands show that the Fab arms can bend relative to the Fc portion. However, such a difference in structure may have functional consequences that are not yet characterized. Different isotypes and subtypes also differ in their ability to engage various effector functions, as will be described in Section 4-19.

Fig. 4.18 The structural organization of the main human immunoglobulin isotype monomers. Both IgM and IgE lack a hinge region but each contains an extra heavy-chain domain. Note the differences in the numbers and locations of the disulfide bonds (black lines) linking the chains. The isotypes also differ in the distribution of *N*-linked carbohydrate groups, shown as turquoise hexagons.

4-17 Mature naive B cells express both IgM and IgD at their surface.

The immunoglobulin C_H genes form a large cluster spanning about 200 kb to the 30side of the J_H gene segments (Fig. 4.19). Each C_H gene is split into several exons (not shown in the figure), each corresponding to an individual immunoglobulin domain in the folded C region. The gene encoding the μ C region lies closest to the J_H gene segments, and therefore closest to the assembled V-region exon after DNA rearrangement. A complete μ heavy-chain transcript is produced from the newly rearranged gene. Any J_H gene segments remaining between the assembled V gene and the $C_μ$ gene are removed during RNA processing to generate the mature mRNA. μ heavy chains are therefore the first to be expressed and IgM is the first immunoglobulin isotype to be expressed during B-cell development.

Immediately 30to the μ gene lies the δ gene, which encodes the C region of the IgD heavy chain. IgD is coexpressed with IgM on the surface of almost all mature B cells, although this isotype is secreted in only small amounts and its function is unknown. Indeed, mice lacking the $C_δ$ exons seem to have essentially normal immune systems. B cells expressing IgM and IgD have not

Fig. 4.19 The organization of the immunoglobulin heavy-chain C-region genes in mice and humans (not to scale). In humans, the cluster shows evidence of evolutionary duplication of a unit consisting of two γ genes, an ε gene, and an α gene. One of the ε genes is a pseudogene (ψ); hence only one subtype of IgE is expressed. For simplicity, other pseudogenes are not illustrated, and the exon details within each C gene are not shown. The classes of immunoglobulins found in mice are called IgM, IgD, IgG1, IgG2a, IgG2b, IgG3, IgA, and IgE.

Fig. 4.20 Coexpression of IgD and IgM is regulated by RNA processing. In mature B cells, transcription initiated at the V_H promoter extends through both C_μ and C_δ exons. This long primary transcript is then processed by cleavage and polyadenylation (AAA), and by splicing. Cleavage and polyadenylation at the µ site (pA1) and splicing between C_μ exons yields an mRNA encoding the µ heavy chain (left panel). Cleavage and polyadenylation at the δ site (pA2) and a different pattern of splicing that removes the C_μ exons yields mRNA encoding the δ heavy chain (right panel). For simplicity we have not shown all the individual C-region exons.

undergone isotype switching, which, as we will see, entails an irreversible change in the DNA. Instead, these cells produce a long primary mRNA transcript that is differentially cleaved and spliced to yield one of two distinct mRNA molecules. In one of these, the VDJ exon is linked to the C_μ exons to encode a µ heavy chain, and in the other the VDJ exon is linked to the C_δ exons to encode a δ heavy chain (Fig. 4.20). The differential processing of the long mRNA transcript is developmentally regulated, with immature B cells making mostly the µ transcript and mature B cells making mostly the δ form along with some of the µ transcript.

When a B cell is activated it ceases to coexpress IgD with IgM, either because µ and δ sequences have been removed as a consequence of an isotype switch or, in IgM-secreting plasma cells, because transcription from the V_H promoter no longer extends through the C_δ exons.

4-18 Isotype switching enables the same assembled V_H exon to be associated with different C_H genes in the course of an immune response.

The V_H-region exons expressed by any given B cell are determined during its early differentiation in the bone marrow (see Chapter 7) and, although they may subsequently be modified by somatic hypermutation, no further V(D)J recombination occurs. All the progeny of that B cell will therefore express the same assembled V_H gene. By contrast, several different C-region genes can be expressed in the B cell's progeny as the cells mature and proliferate in the course of an immune response. Every B cell begins by expressing IgM as its B-cell receptor, and the first antibody produced in an immune response is always IgM. We have already seen how IgM and IgD are expressed simultaneously in naive B cells by means of RNA processing. Later in the immune response, the same assembled V region may be expressed in IgG, IgA, or IgE antibodies. This change is known as **isotype switching** and, unlike the expression of IgD, it involves irreversible DNA recombination. It is stimulated in the course of an immune response by external signals such as cytokines released by T cells or mitogenic signals delivered by pathogens, as we will discuss further in Chapter 9. Here we are concerned with the molecular basis of the isotype switch.

Switching to the other isotypes occurs only after B cells have been stimulated by antigen. It occurs through a specialized nonhomologous DNA recombination mechanism guided by stretches of repetitive DNA known as **switch regions**. Switch regions lie in the intron between the J_H gene segments and the C_μ gene, and at equivalent sites upstream of the genes for each of the other heavy-chain isotypes, with the exception of the δ gene, the expression of which is not dependent on DNA rearrangement (Fig. 4.21, top panel).

When a B cell switches from coexpression of IgM and IgD to expression of an IgG subtype, DNA recombination occurs between S_μ and the S_γ of that IgG subtype. The C_μ and C_δ coding regions are deleted, and γ heavy-chain transcripts are made from the recombined gene. Figure 4.21 (left panels) illustrates switching to γ3 in the mouse. Some of the progeny of this IgG-producing cell may subsequently undergo a further switching event to produce a different isotype, for example IgA, as shown in the bottom panel of Fig. 4.21. Alternatively, as shown in the right panels of Fig. 4.21, the switch

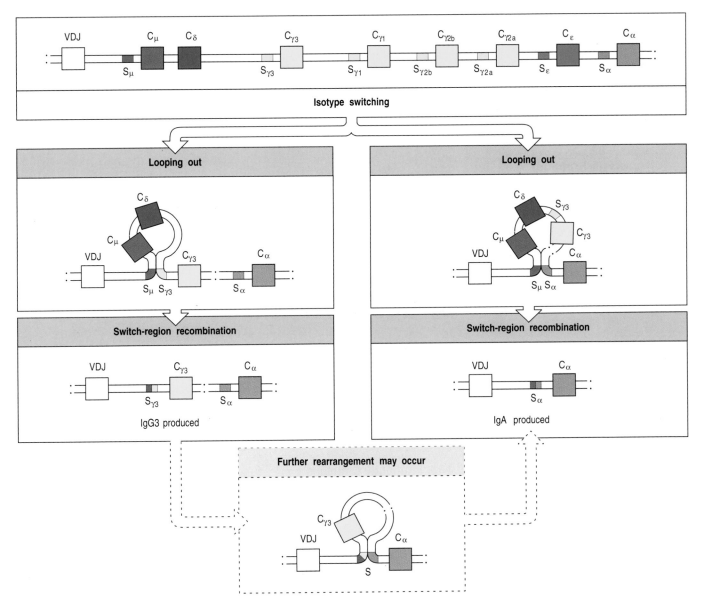

Fig. 4.21 Isotype switching involves recombination between specific switch signals. Repetitive DNA sequences that guide isotype switching are found upstream of each of the immunoglobulin C-region genes, with the exception of the δ gene. The figure illustrates switching in the mouse heavy-chain genes. Switching occurs by recombination between these repetitive sequences, or switch signals, with deletion of the intervening DNA. The initial switching event takes place from the μ switch region; switching to other isotypes can take place subsequently from the recombinant switch region formed after μ switching. S, switch region.

recombination may occur between S_μ and one of the switch regions downstream of the C_γ genes, so that the cell switches from IgM to IgA or IgE (illustrated for IgA only). All switch recombination events produce genes that can encode a functional protein because the switch sequences lie in introns and therefore cannot cause frameshift mutations.

The mechanism of isotype switching itself is not fully worked out. It is known that transcription through the switch regions, initiated from promoters upstream of the switch region, is required for efficient switching, much as transcription is required for somatic hypermutation. Another important clue comes from the switch region sequences themselves. The μ switch region (S_μ) consists of about 150 repeats of the sequence $[(GAGCT)_n(GGGGGT)]$, where n is usually 3 but can be as many as 7. The sequences of the other switch regions (S_γ, S_α, and S_ϵ) differ in detail but all contain repeats of the GAGCT and GGGGGT sequences. It is thought that the repetitive sequences might promote short stretches of homologous alignment that in turn promote DNA recombination. They may also be unique targets for the enzymatic machinery of switching. Recently, it was discovered that a lack of AID completely blocks isotype switching. As mentioned in Section 4-9, this deficiency also blocks somatic hypermutation. A deficiency in this enzyme in humans has now been associated with a form of immunodeficiency known as **hyper IgM type 2 syndrome**, which is characterized by an absence of immunoglobulins other than IgM. It seems likely that AID deaminates G–C base pairs in the switch region in an early step in the reaction, and that transcription makes the switch region accessible to AID. This in turn may allow the recruitment of generic DNA repair enzymes that catalyze the actual nonhomologous recombination required for isotype switching, promoted by the alignment of repetitive sequences shared between switch regions. Indeed, we do know that DNA repair enzymes are involved because switching is markedly reduced in mice lacking Ku proteins; Ku proteins are also essential for the rejoining of DNA during V(D)J joining (see Section 4-5). The complete story of how AID works to promote both somatic hypermutation and isotype switching has yet to be revealed.

Although they both involve DNA rearrangement and some of the same enzymatic machinery, isotype switch recombination is unlike V(D)J recombination in several ways. First, all isotype switch recombination is productive; second, it uses different recombination signal sequences and does not require the RAG enzymes; third, it happens after antigen stimulation and not during B-cell development in the bone marrow; and fourth, the switching process is not random but is directed by external signals such as those provided by T cells, as will be discussed in Chapter 9.

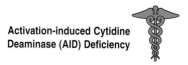

Activation-induced Cytidine Deaminase (AID) Deficiency

4-19 Antibody C regions confer functional specialization.

The secreted antibodies protect the body in a variety of ways, as we briefly outline here and discuss further in Chapter 9. In some cases it is enough for the antibody simply to bind antigen. For instance, by binding tightly to a toxin or virus, an antibody can prevent it from recognizing its receptor on a host cell. The V regions on their own are sufficient for this. The C region is essential, however, for recruiting the help of other cells and molecules to destroy and dispose of pathogens to which the antibody has bound.

The C regions (Fc portions) of antibodies have three main effector functions. First, the Fc portions of certain isotypes are recognized by specialized receptors expressed by immune effector cells. The Fc portions of IgG1 and IgG3 antibodies are recognized by **Fc receptors** present on the surface of phagocytic cells such as macrophages and neutrophils, which can thereby bind and

Fig. 4.22 Protein A of *Staphylococcus aureus* bound to a fragment of the Fc region of IgG. A fragment of the Fc portion of a single IgG heavy chain is complexed with a fragment of the immunoglobulin-binding Protein A from *Staphylococcus aureus*. The Fc fragment has two domains, C_H2 and C_H3, shown in magenta. A carbohydrate chain is attached to an asparagine residue in the C_H2 domain: all the atoms are shown and the surface is outlined in green. The fragment of Protein A (white) is bound between the two domains of the Fc fragment. The amino acids that bind to the complement component C1q (red) lie in the C_H2 domain. Courtesy of C. Thorpe.

engulf pathogens coated with antibodies of these isotypes. The Fc portion of IgE binds to a high-affinity Fcε receptor on mast cells, basophils, and activated eosinophils, enabling these cells to respond to the binding of specific antigen by releasing inflammatory mediators. Second, the Fc portions of antigen:antibody complexes can bind to complement (see Fig. 1.24) and initiate the complement cascade, which helps to recruit and activate phagocytes, aids the engulfment of microbes by phagocytes, and can also directly destroy pathogens. Third, the Fc portion can deliver antibodies to places they would not reach without active transport. These include mucous secretions, tears, and milk (IgA), and the fetal blood circulation by transfer from the pregnant mother (IgG). In both cases, the Fc portion engages a specific receptor that leads to the active transport of the immunoglobulin through cells to reach different body compartments.

The role of the Fc portion in these effector functions has been demonstrated by studying enzymatically treated immunoglobulins that have had one or other domain of the Fc cleaved off (see Section 3-3) or, more recently, by genetic engineering, which permits detailed mapping of the exact amino-acid residues within the Fc that are needed for particular functions. Many kinds of microorganism seem to have responded to the destructive potential of the Fc portion by manufacturing proteins that either bind to it or proteolytically cleave it, and so prevent the Fc region from working. Examples of these are Protein A and Protein G made by species of *Staphylococcus* (Fig. 4.22), and Protein D of *Haemophilus* species. Researchers have exploited these proteins to help to map the Fc and as immunological reagents (see Appendix I, Section A-10). Not all immunoglobulin isotypes or subtypes have the same capacity to engage each of the effector functions. The differential capabilities of each isotype are summarized in Fig. 4.17. For example, IgG1 and IgG3 have a higher affinity than IgG2 for the most common type of Fc receptor.

4-20   IgM and IgA can form polymers.

Although all immunoglobulin molecules are constructed from a basic unit of two heavy and two light chains, both IgM and IgA can form multimers of these basic units (Fig. 4.23). IgM and IgA C regions include a 'tailpiece' of 18 amino acids that contains a cysteine residue essential for polymerization. An additional separate 15 kDa polypeptide chain called the J chain promotes polymerization by linking to the cysteines of this tailpiece, which is found only in the secreted forms of the μ and α chains. (This J chain should not be confused with the immunoglobulin J region encoded by a J gene segment; see Section 4-2.) In the case of IgA, polymerization is required for transport through epithelia, as we discuss in Chapter 9. IgM molecules are found as pentamers, and occasionally hexamers (without J chain), in plasma, whereas IgA in mucous secretions, but not in plasma, is found mainly as a dimer (see Fig. 4.23).

Fig. 4.23 The IgM and IgA molecules can form multimers. IgM and IgA are usually synthesized as multimers in association with an additional polypeptide chain, the J chain. In pentameric IgM, the monomers are crosslinked by disulfide bonds to each other and to the J chain. The top left panel shows an electron micrograph of an IgM pentamer, showing the arrangement of the monomers in a flat disc. IgM can also form hexamers that lack a J chain. In dimeric IgA, the monomers have disulfide bonds to the J chain as well as to each other. The bottom left panel shows an electron micrograph of dimeric IgA. Photographs (× 900,000) courtesy of K.H. Roux and J.M. Schiff.

Pentameric IgM

J chain

Dimeric IgA

J chain

The polymerization of immunoglobulin molecules is also thought to be important in the binding of antibody to repetitive epitopes. The dissociation rate of an individual epitope from an individual antibody-binding site influences the strength of binding, or affinity, of that site: the lower the dissociation rate, the higher the affinity (see Appendix I, Section A-9). An antibody molecule has two or more identical antigen-binding sites, and if it attaches to two or more repeating epitopes on a single target antigen, it will dissociate only when all sites dissociate. The dissociation rate of the whole antibody from the whole antigen will therefore be much slower than the rate for the individual binding sites, giving a greater effective total binding strength, or **avidity**. This consideration is particularly relevant for pentameric IgM, which has 10 antigen-binding sites. IgM antibodies frequently recognize repetitive epitopes such as those expressed by bacterial cell-wall polysaccharides, but the binding of individual sites is often of low affinity because IgM is made early in immune responses, before somatic hypermutation and affinity maturation. Multisite binding makes up for this, markedly improving the overall functional binding strength.

4-21   Various differences between immunoglobulins can be detected by antibodies.

When an immunoglobulin is used as an antigen to immunize a different species of animal, it will be treated like any other foreign protein and will elicit an antibody response. Anti-immunoglobulin antibodies can be made that recognize the amino acids that characterize the isotype of the injected antibody. Such anti-isotypic antibodies recognize all immunoglobulins of the same isotype in all members of the species from which the injected antibody came.

It is also possible to raise antibodies that recognize differences in immunoglobulins from members of the same species that are due to the presence of multiple alleles of the individual C genes in the population (genetic polymorphism). Such allelic variants are called **allotypes**. In contrast to anti-isotypic antibodies, anti-allotypic antibodies will recognize immunoglobulin of a particular isotype only in some members of a species. Finally, as individual antibodies differ in their V regions, one can raise antibodies against unique features of the antigen-binding site, which are called **idiotypes**.

A schematic picture of the differences between idiotypes, allotypes, and isotypes is given in Fig. 4.24. Historically, the main features of immunoglobulins were defined by using isotypic and allotypic genetic markers identified by antisera raised in different species or in genetically distinct members of the same species (see Appendix I, Section A-10). The independent segregation of allotypic and isotypic markers revealed the existence of separate heavy-chain, κ, and λ genes. Such anti-idiotypic, allotypic, and isotypic antibodies are still enormously useful in detecting antibodies and B cells in scientific experimentation and medical diagnostics.

Fig. 4.24 Different types of variation between immunoglobulins. Differences between constant regions due to usage of different C-region genes are called isotypes; differences due to different alleles of the same C gene are called allotypes; differences due to particular rearranged V_H and V_L genes are called idiotypes.

Summary.

The isotypes of immunoglobulins are defined by their heavy-chain C regions, each isotype being encoded by a separate C-region gene. The heavy-chain C-region genes lie in a cluster 3′ to the V and J gene segments. A productively rearranged V-region exon is initially expressed in association with μ and δ C_H regions, which are coexpressed via alternative mRNA splicing. The same V-region exon can subsequently be associated with any one of the other isotypes by the process of isotype switching, in which the DNA is rearranged to place the V region 5′ to a different C-region gene. Unlike V(D)J recombination, isotype switching is always productive and occurs only in B cells activated by antigen. The immunological functions of the various isotypes differ; thus, isotype switching varies the effector response to the same antigen at different times or under different conditions. Immunoglobulin RNA can be processed in two different ways to produce either membrane-bound immunoglobulin, which acts as the B-cell receptor for antigen, or secreted antibody. In this way, the B-cell antigen receptor has the same specificity as the antibody that the B cell secretes upon activation.

Summary to Chapter 4.

Lymphocyte receptors are remarkably diverse, and developing B cells and T cells use the same basic mechanism to achieve this diversity. In each cell, functional genes for the immunoglobulin and T-cell receptor chains are assembled by somatic recombination from sets of separate gene segments that together encode the V region. The substrates for the joining process, arrays of V, D, and J gene segments, are similar among all the receptor loci, though there are some important differences in the details of their arrangement. The lymphoid-specific proteins RAG-1 and RAG-2 direct the V(D)J recombination process in both T and B cells. These genes function in concert with ubiquitous DNA-modifying enzymes and at least one other lymphoid-specific enzyme, TdT, to complete the joining process. As each type of gene segment is present in multiple, slightly different, versions, the random selection of gene segments for assembly is the source of substantial potential diversity. During the process of assembly, a high degree of functionally important diversity is introduced at the gene segment junctions through imprecise joining mechanisms. This diversity is concentrated in the DNA encoding the CDR3 loops of the receptors, which lie at the center of the antigen-binding site. The independent association of the two chains of immunoglobulins or T-cell receptors multiplies the overall diversity of the complete antigen receptor. In addition, mature B cells that are activated by antigen initiate a process of somatic point mutation of the V-region DNA, which creates numerous variants of the original assembled V regions.

An important difference between immunoglobulins and T-cell receptors is that immunoglobulins exist in both membrane-bound forms (B-cell receptors) and secreted forms (antibodies). The ability to express both a secreted and a membrane-bound form of the same molecule is due to differential splicing of mRNA to include exons that encode either the hydrophobic membrane anchor or the secreted tailpiece. Heavy-chain C regions contain three or four immunoglobulin domains, whereas the T-cell receptor chains have only one. Antibodies also have a variety of effector functions that are mediated by their C regions. Moreover, there are several alternative heavy-chain C regions for immunoglobulins, each with different effector functions. The same V region can be expressed along with different C regions through a process known as isotype switching. In this way, the progeny of a single B cell can express multiple different isotypes, thus maximizing the possible effector functions of any given antigen-specific antibody. The changes in immunoglobulin and T-cell receptor genes that occur during B-cell and T-cell development are summarized in Fig. 4.25.

Event	Process	Nature of change	Process occurs in:	
			B cells	T cells
V-region assembly	Somatic recombination of DNA	Irreversible	Yes	Yes
Junctional diversity	Imprecise joining, N-sequence insertion in DNA	Irreversible	Yes	Yes
Transcriptional activation	Activation of promoter by proximity to the enhancer	Irreversible but regulated	Yes	Yes
Switch recombination	Somatic recombination of DNA	Irreversible	Yes	No
Somatic hypermutation	DNA point mutation	Irreversible	Yes	No
IgM, IgD expression on surface	Differential splicing of RNA	Reversible, regulated	Yes	No
Membrane vs secreted form	Differential splicing of RNA	Reversible, regulated	Yes	No

Fig. 4.25 Changes in immunoglobulin and T-cell receptor genes that occur during B-cell and T-cell development and differentiation. Those changes that establish immunological diversity are all irreversible, as they involve changes in B-cell or T-cell DNA. Certain changes in the organization of DNA or in its transcription are unique to B cells. Somatic hypermutation has not been observed in functional T-cell receptors. The B-cell-specific processes, such as switch recombination, allow the same variable (V) region to be attached to several functionally distinct heavy-chain C regions, and thereby create functional diversity in an irreversible manner. By contrast, the expression of IgM versus IgD, and of membrane-bound versus secreted forms of all immunoglobulin types, can in principle be reversibly regulated.

Chapter 4 questions.

4.1   (a) What are the two kinds of somatic rearrangements of DNA that occur in the immunoglobulin gene locus? (b) Compare and contrast the mechanisms.

4.2   (a) What are the critical lymphocyte-specific genes involved in V(D)J recombination? (b) What are their main enzymatic activities?

4.3   Discuss two nonspecific (ie, ubiquitously expressed) enzymatic activities that are required for completion of V(D)J joining.

4.4   (a) Discuss the four main processes that generate diversity of the lymphocyte repertoire. (b) Which of these is not shared by both B and T cells?

4.5   What are the physiologic functions of antibody gene class switching?

General references.

Casali, P., and Silberstein, L.E.S. (eds): **Immunoglobulin gene expression in development and disease.** *Ann. N.Y. Acad. Sci.* 1995, **764**.

Fugmann, S.D., Lee, A.I., Shockett, P.E., Villey, I.J., and Schatz, D.G.: **The RAG proteins and V(D)J recombination: complexes, ends, and transposition.** *Annu. Rev. Immunol.* 2000, **18**:495–527.

Papavasiliou, F.N. and Schatz, D.G.: **Somatic hypermutation of immunoglobulin genes: merging mechanisms for genetic diversity.** *Cell* 2002, **109** Suppl:S35–S44.

Section references.

4-1   Immunoglobulin genes are rearranged in antibody-producing cells.

Hozumi, N., and Tonegawa, S.: **Evidence for somatic rearrangement of immunoglobulin genes coding for variable and constant regions.** *Proc. Natl. Acad. Sci. USA* 1976, **73**:3628–3632.

Tonegawa, S., Brack, C., Hozumi, N., and Pirrotta, V.: **Organization of immunoglobulin genes.** *Cold Spring Harbor Symp. Quant. Biol.* 1978, **42**:921–931.

Waldmann, T.A.: **The arrangement of immunoglobulin and T-cell receptor genes in human lymphoproliferative disorders.** *Adv. Immunol.* 1987, **40**:247–321.

4-2   Complete genes that encode a V region are generated by the somatic recombination of separate gene segments.

Early, P., Huang, H., Davis, M., Calame, K., and Hood, L.: **An immunoglobulin heavy chain variable region gene is generated from three segments of DNA: VH, D and JH.** *Cell* 1980, **19**:981–992.

Tonegawa, S., Maxam, A.M., Tizard, R., Bernard, O., and Gilbert, W.: **Sequence of a mouse germ-line gene for a variable region of an immunoglobulin light chain.** *Proc. Natl. Acad. Sci. USA* 1978, **75**:1485–1489.

4-3   For each immunoglobulin chain, multiple contiguous V-region gene segments are present on a stretch of chromosome.

Cook, G.P., and Tomlinson, I.M.: **The human immunoglobulin V-H repertoire.** *Immunol. Today* 1995, **16**:237–242.

Kofler, R., Geley, S., Kofler, H., and Helmberg, A.: **Mouse variable-region gene families—complexity, polymorphism, and use in nonautoimmune responses.** *Immunol. Rev.* 1992, **128**:5–21.

Maki, R., Traunecker, A., Sakano, H., Roeder, W., and Tonegawa, S.: **Exon shuffling generates an immunoglobulin heavy chain gene.** *Proc. Natl. Acad. Sci. USA* 1980, **77**:2138–2142.

Matsuda, F., and Honjo, T.: **Organization of the human immunoglobulin heavy-chain locus.** *Adv. Immunol.* 1996, **62**:1–29.

Thiebe, R., Schable, K.F., Bensch, A., Brensing-Kuppers, J., Heim, V., Kirschbaum, T., Mitlohner, H., Ohnrich, M., Pourrajabi, S., Roschenthaler, F., Schwendinger, J., Wichelhaus, D., Zocher, I., and Zachau, H.G.: **The variable genes and gene families of the mouse immunoglobulin kappa locus.** *Eur. J. Immunol.* 1999, **29**:2072–2081.

4-4   Rearrangement of V, D, and J gene segments is guided by flanking DNA sequences.

Grawunder, U., West, R.B., and Lieber, M.R.: **Antigen receptor gene rearrangement.** *Curr. Opin. Immunol.* 1998, **10**:172–180.

Max, E.E., Seidman, J.G., and Leder, P.: **Sequences of five potential recombination sites encoded close to an immunoglobulin kappa constant region gene.** *Proc. Natl. Acad. Sci. USA* 1979, **76**:3450–3454.

Sakano, H., Huppi, K., Heinrich, G., and Tonegawa, S.: **Sequences at the somatic recombination sites of immunoglobulin light-chain genes.** *Nature* 1979, **280**:288–294.

4-5   The reaction that recombines V, D, and J gene segments involves both lymphocyte-specific and ubiquitous DNA-modifying enzymes.

Agrawal, A., and Schatz, D.G.: **RAG1 and RAG2 form a stable postcleavage synaptic complex with DNA containing signal ends in V(D)J recombination.** *Cell* 1997, **89**:43–53.

Blunt, T., Finnie, N.J., Taccioli, G.E., Smith, G.C.M., Demengeot, J., Gottlieb, T.M., Mizuta, R., Varghese, A.J., Alt, F.W., Jeggo, P.A., and Jackson, S.P.: **Defective DNA-dependent protein kinase activity is linked to V(D)J recombination and DNA-repair defects associated with the murine–scid mutation.** *Cell* 1995, **80**:813–823.

Gu, Z., Jin, S., Gao, Y., Weaver, D.T., and Alt, F.W.: **Ku70-deficient embryonic stem cells have increased ionizing radiosensitivity, defective DNA end-binding activity, and inability to support V(D)J recombination.** *Proc. Natl. Acad. Sci. USA* 1997, **94**:8076–8081.

Li, Z.Y., Otevrel, T., Gao, Y.J., Cheng, H.L., Seed, B., Stamato, T.D., Taccioli, G.E., and Alt, F.W.: **The XRCC4 gene encodes a novel protein involved in DNA double-strand break repair and V(D)J recombination.** *Cell* 1995, **83**:1079–1089.

Moshous, D., Callebaut, I., de Chasseval, R., Corneo, B., Cavazzana-Calvo, M., Le Deist, F., Tezcan, I., Sanal, O., Bertrand, Y., Philippe, N., Fischer, A., and de Villartay, J.P.: **Artemis, a novel DNA double-strand break repair/V(D)J recombination protein, is mutated in human severe combined immune deficiency.** *Cell* 2001, **105**:177–186.

Oettinger, M.A., Schatz, D.G., Gorka, C., and Baltimore, D.: **RAG-1 and RAG-2, adjacent genes that synergistically activate V(D)J recombination.** *Science* 1990, **248**:1517–1523.

4-6   The diversity of the immunoglobulin repertoire is generated by four main processes.

Fanning, L.J., Connor, A.M., and Wu, G.E.: **Development of the immunoglobulin repertoire.** *Clin. Immunol. Immunopathol.* 1996, **79**:1–14.

Weigert, M., Perry, R., Kelley, D., Hunkapiller, T., Schilling, J., and Hood, L.: **The joining of V and J gene segments creates antibody diversity.** *Nature* 1980, **283**:497–499.

4-7   The multiple inherited gene segments are used in different combinations.

Lee, A., Desravines, S., and Hsu, E.: **IgH diversity in an individual with only one million B lymphocytes.** *Develop. Immunol.* 1993, **3**:211–222.

4-8   Variable addition and subtraction of nucleotides at the junctions between gene segments contributes to the diversity in the third hypervariable region.

Gauss, G.H., and Lieber, M.R.: **Mechanistic constraints on diversity in human V(D)J recombination.** *Mol. Cell. Biol.* 1996, **16**:258–269.

Komori, T., Okada, A., Stewart, V., and Alt, F.W.: **Lack of N regions in antigen receptor variable region genes of TdT-deficient lymphocytes.** *Science* 1993, **261**:1171–1175.

Weigert, M., Gatmaitan, L., Loh, E., Schilling, J., and Hood, L.: **Rearrangement of genetic information may produce immunoglobulin diversity.** *Nature* 1978, **276**:785–790.

4-9   Rearranged V genes are further diversified by somatic hypermutation.

Betz, A.G., Rada, C., Pannell, R., Milstein, C., and Neuberger, M.S.: **Passenger transgenes reveal intrinsic specificity of the antibody hypermutation** mechanism: clustering, polarity, and specific hot spots. *Proc. Natl. Acad. Sci. USA* 1993, **90**:2385–2388.

Di Noia, J. and Neuberger, M.S.: **Altering the pathway of immunoglobulin hypermutation by inhibiting uracil-DNA glycosylase.** *Nature* 2002, **419**:43–48.

McKean, D., Huppi, K., Bell, M., Straudt, L., Gerhard, W., and Weigert, M.: **Generation of antibody diversity in the immune response of BALB/c mice to influenza virus hemagglutinin.** *Proc. Natl. Acad. Sci. USA* 1984, **81**:3180–3184.

Muramatsu, M., Kinoshita, K., Fagarasan, S., Yamada, S., Shinkai, Y., and Honjo, T.: **Class switch recombination and hypermutation require activation-induced cytidine deaminase (AID), a potential RNA editing enzyme.** *Cell* 2000, **102**:553–563.

Petersen-Mahrt, S.K., Harris, R.S., and Neuberger, M.S.: **AID mutates *E. coli* suggesting a DNA deamination mechanism for antibody diversification.** *Nature* 2002, **418**:99–103.

Weigert, M.G., Cesari, I.M., Yonkovich, S.J., and Cohn, M.: **Variability in the lambda light chain sequences of mouse antibody.** *Nature* 1970, **228**:1045–1047.

4-10 In some species most immunoglobulin gene diversification occurs after gene rearrangement.

Harris, R.S., Sale, J.E., Petersen-Mahrt, S.K., and Neuberger, M.S.: **AID is essential for immunoglobulin V gene conversion in a cultured B cell line.** *Curr. Biol.* 2002, **12**:435–438.

Knight, K.L., and Crane, M.A.: **Generating the antibody repertoire in rabbit.** *Adv. Immunol.* 1994, **56**:179–218.

Reynaud, C.A., Bertocci, B., Dahan, A., and Weill, J.C.: **Formation of the chicken B-cell repertoire—ontogeny, regulation of Ig gene rearrangement, and diversification by gene conversion.** *Adv. Immunol.* 1994, **57**:353–378.

Reynaud, C.A., Garcia, C., Hein, W.R., and Weill, J.C.: **Hypermutation generating the sheep immunoglobulin repertoire is an antigen independent process.** *Cell* 1995, **80**:115–125.

Vajdy, M., Sethupathi, P., and Knight, K.L.: **Dependence of antibody somatic diversification on gut-associated lymphoid tissue in rabbits.** *J. Immunol.* 1998, **160**:2725–2729.

4-11 The T-cell receptor gene segments are arranged in a similar pattern to immunoglobulin gene segments and are rearranged by the same enzymes.

Rowen, L., Koop, B.F., and Hood, L.: **The complete 685-kilobase DNA sequence of the human β T cell receptor locus.** *Science* 1996, **272**:1755–1762.

Shinkai, Y., Rathbun, G., Lam, K.P., Oltz, E.M., Stewart, V., Mendelsohn, M., Charron, J., Datta, M., Young, F., Stall, A.M., and Alt, F.W.: **RAG-2 deficient mice lack mature lymphocytes owing to inability to initiate V(D)J rearrangement.** *Cell* 1992, **68**:855–867.

4-12 T-cell receptors concentrate diversity in the third hypervariable region.

Davis, M.M., and Bjorkman, P.J.: **T-cell antigen receptor genes and T-cell recognition.** *Nature* 1988, **334**:395–402.

Garboczi, D.N., Ghosh, P., Utz, U., Fan, Q.R., Biddison, W.E., and Wiley, D.C.: **Structure of the complex between human T-cell receptor, viral peptide and HLA-A2.** *Nature* 1996, **384**:134–141.

Hennecke, J., Carfi, A., and Wiley, D.C.: **Structure of a covalently stabilized complex of a human alphabeta T-cell receptor, influenza HA peptide and MHC class II molecule, HLA-DR1.** *EMBO J.* 2000, **19**:5611–5624.

Hennecke, J., and Wiley, D.C.: **T cell receptor-MHC interactions up close.** *Cell* 2001, **104**:1–4.

Jorgensen, J.L., Esser, U., Fazekas de St. Groth, B., Reay, P.A., and Davis, M.M.: **Mapping T-cell receptor-peptide contacts by variant peptide immunization of single-chain transgenics.** *Nature* 1992, **355**:224–230.

4-13 γ:δ T-cell receptors are also generated by gene rearrangement.

Chien, Y.H., Iwashima, M., Kaplan, K.B., Elliott, J.F., and Davis, M.M.: **A new T-cell receptor gene located within the alpha locus and expressed early in T-cell differentiation.** *Nature* 1987, **327**:677–682.

Hayday, A.C., Saito, H., Gillies, S.D., Kranz, D.M., Tanigawa, G., Eisen, H.N., and Tonegawa, S.: **Structure, organization, and somatic rearrangement of T cell gamma genes.** *Cell* 1985, **40**:259–269.

Lafaille, J.J., DeCloux, A., Bonneville, M., Takagaki, Y., and Tonegawa, S.: **Junctional sequences of T cell receptor gamma delta genes: implications for gamma delta T cell lineages and for a novel intermediate of V-(D)-J joining.** *Cell* 1989, **59**:859–870.

Tonegawa, S., Berns, A., Bonneville, M., Farr, A.G., Ishida, I., Ito, K., Itohara, S., Janeway, C.A., Jr., Kanagawa, O., Kubo, R., et al.: **Diversity, development, ligands, and probable functions of gamma delta T cells.** *Adv. Exp. Med. Biol.* 1991, **292**:53–61.

4-14 Somatic hypermutation does not generate diversity in T-cell receptors.

Zheng, B., Xue, W., and Kelsoe, G.: **Locus-specific somatic hypermutation in germinal centre T cells.** *Nature* 1994, **372**:556–559.

4-15 Transmembrane and secreted forms of immunoglobulin are generated from alternative heavy-chain transcripts.

Early, P., Rogers, J., Davis, M., Calame, K., Bond, M., Wall, R., and Hood, L.: **Two mRNAs can be produced from a single immunoglobulin μ gene by alternative RNA processing pathways.** *Cell* 1980, **20**:313–319.

Peterson, M.L., Gimmi, E.R., and Perry, R.P.: **The developmentally regulated shift from membrane to secreted μ mRNA production is accompanied by an increase in cleavage-polyadenylation efficiency but no measurable change in splicing efficiency.** *Mol. Cell. Biol.* 1991, **11**:2324–2327.

Rogers, J., Early, P., Carter, C., Calame, K., Bond, M., Hood, L., and Wall, R.: **Two mRNAs with different 3′ ends encode membrane-bound and secreted forms of immunoglobulin mu chain.** *Cell* 1980, **20**:303–312.

4-16 The immunoglobulin heavy-chain isotypes are distinguished by the structure of their constant regions.

Davies, D.R., and Metzger, H.: **Structural basis of antibody function.** *Annu. Rev. Immunol.* 1983, **1**:87–117.

4-17 Mature naive B cells express both IgM and IgD at their surface.

Abney, E.R., Cooper, M.D., Kearney, J.F., Lawton, A.R., and Parkhouse, R.M.: **Sequential expression of immunoglobulin on developing mouse B lymphocytes: a systematic survey that suggests a model for the generation of immunoglobulin isotype diversity.** *J. Immunol.* 1978, **120**:2041–2049.

Blattner, F.R. and Tucker, P.W.: **The molecular biology of immunoglobulin D.** *Nature* 1984, **307**:417–422.

Goding, J.W., Scott, D.W., and Layton, J.E.: **Genetics, cellular expression and function of IgD and IgM receptors.** *Immunol. Rev.* 1977, **37**:152–186.

4-18 Isotope switching enables the same assembled V$_H$ exon to be associated with different C$_H$ genes in the course of an immune response.

Jung, S., Rajewsky, K., and Radbruch, A.: **Shutdown of class switch recombination by deletion of a switch region control element.** *Science* 1993, **259**:984.

Revy, P., Muto, T., Levy, Y., Geissmann, F., Plebani, A., Sanal, O., Catalan, N., Forveille, M., Dufourcq-Lagelouse, R., Gennery, A., Tezcan, I., Ersoy, F., Kayserili, H., Ugazio, A.G., Brousse, N., Muramatsu, M., Notarangelo, L.D., Kinoshita, K., Honjo, T., Fischer, A., and Durandy, A.: **Activation-induced cytidine deaminase (AID) deficiency causes the autosomal recessive form of the hyper-IgM syndrome (HIGM2).** *Cell* 2000, **102**:565–575.

Sakano, H., Maki, R., Kurosawa, Y., Roeder, W., and Tonegawa, S.: **Two types of somatic recombination are necessary for the generation of complete immunoglobulin heavy-chain genes.** *Nature* 1980, **286**:676–683.

Stavnezer, J.: **Immunoglobulin class switching.** *Curr. Opin. Immunol.* 1996, **8**:199–205.

Shinkura, R., Tian, M., Smith, M., Chua, K., Fujiwara, Y., and Alt, F.W.: **The influence of transcriptional orientation on endogenous switch region function.** *Nat. Immunol.* 2003, **4**:435–441.

4-19   Antibody C regions confer functional specialization.

Helm, B.A., Sayers, I., Higginbottom, A., Machado, D.C., Ling, Y., Ahmad, K., Padlan, E.A., and Wilson, A.P.M.: **Identification of the high affinity receptor binding region in human IgE.** *J. Biol. Chem.* 1996, **271**:7494–7500.

Jefferis, R., Lund, J., and Goodall, M.: **Recognition sites on human IgG for Fcγ receptors—the role of glycosylation.** *Immunol. Lett.* 1995, **44**:111–117.

Sensel, M.G., Kane, L.M., and Morrison, S.L.: **Amino acid differences in the N-terminus of CH2 influence the relative abilities of IgG2 and IgG3 to activate complement.** *Mol. Immunol.* **34**:1019–1029.

4-20   IgM and IgA can form polymers.

Hendrickson, B.A., Conner, D.A., Ladd, D.J., Kendall, D., Casanova, J.E., Corthesy, B., Max, E.E., Neutra, M.R., Seidman, C.E., and Seidman, J.G.: **Altered hepatic transport of IgA in mice lacking the J chain.** *J. Exp. Med.* 1995, **182**:1905–1911.

Niles, M.J., Matsuuchi, L., and Koshland, M.E.: **Polymer IgM assembly and secretion in lymphoid and nonlymphoid cell-lines—evidence that J chain is required for pentamer IgM synthesis.** *Proc. Natl. Acad. Sci. USA* 1995, **92**:2884–2888.

4-21   Various differences between immunoglobulins can be detected by antibodies.

Capra, J.D., and Kehoe, J.M.: **Structure of antibodies with shared idiotypy: the complete sequence of the heavy chain variable regions of two immunoglobulin M anti-gamma globulins.** *Proc. Natl. Acad. Sci. USA* 1974, **71**:4032–4036.

Fields, B.A., Goldbaum, F.A., Ysern, X., Poljak, R.J., and Mariuzza, R.A.: **Molecular basis of antigen mimicry by an anti idiotope.** *Nature* 1995, **374**:739–742.

Wu, T.T., Kabat, E.A., and Bilofsky, H.: **Similarities among hypervariable segments of immunoglobulin chains.** *Proc. Natl. Acad. Sci. USA* 1975, **72**:5107–5110.

Antigen Presentation to T Lymphocytes

In an adaptive immune response, antigen is recognized by two distinct sets of highly variable receptor molecules—the immunoglobulins that serve as antigen receptors on B cells and the antigen-specific receptors of T cells. As we saw in Chapter 3, T cells only recognize antigens that are displayed on cell surfaces. These antigens may be derived from pathogens that replicate within cells, such as viruses or intracellular bacteria, or from pathogens or their products that cells internalize by endocytosis from the extracellular fluid. T cells can detect the presence of intracellular pathogens because infected cells display on their surface peptide fragments derived from the pathogens' proteins. These foreign peptides are delivered to the cell surface by specialized host-cell glycoproteins, the **MHC molecules**, which are also described in Chapter 3. The MHC glycoproteins are encoded in a large cluster of genes that were first identified by their potent effects on the immune response to transplanted tissues. For that reason, the gene complex was termed the **major histocompatibility complex (MHC)**. We now know that within this region of the genome, in addition to those genes encoding the MHC molecules themselves, are many genes whose products are involved in the production of the MHC:peptide complexes.

We will begin by discussing the mechanisms of antigen processing and presentation, whereby protein antigens are degraded into peptides inside cells and the peptides are then carried to the cell surface bound to MHC molecules. We will see that the two different classes of MHC molecule, known as MHC class I and MHC class II, deliver peptides from different cellular compartments to the surface of the infected cell. Peptides from the cytosol are bound to MHC class I molecules and are recognized by CD8 T cells, whereas peptides generated in intracellular vesicles are bound to MHC class II molecules and recognized by CD4 T cells. The two functional subsets of T cells are thereby activated to initiate the destruction of pathogens resident in these two different cellular compartments. Some CD4 T cells activate naive B cells that have internalized specific antigen, and thus also stimulate the production of antibodies against extracellular pathogens and their products.

In the second part of this chapter we will see that there are several genes for each class of MHC molecule: that is, the MHC is polygenic. Each of these genes has many variants: that is, the MHC is also highly polymorphic. Indeed, the most remarkable feature of the MHC class I and II genes is their genetic variability. MHC polymorphism has a profound effect on antigen recognition by T cells, and the combination of polygeny and polymorphism greatly extends the range of peptides that can be presented to T cells by each individual and each population at risk from an infectious pathogen.

The generation of T-cell receptor ligands.

The protective function of T cells depends on their ability to recognize cells that are harboring pathogens or that have internalized pathogens or their products. T cells do this by recognizing peptide fragments of pathogen-derived proteins in the form of complexes of peptides and MHC molecules on the cell surface. Because the generation of peptides from an intact antigen involves modification of the native protein, it is commonly referred to as **antigen processing**, whereas the display of the peptide at the cell surface by the MHC molecule is referred to as **antigen presentation**. We have already described the structure of MHC molecules and seen how they bind peptide antigens in a cleft on their outer surface (see Sections 3-15 to 3-18). In this chapter we will look at how peptides are generated from pathogens present in the cytosol or in the vesicular compartment of cells and loaded onto MHC class I or MHC class II molecules, respectively, at different sites inside the cell. Both classes of MHC molecule must combine with a peptide before they can be stably expressed at the cell surface. Peptide binding completes the folding and assembly of newly synthesized MHC class I molecules in the endoplasmic reticulum, while MHC class II molecules are prevented from binding peptides in the endoplasmic reticulum and are instead escorted to an endosomal compartment where loading with vesicular peptides occurs.

5-1   The MHC class I and class II molecules deliver peptides to the cell surface from two distinct intracellular compartments.

Infectious agents can replicate in either of two distinct intracellular compartments (Fig. 5.1). Viruses and certain bacteria replicate in the cytosol or in the contiguous nuclear compartment (Fig. 5.2, left panel), whereas many pathogenic bacteria and some eukaryotic parasites replicate in the endosomes and lysosomes that form part of the vesicular system (Fig. 5.2, center panel). The immune system has different strategies for eliminating pathogens from these two sites. Cells infected with viruses or with bacteria that live in the cytosol are eliminated by cytotoxic T cells; as mentioned in Chapter 3, these T cells are distinguished by the co-receptor molecule CD8. The function of **CD8 T cells** is to kill infected cells; this is an important means of eliminating sources of new viral particles and obligate cytosolic bacteria, thus freeing the host from infection.

Pathogens and their products in the vesicular compartments of cells are detected by a different class of T cell, distinguished by the co-receptor molecule CD4 (see Chapter 3). **CD4 T cells are specialized to activate other cells**, and fall into two functional classes: T$_H$1 cells (sometimes known as inflammatory T cells), whose main function is to activate macrophages to kill the intravesicular pathogens they harbor; and T$_H$2 cells, which activate B cells to make antibody. Microbial antigens may enter the vesicular compartment in either of two ways. Some bacteria, including the mycobacteria that cause tuberculosis and leprosy, invade macrophages and flourish in intracellular vesicles. Other bacteria proliferate outside cells, where they cause pathology by secreting toxins and other proteins. These bacteria and their toxic products can be internalized by phagocytosis, endocytosis, or macropinocytosis into the intracellular vesicles of cells that then present antigen to T cells. These include the dendritic cells that specialize in initiating T-cell responses (see Section 1-6), macrophages that specialize in taking up particulate material (see Section 2-3), and B cells that efficiently internalize specific antigen by receptor-mediated endocytosis of the antigen bound to their surface immunoglobulin (Fig. 5.2, right panel).

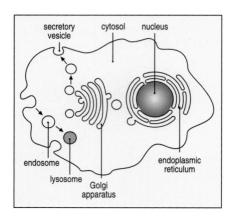

secretory vesicle   cytosol   nucleus

endosome

lysosome   Golgi apparatus

endoplasmic reticulum

Fig. 5.1 There are two major intracellular compartments, separated by membranes. The first is the cytosol, which also communicates with the nucleus via the nuclear pores in the nuclear membrane. The second is the vesicular system, which comprises the endoplasmic reticulum, Golgi apparatus, endosomes, lysosomes, and other intracellular vesicles. The vesicular system can be thought of as continuous with the extracellular fluid. Secretory vesicles bud off from the endoplasmic reticulum and are transported via fusion with Golgi membranes to move vesicular contents out of the cell, whereas extracellular material is taken up by endocytosis into endosomes, which move it eventually into lysosomes, where it is degraded.

	Cytosolic pathogens	Intravesicular pathogens	Extracellular pathogens and toxins
	any cell	macrophage	B cell
Degraded in	Cytosol	Endocytic vesicles (low pH)	Endocytic vesicles (low pH)
Peptides bind to	MHC class I	MHC class II	MHC class II
Presented to	CD8 T cells	CD4 T cells	CD4 T cells
Effect on presenting cell	Cell death	Activation to kill intravesicular bacteria and parasites	Activation of B cells to secrete Ig to eliminate extracellular bacteria/toxins

Fig. 5.2 Pathogens and their products can be found in either the cytosolic or the vesicular compartment of cells. Left panel: all viruses and some bacteria replicate in the cytosolic compartment. Their antigens are presented by MHC class I molecules to CD8 T cells. Center panel: other bacteria and some parasites are taken up into endosomes, usually by specialized phagocytic cells such as macrophages. Here they are killed and degraded, or in some cases are able to survive and proliferate within the vesicle. Their antigens are presented by MHC class II molecules to CD4 T cells. Right panel: proteins derived from extracellular pathogens may enter the vesicular system of cells by binding to surface molecules followed by endocytosis. This is illustrated for proteins bound by the surface immunoglobulin of B cells (the endoplasmic reticulum and Golgi apparatus have been omitted, for simplicity). The B cells present these antigens to CD4 helper T cells, which can then stimulate the B cells to produce antibody. Other types of cell that bear receptors for the Fc regions of antibody molecules can also internalize antigens in this way and are able to activate T cells.

To produce an appropriate response to infectious microorganisms, T cells need to be able to detect the presence of intracellular pathogens and to distinguish between foreign material coming from the cytosolic and vesicular compartments. This is achieved through the use of the different classes of MHC molecule. MHC class I molecules deliver peptides originating in the cytosol to the cell surface, where they are recognized by CD8 T cells. MHC class II molecules deliver peptides originating in the vesicular system to the cell surface, where they are recognized by CD4 T cells. As we saw in Section 3-12, CD8 and CD4 bind MHC class I and MHC class II molecules, respectively, and so help to ensure that the appropriate type of T cell is activated in response to a given pathogen.

5-2 Peptides that bind to MHC class I molecules are actively transported from the cytosol to the endoplasmic reticulum.

The antigen fragments that bind to MHC class I molecules are typically derived from viruses that take over the cell's biosynthetic mechanisms to make their own proteins. All proteins are made in the cytosol. The polypeptide chains of proteins destined for the cell surface, which include both classes of MHC molecule, are translocated during synthesis into the lumen of the endoplasmic reticulum. Here, the chains must fold correctly and assemble with each other, before the complete protein can be transported to the cell surface. Thus the peptide-binding site of the MHC class I molecule is formed in the lumen of the endoplasmic reticulum and is never exposed to the cytosol. This raised the question—how are peptides derived from viral proteins in the cytosol able to bind to MHC class I molecules for delivery to the cell surface?

The first clues came from mutant cells with a defect in antigen presentation by MHC class I molecules. Although both chains of MHC class I molecules are synthesized normally in these cells, the MHC class I proteins are present at abnormally low levels on the cell surface. This defect can be corrected by the addition of synthetic peptides to the medium bathing the cells, suggesting both that the mutation affects the supply of peptides to MHC class I molecules and that peptide is required for their maintenance at the cell surface. This was the first indication that MHC molecules are unstable in the absence of bound peptide.

Fig. 5.3 TAP1 and TAP2 form a peptide transporter in the endoplasmic reticulum membrane. All transporters of the ATP-binding cassette (ABC) family are composed of four domains as shown in the upper panel of this figure: two hydrophobic transmembrane domains that have multiple transmembrane regions, and two ATP-binding domains. *TAP1* and *TAP2* each encode a polypeptide chain with one hydrophobic and one ATP-binding domain; the two chains assemble into a heterodimer to form a four-domain transporter. From similarities between the TAP molecules and other members of the ABC-transporter family, it is believed that the ATP-binding domains lie within the cytosol, whereas the hydrophobic domains project through the membrane into the lumen of the endoplasmic reticulum (ER) to form a channel through which peptides can pass, as shown in the lower panel in an electron microscopic reconstruction of the structure of the TAP1:TAP2 heterodimer. View a shows the ER luminal surface of the TAP transporter, looking down onto the top of the transmembrane domains, while view b shows the molecule in the plane of the membrane. The ATP-binding domains form two lobes beneath the transmembrane domains and are not visible in this view. Bottom panel courtesy of G. Velarde.

Analysis of the DNA of the mutant cells showed that two genes encoding members of the ATP-binding cassette, or ABC, family of proteins are mutant or absent in these cells. ABC proteins mediate ATP-dependent transport of ions, sugars, amino acids, and peptides across membranes in many types of cells, including bacteria. The two ABC proteins missing in the mutant cells are normally associated with the endoplasmic reticulum membrane. Transfection of the mutant cells with both genes restores presentation of peptides by the cell's MHC class I molecules. These proteins are now called **transporters associated with antigen processing-1 and -2** (**TAP1** and **TAP2**). The two TAP proteins form a heterodimer (Fig. 5.3) and mutations in either TAP gene can prevent antigen presentation by MHC class I molecules. The genes *TAP1* and *TAP2* map within the MHC itself (see Section 5-9) and are inducible by interferons, which are produced in response to viral infection.

In assays *in vitro* using normal cell fractions, microsomal vesicles that mimic the endoplasmic reticulum will internalize peptides, which then bind to MHC class I molecules already present in the microsome lumen. Vesicles from TAP1- or TAP2-deficient cells do not transport peptides. Peptide transport into the normal microsomes requires ATP hydrolysis, proving that the TAP1:TAP2 complex is an ATP-dependent peptide transporter. Such experiments have also shown that the TAP complex has some specificity for the peptides it will transport. It prefers peptides of between 8 and 16 amino acids with hydrophobic or basic residues at the carboxy terminus—the exact features of peptides that bind MHC class I molecules—and has a bias against proline in the first three amino-terminal residues. The TAP transporter provides the answer to the question of how viral peptides gain access to the lumen of the endoplasmic reticulum in order to bind to MHC class I molecules, but leaves open the question of how these peptides are generated.

5-3 Peptides for transport into the endoplasmic reticulum are generated in the cytosol.

Proteins in cells are continually being degraded and replaced with newly synthesized proteins. Much cytosolic protein degradation is carried out by a large, multicatalytic protease complex called the **proteasome** (Fig. 5.4). This is a large cylindrical complex of some 28 subunits, arranged in four stacked rings, each of seven subunits. It has a hollow core lined by the active sites of the proteolytic subunits. Proteins to be degraded are introduced into the core of the proteasome, are there broken down into short peptides, and are then released.

Various lines of evidence implicate the proteasome in the production of peptide ligands for MHC class I molecules. For example, the proteasome is part of the ubiquitin-dependent degradation pathway for cytosolic proteins, and experimentally tagging proteins with ubiquitin also results in more efficient presentation of their peptides by MHC class I molecules. Moreover, inhibitors of the proteolytic activity of the proteasome also inhibit antigen presentation by MHC class I molecules. Whether the proteasome is the only cytosolic protease capable of generating peptides for transport into the endoplasmic reticulum is not known.

Two subunits of the proteasome, called b1i (previously known as LMP2) and b5i (previously LMP7), are encoded within the MHC near *TAP1* and *TAP2*. Along with MHC class I and TAP molecules, their expression is induced by interferons, which are produced in response to viral infections. The b1i and b5i subunits substitute for two constitutively expressed subunits of the proteasome. A third subunit, b2i (previously MECL-1), which is not encoded within the MHC, is also induced by interferons and also displaces a constitutive proteasome subunit. The proteasome can therefore exist in two forms—the constitutive proteasome, found in all cells, and the **immunoproteasome**, found in cells stimulated with interferons. The three inducible subunits of the immunoproteasome and their constitutive counterparts are thought to be the active proteases of the proteasome. The replacement of the constitutive components by their interferon-inducible counterparts in the immunoproteasome seems to change the specificity of the proteasome such that there is increased cleavage of polypeptides after hydrophobic residues, and reduced cleavage after acidic residues. This produces peptides with carboxy-terminal residues that are preferred anchor residues for binding to most MHC class I molecules and are also the preferred structures for transport by TAP.

The production of antigenic peptides by the proteasome is enhanced by a further modification of the proteasome induced by interferon-γ (IFN-γ). The PA28 proteasome-activator molecule is a six- or seven-membered ring composed of two protein molecules, PA28α and PA28β, both of which are induced by IFN-γ. The PA28 rings can bind to either or both ends of the proteasome cylinder and, by opening up the ends of the cylinder, increase the rate at which peptides can be released from the proteasome (Fig. 5.5). Moreover, this increased efflux of peptides from the proteasome will allow potentially antigenic peptides that might be cleaved further by the proteasome to escape this additional processing.

MHC class I molecules also present peptides derived from membrane and secreted proteins, for example the glycoproteins of viral envelopes. Membrane and secreted proteins are normally translocated into the lumen of the endoplasmic reticulum during their biosynthesis. Yet the peptides bound by MHC class I molecules bear evidence that such proteins are degraded in the cytosol. Asparagine-linked carbohydrate moieties commonly present on membrane-bound or secreted proteins can be removed in the cytosol by an enzyme reaction that changes the asparagine residue into aspartic acid, and this diagnostic sequence change can be seen in some peptides presented by MHC class I molecules. It now seems that endoplasmic reticulum proteins can be returned to the cytosol by the same translocation system that transported them into the endoplasmic reticulum in the first place. This newly discovered mechanism, known as retrograde translocation, may be the normal mechanism by which proteins in the endoplasmic reticulum are turned over, and by which misfolded proteins in the endoplasmic reticulum are removed and degraded. Once in the cytosol, the polypeptides are degraded by the proteasome. The resulting peptides can then be transported back into the lumen of the endoplasmic reticulum via TAP and loaded onto MHC class I molecules.

Fig. 5.4 The structure of the proteasome. Proteasomes are found throughout the eukaryotes and the archaea, and their structure and function are highly conserved. The structure shown here is from an archaebacterium, as the detailed structure of a mammalian proteasome has not yet been determined. The proteasome contains 28 subunits arranged to form a cylindrical structure composed of four rings, each of seven subunits. Panel a shows a horizontal cross-section through the proteasome, showing the arrangement of the seven subunits that comprise each ring; panel b shows a longitudinal section, in which the surface of the proteasome can be seen. The subunits that form the two central rings of the archaebacterial proteasome contain the proteolytic activity, and the active sites (seven in each ring) are indicated in green in panel a and in gold in panel b. Thus it is thought that proteins have to unfold and pass through the center of the cylinder in order to be degraded to peptides. It is not known exactly how the mammalian proteasome functions; it has six proteolytic sites, three in each of the two central rings, and these sites also lie in the center of the cylinder. It is therefore likely that its mechanism of action is very similar to that of the archaebacterial proteasome. Courtesy of W. Baumeister (× 667,000).

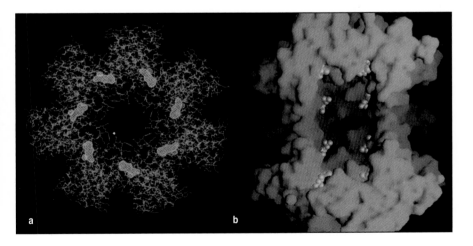

Fig. 5.5 The PA28 proteasome activator binds to either end of the proteasome. Panel a: the hexamer or heptamer rings of the PA28 proteasome activator (yellow) interact with the end of the proteasome, a part of the proteasome composed of α subunits (pink; β subunits are colored blue). Within this region is the α-annulus (green), a narrow ring-like opening that is normally blocked by other parts of the α subunits that are shown in red. Panel b: close-up view of the α-annulus. Panel c: binding of PA28 (not shown, for simplicity) to the proteasome changes the conformation of the α subunits, moving those parts of the molecule that block the α-annulus and thus opening the end of the cylinder. Courtesy of F. Whitby.

Cleavage in the proteasome may not be the only peptide cleavage that takes place in the generation of peptide ligands for MHC class I molecules. There is very good evidence that the carboxy-terminal ends of the peptides bound by MHC class I molecules are those produced by the proteasome cleavage step. However, peptides that are longer than those that bind to MHC class I molecules can be transported into the lumen of the endoplasmic reticulum where they can be trimmed by an aminopeptidase, an enzyme that removes residues from the amino-terminal end of a polypeptide. Such an enzyme has been characterized in cells and has been called the **endoplasmic reticulum aminopeptidase associated with antigen processing**, or **ERAAP**. Like other components of the antigen-processing pathway, ERAAP is upregulated by IFN-γ.

MHC Class I
Deficiency

5-4 Newly synthesized MHC class I molecules are retained in the endoplasmic reticulum until they bind peptide.

Binding of peptide is an important step in the assembly of stable MHC class I molecules. When the supply of peptides into the endoplasmic reticulum is disrupted, as in *TAP* mutant cells, newly synthesized MHC class I molecules are held in the endoplasmic reticulum in a partly folded state. This explains why cells with mutations in *TAP1* or *TAP2* fail to express MHC class I molecules at the cell surface. The folding and assembly of a complete MHC class I molecule (see Fig. 3.20) depends on the association of the MHC class I α chain first with β_2-microglobulin and then with peptide, and this process involves a number of accessory proteins with a chaperone-like function. Only after peptide has bound is the MHC class I molecule released from the endoplasmic reticulum and allowed to reach the cell surface.

In humans, newly synthesized MHC class I α chains that enter the endoplasmic reticulum membranes bind to a chaperone protein, **calnexin**, which retains the MHC class I molecule in a partly folded state in the endoplasmic reticulum (Fig. 5.6). Calnexin also associates with partly folded T-cell receptors, immunoglobulins, and MHC class II molecules, and so has a central role in the assembly of many immunological proteins. When β$_2$-microglobulin binds to the α chain, the partly folded α:β$_2$-microglobulin heterodimer dissociates from calnexin and now binds to a complex of proteins, called the MHC class I loading complex, one component of which—**calreticulin**—is similar to calnexin and probably carries out a similar chaperone function. A second component of the complex is the TAP-associated protein **tapasin**, also encoded by a gene that lies within the MHC. Tapasin forms a bridge between MHC class I molecules and TAP, allowing the partly folded α:β$_2$-microglobulin heterodimer to await the transport of a suitable peptide from the cytosol. A third component of this complex is the chaperone molecule **Erp57**, a thiol oxidoreductase that may have a role in breaking and reforming the disulfide bond in the MHC class I α$_2$ domain during peptide loading. Calnexin, Erp57, and calreticulin bind to a number of glycoproteins during their assembly in the endoplasmic reticulum and seem to be part of the cell's general quality-control mechanism.

The final component of this complex is the TAP molecule itself. The exact role of each of the components of this complex has not been fully defined, perhaps with the exception of TAP. The other components seem to be essential both to maintain the MHC class I molecule in a state where it is receptive to

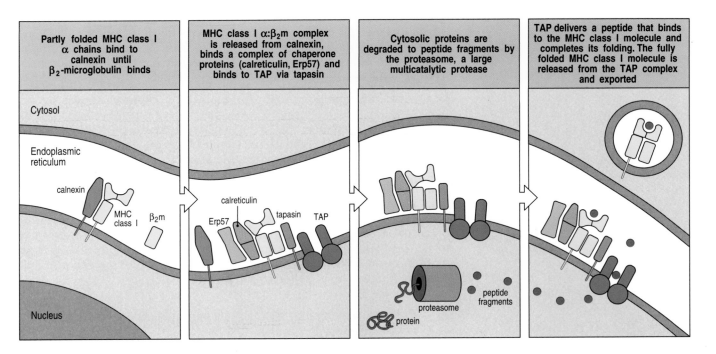

Fig. 5.6 MHC class I molecules do not leave the endoplasmic reticulum unless they bind peptides.
Newly synthesized MHC class I α chains assemble in the endoplasmic reticulum with a membrane-bound protein, calnexin. When this complex binds β$_2$-microglobulin (β$_2$m), the MHC class I α:β$_2$m dimer dissociates from calnexin, and the partly folded MHC class I molecule then binds to the peptide transporter TAP by interacting with one molecule of the TAP-associated protein tapasin. The chaperone molecules calreticulin and Erp57 also bind to form part of this complex. The MHC class I molecule is retained within the endoplasmic reticulum until released by the binding of a peptide, which completes the folding of the MHC molecule. Peptides generated by the degradation of proteins in the cytoplasm are transported into the lumen of the endoplasmic reticulum by TAP. Once peptide has bound to the MHC molecule, the peptide:MHC complex leaves the endoplasmic reticulum and is transported through the Golgi apparatus to the cell surface.

peptide, and also to carry out a peptide-editing function, allowing the exchange of low-affinity peptides bound to the MHC class I molecule for peptides of higher affinity. Certainly, cells defective in either calreticulin or tapasin show defects in the assembly of class I molecules and express MHC class I complexes at the cell surface that contain suboptimal, low-affinity peptides. Finally, the binding of a peptide to the partly folded heterodimer releases it from the complex of TAP:tapasin:calreticulin:Erp57. The fully folded MHC class I molecule and its bound peptide are now able to leave the endoplasmic reticulum and are transported to the cell surface.

Most of the peptides transported by TAP will not bind to the MHC molecules in that cell and are rapidly cleared out of the endoplasmic reticulum; there is evidence that they are transported back into the cytosol by an ATP-dependent transport mechanism distinct from that of TAP. It is not yet clear whether the TAP:tapasin complex directly loads peptides onto MHC class I molecules or whether binding to the TAP complex merely allows the MHC class I molecule to scan the transported peptides before they diffuse through the lumen of the endoplasmic reticulum and are transported back into the cytosol.

In cells with mutant TAP genes, the MHC class I molecules in the endoplasmic reticulum are unstable and are eventually translocated back into the cytosol, where they are degraded. Thus, the MHC class I molecule must bind a peptide to complete its folding and be transported onward from the endoplasmic reticulum. In uninfected cells, peptides derived from self proteins fill the peptide-binding cleft of the mature MHC class I molecules and are carried to the cell surface. In normal cells, MHC class I molecules are retained in the endoplasmic reticulum for some time, which suggests that they are present in excess of peptide. This is very important for the function of MHC class I molecules because they must be immediately available to transport viral peptides to the cell surface if the cell becomes infected. When a cell is infected by a virus, the presence of excess MHC class I molecules in the endoplasmic reticulum allows the rapid appearance of pathogen-derived peptides at the cell surface.

Because the presentation of viral peptides by MHC class I molecules signals CD8 T cells to kill the infected cell, some viruses have evolved means of evading recognition by preventing the appearance of peptide:MHC class I complexes at the cell surface. The herpes simplex virus prevents the transport of viral peptides into the endoplasmic reticulum by producing a protein that binds to and inhibits TAP. Adenoviruses, in contrast, encode a protein that binds to MHC class I molecules and retains them in the endoplasmic reticulum. Cytomegalovirus accelerates the retrograde translocation of MHC class I molecules back into the cytosol, where they are degraded. The advantage to a virus of blocking the recognition of infected cells is so great that it would not be surprising if other steps in the formation of MHC:peptide complexes, for example the association of the MHC class I:chaperone complex with TAP, were also found to be inhibited by some viruses.

5-5   Peptides presented by MHC class II molecules are generated in acidified endocytic vesicles.

Several classes of pathogen, including the protozoan parasite *Leishmania* and the mycobacteria that cause leprosy and tuberculosis, replicate inside intracellular vesicles in macrophages. Because they reside in membrane-bounded vesicles, the proteins of these pathogens are not accessible to proteasomes in the cytosol. Instead, after activation of the macrophage, proteins in vesicles are degraded by proteases within the vesicles into peptide fragments that bind to MHC class II molecules. In this way they are delivered to the cell surface, where they can be recognized by CD4 T cells. Extracellular pathogens and proteins that are internalized into endocytic vesicles are also processed by this pathway and their peptides are presented to CD4 T cells (Fig. 5.7).

Most of what we know about protein processing in the endocytic pathway has come from experiments in which simple proteins are fed to macrophages and are taken up by endocytosis; in this way the processing of added antigen can be quantified. Proteins that bind to surface immunoglobulin on B cells and are internalized by receptor-mediated endocytosis are processed by the same pathway. Proteins that enter cells through endocytosis are delivered to endosomes, which become increasingly acidic as they progress into the interior of the cell, eventually fusing with lysosomes. The endosomes and lysosomes contain proteases, known as acid proteases, that are activated at low pH and eventually degrade the protein antigens contained in the vesicles. Larger particulate material internalized by phagocytosis or macropinocytosis can also be handled by this pathway of antigen processing.

Drugs such as chloroquine that raise the pH of endosomes, making them less acid, inhibit the presentation of antigens that enter the cell in this way, suggesting that acid proteases are responsible for processing internalized antigen. Among these acid proteases are the cysteine proteases cathepsins B, D, S, and L, the last of which is the most active enzyme in this family. Antigen processing can be mimicked to some extent by digestion of proteins with these enzymes in vitro at acid pH. Cathepsins S and L may be the predominant proteases involved in the processing of vesicular antigens; mice that lack cathepsin B or cathepsin D show normal antigen processing, whereas mice with no cathepsin S show some deficiencies in antigen processing. Other proteases do have a role, however, and are important for the presentation of at least some antigens; the newly discovered protease asparaginyl endopeptidase is required for the production of epitopes from tetanus toxin. It is likely that the overall repertoire of peptides produced within the endosomal pathway reflects the activities of the many proteases that are found in the endosomal and lysosomal compartments.

Fig. 5.7 Peptides that bind to MHC class II molecules are generated in acidified endocytic vesicles. In the case illustrated here, extracellular foreign antigens, such as bacteria or bacterial antigens, have been taken up by an antigen-presenting cell such as a macrophage or immature dendritic cell. In other cases, the source of the peptide antigen may be bacteria or parasites that have invaded the cell to replicate in intracellular vesicles. In both cases the antigen-processing pathway is the same. The pH of the endosomes containing the engulfed pathogens progressively decreases, activating proteases that reside within the vesicles to degrade the engulfed material. At some point on their pathway to the cell surface, newly synthesized MHC class II molecules pass through such acidified vesicles and bind peptide fragments of the antigen, transporting the peptides to the cell surface.

Disulfide bonds, particularly intramolecular disulfide bonds, may need to be reduced before proteins that contain them can be digested in endosomes. An IFN-γ-induced thiol reductase present in the endosomal compartment—gamma interferon-induced lysosomal thiol reductase, or GILT—carries out this role in the antigen-processing pathway.

5-6 The invariant chain directs newly synthesized MHC class II molecules to acidified intracellular vesicles.

The function of MHC class II molecules is to bind peptides generated in the intracellular vesicles of macrophages, immature dendritic cells, B cells, and other antigen-presenting cells and to present these peptides to CD4 T cells. However, the biosynthetic pathway for MHC class II molecules, like that of other cell-surface glycoproteins, starts with their translocation into the endoplasmic reticulum, and they therefore be prevented from binding prematurely to peptides transported into the endoplasmic reticulum lumen or to the cell's own newly synthesized polypeptides. Because the endoplasmic reticulum is richly endowed with unfolded and partly folded polypeptide chains, a general mechanism is needed to prevent their binding in the open-ended MHC class II molecule peptide-binding groove.

Binding is prevented by the assembly of newly synthesized MHC class II molecules with a protein known as the MHC class II-associated **invariant chain** (**Ii**). The invariant chain forms trimers, with each subunit binding noncovalently to an MHC class II α:β heterodimer (Fig. 5.8). Ii binds to the MHC class II molecule with part of its polypeptide chain lying within the peptide-binding groove, thus blocking the groove and preventing the binding of either peptides or partly folded proteins. While this complex is being assembled in the endoplasmic reticulum, its component parts are associated with calnexin. Only when assembly is completed to produce a nine-chain complex is the complex released from calnexin for transport out of the endoplasmic reticulum. When it is part of the nine-chain complex, the MHC class II molecule cannot bind

Fig. 5.8 The invariant chain is cleaved to leave a peptide fragment, CLIP, bound to the MHC class II molecule. A model of the trimeric invariant chain bound to MHC class II α:β heterodimers is shown on the left. The CLIP portion is shown in red, the rest of the invariant chain in green, and the MHC class II molecules in yellow. In the endoplasmic reticulum, the invariant chain (Ii) binds to MHC class II molecules with the CLIP section of its polypeptide chain lying along the peptide-binding groove (model and left of three panels). After transport into an acidified vesicle, Ii is cleaved, initially just at one side of the MHC class II molecule (center panel). The remaining portion of Ii (known as the leupeptin-induced peptide or LIP fragment) retains the transmembrane and cytoplasmic segments that contain the signals that target Ii:MHC class II complexes to the endosomal pathway. Subsequent cleavage (right panel) of LIP leaves only a short peptide still bound by the class II molecule; this peptide is the CLIP fragment. Model structure courtesy of P. Cresswell.

peptides or unfolded proteins, so that peptides present in the endoplasmic reticulum are not usually presented by MHC class II molecules. There is evidence that in the absence of invariant chains many MHC class II molecules are retained in the endoplasmic reticulum as complexes with misfolded proteins.

The invariant chain has a second function, which is to target delivery of the MHC class II molecules to a low-pH endosomal compartment where peptide loading can occur. The complex of MHC class II α:β heterodimers with invariant chain is retained for 2–4 hours in this compartment. During this time, the invariant chain is cleaved by acid proteases such as cathepsin S in several steps, as shown in Fig. 5.8. The initial cleavages generate a truncated form of the invariant chain that remains bound to the MHC class II molecule and retains it within the proteolytic compartment. A subsequent cleavage releases the MHC class II molecule from the membrane-associated fragment of Ii, leaving a short fragment of Ii, called CLIP (for *class* II-associated *invariant-chain peptide*) still bound to the MHC class II molecule. MHC class II molecules associated with CLIP cannot bind other peptides. CLIP must either dissociate or be displaced to allow a peptide to bind to the MHC molecule and enable the complex to be delivered to the cell surface. Cathepsin S cleaves Ii in most MHC class II-positive cells, including antigen-presenting cells, whereas cathepsin L seems to substitute for cathepsin S in thymic cortical epithelial cells.

The endosomal compartment in which invariant chain is cleaved and MHC class II molecules encounter peptide is not yet clearly defined. Most newly synthesized MHC class II molecules are brought toward the cell surface in vesicles, which at some point fuse with incoming endosomes. However, there is also evidence that some MHC class II:Ii complexes are first transported to the cell surface and then reinternalized into endosomes. In either case, MHC class II:Ii complexes enter the endosomal pathway and there encounter and bind peptides derived from self proteins. Immunoelectron-microscopy using antibodies tagged with gold particles to localize Ii and MHC class II molecules within cells suggests that Ii is cleaved and peptides bind to MHC class II molecules in a particular endosomal compartment called the MIIC (MHC *class II compartment*), late in the endosomal pathway (Fig. 5.9).

As with MHC class I molecules, MHC class II molecules in uninfected cells bind peptides derived from self proteins. MHC class II molecules that do not bind peptide after dissociation from the invariant chain are unstable; in the acidic pH of the endosome they aggregate and are rapidly degraded. It is therefore not surprising that peptides derived from MHC class II molecules form a large proportion of the self peptides presented by MHC class II molecules in normal uninfected cells. This suggests that, as for MHC class I molecules, MHC class II molecules are produced in excess. Thus, when a cell is infected by pathogens that proliferate in intracellular vesicles, when a phagocyte engulfs a pathogen, or when pathogen-derived proteins are internalized by B cells, the peptides generated from the pathogen proteins find plentiful empty MHC class II molecules to which they can bind.

5-7 A specialized MHC class II-like molecule catalyzes loading of MHC class II molecules with peptides.

An unsuspected component of the vesicular antigen-processing pathway has been revealed by analysis of mutant human B-cell lines with a defect in antigen presentation. MHC class II molecules in these cell lines assemble correctly with the invariant chain and seem to follow the normal vesicular route. However, they fail to bind peptides derived from internalized proteins and often arrive at the cell surface with the CLIP peptide still bound.

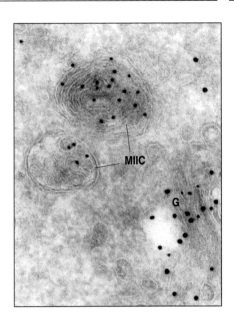

Fig. 5.9 MHC class II molecules are loaded with peptide in a specialized intracellular compartment. MHC class II molecules are transported from the Golgi apparatus (labeled G in this electron micrograph of an ultrathin section of a B cell) to the cell surface via specialized intracellular vesicles called the *M*HC class *II c*ompartment (MIIC). These have a complex morphology, showing internal vesicles and sheets of membrane. Antibodies labeled with different-sized gold particles identify the presence of both MHC class II molecules (small gold particles) and the invariant chain (large gold particles) in the Golgi, whereas only MHC class II molecules are detectable in the MIIC. This compartment is thus thought to be the one in which the invariant chain is cleaved and peptide loading occurs. Photograph (× 135,000) courtesy of H.J. Geuze.

The defect in these cells lies in an MHC class II-like molecule called **HLA-DM** in humans (H-2M in mice). The HLA-DM genes are found near the TAP and LMP genes in the MHC class II region (see Fig. 5.11); they encode an α chain and a β chain that closely resemble those of other MHC class II molecules. The HLA-DM molecule is not expressed at the cell surface, however, but is found predominantly in the MIIC compartment. HLA-DM binds to and stabilizes empty MHC class II molecules that would otherwise aggregate; in addition, it catalyzes both the release of the CLIP fragment from MHC class II:CLIP complexes and the binding of other peptides to the empty MHC class II molecule (Fig. 5.10). However, the HLA-DM molecule itself does not bind peptides and the open groove found in other MHC class II molecules is closed in the structure of HLA-DM.

HLA-DM also catalyzes the release of unstably bound peptides from MHC class II molecules. In the presence of a mixture of peptides capable of binding to MHC class II molecules, as occurs in the MIIC, HLA-DM continuously binds and rebinds to peptide:MHC class II complexes, removing weakly bound peptides and allowing other peptides to replace them. Antigens presented by MHC class II molecules may have to persist on the surface of antigen-presenting cells for some days before encountering T cells able to recognize them. The ability of HLA-DM to remove unstably bound peptides, sometimes called 'peptide editing,' ensures that the peptide:MHC class II complexes displayed on the surface of the antigen-presenting cell survive long enough to stimulate the appropriate CD4 cells.

A second atypical MHC class II molecule, called **HLA-DO** (H-2O in mice), is produced in thymic epithelial cells and B cells. This molecule is a heterodimer

| Invariant chain (Ii) forms a complex with MHC class II molecule, blocking the binding of peptides and misfolded proteins | Ii is cleaved in an acidified endosome, leaving a short peptide fragment, CLIP, still bound to the MHC class II molecule | Endocytosed antigens are degraded to peptides in endosomes, but the CLIP peptide blocks the binding of peptides to MHC class II molecules | HLA-DM binds to the MHC class II molecule, releasing CLIP and allowing other peptides to bind. The MHC class II molecule then travels to the cell surface |

Fig. 5.10 HLA-DM facilitates the loading of antigenic peptides onto MHC class II molecules. The invariant chain binds to newly synthesized MHC class II molecules and blocks the binding of peptides and unfolded proteins in the endoplasmic reticulum and during the transport of the MHC class II molecule into acidified endocytic vesicles (first panel). In such vesicles, proteases cleave the invariant chain, leaving the CLIP peptide bound to the MHC class II molecule (second panel). Pathogens and their proteins are broken down into peptides within acidified endosomes, but these peptides cannot bind to MHC class II molecules that are occupied by CLIP (third panel). The class II-like molecule, HLA-DM, binds to MHC class II:CLIP complexes, catalyzing the release of CLIP and the binding of antigenic peptides (fourth panel).

of the HLA-DNα chain and the HLA-DOβ chain (see Fig. 5.11). HLA-DO is not present at the cell surface, being found only in intracellular vesicles, and it does not seem to bind peptides. Instead, it acts as a negative regulator of HLA-DM, binding to it and inhibiting both the HLA-DM-catalyzed release of CLIP from, and the binding of other peptides to, MHC class II molecules. Expression of the HLA-DOβ chain is not increased by IFN-γ, whereas the expression of HLA-DM is. Thus, during inflammatory responses, in which IFN-γ is produced by T cells and NK cells (see Section 2-27), the increased expression of HLA-DM is able to overcome the inhibitory effects of HLA-DO. Why the antigen-presenting ability of thymic epithelial cells and B cells should be regulated in this way is not known; in thymic epithelial cells the purpose may be to select developing CD4 T cells by using a repertoire of self peptides different from those to which they will be exposed as mature T cells.

The role of HLA-DM in facilitating the binding of peptides to MHC class II molecules parallels that of TAP in facilitating peptide binding to MHC class I molecules. Thus it seems likely that specialized mechanisms of delivering peptides have coevolved with the MHC molecules themselves. It is also likely that pathogens have evolved strategies to inhibit the loading of peptides onto MHC class II molecules, much as viruses have found ways of subverting antigen processing and presentation through the MHC class I molecules.

5-8   Stable binding of peptides by MHC molecules provides effective antigen presentation at the cell surface.

For MHC molecules to perform their essential function of signaling intracellular infection, the peptide:MHC complex must be stable at the cell surface. If the complex were to dissociate too readily, the pathogen in the infected cell could escape detection. In addition, MHC molecules on uninfected cells could pick up peptides released by MHC molecules on infected cells and falsely signal to cytotoxic T cells that a healthy cell is infected, triggering its unwarranted destruction. The tight binding of peptides by MHC molecules makes both of these undesirable outcomes unlikely.

The persistence of a peptide:MHC complex on a cell can be measured by its ability to stimulate T cells, while the fate of the MHC molecules themselves can be directly followed by specific staining. In this way it can be shown that specific peptide:MHC complexes on living cells are lost from the surface and reinternalized as part of natural protein turnover at the same rate as the MHC molecules themselves, indicating that peptide binding is essentially irreversible. This stable binding enables even rare peptides to be transported efficiently to the cell surface by MHC molecules, and allows long-term display of these complexes on the surface of the infected cell. This fulfills the first of the requirements for effective antigen presentation.

The second requirement is that if a peptide should dissociate from a cell-surface MHC molecule, peptides from the surrounding extracellular fluid would not be able to bind to the empty peptide-binding site. In fact, removal of the peptide from a purified MHC class I molecule has been shown to require denaturation of the protein. When peptide dissociates from an MHC class I molecule at the surface of a living cell, the molecule changes conformation, the β_2-microglobulin dissociates, and the α chain is internalized and rapidly degraded. Thus, most empty MHC class I molecules are quickly lost from the cell surface.

At neutral pH, empty MHC class II molecules are more stable than empty MHC class I molecules, yet empty MHC class II molecules are also removed from the cell surface. They aggregate readily, and internalization of such aggregates may account for their loss from the surface. Moreover, peptide loss from MHC class II molecules is most likely when the molecules transit through acidified endosomes as part of the normal process of cell-membrane recycling. At acidic pH, MHC class II molecules are able to bind peptides that are present in the vesicles, but those that fail to do so are rapidly degraded.

Thus, both MHC class I and class II molecules are effectively prevented from acquiring peptides from the surrounding extracellular fluid. This ensures that T cells act selectively on infected cells or on cells specialized for pathogen ingestion and display, while sparing surrounding healthy cells.

Summary.

The most distinctive feature of antigen recognition by T cells is the form of the ligand recognized by the T-cell receptor. This comprises a peptide derived from a foreign antigen and bound to an MHC molecule. MHC molecules are cell-surface glycoproteins with a peptide-binding groove that can bind a wide variety of different peptides. The MHC molecule binds the peptide in an intracellular location and delivers it to the cell surface, where the combined ligand can be recognized by a T cell. There are two classes of MHC molecule, MHC class I and MHC class II, which bind peptides from proteins degraded in different intracellular sites. MHC class I molecules bind peptides from proteins degraded in the cytosol, where a multicatalytic protease, the proteasome, degrades both normal cytosolic proteins and proteins that have been transported back into the cytosol from the endoplasmic reticulum. Peptides produced by proteasomes are transported into the endoplasmic reticulum by a heterodimeric ATP-binding protein called TAP and are then available for binding by partly folded MHC class I molecules that are held tethered to TAP. Peptide binding is an integral part of MHC class I molecule assembly, and must occur before the MHC class I molecule can complete its folding and leave the endoplasmic reticulum for the cell surface. By binding stably to peptides from proteins degraded in the cytosol, MHC class I molecules on the surface of cells infected with viruses or other cytosolic pathogens display peptides from these pathogens. In contrast, MHC class II molecules are prevented from binding to peptides in the endoplasmic reticulum by their early association with the invariant chain, which fills and blocks their peptide-binding groove. They are targeted by the invariant chain to an acidic endosomal compartment where—in the presence of active proteases, in particular cathepsin S, and with the help of a specialized MHC class II-like molecule, which catalyzes peptide loading—the invariant chain is released and other peptides are bound. MHC class II molecules thus bind peptides from proteins that are degraded in endosomes. There they can capture peptides from pathogens that have entered the vesicular system of macrophages, or from antigens internalized by immature dendritic cells or the immunoglobulin receptors of B cells. Different types of T cell are activated on recognizing foreign peptides presented by the different classes of MHC molecule. The CD8 T cells that recognize MHC class I:peptide complexes are specialized to kill any cells displaying foreign peptides and so rid the body of cells infected with viruses and other cytosolic pathogens. The CD4 T cells that recognize MHC class II:peptide complexes are specialized to activate other effector cells of the immune system; macrophages, for example, are activated to kill the intravesicular pathogens they harbor, and B cells to secrete immunoglobulins against foreign molecules. Thus, the two classes of MHC molecule deliver peptides from different cellular compartments to the cell surface, where they are recognized by T cells mediating distinct and appropriate effector functions.

The major histocompatibility complex and its functions.

The function of MHC molecules is to bind peptide fragments derived from pathogens and display them on the cell surface for recognition by the appropriate T cells. The consequences are almost always deleterious to the pathogen—virus-infected cells are killed, macrophages are activated to kill bacteria living in their intracellular vesicles, and B cells are activated to produce antibodies that eliminate or neutralize extracellular pathogens. Thus, there is strong selective pressure in favor of any pathogen that has mutated in such a way that it escapes presentation by an MHC molecule.

Two separate properties of the MHC make it difficult for pathogens to evade immune responses in this way. First, the MHC is **polygenic**: it contains several different MHC class I and MHC class II genes, so that every individual possesses a set of MHC molecules with different ranges of peptide-binding specificities. Second, the MHC is highly **polymorphic**; that is, there are multiple variants of each gene within the population as a whole. The MHC genes are, in fact, the most polymorphic genes known. In this section we will describe the organization of the genes in the MHC and discuss how the variation in MHC molecules arises. We will also see how the effect of polygeny and polymorphism on the range of peptides that can be bound contributes to the ability of the immune system to respond to the multitude of different and rapidly evolving pathogens.

5-9 Many proteins involved in antigen processing and presentation are encoded by genes within the major histocompatibility complex.

The major histocompatibility complex is located on chromosome 6 in humans and chromosome 17 in the mouse and extends over some 4 centimorgans of DNA, about 4×10^6 base pairs. In humans it contains more than 200 genes. As work continues to define the genes within and around the MHC, both its extent and the number of genes are likely to grow; in fact, recent studies suggest that the MHC may span at least 7×10^6 base pairs. The genes encoding the α chains of MHC class I molecules and the α and β chains of MHC class II molecules are linked within the complex; the genes for β_2-microglobulin and the invariant chain are on different chromosomes (chromosomes 15 and 5, respectively, in humans, and chromosomes 2 and 18 in the mouse). Figure 5.11 shows the general organization of the MHC class I and II genes in human and mouse. In humans these genes are called *human leukocyte antigen* or HLA genes, as they were first discovered through antigenic differences between white blood cells from different individuals; in the mouse they are known as the **H-2** genes.

There are three class I α-chain genes in humans, called HLA-A, -B, and -C. There are also three pairs of MHC class II α- and β-chain genes, called HLA-DR, -DP, and -DQ. However, in many cases the HLA-DR cluster contains an extra β-chain gene whose product can pair with the DRα chain. This means that the three sets of genes can give rise to four types of MHC class II molecule. All the MHC class I and class II molecules can present peptides to T cells, but each protein binds a different range of peptides (see Sections 3-16 and 3-17). Thus, the presence of several different genes of each MHC class means that any one individual is equipped to present a much broader range of peptides than if only one MHC molecule of each class were expressed at the cell surface.

Fig. 5.11 The genetic organization of the major histocompatibility complex (MHC) in human and mouse. The organization of the principal MHC genes is shown for both humans (where the MHC is called HLA and is on chromosome 6) and mice (in which the MHC is called H-2 and is on chromosome 17). The organization of the MHC genes is similar in both species. There are separate clusters of MHC class I genes (red) and MHC class II genes (yellow), although in the mouse an MHC class I gene (H-2K) seems to have translocated relative to the human MHC so that the class I region in mice is split in two. In both species there are three main class I genes, which are called HLA-A, -B, and -C in humans, and H2-K, -D, and -L in the mouse. The gene for β_2-microglobulin, although it encodes part of the MHC class I molecule, is located on a different chromosome, chromosome 15 in humans and chromosome 2 in the mouse. The class II region includes the genes for the α and β chains of the antigen-presenting MHC class II molecules HLA-DR, -DP, and -DQ (H-2A and -E in the mouse). In addition, the genes for the TAP1:TAP2 peptide transporter, the LMP genes that encode proteasome subunits, the genes encoding the DMα and DMβ chains, the genes encoding the α and β chains of the DO molecule (DNα and DOβ, respectively), and the gene encoding tapasin (TAPBP) are also in the MHC class II region. The so-called class III genes encode various other proteins with functions in immunity (see Fig. 5.12).

The two *TAP* genes lie in the MHC class II region, in close association with the *LMP* genes that encode components of the proteasome, whereas the gene encoding tapasin (TAPBP), which binds to both TAP and empty MHC class I molecules, lies at the edge of the MHC nearest the centromere (see Fig. 5.11). The genetic linkage of the MHC class I genes (whose products deliver cytosolic peptides to the cell surface) with the *TAP*, tapasin, and proteasome genes (which encode the molecules that generate peptides in the cytosol and transport them into the endoplasmic reticulum) suggests that the entire MHC has been selected during evolution for antigen processing and presentation.

When cells are treated with the interferons IFN-α, -β, or -γ, there is a marked increase in transcription of MHC class I α-chain and β_2-microglobulin genes, and of the proteasome, tapasin, and *TAP* genes. Interferons are produced early in viral infections as part of the innate immune response, as described in Chapter 2, and so this effect increases the ability of cells to process viral proteins and present the resulting virus-derived peptides at the cell surface. This helps to activate the appropriate T cells and initiate the adaptive immune response in response to the virus. The coordinated regulation of the genes encoding these components may be facilitated by the linkage of many of them in the MHC.

The *HLA-DM* genes, which encode the DM molecule, whose function is to catalyze peptide binding to MHC class II molecules (see Section 5-7), are clearly related to the MHC class II genes. The DNα and DOβ genes, which encode the DO molecule, a negative regulator of DM, are also clearly related to the MHC class II genes. The classical MHC class II genes, along with the invariant-chain gene and the genes encoding DMα, DMβ, and DNα, but not DOβ, are coordinately regulated. This distinct regulation of MHC class II genes by IFN-γ, which is made by activated T cells of the T_H1 type as well as by activated CD8 and NK cells, allows T cells responding to bacterial infections to increase the expression of those molecules concerned with the processing and presentation of intravesicular antigens. Expression of all these molecules is induced by IFN-γ (but not by IFN-α or -β), via the production of

**MHC Class II
Deficiency**

a transcriptional activator known as **MHC class II transactivator** (CIITA). An absence of CIITA causes severe immunodeficiency due to nonproduction of MHC class II molecules.

5-10 A variety of genes with specialized functions in immunity are also encoded in the MHC.

Although the most important known function of the gene products of the MHC is the processing and presentation of antigens to T cells, many other genes map within this region; some of these are known to have other roles in the immune system, but many have yet to be characterized functionally. Figure 5.12 shows the detailed organization of the human MHC.

Fig. 5.12 Detailed map of the human MHC. The organization of the class I, class II, and class III regions of the human MHC are shown, with approximate genetic distances given in thousands of base pairs (kbp). Most of the genes in the class I and class II regions are mentioned in the text. The additional genes indicated in the class I region (for example, E, F, and G) are class I-like genes, encoding class IB molecules; the additional class II genes are pseudogenes. The genes shown in the class III region encode the complement proteins C4 (two genes, shown as C4A and C4B), C2, and factor B (shown as Bf) as well as genes that encode the cytokines tumor necrosis factor-α (TNF) and lymphotoxin (LTA, LTB). Closely linked to the C4 genes is the gene encoding 21-hydroxylase (shown as CYP 21B), an enzyme involved in steroid biosynthesis. Genes shown in dark gray and named in italic are pseudogenes. The genes are color coded, with the MHC class I genes being shown in red, except for the MIC genes, which are shown in blue; these are distinct from the other class I-like genes and are under different transcriptional control. The MHC class II genes are shown in yellow. Genes in the MHC region that have immune functions but are not related to the MHC class I and class II genes are shown in purple.

In addition to the highly polymorphic 'classical' MHC class I and class II genes, there are many genes encoding MHC class I-type molecules that show little polymorphism; most of these have yet to be assigned a function. They are linked to the class I region of the MHC and their exact number varies greatly between species and even between members of the same species. These genes have been termed **MHC class IB** genes; like MHC class I genes, they encode β_2-microglobulin-associated cell-surface molecules. Their expression on cells is variable, both in the amount present at the cell surface and in the tissue distribution.

One of the mouse MHC class IB molecules, H2-M3, can present peptides with N-formylated amino termini, which is of interest because all bacteria initiate protein synthesis with N-formylmethionine. Cells infected with cytosolic bacteria can be killed by CD8 T cells that recognize N-formylated bacterial peptides bound to H2-M3. Whether an equivalent MHC class IB molecule exists in humans is not known. The large number of MHC class IB genes (50 or more in the mouse) means that many different MHC class IB molecules can exist in a single animal. They may, like the protein that presents N-formylmethionyl peptides, have specialized roles in antigen presentation. Some of them are known to be recognized by NK-cell receptors, as we discuss further below.

Yet other MHC class IB genes have functions unrelated to the immune system. The HFE gene lies some 3×10^6 base pairs from HLA-A. Its protein product is expressed on cells in the intestinal tract, and has a function in iron metabolism, regulating the uptake of dietary iron into the body, most probably through interactions with the transferrin receptor. Individuals defective for this gene have an iron-storage disease, hereditary hemochromatosis, in which an abnormally high level of iron is retained in the liver and other organs. Mice lacking β_2-microglobulin, and hence being defective in the expression of all class I molecules, have a similar iron overload. Exactly how this protein regulates the levels of iron within the body is not known, but it is unlikely to involve an immunological mechanism.

The other genes that map within the MHC include some that encode complement components (for example, C2, C4, and factor B) and some that encode cytokines—for example, tumor necrosis factor-α (TNF-α) and lymphotoxin (TNF-β)—all of which have important functions in immunity. These have been termed MHC class III genes, and are shown in Fig. 5.12. The functions of these genes are discussed in Chapter 2.

Many studies have established associations between susceptibility to certain diseases and particular alleles of MHC genes, and we now have considerable insight into how polymorphism in the classical MHC class I and class II genes can affect resistance or susceptibility. But although most of these MHC-influenced diseases are known or suspected to have an immune etiology, this is not true of all of them, and it is important to remember that there are many genes lying within the MHC that have no known or suspected immunological function. One of these is the enzyme 21-hydroxylase, which, when deficient, causes congenital adrenal hyperplasia and, in severe cases, salt-wasting syndrome. Even where a disease-related gene is clearly homologous to immune-system genes, as is the case with *HFE*, the disease mechanism may not be immune related. Disease associations mapping to the MHC must therefore be interpreted with caution, in the light of a detailed understanding of its genetic structure and the functions of its individual genes. Much remains to be learned about the latter and about the significance of all the genetic variation localized within the MHC. For instance, the C4 genes are highly polymorphic, but the adaptive significance of this genetic variability is not well understood.

5-11 Specialized MHC class I molecules act as ligands for the activation and inhibition of NK cells.

Some class IB genes, for example the members of the **MIC** gene family, are under a different regulatory control from the classical MHC class I genes and are induced in response to cellular stress (such as heat shock). There are five MIC genes, but only two—*MICA* and *MICB*—are expressed and produce protein products. They are expressed in fibroblasts and epithelial cells, particularly in intestinal epithelial cells, and may have a role in innate immunity or in the induction of immune responses in circumstances in which interferons are not produced. The MICA and MICB molecules are recognized by a receptor that is present on NK cells, γ:δ T cells, and some CD8 T cells, and can activate these cells to kill MIC-expressing targets. The MIC receptor is composed of two chains. One is NKG2D, an 'activating' member of the NKG2 family of NK-cell receptors; its cytoplasmic domain lacks an inhibitory sequence motif found in other members of this family, which act as inhibitory receptors (see Section 2-28). The other is a protein called DAP10, which transmits the signal into the interior of the cell by interacting with and activating intracellular phosphatidyl-inositol-3 kinase or PI-3K (see Chapter 6).

Even more distantly related to MHC class I genes are a small family of proteins known in humans as the UL16- binding proteins or ULBP; the homologous proteins in mice are known as Rae1. These also bind the NKG2D receptor and can also co-stimulate NK cells, γ:δ T cells and CD8 α:β T cells.

Other MHC class IB molecules may inhibit cell killing by NK cells, as described in Chapter 2. Such a role has been suggested for the MHC class IB molecule HLA-G, which is expressed on fetus-derived placental cells that migrate into the uterine wall. These cells express no classical MHC class I molecules and cannot be recognized by CD8 T cells but, unlike other cells lacking classical MHC class I molecules, they are not killed by NK cells. This seems to be because HLA-G is recognized by an inhibitory receptor, ILT-2, on the NK cell, which prevents the NK cell from killing placental cells.

Another MHC class IB molecule, HLA-E, also has a specialized role in cell recognition by NK cells. HLA-E binds a very restricted subset of peptides, derived from the leader peptides of other HLA class I molecules. These peptide:HLA-E complexes can bind to the receptor NKG2A, which is present on NK cells in a complex with the cell-surface molecule CD94. NKG2A is an inhibitory member of the NKG2 family, and on stimulation inhibits the cytotoxic activity of the NK cell. Thus a cell that expresses either HLA-E or HLA-G is not killed by NK cells.

5-12 The protein products of MHC class I and class II genes are highly polymorphic.

Because of the polygeny of the MHC, every person will express at least three different antigen-presenting MHC class I molecules and three (or sometimes four) MHC class II molecules on his or her cells (see Section 5-9). In fact, the number of different MHC molecules expressed on the cells of most people is greater because of the extreme polymorphism of the MHC and the codominant expression of MHC gene products.

The term **polymorphism** comes from the Greek *poly*, meaning many, and *morphe*, meaning shape or structure. As used here, it means within-species variation at a gene locus, and thus in its protein product; the variant genes that can occupy the locus are termed **alleles**. There are more than 400 alleles of some human MHC class I and class II genes (Fig. 5.13), each allele being present at a relatively high frequency in the population. So there is only a

Fig. 5.13 Human MHC genes are highly polymorphic. With the notable exception of the DRα locus, which is functionally monomorphic, each locus has many alleles. The numbers of different alleles are shown in this figure by the heights of the bars. The figures are the numbers of HLA alleles currently officially assigned by the WHO Nomenclature Committee for Factors of the HLA System as of January 2004.

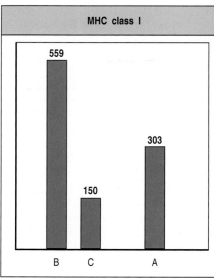

small chance that the corresponding MHC locus on both the homologous chromosomes of an individual will have the same allele; most individuals will be **heterozygous** at MHC loci. The particular combination of MHC alleles found on a single chromosome is known as an **MHC haplotype.** Expression of MHC alleles is codominant, with the protein products of both the alleles at a locus being expressed in the cell, and both gene products being able to present antigens to T cells (Fig. 5.14). The extensive polymorphism at each locus thus has the potential to double the number of different MHC molecules expressed in an individual and thereby increases the diversity already available through polygeny (Fig. 5.15).

Fig. 5.14 Expression of MHC alleles is codominant. The MHC is so polymorphic that most individuals are likely to be heterozygous at each locus. Alleles are expressed from both MHC haplotypes in any one individual, and the products of all alleles are found on all expressing cells. In any mating, four possible combinations of haplotypes can be found in the offspring; thus siblings are also likely to differ in the MHC alleles they express, there being one chance in four that an individual will share both haplotypes with a sibling. One consequence of this is the difficulty of finding suitable donors for tissue transplantation.

Fig. 5.15 Polymorphism and polygeny both contribute to the diversity of MHC molecules expressed by an individual. The high polymorphism of the classical MHC loci ensures a diversity in MHC gene expression in the population as a whole. However, no matter how polymorphic a gene, no individual can express more than two alleles at a single gene locus. Polygeny, the presence of several different related genes with similar functions, ensures that each individual produces a number of different MHC molecules. Polymorphism and polygeny combine to produce the diversity of MHC molecules seen both within an individual and in the population at large.

Polymorphism

Polygeny

Polymorphism and polygeny

Thus, with three MHC class I genes and a possible four sets of MHC class II genes on each chromosome 6, a human typically expresses six different MHC class I molecules and eight different MHC class II molecules on his or her cells. For the MHC class II genes, the number of different MHC molecules may be increased still further by the combination of α and β chains encoded by different chromosomes (so that two α chains and two β chains can give rise to four different proteins, for example). In mice it has been shown that not all combinations of α and β chains can form stable dimers and so, in practice, the exact number of different MHC class II molecules expressed depends on which alleles are present on each chromosome.

All MHC class I and II proteins are polymorphic to a greater or lesser extent, with the exception of the DRα chain and its mouse homolog Eα. These chains do not vary in sequence between different individuals and are said to be **monomorphic**. This might indicate a functional constraint that prevents variation in the DRα and Eα proteins, but no such special function has been found. Many mice, both domestic and wild, have a mutation in the Eα gene that prevents synthesis of the Eα protein. They thus lack cell-surface H-2E molecules, so if H2-E molecules do have a special function it is unlikely to be essential.

5-13   MHC polymorphism affects antigen recognition by T cells by influencing both peptide binding and the contacts between T-cell receptor and MHC molecule.

The products of individual MHC alleles can differ from one another by up to 20 amino acids, making each variant protein quite distinct. Most of the differences are localized to exposed surfaces of the extracellular domain furthest from the membrane, and to the peptide-binding groove in particular (Fig. 5.16). The polymorphic residues that line the peptide-binding groove determine the peptide-binding properties of the different MHC molecules.

We have seen that peptides bind to MHC class I molecules through specific anchor residues (see Section 3-16), and that the amino-acid side chains of these residues anchor the peptide by binding in pockets that line the peptide-binding groove. Polymorphism in MHC class I molecules affects which amino acids line these pockets and thus the pockets' binding specificities. In consequence, the anchor residues of peptides that bind to each allelic variant are different. The set of anchor residues that allows binding to a given MHC class I molecule is called a sequence motif. These sequence motifs make it possible to identify peptides within a protein that can potentially bind the appropriate MHC molecule, which may be very important in designing peptide vaccines. Different allelic variants of MHC class II molecules also bind different peptides, but the more open structure of the MHC class II peptide-binding groove and the greater length of the peptides bound in it allow greater flexibility in peptide binding (see Section 3-17). It is therefore more difficult to predict which peptides will bind to MHC class II molecules.

Fig. 5.16 Allelic variation occurs at specific sites within MHC molecules. Variability plots of the amino acid sequences of MHC molecules show that the variation arising from genetic polymorphism is restricted to the amino-terminal domains (α_1 and α_2 domains of class I molecules, and α_1 and β_1 domains of MHC class II molecules). These are the domains that form the peptide-binding cleft. Moreover, allelic variability is clustered in specific sites within the amino-terminal domains, lying in positions that line the peptide-binding cleft, either on the floor of the groove or directed inward from the walls. For the MHC class II molecule, the variability of the HLA-DR alleles is shown. For HLA-DR, and its homologs in other species, the α chain is essentially invariant and only the β chain shows significant polymorphism.

In rare cases, processing of a protein will not generate any peptides with a suitable motif for binding to any of the MHC molecules expressed by an individual. When this happens, the individual fails to respond to the antigen. Such failures in responsiveness to simple antigens were first reported in inbred animals, where they were called **immune response (Ir) gene defects**. These defects were identified and mapped to genes within the MHC long before the function of MHC molecules was understood. Indeed, they were the first clue to the antigen-presenting function of MHC molecules, although it was only much later that the 'Ir genes' were shown to encode MHC class II molecules. Ir gene defects are common in inbred strains of mice because the mice are homozygous at all their MHC loci and therefore express only one type of MHC molecule from each gene locus. This limits the range of peptides they can present to T cells. Ordinarily, MHC polymorphism guarantees a sufficient number of different MHC molecules in a single individual to make this type of nonresponsiveness unlikely, even to relatively simple antigens such as small toxins. This has obvious importance for host defense.

Initially, the only evidence linking Ir gene defects to the MHC was genetic—mice of one MHC genotype could make antibody in response to a particular antigen, whereas mice of a different MHC genotype, but otherwise genetically identical, could not. The MHC genotype was somehow controlling the ability of the immune system to detect or respond to specific antigens, but it was not clear at the time that direct recognition of MHC molecules was involved.

Later experiments showed that the antigen specificity of T-cell recognition was controlled by MHC molecules. The immune responses affected by the Ir genes were known to be dependent on T cells, and this led to a series of experiments in mice to ascertain how MHC polymorphism might control T-cell responses. The earliest of these experiments showed that T cells could be activated only by macrophages or B cells that shared MHC alleles with the mouse in which the T cells originated. This was the first evidence that antigen recognition by T cells depends on the presence of specific MHC molecules in the antigen-presenting cell. The clearest example of this feature of T-cell recognition came, however, from studies of virus-specific cytotoxic T cells, for which Peter Doherty and Rolf Zinkernagel were awarded the Nobel Prize in 1996.

When mice are infected with a virus, they generate cytotoxic T cells that kill self cells infected with the virus, while sparing uninfected cells or cells infected with unrelated viruses. The cytotoxic T cells are thus virus-specific. A particularly striking outcome of these experiments was that the specificity of the cytotoxic T cells was also affected by the polymorphism of MHC molecules. Cytotoxic T cells induced by viral infection in mice of MHC genotype a (MHC^a) would kill any MHC^a cell infected with that virus but would not kill cells of MHC genotype b, or c, and so on, even if they were infected with the same virus. Because the MHC genotype restricts the antigen specificity of T cells, this effect is called MHC restriction. Together with the earlier studies on both B cells and macrophages, this work showed that MHC restriction is a critical feature of antigen recognition by all functional classes of T cells.

Because different MHC molecules bind different peptides, MHC restriction in immune responses to viruses and other complex antigens can largely be explained solely on this indirect basis. However, it can be seen from Fig. 5.16 that some of the polymorphic amino acids in MHC molecules are located in the α helices flanking the peptide-binding cleft in such a way that they are exposed on the outer surface of the peptide:MHC complex and can be directly contacted by the T-cell receptor (see Fig. 3.27). It is therefore not surprising that when T cells are tested for their ability to recognize the same peptide bound to different MHC molecules, they readily distinguish the peptide bound to MHC^a from the same peptide bound to MHC^b. Thus, the specificity of a T-cell receptor is defined both by the peptide it recognizes and by the MHC molecule bound to it (Fig. 5.17). This restricted recognition may sometimes be caused by differences in the conformation of the bound peptide imposed by the different MHC molecules rather than by direct recognition of polymorphic amino acids in the MHC molecule itself. MHC restriction in antigen recognition therefore reflects the combined effect of differences in peptide binding and of direct contact between the MHC molecule and the T-cell receptor.

Fig. 5.17 T-cell recognition of antigens is MHC restricted. The antigen-specific T-cell receptor (TCR) recognizes a complex of an antigenic peptide and a molecule of self MHC. One consequence of this is that a T cell specific for peptide x and a particular MHC allele, MHC^a (left panel), will not recognize the complex of peptide x with a different MHC allele, MHC^b (center panel), or the complex of peptide y with MHC^a (right panel). The co-recognition of a foreign peptide and MHC molecule is known as MHC restriction because the MHC molecule is said to restrict the ability of the T cell to recognize antigen. This restriction may either result from direct contact between the MHC molecule and T-cell receptor or be an indirect effect of MHC polymorphism on the peptides that bind or on their bound conformation.

5-14   Nonself MHC molecules are recognized by 1–10% of T cells.

The discovery of MHC restriction, by revealing the physiological function of the MHC molecules, also helped to explain the otherwise puzzling phenomenon of recognition of nonself MHC in the rejection of organs and tissues transplanted between members of the same species. Transplanted organs from donors bearing MHC molecules that differ from those of the recipient—even by as little as one amino acid—are invariably rejected. The rapid and very potent cell-mediated immune response to the transplanted tissue results from the presence in any individual of large numbers of T cells that are specifically reactive to nonself, or **allogeneic**, MHC molecules. Early studies on T-cell responses to allogeneic MHC molecules used the **mixed lymphocyte reaction**. In this reaction T cells from one individual are mixed with lymphocytes from a second individual. If the T cells of this individual recognize the other individual's MHC molecules as 'foreign,' the T cells will divide and proliferate. (The lymphocytes from the second individual are usually prevented from dividing by irradiation or treatment with the cytostatic drug mitomycin C.) Such studies have shown that roughly 1–10% of all T cells in an individual will respond to stimulation by cells from another, unrelated, member of the same species. This type of T-cell response is called an **alloreaction** or **alloreactivity** because it represents the recognition of allelic polymorphism in allogeneic MHC molecules.

Before the role of the MHC molecules in antigen presentation was understood, it was a mystery why so many T cells should recognize nonself MHC molecules, as there is no reason that the immune system should have evolved a defense against tissue transplants. However, once it was realized that T-cell receptors have evolved to recognize foreign peptides in combination with polymorphic MHC molecules, alloreactivity became easier to explain. From experiments in which T cells from animals lacking MHC class I and class II molecules have been artificially driven to mature, it has been shown that the ability to recognize MHC molecules is inherent in the genes that encode the T-cell receptor, rather than being dependent on selection for MHC recognition during T-cell development. The high frequency of alloreactive T cells clearly reflects the commitment of the T-cell receptor to the recognition of MHC molecules in general.

Mature T cells have, however, survived a stringent selection process for the ability to respond to foreign peptides bound to self MHC molecules, but not to self peptides presented by these same molecules. It is therefore thought that the alloreactivity of mature T cells reflects the cross-reactivity of T-cell receptors normally specific for a variety of foreign peptides bound by self MHC molecules. Given a T-cell receptor that normally binds a foreign peptide displayed by a self MHC molecule (Fig. 5.18, left panel), there are two ways in which it may bind to nonself MHC molecules. In some cases the peptide bound by the nonself MHC molecule interacts strongly with the T-cell receptor, and the T cells bearing this receptor are stimulated to respond. This type of cross-reactive recognition arises because the spectrum of peptides bound by nonself MHC molecules on the transplanted tissues differs from those bound by the host's own MHC, and it is known as peptide-dominant binding (Fig. 5.18, center panel). In a second type of cross-reactive recognition, known as MHC-dominant binding, alloreactive T cells respond because of direct binding of the T-cell receptor to distinctive features of the nonself MHC molecule (Fig. 5.18, right panel). In these cases the recognition is less dependent on the particular peptide bound; T-cell receptor binding to unique features of the nonself MHC molecule generates a strong signal because of the high concentration of the nonself MHC molecule on the surface of the presenting cell. Both these mechanisms may contribute to the high frequency of T cells that can respond to nonself MHC molecules on transplanted tissue.

Fig. 5.18 Two modes of cross-reactive recognition that may explain alloreactivity. A T cell that is specific for a nonself or foreign peptide:self MHC combination (left panel) may cross-react with peptides presented by other, nonself (allogeneic), MHC molecules. This may come about in either of two ways. Most commonly, the peptides bound to the allogeneic MHC molecule fit well to the T-cell receptor (TCR), allowing binding even if there is not a good fit with the MHC molecule (center panel). Alternatively, but less often, the allogeneic MHC molecule may provide a better fit to the T-cell receptor, giving a tight binding that is thus less dependent on the peptide that is bound to the MHC molecule (right panel).

5-15 Many T cells respond to superantigens.

Superantigens are a distinct class of antigens that stimulate a primary T-cell response similar in magnitude to a response to allogeneic MHC molecules. Such responses were first observed in mixed lymphocyte reactions using lymphocytes from strains of mice that were MHC identical but otherwise genetically distinct. The antigens provoking this reaction were originally designated minor lymphocyte stimulating (Mls) antigens, and it seemed reasonable to suppose that they might be functionally similar to the MHC molecules themselves. We now know that this is not true, however. The Mls antigens found in these mouse strains are encoded by retroviruses that have become stably integrated at various sites into the mouse chromosomes. They act as superantigens because they have a distinctive mode of binding to both MHC and T-cell receptor molecules that enables them to stimulate very large numbers of T cells. Superantigens are produced by many different pathogens, including bacteria, mycoplasmas, and viruses, and the responses they provoke are helpful to the pathogen rather than the host.

Superantigens are unlike other protein antigens, in that they are recognized by T cells without being processed into peptides that are captured by MHC molecules. Indeed, fragmentation of a superantigen destroys its biological activity, which depends on binding as an intact protein to the outside surface of an MHC class II molecule that has already bound peptide. In addition to binding MHC class II molecules, superantigens are able to bind the V_β region of many T-cell receptors (Fig. 5.19). Bacterial superantigens bind mainly to the V_β CDR2 loop, and to a smaller extent to the V_β CDR1 loop and an additional loop called the hypervariable 4 or HV4 loop. The HV4 loop is the predominant binding site for viral superantigens, at least for the Mls antigens encoded by the endogenous mouse mammary tumor viruses. Thus, the α-chain V region and the CDR3 of the β chain of the T-cell receptor have little effect on superantigen recognition, which is determined largely by the germline-encoded V gene segments that encode the expressed V_β chain. Each superantigen is specific for one or a few of the different V_β gene products, of which there are 20–50 in mice and humans; a superantigen can thus stimulate 2–20% of all T cells.

MHCα

MHC β

SE

Vα   peptide

Vβ

Cβ

Toxic Shock
Syndrome

Fig. 5.19 Superantigens bind directly to T-cell receptors and to MHC molecules. Superantigens can bind independently to MHC class II molecules and to T-cell receptors, binding to the Vβ domain of the T-cell receptor (TCR), away from the complementarity-determining regions, and to the outer faces of the MHC class II molecule, outside the peptide-binding site (top panels). The bottom panel shows a reconstruction of the interaction between a T-cell receptor, an MHC class II molecule and a staphylococcal enterotoxin (SE) superantigen, produced by superimposing separate structures of an enterotoxin:MHC class II complex onto an enterotoxin:T-cell receptor complex. The two enterotoxin molecules (actually SEC3 and SEB) are shown in turquoise and blue, binding to the α chain of the class II molecule (yellow) and to the β chain of the T-cell receptor (colored gray for the Vβ domain and pink for the Cβ domain). Molecular model courtesy of H.M. Li, B.A. Fields, and R.A. Mariuzza.

This mode of stimulation does not prime an adaptive immune response specific for the pathogen. Instead, it causes a massive production of cytokines by CD4 T cells, the predominant responding population of T cells. These cytokines have two effects on the host: systemic toxicity and suppression of the adaptive immune response. Both these effects contribute to microbial pathogenicity. Among the bacterial superantigens are the **staphylococcal enterotoxins** (**SEs**), which cause food poisoning, and the **toxic shock syndrome toxin-1** (**TSST-1**), the etiologic principle in toxic shock syndrome.

The role of viral superantigens in human disease is less clear. The T-cell responses to rabies virus and the Epstein–Barr virus indicate the existence of superantigens in these human pathogens, but the genes encoding them have not yet been identified. The best characterized viral superantigens remain the mouse mammary tumor virus superantigens, which are common as endogenous antigens in mice.

5-16   MHC polymorphism extends the range of antigens to which the immune system can respond.

Most polymorphic genes encode proteins that vary by only one or a few amino acids, whereas the different allelic variants of MHC proteins differ by up to 20 amino acids. The extensive polymorphism of the MHC proteins has almost certainly evolved to outflank the evasive strategies of pathogens. Pathogens can avoid an immune response either by evading detection or by suppressing the ensuing response. The requirement that pathogen antigens must be presented by an MHC molecule provides two possible ways of evading detection. One is through mutations that eliminate from the pathogen's proteins all peptides able to bind MHC molecules. The Epstein–Barr virus provides an example of this strategy. In regions of south-east China and in Papua New Guinea there are small isolated populations in which about 60% of the people carry the HLA-A11 allele. Many isolates of the Epstein–Barr virus obtained from these populations have mutations in a dominant peptide epitope normally presented by HLA-A11; the mutant peptides no longer bind to HLA-A11 and cannot be recognized by HLA-A11-restricted T cells. This strategy is plainly much more difficult to follow if there are many different MHC molecules, and the presence of different loci encoding functionally related proteins may have been an evolutionary adaptation by hosts to this strategy by pathogens.

In large outbred populations, polymorphism at each locus can potentially double the number of different MHC molecules expressed by an individual, as most individuals will be heterozygotes. Polymorphism has the additional advantage that individuals in a population will differ in the combinations of MHC molecules that they express and will therefore present different sets of peptides from each pathogen. This makes it unlikely that all individuals in a population will be equally susceptible to a given pathogen and its spread will therefore be limited. That exposure to pathogens over an evolutionary timescale can select for the expression of particular MHC alleles is indicated by the strong association of the HLA-B53 allele with recovery from a potentially lethal form of malaria. This allele is very common in people from West Africa, where malaria is endemic, and rare elsewhere, where lethal malaria is uncommon.

Similar arguments apply to a second strategy for evading recognition. If pathogens can develop mechanisms to block the presentation of their peptides by MHC molecules, they can avoid the adaptive immune response. Adenoviruses encode a protein that binds to MHC class I molecules in the endoplasmic reticulum and prevents their transport to the cell surface, thus preventing the recognition of viral peptides by CD8 cytotoxic T cells. This MHC-binding protein must interact with a polymorphic region of the MHC class I molecule, because some allelic variants are retained in the endoplasmic reticulum by the adenoviral protein whereas others are not. Increasing the variety of MHC molecules expressed therefore reduces the likelihood that a pathogen will be able to block presentation by all of them and completely evade an immune response.

These arguments raise a question: if having three MHC class I loci is better than having one, why are there not far more? The probable explanation is that each time a distinct MHC molecule is added to the repertoire, all T cells that can respond against that self peptide bound to that MHC molecule must be removed to maintain self tolerance. It seems that the number of MHC loci present in humans and mice is about optimal to balance out the advantages of presenting an increased range of foreign peptides and the disadvantages of an increased loss of T cells from the repertoire.

5-17   MHC polymorphism is generated by several different genetic processes.

MHC polymorphism seems to have been strongly selected by evolutionary pressures. However, for selection to work efficiently in organisms that reproduce slowly, such as humans, there must also be powerful mechanisms for generating the variability on which selection can act. The generation of polymorphism in MHC molecules is an evolutionary problem not easily analyzed in the laboratory; however, it is clear that several genetic mechanisms contribute to the generation of new alleles. Some new alleles are the result of point mutations, but many arise from the combination of sequences from different alleles either by genetic recombination or by **gene conversion**, a process in which one sequence is replaced, in part, by another from a different gene (Fig. 5.20).

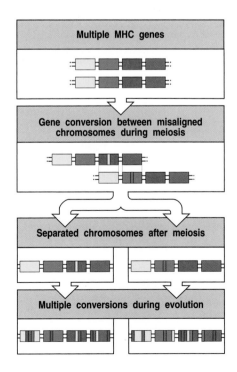

Fig. 5.20 Gene conversion can create new alleles by copying sequences from one MHC gene to another. Sequences can be transferred from one gene to a similar but different gene by a process known as gene conversion. For this to happen, the two genes must become apposed during meiosis. This can occur as a consequence of the misalignment of the two paired homologous chromosomes when there are many copies of similar genes arrayed in tandem—somewhat like buttoning in the wrong buttonhole. During the process of crossing-over and DNA recombination, a DNA sequence from one chromosome is sometimes copied to the other, replacing the original sequence. In this way, several nucleotide changes can be inserted all at once into a gene and can cause several simultaneous amino-acid changes between the new gene sequence and the original gene. Because of the similarity of the MHC genes to each other and their close linkage, gene conversion has occurred many times in the evolution of MHC alleles.

Polymorphic regions in alleles from closely related mouse strains

Strain 1
Strain 2
Strain 3
Strain 4

Polymorphic regions in alleles from distantly related mouse strains

Strain 5
Strain 6
Strain 7
Strain 8

Position of polymorphic regions in one domain of MHC structure

Strain 1

Position of polymorphic regions in one domain of MHC structure

Strain 8

Fig. 5.21 Genetic recombination can create new MHC alleles by DNA exchange between different alleles of the same gene. Conventional meiotic recombination differs from gene conversion in that DNA segments are exchanged between alleles on the two homologous chromosomes rather than, as in gene conversion, being copied in one direction only. Analysis of many MHC allele sequences has shown that the swapping of segments of DNA has occurred many times in the evolution of MHC alleles. Closely related strains of mice have MHC genes in which only one or two segments have been swapped between alleles (first panel), whereas more distantly related strains show a patchwork effect that results from the accumulation of many such recombination events (second panel). The variable parts of MHC molecules correspond to segments of the structure around the peptide-binding groove, such as the β strands or parts of the α helix, as shown in the bottom panels.

Evidence for gene conversion comes from studies of the sequences of different MHC alleles. These reveal that some changes involve clusters of several amino acids in the MHC molecule and require multiple nucleotide changes in a contiguous stretch of the gene. Even more significantly, the sequences that have been changed are frequently derived from other MHC genes on the same chromosome, which is a typical signature of gene conversion. Genetic recombination between different alleles at the same locus may, however, have been more important than gene conversion in generating MHC polymorphism. A comparison of sequences of MHC alleles shows that many different alleles could represent recombination events between a relatively small set of hypothetical ancestral alleles (Fig. 5.21).

The effects of selective pressure in favor of polymorphism can be seen clearly in the pattern of point mutations in the MHC genes. Point mutations can be classified as replacement substitutions, which change an amino acid, or silent substitutions, which simply change the codon but leave the amino acid the same. Replacement substitutions occur within the MHC at a higher frequency relative to silent substitutions than would be expected, providing evidence that polymorphism has been actively selected for in the evolution of the MHC.

5-18   Some peptides and lipids generated in the endocytic pathway can be bound by MHC class I-like molecules that are encoded outside the MHC.

Some MHC class I-like genes map outside the MHC region. One small family of such genes is called CD1 and is expressed on dendritic cells and monocytes as well as some thymocytes. CD1 molecules can present antigens to T cells, but they have two features that distinguish them from classical MHC class I molecules. The first is that the CD1 molecule, although similar to MHC class I molecules in its subunit organization and association with β₂-microglobulin, behaves like an MHC class II molecule. It is not retained within the endoplasmic reticulum by association with the TAP complex but is targeted to vesicles, where it binds its peptide ligand. The peptide antigens bound by CD1 are therefore derived from the breakdown of extracellular proteins within acidified endosomal compartments and, like the peptides that bind to MHC class II molecules, tend to be longer than the peptides that bind to classical MHC class I molecules.

The second unusual feature of CD1 is that it can bind and present glycolipids, in particular the mycobacterial membrane components mycolic acid, glucose monomycolate, phosphoinositol mannosides, and lipoarabinomannan. These are derived either from internalized mycobacteria or from the receptor-mediated ingestion of lipoarabinomannans mediated by the mannose receptor, which is expressed by many phagocytic cells (see Section 2-5). These ligands will thus be delivered into the endocytic pathway, where they can be bound by CD1 molecules. The relationship between the peptide-binding and lipid-binding capacities of CD1 is not clear. Structural studies show that the CD1 molecule has a deep binding groove into which the glycolipid antigens bind. It seems that the CD1 proteins have evolved as a separate lineage of antigen-presenting molecules able to present microbial lipids and glycolipids to T cells.

Summary.

The major histocompatibility complex (MHC) of genes consists of a linked set of genetic loci encoding many of the proteins involved in antigen presentation to T cells, most notably the MHC class I and class II glycoproteins (the MHC molecules) that present peptides to the T-cell receptor. The outstanding feature of the MHC molecules is their extensive polymorphism. This polymorphism is of critical importance in antigen recognition by T cells. A T cell recognizes antigen as a peptide bound by a particular allelic variant of an MHC molecule, and will not recognize the same peptide bound to other MHC molecules. This behavior of T cells is called MHC restriction. Most MHC alleles differ from one another by multiple amino-acid substitutions, and these differences are focused on the peptide-binding site and adjacent regions that make direct contact with the T-cell receptor. At least three properties of MHC molecules are affected by MHC polymorphism: the range of peptides bound; the conformation of the bound peptide; and the direct interaction of the MHC molecule with the T-cell receptor. Thus the highly polymorphic nature of the MHC has functional consequences, and the evolutionary selection for this polymorphism suggests that it is critical to the role of the MHC molecules in the immune response. Powerful genetic mechanisms generate the variation that is seen among MHC alleles, and a compelling argument can be made that selective pressure to maintain a wide variety of MHC molecules in the population comes from infectious agents.

Summary to Chapter 5.

Normally, the antigen receptors on T cells recognize different self peptides that are bound by self MHC molecules. During an infection, the antigen receptors on T cells recognize complexes of pathogen-derived peptides bound to MHC molecules on a target cell surface. There are two classes of MHC molecule—MHC class I molecules, which bind stably to peptides derived from proteins synthesized and degraded in the cytosol, and MHC class II molecules, which bind stably to peptides derived from proteins degraded in endocytic vesicles. In addition to being bound by the T-cell receptor, the two classes of MHC molecule are differentially recognized by the two co-receptor molecules, CD8 and CD4, which characterize the two major subsets of T cells. CD8 T cells recognize MHC class I:peptide complexes and are activated to kill cells displaying foreign peptides derived from cytosolic pathogens, such as viruses. CD4 T cells recognize MHC class II:peptide complexes and are specialized to activate other immune effector cells, for example B cells or macrophages, to act against the foreign antigens or pathogens that they have taken up. Thus, the two classes of MHC molecule deliver peptides from different intracellular compartments to the cell surface, where they are recognized by different types of T cells that perform the appropriate effector function. There are several genes for each class of MHC molecule, arranged in clusters within a larger region known as the major histocompatibility complex (MHC). Within the MHC, the genes for the MHC molecules are closely linked to genes involved in the degradation of proteins into peptides, the formation of the complex of peptide and MHC molecule, and the transport of these complexes to the cell surface. Because the several different genes for the MHC class I and class II molecules are highly polymorphic and are expressed in a codominant fashion, each individual expresses a number of different MHC class I and class II molecules. Each different MHC molecule can bind stably to a range of different peptides, and thus the MHC repertoire of each individual can recognize and bind many different peptide antigens. Because the T-cell receptor binds a combined peptide:MHC ligand, T cells show MHC-restricted antigen recognition, such that a given T cell is specific for a particular peptide bound to a particular MHC molecule. The genes encoding the T-cell receptors seem to have evolved to recognize MHC molecules, thus accounting for the high frequency of T cells that respond to allogeneic MHC molecules, such as those on an organ transplant from an unrelated donor.

Chapter 5 questions.

5.1 MHC class I and class II molecules are structurally and functionally homologous, yet have dissimilar pathways of assembly and delivery to the cell surface. Describe how these are integrated with the different functions of class I and class II molecules.

5.2 "The MHC is an antigen presentation operon." To what extent is this statement an accurate description of the MHC, and what factors may have been responsible for this organization?

5.3 Many of the proteins encoded within the MHC exist in the population in multiple forms. (a) What genetic events give rise to this variation and what are its functional consequences? (b) In some cases, particular combinations of alleles of the different MHC genes are found to be present at a far higher frequency than chance would predict. What are the possible mechanisms that might explain this finding?

General references.

Bodmer, J.G., Marsh, S.G.E., Albert, E.D., Bodmer, W.F., DuPont, B., Erlich, H.A., Mach, B., Mayr, W.R., Parham, P., Saszuki, T., et al.: **Nomenclature for factors of the HLA system, 1991.** *Tissue Antigens* 2000, **56**:289–290.

Germain, R.N.: **MHC-dependent antigen processing and peptide presentation: providing ligands for T lymphocyte activation.** *Cell* 1994, **76**:287–299.

Klein, J.: *Natural History of the Major Histocompatibility Complex.* New York, J. Wiley & Sons, 1986.

Moller, G. (ed): **Origin of major histocompatibility complex diversity.** *Immunol. Rev.* 1995, **143**:5–292.

Section references.

5-1   The MHC class I and class II molecules deliver peptides to the cell surface from two distinct intracellular compartments.

Brocke, P., Garbi, N., Momburg, F., and Hammerling, G.J.: **HLA-DM, HLA-DO and tapasin: functional similarities and differences.** *Curr. Opin. Immunol.* 2002, **14**:22–29.

Gromme, M., and Neefjes, J.: **Antigen degradation or presentation by MHC class I molecules via classical and non-classical pathways.** *Mol. Immunol.* 2002, **39**:181–202.

Villadangos, J.A.: **Presentation of antigens by MHC class II molecules: getting the most out of them.** *Mol. Immunol.* 2001, **38**:329–346.

Williams, A., Peh, C.A., and Elliott, T.: **The cell biology of MHC class I antigen presentation.** *Tissue Antigens* 2002, **59**:3–17.

5-2   Peptides that bind to MHC class I molecules are actively transported from the cytosol to the endoplasmic reticulum.

Gorbulev, S., Abele, R., and Tampe, R.: **Allosteric crosstalk between peptide-binding, transport, and ATP hydrolysis of the ABC transporter TAP.** *Proc. Natl. Acad. Sci. USA* 2001, **98**:3732–3737.

Lankat-Buttgereit, B., and Tampe, R.: **The transporter associated with antigen processing: function and implications in human diseases.** *Physiol. Rev.* 2002, **82**:187–204.

Townsend, A., Ohlen, C., Foster, L., Bastin, J., Lunggren, H.G., and Karre, K.: **A mutant cell in which association of class I heavy and light chains is induced by viral peptides.** *Cold Spring Harbor Symp. Quant. Biol.* 1989, **54**:299–308.

Uebel, S., and Tampe, R.: **Specificity of the proteasome and the TAP transporter.** *Curr. Opin. Immunol.* 1999, **11**:203–208.

5-3   Peptides for transport into the endoplasmic reticulum are generated in the cytosol.

Goldberg, A.L., Cascio, P., Saric, T., and Rock, K.L.: **The importance of the proteasome and subsequent proteolytic steps in the generation of antigenic peptides.** *Mol. Immunol.* 2002, **39**:147–164.

Rock, K.L., York, I.A., Saric, T., and Goldberg, A.L.: **Protein degradation and the generation of MHC class I-presented peptides.** *Adv. Immunol.* 2002, **80**:1–70.

Serwold, T., Gonzalez, F., Kim, J., Jacob, R., and Shastri, N.: **ERAAP customizes peptides for MHC class I molecules in the endoplasmic reticulum.** *Nature* 2002, **419**:480–483.

Shastri, N., Schwab, S., and Serwold, T.: **Producing nature's gene-chips: the generation of peptides for display by MHC class I molecules.** *Annu. Rev. Immunol.* 2002, **20**:463–493.

Sijts, A., Sun, Y., Janek, K., Kral, S., Paschen, A., Schadendorf, D., and Kloetzel, P.M.: **The role of the proteasome activator PA28 in MHC class I antigen processing.** *Mol. Immunol.* 2002, **39**:165–169.

5-4   Newly synthesized MHC class I molecules are retained in the endoplasmic reticulum until they bind peptide.

Bouvier, M.: **Accessory proteins and the assembly of human class I MHC molecules: a molecular and structural perspective.** *Mol. Immunol.* 2003, **39**:697–706.

Gao, B., Adhikari, R., Howarth, M., Nakamura, K., Gold, M.C., Hill, A.B., Knee, R., Michalak, M., and Elliott, T.: **Assembly and antigen-presenting function of MHC class I molecules in cells lacking the ER chaperone calreticulin.** *Immunity* 2002, **16**:99–109.

Grandea, A.G., III, and Van Kaer, L.: **Tapasin: an ER chaperone that controls MHC class I assembly with peptide.** *Trends Immunol.* 2001, **22**:194–199.

Van Kaer, L.: **Accessory proteins that control the assembly of MHC molecules with peptides.** *Immunol. Res.* 2001, **23**:205–214.

Williams, A., Peh, C.A., and Elliott, T.: **The cell biology of MHC class I antigen presentation.** *Tissue Antigens* 2002, **59**:3–17.

Williams, A.P., Peh, C.A., Purcell, A.W., McCluskey, J., and Elliott, T.: **Optimization of the MHC class I peptide cargo is dependent on tapasin.** *Immunity* 2002, **16**:509–520.

5-5   Peptides presented by MHC class II molecules are generated in acidified endocytic vesicles.

Godkin, A.J., Smith, K.J., Willis, A., Tejada-Simon, M.V., Zhang, J., Elliott, T., and Hill, A.V.: **Naturally processed HLA class II peptides reveal highly conserved immunogenic flanking region sequence preferences that reflect antigen processing rather than peptide–MHC interactions.** *J. Immunol.* 2001, **166**:6720–6727.

Hiltbold, E.M., and Roche, P.A.: **Trafficking of MHC class II molecules in the late secretory pathway.** *Curr. Opin. Immunol.* 2002, **14**:30–35.

Hsieh, C.S., deRoos, P., Honey, K., Beers, C., and Rudensky, A.Y.: **A role for cathepsin L and cathepsin S in peptide generation for MHC class II presentation.** *J. Immunol.* 2002, **168**:2618–2625.

Lennon-Dumenil, A.M., Bakker, A.H., Wolf-Bryant, P., Ploegh, H.L., and Lagaudriere-Gesbert, C.: **A closer look at proteolysis and MHC-class-II-restricted antigen presentation.** *Curr. Opin. Immunol.* 2002, **14**:15–21.

Maric, M., Arunachalam, B., Phan, U.T., Dong, C., Garrett, W.S., Cannon, K.S., Alfonso, C., Karlsson, L., Flavell, R.A., and Cresswell, P.: **Defective antigen processing in GILT-free mice.** *Science* 2001, **294**:1361–1365.

Pluger, E.B., Boes, M., Alfonso, C., Schroter, C.J., Kalbacher, H., Ploegh, H.L., and Driessen, C.: **Specific role for cathepsin S in the generation of antigenic peptides in vivo.** *Eur. J. Immunol.* 2002, **32**:467–476.

Schwarz, G., Brandenburg, J., Reich, M., Burster, T., Driessen, C., and Kalbacher, H.: **Characterization of legumain.** *Biol. Chem.* 2002, **383**:1813–1816.

5-6   The invariant chain directs newly synthesized MHC class II molecules to acidified intracellular vesicles.

Gregers, T.F., Nordeng, T.W., Birkeland, H.C., Sandlie, I., and Bakke, O.: **The cytoplasmic tail of invariant chain modulates antigen processing and presentation.** *Eur. J. Immunol.* 2003, **33**:277–286.

Hiltbold, E.M., and Roche, P.A.: **Trafficking of MHC class II molecules in the late secretory pathway.** *Curr. Opin. Immunol.* 2002, **14**:30–35.

Kleijmeer, M., Ramm, G., Schuurhuis, D., Griffith, J., Rescigno, M., Ricciardi-Castagnoli, P., Rudensky, A.Y., Ossendorp, F., Melief, C.J., Stoorvogel, W., and Geuze, H.J.: **Reorganization of multivesicular bodies regulates MHC class II antigen presentation by dendritic cells.** *J. Cell Biol.* 2001, **155**:53–63.

van Lith, M., van Ham, M., Griekspoor, A., Tjin, E., Verwoerd, D., Calafat, J., Janssen, H., Reits, E., Pastoors, L., and Neefjes, J.: **Regulation of MHC class II antigen presentation by sorting of recycling HLA-DM/DO and class II within the multivesicular body.** *J. Immunol.* 2001, **167**:884–892.

5-7   A specialized MHC class II-like molecule catalyzes loading of MHC class II molecules with peptides.

Pathak, S.S., Lich, J.D., and Blum, J.S.: **Cutting edge: editing of recycling** class II:peptide complexes by HLA-DM. *J. Immunol.* 2001, **167**:632–635.

Qi, L., and Ostrand-Rosenberg, S.: **H2-O inhibits presentation of bacterial superantigens, but not endogenous self antigens.** *J. Immunol.* 2001, **167**:1371–1378.

Van Kaer, L.: **Accessory proteins that control the assembly of MHC molecules with peptides.** *Immunol. Res.* 2001, **23**:205–214.

Zarutskie, J.A., Busch, R., Zavala-Ruiz, Z., Rushe, M., Mellins, E.D., and Stern, L.J.: **The kinetic basis of peptide exchange catalysis by HLA-DM.** *Proc. Natl. Acad. Sci. USA* 2001, **98**:12450–12455.

5-8 Stable binding of peptides by MHC molecules provides effective antigen presentation at the cell surface.

Apostolopoulos, V., McKenzie, I.F., and Wilson, I.A.: **Getting into the groove: unusual features of peptide binding to MHC class I molecules and implications in vaccine design.** *Front. Biosci.* 2001, **6**: D1311–D1320.

Buslepp, J., Zhao, R., Donnini, D., Loftus, D., Saad, M., Appella, E., and Collins, E.J.: **T cell activity correlates with oligomeric peptide-major histocompatibility complex binding on T cell surface.** *J. Biol. Chem.* 2001, **276**:47320–47328.

Hill, J.A., Wang, D., Jevnikar, A.M., Cairns, E., and Bell, D.A.: **The relationship between predicted peptide-MHC class II affinity and T-cell activation in a HLA-DRbeta1*0401 transgenic mouse model.** *Arthritis. Res. Ther.* 2003, 5:R40–R48.

Su, R.C., and Miller, R.G.: **Stability of surface H-2K(b), H-2D(b), and peptide-receptive H-2K(b) on splenocytes.** *J. Immunol.* 2001, **167**:4869–4877.

5-9 Many proteins involved in antigen processing and presentation are encoded by genes within the major histocompatibility complex.

Aguado, B., Bahram, S., Beck, S., Campbell, R.D., Forbes, S.A., Geraghty, D., Guillaudeux, T., Hood, L., Horton, R., Inoko, H., et al. (The MHC Sequencing Consortium): **Complete sequence and gene map of a human major histocompatibility complex.** *Nature* 1999, **401**:921–923.

Chang, C.H., Gourley, T.S., and Sisk, T.J.: **Function and regulation of class II transactivator in the immune system.** *Immunol. Res.* 2002, **25**:131–142.

Kumanovics, A., Takada, T., and Lindahl, K.F.: **Genomic organization of the mammalian MHC.** *Annu. Rev. Immunol.* 2003, **21**:629–657.

Lefranc, M.P.: **IMGT, the international ImMunoGeneTics database.** *Nucleic Acids Res.* 2003, **31**:307–310.

5-10 A variety of genes with specialized functions in immunity are also encoded in the MHC.

Alfonso, C., and Karlsson, L.: **Nonclassical MHC class II molecules.** *Annu. Rev. Immunol.* 2000, **18**:113–142.

Allan, D.S., Lepin, E.J., Braud, V.M., O'Callaghan, C.A., and McMichael, A.J.: **Tetrameric complexes of HLA-E, HLA-F, and HLA-G.** *J. Immunol. Methods* 2002, **268**:43–50.

Braud, V.M., Allan, D.S., and McMichael, A.J.: **Functions of nonclassical MHC and non-MHC-encoded class I molecules.** *Curr. Opin. Immunol.* 1999, **11**:100–108.

Gao, G.F., Willcox, B.E., Wyer, J.R., Boulter, J.M., O'Callaghan, C.A., Maenaka, K., Stuart, D.I., Jones, E.Y., Van Der Merwe, P.A., Bell, J.I., and Jakobsen, B.K.: **Classical and nonclassical class I major histocompatibility complex molecules exhibit subtle conformational differences that affect binding to CD8αα.** *J. Biol. Chem.* 2000, **275**:15232–15238.

Powell, L.W., Subramaniam, V.N., and Yapp, T.R.: **Haemochromatosis in the new millennium.** *J. Hepatol.* 2000, **32**:48–62.

5-11 Specialized MHC class I molecules act as ligands for the activation and inhibition of NK cells.

Borrego, F., Kabat, J., Kim, D.K., Lieto, L., Maasho, K., Pena, J., Solana, R., and Coligan, J.E.: **Structure and function of major histocompatibility complex (MHC) class I specific receptors expressed on human natural killer (NK) cells.** *Mol. Immunol.* 2002, **38**:637–660.

Boyington, J.C., Riaz, A.N., Patamawenu, A., Coligan, J.E., Brooks, A.G., and Sun, P.D.: **Structure of CD94 reveals a novel C-type lectin fold: implications for the NK cell-associated CD94/NKG2 receptors.** *Immunity* 1999, **10**:75–82.

Braud, V.M., and McMichael, A.J.: **Regulation of NK cell functions through interaction of the CD94/NKG2 receptors with the nonclassical class I molecule HLA-E.** *Curr. Top. Microbiol. Immunol.* 1999, **244**:85–95.

Lopez-Botet, M., and Bellon, T.: **Natural killer cell activation and inhibition by receptors for MHC class I.** *Curr. Opin. Immunol.* 1999, **11**:301–307.

Lopez-Botet, M., Bellon, T., Llano, M., Navarro, F., Garcia, P., and de Miguel, M.: **Paired inhibitory and triggering NK cell receptors for HLA class I molecules.** *Hum. Immunol.* 2000, **61**:7–17.

Lopez-Botet, M., Llano, M., Navarro, F., and Bellon, T.: **NK cell recognition of non-classical HLA class I molecules.** *Semin. Immunol.* 2000, **12**:109–119.

Vales-Gomez, M., Reyburn, H., and Strominger, J.: **Interaction between the human NK receptors and their ligands.** *Crit. Rev. Immunol.* 2000, **20**:223–244.

Vales-Gomez, M., Reyburn, H., and Strominger, J.: **Molecular analyses of the interactions between human NK receptors and their HLA ligands.** *Hum. Immunol.* 2000, **61**:28–38.

5-12 The protein products of MHC class I and class II genes are highly polymorphic.

Marsh, S.G.: **Nomenclature for factors of the HLA system, update December 2002.** *Eur. J. Immunogenet.* 2003, **30**:167–169.

Robinson, J., and Marsh, S.G.: **HLA informatics. Accessing HLA sequences from sequence databases.** *Methods Mol. Biol.* 2003, **210**:3–21.

Robinson, J., Waller, M.J., Parham, P., de Groot, N., Bontrop, R., Kennedy, L.J., Stoehr, P., and Marsh, S.G.: **IMGT/HLA and IMGT/MHC: sequence databases for the study of the major histocompatibility complex.** *Nucleic Acids Res.* 2003, **31**:311–314.

5-13 MHC polymorphism affects antigen recognition by T cells by influencing both peptide binding and the contacts between T-cell receptor and MHC molecule.

Garcia, K.C., Degano, M., Speir, J.A., and Wilson, I.A.: **Emerging principles for T cell receptor recognition of antigen in cellular immunity.** *Rev. Immunogenet.* 1999, **1**:75–90.

Hillig, R.C., Coulie, P.G., Stroobant, V., Saenger, W., Ziegler, A., and Hulsmeyer, M.: **High-resolution structure of HLA-A*0201 in complex with a tumour-specific antigenic peptide encoded by the MAGE-A4 gene.** *J. Mol. Biol.* 2001, **310**:1167–1176.

Katz, D.H., Hamaoka, T., Dorf, M.E., Maurer, P.H., and Benacerraf, B.: **Cell interactions between histoincompatible T and B lymphocytes. IV. Involvement of immune response (Ir) gene control of lymphocyte interaction controlled by the gene.** *J. Exp. Med.* 1973, **138**:734–739.

Kjer-Nielsen, L., Clements, C.S., Brooks, A.G., Purcell, A.W., Fontes, M.R., McCluskey, J., and Rossjohn, J.: **The structure of HLA-B8 complexed to an immunodominant viral determinant: peptide-induced conformational changes and a mode of MHC class I dimerization.** *J. Immunol.* 2002, **169**:5153–5160.

Rosenthal, A.S., and Shevach, E.M.: **Function of macrophages in antigen recognition by guinea pig T lymphocytes. I. Requirement for histocompatible macrophages and lymphocytes.** *J. Exp. Med.* 1973, **138**:1194–1212.

Wang, J.H., and Reinherz, E.L.: **Structural basis of T cell recognition of peptides bound to MHC molecules.** *Mol. Immunol.* 2002, **38**:1039–1049.

Zinkernagel, R.M., and Doherty, P.C.: **Restriction of *in vivo* T-cell mediated cytotoxicity in lymphocytic choriomeningitis within a syngeneic or semiallogeneic system.** *Nature* 1974, **248**:701–702.

5-14 Nonself MHC molecules are recognized by 1–10% of T cells.

Hennecke, J., and Wiley, D.C.: **Structure of a complex of the human alpha/beta T cell receptor (TCR) HA1.7, influenza hemagglutinin peptide, and major histocompatibility complex class II molecule, HLA-DR4 (DRA*0101 and**

DRB1*0401): insight into TCR cross-restriction and alloreactivity. *J. Exp. Med.* 2002, **195**:571–581.

Jankovic, V., Remus, K., Molano, A., and Nikolich-Zugich, J.: **T cell recognition of an engineered MHC class I molecule: implications for peptide-independent alloreactivity.** *J. Immunol.* 2002, **169**:1887–1892.

Merkenschlager, M., Graf, D., Lovatt, M., Bommhardt, U., Zamoyska, R., and Fisher, A.G.: **How many thymocytes audition for selection?** *J. Exp. Med.* 1997, **186**:1149–1158.

Nesic, D., Maric, M., Santori, F.R., and Vukmanovic, S.: **Factors influencing the patterns of T lymphocyte allorecognition.** *Transplantation* 2002, **73**:797–803.

Reiser, J.B., Darnault, C., Guimezanes, A., Gregoire, C., Mosser, T., Schmitt-Verhulst, A.M., Fontecilla-Camps, J.C., Malissen, B., Housset, D., and Mazza, G.: **Crystal structure of a T cell receptor bound to an allogeneic MHC molecule.** *Nat. Immunol.* 2000, **1**:291–297.

Speir, J.A., Garcia, K.C., Brunmark, A., Degano, M., Peterson, P.A., Teyton, L., and Wilson, I.A.: **Structural basis of 2C TCR allorecognition of H-2Ld peptide complexes.** *Immunity* 1998, **8**:553–562.

Zerrahn, J., Held, W., and Raulet, D.H.: **The MHC reactivity of the T cell repertoire prior to positive and negative selection.** *Cell* 1997, **88**:627–636.

5-15   Many T cells respond to superantigens.

Acha-Orbea, H., Finke, D., Attinger, A., Schmid, S., Wehrli, N., Vacheron, S., Xenarios, I., Scarpellino, L., Toellner, K.M., MacLennan, I.C., and Luther, S.A.: **Interplays between mouse mammary tumor virus and the cellular and humoral immune response.** *Immunol. Rev.* 1999, **168**:287–303.

Alam, S.M., and Gascoigne, N.R.: **Binding kinetics of superantigen with TCR and MHC class II.** *Methods Mol. Biol.* 2003, **214**:65–85.

Alouf, J.E., and Muller-Alouf, H.: **Staphylococcal and streptococcal superantigens: molecular, biological and clinical aspects.** *Int. J. Med. Microbiol.* 2003, **292**:429–440.

Krakauer, T.: **Immune response to staphylococcal superantigens.** *Immunol. Res.* 1999, **20**:163–173.

Macphail, S.: **Superantigens: mechanisms by which they may induce, exacerbate and control autoimmune diseases.** *Int. Rev. Immunol.* 1999, **18**:141–180.

Sundberg, E.J., Li, H., Llera, A.S., McCormick, J.K., Tormo, J., Schlievert, P.M., Karjalainen, K., and Mariuzza, R.A.: **Structures of two streptococcal superantigens bound to TCR beta chains reveal diversity in the architecture of T cell signaling complexes.** *Structure* 2002, **10**:687–699.

Torres, B.A., Perrin, G.Q., Mujtaba, M.G., Subramaniam, P.S., Anderson, A.K., and Johnson, H.M.: **Superantigen enhancement of specific immunity: antibody production and signaling pathways.** *J. Immunol.* 2002, **169**:2907–2914.

5-16   MHC polymorphism extends the range of antigens to which the immune system can respond.

Franco, A., Ferrari, C., Sette, A., and Chisari, F.V.: **Viral mutations, TCR antagonism and escape from the immune response.** *Curr. Opin. Immunol.* 1995, **7**:525–531.

Grosberg, R.K., and Hart, M.W.: **Mate selection and the evolution of highly polymorphic self/nonself recognition genes.** *Science* 2000, **289**:2111–2114.

Hill, A.V., Elvin, J., Willis, A.C., Aidoo, M., Allsopp, C.E.M., Gotch, F.M., Gao, X.M., Takiguchi, M., Greenwood, B.M., Townsend, A.R.M., et al.: **Molecular analysis of the association of B53 and resistance to severe malaria.** *Nature* 1992, **360**:435–440.

Potts, W.K., and Slev, P.R.: **Pathogen-based models favouring MHC genetic diversity.** *Immunol. Rev.* 1995, **143**:181–197.

5-17   MHC polymorphism is generated by several different genetic processes.

Gaur, L.K., and Nepom, G.T.: **Ancestral major histocompatibility complex DRB genes beget conserved patterns of localized polymorphisms.** *Proc. Natl. Acad. Sci. USA* 1996, **93**:5380–5383.

5-18   Some peptides and lipids generated in the endocytic pathway can be bound by MHC class I-like molecules that are encoded outside the MHC.

Gadola, S.D., Zaccai, N.R., Harlos, K., Shepherd, D., Castro-Palomino, J.C., Ritter, G., Schmidt, R.R., Jones, E.Y., and Cerundolo, V.: **Structure of human CD1b with bound ligands at 2.3 Å, a maze for alkyl chains.** *Nat. Immunol.* 2002, **3**:721–726.

Gumperz, J.E., and Brenner, M.B.: **CD1-specific T cells in microbial immunity.** *Curr. Opin. Immunol.* 2001, **13**:471–478.

Jayawardena-Wolf, J., and Bendelac, A.: **CD1 and lipid antigens: intracellular pathways for antigen presentation.** *Curr. Opin. Immunol.* 2001, **13**:109–113.

MacDonald, H.R.: **Development and selection of NKT cells.** *Curr. Opin. Immunol.* 2002, **14**:250–254.

Moody, D.B., and Besra, G.S.: **Glycolipid targets of CD1-mediated T-cell responses.** *Immunology* 2001, **104**:243–251.

Moody, D.B., and Porcelli, S.A.: **CD1 trafficking: invariant chain gives a new twist to the tale.** *Immunity* 2001, **15**:861–865.

Moody, D.B., and Porcelli, S.A.: **Intracellular pathways of CD1 antigen presentation.** *Nat. Rev. Immunol.* 2003, **3**:11–22.

PART III

THE DEVELOPMENT OF MATURE LYMPHOCYTE RECEPTOR REPERTOIRES

Chapter 6   Signaling Through Immune System Receptors

General principles of transmembrane signaling.

Antigen receptor structure and signaling pathways.

Other signaling pathways that contribute to lymphocyte behavior.

Chapter 7   The Development and Survival of Lymphocytes

Generation of lymphocytes in bone marrow and thymus.

The rearrangement of antigen-receptor gene segments controls lymphocyte development.

Interaction with self antigens selects some lymphocytes for survival but eliminates others.

Survival and maturation of lymphocytes in peripheral lymphoid tissues.

Signaling Through Immune System Receptors

6

Cells communicate with their environment through a variety of cell-surface receptors that recognize and bind molecules present in the extracellular environment. The main function of T and B lymphocytes is to respond to antigen and so, in their case, the receptors for antigen are the most important and the best studied. Binding of antigen to these receptors generates intracellular signals that alter the cells' behavior, and the mechanisms that bring this about are the main topic of this chapter. Because of the diversity of antigen receptors in the normal lymphocyte population, most of our information on intracellular signaling in lymphocytes comes from tumor-derived lymphoid cell lines that are activated when their antigen receptors are stimulated by anti-receptor antibodies. However, more information is increasingly being derived from studies on normal cells from transgenic animals that express a single type of antigen receptor on their B or T cells. We will use this information to infer the signaling pathways generated when a mature naive lymphocyte binds its specific antigen and is activated to undergo clonal expansion followed by differentiation to a functional effector cell. We will, however, also consider how signaling via the antigen receptor and other lymphocyte receptors can lead to other responses such as inactivation or cell death, depending on the stage of development of the cell and the nature of the ligand.

The antigen receptors of B and T lymphocytes are present at the cell surface as multiprotein complexes. These are composed of clonally variable antigen-binding chains associated with invariant accessory chains that have signaling function. The B-cell and T-cell antigen receptors are formed from different proteins and have different recognition properties, which have been described in Chapters 3 and 4. After these receptors bind their ligand, however, the intracellular signaling pathways leading from the receptor are remarkably similar in B and T cells. In both cases they lead to the nucleus and to changes in gene expression that dictate the lymphocyte's response.

We start this chapter by discussing some general principles of cell signaling, and introduce some of the common mechanisms used in intracellular signaling pathways, with particular reference to the antigen-receptor signaling pathways. In the second part of the chapter we outline the signaling pathways from the antigen receptors to the nucleus, and consider how these can be supplemented or inhibited by signals simultaneously received from other receptors. Other signals act through different receptors at different times to influence the development, survival, and responses of lymphocytes and other immune system cells, and these are considered in the third and final part of the chapter.

General principles of transmembrane signaling.

The challenge that faces all cells that respond to external stimuli is how the recognition of a stimulus, usually by receptors on the outer surface of the cell, is able to effect changes within the cell. Extracellular signals are transmitted across the plasma membrane by receptor proteins, which are instrumental in converting extracellular ligand binding into an intracellular biochemical event. Conversion of a signal from one form into another is known as **signal transduction**, and in this part of the chapter we consider several different mechanisms of signal transduction in cell signaling. Cell-surface receptors activate intracellular signaling pathways and so convert an extracellular signal into an intracellular one that then transmits the signal onward. The signal is converted into different biochemical forms, distributed to different sites in the cell, and sustained and amplified as it proceeds toward its various destinations. One result of intracellular signaling may be changes in the cytoskeleton and secretory apparatus. This is seen in the activation of effector T cells, which direct the release of secretory vesicles to the site where the antigen receptor is bound to antigen on the target cell. The final destination of intracellular signaling is usually the nucleus, where the activation of transcription factors turns on new gene expression and cell division may be induced.

6-1 Binding of antigen leads to clustering of antigen receptors on lymphocytes.

All cell-surface receptors that have a signaling function are either transmembrane proteins themselves or form parts of protein complexes that link the exterior and interior of the cell. Many receptors undergo a change in protein conformation on binding their ligand. In some types of receptor this conformational change opens an ion channel into the cell, and the resulting change in the concentration of important ions within the cell acts as the intracellular signal, which is then converted into an intracellular response. In other receptors the conformational change affects the cytoplasmic portion of the receptor, enabling it to associate with and activate intracellular signaling proteins and enzymes.

The antigen receptors on lymphocytes transmit a signal when they bind a ligand, that causes them to cluster together on the cell surface. The requirement for receptor clustering was first shown experimentally in somewhat artificial systems by using antibodies against the extracellular portion of the receptor to mimic antigen binding. Antibodies specific for the B-cell receptor or the T-cell receptor activate signaling by inducing clustering of the receptor complexes. This is a very convenient system for the analysis of early events after activation, as all the cells in a sample are stimulated at the same time, making the course of the response easier to follow.

Antigen receptor clustering occurs when the receptors are cross-linked to each other. The importance of cross-linking was shown by comparing the response to stimulation with antibody $F(ab')_2$ fragments, which have two binding sites, and with Fab fragments, which have only one (see Fig. 3.3). On lymphocytes treated with Fab fragments the antigen receptors do not cluster and the cells make no response, whereas on lymphocytes treated with $F(ab')_2$ fragments the receptors become dimerized and the cells respond, although they may respond only weakly. The response is strongest when the $F(ab')_2$ cross-linked dimers are further clustered by using anti-immunoglobulin sera directed against the $F(ab')_2$ fragments. The extensive cross-linking of the antigen receptors that then occurs delivers a very strong signal to the cell (Fig. 6.1).

Fab fragments of antibodies bind to BCR but do not signal

Fab

BCR

B cell

F(ab')₂ fragments cross-link BCR and can produce a signal

F(ab')₂

Anti-F(ab')₂ antibodies cause extensive cross-linking and a strong signal

rabbit anti-F(ab')₂ antibody

Fig. 6.1 Cross-linking of antigen receptors is the first step in lymphocyte activation. The requirement for receptor cross-linking is illustrated by the use of anti-immunoglobulin antibodies to activate the B-cell antigen receptor (BCR). As shown in the left panel, Fab fragments of an anti-immunoglobulin can bind to the receptors but cannot cross-link them; they also fail to activate B cells. F(ab')₂ fragments of the same anti-immunoglobulin, which have two binding sites, can bridge two receptors (center panel), and thus signal, albeit weakly, o the B cell. The most effective activation occurs when receptors are extensively cross-linked by first adding the F(ab')₂ fragments and then rabbit antibody molecules that bind and cross-link the bound F(ab')₂ fragments (right panel). The use of antibodies generally to stimulate receptors is described in Appendix I, Section A-19.

How antigen receptors are clustered *in vivo* when B and T cells encounter their specific antigens is not yet completely understood. T-cell receptors are presumed to undergo clustering in response to contact with another cell surface bearing multiple copies of the specific MHC:peptide complex that they recognize. B-cell receptors can be cross-linked by pathogens such as intact bacteria and viruses that have repetitive epitopes on their surfaces. Complex molecules that contain regularly repeated identical epitopes will have the same effect. However, it is still uncertain how B-cell receptors can be clustered by soluble monomeric antigens, such as most of the experimental antigens that immunologists use to study immune responses. An inability, or limited ability, of soluble monomeric antigens to induce receptor clustering might explain why the activation of naive B cells in response to these antigens depends on receiving activating signals from antigen-specific T cells. As we will see in Chapter 9, the binding of soluble monomeric antigen by the B-cell receptor triggers receptor-mediated endocytosis but is not sufficient by itself to stimulate cell division and differentiation. However, receptor-mediated uptake allows the antigen to be processed and displayed as peptide fragments bound to MHC class II molecules at the cell surface. The B cell can then be recognized by an antigen-specific CD4 effector T cell, which can deliver activating signals that drive clonal expansion and differentiation.

Understanding how the binding of antigen leads to receptor clustering and signaling in lymphocytes is complicated by the diversity of antigen receptors and their ligands. In addition, co-receptors for antigen-linked molecules also cluster with the receptor and contribute to the initiation of intracellular signaling. As we will see in Chapter 8, the clustering of T-cell or B-cell receptors leads to the formation of an organized structure, called the **supramolecular adhesion complex**, or **SMAC**, in which the antigen receptors are—as we will see in Section 6-9—co-localized with other cell-surface signaling and adhesion molecules. How these clusters are formed and organized is poorly understood but is thought to involve both the redistribution of molecules in the B-cell and T-cell membranes and changes in the cytoskeleton of the cells as a result of the signaling process. In T cells, whose antigen is present on the surface of other cells, the formation of the SMAC leads to the clustering on the surface of the antigen-presenting cell of the ligands for the T-cell receptor, co-receptors, and adhesion molecules present in the SMAC. The contact between T cell and antigen-presenting cell is therefore a highly organized interface, which has been referred to as the **immunological synapse**. In this interface both the spatial organization of the signaling molecules and their temporal organization—the rate and order in which molecules are recruited to the immunological synapse—contribute to the overall signal that is generated on antigen recognition.

Kit (CD117), a hematopoietic growth factor receptor, has an extracellular ligand-binding domain and an intracellular kinase domain

Kit

kinase domain

Kit undergoes dimerization upon binding to its ligand, stem-cell factor (SCF)

SCF

The juxtaposed kinase domains phosphorylate and so activate each other

ATP

ADP

Fig. 6.2 Ligand binding to the growth factor receptor Kit induces receptor dimerization and transphosphorylation of its cytoplasmic tyrosine kinase domains. Kit (CD117) is a transmembrane protein with an external ligand-binding domain specific for stem-cell factor (SCF) and a cytoplasmic domain with intrinsic tyrosine kinase activity. In the unbound state, the kinase part of the receptor is inactive (top panel). When SCF binds to Kit, it causes the receptor proteins to dimerize; this allows the two tyrosine kinase domains to phosphorylate one another and so become activated (center and bottom panels). Transactivation of protein kinases by transphosphorylation is an important step in signaling from many cell-surface kinases.

6-2   Clustering of antigen receptors leads to activation of intracellular signal molecules.

Most of the receptors discussed in this chapter initiate intracellular signaling by the activation of **protein tyrosine kinases**, enzymes that affect the activity of other proteins by adding a phosphate group to certain tyrosine residues. The receptors for some growth factors provide the simplest example of this type of receptor. They have cytoplasmic domains that contain an intrinsic tyrosine kinase activity. These enzyme domains are normally inactive, but when brought together by receptor clustering they are able to activate each other by transphosphorylation (Fig. 6.2). Once activated, these tyrosine kinases can phosphorylate and activate other cytoplasmic signaling molecules.

The situation in the antigen receptors is somewhat more complex. As we will see in a later section, they do not themselves have intrinsic tyrosine kinase activity. Instead, the cytoplasmic portions of some of the receptor components interact with intracellular protein tyrosine kinases, which are therefore known as **receptor-associated tyrosine kinases** or, because they have no extracellular receptor domains, as **nonreceptor tyrosine kinases**. When the antigen receptors cluster, these enzymes are brought together and act on each other and on the antigen receptor cytoplasmic tails to initiate the signaling process as in the example above.

In the antigen receptors, the first tyrosine kinases associated with the receptor are members of the Src (pronounced 'Sark') family of tyrosine kinases. The Src-family kinases are common components of signaling pathways concerned with the control of cell division and differentiation in vertebrates and other animals. The prototypic family member Src was initially discovered as the **oncogene** v-*src*, which is responsible for the ability of the Rous sarcoma virus to produce tumors in chickens. This viral gene was subsequently shown to be a modified form of a normal cellular gene called c-*src* that the virus had picked up from its host cell at some time in the past. Several other common components of signaling pathways that regulate cell growth and division were also first discovered through their oncogenic action when mutated or removed from their normal controls.

The receptor-associated Src-family kinases have a key role in transducing signals across the lymphocyte membrane; their activation informs the cell interior that the receptor has encountered its antigen. But this is just the first step in a multistep process. When a cell is signaled by the binding of ligand to a kinase-coupled receptor, kinase activation initiates a cascade of intracellular signaling that transfers the signal to other molecules and eventually carries it to the nucleus.

6-3   Receptors and signaling molecules concentrate in specialized regions of the cell membrane.

The cell membrane of eukaryotic cells is not the simple, uniformly distributed array of lipids initially proposed as the 'fluid mosaic' model, in which proteins either float or remain anchored through contacts with the underlying cytoskeleton. It has become clear that within the membrane are specialized compartments, or microdomains, enriched in particular lipids and with which different membrane proteins associate preferentially. One of these types of microdomain that seems to be important in signaling has been variously called the glycolipid-enriched microdomain (GEM), detergent-insoluble glycolipid-rich domain (DIG), or, more simply, **lipid raft**. Lipid rafts are small, cholesterol-rich areas in the cell membrane that are relatively resistant to solubilization by mild detergents. In these regions the outer leaflet of the lipid bilayer is enriched in particular lipids, notably sphingolipids and cholesterol, that make it more rigid than the surrounding membrane (Fig. 6.3). A better analogy than a raft might be an ice floe because, like ice floes, lipid rafts are dynamic structures that can coalesce to form larger rafts or can break down to smaller structures.

Some proteins are found preferentially in lipid rafts, notably those proteins that have lipid attachments to the membrane rather than hydrophobic transmembrane polypeptide anchors. Thus, glycosylphosphatidylinositol (GPI)-linked proteins are found in lipid rafts, as are intracellular proteins that are attached to the membrane by a fatty-acid or prenyl link. None of these proteins is exclusively associated with rafts, however; they are found in other regions of the membrane as well. The lipid raft is a dynamic rather than a static structure and membrane proteins can move in and out of them, thus changing the properties of the proteins in their immediate environment. In some cases, the preference of individual proteins for rafts is quite weak but can become significant if the protein is aggregated; this is true of the antigen receptors of B and T cells, which can become associated with lipid rafts on cross-linking. Receptor-associated Src-family kinases with a role in immune-cell signaling are found in lipid rafts, as are other important intracellular signaling proteins. Thus, when T-cell and B-cell antigen receptors migrate into lipid rafts they are moving into an environment that enables signaling from the receptors to occur. The importance of this can be demonstrated by disrupting lipid rafts (this is usually done by depleting the cell of cholesterol), which inhibits T-cell signaling.

Fig. 6.3 Signaling molecules are associated with specialized regions of the membrane called lipid rafts. Cell membranes contain phospholipids that have saturated fatty-acid chains and those that have both saturated and unsaturated fatty-acid chains (top panel). Saturated phospholipids can pack more closely together, so that regions of the membrane enriched for saturated phospholipids are more rigid than those that have more unsaturated phospholipids. Such regions also contain a higher proportion of cholesterol than the rest of the membrane, which also increases membrane rigidity. Such specialized membrane microdomains are called 'lipid rafts', on account of their relatively rigid nature. Lipid rafts are enriched for other saturated lipids such as sphingolipids and glycolipids. These are restricted to the external face of the membrane. The phospholipid phosphatidylinositol is enriched in the inner leaflet of the bilayer of these lipid rafts. Various proteins are associated with lipid rafts, such as GPI-linked proteins and those intracellular proteins that have acyl modifications (palmitoylation, myristoylation, isoprenylation), such as the palmitoyl-linked Src-family kinases. Other proteins can migrate into the rafts. Receptors that are found outside lipid rafts can migrate into rafts once the receptor has been oligomerized by binding ligand (bottom panel), changing a weak preference for rafts into a strong one.

Lipid rafts are specialized regions of the cell membrane enriched for saturated lipids and cholesterol. GPI-linked proteins and acylated proteins such as Src-family kinases are found in lipid rafts

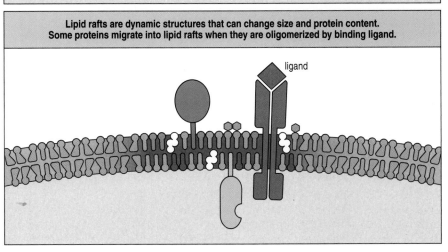

Lipid rafts are dynamic structures that can change size and protein content. Some proteins migrate into lipid rafts when they are oligomerized by binding ligand.

6-4 Phosphorylation of receptor cytoplasmic tails by tyrosine kinases concentrates intracellular signaling molecules around the receptors.

Phosphorylation of enzymes and other proteins by protein kinases is a common general mechanism by which cells regulate their biochemical activity, and it has many advantages as a control mechanism. It is rapid, not requiring new protein synthesis or protein degradation to change the biochemical activity of a cell. It can also be easily reversed by the action of **protein phosphatases**, which remove the phosphate group. Many enzymes become active when phosphorylated and inactive when dephosphorylated, or vice versa; the activity of many of the protein kinases involved in signaling is regulated in this way.

Another and equally important outcome of protein phosphorylation is the creation of a binding site for other proteins. This does not alter the intrinsic activity of the phosphorylated molecule. In this case, phosphorylation is used as a tag, allowing the recruitment of other proteins that bind to the phosphorylated site. For example, many kinases involved in signaling are associated with the inner surface of the cell membrane and can act only inefficiently upon their target proteins when these are free in the cytosol. Receptor activation and the phosphorylation of membrane-associated proteins can, however, create binding sites for these target proteins. Cytosolic proteins that bind to phosphorylated sites at the membrane are thus concentrated near to the kinase, and can in their turn be phosphorylated and activated (Fig. 6.4). They can also, in some cases, be activated simply by binding to phosphotyrosine. This is an example of allosteric activation, because binding the phosphotyrosine leads to an alteration in the protein's molecular conformation.

Proteins can be phosphorylated on three classes of amino acid—tyrosine, serine or threonine, or histidine. Each of these requires a separate class of kinases to add phosphate groups; only the first two are currently known to be relevant to signaling within the immune system. As we have seen, the early events of signaling, associated with the clustering of the antigen receptors, predominantly involve protein tyrosine kinases; the later events also involve protein serine/threonine kinases.

In antigen receptor signaling, the phosphotyrosines generated by the action of tyrosine kinase form binding sites for a protein domain known as an **SH2 domain** (Src homology 2 domain). This is found in many intracellular signaling proteins, including the Src-family kinases in which SH2 domains were first discovered. Binding of SH2 domains to phosphotyrosines is a crucial mechanism for recruiting intracellular signaling molecules to an activated receptor. As well as the SH2 domain, Src-family kinases possess another binding domain known as SH3 or Src homology 3. This domain, which is also found in other proteins, binds to proline-rich regions in diverse proteins and can thus recruit these pro-

Fig. 6.4 Receptor activation recruits cytosolic proteins to the signaling pathway. Receptor-associated protein kinases are localized at the inner surface of the cell membrane and cannot activate their cytosolic targets efficiently unless these are brought to the membrane. However, another membrane-associated protein functions as an adaptor, being phosphorylated by the active kinase to create a binding site for the cytosolic target, bringing the target molecules to the membrane. These proteins can then be phosphorylated, and thus activated, by the membrane-associated kinase.

teins into the signaling pathway, as we will see in a later section. Src-family kinases are usually anchored to the cell membrane by a lipid moiety attached to their amino-terminal region. They are distributed over the inner surface of the cell membrane; during cell activation they become localized to sites of receptor signaling either by binding to phosphotyrosine residues at the receptor site via their SH2 domains or by being associated with other membrane proteins that are themselves recruited to the site of signaling.

As a signaling mechanism, phosphorylation also has the advantage that it is easily and rapidly reversible by protein phosphatases that specifically remove the phosphate groups added by the protein kinases. It is crucial that components of signaling pathways can be readily returned to their unstimulated state; not only does this make the signaling pathway ready to receive another signal but it sets a limit on the time for which any individual signal is active, preventing cellular responses from running out of control. It is therefore not surprising that the signaling pathways that link the cell surface to changes in gene expression use protein phosphorylation and dephosphorylation to regulate the activity of many of their components.

6-5   Intracellular signaling components recruited to activated receptors transmit the signal onward from the membrane and amplify it.

Several classes of protein are typically recruited to the plasma membrane by the activated receptors and participate in signal propagation. The enzyme **phospholipase C-γ (PLC-γ)** contains two SH2 domains through which it can bind to phosphotyrosine, and also an SH3 domain that allows it to bind to proline-rich regions of other signaling proteins; it is thus recruited to the site of receptor-associated tyrosine kinase activity at the plasma membrane. PLC-γ has a crucial role in propagating the signal onward from the membrane and amplifying it. Phosphorylation of tyrosine residues in PLC-γ activates the enzyme, which then cleaves molecules of the membrane phospholipid **phosphatidylinositol bisphosphate (PIP$_2$)** into two parts, **inositol trisphosphate (IP$_3$)** and **diacylglycerol (DAG)** (Fig. 6.5). Because one molecule of PLC-γ can generate many molecules of DAG and IP$_3$, this and similar enzymatic steps serve to amplify and sustain the signal. The production of DAG and IP$_3$ by activated PLC-γ is a common step in pathways from many types of receptor.

The interaction of IP$_3$ with its receptors in the endoplasmic reticulum causes the release of Ca^{2+} into the cytosol from this intracellular storage site, immediately raising intracellular free Ca^{2+} levels severalfold. Depletion of the endoplasmic reticulum calcium stores triggers the opening of calcium channels in

Phospholipase C-γ (PLC-γ) cleaves phosphatidylinositol bisphosphate (PIP$_2$) into diacylglycerol (DAG) and inositol trisphosphate (IP$_3$)

IP$_3$ opens calcium channels to allow Ca^{2+} entry from the endoplasmic reticulum and extracellular fluid. Ca^{2+} activates calmodulin and, with DAG, PKC

Fig. 6.5 The enzyme phospholipase C-γ cleaves inositol phospholipids to generate two important signaling molecules. Phosphatidylinositol bisphosphate (PIP$_2$) is a component of the inner leaflet of the plasma membrane. When phospholipase C-γ (PLC-γ) is activated by phosphorylation, it cleaves PIP$_2$ into two parts, inositol trisphosphate (IP$_3$), which diffuses away from the membrane, and diacylglycerol (DAG), which stays in the membrane. Both these molecules are important in signaling. IP$_3$ binds to calcium channels in the endoplasmic reticulum (ER) membrane, opening the channels and allowing Ca^{2+} to enter the cytosol from stores in the ER. The depletion of Ca^{2+} from the ER in turn triggers the opening of channels in the plasma membrane, allowing Ca^{2+} in from the external fluid. DAG attracts a protein kinase C (PKC) to the cell membrane, where it is activated, often with the help of the increased level of Ca^{2+}. The active forms of protein kinase C are serine/threonine kinases with several roles in cell activation. Raised Ca^{2+} levels also activate a protein known as calmodulin, a ubiquitous Ca^{2+}-binding protein that is responsible for activating other Ca^{2+}-dependent enzymes within the cell.

the plasma membrane that let more Ca^{2+} into the cell, thus sustaining the signal (see Fig. 6.5). Increased intracellular free Ca^{2+} leads to the activation of the Ca^{2+}-binding protein calmodulin, which in turn binds to and regulates the activity of several other proteins and enzymes in the cell, transmitting the signal onward along pathways that eventually converge on the nucleus. One protein that is regulated by the calcium pathway is the nuclear factor of activated T cells (NFAT), a transcription factor we will discuss further in Section 6-12.

The other product of PIP_2 cleavage is DAG, which remains associated with the inner surface of the plasma membrane. DAG helps to activate members of the **protein kinase C (PKC)** family (see Fig. 6.5). These are serine/threonine protein kinases that are thought to initiate several signaling pathways leading to the nucleus. Some isoforms of PKC are further activated by the Ca^{2+} released by IP_3 action. Thus, the two products of the cleavage of PIP_2 reinforce each other in activating PKC as well as having their own independent effects.

Many of the cellular processes that are activated in lymphocytes when antigen binds to its receptor are common to many cell types. For example, resting lymphocytes proliferate when exposed to antigen, whereas other cell types proliferate in response to particular growth factors; what differs in each case is the receptor that initiates the common response pathway in the different cell types. Specialized **adaptor proteins** link these different receptors to common intracellular signaling components.

In lymphocytes, the adaptor proteins that bind to the antigen receptors contain two or more domains, for example, SH2 and SH3 domains, that mediate protein–protein interactions. These proteins do not have kinase activity themselves and their function in general is to recruit other molecules to the activated receptor. Such a protein can bind to a phosphotyrosine residue via its SH2 domain and to other proteins containing proline-rich motifs via its SH3 domains (Fig. 6.6). Binding to an adaptor protein positions these other

| Adaptor proteins contain SH2 and SH3 domains, often arranged as shown | Ligand binding clusters receptors, activating tyrosine kinases and leading to the phosphorylation of receptor cytoplasmic domains | Adaptor proteins bind to phosphotyrosine via their SH2 domains | Other signaling proteins bind to the adaptor protein via proline-rich sequences, becoming concentrated around the activated receptor |

Fig. 6.6 Signals are propagated from the receptor through adaptor proteins, which recruit other signaling proteins to the receptor. Adaptor proteins are specialized signaling molecules that usually have no enzymatic activity themselves. Instead, they allow other molecules to become associated with the activated receptors. Adaptors, as shown in the first panel, often contain SH2 domains flanked by SH3 domains. Once a receptor, in this case Kit, has been activated and transphosphorylated (second panel), adaptors can bind to the phosphotyrosines through their SH2 domains (third panel). Other molecules that contain proline-rich regions can now bind to the adaptors through the SH3 domains and be activated by the receptor-associated kinases (fourth panel).

proteins at or near the cell membrane, where they can in turn be phosphorylated and activated by the tyrosine kinases associated with the receptor. One important family of proteins whose members are bound by adaptors and activated during signaling are the guanine-nucleotide exchange factors, which pass the signal on to another common central component of many signaling pathways, the small G proteins.

6-6 Small G proteins activate a protein kinase cascade that transmits the signal to the nucleus.

Small GTP-binding proteins or **small G proteins** are another class of protein that serves to propagate signals from tyrosine kinase-associated receptors. The family of small single-chain GTP-binding proteins is distinct from the heterotrimeric G proteins that associate with seven-span transmembrane receptors such as the anaphylatoxin or chemokine receptors (see Section 6-18). The best-known small G protein is **Ras**. Like the Src-family kinases, Ras was discovered through its effects on cell growth. A gene encoding a mutated form of Ras was found in various animal retroviruses that cause tumors, and the corresponding cellular *ras* gene (c-*ras*) was subsequently found to be mutated in many different human tumors. The frequent discovery of mutant c-*ras* in tumors indicated that the normal *ras* gene had a crucial role in the control of cell growth and focused attention on the physiological function of Ras. This protein has been highly conserved throughout evolution. Ras proteins are found in all eukaryotic cells and are activated in response to many different cell-activating ligands.

Small G proteins such as Ras exist in two states, depending on whether they are bound to GTP or to GDP. The GTP-bound form of Ras is active, but it can be converted into an inactive GDP-bound form by an intrinsic Ras-GTPase activity, which removes a phosphate group from the bound GTP. This reaction is accelerated by regulatory cofactors, and small G proteins do not normally stay permanently activated; instead they eventually turn themselves off. Thus, the small G proteins are usually found in the inactive GDP-containing state and are activated only transiently in response to activating ligands. However, mutation at a single residue can lock them in the active state, causing them to become oncogenic.

The activation of small G proteins is mediated by **guanine-nucleotide exchange factors** (**GEFs**), which exchange GDP for GTP (Fig. 6.7). The GEFs are recruited to the site of receptor activation indirectly by binding to adaptor proteins. Once recruited to the cell membrane, they are able to activate Ras and other small G proteins, which themselves are localized to the inner surface of the plasma membrane via covalently attached lipids. Thus, G proteins can act as molecular switches, becoming switched on only when the cell-surface receptor is activated.

Fig. 6.7 Small G proteins are switched from inactive to active states by guanine-nucleotide exchange factors. Ras is a small GTP-binding protein with intrinsic GTPase activity. In its GTP-bound state, it is active (first panel), whereas in the GDP-bound state it is inactive. Most of the time it is in the inactive state owing to its intrinsic GTPase activity (second panel). Receptor signaling activates guanine-nucleotide exchange factors (GEFs), which can bind to small G proteins such as Ras and displace GDP, allowing GTP to bind in its place (right panel). In the time before the intrinsic GTPase activity converts GTP to GDP, the Ras protein is active and transmits the signal onward.

| Small G proteins like Ras are active when they bind GTP | Small G proteins cleave bound GTP to GDP, becoming inactive | Guanine-nucleotide exchange factors (GEFs) displace GDP from small G proteins and allow GTP to bind |

Once activated, small G proteins activate, among other things, a cascade of protein kinases known as the **mitogen-activated protein kinase** (**MAP kinase**) cascade. This cascade is found in all multicellular animals and is responsible for many of the effects of activating ligands. The MAP kinase cascade leads directly to the phosphorylation and activation of transcription factors in the nucleus. In particular, the AP-1 family of transcription factors, which are heterodimers of the Fos and Jun proteins, the products of the potential oncogenes *fos* and *jun*, are activated through MAP kinase cascades. We will discuss these activation pathways in more detail in the next part of the chapter, where the structures of the lymphocyte antigen–receptor complexes are described and we look at the particular signals generated by the antigen receptors and the co-receptors that cluster with them.

Summary.

Lymphocyte antigen receptors signal for cell activation using signal transduction mechanisms common to many intracellular signaling pathways. On ligand binding, antigen receptor clustering within specialized regions of the cell membrane called lipid rafts leads to the activation of receptor-associated protein tyrosine kinases at the cytoplasmic face of the plasma membrane. These initiate intracellular signaling by phosphorylating tyrosine residues in the clustered receptor tails. The phosphorylated tyrosines act as binding sites for additional kinases and other signaling molecules that amplify the signal and transmit it onward. The enzyme phospholipase C-γ is recruited in this way and initiates two major pathways of intracellular signaling that are common to many other receptors. Cleavage of the membrane phospholipid PIP_2 by this enzyme produces the diffusible messenger inositol trisphosphate (IP_3) and membrane-bound DAG. The action of IP_3 leads to a sharp increase in the level of intracellular free Ca^{2+}, which activates various calcium-dependent enzymes. Together with Ca^{2+}, DAG initiates a second signaling pathway by activating members of the protein kinase C family. A third pathway involves small G proteins, proteins with GTPase activity that are activated by binding GTP but then hydrolyze the GTP to GDP and become inactive. Small G proteins are recruited to the signaling pathway and activated by guanine-nucleotide exchange factors (GEFs), which catalyze the exchange of GDP for GTP. GEFs and other signaling molecules are linked to the activated receptors by adaptor proteins that bind to phosphorylated tyrosines through one protein domain, the SH2 domain, and to other signaling molecules through other domains including SH3. All these signaling pathways eventually converge on the nucleus to alter patterns of gene transcription.

Antigen receptor structure and signaling pathways.

The antigen receptors on B cells (the **B-cell receptor** or **BCR**) and T cells (the **T-cell receptor** or **TCR**) are multiprotein complexes made up of clonally variable antigen-binding chains—the heavy and light immunoglobulin chains in the B-cell receptor, and the TCRα and TCRβ chains in the T-cell receptor—that are associated with invariant accessory proteins. The invariant chains are required both for transport of the receptors to the cell surface and, most importantly, for initiating signaling when the receptors bind to an extracellular ligand. Antigen binding to the receptor generates signals leading ultimately to the activation of nuclear transcription factors that turn on new gene expression and turn off genes typically expressed only in resting cells. In this part of the chapter we also see how clustering of the antigen receptors with co-receptors helps to generate these signals.

6-7   The variable chains of lymphocyte antigen receptors are associated with invariant accessory chains that perform the signaling function of the receptor.

The antigen-binding portion of the B-cell receptor complex is a cell-surface immunoglobulin that has the same antigen specificity as the secreted antibodies that the B cell will eventually produce. Indeed, it is identical to a secreted monomeric immunoglobulin, except that it is attached to the membrane through the carboxy termini of the paired heavy chains. The mRNA for the cell-surface heavy chain is spliced in such a way that the carboxy terminus of the protein is made up of a transmembrane domain and a very short cytoplasmic tail (see Fig. 4.16). The heavy and light chains do not by themselves make up a complete cell-surface receptor, however. When cells were transfected with heavy- and light-chain cDNA derived from a cell expressing surface immunoglobulin, the immunoglobulin that was synthesized remained inside the transfected cell rather than appearing on the surface. This implied that other molecules were required for the immunoglobulin receptor to be expressed on the cell surface. Two proteins associated with heavy chains on the B-cell surface were subsequently identified and called **Igα** and **Igβ**. Transfection of Igα and Igβ cDNA along with that for the immunoglobulin chains results in the appearance of a B-cell receptor on the cell surface.

Igα and Igβ form disulfide-linked heterodimers that are noncovalently associated with each surface immunoglobulin molecule. Thus the complete B-cell receptor is thought to be a complex of six chains—two identical light chains, two identical heavy chains, one Igα, and one Igβ (Fig. 6.8). The Igα and Igβ genes encode proteins composed of a single amino-terminal immunoglobulin-like domain connected via a transmembrane domain to a cytoplasmic tail. Igα and Igβ provide the only substantial cytoplasmic domains present in the receptor complex and are crucial for signaling. The transmembrane form of the immunoglobulin heavy chain has a very short cytoplasmic tail and it was hard to understand how this could signal into the cell that the surface immunoglobulin was ligated. The discovery of Igα and Igβ solved this conceptual problem.

Signaling from the B-cell receptor complex depends on the presence in Igα and Igβ of amino acid sequences called **immunoreceptor tyrosine-based activation motifs** (**ITAMs**). These motifs were originally identified in the cytoplasmic tails of CD3, the accessory molecules of the T-cell antigen receptor that we will describe later, but are also present in Igα and Igβ, and are now known to be present in the accessory chains involved in signaling from natural killer (NK) cell receptors, and in the Fc receptors on mast cells, macrophages, monocytes, and NK cells that bind antibody constant regions. ITAMs are composed of two tyrosine residues separated by about 9–12 amino acids; the canonical ITAM sequence is …YXX[L/I]X_{6-9}YXX[L/I]…, where Y is tyrosine, L is leucine, I is isoleucine, and X represents any amino acid. Igα and Igβ each have a single ITAM in their cytosolic tails, giving the B-cell receptor a total of two ITAMs. When antigen binds, the tyrosines in these ITAMs become phosphorylated by receptor-associated Src-family tyrosine kinases Blk, Fyn, or Lyn. The ITAMs, by virtue of their two precisely spaced tyrosines, are then able to bind with high affinity to the tandem SH2 domains of members of a second family of protein tyrosine kinases. These kinases—Syk in B cells and ZAP-70 in T cells—are important in transmitting the signal onward.

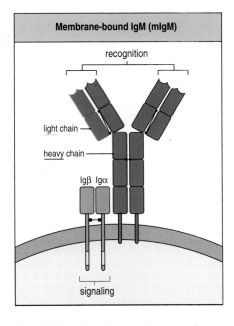

Fig. 6.8 The B-cell receptor complex is made up of cell-surface immunoglobulin with one each of the invariant proteins Igα and Igβ. The immunoglobulin recognizes and binds antigen but cannot itself generate a signal. It is associated with antigen-nonspecific signaling molecules—Igα and Igβ. These each have a single immunoreceptor tyrosine-based activation motif (ITAM), shown as a yellow segment, in their cytosolic tails that enables them to signal when the B-cell receptor is ligated with antigen. Igα and Igβ form a disulfide-linked heterodimer that is associated with the heavy chains, but it is not known which binds to the heavy chain.

Fig. 6.9 The T-cell receptor complex is made up of antigen-recognition proteins and invariant signaling proteins. The T-cell receptor α:β heterodimer (TCR) recognizes and binds its peptide:MHC ligand, but cannot signal to the cell that antigen has bound. In the functional receptor complex, α:β heterodimers are associated with a complex of four other signaling chains (two ε, one δ, one γ) collectively called CD3, which are required for the cell-surface expression of the antigen-binding chains and for signaling. The cell-surface receptor complex is also associated with a homodimer of ζ chains, which signal to the interior of the cell upon antigen binding. Each CD3 chain has one ITAM (yellow segment), whereas each ζ chain has three. The transmembrane regions of each chain have either a net positive or negative charge as shown. It is thought that each complete receptor complex contains two α:β heterodimers associated with the six accessory chains shown in the figure, in which case the charges would balance.

The complete α:β T-cell antigen receptor complex contains several different accessory chains in addition to the highly variable TCRα and TCRβ chains, which form heterodimers containing a single antigen-binding site (see Chapter 4). The invariant accessory chains are CD3γ, CD3δ, and CD3ε, which make up the **CD3 complex**, and the ζ chain, which is present as a largely intracytoplasmic homodimer. Although the exact stoichiometry of the T-cell receptor complex is not definitively established, it seems likely that two α:β heterodimers are associated at the cell surface with one CD3γ, one CD3δ, two CD3ε, and one ζ homodimer (Fig. 6.9, one α:β heterodimer omitted). The three CD3 proteins are encoded in adjacent genes that are regulated as a unit and are required for surface expression of the α:β heterodimers and for signaling via the receptor. Optimal expression and maximum signaling, however, also require the ζ chain, which is encoded elsewhere in the genome.

The CD3 proteins resemble Igα and Igβ in having an extracellular immunoglobulin-like domain and a single ITAM in their cytoplasmic tails. The ζ chain is distinct in having only a short extracellular domain, but it has three ITAMs in its cytoplasmic domain. The CD3 chains have negatively charged acidic residues in their transmembrane domains, which are able to interact with the positive charges of the α and β chains, as shown in Fig. 6.9. In total, the T-cell receptor complex is equipped with 10 ITAMs, which might give it greater flexibility in signaling compared with the B-cell receptor, as discussed later in this chapter.

Thus, the antigen receptors of B and T lymphocytes are made from distinct sets of proteins but are similarly constructed. Both are molecular complexes made up of two types of functional component: variable chains that recognize the individual antigens, and invariant chains that have a role both in the surface expression of the receptors and in transmitting signals to the cell's interior, enabling antigen recognition to be translated into action.

6-8   The ITAMs associated with the B-cell and T-cell receptors are phosphorylated by protein tyrosine kinases of the Src family.

Phosphorylation of the tyrosines in ITAMs serves as the first intracellular signal indicating that the lymphocyte has detected its specific antigen. In B cells, three protein tyrosine kinases of the Src family—Fyn, Blk, and Lyn—are thought to be responsible for this. These Src-family kinases can associate with resting receptors through a low-affinity interaction with an unphosphorylated ITAM, to which they bind through a site in their amino-terminal domain. When the receptors cluster after antigen binding, the receptor-associated kinases phosphorylate and activate each other and are then thought to phosphorylate the tyrosine residues in the ITAMs of the cytoplasmic tails of Igβ and Igα. Phosphorylation of a single tyrosine in an ITAM allows the binding of a Src-family kinase through its SH2 domains, and kinases bound in this way are in turn activated to phosphorylate further ITAM tyrosine residues (Fig. 6.10). It is also possible that the Syk kinase, which binds to the phosphorylated ITAMs in B cells and is responsible for further signaling, can itself phosphorylate the Igα and β ITAMs.

The initial events in T-cell receptor signaling are also implemented by two Src-family kinases—**Lck**, which is constitutively associated with the cytoplasmic domain of the co-receptor molecules CD4 and CD8 (see Section 3-12), and Fyn, which associates with the cytoplasmic domains of the ζ and CD3ε chains upon receptor clustering. In the next section we discuss how CD4 or CD8 is clustered together with the antigen receptor when the receptor binds to its peptide:MHC ligand. Thus antigen recognition allows both Fyn and Lck to phosphorylate specific ITAMs on the accessory chains of the T-cell receptor complex.

Fig. 6.10 Src-family kinases are associated with antigen receptors and phosphorylate the tyrosines in ITAMs. The membrane-bound Src-family kinases Fyn, Blk, and Lyn associate with the B-cell antigen receptor by binding to ITAMs, either through their amino-terminal domains or, as shown in the figure, by binding a single phosphorylated tyrosine through their SH2 domains. After ligand binding and receptor clustering, they phosphorylate tyrosines in the ITAMs on the cytoplasmic tails of Igα and Igβ.

The enzyme activity of the Src-family kinases is itself regulated by the phosphorylation status of the kinase domain and the carboxy-terminal region, each of which has regulatory tyrosine residues. Phosphorylation of the tyrosine in the kinase domain is activatory, whereas phosphorylation of a tyrosine at the carboxy terminus is inhibitory. Even after being phosphorylated at the activating tyrosine, Src-family kinases can be kept inactive by a protein tyrosine kinase called **Csk** (C-terminal Src kinase), which phosphorylates the inhibitory tyrosine (Fig. 6.11). As Csk activity is constitutive in resting cells, the Src proteins are generally inactive. The Src-family kinases are bound to the inner face of the plasma membrane by covalently attached palmitoyl or myristoyl lipids, so for Csk to inactivate these kinases it must first be recruited to the membrane. This task is performed by Cbp (Csk-binding protein), a transmembrane protein whose cytoplasmic domain contains multiple tyrosine residues that can be phosphorylated by Src-family kinases. Phosphorylated Cbp binds Csk, recruiting it to the membrane where it can phosphorylate and thus inactivate Src-family kinases. In this way Cbp and Csk create a negative feedback loop that regulates the Src-family kinase activity within the cell.

An agent that counteracts the effects of Csk is the transmembrane protein tyrosine phosphatase **CD45**, also known as leukocyte common antigen, which is required for receptor signaling in lymphocytes and other cells. CD45 can remove the phosphate from phosphotyrosines, especially from the inhibitory tyrosine residue of Src-family kinases (see Fig. 6.11). Thus, the balance between Csk, which prevents the activation of Src-family kinases, and CD45, which restores their potential for being activated, determines the signaling activity of Src-family kinases in response to receptor aggregation. This is one way in which the threshold for initiating receptor signaling is regulated in lymphocytes. For example, as we will see in Chapter 10, activated effector T lymphocytes and memory T lymphocytes express an isoform of CD45 that associates with the T-cell receptor complex, thus facilitating signaling through the receptor. By contrast, naive T cells express a CD45 isoform that does not have this property.

The activity of Src-family kinases can also be regulated by controlling their level in the cell. They can be modified by covalent attachment of ubiquitin, a signal that targets proteins for degradation by the proteasome, and this degradation pathway is controlled through association with a regulatory protein, Cbl. Cbl itself does not seem to add the ubiquitin to the Src-family kinases; rather, it acts as an adaptor between the kinases and ubiquitin ligase enzymes.

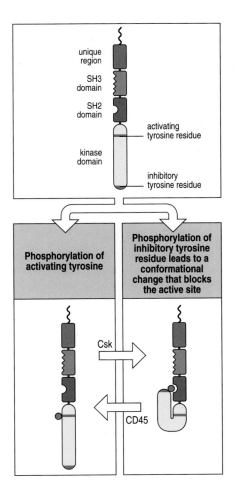

Fig. 6.11 Regulation of Src-family kinase activity. Src-family kinases contain two tyrosine residues (red bars) that are targets for phosphorylation. Phosphorylation of the tyrosine in the amino-terminal part of the kinase domain (bottom left panel) stimulates kinase activity, and this tyrosine is a target for phosphorylation by receptor-associated tyrosine kinases. The second tyrosine lies near the carboxy terminus and has a regulatory function. When it has been phosphorylated, the kinase is inactive as a result of an interaction between the inhibitory phosphotyrosine and the SH2 domain, as shown in the lower right panel.

This process may be used to set a maximum level of response by limiting the concentration of kinases within the cell. However, Cbl is itself a target of tyrosine phosphorylation after receptor aggregation, and it seems more likely that its role is to switch off cascades of activated Src-family kinases after the cell has become activated. Cbl might also be involved in the ubiquitin labeling of other cellular proteins, including components of the T-cell receptor itself, and thus be involved in a more general regulation of cell signaling.

In signaling from the antigen receptor, the activation of Src-family kinases is the first step in a pathway that passes the signal on to many different molecules. Before we consider how signals generated by Src-family kinases are transmitted onward, we will look at how antigen binding by B cells and T cells activates, directly or indirectly, co-receptor molecules that are essential for producing a strong and effective intracellular signal.

6-9 Antigen receptor signaling is enhanced by co-receptors that bind the same ligand.

Optimal signaling through the T-cell receptor complex occurs only when it clusters with the co-receptors CD4 or CD8. This is why most T cells with MHC class II-restricted T-cell receptors express CD4, which binds to the membrane-proximal domain of MHC class II molecules, whereas most T cells with MHC class I-restricted T-cell receptors express CD8, which binds MHC class I molecules. Expression of the appropriate co-receptor means that the MHC:peptide complex bound by the antigen receptor can be simultaneously bound by a co-receptor molecule. Between 10 and 100 identical specific MHC:peptide complexes expressed on a target cell can trigger a T cell expressing the appropriate co-receptor, but in the absence of the co-receptor 10,000 identical complexes (about 10% of all the MHC molecules on a cell) are required for optimal T-cell activation. This density is rarely, if ever, achieved *in vivo*.

Aggregation of the T-cell receptor with the appropriate co-receptor helps to activate the T cell by bringing the Lck tyrosine kinase associated with the cytoplasmic domain of the co-receptor together with the ITAMs and other targets associated with the cytoplasmic domains of the T-cell receptor complex (Fig. 6.12). One of the principal targets of Lck in T cells is another kinase, the ζ-chain-associated protein or ZAP-70, which is important in propagating the signal onward.

B-cell receptor signaling is also enhanced by aggregation with a co-receptor. The **B-cell co-receptor** is expressed on mature B cells as a complex of the cell-surface molecules CD19, CD21, and CD81. One way in which this complex can be co-ligated with the B-cell receptor is through recognition of an antigen that has activated complement. CD21 (also known as complement receptor 2, CR2) is a receptor for the C3d fragment of complement, so antigens, such as pathogens, that have activated complement directly (see Chapter 2) or through the activation of antibody can cross-link the B-cell receptor with CD21 and its associated proteins. This induces phosphorylation of the cytoplasmic tail of CD19 by B-cell receptor-associated tyrosine kinases, which in turn leads to the binding of Src-family kinases and the recruitment of a lipid kinase called phosphatidylinositol 3-OH kinase (PI 3-kinase) (Fig. 6.13). Co-ligation of the B-cell receptor with its CD19/CD21/CD81 co-receptor increases signaling 1000- to 10,000-fold. The role of the third component of the B-cell receptor complex, CD81 (TAPA-1), is as yet unknown.

CD19 is expressed on all B cells from an early stage in their development, before CD21 and CD81 are expressed, and it seems to contribute to signaling through the B-cell receptor even in the absence of co-ligation through CD21.

| In the resting T cell the ITAMs are not phosphorylated | Binding of ligand to the receptor leads to phosphorylation of the ITAMs by Lck when the co-receptor binds to the MHC ligand | ZAP-70 binds to the phosphorylated ζ chain ITAMs and is phosphorylated and activated |

Fig. 6.12 Clustering of the T-cell receptor and a co-receptor initiates signaling within the T cell. When T-cell receptors and co-receptors become clustered on binding MHC:peptide complexes on the surface of an antigen-presenting cell, recruitment of the co-receptor-associated kinase Lck and activation of receptor-associated kinases such as Fyn lead to phosphorylation of the CD3γ, δ, and ε ITAMs as well as those on the ζ chain. The tyrosine kinase ZAP-70 binds to the phosphorylated ITAMs of the ζ chain and is subsequently phosphorylated and activated by Lck.

Thus, B-cell activation that is experimentally induced by cross-linking the B-cell receptor with anti-receptor antibodies is accompanied by co-capping of CD19, the tyrosine phosphorylation of its cytoplasmic tail, and the activation of PI 3-kinase. By contrast, B cells from mice that lack CD19 fail to proliferate in response to B-cell receptor cross-linking and do not fully activate the intracellular signaling pathways normally generated when the B-cell receptor is cross-linked. These experiments suggest that CD19 can associate with the B-cell receptor, either constitutively or after receptor activation, and contribute to signaling even when the co-receptor has not been engaged through CD21 binding to complement. The physiological importance of CD19 is demonstrated by genetically engineered mice that lack this molecule; these mice make deficient B-cell responses to most antigens.

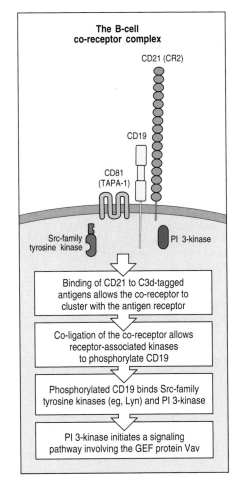

Fig. 6.13 B-cell antigen receptor signaling is modulated by a co-receptor complex of at least three cell-surface molecules, CD19, CD21, and CD81. Binding of the cleaved complement fragment C3d to antigen allows the tagged antigen to bind to both the B-cell receptor and the cell-surface protein CD21 (complement receptor 2, CR2), a component of the B-cell co-receptor complex. Cross-linking and clustering of the co-receptor with the antigen receptor results in phosphorylation of tyrosine residues in the cytoplasmic domain of CD19 by protein kinases associated with the B-cell receptor; other Src-family kinases can bind to phosphorylated CD19 and so augment signaling through the B-cell receptor. Phosphorylated CD19 can also bind the enzyme phosphatidylinositol 3-OH kinase (PI 3-kinase), which is instrumental in recruiting the guanine-nucleotide exchange factor (GEF) Vav to the receptor complex.

Fig. 6.14 Full phosphorylation of the ITAMs on clustered Igα or β chains associated with the B-cell receptor creates binding sites for Syk and Syk activation via transphosphorylation. On clustering of the receptors, the receptor-associated tyrosine kinases Blk, Fyn, and Lyn phosphorylate the ITAMs on the cytoplasmic tails of Igα and Igβ (shown in pale blue and orange, respectively). Subsequently, Syk binds to the phosphorylated ITAMs of the Igβ chain. Because there are at least two receptor complexes in each cluster, Syk molecules become bound in close proximity and can activate each other by transphosphorylation, thus initiating further signaling.

(In figure, top panel:) Clustering of antigen receptors allows receptor-associated kinases to phosphorylate the ITAMs

(labels:) Blk, Fyn, or Lyn   Syk

(bottom panel:) Syk binds to doubly phosphorylated ITAMs and is activated on binding

6-10 Fully phosphorylated ITAMs bind the protein tyrosine kinases Syk and ZAP-70 and enable them to be activated.

Once the ITAMs in the receptor cytoplasmic tails have been phosphorylated, they can recruit the next players in the signaling cascade, the protein tyrosine kinases **Syk** in B cells and **ZAP-70** (ζ-**chain-associated protein**) in T cells. These two proteins define a second family of protein tyrosine kinases expressed mainly in hematopoietic cells (Syk) or mainly in T lymphocytes (ZAP-70); they have two SH2 domains in their amino-terminal halves and a carboxy-terminal kinase domain. Because each SH2 domain binds to one phosphotyrosine, these proteins bind preferentially to motifs with two phosphotyrosines spaced a precise distance apart; tyrosines spaced correctly are found in the ITAM. Thus, ZAP-70 or Syk molecules are recruited to the receptor complex upon full phosphorylation of the ITAMs.

Until Syk has bound to the doubly phosphorylated ITAM in the B-cell receptor, it is inactive enzymatically. To become active it must itself be phosphorylated, and this is thought to occur by transphosphorylation mediated by Syk itself or by Src kinases. Each B-cell receptor complex contains two molecules of Syk, bound to the Igα and Igβ chains. Once the receptors are clustered, these receptor-associated kinases are brought into contact with each other and are thus able to phosphorylate, and hence activate, each other (Fig. 6.14). Once activated, Syk phosphorylates target proteins to initiate a cascade of intracellular signaling molecules.

ZAP-70 is not activated by transphosphorylation after binding to the ITAMs in the ζ chain; instead, it is activated by the co-receptor-associated Src kinase Lck (see Fig. 6.12). Once activated, ZAP-70 phosphorylates the substrate **LAT (linker of activation in T cells)** and a protein called SLP-76, a second linker or adaptor protein in T cells. LAT is a transmembrane protein with a cytoplasmic domain containing multiple tyrosines. It associates with the inside face of the plasma membrane through palmitoylation on cysteine residues. LAT is found within lipid rafts in the membrane and this association is essential for recruitment of a signaling complex and the propagation of signals away from the membrane and into the interior of the cell. By virtue of its many tyrosine residues, phosphorylated LAT is able to recruit proteins that bind through their SH2 domains and transmit the signal from the T-cell membrane to downstream targets. A protein serving the same function in B cells has recently been identified as SLP-65 or **BLNK**, for B-cell linker protein. This, again, has multiple sites for tyrosine phosphorylation, and interacts with many of the same proteins as LAT and SLP-76, to which it has strong sequence similarity. How BLNK is associated with the cell membrane is not yet known.

6-11 Downstream events are mediated by proteins that associate with the phosphorylated tyrosines, and bind to and activate other proteins.

Once ZAP-70 tyrosine kinase has been activated in T cells, and LAT and SLP-76 have been phosphorylated, the next steps in the signaling pathway propagate the signal at the cell membrane, and eventually communicate it to the nucleus. A very similar signaling pathway exists in B cells, made up of activated Syk acting on BLNK, and again propagating the signal from the cell membrane into the nucleus. Signal propagation involves various proteins that bind to phosphotyrosine via SH2 domains, and proteins that are targets for protein tyrosine kinases. Several classes of protein participate in signal propagation. These include the enzyme PLC-γ (see Section 6-5), which initiates two of the main signaling pathways that lead to the nucleus. The third main pathway is generated by activation of the small G protein Ras. These three pathways propagate the signal from the activated receptors at the plasma membrane and carry it to the nucleus, as illustrated schematically in Fig. 6.15 for B cells and Fig. 6.16 for T cells.

Activation of PLC-γ is linked to activation of the antigen receptor through a family of Src-like tyrosine kinases called **Tec kinases**, after a member of the family expressed in T cells and B cells. Other Tec kinases with important roles in lymphocytes are Btk, which is expressed in B lymphocytes, and Itk, which is expressed in T lymphocytes. These kinases contain a domain, called a pleckstrin-homology (PH) domain, that allows them to interact with phosphorylated lipids on the inner face of the cell membrane. They also carry SH2 and SH3 domains that allow them to interact with the adaptor proteins LAT, SLP-76, and BLNK. These interactions allow Tec kinases to cluster around the activated antigen receptor, where they are phosphorylated and activated by other Src-family tyrosine kinases. Once activated, Tec kinases phosphorylate

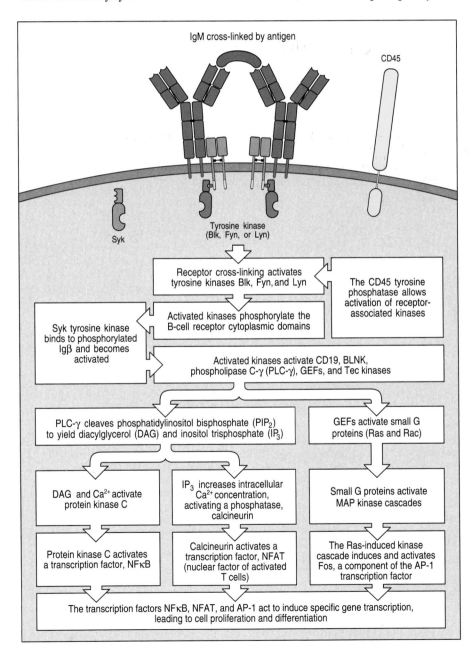

Fig. 6.15 Simplified outline of the intracellular signaling pathways initiated by cross-linking of B-cell receptors by antigen. Cross-linking of surface immunoglobulin molecules activates the receptor-associated Src-family protein tyrosine kinases Blk, Fyn, and Lyn. The CD45 phosphatase can remove an inhibitory phosphate from these kinases, thus allowing their activation. The receptor-associated kinases phosphorylate the ITAMs in the receptor complex, which bind and activate the cytosolic protein kinase Syk, whose activation has been described in Fig. 6.14. Syk then phosphorylates other targets, including the adaptor protein BLNK, which help to recruit Tec kinases that in turn phosphorylate and activate the enzyme phospholipase C-γ. PLC-γ cleaves the membrane phospholipid PIP_2 into IP_3 and DAG, thus initiating two of the three main signaling pathways to the nucleus. IP_3 releases Ca^{2+} from intracellular and extracellular sources, and Ca^{2+}-dependent enzymes are activated, whereas DAG activates protein kinase C with the help of Ca^{2+}. The third main signaling pathway is initiated by guanine-nucleotide exchange factors (GEFs) that become associated with the receptor and activate small GTP-binding proteins such as Ras. These in turn trigger protein kinase cascades (MAP kinase cascades) that lead to the activation of MAP kinases that move into the nucleus and phosphorylate proteins that regulate gene transcription. This scheme is a simplification of the events that actually occur during signaling, showing only the main events and pathways.

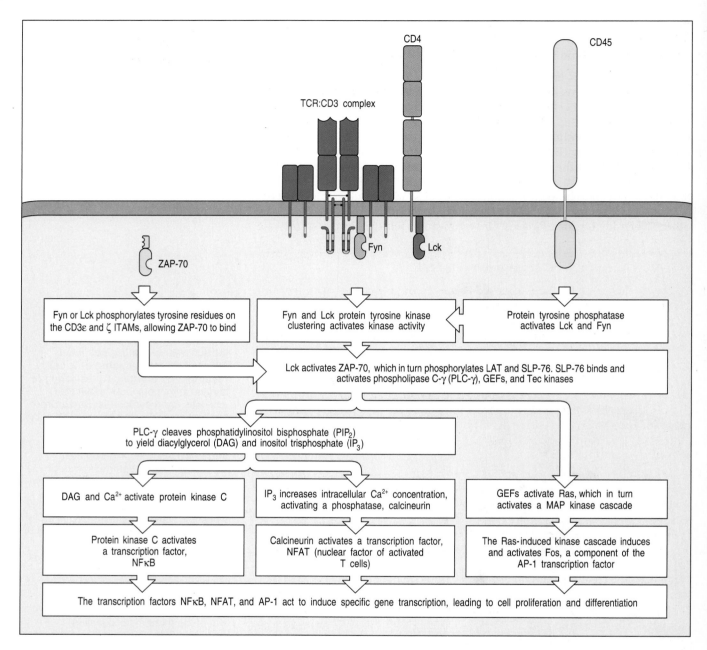

Fig. 6.16 Simplified outline of the intracellular signaling pathways initiated by the T-cell receptor complex and its co-receptor. The T-cell receptor complex and co-receptor (in this example the CD4 molecule) are associated with Src-family protein kinases Fyn and Lck, respectively. It is thought that binding of a peptide:MHC ligand to the T-cell receptor and co-receptor brings together CD4, the T-cell receptor complex, and CD45. This allows the CD45 tyrosine phosphatase to remove inhibitory phosphate groups and thereby allow the activation of Lck and Fyn. Phosphorylation of the ζ chains enables them to bind the cytosolic tyrosine kinase ZAP-70. In freshly isolated T cells, inactive ZAP-70 is already bound to the ζ chain, so this step is thought to occur before stimulation with specific antigen. The subsequent activation of bound ZAP-70 by phosphorylation leads to three important signaling pathways. ZAP-70 phosphorylates the adaptor proteins LAT and SLP-76, which in turn leads to the activation of PLC-γ by Tec kinases and the activation of Ras by guanine-nucleotide exchange factors (GEFs). As illustrated, activated PLC-γ and Ras initiate three important signaling pathways that culminate in the activation of transcription factors in the nucleus. Together, NFκB, NFAT, and AP-1 act on the T-cell chromosomes, initiating new gene transcription that results in the differentiation, proliferation and effector actions of T cells. As with Fig. 6.15, this model is a simplified version showing the main events only.

and activate PLC-γ, which cleaves inositol phospholipids to generate the intracellular second messengers DAG and IP$_3$ (see Section 6-5). The importance of the Tec kinases in lymphocytes can be seen from inherited deficiencies in these enzymes. The human immunodeficiency disease X-linked agammaglobulinemia (XLA), in which B cells fail to mature (see Section 11-8), results from a mutation of Btk, while the same gene mutated in mice leads to a similar immunodeficiency called *xid*.

X-linked Agammaglobulinemia

The activation of Ras is achieved by adaptor proteins and GEFs (see Section 6-6) recruited to the phosphorylated receptors. In B lymphocytes, the adaptor protein Shc binds to tyrosine residues that have been phosphorylated by the receptor-associated tyrosine kinases. Another adaptor protein, Grb2, which has an SH2 domain flanked on both sides by SH3 domains, forms a complex with Shc and this complex binds the guanine-nucleotide exchange factor SOS. SOS, in turn, is involved in activating Ras by the mechanism shown in Fig. 6.7. In T lymphocytes the adaptor protein GADS, a homolog of Grb2, is recruited by phosphorylated LAT, which again uses SOS to recruit Ras to the pathway. Adaptor proteins thus form the scaffolding of a signaling complex, associated with lipid rafts, that links ligand binding by the antigen receptor at the cell surface to the activation of Ras, which then triggers further signaling events downstream.

A second route for the activation of Ras is through another guanine-nucleotide exchange factor, the Ras guanyl-releasing protein, Ras-GRP. The Ras-GRP exchange factor is activated by the binding of lipid second messengers, such as DAG, and also by phorbol esters. Ras-GRP thus links the activation of PLC-γ to the activation of MAP kinase pathways. As described in Section 6-5, activation of PLC-γ produces two independent second messengers, DAG and IP$_3$, which in turn induces a further 'second messenger'—intracellular Ca^{2+} ions. The combination of phorbol esters and calcium ionophores mimics this combination of intracellular messages; the ability of phorbol esters to activate MAP kinases through Ras-GRP underlies the experimental use of combinations of phorbol esters and calcium ionophores to induce T-cell activation and proliferation.

Another small G protein that has a role in both B-cell and T-cell activation is Vav, a multifunctional intracellular adaptor protein that also contains GEF activity. In B cells, Vav is activated via the B-cell co-receptor complex (see Section 6-9). Phosphorylated CD19 binds Vav, which subsequently activates the small G protein **Rac**. In T cells, Vav is recruited to the activated receptor by binding to adaptor proteins SLP-76 and LAT, and again activates Rac. Small G proteins such as Ras and Rac activate a cascade of protein kinases that leads directly to the phosphorylation and activation of transcription factors. Vav and Rac can also influence changes in the actin cytoskeleton, thus linking signaling through cell-surface receptors to changes in cell shape and motility. Changes in the cytoskeleton can also result in the redistribution of cell-surface molecules that contact the cytoskeleton and in the reorientation of the secretory apparatus of the cell, allowing, for example, the targeted release of proteins from the cell at the site of contact with another cell.

Thus, as we have seen so far, a signal originating from activated tyrosine kinases at the cell membrane can be propagated through several different pathways involving many intracellular proteins. We now turn to the question of how signals are transmitted to the nucleus, there to activate transcription factors that can regulate specific genes.

6-12 Antigen recognition leads ultimately to the induction of new gene synthesis by activating transcription factors.

The ultimate response of lymphocytes to extracellular signals is the induction of the expression of new genes. This is achieved through the activation of transcription factors—proteins that control the initiation of transcription by binding to regulatory sites in the DNA. Several important transcription

Fig. 6.17 MAP kinase cascades activate transcription factors.
All MAP kinase cascades share the same general features. They are initiated by a small G protein, which is switched from an inactive state to an active state by a guanine-nucleotide exchange factor (GEF). The small G protein activates the first enzyme of the cascade, a protein kinase called a MAP kinase kinase kinase (MAPKKK). As expected from its name, MAPKKK phosphorylates a second enzyme, MAP kinase kinase (MAPKK), which phosphorylates and activates the mitogen-activated protein kinase (MAP kinase, MAPK) on two sites, a tyrosine and a threonine separated by a single amino acid. This MAP kinase, when doubly phosphorylated, is both activated as a kinase and enabled to translocate from the cytosol into the nucleus, where it can phosphorylate and activate nuclear transcription factors.

factors involved in lymphocyte responses to antigen are activated as a consequence of phosphorylation by the MAP kinases (see Section 6-6). These kinases are themselves activated by phosphorylation; in the inactive, unphosphorylated state they are resident in the cytoplasm, but when activated by phosphorylation they translocate into the nucleus.

Transcription factors are activated by MAP kinases by the general pathway shown in Fig. 6.17. In lymphocytes, the MAP kinases that are thought to activate transcription factors in response to antigen-receptor ligation are called Erk1 (for extracellular-regulated kinase-1) and Erk2. MAP kinases are unusual in that their full activation requires phosphorylation on both a tyrosine and a threonine residue, which are separated in the protein by a single amino acid. This can be done only by MAP kinase kinases, enzymes with dual specificity for tyrosine and serine/threonine residues. In the context of antigen-receptor signaling, the MAP kinase kinases that activate Erk1 and Erk2 are called Mek1 and Mek2. MAP kinase kinases are themselves activated by phosphorylation by a MAP kinase kinase kinase, which is the first kinase in the cascade. It is thought that in lymphocytes this MAP kinase kinase kinase is the serine/threonine kinase **Raf** (Fig. 6.18, left panel). The antigen receptor activates this cascade through the activation of Raf by the GTP-bound form of Ras.

The activation of transcription factors through a MAP kinase cascade is a crucial part of many cell signaling pathways. How the signal is individualized for different stimuli is not yet known, although the existence of variant components at each level of the pathway may allow this to occur. For example, the MAP kinase cascade triggered by signals from the B-cell co-receptor through Vav and Rac uses different kinases from those in the antigen-receptor pathway, and activates different transcription factors (Fig. 6.18, right panel). The MAP kinase cascade activated by the antigen receptor activates the transcription factor Elk, which in turn increases the synthesis of the transcription factor Fos. By contrast, the MAP kinase pathway activated by co-ligation of the B-cell co-receptor activates the transcription factor Jun. These pathways can combine in their effects because heterodimers of Fos and Jun form AP-1 transcription factors, which regulate the expression of many genes involved in cell growth. It seems that both pathways are required to drive the clonal expansion of naive lymphocytes. In T cells, the MAP kinase pathway that activates Jun is activated through a cell-surface molecule known as CD28, which interacts with co-stimulatory molecules that are induced on the surface of antigen-presenting cells during the innate immune response to infection (see Section 2-9). Thus, this second MAP kinase pathway seems to convey to the cell that the antigen is part of a pathogen that has already been recognized by the innate immune system.

A transcription factor that is activated through antigen-receptor signaling, but by a different pathway, is **NFAT (nuclear factor of activated T cells)**. This is something of a misnomer, because NFAT transcription factors are found not only in T cells but also in B cells, NK cells, mast cells, and monocytes, as well as in some nonhematopoietic cells. The function of NFAT is regulated by its intracellular location. NFAT contains amino acid sequence motifs specifying a nuclear localization signal, which enables it to be translocated into the nucleus, and a nuclear export signal, which directs the movement of NFAT back into the cytosol. In unstimulated cells, the nuclear localization signal is rendered inoperative by phosphorylation at serine/threonine residues; hence, NFAT is retained in the cytosol after its synthesis. In addition, should any NFAT make its way to the nucleus, the nuclear export sequence also becomes phosphorylated by a kinase, glycogen synthase kinase 3 (GSK3), which resides primarily within the nucleus. The phosphorylated NFAT is then rapidly exported from the nucleus. The sum of these two effects is that all the NFAT in a resting cell is found in the cytosol.

NFAT is released from the cytosol by the action of the enzyme **calcineurin**, a serine/threonine protein phosphatase. Calcineurin is itself activated by the increase in intracellular free Ca^{2+} that accompanies lymphocyte activation (see Figs. 6.15 and 6.16); the calcium is bound by calmodulin within the cell and the Ca^{2+}–calmodulin complex binds to and activates calcineurin. Once NFAT has been dephosphorylated by calcineurin it enters the nucleus, where it can act as a transcriptional regulatory protein. However, activation of calcineurin alone is insufficient to allow NFAT to function within the nucleus. In the absence of other signals, the NFAT is phosphorylated by GSK3 and exported back out of the nucleus again. Other signals mediated through the T-cell receptor are required to downregulate the activity of GSK3 and permit NFAT to remain in the nucleus. These other signals, and signals generated through co-stimulation, may contribute to NFAT function in another way, because NFAT acts as a transcriptional regulator in combination with AP-1 transcription factors, which, as we have seen above, are dimers of Fos and Jun. In lymphocytes, NFAT interacts with Fos:Jun heterodimers that have been activated by the MAP kinase known as Jnk (commonly pronounced 'Junk') (see Fig. 6.18, right panel). This illustrates how complex the process of signal transduction can be, and how proteins that regulate transcription can integrate signals that come from different pathways.

The importance of NFAT in T-cell activation is illustrated by the effects of the selective inhibitors of NFAT called cyclosporin A and FK506 (tacrolimus). These drugs inhibit calcineurin and hence prevent the formation of active NFAT. T cells express low levels of calcineurin, so they are more sensitive to inhibition of this pathway than are many other cell types. Both cyclosporin A and FK506 thus act as effective inhibitors of T-cell activation with only limited side-effects (see Chapter 14). These drugs are widely used to prevent graft rejection, which they do by inhibiting the activation of alloreactive T cells.

Fig. 6.18 Initiation of MAP kinase cascades by guanine-nucleotide exchange factors is involved in both antigen receptor and co-stimulatory signaling. Signaling through the antigen receptors of both B and T cells (left panel) leads to the activation of the guanine-nucleotide exchange factor SOS, which activates the small G protein Ras. Ras activates the MAP kinase cascade, in which Raf, Mek, and Erk activate each other in turn. Erk finally phosphorylates and activates the transcription factor Elk, which enters the nucleus to initiate new gene transcription, particularly of the *fos* gene. Signaling through the B-cell co-receptor or through the co-stimulatory receptor CD28 on T cells leads to the recruitment and activation of a different guanine-nucleotide exchange factor, Vav (right panel). Activation of Vav initiates a second MAP kinase cascade as Vav activates the small G protein Rac, which initiates the sequential activation of Mekk, Jnkk, and Jnk. Finally, Jnk (which stands for Jun N-terminal kinase) phosphorylates and activates Jun, which, together with Fos, forms the AP-1 transcription factor.

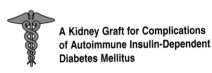

A Kidney Graft for Complications of Autoimmune Insulin-Dependent Diabetes Mellitus

6-13 Signals from the antigen receptor alter the cytoskeleton to produce changes in cell shape, motility, and secretion.

As well as changing the pattern of transcription within cells, signals from cell-surface receptors change cells' behavior in other ways. We have seen that phagocytes actively engulf pathogens that bind to appropriate cell-surface receptors, and that many immune cells can squeeze through vascular endothelia and migrate towards sources of chemokines. Later, in Chapter 8, we will also describe how the secretory apparatus of T cells becomes redirected towards the immune synapse, allowing directed secretion of cytokines or, in CD8 T cells and NK cells, cytotoxic effector molecules, directly into the interface with the target cell. The generation of the organized immune synapse itself requires changes in the distribution of cell-surface molecules that are mediated through contacts with the cytoskeleton of the cell. Thus, signaling often produces a physical change in the cell.

Wiskott–Aldrich Syndrome

The interaction of the signaling pathway with the cytoskeleton is mediated primarily through the adaptor proteins, which transduce signals from the activated receptor through three separate pathways to effect changes in cell shape and behavior. The first of these pathways involves the adaptor protein SLP-76. In T cells, SLP-76 is recruited to LAT by binding to another adaptor, Gads. SLP-76 is phosphorylated by ZAP-70 and then binds a protein called the **adhesion and degranulation promoting protein**, or **ADAP**, which is thought to be involved in cytoskeletal rearrangements and in the increase in integrin affinity—the so-called 'inside-out signaling'—that occurs after low-affinity integrin interactions have allowed initial signaling events to take place. The second pathway of signal transduction to the cytoskeleton also involves SLP-76, serving as the binding site for another adaptor protein, Nck, which in turn binds **WASP**, the **Wiskott–Aldrich Syndrome protein**. Defects in WASP cause an immune deficiency syndrome characterized by thrombocytopenia and impaired cellular and humoral immunity (see Section 11-13). WASP has a key role in transducing signals to the cytoskeletal framework of the cell, because it activates the Arp2/3 complex, an essential component of the actin-polymerization machinery responsible for nucleating actin polymerization.

A third pathway to the cytoskeleton involves the activation of Vav by ZAP-70. To send signals to the cytoskeleton, Vav acts as a GEF for the small G proteins Rac and Rho. These two proteins act in a complementary fashion in regulating cell movement. Rac proteins are involved in the creation of new actin fibers at the leading edge of a moving cell, whereas Rho proteins have a role in the reorganization of the existing cytoskeleton at the trailing edge. A Rac-related G protein, Cdc42, is also activated by Vav and is able to regulate the polarization of activated T cells towards their antigen-presenting targets.

6-14 Not all ligands for the T-cell receptor produce a similar response.

So far, we have assumed that all MHC:peptide complexes that are recognized by a given T-cell receptor will activate the T cell equally—that is, that the T-cell receptor is a binary switch with only two settings, 'on' and 'off.' Peptides that trigger the 'on' setting are called **agonist peptides**, by analogy with the agonist drugs that activate other types of receptor. However, experiments originally designed to explore the structural basis for antigen recognition by T cells by exhaustive mutagenesis of peptides to generate **altered peptide ligands** showed unexpectedly that recognition does not necessarily lead to activation. Indeed, some variant MHC:peptide complexes that do not themselves activate a given T cell can actually inhibit its response to the agonist MHC:peptide complex. These peptides are usually called **antagonist peptides**, because they antagonize the action of the agonist peptide. Other peptides that can trigger only a part of the program activated by the agonist peptide are called **partial agonists**. Such ligands can, for instance, induce the lymphocyte to secrete cytokines but not to proliferate. Most of the antagonist and partial agonist peptides that have been described are closely related in sequence to the agonist peptide, although this is not always so.

Several studies have suggested that the binding interactions between T-cell receptors and these variant MHC:peptide complexes are of a lower affinity than the binding interactions between a T-cell receptor and its agonist peptide:MHC ligand. In many cases the lower affinity results from an increased dissociation rate of the T-cell receptor from the MHC:peptide complex; the dissociation rate might be more important than the overall affinity because T-cell activation through the T-cell receptor is a nonequilibrium process. For MHC:peptide complexes with a fast dissociation rate, the complex with the T-cell receptor might not persist long enough to deliver a full activating signal.

The extent to which antagonist peptides and altered peptide ligands influence physiological immune responses is not known, although they might contribute to the persistence of some viral infections. For example, mutant peptides of epitopes on cells infected with human immunodeficiency virus (HIV) can inhibit the activation of CD8 T cells specific for the original agonist epitope at a 1:100 ratio of mutant to agonist. This sort of effect could allow cells infected with a mutant virus, which arise commonly during the course of HIV infection, to inhibit virus-specific cytotoxic T cells and thereby promote the survival of all infected cells.

Differential signaling by variants of agonist peptides is thought to be important for the development of T cells in the thymus and their subsequent maintenance in the periphery. As we will discuss in Chapter 7, T cells are selected for their potential to be activated by foreign peptide antigens in the context of self MHC molecules through interactions with self-MHC:self-peptide complexes. This process seems to require the receipt of survival signals from self-MHC:self-peptide complexes that are related to, but not identical with, the self-MHC:foreign-peptide complexes that the mature T cell will recognize.

The basis of the incomplete activating signal delivered by altered peptide ligands is unknown, but it has been shown that the recognition of these ligands leads to altered phosphorylation of CD3ε and ζ chains, and to recruitment of the inactive form of ZAP-70 tyrosine kinase to the T-cell receptor. Cross-linking the T-cell receptor alone, without any co-receptor engagement, can also generate the same partial phosphorylation events within the cell. Thus, the incomplete signal generated by altered peptide ligands might reflect a failure to recruit the co-receptors or a failure of the T-cell receptor to interact with the co-receptor productively. Also, because the affinity of the T-cell receptor for the altered peptide ligand:MHC complex is lower than that for the activating complex, the T-cell receptor might dissociate too quickly from its ligand for a full activating signal to be delivered. Another possibility is that conformational changes in the T-cell receptor can contribute to the life-span of the signaling complex and its ability to recruit Lck, and that altered peptide ligands fail to trigger these conformational changes. Antagonist signaling also recruits the tyrosine phosphatase SHP-1 to the T-cell receptor signaling complex, where it can dephosphorylate the signaling complex. This recruitment, which is seen late in activation by agonist peptides, occurs within 1 minute in T cells recognizing antagonist peptides.

Receptors other than antigen receptors also associate with ITAM-containing chains that deliver activating signals		
NK cells Macrophages Neutrophils	NK cells	Mast cells Basophils
FcγRIII (CD16)	KAR	FcεRI
γ or ζ	DAP12	γ

Fig. 6.19 Other receptors that pair with ITAM-containing chains can deliver activating signals. Cells other than B and T cells have receptors that pair with accessory chains containing ITAMs, which are phosphorylated when the receptor is cross-linked. These receptors deliver activating signals. The Fcγ receptor III (CD16) is found on NK cells, macrophages, and neutrophils. Binding of IgG to this receptor activates the killing function of the NK cell, leading to the process known as antibody-dependent cell-mediated cytotoxicity (ADCC). Killer-activating receptors (KAR) are also found on NK cells. The Fcε receptor (FcεRI) is found on mast cells and basophils. It binds to IgE antibodies with very high affinity. When antigen subsequently binds to the IgE, the mast cell is triggered to release granules containing inflammatory mediators. The γ chain associated with the Fc receptors, and the DAP12, or similar DAP10, chain that associates with the NK killer-activating receptors contain one ITAM per chain and are present as homodimers.

6-15 Other receptors on leukocytes also use ITAMs to signal activation.

Although this chapter is focused on lymphocyte antigen receptors, which are the signaling machines that regulate adaptive immunity, other receptors on immune-system cells also use the ITAM to transduce activating signals (Fig. 6.19). One example is FcγRIII (CD16); this is a receptor for IgG that triggers antibody-dependent cell-mediated cytotoxicity (ADCC) by NK cells, which we will consider in Chapter 9; it is also found on macrophages and neutrophils, where it facilitates the uptake and destruction of antibody-bound pathogens. FcγRIII is associated with either an ITAM-containing ζ chain like those found in the T-cell receptor complex or with a second member of the same protein family known as the γ chain. The γ chain is also associated with another type of receptor—the Fcε receptor I (FcεRI) on mast cells. As we will discuss in Chapter 12, this receptor binds IgE antibodies and on cross-linking by allergens it triggers the degranulation of mast cells.

Other members of the ζ-chain family have recently been discovered in NK cells. These proteins, called DAP10 and DAP12, are similar to ζ chains and can form ζ-like homodimers in the NK-cell membrane. Both DAP10 and DAP12 associate with receptors that activate NK cells to kill infected or abnormal target cells (see Section 2-28). DAP12 contains a single ITAM sequence, which when phosphorylated recruits the Syk kinase. DAP10 does not contain an ITAM sequence and instead recruits PI 3-kinase to activate a signaling pathway related to that activated by the co-stimulatory receptor CD28. Both DAP10 and DAP12 are able to signal for the release of the cytotoxic granules by which NK cells kill their targets. DAP10-linked receptors are also present on CD8 T cells, and signaling through DAP10 in these cells delivers co-stimulatory signals that enhance responses to T-cell receptor:MHC:peptide interactions.

Several viral pathogens seem to have acquired ITAM-containing receptors from their hosts. These include the Epstein–Barr virus (EBV), whose *LMP2A* gene has a cytoplasmic tail that encodes an ITAM. This allows EBV to trigger B-cell proliferation by using the downstream signaling molecules that we discussed in Sections 6-10 to 6-12. Other viruses also express genes that encode proteins with ITAMs in their transmembrane regions and also induce transformation. An example is the Kaposi sarcoma herpes virus (KSHV or HHV8).

6-16 Antigen-receptor signaling can be inhibited by receptors associated with ITIMs.

Both B and T cells receive signals that can counteract and modify the activating signals delivered through antigen receptors and co-receptors. These inhibitory signals usually block the response by raising the threshold at which signal transduction can occur. Most of these modifying signals are received through receptors that bear a distinct motif called an **immunoreceptor tyrosine-based inhibitory motif** (**ITIM**) in their cytoplasmic tails. In this motif, a large hydrophobic residue such as isoleucine or valine occurs two residues upstream of a tyrosine that is followed by two amino acids and a leucine to give the amino acid sequence …[I/V]XYXXL… (Fig. 6.20).

The ITIM is found in several receptors that modulate activation signals in lymphocytes. It functions by recruiting one or other of the inhibitory phosphatases SHP-1 (see Section 6-14) and SHIP. These phosphatases carry one or more SH2 domains that preferentially bind the phosphorylated tyrosines in the ITIM. SHP-1 is a protein tyrosine phosphatase and removes the phosphate groups added by tyrosine kinases. SHIP is an inositol phosphatase and removes the 5′ phosphate from phosphatidylinositol trisphosphate (PI-3,4,5-P); the exact mechanism by which SHIP regulates signaling is not known, but it is thought to inhibit the activation of PLC-γ by inhibiting the recruitment of the Tec family of kinases, including Btk and Itk, to the cell membrane and thus inhibiting the production of DAG and IP$_3$ and the associated mobilization of calcium.

One example of an ITIM-containing receptor that inhibits lymphocyte activation is the B-cell Fc receptor for IgG known as FcγRIIB-1. It has long been known that the activation of naive B cells in response to antigen can be inhibited by soluble IgG antibodies that recognize the same antigen and therefore co-ligate the B-cell receptor with this Fc receptor. It was only recently, however, that the FcγRIIB-1 ITIM was defined and shown to function by drawing SHIP into a complex with the B-cell receptor.

Several other receptors on B and T cells contain the ITIM and inhibit cell activation when they are ligated along with the antigen receptors. One example is CD22, a B-cell transmembrane protein that inhibits B-cell signaling. PIR-B, the paired immunoglobulin-like receptor, also expressed on B cells, contains an ITIM that allows it to interact with the tyrosine phosphatase SHP-1. In T cells the transmembrane protein CTLA-4 is induced by activation and then has a crucial role in regulating T-cell signaling; it binds to the same co-stimulatory molecules as CD28 and inhibits signaling through the T-cell receptor by recruiting the tyrosine phosphatase SHP-2. Antibodies that block the recognition by CTLA-4 of its ligands lead to massive increases in T-cell effector function. We will return to the therapeutic consequences of this in Chapter 14, when we look at how T cells can be induced to reject established tumors. The killer inhibitory receptors on NK cells and T cells also have ITIMs; they recognize MHC class I molecules and transmit signals that inhibit the release of cytotoxic granules when NK cells recognize healthy uninfected cells (see Section 2-28). These examples illustrate how the ITIM is able to modify signals originating from the B-cell receptor, the T-cell receptor, Fc receptors, and NK-cell receptors, even to the extent of completely negating them.

Summary.

Lymphocyte antigen receptors are multiprotein complexes made up of variable antigen-binding chains and invariant chains that transmit the signal that antigen has bound. The cytoplasmic tails of the invariant chains contain amino acid motifs called ITAMs, each possessing two tyrosine residues, which are targeted by receptor-associated protein tyrosine kinases of the Src family upon receptor aggregation. The B-cell receptor complex is associated with two such ITAMs, whereas the T-cell receptor complex is associated with 10 ITAMs, the larger number allowing the T-cell receptor a greater flexibility in signaling. Once the ITAMs have been phosphorylated by a Src-family kinase, the Syk-family kinases—Syk in B cells and ZAP-70 in T cells—bind and become activated. Linker and adaptor proteins are subsequently phosphorylated and serve to recruit enzymes that are activated by relocalization to the plasma membrane, by phosphorylation, or by both. Receptor phosphorylation initiates several signaling pathways, including those propagated through phospholipase C-γ and the small G proteins. These pathways converge on the nucleus and result in new patterns of gene expression. The small G proteins activate a cascade of serine/threonine protein kinases known as a MAP kinase cascade, which leads to the phosphorylation and activation of transcription factors. Signaling through the antigen receptors can be enhanced by signaling through the B-cell co-receptor on B cells or the CD4 and CD8 co-receptor molecules on T cells; signaling through the co-stimulatory receptor CD28 on T cells also contributes to activating naive T cells. Activating signals can be modulated or inhibited by signals from inhibitory receptors that are associated with chains containing a different motif, ITIM,

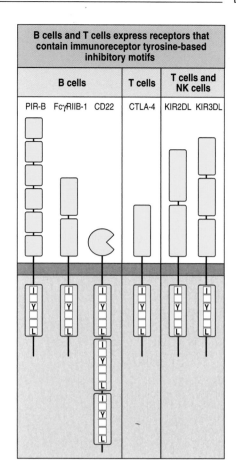

Fig. 6.20 Some lymphocyte cell-surface receptors contain motifs involved in downregulating activation. Several receptors that transduce signals that inhibit lymphocyte or NK-cell activation contain ITIMs (immunoreceptor tyrosine-based inhibitory motifs) in their cytoplasmic tails. These bind to various phosphatases that, when activated, inhibit signals derived from ITAM-containing receptors. Analysis of the mode of action of these receptors has implicated lipid and protein phosphatases that contain SH2 domains.

in their cytoplasmic tails. This provides a mechanism for tuning the on/off threshold according to external stimuli or the state of development of the cell, allowing the modulation of the adaptive immune response. Signaling through the T-cell receptor also occurs in response to altered peptide or antagonist ligands, leading to a state of partial activation that can affect cell survival and the response to agonist ligands.

Other signaling pathways that contribute to lymphocyte behavior.

Lymphocytes are normally studied in terms of their responsiveness to antigen. However, they bear numerous other receptors that make them aware of events occurring both in their immediate neighborhood and at distant sites. Among these are receptors that detect the presence of infection and receptors that bind cytokines produced by the cell itself or reaching it from elsewhere. In the absence of infection, lymphocyte populations are also kept remarkably constant in numbers. This **homeostasis** is achieved by a host of extracellular factors that interact with receptors on lymphocytes, the most important of which is the antigen receptor. Other receptors and ligands that come into play include Fas and its ligand, various cytokine receptors and their ligands, and intracellular proteins such as Bcl-2 that modulate survival.

6-17 Microbes and their products release NFκB from its site in the cytosol through an ancient pathway of host defense against infection.

As we saw in Chapter 2, pathogens that infect the body are detected by the germline-encoded receptors of the innate immune system. One of these families of receptors is the Toll family. The original Toll receptor was first identified in the fruitfly *Drosophila melanogaster* on account of its role in determining dorsoventral body pattern during fly embryogenesis. Later, it was also found to participate in signaling in response to infection in adult flies. Close homologs of Toll have been identified in mammals (see Fig. 2.12), and similar proteins are also used by plants in their defense against viruses, indicating that the Toll pathway is an ancient signaling pathway that is used in innate defenses in most multicellular organisms.

In mammals, the Toll pathway leads to the activation of a transcription factor known as NFκB. Microbial substances such as lipopolysaccharide (LPS), a component of the cell wall of Gram-negative bacteria, and many other microbes and their products can activate NFκB in lymphocytes and other cells through this pathway. LPS signals through a mammalian Toll-like receptor known as TLR-4, with which it interacts indirectly, through association with another cellular receptor (CD14) for LPS (see Section 2-8). Other microbial substances can interact directly with other Toll-like receptors; Gram-positive bacteria, for example, interact with TLR-2. Toll-like receptors signal for NFκB activation through a pathway that seems to operate in most multicellular organisms. The cytoplasmic domain of the Toll receptor is known as a TIR domain because it is also found in the cytoplasmic tail of the receptor for the cytokine interleukin-1 (IL-1R). Ligand binding to the extracellular portion of the Toll receptor induces the TIR domain to bind and activate an adaptor protein known as MyD88. The IL-1 receptor also binds and activates MyD88 on binding IL-1. As the ligands recognized by the various Toll-like receptors and their downstream

| The components of the Toll-like receptor signaling pathway | TLR-4 bound to LPS and LBP binds the adaptor protein MyD88 | MyD88 binds and activates SIIK, which initiates a cascade of TRAF6 and the kinase Iκk | Iκk phosphorylates IκB | Phosphorylated IκB is degraded, releasing NFκB to migrate into the nucleus and activate gene transcription |

connections are now fully worked out, we illustrate this pathway in Fig. 6.21 and describe it below; the pathway from the IL-1R is very similar.

At one end, the MyD88 protein also has a TIR domain through which it interacts with the TIR domain of Toll or IL-1R. At the other end of the MyD88 protein is another domain that mediates protein–protein interactions. This is known as a **death domain** because it was first found in proteins involved in programmed cell death. Through this death domain, the bound adaptor protein interacts with another death domain on a serine/threonine innate immunity kinase (SIIK) known as IRAK, or the IL-1R-associated kinase. This initiates a kinase activation cascade, initially activating two kinases, known as Iκkα and Iκkβ, that dimerize to form part of a multimeric IκB kinase (Iκk), which in turn phosphorylates an inhibitory protein known as IκB. This protein is bound in a complex in the cytosol with the transcription factor NFκB and inhibits its action by retaining it there. When IκB is phosphorylated, it dissociates from the complex and is rapidly targeted for ubiquitination; it is subsequently degraded by proteasomes. After removal of IκB, NFκB enters the nucleus and binds to various promoters, activating genes that contribute to adaptive immunity and the secretion of pro-inflammatory cytokines. Also activated is the gene for IκB itself, which is rapidly synthesized and inactivates the NFκB signal.

The responses activated by this pathway depend on the cell type and organism concerned: in adult *Drosophila*, Toll-family receptors induce the expression of antimicrobial peptides in response to bacterial or fungal infection. In mammals, the Toll signaling pathway contributes to the initiation of an adaptive immune response by inducing the expression of co-stimulatory molecules on tissue dendritic cells and the migration of these cells from a site of infection to a local lymph node (see Chapter 2). Here they can function as antigen-presenting cells and provide a naive lymphocyte that recognizes its antigen with a co-stimulatory signal that combines with the antigen-receptor signal to drive clonal expansion and differentiation.

Fig. 6.21 The transcription factor NFκB is activated by signals from receptors of the Toll-like receptor (TLR) family. The cytoplasmic domain of TLR-4 is homologous to that of the receptor for the cytokine IL-1 and is called a TIR (Toll/IL-1R) domain. This domain can interact with other TIR domains, including that found in the adaptor protein MyD88. MyD88 also contains a death domain through which it interacts with the death domain in a serine/threonine innate immunity kinase (SIIK), which in turn activates TRAF6. TRAF6 activates Iκ kinase-α and Iκ kinase-β, which form the dimer Iκk. Iκk phosphorylates IκB, a cytosolic protein that is retaining the transcription factor NFκB in the cytoplasm. Once phosphorylated, IκB dissociates from its complex with NFκB, allowing NFκB to enter the nucleus and activate genes involved in host defense against infection. The released IκB is subsequently degraded in a ubiquitin-dependent process.

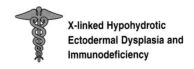

X-linked Hypohydrotic Ectodermal Dysplasia and Immunodeficiency

6-18   Bacterial peptides, mediators of inflammatory responses, and chemokines signal through members of the G-protein-coupled receptor family.

Another way in which cells in the innate immune system are able to detect the presence of infection is by binding bacterial peptides containing *N*-formyl-methionine, or fMet, a modified amino acid that initiates all proteins synthesized in prokaryotes. The receptor that recognizes these peptides is known as the fMet-Leu-Phe (fMLP) receptor, after a tripeptide for which it has a high affinity, although it is not restricted to binding just this tripeptide. The fMLP receptor belongs to an ancient and widely distributed family of receptors that have seven membrane-spanning segments; the best-characterized members of this family are the photoreceptors rhodopsin and bacteriorhodopsin. In the immune system, members of this family of receptors have several essential roles; the receptors for the anaphylatoxins (see Section 2-17) and for chemokines (see Section 2-21) belong to this family.

All receptors of this family use the same mechanism of signaling; ligand binding activates a member of a class of GTP-binding proteins called **G proteins**. These are sometimes called 'large G proteins'—to distinguish them from the smaller Ras-like family of GTP-binding proteins—or 'heterotrimeric G proteins,' because each is made up of three subunits: Gα, Gβ, and Gγ. Roughly 20 different heterotrimeric G proteins are known, each interacting with different cell-surface receptors and transmitting signals to different intracellular pathways. In the resting state, the G protein is inactive, not associated with the receptor and has a molecule of GDP bound to the α subunit. When the receptor binds its ligand, a conformational change in the receptor allows it now to bind the G protein, displacing the GDP molecule from the G protein and replacing it with a molecule of GTP. The G protein now dissociates into two components, the α subunit and the combined βγ subunits; each of these components is capable of interacting with other cellular components to transmit and amplify the signal. Binding of the α subunit to its ligand activates the GTPase activity of this subunit, cleaving the molecule of GTP to GDP, and thus allowing the α and βγ subunits to reassociate (Fig. 6.22).

Fig. 6.22 Seven-transmembrane-domain receptors signal by coupling with trimeric GTP-binding proteins. Seven-transmembrane-domain receptors such as the chemokine receptors signal through trimeric GTP-binding proteins known as large G proteins. In the inactive state, the G protein is bound to GDP. When the receptor binds its ligand, the G protein binds to the receptor and the GDP is replaced by GTP. This triggers the dissociation of the trimeric G protein into α and βγ subunits, both of which can activate other proteins at the inner surface of the cell membrane. The activated response ceases when the α subunit, which contains intrinsic GTPase activity, cleaves GTP to GDP, allowing the α and βγ subunits to reassociate.

Important targets for the activated G protein subunits are adenylate cyclase and phospholipase C, whose activation gives rise to the second messengers cyclic AMP, IP$_3$ and Ca^{2+}. These in turn activate a variety of intracellular pathways that affect cell metabolism, motility, gene expression, and cell division. Thus, activation of G-protein-coupled receptors can have a wide variety of effects depending on the exact nature of the receptor and the G proteins that it interacts with, as well as the different downstream pathways that are activated in different cell types.

6-19 Cytokines signal lymphocytes by binding to cytokine receptors and triggering Janus kinases to phosphorylate and activate STAT proteins.

Cytokines, which we encountered in Chapter 2, are small proteins (with a molecular weight of around 20–25 kDa) that each act on a specific receptor. They are secreted by a variety of cells, usually in response to an external stimulus, and they can then act on the cells that produce them (autocrine action), on other cells in the immediate vicinity (paracrine action), or on cells at a distance (endocrine action) after being carried in blood or tissue fluids. Cytokines affect cell behavior in a variety of ways and, as we will see in subsequent chapters, they have key roles in controlling the growth, development, and functional differentiation of lymphocytes, and as effector molecules of activated T cells. Many cytokines bind to receptors that use a particularly rapid and direct signaling pathway to effect changes in gene expression in the nucleus.

Cytokine binding to such receptors activates receptor-associated tyrosine kinases of the **Janus kinase** family (**JAKs**), so called because they have two symmetrical kinase-like domains and thus resemble the two-headed mythical Roman god Janus. These kinases then phosphorylate cytosolic proteins called **signal transducers and activators of transcription** (**STATs**). Phosphorylation of STAT proteins leads to their homodimerization and heterodimerization through interactions involving their SH2 domains; STAT dimers can then translocate to the nucleus, where they activate various genes (Fig. 6.23). The proteins encoded by these genes contribute to the growth and differentiation of particular subsets of lymphocytes.

Fig. 6.23 Many cytokine receptors signal by a rapid pathway using receptor-associated kinases to activate specific transcription factors. Many cytokines act via receptors that are associated with cytoplasmic Janus kinases (JAKs). The receptor consists of at least two chains, each associated with a specific JAK (first panel). Ligand binding and dimerization of the receptor chains brings together the JAKs, which can transactivate each other, subsequently phosphorylating tyrosines in the receptor tails (second panel). Members of the STAT (signal transducers and activators of transcription) family of proteins bind to the phosphorylated receptors and are themselves phosphorylated by the JAKs (third panel). On phosphorylation, STAT proteins dimerize by binding phosphotyrosine residues in SH2 pockets and go rapidly to the nucleus (last panel), where they bind to and activate the transcription of a variety of genes important for adaptive immunity.

| Cytokine receptors consist of at least two chains, the cytoplasmic domains of which bind Janus kinases (JAKs) | Cytokine binding dimerizes the receptor, bringing together the cytoplasmic JAKs, which activate each other and phosphorylate the receptor | Transcription factors (STATs) bind to the phosphorylated receptors, and are in turn phosphorylated by the activated JAKs | Phosphorylated STATs form dimers that translocate into the nucleus to initiate new gene transcription |

In this pathway, gene transcription is activated very soon after the cytokine binds to its receptor, and specificity of signaling in response to different cytokines is achieved by using different combinations of JAKs and STATs. This signaling pathway is used by most of the cytokines that are released by T cells in response to antigen. Although cytokines are not in themselves antigen specific, their effects can be targeted in an antigen-specific manner by their directed release in antigen-specific cell–cell interactions and their selective action on the cell that triggers their production, as we will see in Chapter 8.

6-20   Programmed cell death of activated lymphocytes is triggered mainly through the receptor Fas.

When antigen-specific lymphocytes are activated through their antigen receptors in an adaptive immune response, they first undergo blast transformation and begin to increase their numbers exponentially by cell division. This clonal expansion can continue for up to 7 or 8 days, so that lymphocytes specific for the infecting pathogen increase vastly in numbers and can come to predominate in the population. In the response to certain viruses, nearly 50% of the CD8 T cells at the peak of the response are specific for a single virus-derived MHC:peptide class I complex. After clonal expansion, the activated T cells undergo their final differentiation into effector cells; these remove the pathogen from the body, which terminates the antigenic stimulus.

When the infection has terminated, the activated effector T cells are no longer needed, and cessation of the antigenic stimulus prompts them to undergo programmed cell death or apoptosis. Apoptosis can probably be induced by several mechanisms, but one that has been particularly well defined is the interaction of the receptor molecule **Fas** on T cells with its ligand, **Fas ligand**. Fas ligand is a member of the tumor necrosis factor (TNF) family of membrane-associated cytokines, whereas Fas is a member of the TNF receptor family. Both Fas and its ligand are normally induced during the course of an adaptive immune response. TNF and its receptor TNFR-I can act in a similar way to Fas ligand and Fas but their actions are far less significant.

All pathways inducing apoptosis lead to the activation of a series of cysteine proteases that cleave protein chains on the carboxy-terminal side of aspartic acid residues and have therefore been called **caspases**. In activated lymphocytes, apoptosis is initiated by stimulation of either of the receptors Fas or TNFR-I. The receptors and their ligand are both trimeric, and when the ligands bind they induce a conformational change in their trimeric receptors (Fig. 6.24). The cytoplasmic tails of these receptors share a motif known as a death domain, which, as we saw in Section 6-17, is a protein–protein interaction domain. The adaptor proteins that interact with the death domains in the cytosolic tails of Fas and TNFR-I are called FADD and TRADD, respectively. These in turn interact through a second death domain with the protein caspase 8 (also known as FLICE), whose carboxy-terminal domain is a procaspase (the inactive form of a caspase). Binding activates the enzymatic activity of caspase 8, leading to a protease cascade in which activated caspases cleave and activate a succession of downstream caspases. At the end of this pathway a caspase-activated DNase (CAD) enters the nucleus and cleaves DNA to produce the DNA fragments characteristic of an apoptotic cell. These fragments can be labeled by a procedure known as TUNEL (see Appendix I, Section A-32) that selectively stains and detects only those cells that have undergone apoptosis.

Mutations in the genes encoding Fas and Fas ligand have now been identified in both mice and humans. These mutations are associated with an excessive accumulation of abnormal T cells that lack both co-receptor proteins and express the CD45 isoform usually expressed by B cells. It is thought that

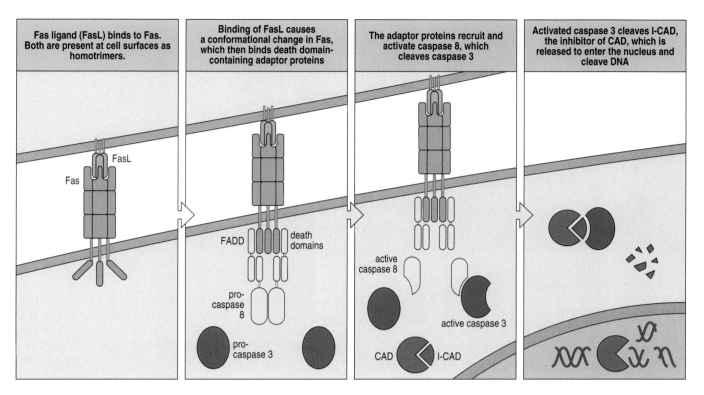

Fig. 6.24 Binding of Fas ligand to Fas initiates the process of apoptosis. When Fas ligand (FasL) binds Fas this produces a signal which results in adaptor proteins binding to the clustered death domains of the Fas trimer. One of these is the protein FADD, which in turn interacts through a second death domain with the protease caspase 8. Clustered caspase 8 can transactivate, cleaving caspase 8 itself to release an active caspase domain that in turn can activate other caspases. The ensuing caspase cascade culminates in the activation of the caspase-activatable DNase (CAD), which is present in all cells in an inactive cytoplasmic form bound to an inhibitory protein called I-CAD. When I-CAD is broken down by caspases, CAD can enter the nucleus, where it cleaves DNA into the 200-base-pair fragments that are characteristic of apoptosis.

these cells have been activated but have subsequently failed to die. The mutations that cause this phenotype are mostly recessive; that is, both copies of the gene for either Fas or Fas ligand must be defective to produce an effect. However, in some cases in humans, the mutant phenotype is seen in heterozygous individuals. The production of an effect in heterozygotes is likely to reflect the need for trimerization of Fas for efficient operation of the interaction between Fas and Fas ligand, and the fact that if one of the members of the trimer is mutant, the trimer cannot transduce a signal.

X-linked Lymphoproliferative Syndrome

6-21 Lymphocyte survival is maintained by a balance between death-promoting and death-inhibiting members of the Bcl-2 family of proteins.

Apoptosis has a major role in the development and maintenance of all multi-cellular organisms. The apoptotic program is present in all cells and can be triggered by an absence of appropriate survival signals as well as by external stimuli as described for Fas-induced cell death above. Thus, it is not surprising that all cells also possess a separate set of proteins that can inhibit programmed cell death.

The first member of this family of proteins was discovered as an oncogene in B cells. When tumors form in the B-cell lineage, they are frequently associated

| In a normal cell, cytochrome *c* is present only in mitochondria | When programmed cell death is induced, the mitochondria swell and leak, releasing cytochrome *c*, which binds to Apaf-1 | The Apaf-1/cytochrome *c* complex activates caspase, which cleaves I-CAD, releasing CAD to enter the nucleus and cleave DNA | Bcl-2 binds to mitochondrial membranes, blocking the swelling and so blocking the process that leads to cell death |

Fig. 6.25 Bcl-2 inhibits the processes that lead to programmed cell death.
In normal cells, cytochrome *c* is confined to the mitochondria (first panel). However, during apoptosis the mitochondria swell, allowing the cytochrome *c* to leak out into the cytosol (second panel). There it interacts with the protein Apaf-1, forming a cytochrome *c*:Apaf-1 complex that can activate caspases. An activated caspase cleaves I-CAD (see Fig. 6.24), which leads to DNA fragmentation (third panel). Bcl-2 interacts with the mitochondrial outer membrane and blocks the mitochondrial swelling that leads to cytochrome *c* release (last panel).

with chromosomal translocations in which the chromosomal DNA is broken and an active immunoglobulin locus is joined to a gene that affects cell growth, usually activating that gene in the process. By cloning the DNA breakpoints, one can isolate the gene that has been activated by the translocation. One such gene is *bcl-2*, which was isolated from the second B-cell lymphoma to have its breakpoint identified. *bcl-2* is homologous with the *Caenorhabditis elegans* gene *ced-9*, which is a cell-death-inhibitory gene. In cultured B cells and in transgenic mice, the expression of *bcl-2* protects against cell death. *bcl-2* is a member of a small family of closely related genes, some of which inhibit cell death whereas others promote it. These genes can be divided into death-inhibiting genes, such as *bcl-2* and *bcl-X$_L$*, and death-promoting genes, such as *Bax* and *Bad*. The proteins encoded by these genes act as dimers, and because Bcl-2 and Bax proteins can dimerize with each other to form heterodimers, the more abundant protein determines whether the cell lives or dies. One way in which Bcl-2 acts to prevent cell death is shown in Fig. 6.25.

The balance between death-promoting and death-inhibiting gene expression is critically important in lymphocytes, because lymphocyte populations are regulated so that a person will, in the absence of infection, maintain a constant level of T and B cells despite the production and death of many lymphocytes each day. The fate of individual lymphocytes is set by signals delivered mainly or entirely through the antigen-specific receptors, as we will see in Chapter 7, which deals with the production of the mature repertoire of receptors on B and T lymphocytes. In the last section of this chapter we will look at the evidence for a continued role of antigen-receptor signaling in maintaining the survival of mature T and B cells.

6-22   Homeostasis of lymphocyte populations is maintained by signals that lymphocytes are continually receiving through their antigen receptors.

Most of what we know about signaling through the B-cell receptor and the T-cell receptor derives from observations in cultured B-cell and T-cell lines. In these cells, the tyrosine kinases Syk and ZAP-70 are recruited as a consequence of receptor clustering and the subsequent phosphorylation of ITAMs in the receptor subunit tails, as discussed in Section 6-10. However, in T cells isolated directly from lymph nodes or the thymus, ZAP-70 is already bound to partly phosphorylated ζ chains but is not yet activated. The same state can be produced in both normal naive T cells and cultured T cells by exposure to altered peptide ligands (see Section 6-14). It therefore seems likely that the phosphorylated ITAMs and bound ZAP-70 seen in mature naive T cells *in vivo* reflect the receipt of signals from self MHC molecules bound to self peptides that behave like altered peptide ligands.

As we will see in Chapter 7, the ability to interact with self-MHC:self-peptide ligands is a criterion for survival during T-cell development in the thymus. Developing T cells are subject to stringent testing once the α:β T-cell receptor is expressed. This selection process retains those cells whose receptors interact effectively with various self-MHC:self-peptide ligands (positive selection), and removes those T cells that either cannot participate in such interactions (death by neglect) or recognize a self-MHC:self-peptide complex so well that they could damage host cells if allowed to mature; such cells are removed by clonal deletion (negative selection). Those T cells that mature and emerge into the periphery have therefore been selected for their ability to recognize self-MHC:self-peptide complexes without being fully activated by them.

Several studies have now shown that naive T cells in the peripheral lymphoid tissues continue to receive signals through interactions with self-MHC:self-peptide complexes. These signals enable the cells to survive and are delivered most effectively by the cells that are most capable of T-cell activation, namely the dendritic cells. Thus, the T cells in mice transgenic for a T-cell receptor that is positively selected on a particular self-MHC:self-peptide complex can survive only if they receive similar signals from self-MHC:self-peptide complexes in the periphery. It seems as though the peripheral T-cell repertoire is maintained by a continuous dialog between dendritic cells presenting self peptides on self MHC molecules and recirculating naive T cells that were positively selected by signals from the same self-MHC:self-peptide molecules during development. This dialog is likely to account for the state of partial phosphorylation of the ζ chains discussed above. A requirement for repeated interaction with dendritic cells resident in peripheral lymphoid tissue could also account for the tight regulation of the numbers of naive CD4 and CD8 cells. For memory T cells, the factors that govern survival are less well defined. It is clear that self-MHC:self-peptide recognition is not required for the survival of memory T cells; in fact, the presence of MHC molecules does not seem to be required at all. Rather, it is likely that the levels of particular cytokines, notably IL-7 and IL-15, serve to maintain the memory T-cell pool.

In B cells it is also clear that signaling through the antigen receptor determines cell survival from the time that it is first expressed on the cell surface. As we will see in Chapter 7, autoreactive B cells are induced to die on binding antigen. However, the expression of a functional B-cell receptor at the cell surface is also essential for cell maturation and survival. The role of the B-cell receptor in signaling for survival in the periphery was demonstrated quite dramatically by using a conditional gene knockout strategy (see Appendix I, Section A-47). Mice were made transgenic for a rearranged immunoglobulin V_H gene flanked by *loxP* sites. This construct was 'knocked-in' to the site at which the rearranged V_H gene normally occurs in such a way that only the transgene could produce the heavy-chain V region. The animals were also made transgenic for the enzyme Cre recombinase, which can excise *loxP*-flanked genes; the transgene encoding the Cre recombinase was made inducible by interferon. After treatment with interferon, the induced Cre recombinase removed the transgenic rearranged V_H gene, preventing the production of a heavy chain. Most of the B cells in the treated animals lost their receptors; these receptor-negative B cells rapidly disappeared. Thus, the B-cell receptor is clearly required to keep recirculating B cells alive and must have a role in perceiving or transmitting survival signals to each B cell. Evidence also shows that receptor specificity can affect this process. However, the ligand or ligands responsible for signaling for B-cell survival are not yet known.

The identity of the ligands responsible for delivering survival signals to T and B cells through their antigen receptors remains an important question in immunology. There is also much to learn about the signaling process itself. Survival signals are likely to regulate the level of proteins in the Bcl-2 family because, as we discussed in Section 6-21, increased levels of Bcl-2 and Bcl-X$_L$ promote the survival of lymphocytes, whereas increased levels of Bax and Bad have an opposing effect. As yet, however, a direct link between antigen-receptor signaling for survival and the regulation of the Bcl-2 family has not been shown.

Summary.

Many different signals govern lymphocyte behavior, only some of which are delivered via the antigen receptor. Lymphocyte development, activation, and longevity are clearly influenced by the antigen receptor, but these processes are also regulated by other extracellular signals. Other signals are delivered in a variety of ways. An ancient signaling pathway with a role in host defense leads rapidly from the IL-1 receptor or a similar receptor called Toll to initiate the detachment and degradation of the inhibitory protein IκB from the transcription factor NFκB, which can then enter the nucleus and activate the transcription of many genes. Many cytokines signal through an express pathway that links receptor-associated JAK kinases to preformed STAT proteins, which after phosphorylation dimerize through their SH2 domains and head for the nucleus. Activated lymphocytes are programmed to die when the Fas receptor that they express binds the Fas ligand. This transmits a death signal, which activates a protease cascade that triggers apoptosis. Lymphocyte apoptosis is inhibited by some members of the intracellular Bcl-2 family and promoted by others. Working out the complete picture of the signals processed by lymphocytes as they develop, circulate, respond to antigen, and die is an immense and exciting prospect.

Summary to Chapter 6.

In adaptive immune responses, signaling through the antigen receptors of naive mature lymphocytes induces the clonal expansion and differentiation of antigen-specific lymphocytes after engagement with foreign antigen, provided that, in the case of T cells, they receive a co-stimulatory signal through CD28. Lymphocyte antigen receptors belong to the general class of receptors that are associated with cytoplasmic protein tyrosine kinases. The antigen-binding chains of the receptors are associated on the cell surface with invariant chains that are responsible for generating an intracellular signal indicating that antigen has bound. These chains contain sequence motifs called ITAMs, which after phosphorylation by receptor-associated tyrosine kinases recruit intracellular signaling molecules to the activated receptor. The intracellular signaling pathway leading from the antigen receptors results in gene activation, new protein synthesis, and the stimulation of cell division. This pathway is subject to regulation at most of its steps; these control points form important checkpoints in the pathways leading to lymphocyte activation and the clonal expansion and differentiation of antigen-specific lymphocytes that occurs during an adaptive immune response. As well as enabling lymphocytes to respond to foreign antigens in an adaptive immune response, signals delivered through the antigen receptors are important in selecting lymphocytes for removal or survival during lymphocyte development in the primary lymphoid organs as well as survival later on in the periphery. The ligands responsible for providing survival signals seem similar to altered peptide ligands in the case of T cells but are unknown in the case of B cells: their identity remains a central question in immunology. Lymphocytes also carry receptors for many other extracellular signals, such as cytokines and Fas ligand. The latter, by interacting with the cell-surface receptor Fas on activated lymphocytes, induces apoptosis and is involved in controlling lymphocyte numbers and in removing activated lymphocytes once an infection has been cleared.

Chapter 6 questions.

6.1   Adaptor proteins link cell-surface receptors to intracellular signaling events. (a) Show, with examples, how adaptor proteins allow different signaling pathways to be activated by the same cell-surface recognition event. (b) How does the cell surface itself function as an adaptor?

6.2   Discuss the role of phosphotyrosine in signal transduction.

6.3   Signals can be transduced either through direct signaling cascades or indirectly through second messenger molecules. (a) Give an example of each type of pathway. (b) What second messengers are involved in immune-cell signaling?

6.4   Cell death reveals how different signaling events can feed into a common pathway. Discuss the different ways in which cell death is initiated by: (a) developmentally programmed cell death; (b) T-cell or NK-cell cytotoxicity (see also Chapter 8); (c) Fas.

General references.

Healy, J.L., and Goodnow, C.C.: **Positive versus negative signaling by lymphocyte antigen receptors.** *Annu. Rev. Immunol.* 1998, **16**:645–670.

Weiss, A., and Littman, D.R.: **Signal transduction by lymphocyte antigen receptors.** *Cell* 1994, **76**:263–274.

Section references.

6-1   Binding of antigen leads to clustering of antigen receptors on lymphocytes.

Bunnell, S.C., Hong, D.I., Kardon, J.R., Yamazaki, T., McGlade, C.J., Barr, V.A., and Samelson, L.E.: **T cell receptor ligation induces the formation of dynamically regulated signaling assemblies.** *J. Cell. Biol.* 2002, **158**:1263–1275.

Cochran, J.R., Aivazian, D., Cameron, T.O., and Stern, L.J.: **Receptor clustering and transmembrane signaling in T cells.** *Trends Biochem. Sci.* 2001, **26**:304–310.

Delon, J., and Germain, R.N.: **Information transfer at the immunological synapse.** *Curr. Biol.* 2000, **10**:R923–R933.

Dustin, M.L., and Chan, A.C.: **Signaling takes shape in the immune system.** *Cell* 2000, **103**:283–294.

Dustin, M.L., and Cooper, J.A.: **The immunological synapse and the actin cytoskeleton: molecular hardware for T cell signaling.** *Nat. Immunol.* 2000, **1**:23–29.

Metzger, H., Chen, H., Goldstein, B., Haleem-Smith, H., Inman, J.K., Peirce, M., Torigoe, C., Vonakis, B., and Wofsy, C.: **A quantitative approach to signal transduction.** *Immunol. Lett.* 1999, **68**:53–57.

Monks, C.R., Freiberg, B.A., Kupfer, H., Sciaky, N., and Kupfer, A.: **Three-dimensional segregation of supramolecular activation clusters in T cells.** *Nature* 1998, **395**:82–86.

Thomason, P.A., Wolanin, P.M., and Stock, J.B.: **Signal transduction: receptor clusters as information processing arrays.** *Curr. Biol.* 2002, **12**:R399–R401.

6-2   Clustering of antigen receptors leads to activation of intracellular signal molecules.

Germain, R.N.: **T-cell signaling: the importance of receptor clustering.** *Curr. Biol.* 1997, **7**:R640-R644.

Klemm, J.D., Schreiber, S.L., and Crabtree, G.R.: **Dimerization as a regulatory mechanism in signal transduction.** *Annu. Rev. Immunol.* 1998, **16**:569–592.

Zhang, W., and Samelson, L.E.: **The role of membrane-associated adaptors in T cell receptor signalling.** *Semin. Immunol.* 2000, **12**:35–41.

6-3   Receptors and signaling molecules concentrate in specialized regions of the cell membrane.

Bini, L., Pacini, S., Liberatori, S., Valensin, S., Pellegrini, M., Raggiaschi, R., Pallini, V., and Baldari, C.T.: **Extensive temporally regulated reorganization of the lipid raft proteome following T-cell antigen receptor triggering.** *Biochem. J.* 2003, **369**:301–309.

Cheng, P.C., Cherukuri, A., Dykstra, M., Malapati, S., Sproul, T., Chen, M.R., and Pierce, S.K.: **Floating the raft hypothesis: the roles of lipid rafts in B cell antigen receptor function.** *Semin. Immunol.* 2001, **13**:107–114.

Cherukuri, A., Dykstra, M., and Pierce, S.K.: **Floating the raft hypothesis: lipid rafts play a role in immune cell activation.** *Immunity* 2001, **14**:657–660.

Ilangumaran, S., He, H.T., and Hoessli, D.C.: **Microdomains in lymphocyte signalling: beyond GPI-anchored proteins.** *Immunol. Today* 2000, **21**:2–7.

Janes, P.W., Ley, S.C., Magee, A.I., and Kabouridis, P.S.: **The role of lipid rafts in T cell antigen receptor (TCR) signalling.** *Semin. Immunol.* 2000, **12**:23–34.

Simons, K., and Toomre, D.: **Lipid rafts and signal transduction.** *Nat. Rev. Mol. Cell Biol.* 2000, **1**:31–39.

van Meer, G.: **Cell biology. The different hues of lipid rafts.** *Science* 2002, **296**:855–857.

6-4   Phosphorylation of receptor cytoplasmic tails by tyrosine kinases concentrates intracellular signaling molecules around the receptors.

Buday, L.: **Membrane-targeting of signalling molecules by SH2/SH3 domain-containing adaptor proteins.** *Biochim. Biophys. Acta* 1999, **1422**:187–204.

Fisher, M.J., Paton, R.C., and Matsuno, K.: **Intracellular signalling proteins as smart agents in parallel distributed processes.** *Biosystems* 1999, **50**:159–171.

Kholodenko, B.N., Hoek, J.B., and Westerhoff, H.V.: **Why cytoplasmic signalling proteins should be recruited to cell membranes.** *Trends Cell Biol.* 2000, **10**:173–178.

6-5   Intracellular signaling components recruited to activated receptors transmit the signal onward from the membrane and amplify it.

Janssen, E., and Zhang, W.: **Adaptor proteins in lymphocyte activation.** *Curr. Opin. Immunol.* 2003, **15**:269–276.

Jordan, M.S., Singer, A.L., and Koretzky, G.A.: **Adaptors as central mediators of signal transduction in immune cells.** *Nat. Immunol.* 2003, **4**:110–116.

Peterson, E.J., Clements, J.L., Fang, N., and Koretzky, G.A.: **Adaptor proteins in lymphocyte antigen receptor signaling.** *Curr. Opin. Immunol.* 1998, **10**:337–344.

6-6   Small G proteins activate a protein kinase cascade that transmits the signal to the nucleus.

Cantrell, D.A.: **T-cell antigen receptor signal transduction.** *Immunology* 2002, **105**:369–374.

Cantrell, D.A.: **GTPases and T cell activation.** *Immunol. Rev.* 2003, **192**:122–130.

Cantrell, D.A.: **Regulation and function of serine kinase networks in lymphocytes.** *Curr. Opin. Immunol.* 2003, **15**:294–298.

Dong, C., Davis, R.J., and Flavell, R.A.: **MAP kinases in the immune response.** *Annu. Rev. Immunol.* 2002, **20**:55–72.

Turner, M., and Billadeau, D.D.: **VAV proteins as signal integrators for multi-subunit immune-recognition receptors.** *Nat. Rev. Immunol.* 2002, **2**:476–486.

6-7   The variable chains of lymphocyte antigen receptors are associated with invariant accessory chains that perform the signaling function of the receptor.

Borst, J., Jacobs, H., and Brouns, G.: **Composition and function of T-cell receptor and B-cell receptor complexes on precursor lymphocytes.** *Curr. Opin. Immunol.* 1996, **8**:181–190.

Gobel, T.W., and Bolliger, L.: **Evolution of the T cell receptor signal transduction units.** *Curr. Top. Microbiol. Immunol.* 2000, **248**:303–320.

Malissen, B., Ardouin, L., Lin, S.Y., Gillet, A., and Malissen, M.: **Function of the CD3 subunits of the pre-TCR and TCR complexes during T cell development.** *Adv. Immunol.* 1999, **72**:103–148.

Pitcher, L.A., and van Oers, N.S.: **T-cell receptor signal transmission: who gives an ITAM?** *Trends Immunol.* 2003, **24**:554–560.

6-8   The ITAMs associated with the B-cell and T-cell receptors are phosphorylated by protein tyrosine kinases of the Src family.

Cornall, R.J., Cheng, A.M., Pawson, T., and Goodnow, C.C.: **Role of Syk in B-cell development and antigen-receptor signaling.** *Proc. Natl Acad. Sci. USA* 2000, **97**:1713–1718.

Hegedus, Z., Chitu, V., Toth, G.K., Finta, C., Varadi, G., Ando, I., and Monostori, E.: **Contribution of kinases and the CD45 phosphatase to the generation of** tyrosine phosphorylation patterns in the T-cell receptor complex zeta chain. *Immunol. Lett.* 1999, **67**:31–39.

Lin, J., and Weiss, A.: **T cell receptor signalling.** *J. Cell Sci.* 2001, **114**:243–244.

Sohn, H.W., Gu, H., and Pierce, S.K.: **Cbl-b negatively regulates B cell antigen receptor signaling in mature B cells through ubiquitination of the tyrosine kinase Syk.** *J. Exp. Med.* 2003, **197**:1511–1524.

Turner, M., Schweighoffer, E., Colucci, F., Di Santo, J.P., and Tybulewicz, V.L.: **Tyrosine kinase SYK: essential functions for immunoreceptor signalling.** *Immunol. Today* 2000, **21**:148–154.

Yokozeki, T., Adler, K., Lankar, D., and Bonnerot, C.: **B cell receptor-mediated Syk-independent activation of phosphatidylinositol 3-kinase, Ras, and mitogen-activated protein kinase pathways.** *J. Immunol.* 2003, **171**:1328–1335.

6-9   Antigen receptor signaling is enhanced by co-receptors that bind the same ligand.

Denny, M.F., Patai, B., and Straus, D.B.: **Differential T-cell antigen receptor signaling mediated by the Src family kinases Lck and Fyn.** *Mol. Cell. Biol.* 2000, **20**:1426–1435.

Filipp, D., Zhang, J., Leung, B.L., Shaw, A., Levin, S.D., Veillette, A., and Julius, M.: **Regulation of Fyn through translocation of activated Lck into lipid rafts.** *J. Exp. Med.* 2003, **197**:1221–1227.

Kim, P.W., Sun, Z.Y., Blacklow, S.C., Wagner, G., and Eck, M.J.: **A zinc clasp structure tethers Lck to T cell coreceptors CD4 and CD8.** *Science* 2003, **301**:1725–1728.

Lefebvre, D.C., Felberg, J., Cross, J.L., and Johnson, P.: **The noncatalytic domains of Lck regulate its dephosphorylation by CD45.** *Biochim. Biophys. Acta* 2003, **1650**:40–49.

6-10   Fully phosphorylated ITAMs bind the protein tyrosine kinases Syk and ZAP-70 and enable them to be activated.

Chitu, V., Fajka-Boja, R., Toth, G.K., Varadi, G., Hegedus, Z., Franko, A., Szucs, K.S., and Monostori, E.: **Comparative study on the effect of phosphorylated TCR zeta chain ITAM sequences on early activation events in Jurkat T cells.** *Peptides* 2001, **22**:1963–1971.

Pao, L.I., and Cambier, J.C.: **Syk, but not Lyn, recruitment to B cell antigen receptor and activation following stimulation of CD45 B cells.** *J. Immunol.* 1997, **158**:2663–2669.

Visco, C., Magistrelli, G., Bosotti, R., Perego, R., Rusconi, L., Toma, S., Zamai, M., Acuto, O., and Isacchi, A.: **Activation of Zap-70 tyrosine kinase due to a structural rearrangement induced by tyrosine phosphorylation and/or ITAM binding.** *Biochemistry* 2000, **39**:2784–2791.

6-11   Downstream events are mediated by proteins that associate with the phosphorylated tyrosines, and bind to and activate other proteins.

Blanchard, N., Di Bartolo, V., and Hivroz, C.: **In the immune synapse, ZAP-70 controls T cell polarization and recruitment of signaling proteins but not formation of the synaptic pattern.** *Immunity* 2002, **17**:389–399.

Chu, P., Pardo, J., Zhao, H., Li, C.C., Pali, E., Shen, M.M., Qu, K., Yu, S.X., Huang, B.C., Yu, P., Masuda, E.S., Molineaux, S.M., Kolbinger, F., Aversa, G., De Vries, J., Payan, D.G., and Liao, X.C.: **Systematic identification of regulatory proteins critical for T-cell activation.** *J. Biol.* 2003, **2**:21.

Janssen, E., and Zhang, W.: **Adaptor proteins in lymphocyte activation.** *Curr. Opin. Immunol.* 2003, **15**:269–276.

Jordan, M.S., Singer, A.L., and Koretzky, G.A.: **Adaptors as central mediators of signal transduction in immune cells.** *Nat. Immunol.* 2003, **4**:110–116.

Samelson, L.E.: **Signal transduction mediated by the T cell antigen receptor: the role of adapter proteins.** *Annu. Rev. Immunol.* 2002, **20**:371–394.

Wienands, J.: **Signal transduction elements of the B cell antigen receptor and their role in immunodeficiencies.** *Immunobiology* 2000, **202**:120–133.

Wienands, J.: **The B-cell antigen receptor: formation of signaling complexes and the function of adaptor proteins.** *Curr. Top. Microbiol. Immunol.* 2000, **245**:53–76.

Yokozeki, T., Adler, K., Lankar, D., and Bonnerot, C.: **B cell receptor-mediated Syk-independent activation of phosphatidylinositol 3-kinase, Ras, and mitogen-activated protein kinase pathways.** *J. Immunol.* 2003, **171**:1328–1335.

6-12   Antigen recognition leads ultimately to the induction of new gene synthesis by activating transcription factors.

Ballard, D.W.: **Molecular mechanisms in lymphocyte activation and growth.** *Immunol. Res.* 2001, **23**:157–166.

Ma, P., Magut, M., Faller, D.V., and Chen, C.Y.: **The role of Ras in T lymphocyte activation.** *Cell Signal.* 2002, **14**:849–859.

Matsuda, S., and Koyasu, S.: **Regulation of MAPK signaling pathways through immunophilin-ligand complex.** *Curr. Top. Med. Chem.* 2003, **3**:1358–1367.

Rincon, M., Flavell, R.A., and Davis, R.J.: **Signal transduction by MAP kinases in T lymphocytes.** *Oncogene* 2001, **20**:2490–2497.

Ruland, J., and Mak, T.W.: Transducing signals from antigen receptors to nuclear factor κB. *Immunol. Rev.* 2003, **193**:93–100.

6-13   Signals from the antigen receptor alter the cytoskeleton to produce changes in cell shape, motility, and secretion.

Acuto, O., and Cantrell, D.: **T cell activation and the cytoskeleton.** *Annu. Rev. Immunol.* 2000, **18**:165–184.

Miletic, A.V., Swat, M., Fujikawa, K., and Swat, W.: **Cytoskeletal remodeling in lymphocyte activation.** *Curr. Opin. Immunol.* 2003, **15**:261–268.

Samstag, Y., Eibert, S.M., Klemke, M., and Wabnitz, G.H.: **Actin cytoskeletal dynamics in T lymphocyte activation and migration.** *J. Leukoc. Biol.* 2003, **73**:30–48.

Sancho, D., Vicente-Manzanares, M., Mittelbrunn, M., Montoya, M.C., Gordon-Alonso, M., Serrador, J.M., and Sanchez-Madrid, F.: **Regulation of microtubule-organizing center orientation and actomyosin cytoskeleton rearrangement during immune interactions.** *Immunol. Rev.* 2002, **189**:84–97.

Vigorito, E., Billadeu, D.D., Savoy, D., McAdam, S., Doody, G., Fort, P., and Turner, M.: **RhoG regulates gene expression and the actin cytoskeleton in lymphocytes.** *Oncogene* 2003, **22**:330–342.

6-14   Not all ligands for the T-cell receptor produce a similar response.

Baker, B.M., Gagnon, S.J., Biddison, W.E., and Wiley, D.C.: **Conversion of a T cell antagonist into an agonist by repairing a defect in the TCR/peptide/MHC interface: implications for TCR signaling.** *Immunity* 2000, **13**:475–484.

Smyth, L.A., Ardouin, L., Williams, O., Norton, T., Tybulewicz, V., and Kioussis, D.: **Inefficient clustering of tyrosine-phosphorylated proteins at the immunological synapse in response to an antagonist peptide.** *Eur. J. Immunol.* 2002, **32**:3386–3394.

Stefanova, I., Dorfman, J.R., and Germain, R.N.: **Self-recognition promotes the foreign antigen sensitivity of naive T lymphocytes.** *Nature* 2002, **420**:429–434.

Stefanova, I., Dorfman, J.R., Tsukamoto, M., and Germain, R.N.: **On the role of self-recognition in T cell responses to foreign antigen.** *Immunol. Rev.* 2003, **191**:97–106.

6-15   Other receptors on leukocytes also use ITAMs to signal activation.

Billadeau, D.D., Upshaw, J.L., Schoon, R.A., Dick, C.J., and Leibson, P.J.: **NKG2D-DAP10 triggers human NK cell-mediated killing via a Syk-independent regulatory pathway.** *Nat. Immunol.* 2003, **4**:557–564.

Foster, C.E., Colonna, M., and Sun, P.D.: **Crystal structure of the human NK cell activating receptor NKp46 reveals structural relationship to other leukocyte receptor complex immunoreceptors.** *J. Biol. Chem.* 2003, **278**:46081–46086.

Goldstein, B., Faeder, J.R., Hlavacek, W.S., Blinov, M.L., Redondo, A., and Wofsy, C.: **Modeling the early signaling events mediated by FcεRI.** *Mol. Immunol.* 2002, **38**:1213–1219.

Lanier, L.L.: **On guard—activating NK cell receptors.** *Nat. Immunol.* 2001, **2**:23–27.

Lanier, L.L., and Bakker, A.B.: **The ITAM-bearing transmembrane adaptor DAP12 in lymphoid and myeloid cell function.** *Immunol. Today* 2000, **21**:611–614.

Lopez-Botet, M., Bellon, T., Llano, M., Navarro, F., Garcia, P., and de Miguel, M.: **Paired inhibitory and triggering NK cell receptors for HLA class I molecules.** *Hum. Immunol.* 2000, **61**:7–17.

Monteiro, R.C., and Van De Winkel, J.G.: **IgA Fc receptors.** *Annu. Rev. Immunol.* 2003, **21**:177–204.

6-16 Antigen-receptor signaling can be inhibited by receptors associated with ITIMs.

Augugliaro, R., Parolini, S., Castriconi, R., Marcenaro, E., Cantoni, C., Nanni, M., Moretta, L., Moretta, A., and Bottino, C.: **Selective cross-talk among natural cytotoxicity receptors in human natural killer cells.** *Eur. J. Immunol.* 2003, **33**:1235–1241.

Kabat, J., Borrego, F., Brooks, A., and Coligan, J.E.: **Role that each NKG2A immunoreceptor tyrosine-based inhibitory motif plays in mediating the human CD94/NKG2A inhibitory signal.** *J. Immunol.* 2002, **169**:1948–1958.

McVicar, D.W., and Burshtyn, D.N.: **Intracellular signaling by the killer immunoglobulin-like receptors and Ly49.** *Sci.* http://stke.sciencemag.org/cgi/content/full/OC-sigtrans;2001/75/re1, 2001, RE1.

Moretta, A., Biassoni, R., Bottino, C., and Moretta, L.: **Surface receptors delivering opposite signals regulate the function of human NK cells.** *Semin. Immunol.* 2000, **12**:129–138.

Sinclair, N.R.: **Immunoreceptor tyrosine-based inhibitory motifs on activating molecules.** *Crit. Rev. Immunol.* 2000, **20**:89–102.

Tomasello, E., Blery, M., Vely, F., and Vivier, E.: **Signaling pathways engaged by NK cell receptors: double concerto for activating receptors, inhibitory receptors and NK cells.** *Semin. Immunol.* 2000, **12**:139–147.

Yusa, S., Catina, T.L., and Campbell, K.S.: **SHP-1- and phosphotyrosine-independent inhibitory signaling by a killer cell Ig-like receptor cytoplasmic domain in human NK cells.** *J. Immunol.* 2002, **168**:5047–5057.

6-17 Microbes and their products release NFκB from its site in the cytosol through an ancient pathway of host defense against infection.

Barton, G.M., and Medzhitov, R.: **Toll-like receptor signaling pathways.** *Science* 2003, **300**:1524–1525.

Ruland, J., and Mak, T.W.: **Transducing signals from antigen receptors to nuclear factor κB.** *Immunol. Rev.* 2003, **193**:93–100.

Schjetne, K.W., Thompson, K.M., Nilsen, N., Flo, T.H., Fleckenstein, B., Iversen, J.G., Espevik, T., and Bogen, B.: **Cutting edge: link between innate and adaptive immunity: Toll-like receptor 2 internalizes antigen for presentation to CD4+ T cells and could be an efficient vaccine target.** *J. Immunol.* 2003, **171**:32–36.

Takeda, K., Kaisho, T., and Akira, S.: **Toll-like receptors.** *Annu. Rev. Immunol.* 2003, **21**:335–376.

Ulevitch, R.J.: **Regulation of receptor-dependent activation of the innate immune response.** *J. Infect. Dis.* 2003, **187** Suppl. 2: S351–S355.

Vercelli, D.: **Innate immunity: sensing the environment and regulating the regulators.** *Curr. Opin. Allergy Clin. Immunol.* 2003, **3**:343–346.

6-18 Bacterial peptides, mediators of inflammatory responses, and chemokines signal through members of the G-protein-coupled receptor family.

Gerber, B.O., Meng, E.C., Dotsch, V., Baranski, T.J., and Bourne, H.R.: **An activation switch in the ligand binding pocket of the C5a receptor.** *J. Biol. Chem.* 2001, **276**:3394–3400.

Proudfoot, A.E.: **Chemokine receptors: multifaceted therapeutic targets.** *Nat. Rev. Immunol.* 2002, **2**:106–115.

6-19 Cytokines signal lymphocytes by binding to cytokine receptors and triggering Janus kinases to phosphorylate and activate STAT proteins.

Aaronson, D.S., and Horvath, C.M.: **A road map for those who don't know JAK-STAT.** *Science* 2002, **296**:1653–1655.

Heinrich, P.C., Behrmann, I., Haan, S., Hermanns, H.M., Muller-Newen, G., and Schaper, F.: **Principles of interleukin (IL)-6-type cytokine signalling and its regulation.** *Biochem. J.* 2003, **374**:1–20.

Kerr, I.M., Costa-Pereira, A.P., Lillemeier, B.F., and Strobl, B.: **Of JAKs, STATs, blind watchmakers, jeeps and trains.** *FEBS Lett.* 2003, **546**:1–5.

Khaled, A.R., and Durum, S.K.: **Death and Baxes: mechanisms of lymphotrophic cytokines.** *Immunol. Rev.* 2003, **193**:48–57.

Kisseleva, T., Bhattacharya, S., Braunstein, J., and Schindler, C.W.: **Signaling through the JAK/STAT pathway, recent advances and future challenges.** *Gene* 2002, **285**:1–24.

6-20 Programmed cell death of activated lymphocytes is triggered mainly through the receptor Fas.

Dempsey, P.W., Doyle, S.E., He, J.Q., and Cheng, G.: **The signaling adaptors and pathways activated by TNF superfamily.** *Cytokine Growth Factor Rev.* 2003, **14**:193–209.

Green, D.R., and Ferguson, T.A.: **The role of Fas ligand in immune privilege.** *Nat. Rev. Mol. Cell Biol.* 2001, **2**:917–924.

Wajant, H.: **The Fas signaling pathway: more than a paradigm.** *Science* 2002, **296**:1635–1636.

Zhou, T., Mountz, J.D., and Kimberly, R.P.: **Immunobiology of tumor necrosis factor receptor superfamily.** *Immunol. Res.* 2002, **26**:323–336.

6-21 Lymphocyte survival is maintained by a balance between death-promoting and death-inhibiting members of the Bcl-2 family of proteins.

Borner, C.: **The Bcl-2 protein family: sensors and checkpoints for life-or-death decisions.** *Mol. Immunol.* 2003, **39**:615–647.

Hildeman, D.A., Zhu, Y., Mitchell, T.C., Kappler, J., and Marrack, P.: **Molecular mechanisms of activated T cell death in vivo.** *Curr. Opin. Immunol.* 2002, **14**:354–359.

Marsden, V.S., and Strasser, A.: **Control of apoptosis in the immune system: Bcl-2, BH3-only proteins and more.** *Annu. Rev. Immunol.* 2003, **21**:71–105.

Nopora, A., and Brocker, T.: **Bcl-2 controls dendritic cell longevity in vivo.** *J. Immunol.* 2002, **169**:3006–3014.

6-22 Homeostasis of lymphocyte populations is maintained by signals that lymphocytes are continually receiving through their antigen receptors.

Ferreira, C., Barthlott, T., Garcia, S., Zamoyska, R., and Stockinger, B.: **Differential survival of naive CD4 and CD8 T cells.** *J. Immunol.* 2000, **165**:3689–3694.

Guzman-Rojas, L., Sims-Mourtada, J.C., Rangel, R., and Martinez-Valdez, H.: **Life and death within germinal centres: a double-edged sword.** *Immunology* 2002, **107**:167–175.

Kassiotis, G., Zamoyska, R., and Stockinger, B.: **Involvement of avidity for major histocompatibility complex in homeostasis of naive and memory T cells.** *J. Exp. Med.* 2003, **197**:1007–1016.

Khaled, A.R., and Durum, S.K.: **Death and Baxes: mechanisms of lymphotrophic cytokines.** *Immunol. Rev.* 2003, **193**:48–57.

Lodolce, J., Burkett, P., Koka, R., Boone, D., Chien, M., Chan, F., Madonia, M., Chai, S., and Ma, A.: **Interleukin-15 and the regulation of lymphoid homeostasis.** *Mol. Immunol.* 2002, **39**:537–544.

Plas, D.R., Rathmell, J.C., and Thompson, C.B.: **Homeostatic control of lymphocyte survival: potential origins and implications.** *Nat. Immunol.* 2002, **3**:515–521.

Seddon, B., and Zamoyska, R.: **Regulation of peripheral T-cell homeostasis by receptor signalling.** *Curr. Opin. Immunol.* 2003, **15**:321–324.

Seddon, B., Tomlinson, P., and Zamoyska, R.: **Interleukin 7 and T cell receptor signals regulate homeostasis of CD4 memory cells.** *Nat. Immunol.* 2003, **4**:680–686.

The Development and Survival of Lymphocytes

7

As described in Chapters 3 and 4, the antigen receptors carried by B and T lymphocytes are immensely variable in their antigen specificity, enabling an individual to make immune responses against the wide range of pathogens encountered during a lifetime. This diverse repertoire of **B-cell receptors** and **T-cell receptors** is generated during the development of B cells and T cells from their uncommitted precursors. The production of new lymphocytes, or **lymphopoiesis**, takes place in specialized lymphoid tissues—the **central lymphoid tissues**—which are the bone marrow for most B cells and the thymus for most T cells. Like all hematopoietic cells, lymphocyte precursors originate in the bone marrow, but whereas B cells complete most of their development there, T cells are generated in the thymus from precursor cells that migrate from the bone marrow. In the fetus, B cells also develop in the liver. Some T cells destined to form specialized populations within the gut epithelium may develop directly in sites called 'cryptopatches' just under the intestinal epithelial crypts. We will mainly focus here on the development of bone marrow derived B cells and thymus-derived T cells.

The antigen specificity of an individual lymphocyte is determined early in its differentiation, when the DNA sequences encoding the variable regions of immunoglobulins in B cells and T-cell receptors in T cells are assembled from gene segments, as described in Chapter 4. Because of this requirement for gene segment rearrangement, the early stages of B-cell and T-cell development proceed along broadly similar lines. In both B cells and T cells this aspect of development is regulated in similar ways to ensure both the diversity of the lymphocyte repertoire as a whole and the unique antigen specificity of the individual lymphocyte.

The expression of an antigen receptor on the surface of a lymphocyte marks a watershed in its development, as it can now detect ligands that bind to this receptor. In the next phase of lymphocyte development, the receptor is tested for its antigen-recognition properties against molecules present in the immediate environment. The specificity and affinity of the receptor for these ligands determines the fate of the immature lymphocyte; that is, whether the cell is selected to survive and develop further, or whether it dies without reaching maturity.

In general, it seems that developing lymphocytes whose receptors interact weakly with self antigens, or bind self antigens in a particular way, receive a signal that enables them to survive; this type of selection is known as **positive selection**. Positive selection is particularly critical in the development of α:β T cells, which recognize antigen as peptides bound to MHC molecules (see Chapter 3). Because T cells that cannot recognize peptides bound to the body's own MHC molecules would not be able to mount an immune response against any antigen, positive selection ensures that an individual will have a repertoire of T cells that can respond to peptides bound to his or her MHC molecules. Although the initial selecting peptides are self-derived, they allow the selection of T cells that will also react with self MHC molecules carrying foreign antigenic peptides that are generated during an infection.

In contrast, lymphocytes whose receptors bind strongly to self antigens receive signals that lead to their death: this is termed **negative selection**. Strongly self-reactive lymphocytes are therefore removed from the repertoire before they become fully mature and might initiate damaging autoimmune reactions. In this way, immunological **tolerance** is established to ubiquitous self antigens. The default fate of developing lymphocytes, in the absence of any signal being received from the receptor, is death and, as we will see, the vast majority of developing lymphocytes die either before emerging from the central lymphoid organs or before completing maturation in the peripheral lymphoid organs.

The lymphocytes that survive to form the mature lymphocyte population are thus only a small fraction of those generated in the bone marrow or thymus. Nonetheless, these cells express a large repertoire of receptors capable of responding to a virtually unlimited variety of nonself structures. This repertoire provides the raw material on which clonal selection acts in an adaptive immune response.

In this chapter we will describe the different stages of the development of B cells and T cells in mice and humans, from the uncommitted stem cell up to the mature, functionally specialized lymphocyte with its unique antigen receptor ready to respond to a foreign antigen. The final stages in the life history of a mature lymphocyte, in which an encounter with a foreign antigen activates it to become an effector or memory lymphocyte, are discussed in Chapters 8–10. In the first two parts of the chapter we define the stages through which lymphocytes develop in the central lymphoid organs and how the unselected primary receptor repertoire is generated. We then discuss what is known of the mechanisms by which positive selection and tolerance to self occur once a cell expresses an antigen receptor at the surface.

In the last part of the chapter we follow the fate of newly generated lymphocytes as they leave the central lymphoid organs and migrate to the peripheral lymphoid tissues, where further maturation occurs. Mature lymphocytes continually recirculate between the blood and peripheral lymphoid tissues and, in the absence of infection, their numbers remain relatively constant, despite the continual production of new lymphocytes. We look at the factors that govern the survival of naive lymphocytes in the peripheral lymphoid organs, and thus the maintenance of lymphocyte homeostasis.

The main phases of a lymphocyte's life history are shown for B cells in Fig. 7.1 and for T cells in Fig. 7.2. The last part of this chapter includes a discussion of the lymphoid tumors; these represent cells that have escaped from the normal controls on cell proliferation and are also of interest because they capture features of the different developmental stages of B cells and T cells.

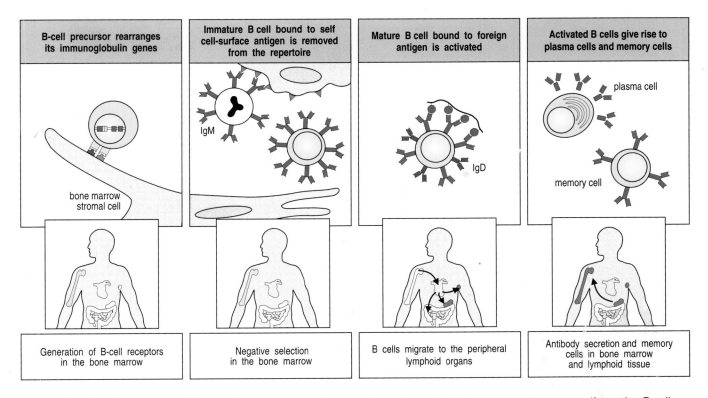

Fig. 7.1 B cells originate from a lymphoid progenitor in the bone marrow. In the first phase of development, progenitor B cells in the bone marrow rearrange their immunoglobulin genes. This phase is independent of antigen but is dependent on interactions with bone marrow stromal cells (first panels). It ends in an immature B cell that carries an antigen receptor in the form of cell-surface IgM and can now interact with antigens in its environment. Immature B cells that are strongly stimulated by antigen at this stage either die or are inactivated in a process of negative selection, thus removing many self-reactive B cells from the repertoire (second panels). In the third phase of development, the surviving immature B cells emerge into the periphery and mature to express IgD as well as IgM. They can now be activated by encounter with their specific foreign antigen in a secondary lymphoid organ (third panels). Activated B cells proliferate, and differentiate into antibody-secreting plasma cells and long-lived memory cells (fourth panels).

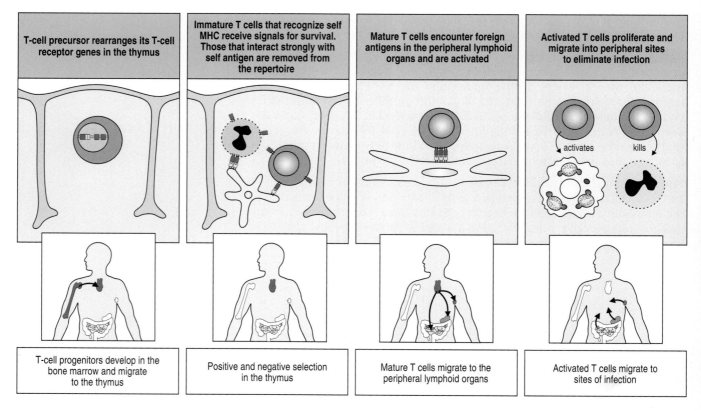

Fig. 7.2 The development of T cells. T-cell development follows broadly similar lines to that of B cells. T-cell precursors migrate from the bone marrow to the thymus where the T-cell receptor genes are rearranged (first panels); α:β T-cell receptors that are compatible with self MHC molecules transmit a survival signal on interacting with thymic epithelium, leading to positive selection of the cells that bear them. Self-reactive receptors transmit a signal that leads to cell death and are thus removed from the repertoire in a process of negative selection (second panels). T cells that survive selection mature and leave the thymus to circulate in the periphery; they repeatedly leave the blood to migrate through the peripheral lymphoid organs, where they may encounter their specific foreign antigen and become activated (third panels). Activation leads to clonal expansion and differentiation into effector T cells. These are attracted to sites of infection, where they can kill infected cells or activate macrophages (fourth panels); others are attracted into B-cell areas, where they help to activate an antibody response (not shown).

Generation of lymphocytes in bone marrow and thymus.

The greater part of lymphocyte development in mammals occurs in the specialized environments of the central lymphoid organs—the bone marrow (and the liver in the fetus) for B cells and the thymus for T cells. In the fetus and the juvenile these tissues are the source of large numbers of new lymphocytes, which migrate to populate the peripheral lymphoid tissues. In mature individuals, the development of new T cells in the thymus slows down and T-cell numbers are maintained through long-lived individual T cells together with the division of mature T cells outside the central lymphoid organs. New B cells, in contrast, are continually produced from the bone marrow, even in adults.

In this part of the chapter we describe the nature of these primary lymphopoietic environments and the developmental stages through which lymphocytes pass. These stages are defined mainly by the various steps in the assembly and expression of functional antigen-receptor genes, and by the appearance of features that distinguish the different functional types of B and T cells. At each step of lymphocyte development, the progress of gene rearrangement is monitored. The major recurring theme is that successful gene rearrangement leads to the production of a protein chain that serves as a signal for the cell to progress to the next stage of development.

T-cell development is more complicated than B-cell development because it has to accommodate the production of two distinct lineages of T cells with different types of T-cell receptor—α:β and γ:δ (see Section 4-13). The α:β and γ:δ T cells diverge early in T-cell development. There is a further division of the α:β T cells into CD4 and CD8 T cells (see Section 3-12), which occurs in immature T cells after the T-cell receptor genes have been assembled and expressed.

7-1 Lymphocyte development occurs in specialized environments and is regulated by signals from the environment along with the somatic rearrangement of the antigen-receptor genes.

Certain basic principles apply to the process by which precursor cells develop into committed B or T cells expressing antigen-specific receptors. Lymphocytes develop from undifferentiated precursors or stem cells that reside in the bone marrow and are probably the descendants of pluripotent hematopoietic stem cells. The weight of evidence suggests that lymphocytes derive from a 'common lymphoid precursor'—a cell that could give rise to T cells, B cells, and NK cells but not to other cell types (Fig. 7.3). Development involves the successive acquisition of properties that are essential for the function of the mature cell along with the loss of properties that are more characteristic of the immature cell. As the cell acquires properties that define it as part of the B-cell or T-cell lineage, it becomes committed to that lineage and can no longer differentiate along the alternative ones.

The ordered stages of lymphocyte development are marked by successive steps in the rearrangement of the antigen-receptor genes and expression of their protein products, as well as by changes in the expression of other cell-surface and intracellular proteins. The successful execution of this intrinsic developmental program requires signals from the specialized microenvironments in which lymphocytes develop—bone marrow and fetal liver for B cells, and thymus and intestinal cryptopatches for T cells. These tissues provide a network of specialized nonlymphoid **stromal cells** that interact intimately with developing lymphocytes, providing signals through secreted growth factors and cell-surface molecules that bind to receptors on the lymphocyte precursor cells.

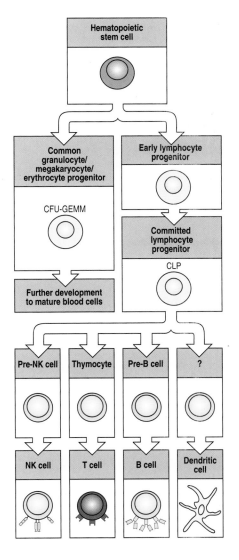

Fig. 7.3 All the cellular components of the immune system derive from a pluripotent hematopoietic stem cell. In the bone marrow or other hematopoietic sites, the pluripotent stem cell gives rise to cells with progressively more limited potential. The first branch leads to cells of myeloid and erythroid potential on the one hand and lymphoid potential on the other. The former give rise to all nonlymphoid cellular blood elements. These include circulating monocytes and granulocytes and also the macrophages and dendritic cells that reside in tissues and secondary lymphoid organs (not shown). The lymphocyte progenitor can give rise to NK cells, T cells or B cells through successive stages of differentiation in either the bone marrow or thymus. There may be considerable plasticity in these pathways, in that in certain circumstances progenitor cells may switch their commitment. For example, a progenitor cell may give rise to either B cells or macrophages; however, for simplicity these alternative pathways are not shown. Some dendritic cells are also thought to be derived from the lymphoid progenitor.

The antigen specificity of each individual lymphocyte is determined through the assembly of V, D, and J gene segments to generate rearranged V gene exons encoding the antigen-receptor variable (V) region (see Sections 4-2 and 4-11). The expression of a complete antigen receptor requires the successful rearrangement of two different genetic loci so as to produce the protein chains of the antigen receptor—the heavy and light chains of immunoglobulins or the α and β chains (or γ and δ chains) of the T-cell receptor. Because of the imprecision in the recombination process, not all rearrangements produce a complete in-frame DNA sequence that can be translated into protein. Unsuccessful rearrangements that do not result in a protein are termed **nonproductive rearrangements**, and if no further rearrangement can occur, the lymphocyte dies. However, most of these loci can undergo successive rearrangements, replacing a nonproductive rearrangement with an new V and (D)J. In all cases, a nonproductive rearrangement can be rescued by a successful rearrangement on the other chromosome. Cells remain in a particular stage of differentiation, performing successive rearrangements of the stage-specific locus until a successful rearrangement is made or the cell dies. A successful rearrangement, termed a **productive rearrangement**, leads to the synthesis of the protein product; this is the signal for the cell to progress to the next stage of development.

To survive these first stages of development, therefore, B cells must make a productive rearrangement at the immunoglobulin heavy-chain locus and at one of the two light-chain loci—κ or λ. T cells must make productive rearrangements at either the α-chain locus and the β-chain locus, to produce an α:β T cell, or at the γ-chain and δ-chain loci, to produce a γ:δ T cell. Those cells that fail to make productive rearrangements die *in situ* by apoptosis.

The events that lead to a B cell with an immunoglobulin B-cell receptor and a T cell with an α:β T-cell receptor have a very close correspondence, and we will discuss these here, leaving aside the complicating factor of rearrangements at the γ and δ loci that are also occurring in the earliest T-cell precursors; we will return to these later in the chapter.

Only one gene locus is rearranged at a time, in a fixed sequence. Both B cells and T cells rearrange the locus that contains D gene segments first: for B cells this is the immunoglobulin heavy-chain locus; for T cells it is the T-cell receptor β-chain locus. Only if a productive rearrangement is made do developing B cells go on to rearrange a light-chain locus, and T cells go on to rearrange the α-chain locus.

The protein product of each antigen-receptor locus is intended to be expressed paired with another chain; an α and a β chain make up the T-cell receptor, for example (see Fig. 3.12). How, therefore, can a developing T cell test whether a productive rearrangement of a β-chain gene has occurred when it has not yet rearranged the α-chain locus? The solution is that both B cells and T cells produce invariant 'surrogate' partner chains that bear structural homology to the rearranging partner's chain (that is, the light chain for B cells and the α chain for T cells) at this stage in development. These surrogates, encoded by separate and nonrearranging genes, pair with the heavy chain or the β chain to produce 'receptors' that can be expressed at the cell surface. Formation of these receptors generates signals that result in the cessation of VDJ rearrangement. This is followed by several rounds of cell division before the cells proceed to the next stage of development, which is V-to-J rearrangement at a light-chain locus in B cells and at the α-chain locus in T cells. If this rearrangement is productive, the lymphocyte can then express a *bona fide* immunoglobulin or T-cell receptor at the surface.

7-2   B cells develop in the bone marrow with the help of stromal cells and achieve maturity in peripheral lymphoid organs.

B-cell development is dependent on the nonlymphoid stromal cells of the bone marrow; stem cells isolated from the bone marrow and grown in culture fail to differentiate into B cells unless bone marrow stromal cells are also present. The contribution of the stromal cells is twofold. First, they form specific adhesive contacts with the developing B-lineage cells by interactions between cell-adhesion molecules and their ligands. Second, they provide soluble factors that control lymphocyte differentiation and proliferation (Fig. 7.4).

Several factors secreted by bone marrow have been identified and their functions elucidated. The growth of early B-lineage cells is stimulated by stem-cell factor (SCF), a membrane-bound cytokine present on stromal cells, which interacts with the cell-surface receptor tyrosine kinase Kit on B-cell precursors. Developing B cells in mice (but not in humans) need the secreted

Fig. 7.4 The early stages of B-cell development are dependent on bone marrow stromal cells. The upper panels show the interactions between precursor B cells and stromal cells that are required for the development to the immature B-cell stage. The designations pro-B cell and pre-B cell refer to defined phases of B-cell development as described in Fig. 7.6. Lymphoid progenitor cells and early pro-B cells bind to the adhesion molecule VCAM-1 on stromal cells through the integrin VLA-4 and also interact through other cell-adhesion molecules (CAMs). These adhesive interactions promote the binding of the receptor tyrosine kinase Kit (CD117) on the surface of the pro-B cell to stem-cell factor (SCF) on the stromal cell, which activates the kinase and induces the proliferation of the B-cell progenitors. The receptor for interleukin-7 (IL-7) is present from the common lymphoid progenitor stage, and is required for the proliferation and further development of these cells in the B lineage. Panel a: light micrograph showing small round cells, which are the B-lymphoid progenitors, in intimate contact with cultured stromal cells, which have extended processes fastening them to the plastic dish on which they are grown. Panel b: high-magnification electron micrograph of a similar cell culture in which two lymphoid cells are seen adhering to a flattened stromal cell. Photographs courtesy of A. Rolink (a); P. Kincade and P.L. Witte (b).

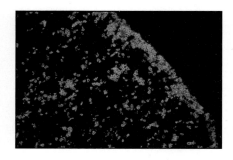

Fig. 7.5 B-lineage cells move within the bone marrow toward its central axis as they mature. Part of a transverse section of a rat femur photographed through a fluorescence microscope to identify cells (green) stained for the enzyme terminal deoxynucleotidyl transferase (TdT), which marks the pro-B stage (see Fig. 7.6). Early pro-B cells expressing TdT are concentrated near the endosteum (the inner bone surface), as seen toward the upper right of the picture. As development proceeds, cells of the B-cell lineage lose TdT and pass toward the center of the marrow cavity (lower left), where they wait in sinuses ready for export. Photograph courtesy of D. Opstelten and M. Hermans.

cytokine interleukin-7 (IL-7) at early stages. The chemokine CXCL12 (stromal cell-derived factor 1; SDF-1) is important in the early stages of B-cell development, as shown by the failure of B cells to develop in mice lacking the gene encoding CXCL12. CXCL12 is produced constitutively by the stromal cells, and one of its roles may be to retain developing B-cell precursors in the marrow microenvironment. Other adhesion molecules and growth factors produced by stromal cells are known to have roles in B-cell development. Steroid hormones have recently been shown to limit the production of B cells in adult life. A full understanding of the factors that regulate B-cell differentiation has yet to be achieved and it remains an active area of research.

As B-lineage cells mature, they migrate within the marrow, remaining in contact with the stromal cells. The earliest stem cells lie in a region called the subendosteum, which is adjacent to the inner bone surface. As maturation proceeds, B-lineage cells move toward the central axis of the marrow cavity (Fig. 7.5). Later stages of maturation become less dependent on contact with stromal cells, and the final stages of development of immature B cells into mature B cells occur in peripheral lymphoid organs such as the spleen.

7-3   Stages in B-cell development are distinguished by the expression of immunoglobulin chains and particular cell-surface proteins.

The stages in primary B-cell development are defined by the sequential rearrangement and expression of heavy- and light-chain immunoglobulin genes (Fig. 7.6). The first classification of B-lineage cells into different developmental stages was made according to whether they expressed no immunoglobulin chains, the immunoglobulin heavy chain only, or both heavy and light chains. Subsequently, intermediate differentiation stages have been distinguished on the basis of the expression of other cell-surface proteins, together with direct DNA analysis of the state of the immunoglobulin gene loci.

The earliest B-lineage cells are known as **pro-B cells**, because they are progenitor cells committed to the B-cell lineages. They are derived from pluripotent hematopoietic stem cells and are identified by the appearance of cell-surface proteins characteristic of early B-lineage cells. Rearrangement of the immunoglobulin heavy-chain locus takes place in pro-B cells; D_H to J_H joining at the **early pro-B cell** stage is followed by V_H to DJ_H joining at the **late pro-B cell** stage.

Productive VDJ_H joining leads to the expression of an intact μ heavy chain, which is the hallmark of the next main stage of development, the **pre-B cell** stage. The μ chain in **large pre-B cells** is expressed intracellularly and possibly in small amounts at the cell surface, in combination with a surrogate light chain, to form the **pre-B-cell receptor**. Expression of the pre-B-cell receptor signals the cell to halt rearrangement of the heavy-chain locus and production of the surrogate light chain, and to divide several times before giving rise to **small pre-B cells**, in which light-chain rearrangements begin. Once a light-chain gene is assembled and a complete IgM molecule is expressed on the cell surface, the cell is defined as an **immature B cell**. The expression of the immunoglobulin heavy and light chains are key milestones in this differentiation pathway; the expression of an intact heavy chain, and later of a complete immunoglobulin molecule, actively regulates progression from one stage to the next.

All development up to this point has taken place in the bone marrow and is independent of antigen. Immature B cells now undergo selection for self tolerance and subsequently for the ability to survive in the peripheral lymphoid tissues. B cells that survive in the periphery undergo further differentiation to

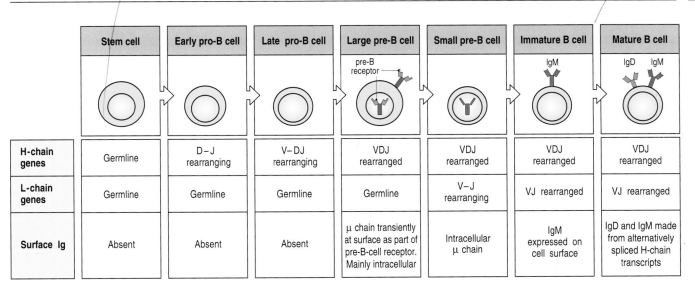

	Stem cell	Early pro-B cell	Late pro-B cell	Large pre-B cell	Small pre-B cell	Immature B cell	Mature B cell
H-chain genes	Germline	D–J rearranging	V–DJ rearranging	VDJ rearranged	VDJ rearranged	VDJ rearranged	VDJ rearranged
L-chain genes	Germline	Germline	Germline	Germline	V–J rearranging	VJ rearranged	VJ rearranged
Surface Ig	Absent	Absent	Absent	µ chain transiently at surface as part of pre-B-cell receptor. Mainly intracellular	Intracellular µ chain	IgM expressed on cell surface	IgD and IgM made from alternatively spliced H-chain transcripts

Fig. 7.6 The development of a B-lineage cell proceeds through several stages marked by the rearrangement and expression of the immunoglobulin genes. The stem cell has not yet begun to rearrange its immunoglobulin (Ig) gene segments; they are in the germline configuration as found in all nonlymphoid cells. The heavy-chain (H-chain) locus rearranges first. Rearrangement of a D gene segment to a J_H gene segment occurs in early pro-B cells, generating late pro-B cells in which V_H to DJ_H rearrangement occurs. A successful VDJ_H rearrangement leads to the expression of a complete immunoglobulin heavy chain as part of the pre-B-cell receptor, which is found mainly in the cytoplasm and to some degree on the surface of the cell.

Once this occurs the cell is stimulated to become a large pre-B cell, which actively divides. Large pre-B cells then cease dividing and become small resting pre-B cells, at which point they cease expression of the surrogate light chains and express the µ heavy chain alone in the cytoplasm. When the cells are again small, they reexpress the RAG proteins and start to rearrange the light-chain (L-chain) genes. Upon successfully assembling a light-chain gene, a cell becomes an immature B cell that expresses a complete IgM molecule at the cell surface. Mature B cells produce a δ heavy chain as well as a µ heavy chain, by a mechanism of alternative mRNA splicing, and are marked by the additional appearance of IgD on the cell surface.

become **mature B cells** that express IgD in addition to IgM. These cells, also called **naive B cells**, recirculate through peripheral lymphoid tissues, where they may encounter and be activated by the appropriate foreign antigen.

As B cells develop from pro-B cells to mature B cells, they express proteins other than immunoglobulin that are characteristic of each stage. Many of these proteins are expressed on the cell surface and are useful markers for B-lineage cells at different developmental stages. Fig. 7.7 summarizes their patterns of expression. The functions of some of these proteins are understood, whereas others serve at present simply as useful signposts for the study of B-cell development. One of the first identifiable proteins expressed on the surface of B-lineage cells is CD45R (known in mice as B220). This is a B-cell-specific form of the CD45 protein originally known as the common leukocyte antigen; T cells, monocytes, and neutrophils express other variants of this protein. CD45R, which is expressed throughout B-cell development from pro-B cells right up to the antibody-secreting plasma cells, is a protein tyrosine phosphatase that functions in B-cell receptor signaling (see Section 6-8). Another protein that is expressed throughout B-cell development is CD19, which also participates in B-cell receptor signaling. Because signaling through the pre-B-cell and B-cell receptors guides B-cell development, the earliest B-cell precursors begin to assemble the signaling components of the receptor complex, including CD45R and CD19. The earliest precursors also express the receptor for IL-7, which is essential for the growth and survival of developing B cells in mice, and of T cells in mice and humans. In mice, blocking signaling by the infusion of an anti-IL-7 antibody will block all B-cell development from the earliest identifiable B-lineage stage, as will mutations that inactivate either IL-7 or its receptor.

Fig. 7.7 The correlation of the stages of B-cell development with immunoglobulin gene segment rearrangement and the expression of cell-surface proteins. Stages of B-cell development are defined by which gene segments are undergoing rearrangement as well as by cell-surface proteins. The earliest B-lineage surface markers are CD19 and CD45R (B220 in the mouse). The expression of these persists throughout B-cell development. A pro-B cell is also distinguished by the expression of CD43, Kit (CD117), and the IL-7 receptor. An early pro-B cell is rearranging D to J_H, and a late pro-B cell V_H to DJ_H. A late pro-B cell starts to express CD24 and CD25. When a late pro-B cell makes a successful VDJ join, it can then express an immunoglobulin heavy chain, which defines it as a pre-B cell. A pre-B cell is phenotypically distinguished by the expression of BP-1, whereas Kit and the IL-7 receptor are no longer expressed. Before going on to rearrange a light-chain locus, a pre-B cell enlarges and undergoes several cycles of cell division. It then becomes a small pre-B cell, which can rearrange light-chain gene segments, first at the κ locus and, if no κ light chain is produced, then at the λ light-chain locus. A cell that has made a productive light chain becomes an immature B cell expressing surface IgM. It then migrates to the spleen, where it acquires IgD expression and thereby completes the antigen-independent phase of B-cell development as a mature resting B cell.

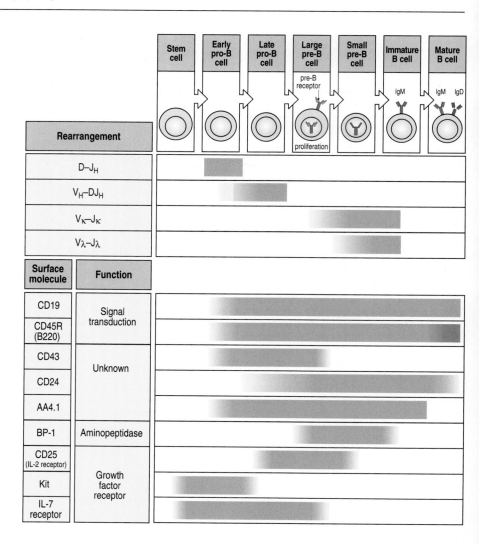

Another cell-surface protein first detected at the pro-B cell stage is CD43 (the mucin leukosialin), but this is lost as cells progress to become immature B cells. CD43 functions both as an adhesion molecule that may guide cell–cell interactions—for example those of B-cell precursors with stromal cells—and also as a signaling molecule, although not as part of the B-cell receptor complex. Exactly why CD43 is expressed at these early stages of B-cell development, but not later, is not yet known. Other cell-surface molecules expressed during early stages of murine B-cell development include the heat-stable antigen (HSA, CD24), the aminopeptidase BP-1, and an antigen called AA4.1, which is expressed on very early B-cell precursors through to the immature B-cell stage but is no longer expressed in mature B cells. The functions of these molecules in B-cell development are unknown, although B cells apparently develop normally in mice lacking BP-1. Kit (CD117), the receptor for SCF, is highly expressed on stem cells and its expression wanes at the later pro-B cell stage. Signals transduced by Kit stimulate both lymphoid and myeloid development in the bone marrow. After Kit is turned off, at the large pre-B cell stage, the high-affinity IL-2 receptor CD25 is expressed. Signaling through Kit, in concert with IL-7 and other stromal-derived signals, promotes the proliferation of pro-B cells and pre-B cells (see Fig. 7.4).

7-4 T cells also originate in the bone marrow, but all the important events in their development occur in the thymus.

The thymus is situated in the upper anterior thorax, just above the heart. It consists of numerous lobules, each clearly differentiated into an outer cortical region—the **thymic cortex**—and an inner **medulla** (Fig. 7.8). In young individuals, the thymus contains large numbers of developing T-cell precursors embedded in a network of epithelia known as the **thymic stroma**, which provides a unique microenvironment for T-cell development analogous to that provided for B cells by the stromal cells of the bone marrow. T lymphocytes develop from a common lymphoid progenitor in the bone marrow that also gives rise to B lymphocytes. Some of these progenitors leave the bone marrow and migrate to the thymus (see Fig. 7.2). In the thymus, the progenitor cell receives a signal, most probably from stromal cells, that is transduced through a receptor called Notch1. Notch signaling is widely used in animal development to specify tissue differentiation; in this case, the Notch signal instructs the precursor to commit to the T-cell lineage rather than the B-cell lineage. This commitment in the thymus is the reason that this lineage of lymphocytes is called thymus-dependent (T) lymphocytes or T cells.

Fig. 7.8 The cellular organization of the human thymus. The thymus, which lies in the midline of the body, above the heart, is made up of several lobules, each of which contains discrete cortical (outer) and medullary (central) regions. As shown in the diagram on the left, the cortex consists of immature thymocytes (dark blue), branched cortical epithelial cells (pale blue), with which the immature cortical thymocytes are closely associated, and scattered macrophages (yellow), which are involved in clearing apoptotic thymocytes. The medulla consists of mature thymocytes (dark blue) and medullary epithelial cells (orange), along with macrophages (yellow) and dendritic cells (yellow) of bone marrow origin. Hassall's corpuscles are probably also sites of cell destruction. The thymocytes in the outer cortical cell layer are proliferating immature cells, whereas the deeper cortical thymocytes are mainly immature T cells undergoing thymic selection. The photograph shows the equivalent section of a human thymus, stained with hematoxylin and eosin. The cortex is darkly staining, whereas the medulla is lightly stained. The large body in the medulla is a Hassall's corpuscle. Photograph courtesy of C.J. Howe.

Fig. 7.9 The epithelial cells of the thymus form a network surrounding developing thymocytes. In this scanning electron micrograph of the thymus, the developing thymocytes (the spherical cells) occupy the interstices of an extensive network of epithelial cells. Photograph courtesy of W. van Ewijk.

The thymic stroma arises early in embryonic development from the endodermal and ectodermal layers of embryonic structures known as the third pharyngeal pouch and the third branchial cleft. Together these epithelial tissues form a rudimentary thymus, or **thymic anlage**. The thymic anlage then attracts cells of hematopoietic origin, which colonize it; these give rise to large numbers of **thymocytes**, which are committed to the T-cell lineage, and the **intrathymic dendritic cells**. The thymocytes are not simply passengers within the thymus: they influence the arrangement of the thymic epithelial cells on which they depend for survival, inducing the formation of a reticular epithelial structure that surrounds the developing thymocytes (Fig. 7.9). The thymus is independently colonized by numerous macrophages, also of bone marrow origin.

The cellular architecture of the human thymus is illustrated in Fig. 7.8. Bone marrow derived cells are differentially distributed between the thymic cortex and medulla; the cortex contains only immature thymocytes and scattered macrophages, whereas more mature thymocytes, along with dendritic cells and macrophages, are found in the medulla. This reflects the different developmental events that occur in these two compartments.

The importance of the thymus in immunity was first discovered through experiments on mice, and indeed, most of our knowledge of T-cell development in the thymus comes from the mouse. It was found that surgical removal of the thymus (**thymectomy**) at birth resulted in immunodeficient mice, focusing interest on this organ at a time when the difference between T and B lymphocytes in mammals had not been defined. Much evidence has accumulated since to establish the importance of the thymus in T-cell development, including observations on immunodeficient children. Thus, for example, in **DiGeorge's syndrome** in humans (a complex combination of cardiac, facial, endocrine, and immune defects associated with deletions of chromosome 22q11), and in mice with the **nude** mutation (a defect in the *whn* gene, a forkhead/winged-helix transcription factor required for terminal epithelial differentiation; the name arose since this mutation also causes hairlessness), the thymus does not form and the affected individual produces B lymphocytes but few T lymphocytes.

The crucial role of the thymic stroma in inducing the differentiation of bone marrow derived precursor cells can be demonstrated by tissue grafts between two mutant mice, each lacking mature T cells for a different reason. In *nude* mice the thymic epithelium fails to differentiate, whereas in *scid* mice B and T lymphocytes fail to develop because of a defect in antigen-receptor gene rearrangement (see Section 4-5). Reciprocal grafts of thymus and bone marrow between these immunodeficient strains show that *nude* bone marrow precursors develop normally in a *scid* thymus (Fig. 7.10). Thus, the defect in *nude* mice is in the thymic stromal cells. Transplanting a *scid* thymus into *nude* mice leads to T-cell development. However, *scid* bone marrow cannot develop T cells, even in a wild-type recipient.

In mice, the thymus continues to develop for 3 to 4 weeks after birth, whereas in humans it is fully developed at birth. The rate of T-cell production by the thymus is greatest before puberty. After puberty, the thymus begins to shrink and the production of new T cells in adults is lower, although it does continue throughout life. In both mice and humans, removal of the thymus after puberty is not accompanied by any notable loss of T-cell function or numbers. Thus, it seems that once the T-cell repertoire is established, immunity can be sustained without the production of significant numbers of new T cells; the pool of peripheral T cells is instead maintained by long-lived T cells and also by some division of mature T cells.

Fig. 7.10 The thymus is critical for the maturation of bone marrow derived cells into T cells. Mice with the *scid* mutation (upper left photograph) have a defect that prevents lymphocyte maturation, whereas mice with the *nude* mutation (upper right photograph) have a defect that affects the development of the cortical epithelium of the thymus. T cells do not develop in either strain of mouse: this can be demonstrated by staining spleen cells with antibodies specific for mature T cells and analyzing them in a flow cytometer (see Appendix I, Section A-22), as represented by the blue line in the graphs in the bottom panels. Bone marrow cells from *nude* mice can restore T cells to *scid* mice (red line in graph on left), showing that, in the right environment, the *nude* bone marrow cells are intrinsically normal and capable of producing T cells. Thymic epithelial cells from *scid* mice can induce the maturation of T cells in *nude* mice (red line in graph on right), demonstrating that the thymus provides the essential microenvironment for T-cell development.

7-5 T-cell precursors proliferate extensively in the thymus but most die there.

T-cell precursors arriving in the thymus from the bone marrow spend up to a week differentiating there before they enter a phase of intense proliferation. In a young adult mouse the thymus contains around 10^8 to 2×10^8 thymocytes. About 5×10^7 new cells are generated each day; however, only about 10^6 to 2×10^6 (roughly 2–4%) of these leave the thymus each day as mature T cells. Despite the disparity between the numbers of T cells generated daily in the thymus and the number leaving, the thymus does not continue to grow in size or cell number. This is because approximately 98% of the thymocytes that develop in the thymus also die within the thymus. No widespread damage is seen, indicating that death is occurring by apoptosis rather than by necrosis (see Section 1-12).

Fig. 7.11 Developing T cells that undergo apoptosis are ingested by macrophages in the thymic cortex. Panel a shows a section through the thymic cortex and part of the medulla in which cells have been stained for apoptosis with a red dye. Thymic cortex is to the right of the photograph. Apoptotic cells are scattered throughout the cortex but are rare in the medulla. Panel b shows a section of thymic cortex at higher magnification that has been stained red for apoptotic cells and blue for macrophages. The apoptotic cells can be seen within macrophages. Magnifications: panel a, × 45; panel b, × 164. Photographs courtesy of J. Sprent and C. Surh.

Changes in the plasma membrane of cells undergoing apoptosis lead to their rapid phagocytosis, and apoptotic bodies, which are the residual condensed chromatin of apoptotic cells, are seen inside macrophages throughout the thymic cortex (Fig. 7.11). This apparently profligate waste of thymocytes is a crucial part of T-cell development because it reflects the intensive screening that each thymocyte undergoes for the ability to recognize self-peptide:self-MHC complexes and for self tolerance.

7-6   Successive stages in the development of thymocytes are marked by changes in cell-surface molecules.

Like developing B cells, developing thymocytes pass through a series of distinct phases that are marked by changes in the status of T-cell receptor genes and in the expression of the T-cell receptor, and by changes in expression of cell-surface proteins such as the CD3 complex (see Section 6-7) and the co-receptor proteins CD4 and CD8 (see Section 3-12). These surface changes reflect the state of functional maturation of the cell. Particular combinations of cell-surface proteins can thus be used as markers for T cells at different stages of differentiation. The principal stages are summarized in Fig. 7.12. Two distinct lineages of T cells—α:β and γ:δ, which have different types of T-cell receptor—are produced early in T-cell development. Later, α:β T cells develop into two distinct functional subsets, CD4 and CD8 T cells. We will return later in this chapter to the question of how these subsets differentiate in coordination with their T-cell receptor specificity.

When progenitor cells first enter the thymus from the bone marrow, they lack most of the surface molecules characteristic of mature T cells, and their receptor genes are unrearranged. These cells give rise to the major population of α:β T cells and the minor population of γ:δ T cells. If injected into the peripheral circulation, these lymphoid progenitors can even give rise to B cells and NK cells (see Section 1-1). Interactions with the thymic stroma trigger an initial phase of differentiation along the T-cell lineage pathway followed by cell proliferation and the expression of the first cell-surface molecules specific for T cells, for example CD2 and (in mice) Thy-1. At the end of this phase, which can last about a week, the thymocytes bear distinctive markers of the T-cell lineage but do not express any of the three cell-surface markers that define mature T cells. These are the CD3:T-cell receptor complex and the co-receptors CD4 or CD8. Because of the absence of CD4 and CD8 such cells are called **'double-negative' thymocytes** (see Fig. 7.12).

In the fully developed thymus, these immature double-negative T cells form approximately 60% of all of the thymocytes that lack both CD4 and CD8. This pool (about 5% of total thymocytes) also includes two populations of more mature T cells that belong to minority lineages. One of these, representing about 20% of all the double-negative cells in the thymus, comprises cells that have rearranged and are expressing the genes encoding the γ:δ T-cell receptor; we will return to these cells in Section 7-15. The second, representing another 20% of all double-negative thymocytes, includes cells bearing α:β T-cell receptors of a very limited diversity. These cells also express the NK1.1 receptor commonly found on NK cells; they are therefore known as **NK T cells**. NK T cells are activated as part of the early response to many infections; they differ from the major lineage of α:β T cells in recognizing CD1 molecules rather than MHC class I or MHC class II molecules (see Section 5-18) and they are not shown in Fig. 7.12. In this and subsequent discussions, we reserve the term double-negative thymocytes for the immature thymocytes that do not yet express a complete T-cell receptor molecule. These cells give rise to both γ:δ and α:β T cells (see Fig. 7.12), although most of them develop along the α:β pathway.

Fig. 7.12 Changes in cell-surface molecules allow thymocyte populations at different stages of maturation to be distinguished. The most important cell-surface molecules for identifying thymocyte subpopulations are CD4, CD8, and T-cell receptor complex molecules (CD3, and the T-cell receptor α and β chains). The earliest cell population in the thymus does not express any of these. Because these cells do not express CD4 or CD8 they are called 'double-negative' thymocytes. These precursor cells give rise to two T-cell lineages: the minority population of γ:δ T cells (which lack CD4 or CD8 even when mature), and the majority α:β T-cell lineage. The development of prospective α:β T cells proceeds through stages in which both CD4 and CD8 are expressed by the same cell; these are known as 'double-positive' thymocytes. At first, double-positive cells express the pre-T-cell receptor (pTα:β). These cells enlarge and divide. Later, they become small resting double-positive cells in which low levels of the T-cell receptor (α:β) itself are expressed. Most thymocytes (about 98%) die within the thymus after becoming small double-positive cells. Those cells whose receptors can interact with self-peptide:self-MHC molecular complexes lose expression of either CD4 or CD8 and increase the level of expression of the T-cell receptor. The outcome of this process is the 'single-positive' thymocytes, which, after maturation, are exported from the thymus as mature single-positive CD4 or CD8 T cells.

The α:β pathway is shown in more detail in Fig. 7.13. The double-negative stage can be subdivided on the basis of expression of the adhesion molecule CD44, CD25 (the α chain of the IL-2 receptor), and Kit, the receptor for SCF (see Section 7-2). At first, double-negative thymocytes express Kit and CD44 but not CD25; in these cells, the genes encoding both chains of the T-cell receptor are in the germline configuration. As the thymocytes mature further, they begin to express CD25 on their surface and, later still, expression of CD44 and Kit is reduced. In these latter cells, which are known as CD44^{low} CD25$^+$ cells, rearrangement of the T-cell receptor β-chain locus occurs. Cells that fail to make a successful rearrangement of the T-cell receptor β-chain locus remain in the CD44^{low} CD25$^+$ stage and soon die, whereas cells that make productive β-chain gene rearrangements and express the β chain lose expression of CD25 once again. The functional significance of the transient expression of CD25 is unclear: T cells develop normally in mice in which the IL-2 gene has been deleted by gene knockout (see Appendix I, Section A-47); however, another cytokine, IL-15, also binds to the IL-2 receptor and may be able to compensate for the loss of IL-2. By contrast, Kit is quite important for the development of the earliest double-negative thymocytes, in that mice lacking Kit have a markedly reduced number of double-negative T cells. In addition, the IL-7 receptor is also essential for early T-cell development, because there is a severe block to T-cell development when this receptor is defective.

The β chains expressed by CD44^{low} CD25$^+$ thymocytes pair with a surrogate pre-T-cell receptor α chain called **pTα** (pre-T-cell α), which allows them to assemble a complete **pre-T-cell receptor** that is analogous in structure and function to the pre-B-cell receptor. The pre-T-cell receptor is expressed on the cell surface in a complex with the CD3 molecules that provide the signaling components of T-cell receptors (see Section 6-7). The assembly of the CD3:pre-T-cell receptor complex leads to cell proliferation, the arrest of further β-chain gene rearrangements, and the expression of both CD8 and CD4. These **double-positive thymocytes** make up the vast majority of thymocytes. Once the large double-positive thymocytes cease to proliferate and become small double-positive cells, the α-chain locus begins to rearrange. As we will see later in this chapter, the structure of the α locus (Section 4-11) allows multiple successive attempts at rearrangement, so that a successful rearrangement at the α-chain locus is achieved in most developing thymocytes. Thus, most double-positive cells produce an α:β T-cell receptor during their relatively short life-span.

Fig. 7.13 The correlation of stages of α:β T-cell development with T-cell receptor gene rearrangement and the expression of cell-surface proteins in murine thymus. Lymphoid precursors are triggered to proliferate and become thymocytes committed to the T-cell lineage through interactions with the thymic stroma. These negative cells express CD44 and Kit and, at a later stage, the α chain of the IL-2 receptor, CD25. After this, the CD44$^+$ CD25$^+$ cells begin to rearrange the β-chain locus, becoming CD44^{low} and Kit^{low} as this occurs. The cells are arrested in the CD44^{low} CD25$^+$ stage until they productively rearrange the β-chain locus; the in-frame β chain then pairs with the surrogate pTα chain and is expressed on the cell surface, which triggers entry into the cell cycle. Expression of small amounts of pTα:β on the cell surface in association with CD3 triggers rapid proliferation of these cells, which causes the loss of CD25 and the cessation of β-chain gene rearrangement. Eventually, cell proliferation ceases and CD4 and CD8 are expressed. The small CD4$^+$ CD8$^+$ double-positive cells begin efficient rearrangement at the α-chain locus. The cells then express low levels of an α:β T-cell receptor and the associated CD3 complex and are ready for selection. Most cells die by failing to be positively selected or as a consequence of negative selection, but some are selected to mature into CD4 or CD8 single-positive cells and eventually to leave the thymus.

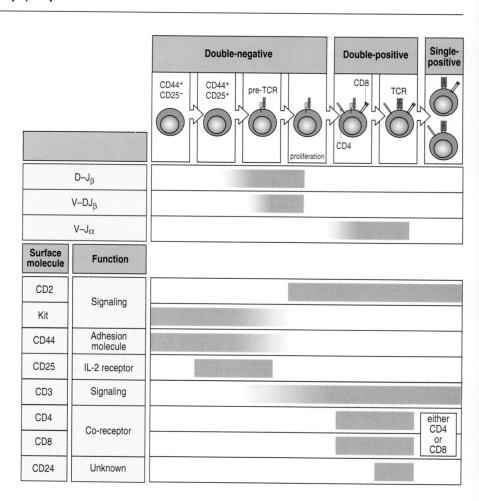

Small double-positive thymocytes initially express low levels of the T-cell receptor. Most of these cells bear receptors that cannot recognize self-peptide:self-MHC molecular complexes; these are destined to fail positive selection and die. In contrast, those double-positive cells that recognize self-peptide:self-MHC and can therefore undergo positive selection go on to mature and express high levels of the T-cell receptor. Concurrently, they cease to express one or other of the two co-receptor molecules, becoming either CD4 or CD8 **single-positive thymocytes.** Thymocytes also undergo negative selection during and after the double-positive stage in development, which eliminates those cells capable of responding to self antigens. Approximately 2% of the double-positive thymocytes survive this dual screening and mature as single-positive T cells that are gradually exported from the thymus to form the peripheral T-cell repertoire. The time between the entry of a T-cell progenitor into the thymus and the export of its mature progeny is estimated to be about 3 weeks in the mouse.

7-7   Thymocytes at different developmental stages are found in distinct parts of the thymus.

The thymus is divided into two main regions, a peripheral cortex and a central medulla (see Fig. 7.8). Most T-cell development takes place in the cortex; only mature single-positive thymocytes are seen in the medulla. Initially, progenitors from the bone marrow enter at the cortico-medullary junction and migrate to the outer cortex. At the outer edge of the cortex, in the subcapsular region of the thymus (Fig. 7.14), large immature double-negative

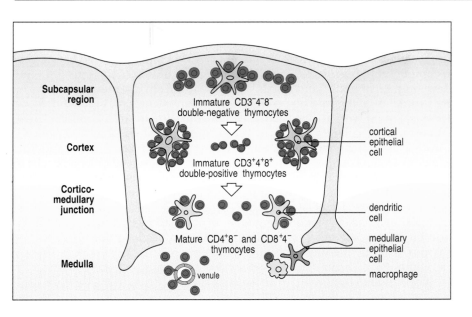

Fig. 7.14 Thymocytes at different developmental stages are found in distinct parts of the thymus. The earliest cells to enter the thymus are found in the subcapsular region of the cortex. As these cells proliferate and mature into double-positive thymocytes, they migrate deeper into the thymic cortex. Finally, the medulla contains only mature single-positive T cells, which eventually leave the thymus and enter the bloodstream.

thymocytes proliferate vigorously; these cells are thought to represent the thymic progenitors and their immediate progeny and will give rise to all subsequent thymocyte populations. Deeper in the cortex, most of the thymocytes are small double-positive cells. The cortical stroma is composed of epithelial cells with long branching processes that express both MHC class II and MHC class I molecules on their surface. The thymic cortex is densely packed with thymocytes, and the branching processes of the thymic cortical epithelial cells make contact with almost all cortical thymocytes (see Fig. 7.9). Contact between the MHC molecules on thymic cortical epithelial cells and the receptors of developing T cells has a crucial role in positive selection, as we will see later in this chapter.

The function of the medulla of the thymus is less well understood. It contains relatively few thymocytes, and those that are present are single-positive cells resembling mature T cells. These cells probably include newly mature T cells that are leaving the thymus through the medulla. In addition, they include other populations of mature T cells that remain within the medulla or return to it from the periphery to perform some specialized function, such as the elimination of infectious agents within the thymus. Before they mature, the developing thymocytes must undergo negative selection to remove self-reactive cells. We will see that this selective process is performed mainly by the dendritic cells, which are particularly numerous at the cortico-medullary junction, and by the macrophages that are scattered in the cortex but are also abundant in the thymic medulla.

Summary.

B cells are generated and develop in the specialized microenvironment of the bone marrow, whereas the thymus provides a specialized and architecturally organized microenvironment for the development of T cells. B cells are produced throughout life, whereas T-cell production from the thymus slows down after puberty. As B cells differentiate from primitive stem cells, they proceed through stages that are marked by the sequential rearrangement of immunoglobulin gene segments to generate a diverse repertoire of antigen receptors. This developmental program also involves changes in the expression of other cellular proteins. Precursors of T cells migrate from the bone marrow and mature in the thymus. This process is similar to that for

B cells, including the sequential rearrangement of antigen-receptor gene segments. Developing T cells pass through a series of stages that can be distinguished by the differential expression of CD44 and CD25, the CD3:T-cell receptor complex proteins, and the co-receptor proteins CD4 and CD8. The development of both T and B cells is guided by the environment, particularly by stromal cells that provide contact-dependent signals and growth factors for developing lymphocytes. Notably, the commitment of a lymphoid progenitor to the T-cell rather than the B-cell lineage involves signals transduced through the Notch1 receptor. There are several ligands for Notch1, and it is not clear which is important for T-lineage commitment and on which cells it might be expressed. However, because Notch1 is expressed from early lymphoid progenitors through to mature T and B cells, the suspicion is that a key ligand is expressed exclusively in the thymus. In T cells the development is compartmentalized, with different types of stromal cells in the thymic cortex and medulla. Most steps in T-cell differentiation occur in the cortex of the thymus. The thymic medulla contains mainly mature T cells. Lymphocyte development is accompanied by extensive cell death, reflecting intense selection and the elimination of those cells that have failed to assemble a receptor or that have receptors with inappropriate specificities.

The rearrangement of antigen-receptor gene segments controls lymphocyte development.

In this part of the chapter we look in more detail at the steps that lead to a mature lymphocyte expressing a unique antigen receptor on its surface. The binding site of this receptor is formed from the variable regions of two different receptor chains and, in general, lymphocyte development is regulated so that each mature cell produces only one of each of these (for example, one immunoglobulin heavy chain and one light chain in B cells) and therefore bears receptors of a single specificity. Production of a complete antigen receptor therefore entails two series of gene segment rearrangements, one for each receptor-chain locus. Each series of rearrangements continues until a protein product is made, at which point the cell moves on to the next stage of development. This process is guided by signals that regulate the expression of the transcription factors and enzymes that control the rearrangement process. Such signals are generated by the expression of a complete antigen receptor and also by the expression of a pre-B-cell or pre-T-cell receptor in which the first receptor chain to be successfully rearranged is combined with a surrogate second chain; these receptors form complexes with accessory chains that have a signaling function. T-cell precursors develop to express either of two mutually exclusive types of T-cell receptor, the α:β receptor or the γ:δ receptor, and we will describe how this occurs.

7-8   B cells undergo a programmed series of gene rearrangements in the bone marrow.

As we saw in Chapter 4, the genes that encode immunoglobulin V regions are initially organized as an array of separate gene segments. These must be rearranged and joined together in the developing B cell to produce a complete V-region exon. The recombination process is imprecise, however, with the random addition of nucleotides at the joins between gene segments (see

Section 4-8). This means that it is a matter of chance whether the juxtaposed J sequence, for example, and the μ constant (C)-region sequence downstream, can be read in the correct reading frame; each time a V gene segment undergoes rearrangement to a J gene segment, or to an already rearranged DJ sequence, there is a roughly two in three chance of generating an out-of-frame sequence downstream from the join. Thus, B-cell development has evolved to preserve and multiply those B cells that have made productive joins and to eliminate cells that have not.

In addition, because there are two alleles for each immunoglobulin locus in the diploid genome, each of which can rearrange, the cell must prevent both alleles from making productive joins, lest the cell express two receptors of different antigen specificities. This is accomplished by checking for productive joins as soon as an allele has rearranged. When a productive join is made, it generally signals the cell to cease the current phase of rearrangement and progress to the next stage. Assembly of the gene segments to produce a complete receptor requires three separate recombination events, which occur at different stages of B-cell development. These are, in the order that they occur: the joining of D to J_H and V_H to DJ_H to produce the functional heavy-chain gene, and the joining of V_L to J_L to produce the functional light-chain gene. The κ-chain locus is generally rearranged before the λ-chain locus, the latter only initiating rearrangement if the κ-locus rearrangements have failed to generate a productive join.

Because only about one in three joins will be successful, and three successful joins are required to express a complete immunoglobulin molecule, a large number of developing B cells are lost because they fail to make a productive rearrangement at one of these stages. The sequence of immunoglobulin gene rearrangements and the points at which nonproductive rearrangements can lead to cell loss are shown in Fig. 7.15. Far fewer cells are expected to be lost because of failure to make productive light-chain gene rearrangements than are lost at the stage of heavy-chain gene rearrangement. This is partly because there are two light-chain loci—κ and λ—that can be rearranged, and partly because the opportunity for successive rearrangement attempts is much greater at each light-chain locus.

Fig. 7.15 The steps in immunoglobulin gene rearrangement at which cells can be lost. The developmental program rearranges the heavy-chain (H-chain) locus first and then the light-chain (L-chain) loci. Cells are allowed to progress to the next stage when a productive rearrangement has been achieved. Each rearrangement has about a one in three chance of being successful, but if the first attempt is nonproductive, development is suspended and there is a chance for one or more further attempts, so by simple mathematics four in nine rearrangements give rise to a heavy chain. The scope for repeated rearrangements is greater at the light-chain loci (see Fig. 7.18), so that fewer cells are lost between the pre-B and immature B cell stages than in the pro-B to pre-B transition.

7-9   Successful rearrangement of heavy-chain immunoglobulin gene segments leads to the formation of a pre-B-cell receptor that halts further V_H to DJ_H rearrangement and triggers the cell to divide.

Immunoglobulin heavy-chain gene rearrangement begins in early pro-B cells with D to J_H joining. This typically occurs at both alleles of the heavy-chain locus, at which point the cell becomes a late pro-B cell. The cell then proceeds to rearrange a V_H gene segment to the DJ_H sequence. Most D to J_H joins in humans are potentially useful, as almost all human D gene segments can be translated in all three reading frames without encountering a stop codon. Thus, there is no need of a special mechanism for distinguishing successful $D–J_H$ joins, and at this early stage there is also no need to ensure that only one allele undergoes rearrangement. Indeed, given the likely rate of failure at later stages, starting off with two successfully rearranged D–J sequences is an advantage.

V_H to DJ_H rearrangement occurs first on only one chromosome. A successful rearrangement causes intact μ chains to be produced, after which V_H to DJ_H rearrangement ceases and the cell progresses to become a pre-B cell. In at least two out of three cases, however, the first rearrangement is nonproductive, and V_H to DJ_H rearrangement continues on the other chromosome, again with a theoretical one in three chance of being productive. A rough estimate of the chance of generating a pre-B cell is thus 55% $(1/3 + (2/3 \times 1/3) = 0.55)$. The actual frequency is somewhat lower because the V gene repertoire contains pseudogenes that can rearrange yet have major defects that prevent the expression of a functional protein. Pro-B cells in which rearrangements at both heavy-chain alleles are nonproductive are eliminated. A considerable proportion (at least 45%) of pro-B cells is therefore lost at this stage.

The large pre-B cell in which a successful heavy-chain gene rearrangement has just occurred stops V_H to DJ_H rearrangement and begins to divide. This change in the cell's state is thought to occur after the transient expression of the rearranged heavy chain as part of a pre-B-cell receptor, which in some way provides the cell with a signal to halt rearrangement and to start proliferation. Pro-B cells in which rearrangements at both heavy-chain alleles are nonproductive are unable to receive this signal, and are eliminated. The signal that results from a productive rearrangement underlies the process of **allelic exclusion**, a term that signifies the expression of only one of the two alleles of a given gene in a diploid cell (Fig. 7.16). Allelic exclusion occurs at both the heavy-chain locus and the light-chain loci. The phenomenon was discovered more than 30 years ago, when it provided one of the original pieces of experimental support for the theory that one lymphocyte expresses one receptor. There are two mechanisms for halting further rearrangements. One is the inactivation of one of the recombinase subunits, RAG-2, by phosphorylation, which targets it for degradation. In addition, synthesis of the mRNAs for both RAG-2 and the other recombinase subunit, RAG-1, is suppressed. A second mechanism must be to make the heavy-chain locus inaccessible to the

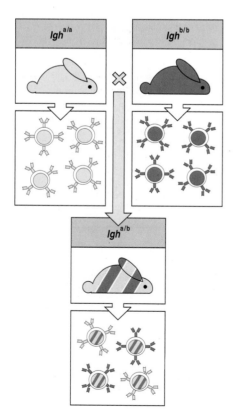

Fig. 7.16 Allelic exclusion in individual B cells. Most species have genetic polymorphisms of the constant regions of their immunoglobulin heavy-chain and light-chain genes; these are known as allotypes (see Section 4-21). In rabbits, for example, all of the B cells in an individual homozygous for the *a* allele of the immunoglobulin heavy-chain locus (*Igh*) will express immunoglobulin of allotype a, whereas in an individual homozygous for the *b* allele all the B cells make immunoglobulin of allotype b. In a heterozygous animal, which carries the *a* allele at one of the *igh* loci and the *b* allele on the other, individual B cells can be shown to carry either a-type or b-type immunoglobulin, but not both. This allelic exclusion reflects the productive rearrangement of only one of the two parental *Igh* alleles.

recombinase machinery, although how and when this happens are not clear. Nonetheless, at later stages of B-cell development, RAG proteins will again be expressed so as to perform light-chain gene segment rearrangements; at this point, the heavy-chain loci do not undergo further rearrangement, presumably because they are no longer accessible.

A major consequence of productive rearrangement in the pro-B cells is formation of the **pre-B-cell receptor,** which is composed of the μ heavy chain and two proteins that are made in pro-B cells, to form a surrogate light chain (Fig. 7.17). One of these is called **λ5** because of its close similarity to the C domain of the λ light chain; the other, called **VpreB,** resembles a light-chain V domain but has an extra amino-terminal region. The signaling capability of the pre-B-cell receptor depends on its further association with Igα and Igβ, two invariant accessory chains that are also associated with the mature B-cell receptor (see Section 6-7). Thus λ5, VpreB, the μ heavy chain, and the attendant Igα and Igβ chains together form a **pre-B-cell receptor complex,** which structurally resembles a mature B-cell receptor complex.

Fig. 7.17 A productively rearranged immunoglobulin gene is expressed immediately as a protein by the developing B cell. In early pro-B cells, heavy-chain gene rearrangement is not yet complete and no functional μ protein is expressed, as shown in the top panel. As soon as a productive heavy-chain gene rearrangement has taken place, μ chains are expressed by the cell in a complex with two other chains, λ5 and VpreB, which together make up a surrogate light chain. The whole immunoglobulin-like complex is known as the pre-B-cell receptor (second panel). It is also associated with two other protein chains, Igα (CD79α) and Igβ (CD79β), in the cell. These associated chains signal the B cell to halt heavy-chain gene rearrangement, and drive the transition to the large pre-B cell stage by inducing proliferation. The progeny of large pre-B cells stop dividing and become small pre-B cells, in which light-chain gene rearrangements commence. Successful light-chain gene rearrangement results in the production of a light chain that binds the μ chain to form a complete IgM molecule, which is expressed together with Igα and Igβ at the cell surface, as shown in the third panel. Signaling via these surface IgM molecules is thought to trigger the cessation of light-chain gene rearrangement.

X-linked
Agammaglobulinemia

The pre-B-cell receptor complex is expressed only transiently, perhaps because the production of λ5 mRNA stops as soon as pre-B-cell receptors begin to be formed. Although the pre-B-cell receptor is expressed at low levels on the surface of pre-B cells, it is not clear whether it interacts with an external ligand. It may simply be the assembly of the receptor, or even its insertion into the endoplasmic reticulum membrane, where most pre-B-cell receptor molecules are found, that generates the signals required for further development. Nevertheless, its formation is an important checkpoint in B-cell development. In mice that either lack λ5 or possess mutant heavy-chain genes that cannot produce the transmembrane domain, the pre-B-cell receptor cannot be formed and B-cell development is blocked after heavy-chain gene segment rearrangement. Because the normal signals that halt V_H to DJ_H rearrangement are not given, λ5 knockout mice have rearrangements of the heavy-chain genes on both chromosomes in all pre-B cells, so that about 10% of the cells have two productive VDJ_H rearrangements. The intracellular tyrosine kinase Btk (see Section 6-11) is thought to have a role in transducing this signal, because in its absence B-cell development is blocked at the pre-B cell stage.

In the mouse, the large pre-B cells divide several times, expanding the population of cells with successful in-frame joins by approximately thirty to sixtyfold before they become resting small pre-B cells. A large pre-B cell with a particular rearranged heavy-chain gene therefore gives rise to numerous progeny. Upon reaching the small pre-B-cell stage, RAG proteins are again produced and each of these progeny can make a different rearranged light-chain gene. Thus cells with many different antigen specificities are generated from a single pre-B cell. This makes an important contribution to B-cell receptor diversity. A similar course of events occurs in the thymus, allowing a diversity of T-cell receptor α chains to be expressed with a successfully rearranged β chain during T-cell development, as we will discuss later in this chapter.

7-10   Rearrangement at the immunoglobulin light-chain locus leads to cell-surface expression of the B-cell receptor.

In mice and humans, the κ light-chain locus tends to rearrange before the λ locus. This was first deduced from the observation that myeloma cells secreting λ light chains generally have both their κ and λ light-chain genes rearranged, whereas in myelomas secreting κ light chains, generally only the κ genes are rearranged. This order is occasionally reversed, however, and λ gene rearrangement does not absolutely require the prior rearrangement of the κ genes.

As with the heavy-chain locus, rearrangements at the light-chain locus generally take place at only one allele at a time. Unlike the case of the heavy-chain genes, however, there is scope for repeated rearrangements of unused V and J gene segments at each allele (Fig. 7.18). Several successive attempts at productive rearrangement of a light-chain gene can therefore be made on one chromosome before initiating any rearrangements on the second chromosome.

The chances of eventually generating an intact light chain are greatly increased by the potential for multiple successive rearrangement events at each allele and by the chance to rearrange either of the two light-chain loci successfully. As a result, many cells that reach the pre-B cell stage succeed in generating progeny that bear intact IgM molecules and can be classified as immature B cells.

Once a light-chain gene has been rearranged successfully, light chains are synthesized and combine with the heavy chain to form intact IgM (see Fig. 7.17). IgM appears at the cell surface together with Igα and Igβ to form the functional B-cell receptor complex. If the newly expressed receptor encoun-

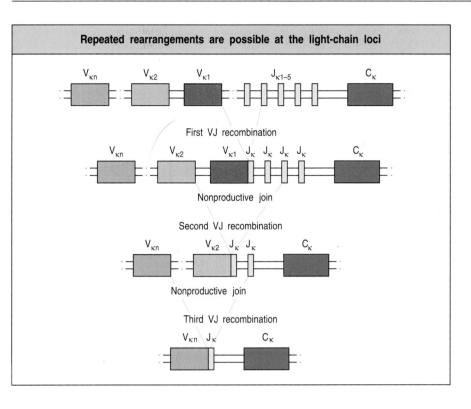

Repeated rearrangements are possible at the light-chain loci

First VJ recombination

Nonproductive join

Second VJ recombination

Nonproductive join

Third VJ recombination

Fig. 7.18 Nonproductive light-chain gene rearrangements can be rescued by further gene rearrangement. The organization of the light-chain loci in mice and humans offers many opportunities for the rescue of pre-B cells that initially make an out-of-frame rearrangement. Light-chain rescue is illustrated for the human κ locus. If the first rearrangement is nonproductive, a 5′ V_κ gene segment can recombine with a 3′ J_κ gene segment to remove the out-of-frame join and replace it. In principle, this can happen up to five times on each chromosome, because there are five functional J_κ gene segments in humans. If all rearrangements of κ-chain genes fail to yield a productive light-chain join, λ-chain gene rearrangement may succeed (not shown, see Fig. 7.15).

ters a strongly cross-linking antigen—that is, if the B cell is strongly self-reactive—development is halted and the cell will not mature further. This is the first negative selection process that B cells undergo. In contrast, if the B-cell receptor is not self-reactive, the cell continues to mature. It is not yet clear how, in the absence of binding to a specific antigen, the B cell senses that a functional immunoglobulin receptor has been expressed and thereby receives signals for further maturation. A role for Igα in signaling at this stage is indicated by a reduction in B-lineage cells in mice that express Igα with a truncated cytoplasmic domain, which therefore cannot signal to the interior of the cell. In such mice, the number of immature B cells in the marrow is reduced fourfold and the number of peripheral B cells is reduced a hundredfold. This shows that an ability to signal through Igα is particularly important in dictating the emigration of B cells from the bone marrow and/or their survival in the periphery once a complete immunoglobulin molecule has been expressed.

Thus, by signaling the completion of a productive rearrangement, the synthesis of an immunoglobulin heavy chain or light chain and its assembly into a receptor (IgM) leads to the further maturation of the B cell and ultimately to the cessation of further rearrangements, which enforces allelic exclusion at the light-chain locus. A similar mechanism underlies **isotypic exclusion**, the production of a light chain from only one of the two light-chain loci—κ or λ—in each individual cell.

In light-chain isotypic exclusion, there is a decided preference for which locus is rearranged first, and the ratios of κ-expressing versus λ-expressing mature B cells vary from one extreme to the other in different species. In mice and rats it is 95% κ to 5% λ, in humans it is typically 65%:35%, and in cats it is 5%:95%, the opposite of that in mice. These ratios correlate most strongly to the number of functional V_κ and V_λ gene segments in the genome of the species. They also reflect the kinetics and efficiency of gene segment rearrangements. The κ:λ ratio in the mature lymphocyte population is useful in clinical diagnostics, as an aberrant κ:λ ratio indicates the dominance of one clone and the presence of a lymphoproliferative disorder, which may be malignant.

7-11   The expression of proteins regulating immunoglobulin gene rearrangement and function is developmentally programmed.

A variety of proteins have a role in the development of B cells, and many of these contribute to regulating and executing the sequential steps in immunoglobulin gene segment rearrangement that mark the different stages in B-cell differentiation. Fig. 7.19 lists some of these proteins and shows how their expression is regulated through the different stages of B-cell development.

Both immunoglobulin gene segment rearrangement and T-cell receptor gene segment rearrangement depend on the proteins RAG-1 and RAG-2. The RAG-1:RAG-2 heterodimer is a component of the V(D)J recombinase (see Section 4-5), which is active at very early stages of lymphoid development. In both B-cell and T-cell lineages there is a later and temporary suppression of *RAG* gene expression after successful rearrangements have been completed at the first of the two rearranging loci, namely the immunoglobulin heavy-chain locus in B cells and the T-cell receptor β locus in T cells. Thus, the RAG proteins are inactive during the burst of cell proliferation that follows these first

Fig. 7.19 The temporal expression of several cellular proteins known to be important for B-cell development. The proteins listed here are a selection of those known to be associated with early B-lineage development and have been included because of their proven importance in the developmental sequence, largely on the basis of studies in mice. Their individual contributions to B-cell development are discussed in the text, with the exception of the Octamer Transcription Factor, Oct-2, which binds the octamer ATGCAAAT found in the heavy-chain promoter and elsewhere, and GATA-2, which is one of the many transcription factors active in several hematopoietic lineages. The *pax-5* gene product, known as B-lineage-specific activator protein (BSAP), is involved in regulating the expression of several of the proteins listed. The tight temporal regulation of the expression of these proteins, and of the immunoglobulin genes themselves, would be expected to impose a strict sequence on the events of B-cell differentiation.

successful rearrangements (see Sections 7-9 and 7-13), but they are resynthesized later when the cells cease dividing and go on to make rearrangements at the second locus.

Another enzyme, **terminal deoxynucleotidyl transferase (TdT)**, contributes to the diversity of both B-cell and T-cell antigen receptor repertoires by adding nontemplated or N-nucleotides at the joints between rearranged gene segments (see Section 4-8). As with the RAG proteins, TdT is expressed in early lymphoid progenitors but, unlike the RAG-1:RAG-2 enzyme, it is not essential to the rearrangement process. Indeed, at the time in fetal development when the peripheral immune system is first being supplied with T and B lymphocytes, TdT is expressed at low levels, if at all. In adult humans it is expressed in pro-B cells but its expression declines at the pre-B cell stage, when heavy-chain gene rearrangement is complete and light-chain gene rearrangement has commenced. This timing explains why N-nucleotides are found in the V–D and D–J joints of nearly all heavy-chain genes but only in about a quarter of human light-chain joints. N-nucleotides are rarely found in mouse light-chain V–J joints, showing that TdT is switched off slightly earlier in the development of mouse B cells.

Proteins required for the formation of a functional receptor complex are also essential for B-cell development. The invariant proteins Igα (CD79α) and Igβ (CD79β) are components of both the pre-B-cell receptor and the B-cell receptor complexes on the cell surface (see Fig. 7.17). As well as enabling immunoglobulins to be transported to the cell surface, Igα and Igβ transduce signals from these receptors by interacting with intracellular tyrosine kinases through their cytoplasmic tails (see Section 6-7). Igα and Igβ are expressed from the pro-B cell stage until the death of the cell or its terminal differentiation into an antibody-secreting plasma cell. Curiously, mice lacking Igβ have a block in B-cell development at the pro-B cell stage, before VDJ$_H$ rearrangements are complete. The requirement for Igβ is thought to be due to the assembly of an Igα:Igβ complex with the chaperone protein calnexin in the normal pro-B cell, which may trigger signals needed for further development.

Other signal transduction proteins with a role in B-cell development are included in Fig. 7.19. Bruton's tyrosine kinase (Btk), a Tec-family kinase (see Section 6-11), has received intense scrutiny because mutations in the *Btk* gene cause a profound B-lineage-specific immune deficiency, **Bruton's X-linked agammaglobulinemia (XLA)**, in which no mature B cells are produced. In humans, the block in B-cell development caused by mutations at the *XLA* locus is almost total, interrupting the transition from pre-B cell to immature B cell. A similar, though less severe, defect called **X-linked immunodeficiency** or **xid** arises from mutations in the corresponding gene in mice.

X-linked
Agammaglobulinemia

Finally, several transcription factors or gene-regulatory proteins are essential for B-cell development, as shown by deficiencies of the B-cell lineage in genetically engineered mice lacking these proteins. At least 10 transcription factors necessary for normal B-lineage development have been described, and there are likely to be others. For several of these factors, such as Ikaros and PU.1, gene deletion leads to no lymphocytes. Such transcription factors are also required for the development of other hematopoietic lineages. Essential transcription factors for B-cell development include the products of the *E2A* gene. These products, which are derived by alternative splicing, induce another transcription factor, the early B-cell factor (EBF), which in turn regulates the transcription of the gene for Igα. In the absence of E2A or EBF, even the earliest identifiable stage in B-cell development, D–J$_H$ joining, fails to occur. Another important transcription factor is the *pax-5* gene product, one isoform of which is the B-lineage-specific activator protein (BSAP). This protein, which may also be induced by EBF, is active in late pro-B cells and enables the proper functioning of the heavy-chain enhancers located 3′ of the heavy-chain C-region genes. It also binds to regulatory sites in the genes for λ5, VpreB, and other B-cell-specific proteins. In the absence of BSAP, pro-B cells fail to develop further down the B-cell pathway but can be induced to give rise to T cells and various myeloid cell types. Thus BSAP is required for the commitment of the pro-B cell to the B-cell lineage.

It seems likely that these regulatory proteins and others like them together direct the developmental program of B-lineage cells. In particular, the proteins involved in the tissue-specific transcriptional regulation of immunoglobulin genes are likely to be important in regulating the order of events in gene rearrangement. The V(D)J recombinase system is not in itself lineage-specific; it operates in both B- and T-lineage cells and uses the same core enzymes. Yet rearrangements of T-cell receptor genes do not occur in B-lineage cells, nor do complete rearrangements of immunoglobulin genes occur in T cells. The ordered rearrangement events that do occur are associated with low-level transcription of the gene segments about to be joined. This is probably because key transcription factors such as BSAP bind to the DNA and 'open' the chromatin, making it accessible to the recombinase enzymes (Fig. 7.20).

Fig. 7.20 Proteins binding to promoter and enhancer elements contribute to the sequence of gene rearrangement and regulate the level of RNA transcription. The immunoglobulin heavy-chain locus is illustrated. First panel: in germline DNA, stem cells, and nonlymphoid cells, the chromatin containing the immunoglobulin genes is in a closed conformation. Second panel: in the early pro-B cell, lineage-specific proteins bind to the Ig enhancer elements (e); for the heavy-chain locus these are in the J–C intron and 3′ to the C exons. The DNA is now in an open conformation, and low-level transcription from promoters (P) upstream of the D and J gene segments occurs. Third panel: the rearrangement of D to J that follows the initiation of transcription of the D and J gene segments sustains transcription from promoters located upstream of the D gene segments. For some D–J joins in the mouse this may result in the expression of a truncated heavy chain (D_μ) at levels sufficient to abort further development, but in most cases it is followed by the initiation of low-level transcription of an upstream V gene segment. Fourth panel: subsequent rearrangement of a V gene segment brings its promoter under the influence of the heavy-chain enhancers, leading to an enhanced production of a μ heavy-chain mRNA in large pre-B cells and their progeny. S_μ represents the switch signal sequence for isotype switching (see Section 4-18).

As a consequence of immunoglobulin gene rearrangement, the promoters that lie upstream of all V gene segments are brought close to the enhancers associated with the C gene segments. This in turn brings transcription factors that have bound the promoter and enhancer into proximity, resulting in a marked increase in transcription of the rearranged gene segments. Thus gene rearrangement can be viewed as a powerful mechanism for regulating gene expression, as well as for generating receptor diversity. In vertebrates, only the immunoglobulin and T-cell receptor genes are known to use gene rearrangement to regulate gene expression.

7-12   T cells in the thymus undergo a series of gene segment rearrangements similar to those of B cells.

Developing T cells face a similar challenge to developing B cells. They must assemble a functional gene for each T-cell receptor chain while ensuring that each T cell expresses a receptor that has only one specificity. Not surprisingly, T cells follow an almost identical strategy to B cells, in that the receptor is assembled in stages, with each stage being checked for correct assembly. Moreover, as in B cells, a productively rearranged gene is expressed as soon as it is made, and the product(s) are assembled into a receptor complex, in this case either a pre-T-cell receptor or a *bona fide* T-cell receptor. Expression of this receptor is instrumental in promoting further development, which ultimately results in shutting down further rearrangement at the locus that has just been active.

Despite the similarities to B-cell development, the control of antigen-receptor assembly during development is more complicated for T cells because there are two different kinds of T cell that could be generated from an undifferentiated precursor—α:β T cells and γ:δ T cells. Different genetic loci are used to make these two types of T-cell receptor, as described in Sections 4-11 and 4-13. Thus, the T-cell developmental program must control which of the two lineages a precursor commits to and must also ensure that a fully developed T cell expresses receptor components of only one or the other lineage. Another key difference between B and T cells is that the final assembly of an immunoglobulin leads to the cessation of gene rearrangement and initiates the further differentiation of the B cell, whereas in T cells rearrangement of the V_α gene segments continues unless there is signaling by a self-peptide:self-MHC complex that positively selects the receptor.

7-13   Successful rearrangement at the β-chain locus and synthesis of a β chain leads to the production of a pre-T-cell receptor that triggers cell proliferation and cessation of β-chain gene rearrangement.

The rearrangement of the β- and α-chain loci during T-cell development follows a sequence that closely parallels the rearrangement of immunoglobulin heavy-chain and light-chain loci during B-cell development (see Section 7-8). As shown in Fig. 7.21, the β-chain gene segments rearrange first, with the D_β gene segments rearranging to J_β gene segments, and this is followed by V_β gene segments to DJ_β gene rearrangement. If no functional β chain can be synthesized from these rearrangements, the cell will not be able to produce a pre-T-cell receptor and will die unless it makes successful rearrangements at both the γ and δ loci (see Section 7-15). However, unlike B cells with nonproductive immunoglobulin heavy-chain gene rearrangements, thymocytes with nonproductive β-chain VDJ rearrangements can be rescued by subsequent rearrangements, which are possible because of the presence of two clusters of D_β and J_β gene segments upstream of two C_β genes (see Fig. 4.11). For this reason, the likelihood of a productive VDJ join at the β locus is somewhat higher than the 55% chance of a productive immunoglobulin heavy-chain gene arrangement.

Fig. 7.21 The stages of gene rearrangement in α:β T cells. The sequence of gene rearrangements is shown, together with an indication of the stage at which the events take place and the nature of the cell-surface receptor molecules expressed at each stage. The β-chain locus rearranges first, in CD4⁻ CD8⁻ double-negative thymocytes expressing CD25 and low levels of CD44. As with immunoglobulin heavy-chain genes, D to J gene segments rearrange before V gene segments rearrange to DJ (second and third panels). It is possible to make up to four attempts to generate a productive rearrangement at the β-chain locus, because there are four D gene segments with two sets of J gene segments associated with each TCR β chain locus (not shown). The productively rearranged gene is expressed initially within the cell and then at low levels on the cell surface. It associates with pTα, a surrogate 33 kDa α chain that is equivalent to λ5 in B-cell development, and this pTα:β heterodimer forms a complex with the CD3 chains (fourth panel). The expression of the pre-T-cell receptor signals the developing thymocytes to halt β-chain gene rearrangement and to undergo multiple cycles of division. At the end of this proliferative burst, the CD4 and CD8 molecules are expressed, the cell ceases cycling, and the α chain is now able to undergo rearrangement. The first α-chain gene rearrangement deletes all δ D, J, and C gene segments on that chromosome, although these are retained as a circular DNA, proving that these are nondividing cells (bottom panel). This permanently inactivates the δ-chain gene. Rearrangements at the α-chain locus can proceed through several cycles, because of the large number of Vα and Jα gene segments, so that productive rearrangements almost always occur. When a functional α chain is produced that pairs efficiently with the β chain, the CD3ˡᵒʷ CD4⁺ CD8⁺ thymocyte is ready to undergo selection for its ability to recognize self peptides in association with self MHC molecules.

Once a productive β-chain gene rearrangement has occurred, the β chain is expressed together with the invariant partner chain pTα and the CD3 molecules (see Fig. 7.21) and is transported to the cell surface. The β:pTα complex is a functional pre-T-cell receptor analogous to the μ:VpreB:λ5 pre-B-cell receptor complex in B-cell development (see Section 7-9). Expression of the pre-T-cell receptor triggers the phosphorylation and degradation of RAG-2, halting β-chain gene rearrangement and thus ensuring allelic exclusion at the β locus. It also induces rapid cell proliferation and eventually the expression of the co-receptor proteins CD4 and CD8. All these events require the cytoplasmic protein tyrosine kinase Lck, which subsequently associates with the co-receptor proteins. In mice genetically deficient in Lck, T-cell development is arrested before the CD4$^+$ CD8$^+$ double-positive stage and no α-chain gene rearrangements can be made.

The role of the expressed β chain in suppressing further β-chain locus rearrangement can be demonstrated in transgenic mice containing a rearranged TCRβ transgene: these mice express the transgenic β chain on virtually 100% of their T cells, showing that rearrangement of the endogenous β-chain genes is strongly suppressed. The importance of pTα has been shown by the hundredfold decrease in α:β T cells and by the absence of allelic exclusion at the β locus in mice deficient in pTα.

During the proliferative phase triggered by expression of the pre-T-cell receptor, the *RAG-1* and *RAG-2* genes are also repressed. Hence, no rearrangement of the α-chain locus occurs until the proliferative phase ends, when *RAG-1* and *RAG-2* are transcribed again, and the functional RAG-1:RAG-2 heterodimer accumulates. This ensures that each cell in which a β-chain gene has been successfully rearranged gives rise to many CD4$^+$ CD8$^+$ double-positive thymocytes. Once the cells stop dividing, each of them can independently rearrange its α-chain genes, so that a single functional β chain can be associated with many different α chains in the progeny cells. During the period of α-chain gene rearrangement, α:β T-cell receptors are first expressed and selection by self-peptide:self-MHC complexes in the thymus can begin.

Along the progression of T cells from the double-negative to the double-positive and finally single-positive stage, there is a distinct pattern of expression of proteins involved in rearrangement and signaling, and also of transcription factors that most probably control developmental fates, as well as the expression of important T-cell loci like those of the T-cell receptor itself. The expression of these molecules through T-cell development is illustrated in Fig. 7.22. The expression of the RAG proteins has already been described. TdT, the protein responsible for the insertion of N-nucleotides at gene segment junctions in both B and T cells, is expressed throughout the developmental period in which thymocytes are rearranging T-cell receptor gene segments; N-nucleotides can be found at the junctions of all rearranged α and β genes. Lck, a Src-family tyrosine kinase, and ZAP-70, another tyrosine kinase, are both expressed from an early stage in thymocyte development. Lck has a key role in signaling of thymocytes at the pre-T cell receptor-positive stage, because mice lacking Lck have a profound loss of cells beyond this stage. Lck is also important for γ:δ T-cell development. In contrast, gene knockout studies (see Appendix I, Section A-47) show that ZAP-70, although expressed from the double-negative stage onward, has a role later: it promotes the development of single-positive thymocytes from double-positive thymocytes. Fyn, a Src-family kinase similar to Lck, is expressed at increasing levels from the double-positive stage onward but is not absolutely essential for thymocyte development as long as Lck is present. The roles of these molecules in mature T-cell signaling are described in Chapter 6.

Finally, a set of transcription factors guides the development of thymocytes from one stage to the next. Several important factors have been identified; in some cases gene knockout studies have shown at which stage of development they are essential. Ikaros and GATA-3 are expressed in early T-cell progenitors; in the absence of either, T-cell development is generally disrupted. Moreover, these molecules also have roles in the normal functioning of mature T cells. In contrast, Ets-1, though also expressed in early progenitors, is not essential for T-cell development, although mice lacking this factor do not make NK cells. TCF1 (T-cell factor-1) is first expressed during the double-

Fig. 7.22 The temporal pattern of expression of some cellular proteins important in early T-cell development. Expression is depicted with respect to the stages of thymocyte development as determined by cell-surface marker expression. The proteins listed here are a selection of those known to be associated with early T-lineage development and have been included because of their proven importance in the developmental sequence, largely on the basis of studies in mice. Their individual contributions to T-cell development are discussed in the text.

negative stage. In its absence, double-negative T cells that make productive β-chain gene rearrangements do not proliferate as usually seen in response to the pre-T-cell receptor signal, preventing the efficient production of double-positive thymocytes. LKLF (lung Kruppel-like factor) is first expressed late in thymocyte development at the single-positive stage; if LKLF is absent, single-positive cells do develop but they are abnormal, displaying a partly activated phenotype. Thus, transcription factors are turned on at various developmental stages and are responsible for normal development through those stages by controlling the expression of important genes. Transcription factors mediate the response to developmental signals by turning on the set of appropriate genes when the factors are activated to bind DNA.

7-14   T-cell α-chain genes undergo successive rearrangements until positive selection or cell death intervenes.

The T-cell receptor α-chain genes are comparable to the immunoglobulin κ and λ light-chain genes in that they do not have D gene segments and are rearranged only after their partner receptor chain has been expressed. As with the immunoglobulin light-chain genes, repeated attempts at rearrangement are possible. Indeed, the presence of multiple V_α gene segments, and about 60 J_α gene segments spread over some 80 kb of DNA, allows many successive V_α to J_α rearrangements to take place. This means that T cells with an initial nonproductive α-gene rearrangement are much more likely to be rescued by a subsequent rearrangement than are B cells with a nonproductive light-chain gene rearrangement (Fig. 7.23).

The potential for many successive rearrangements at both alleles of the α-chain locus virtually guarantees that a functional α chain will be produced in every developing T cell. Moreover, many T cells have in-frame rearrangements on both chromosomes and thus can produce two types of α chain. This is possible because, unlike the situation in B cells, expression of the T-cell receptor is not in itself sufficient to shut off gene rearrangement. Thus, rearrangement of α-chain genes continues even after the production of a T-cell receptor at the cell surface. Continued rearrangements on both chromosomes can allow several different α chains to be produced successively as well as simultaneously in each developing T cell and to be tested for self-peptide:self-MHC recognition in partnership with the same β chain. This phase of gene rearrangement lasts for 3 or 4 days in the mouse and ceases only when positive selection occurs as a consequence of receptor engagement, or when the cell dies. Thus, in the strict sense, T-cell receptor α-chain genes are not subject to allelic exclusion. However, as we will see in the next part of this chapter, only T-cell receptors that are positively selected for self-peptide:self-MHC recognition can function in self-MHC-restricted responses. The regulation of α-chain gene rearrangement by positive selection therefore ensures that each T cell has only a single functional specificity, even if two different α chains are expressed.

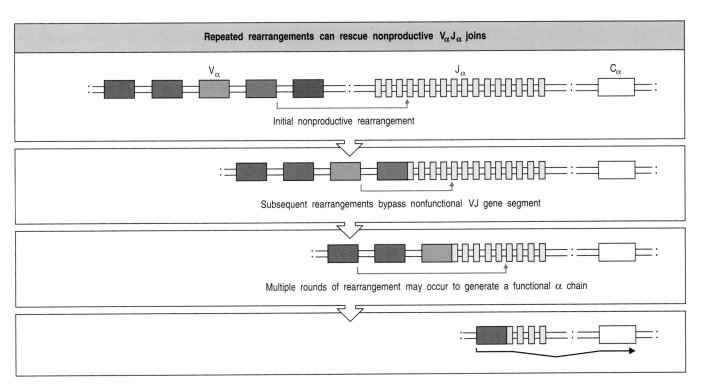

Fig. 7.23 Multiple successive rearrangement events can rescue nonproductive T-cell receptor α-chain gene rearrangements. The multiplicity of V and J gene segments at the α-chain locus allows successive rearrangement events to 'leapfrog' over previously rearranged VJ segments, deleting any intervening gene segments. The α-chain rescue pathway resembles that of the immunoglobulin κ light-chain genes (see Section 7-10), but the number of possible successive rearrangements is greater. α-chain gene rearrangement continues until either a productive rearrangement leads to positive selection or the cell dies.

Clearly, the engagement of any particular T-cell receptor with a self-MHC:self-peptide ligand will depend on the receptor's specificity. The phase of α-chain gene rearrangement therefore marks an important change in the forces shaping the destiny of the T cell. Up to this point, the development of the thymocyte has been independent of antigen; from this point onward, developmental decisions depend on the interaction of the T-cell receptor with its peptide:MHC ligands. Before we consider these ligand-driven events in the development of α:β T cells in the next part of the chapter, we will describe how the minority γ:δ lineage cells develop.

7-15   T cells with α:β or γ:δ receptors arise from a common progenitor.

T cells bearing γ:δ receptors differ from α:β T cells in the types of antigen they recognize, in the pattern of expression of the CD4 and CD8 co-receptors, and in their anatomical distribution in the periphery. The two types of T cell also differ in function, although relatively little is known about the function of γ:δ T cells (see Sections 2-29 and 3-19). The gene rearrangements found in thymocytes and in mature γ:δ and α:β T cells suggest that these two cell lineages diverge from a common precursor after certain gene rearrangements have

Fig. 7.24 Signals through the γ:δ T-cell receptor and the pre-T-cell receptor compete to determine the fate of thymocytes. During the differentiation of T cells in the thymus, at the double-negative stage where they express neither CD4 nor CD8, the developing thymocytes express both a γ:δ T-cell receptor (γ:δ TCR) and the pre-T-cell receptor (pre-TCR) composed of the TCRβ chain and the pre--α chain (pTα, top panel). At this stage, if the thymocyte receives signals through the γ:δ receptor, the cell commits to the γ:δ lineage, switching off expression of the β-chain gene and thus the pre TCR (middle left panel). This cell then matures into a γ:δ T cell and migrates out of the thymus into the peripheral circulation (bottom left panel). In contrast, if the developing thymocyte receives a signal through the pre-TCR (middle right panel), the cell switches off expression of the γ:δ TCR, deletes the δ-chain genes in the process of rearranging the TCRα-chain locus, and goes on to express a mature α:β T-cell receptor (bottom right panel).

already occurred (Fig. 7.24). Mature γ:δ T cells can rearrange β-chain genes, although 80% of these are nonproductive, and mature α:β T cells often contain rearranged, but mostly out-of-frame, γ-chain genes.

The β, γ, and δ loci undergo rearrangement almost simultaneously in developing thymocytes. At present, the factors that regulate lineage commitment of these cells are not known; indeed, commitment to the γ:δ lineage might simply depend on whether productive rearrangements at a γ-chain and a δ-chain gene have occurred in the same cell. In this view, successful rearrangement of a γ and a δ gene leads to the expression of a functional γ:δ T-cell receptor that signals the cell to differentiate along the γ:δ lineage. In most precursors, however, there is a successful rearrangement of a β-chain gene, which results in the production of a functional β-chain protein, before successful rearrangement of both γ and δ has occurred. The β chain pairs with pTα to create a pre-T-cell receptor (β:pTα), thus arresting further gene rearrangement and signaling the thymocyte to proliferate, to express its co-receptor genes, and eventually to start rearranging the α-chain genes. It is known that the β:pTα receptor signals constitutively via the tyrosine kinase Lck and does not seem to need a ligand on thymic stroma. This signaling is crucial for the further development of an α:β T cell (see Section 7-13).

It does seem likely that signals through the pre-T-cell receptor commit the cell to the α:β lineage (see Fig. 7.24). However, one problem with this model is how to explain the mature γ:δ cells that carry productive rearrangements at the β-chain locus. One way to reconcile this is if these cells had committed to the γ:δ rather than α:β lineage because they had received a signal from an assembled γ:δ receptor before having assembled a functional pre-T-cell receptor. This hypothesis requires that the γ:δ T-cell receptor and the pre-T-cell receptor signal differently, which has recently been established. Normally, α-chain gene rearrangements that occur after a pre-T-cell receptor signal delete the intervening δ-chain gene segments as an extrachromosomal circle (see Section 4-13). This further ensures that cells committed to the α:β lineages will not make a complete γ:δ receptor.

7-16 T cells expressing particular γ- and δ-chain V regions arise in an ordered sequence early in life.

We have just described how a precursor T cell that can become either an α:β or a γ:δ T cell becomes directed to one or the other lineage. During the development of the organism these pathways are not equally used; instead, the generation of the various types of T cell—even the particular V region assembled in γ:δ cells—are developmentally controlled. The first T cells to appear during embryonic development carry γ:δ T-cell receptors (Fig. 7.25). In the mouse, where the development of the immune system can be studied in detail, γ:δ T cells first appear in discrete waves or bursts, with the T cells in each wave populating distinct sites in the adult animal.

The first wave of γ:δ T cells populates the epidermis; the T cells become wedged among the keratinocytes and adopt a dendritic-like form that has given them the name of **dendritic epidermal T cells (dETCs)**. The second wave homes to the epithelia of the reproductive tract. Remarkably, given the large number of theoretically possible rearrangements, the receptors expressed by these early waves of γ:δ T cells are essentially invariant. All the cells in each wave assemble the same V_γ and V_δ regions. Each different wave, however, uses a different set of V, D, and J gene segments. Thus, certain V, D, and J gene segments are selected for rearrangement at particular times during embryonic development; the reasons for this limitation are poorly understood. There are no N-nucleotides contributing additional diversity at the junctions between V, D, and J gene segments, reflecting the absence of the enzyme TdT from these fetal T cells.

After these initial waves, T cells are produced continuously rather than in bursts, and α:β T cells predominate, making up more than 95% of thymocytes. The γ:δ T cells produced at this stage are different from those of the early waves. They have a considerably more diverse receptor repertoire, for which several different V gene segments have been used, and the receptor sequences have abundant N-nucleotide additions. Most of these γ:δ T cells, like α:β T cells, are found in peripheral lymphoid tissues rather than in the epithelial sites populated by the early γ:δ T cells.

The developmental changes in V gene segment usage and N-nucleotide addition in murine γ:δ T cells parallel changes in B-cell populations during fetal development, which will be discussed later. Their functional significance is unclear, however, and not all of these changes in the pattern of receptors expressed by γ:δ T cells occur in humans. Certainly, the γ:δ T cells that home to the skin of mice, the dETCs, do not seem to have exact human counterparts, although there are γ:δ T cells in the human reproductive and gastrointestinal tracts. The mouse dETCs may serve as sentinel cells that are activated upon local tissue damage or as cells that regulate inflammatory processes (see Section 2-29).

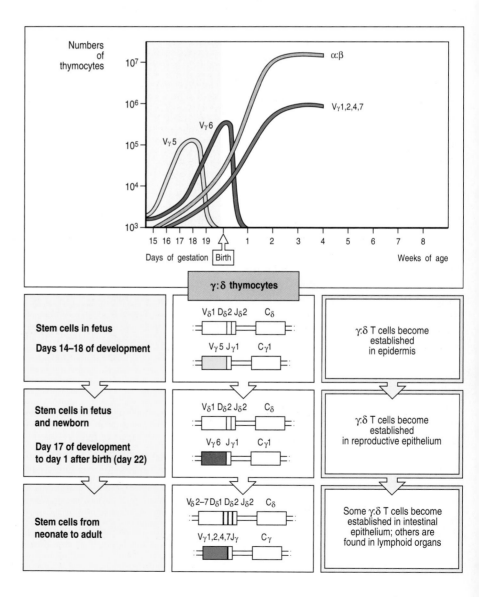

Fig. 7.25 The rearrangement of T-cell receptor γ and δ genes in the mouse proceeds in waves of cells expressing different V$_\gamma$ and V$_\delta$ gene segments. At about 2 weeks of gestation, the C$_\gamma$1 locus is expressed with its closest V gene (V$_\gamma$5). After a few days V$_\gamma$5-bearing cells decline (upper panel) and are replaced by cells expressing the next most proximal gene, V$_\gamma$6. Both these rearranged γ chains are expressed with the same rearranged δ-chain gene, as shown in the lower panels, and there is little junctional diversity in either the V$_\gamma$ or the V$_\delta$ chain. As a consequence, most of the γ:δ T cells produced in each of these early waves have the same specificity, although the antigen recognized in each case is not known. The V$_\gamma$5-bearing cells become established selectively in the epidermis, whereas the V$_\gamma$6-bearing cells become established in the epithelium of the reproductive tract. After birth, the α:β T-cell lineage becomes dominant and, although γ:δ T cells are still produced, they are a much more heterogeneous population, bearing receptors with a great deal of junctional diversity. Note that V$_\gamma$ gene segments are described using the system proposed by Tonegawa.

Summary.

As lymphocytes differentiate from primitive stem cells they proceed through stages that are marked by the sequential rearrangement of the antigen-receptor gene segments at different genetic loci. As each complete receptor-chain gene is generated, the protein it encodes is expressed as part of a receptor, and this signals the developing cell to progress to the next developmental step. For B cells the heavy-chain locus is rearranged first. If rearrangement is successful and a pre-B-cell receptor is made, heavy-chain gene rearrangement ceases and the resulting pre-B cells proliferate, followed by rearrangement at a light-chain locus. If the initial light-chain gene rearrangement is productive, a complete immunoglobulin B-cell receptor is formed, gene rearrangement ceases, and B-cell development proceeds. If not, light-chain gene rearrangement continues until either a new productive rearrangement is made or all available J regions have been used up. If a productive rearrangement is not made, the developing B cell dies.

In developing T cells, receptor loci rearrange according to a defined program similar to that in B cells. There is, however, the added complication that individual precursor T cells can follow one of two distinct lines of development. There are four T-cell receptor gene loci—γ, δ, α, and β. Rearrangement at these loci leads to cells bearing either $\gamma{:}\delta$ T-cell receptors or $\alpha{:}\beta$ T-cell receptors. Early in ontogeny, $\gamma{:}\delta$ T cells predominate, but from birth onward more than 90% of thymocytes express T-cell receptors encoded by rearranged α and β genes. In developing thymocytes, the γ, δ, and β loci rearrange first, and start rearranging virtually simultaneously. Productive rearrangements of both a γ and a δ gene may lead to the production of a functional $\gamma{:}\delta$ T-cell receptor and the development of a $\gamma{:}\delta$ T cell. Most cells, however, enter the $\alpha{:}\beta$ lineage. In these cells the generation of a β-chain gene before both γ and δ have rearranged leads to the expression of a functional β chain and a pre-T-cell receptor. This receptor, like the pre-B-cell receptor, signals the developing cell to proliferate, to arrest β-chain gene rearrangement, to express CD4 and CD8, and eventually to rearrange the α-chain gene. Rearrangement of the α-chain genes continues in these CD4$^+$ CD8$^+$ double-positive thymocytes until positive selection allows the maturation of a single-positive $\alpha{:}\beta$ cell; almost all cells will make productive α-gene rearrangements, but the vast majority of thymocytes die at the CD4$^+$ CD8$^+$ double-positive stage because they are not positively selected.

Thus gene rearrangement follows an ordered sequence in both B and T lineages to produce immature lymphocytes that each bear antigen receptors of a single specificity on their surface. These antigen receptors can now be tested for their antigen-recognition properties and the cells selected accordingly; these selection processes are described in the next part of this chapter.

Interaction with self antigens selects some lymphocytes for survival but eliminates others.

We have followed the development of a lymphocyte from a committed precursor to the point at which a complete antigen receptor is expressed on the cell surface. Development up to this point has been focused on testing for productive gene segment rearrangements and multiplying those cells that are successful, while controlling the rearrangement process so that lymphocytes express only one receptor. Once the cell can express that receptor, however, the focus shifts. Now the fate of the immature lymphocyte will be determined by the specificity of its antigen receptor. Most obviously, lymphocytes with strongly self-reactive receptors should be eliminated to prevent autoimmune reactions; this negative selection is one of the ways in which the immune system is made self-tolerant. In addition, given the incredible diversity of receptors that the rearrangement process can generate, it is important that those lymphocytes that mature are likely to be useful in recognizing and responding to foreign antigens, especially as an individual can only express a small fraction of the total possible receptor repertoire in his or her lifetime. Indeed, certainly for T cells and probably for B cells, a process of positive selection identifies and preserves lymphocytes that are likely to be able to respond to foreign antigens; those that do not pass this test fail to survive. In this part of the chapter we describe how the processes of positive and negative selection shape the mature lymphocyte repertoire.

7-17   Immature B cells that bind self antigens undergo further receptor rearrangement, die, or are inactivated.

Once an immature B cell expresses IgM on its surface (sIgM), its fate is guided by the nature of the signals it receives through its antigen receptor. This was first demonstrated by experiments in which antigen receptors on immature B cells were experimentally stimulated *in vivo* using anti-μ chain antibodies (see Appendix I, Section A-10); the outcome was elimination of the immature B cells. More recent experiments using mice expressing transgenes that enforce the expression of B-cell receptors that bind to self antigens have confirmed these earlier findings, but have also shown that immediate elimination is not the only possible outcome of binding to a self antigen. Instead, there are four possible fates for self-reactive immature B cells, depending on the nature of the ligand they bind (Fig. 7.26). These fates are: cell death by apoptosis; the

Fig. 7.26 Binding to self molecules in the bone marrow can lead to the death or inactivation of immature B cells. Left panels: when developing B cells express receptors that recognize multivalent ligands, for example ubiquitous self cell-surface molecules such as those of the MHC, these receptors are deleted from the repertoire. The B cells either undergo receptor editing (see Fig. 7.27), so that the self-reactive receptor specificity is deleted, or the cells themselves undergo programmed cell death or apoptosis (clonal deletion). Center left panels: immature B cells that bind soluble self antigens able to cross-link the B-cell receptor are rendered unresponsive to the antigen (anergic) and bear little surface IgM. They migrate to the periphery where they express IgD but remain anergic; if in competition with other B cells in the periphery, they are rapidly lost. Center right panels: immature B cells that bind monovalent antigens or soluble self antigens with low affinity do not receive any signal as a result of this interaction and mature normally to express both IgM and IgD at the cell surface. Such cells are potentially self reactive and are said to be clonally ignorant because their ligand is present but is unable to activate them. Right panels: immature B cells that do not encounter antigen mature normally; they migrate from the bone marrow to the peripheral lymphoid tissues where they may become mature recirculating B cells bearing both IgM and IgD on their surface.

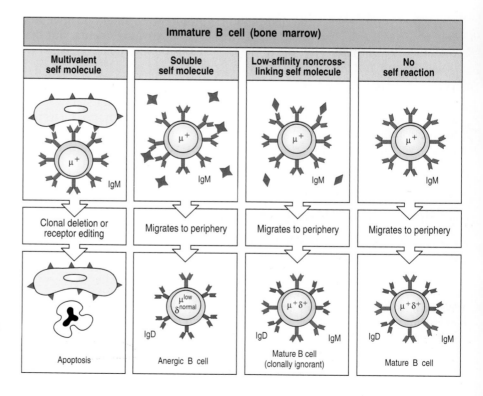

production of a new receptor by receptor editing; the induction of a permanent state of unresponsiveness to antigen; and ignorance. An ignorant cell is defined as one that has affinity for a self antigen but does not sense the self antigen because the antigen either is sequestered, is in low concentration, or does not activate the B-cell receptor. Because ignorant cells can be (and in fact are) activated under certain conditions such as inflammation or when self antigens reach unusually high concentrations, they should not be considered inert, and they are fundamentally different from nonreactive cells that could never be activated by self antigens.

The apoptosis and elimination of immature self-reactive B cells seems to predominate when the interacting self antigen is multivalent. This antigen-induced loss of cells from the B-cell population is known as **clonal deletion**. The effect of an encounter with a multivalent antigen was tested in mice transgenic for both chains of an immunoglobulin specific for H-2K^b MHC class I molecules. In such mice, nearly all the B cells that develop bear the anti-MHC immunoglobulin as sIgM, because the presence of the already re-arranged transgenes inhibits rearrangement of the endogenous immunoglobulin genes (see Sections 7-9 and 7-10). If the transgenic mouse does not express H-2K^b, normal numbers of B cells develop, all bearing transgene-encoded anti-H-2K^b receptors. However, in mice expressing both H-2K^b and the immunoglobulin transgenes, B-cell development is blocked. Normal numbers of pre-B cells and immature B cells are found, but B cells expressing the anti-H-2K^b immunoglobulin as sIgM never mature to populate the spleen and lymph nodes; instead, most of these immature B cells die in the bone marrow by apoptosis. This is because the anti-H-2K^b immunoglobulin on the immature B cells interacts strongly with the H-2K^b molecules on the bone marrow stromal cells.

Closer analysis of this experimental system and others like it revealed the surprising finding that clonal deletion was not the only outcome in these circumstances. There was, in fact, an interval before cell death during which the self-reactive B cell might be rescued by further gene rearrangements that replaced the self-reactive receptor with a new receptor that was not autoreactive. This mechanism for replacing receptors, termed receptor editing, works as follows (Fig. 7.27). When an immature B cell first expresses a light chain, leading to the production of sIgM, the *RAG* genes are still being expressed and RAG protein is being made. If the B cell does not interact with self antigen and there is no strong cross-linking of sIgM, gene rearrangement ceases and the B cell continues its development; RAG protein begins to decline but

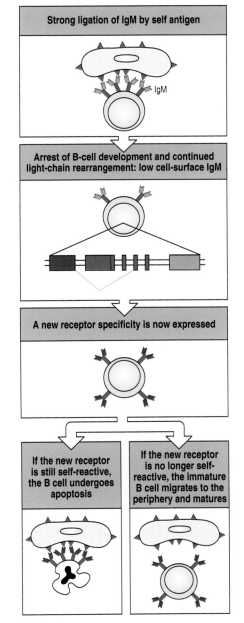

Fig. 7.27 Replacement of light chains by receptor editing can rescue some self-reactive B cells by changing their antigen specificity. When a developing B cell expresses antigen receptors that are strongly cross-linked by multivalent self antigens such as MHC molecules on cell surfaces (top panel), its development is arrested. The cell decreases surface expression of IgM and does not turn off the *RAG* genes (second panel). Continued synthesis of RAG proteins allows the cell to continue light-chain gene rearrangement. This usually leads to a new productive rearrangement and the expression of a new light chain, which combines with the previous heavy chain to form a new receptor (receptor editing; third panel). If this new receptor is not self-reactive, the cell is 'rescued' and continues normal development much like a cell that had never reacted with self (bottom right panel). If the cell remains self-reactive it may be rescued by another cycle of rearrangement, but if it continues to react strongly with self it will undergo programmed cell death or apoptosis and be deleted from the repertoire (clonal deletion; bottom left panel).

Within figure:
Strong ligation of IgM by self antigen

IgM

Arrest of B-cell development and continued light-chain rearrangement: low cell-surface IgM

A new receptor specificity is now expressed

If the new receptor is still self-reactive, the B cell undergoes apoptosis

If the new receptor is no longer self-reactive, the immature B cell migrates to the periphery and matures does not completely disappear until the B cell reaches full maturity in the spleen. However, in self-reactive B cells in which strong cross-linking of sIgM results from an encounter with a self antigen, further development is halted, and *RAG* expression continues at levels similar to those in pre-B cells undergoing light-chain gene rearrangement. As a consequence of the continued presence of recombinase, light-chain gene rearrangement continues, even though the cell has already made one productive rearrangement at this locus. The light-chain loci are able to make numerous successive rearrangements (see Fig. 7.18), and these rearrangements can rescue immature self-reactive B cells by deleting or displacing the rearranged light chain that is part of the self-reactive receptor and replacing it with another sequence. If the light-chain expressed by this new rearrangement does not contribute to an autoreactive receptor, the cell continues normal development. If the receptor remains autoreactive, however, rearrangement continues, provided there are available unused V and J gene segments. If these are exhausted, cells that remain autoreactive undergo apoptosis.

This continuation of light-chain gene rearrangement has parallels with the continuation of α-gene rearrangement in developing T cells, but it should be emphasized that in B cells it occurs only if the receptor encounters a strongly cross-linking antigen. In T cells, by contrast, α-gene rearrangement and 'receptor editing' continue as part of the normal developmental program until the cell is positively selected or dies.

More recently, receptor editing has been shown unambiguously in mice bearing transgenes for autoantibody heavy and light chains that have been placed within the immunoglobulin loci by the homologous recombination method explained in Appendix I, Section A-47. The transgene imitates a primary gene rearrangement and is surrounded by unused endogenous gene segments. In mice that express the antigen recognized by the transgene-encoded receptor, the mature B cells that emerge into the periphery have used these surrounding gene segments for further rearrangements that replace the autoreactive light-chain transgene with a nonautoreactive rearranged gene.

At a light-chain locus, the multiplicity of V and J segments allows the unused V and J gene segments to be selected for multiple further rearrangements. In addition, cells that have exhausted the J_κ regions can rearrange the λ locus. It is not clear whether receptor editing occurs at the heavy-chain locus. There are no available D segments at a rearranged heavy-chain locus, so a new rearrangement cannot simply occur by the normal mechanism and at the same time remove the preexisting one. Instead, a process of V_H replacement may use embedded recombination signal sequences in a recombination event that displaces the V gene segment from the self-reactive rearrangement and replaces it with a new V gene segment. This has been observed in some B-cell tumors, but whether it occurs during normal B-cell development in response to signals from autoreactive B-cell receptors is not certain.

It was originally thought that the successful production of a heavy chain and a light chain caused the almost instantaneous shut down of further light-chain locus rearrangement and that this ensured both allelic and isotypic exclusion (see Section 7-10). The unexpected ability of self-reactive B cells to continue to rearrange their light-chain genes, even after having made a productive rearrangement, has raised questions about this supposed mechanism of allelic exclusion.

Undoubtedly, however, the decline in the level of RAG protein that occurs after a successful non-self-reactive rearrangement is crucial to maintaining allelic exclusion, because it will reduce the chance of a subsequent rearrangement. Furthermore, any additional productive rearrangement that did occur would not necessarily breach allelic exclusion. If it occurred on the same chromosome, it would eliminate the existing productive re-arrangement, whereas if it occurred on the other chromosome it would be nonproductive in two out of three cases. Thus, the observed fall in the level of RAG protein may be sufficient to ensure that a second productive re-arrangement is rarely made, and this could be the principal, if not the sole, mechanism behind allelic exclusion at the light-chain locus. Consistent with this idea, it seems that allelic exclusion is not absolute, because there are rare B cells that express two light chains.

We have so far discussed the fate of newly formed B cells that undergo multi-valent cross-linking of their sIgM. Those immature B cells that encounter more weakly cross-linking self antigens of low valence, such as small soluble proteins, respond differently. In this situation, the self-reactive B cells tend to be inactivated and enter a state of permanent unresponsiveness, or **anergy**, but do not immediately die (see Fig. 7.26). **Anergic** B cells cannot be activated by their specific antigen even with help from antigen-specific T cells. Again, this phenomenon was elucidated using transgenic mice. When hen egg lysozyme (HEL) is expressed in soluble form from a transgene in mice that are also transgenic for high-affinity anti-HEL immunoglobulin, the HEL-spe-cific B cells mature but are unable to respond to antigen. The anergic cells re-tain their IgM within the cell and transport little to the surface. In addition, they develop a partial block in signal transduction so that, despite normal levels of HEL-binding sIgD, the cells cannot be stimulated by cross-linking this receptor. It seems that signal transduction is blocked at a step before the phosphorylation of the Igα and Igβ chains (see Section 6-7), although the exact step is not yet known. The signaling defect may involve the inability of B-cell receptor molecules on tolerant B cells to enter regions of the cell mem-brane in which other important signaling molecules normally segregate so as to transmit a complete signal after antigen binding. Furthermore, cells that have received an anergizing signal may increase the expression of molecules that inhibit signaling.

Anergic B cells are not only impaired in signal transduction and the expres-sion of sIgM. Their migration within peripheral lymphoid organs is altered, and their life-span and ability to compete with immunocompetent B cells are compromised. Mature B cells recirculate through lymphoid follicles through-out their life. In normal circumstances, in which B cells binding a soluble self antigen are rare, anergic B cells that bind soluble antigen with high affinity are detained in the T-cell areas of the peripheral lymphoid tissue and are ex-cluded from lymphoid follicles. Anergic B cells cannot be activated by T cells, because all the T cells will be tolerant to soluble antigens. Instead they die relatively quickly, presumably because they fail to get survival signals from T cells, thus ensuring that the long-lived pool of peripheral B cells is purged of potentially self-reactive cells.

The fourth potential fate of self-reactive immature B cells is that nothing hap-pens to them; they remain in a state of immunological 'ignorance' of their self antigen (see Fig. 7.26). It is clear that some B cells with a weak but definite affinity for a self antigen mature as though they were not self-reactive at all. Such B cells do not respond to the presence of their self antigen because it in-teracts so weakly with the receptor that little, if any, intracellular signal is gen-erated when it binds. Alternatively, some self-reactive B cells may not encounter their antigen at this stage because it is not accessible to B cells de-veloping in the bone marrow and spleen. The fact that such B cells are allowed to mature reflects a balance that the immune system strikes between purging all self-reactivity and maintaining the ability to respond to pathogens. If the elimination of self-reactive cells were too efficient, the receptor repertoire might become too limited and thus unable to recognize a wide variety of pathogens. Some autoimmune disease might be the price of this balance, because it is very likely that these low-affinity self-reactive lymphocytes can be activated and cause disease under certain circumstances. Thus these cells can be thought of as the seeds of autoimmune disease. Normally, however, ignorant B cells will be held in check by a lack of T-cell help, the continued inaccessibility of the self antigen, or the tolerance that can be induced in mature B cells, as described in the next part of the chapter, and in Chapter 13, where autoimmune diseases are discussed.

7-18 The MHC type of the thymic stroma selects a repertoire of mature T cells that can recognize foreign antigens presented by the same MHC type.

As we learned in Chapters 3 and 5, $\alpha{:}\beta$ T-cell receptors recognize intracellular antigens after they have been processed into peptides that can be complexed with self MHC molecules. These antigen-presenting MHC molecules are encoded by a set of highly polymorphic genes at the MHC locus, and their variability extends the range of peptides that can be presented to T cells in any one individual. However, MHC polymorphism also affects antigen recognition by T cells, because the T-cell receptor contacts both the bound peptide and the surrounding polymorphic surface of the MHC molecule itself. Each individual T-cell receptor is specific for a particular combination of MHC molecule and peptide antigen and is thus said to be MHC-restricted in its antigen recognition. Only about 10–30% of the T-cell receptors generated by gene rearrangement will be able to recognize self-MHC:self-peptide complexes and function in self-MHC-restricted responses to foreign antigens; those that have this capability are selected for survival by a process of positive selection that occurs within the thymus.

Positive selection was demonstrated in experiments using mice whose bone marrow had been completely replaced by bone marrow from a mouse of different MHC genotype but otherwise genetically identical. These mice are known as **bone marrow chimeras** (see Appendix I, Section A-43). The recipient mouse is first irradiated to destroy all its own lymphocytes and bone marrow progenitor cells; after bone marrow transplantation, all bone marrow derived cells will be of the donor genotype. These will include all lymphocytes, as well as the antigen-presenting cells they interact with. The rest of the animal's tissues, including the nonlymphoid stromal cells of the thymus, will be of the recipient MHC genotype.

In the experiments that demonstrated positive selection, the donor mice were F_1 hybrids derived from MHC^a and MHC^b parents and thus were of the MHC$^{a\times b}$ genotype. The irradiated recipients were one of the parental strains, either MHC^a or MHC^b. Because of MHC restriction, individual T cells recognize either MHC^a or MHC^b, but not both. In normal circumstances, roughly equal numbers of the MHC$^{a\times b}$ T cells from MHC$^{a\times b}$ F_1 hybrid mice will recognize antigen presented by MHC^a or MHC^b. But in bone marrow chimeras in which T cells of MHC$^{a\times b}$ genotype develop in an MHC^a thymus, T cells immunized to a particular antigen turn out to recognize that antigen mainly, if not exclusively, when it is presented by MHC^a molecules, even though the antigen-presenting cells display antigen bound to both MHC^a and MHC^b (Fig. 7.28). These experiments demonstrated that the MHC molecules present in the environment in which T cells develop, particularly those on the radioresistant cells (MHC^a in this case), determine the MHC restriction of the mature T-cell receptor repertoire. This provided the first evidence for the positive selection of developing T cells.

Fig. 7.28 Positive selection is revealed by bone marrow chimeric mice. As shown in the top two sets of panels, bone marrow from an MHC$^{a \times b}$ F$_1$ hybrid mouse is transferred to a lethally irradiated recipient mouse of either parental MHC type (MHC^a or MHC^b). When these chimeric mice are immunized with antigen, the antigen can be presented by the bone marrow derived MHC$^{a \times b}$ antigen-presenting cells (APCs) in association with both MHC^a and MHC^b molecules. The T cells from an MHC$^{a \times b}$ F$_1$ mouse include cells that respond to antigen presented by APCs from MHC^a mice and cells that respond to APCs from MHC^b mice (not shown). But when immunized T cells from the chimeric animals are tested *in vitro* with APCs bearing MHC^a or MHC^b only, they respond far better to antigen presented by the MHC molecules of the recipient MHC type, as shown in the bottom panels. This shows that the T cells have undergone positive selection for MHC restriction in the recipient thymus.

A second set of experiments involving grafts of thymus tissue demonstrated that the radioresistant component responsible for positive selection is the thymic stroma. In these experiments, the recipient animals were athymic *nude* or thymectomized mice of MHC$^{a \times b}$ genotype who were given thymic stromal grafts of MHC^a genotype. Thus, all of their cells except the thymic stroma carried both MHC^a and MHC^b. The MHC$^{a \times b}$ bone marrow cells of these mice also mature into T cells that recognize antigens presented by MHC^a but not by MHC^b. This result showed that what mature T cells consider to be self MHC is determined by the MHC molecules expressed by the thymic stromal cells that they encounter during intrathymic development. These results also argued that the MHC-restriction phenomenon in the immunized bone marrow chimeras could be mediated in the thymus, presumably by selecting T cells as they develop.

The chimeric mice used to demonstrate positive selection produce normal T-cell responses to foreign antigens. By contrast, chimeras made by injecting MHC^a bone marrow cells into MHC^b animals cannot make normal T-cell responses. This is because most of the T cells in these animals have been selected to recognize peptides when they are presented by MHC^b, whereas most of the antigen-presenting cells that they encounter as mature T cells in the periphery are bone marrow derived MHC^a cells. T cells will therefore fail to recognize antigen presented by antigen-presenting cells of their own MHC type, and T cells can be activated in these animals only if antigen-presenting cells of the MHC^b type are injected together with the antigen. Thus, for a bone marrow graft to reconstitute T-cell immunity, there must be at least one MHC molecule in common between donor and recipient (Fig. 7.29).

Fig. 7.29 Summary of T-cell responses to immunization in bone marrow chimeric mice. A set of bone marrow chimeric mice with different combinations of donor and recipient MHC types were made. These mice were then immunized and their T cells were isolated. These were then tested *in vitro* for a secondary immune reaction by using MHC^a or MHC^b antigen-presenting cells (APCs). The results are indicated in the last two columns. T cells can make antigen-specific immune responses far better if the APCs present in the host at the time of priming share at least one MHC molecule with the thymus in which the T cells developed.

Bone marrow donor	Recipient	Mice contain APC of type:	Secondary T-cell responses to antigen presented *in vitro* by APC of type:	
			MHC^a APC	MHC^b APC
MHC$^{a \times b}$	MHC^a	MHC$^{a \times b}$	Yes	No
MHC$^{a \times b}$	MHC^b	MHC$^{a \times b}$	No	Yes
MHC^a	MHC^b	MHC^a	No	No
MHC^a	MHC^b + MHC^b APC	MHC^a + MHC^b	No	Yes

7-19 Only thymocytes whose receptors interact with self-MHC: self-peptide complexes can survive and mature.

Bone marrow chimeras and thymic grafting provided evidence that MHC molecules in the thymus influence the MHC-restricted T-cell repertoire. However, mice transgenic for rearranged T-cell receptor genes provided the first conclusive evidence that the interaction of the T cell with self-MHC:self-peptide complexes is necessary for the survival of immature T cells and their maturation into naive CD4 or CD8 T cells. For these experiments the re-arranged α- and β-chain genes were cloned from a T-cell line or clone (see Appendix I, Section A-24) whose origin, antigen specificity, and MHC restriction are well characterized. As in B-cell receptor transgenic mice (see Section 7-13), when such genes are introduced into the mouse genome, rearrangement of the endogenous genes is inhibited. β-chain genes are inhibited completely but α-chain genes only incompletely, such that most of the developing T cells express the receptor encoded by the transgenes. By introducing T-cell receptor transgenes into mice of known MHC genotype, the effect of known MHC molecules on the maturation of thymocytes with receptors of known specificity can be directly studied without the need for immunization and analysis of effector function. It was found that thymocytes bearing a transgenic receptor survive and mature only within a thymus that expresses the same self MHC molecule as that on which the original T-cell clone was selected.

Such experiments have also established the fate of T cells that fail positive selection. Rearranged receptor genes from a mature T cell specific for a peptide presented by a particular MHC molecule were introduced into a recipient mouse lacking that MHC molecule, and the fate of the thymocytes was investigated by staining with antibodies specific for the transgenic receptor. Antibodies against other molecules such as CD4 and CD8 were used at the same time to mark the stages of T-cell development. It was found that cells that fail to recognize the MHC molecules present on the thymic epithelium never progress further than the double-positive stage and die in the thymus within 3 or 4 days of their last division.

In a normal thymus the fate of each thymocyte depends on the specificity of the receptor it expresses and, as we saw in Section 7-14, this specificity can undergo several changes as the α-chain genes continue to rearrange. The ability of a single developing thymocyte to express several different re-arranged α-chain genes during the time that it is susceptible to positive selection must increase the yield of useful T cells significantly; without this mechanism many more thymocytes would fail positive selection and die. However, this continued rearrangement of α-chain genes also makes it likely that a significant percentage of T cells will express two receptors, sharing a β chain but differing in their α chains. Indeed, one can predict that if the frequency of positive selection is sufficiently low, roughly one in three mature T cells will express two productively rearranged α chains at the cell surface. This was confirmed recently for both human and mouse T cells.

T cells with dual specificity might be expected to give rise to inappropriate immune responses if the cell is activated through one receptor yet can act upon target cells recognized by the second receptor. However, only one of the two receptors is likely to be able to recognize peptide presented by a self MHC molecule. This is because once the cell has been positively selected, α-chain gene rearrangement ceases. Thus, the existence of cells with two α-chain genes productively rearranged and two α chains expressed at the cell surface does not truly challenge the idea that a single functional specificity is expressed by each cell.

7-20 Positive selection acts on a repertoire of receptors with inherent specificity for MHC molecules.

Positive selection acts on a repertoire of receptors whose specificity is determined by a combination of germline gene segments and junctional regions whose diversity is randomly created as the genes rearrange (see Section 4-8). The unselected receptor repertoire must be capable of recognizing all of the hundreds of different allelic variants of MHC molecules present in the population, because the genes for the T-cell receptor α and β chains segregate in the population independently from those of the MHC. If the binding specificity of the unselected repertoire were completely random, only a very small proportion of thymocytes would be expected to recognize any MHC molecule. However, it seems that the variable CDR1 and CDR2 loops of both chains of the T-cell receptor, which are encoded within the germline V gene segments (see Section 4-12), give the T-cell receptor an intrinsic specificity for MHC molecules. This is evident from the way in which these two regions contact MHC molecules in crystal structures (see Section 3-18). An inherent specificity for MHC molecules has also been shown by examining mature T cells that represent an unselected repertoire of receptors. Such T cells can be generated in fetal thymic organ cultures, using thymuses that do not express either MHC class I or MHC class II molecules, by substituting the binding of anti-β-chain antibodies and anti-CD4 antibodies for the receptor engagement responsible for normal positive selection. When the reactivity of these antibody-selected CD4 T cells is tested, roughly 5% are able to respond to any one MHC class II genotype and, because they developed without selection by MHC molecules, this must reflect a specificity inherent in the germline V gene segments. This germline-encoded specificity for MHC molecules should significantly increase the proportion of receptors that can be positively selected in any one individual.

7-21 Positive selection coordinates the expression of CD4 or CD8 with the specificity of the T-cell receptor and the potential effector functions of the T cell.

At the time of positive selection, the thymocyte expresses both CD4 and CD8 co-receptor molecules. At the end of the selection process, mature thymocytes ready for export to the periphery express only one of these co-receptors. Moreover, almost all mature T cells that express CD4 have receptors that recognize peptides bound to self MHC class II molecules and are programmed to become cytokine-secreting cells. In contrast, most of the cells that express CD8 have receptors that recognize peptides bound to self MHC class I molecules and are programmed to become cytotoxic effector cells. Thus, positive selection also determines the cell-surface phenotype and functional potential of the mature T cell, selecting the appropriate co-receptor for efficient antigen recognition and the appropriate program for the T cell's eventual functional differentiation in an immune response.

Experiments with mice made transgenic for rearranged T-cell receptor genes show clearly that it is the specificity of the T-cell receptor for self-peptide:self-MHC molecule complexes that determines which co-receptor a mature T cell will express. If the T-cell receptor transgenes encode a receptor specific for antigen presented by self MHC class I molecules, mature T cells that express the transgenic receptor are CD8 T cells. Similarly, in mice made transgenic for a receptor that recognizes antigen with self MHC class II molecules, mature T cells that express the transgenic receptor are CD4 T cells (Fig. 7.30).

The importance of MHC molecules in this selection is illustrated by the class of human immunodeficiency diseases known as **bare lymphocyte syndromes**, which are caused by mutations that lead to an absence of MHC molecules on lymphocytes and thymic epithelial cells. People who lack MHC class II molecules have CD8 T cells but only a few, highly abnormal, CD4 T cells; a similar result has been obtained in mice in which MHC class II expression has been eliminated by targeted gene disruption (see Appendix I, Section A-47). Likewise, mice and humans that lack MHC class I molecules lack CD8 T cells. Thus, MHC class II molecules are absolutely required for CD4 T-cell development, whereas MHC class I molecules are similarly required for CD8 T-cell development.

In mature T cells, the co-receptor functions of CD8 and CD4 depend on their respective abilities to bind invariant sites on MHC class I and MHC class II molecules (see Section 3-12). Co-receptor binding to an MHC molecule is also required for normal positive selection, as shown for CD4 in the experiment discussed in the next section. Thus positive selection depends on engagement of both the antigen receptor and co-receptor with an MHC molecule, and determines the survival of single-positive cells that express only the appropriate co-receptor. However, the exact mechanism whereby lineage commitment is coordinated with receptor specificity remains to be established. At present it seems as though the developing thymocyte integrates the signals that it gets from both the antigen receptor and the co-receptor to determine its fate. Co-receptor-associated Lck signals are most effectively delivered when CD4 rather than CD8 is engaged as a co-receptor, and these Lck signals play a large part in the decision to become a CD4 mature cell. The details of lineage commitment are still controversial but it seems that cells that are undergoing positive selection, regardless of whether by MHC class I or MHC class II molecules, first downregulate both CD4 and CD8, after which they reexpress CD4. If the cell is being selected by MHC class II, the reexpression of CD4 first will lead to a sustained signal, mediated in part by Lck. This will signal further differentiation along the CD4 pathway, with the complete loss of CD8. If the cell is being selected by MHC class I,

MHC Class I Deficiency and
MHC Class II Deficiency

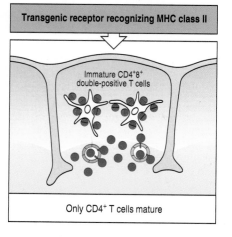

Fig. 7.30 Positive selection determines co-receptor specificity. In mice transgenic for T-cell receptors restricted by an MHC class I molecule (top panel), the only mature T cells to develop have the CD8 (red) phenotype. In mice transgenic for receptors restricted by an MHC class II molecule (bottom panel), all the mature T cells have the CD4 (blue) phenotype. In both cases, normal numbers of immature, double-positive thymocytes are found. The specificity of the T-cell receptor determines the outcome of the developmental pathway, ensuring that the only T cells that mature are those equipped with a co-receptor that is able to bind the same self-MHC molecule as the T-cell receptor.

Fig. 7.31 A molecular map of T-cell development. The top panel shows the result of a FACS analysis of thymocytes with reference to the co-receptor molecules CD4 and CD8. Each gray circle represents a subset of thymocytes at a different stage in development. Cells are believed to develop as indicated by arrows. DN, double-negative; DP, double-positive; SP, single-positive.

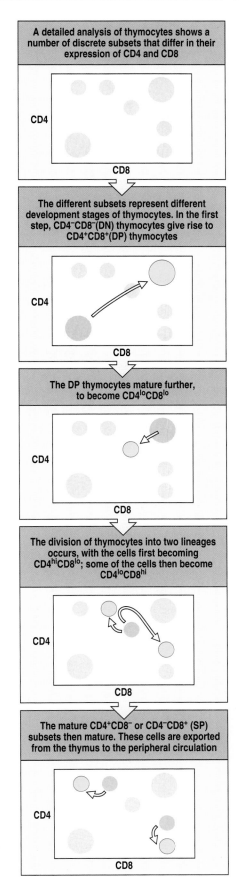

A detailed analysis of thymocytes shows a number of discrete subsets that differ in their expression of CD4 and CD8

The different subsets represent different development stages of thymocytes. In the first step, CD4⁻CD8⁻(DN) thymocytes give rise to CD4⁺CD8⁺(DP) thymocytes

The DP thymocytes mature further, to become CD4^{lo}CD8^{lo}

The division of thymocytes into two lineages occurs, with the cells first becoming CD4^{hi}CD8^{lo}; some of the cells then become CD4^{lo}CD8^{hi}

The mature CD4⁺CD8⁻ or CD4⁻CD8⁺ (SP) subsets then mature. These cells are exported from the thymus to the peripheral circulation

reexpression of CD4 will not lead to any further signaling via Lck; this weak co-receptor signal will in turn determine CD8 commitment, with a subsequent loss of CD4 expression and the reexpression later of CD8 (Fig. 7.31).

Other signaling molecules are clearly important for thymocyte survival and development but seem to be common to the commitment of both lineages. A few of these may, nonetheless, preferentially influence the commitment of thymocytes to one lineage over the other: for example, the MAP kinase signaling pathway initiated by the antigen receptor (see Section 6-11) biases cells toward the CD4 rather than the CD8 lineage. It is a general principle of lineage commitment that different signals must be created to activate lineage-specific factors and generate a divergence of developmental programming. Although much remains to be discovered about this process in developing α:β thymocytes, it is clear that the different signals that are created result in a divergence of functional programming, so that the ability to express genes involved in the killing of target cells, for example, develops in CD8 T cells but not in most CD4 T cells, whereas the potential to express various cytokine genes develops in CD4 T cells and, to a lesser extent, in CD8 T cells.

7-22 Thymic cortical epithelial cells mediate positive selection of developing thymocytes.

The thymic cortical epithelial cell is the stromal cell type critical for positive selection. These cells form a web of cell processes that make close contacts with the double-positive T cells undergoing positive selection (see Fig. 7.9), and T-cell receptors can be seen clustering with MHC molecules at the sites of contact.

That stromal cells were important for positive selection was already suggested by the thymus transplantation studies described in Section 7-18. Direct evidence that thymic cortical epithelial cells mediate positive selection comes from an ingenious manipulation of mice whose MHC class II genes have been eliminated by targeted gene disruption (Fig. 7.32). Mutant mice that lack MHC class II molecules do not normally produce CD4 T cells. To test the role of the thymic epithelium in positive selection, an MHC class II gene was placed under the control of a promoter that restricted its expression to thymic cortical epithelial cells. This was then introduced as a transgene in these mutant mice, which in turn restored CD4 T cell development. A further variant of this experiment shows that, to promote the development of CD4 T cells, the MHC class II molecule on the thymic cortical epithelium must be able to interact effectively with CD4. Thus, when the MHC class II transgene expressed in the thymus contains a mutation that prevents its binding to CD4, very few CD4 T cells develop. Equivalent studies of CD8 interaction with MHC class I molecules show that co-receptor binding is also necessary for normal positive selection of CD8 cells.

The critical role of the thymic cortical epithelium in positive selection raises the question of whether there is anything distinctive about the antigen-presenting properties of these cells. This is not clear at present; however, thymic epithelium may differ from other tissues in the proteases used to degrade the invariant chain (Ii) during the passage of MHC class II molecules to

Normal MHC class II expression	MHC class II-negative mutant	Mutant with MHC class II transgene expressed in thymic epithelium	Mutant with MHC class II transgene expressed that cannot interact with CD4
Both CD8 and CD4 T cells mature	Only CD8 T cells mature	Both CD8 and CD4 T cells mature	Only CD8 T cells mature

Fig. 7.32 Thymic cortical epithelial cells mediate positive selection. The expression of MHC class II molecules in the thymus of normal and mutant strains of mice is shown by coloring the stromal cells only if they are expressing functional MHC class II molecules. In the thymus of normal mice (first panels), which express MHC class II molecules on epithelial cells in the thymic cortex (blue) as well as on medullary epithelial cells (orange) and bone marrow derived cells (yellow), both CD4 (blue) and CD8 (red) T cells mature. Double-positive thymocytes are shown as half red/half blue. The second panels represent mutant mice in which MHC class II expression has been eliminated by targeted gene disruption; in these mice, few CD4 T cells develop, although CD8 T cells develop normally. In MHC class II-negative mice containing an MHC class II transgene engineered so that it is expressed only on the epithelial cells of the thymic cortex (third panels), normal numbers of CD4 T cells mature. The MHC class II molecule needs to be able to interact with the CD4 protein, because mutant MHC class II molecules with a defective CD4 binding site do not allow the positive selection of CD4 T cells (fourth panels). Thus, the cortical epithelial cells are the critical cell type mediating positive selection.

the cell surface (see Section 5-6). The protease cathepsin L dominates in thymic cortical epithelium, whereas cathepsin S seems to be most important in peripheral tissues. Consequently, CD4 T-cell development is severely impaired in cathepsin L knockout mice. Thymic epithelial cells do seem to bear on their cell surfaces a relatively high density of MHC class II molecules that retain the invariant chain-associated peptide (CLIP) (see Fig. 5.8).

Artificial manipulation of the peptides presented by thymic epithelium has a profound effect on positive selection. The effect of selecting thymocytes with a markedly reduced variety of peptides complexed to MHC class II molecules has been demonstrated in experiments in which the α chain of H-2M, the mouse homolog of human HLA-DM, is disrupted (Fig. 7.33). In mice lacking a functional H-2Mα chain, the CLIP fragment of the invariant chain is not released from the newly synthesized MHC class II molecules (see Section 5-7). These CLIP-associated MHC class II molecules are unable to bind the self peptides present in the endosomes, and the main self peptide presented by self MHC class II molecules on the surface of the thymic epithelium is therefore the invariant CLIP peptide. In these mice, the total number of CD4 T cells is reduced by between one-half and two-thirds. The T-cell receptor β-chain repertoire expressed in these cells is still diverse, but it must be severely altered because, when T-cell receptor transgenes recognizing peptide:MHC class II complexes are examined, none is positively selected in H-2Mα knockout mice despite the presence of typical levels of the MHC class II molecules that normally select them.

Thus it seems that a significantly reduced repertoire of T cells is selected in the presence of a predominant peptide:MHC class II complex. In addition, a high proportion of the T cells that are positively selected in H2-M-deficient mice and reach maturity react to the peptide:MHC class II complexes on

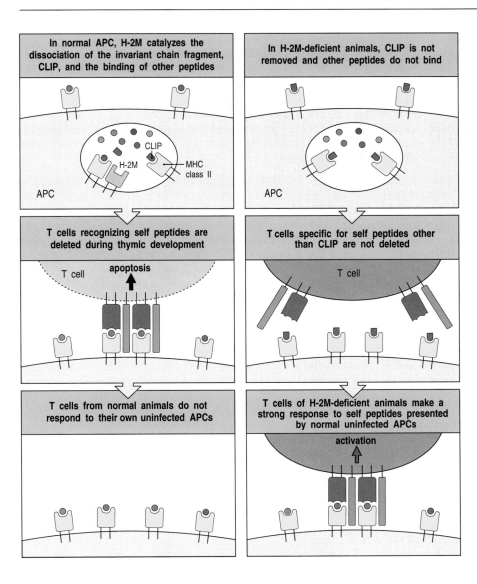

Fig. 7.33 The peptides bound to MHC class II molecules can affect the T-cell receptor repertoire. The left panels show the normal situation, in which a range of peptides is presented by antigen-presenting cells (APCs) to immature T cells in the thymus, with the consequent deletion of self-reactive T cells. The right panels show a case in which a single peptide predominates. Mice with a disrupted H-2Mα gene express MHC class II molecules that predominantly carry the CLIP peptide of the invariant chain (top right panel). Their MHC class II molecules thus present only the CLIP peptide to T cells maturing in the thymus. CD4 T cells mature in the presence of this single dominant peptide:MHC complex but they are reduced in number by between one-half and two-thirds, even though negative selection of MHC class II-restricted T cells will remove only those T cells specific for the CLIP peptide (middle right panel). Mature T cells from such mice respond strongly to MHC-identical APCs that express the normal array of self peptides (bottom right panel). This shows that a majority of the T cells positively selected by this single dominant MHC:peptide complex are reactive with other self peptides complexed with the same MHC molecule. In normal mice, the T cells bearing these receptors would be deleted by negative selection (middle and bottom left panels).

antigen-presenting cells from wild-type mice (see Fig. 7.33). Mice that have intact H-2M have a normal set of self-peptide:self-MHC class II molecules and stimulate strong responses in nearly all the CD4 T cells from mice lacking H-2Mα, presumably because of failed negative selection in H2-M-deficient mice. All these experiments demonstrate that a diversity of bound MHC class II peptides is important for the positive selection of a diverse repertoire of self-MHC-restricted CD4 T cells.

7-23   T cells that react strongly with ubiquitous self antigens are deleted in the thymus.

When the T-cell receptor of a mature naive T cell is ligated by peptide plus MHC antigen displayed by a professional antigen-presenting cell in a peripheral lymphoid organ, the T cell is activated to proliferate and produce effector T cells (see Section 1-13). In contrast, when the T-cell receptor of a developing thymocyte is similarly ligated by antigen on stromal or bone marrow derived cells in the thymus, it dies by apoptosis. This response of immature T cells to stimulation by antigen is the basis of negative selection. Elimination of these T cells in the thymus prevents their potentially harmful activation later on, if they should encounter the same peptides when they are mature T cells. Negative selection has been demonstrated in mice that express a transgenic T-cell receptor specific for a peptide of ovalbumin bound to an MHC class II molecule. As explained in Section 7-19, all the T cells developing in such a mouse will express the transgenic receptor. When these mice are injected with the ovalbumin peptide, the mature CD4 T cells in the periphery become activated, but most of the intrathymic T cells die (Fig. 7.34). Similar results can be obtained in thymic organ culture with T cells from both normal and transgenic mice.

The deletion of developing T cells that recognize self peptides made naturally in the thymus has also been demonstrated experimentally. For example, the negative selection of such thymocytes was observed in mice made transgenic for rearranged genes encoding T-cell receptors specific for self peptides expressed only in male mice. Thymocytes bearing these receptors disappear from the developing T-cell population in male mice at the CD4 CD8 double-positive stage of development, and no single-positive cells bearing the transgenic receptors mature. By contrast, in female mice, which lack the male-specific peptide, the transgenic T cells mature normally. This initial observation has been confirmed by using T-cell receptor transgenes that recognize other antigens, with similar results.

These experiments illustrate the principle that self-peptide:self-MHC complexes encountered in the thymus purge the T-cell repertoire of immature T cells bearing self-reactive receptors. One obvious problem with this scheme is that there are many tissue-specific proteins, such as pancreatic insulin, that would not be expected to be expressed in the thymus. However, it is now clear that many such 'tissue-specific' proteins actually are expressed by some stromal cells present in the thymic medulla; thus, intrathymic negative selection could apply even to proteins that are otherwise restricted to tissues outside the thymus. The expression of these otherwise tissue-specific proteins in the thymic medulla is controlled in an as-yet unknown fashion by a gene called

Fig. 7.34 T cells specific for self antigens are deleted in the thymus. In mice transgenic for a T-cell receptor that recognizes a known peptide antigen complexed with self MHC, all the T cells have the same specificity. In the absence of the peptide, most thymocytes mature and emigrate to the periphery. This can be seen in the bottom left panel, where a normal thymus is stained with antibody to identify the medulla (in green), and by the TUNEL technique (see Appendix I, Section A-32) to identify apoptotic cells (in red). If the mice are injected with the peptide that is recognized by the transgenic T-cell receptor, massive cell death occurs in the thymus, as shown by the increased numbers of apoptotic cells in the right-hand bottom panel. Photographs courtesy of A. Wack and D. Kioussis.

AIRE, the autoimmune regulator. Mutations in AIRE give rise to a widespread autoimmune disease known as autoimmune polyglandular syndrome type I or autoimmune polyendocrinopathy-candidiasis-ectodermal dystrophy (APECED), highlighting the important role that intrathymic expression of tissue-specific proteins plays in maintaining tolerance to self. Nonetheless, not all self proteins are expressed in the thymus, and those that appear exclusively in other tissues, or are expressed at different stages in development, will encounter mature T cells with the potential to respond to them. However, there are several mechanisms operating in the periphery that prevent mature T cells from responding to tissue-specific antigens; these will be discussed in Chapter 13, when we consider the problem of autoimmune responses and their avoidance.

Autoimmune Polyglandular Syndrome

7-24 Negative selection is driven most efficiently by bone marrow derived antigen-presenting cells.

Negative selection in the thymus can be mediated by several different cell types. The most important are the bone marrow derived dendritic cells and macrophages. These are professional antigen-presenting cell types that also activate mature T cells in peripheral lymphoid tissues. The self antigens presented by these cells are therefore the most important source of potential autoimmune responses, and T cells responding to such self peptides must be eliminated in the thymus.

Experiments using bone marrow chimeric mice have clearly shown the role of thymic macrophages and dendritic cells in negative selection. In these experiments, $MHC^{a \times b}$ F_1 bone marrow is grafted into one of the parental strains (MHC^a in Fig. 7.35). The $MHC^{a \times b}$ T cells developing in the grafted animals are thus exposed to the thymic epithelium of the MHC^a host strain. Bone marrow derived dendritic cells and macrophages will, however, express both MHC^a and MHC^b. The bone marrow chimeras will tolerate skin grafts from either MHC^a or MHC^b animals (see Fig. 7.35), and from the acceptance of both types of skin grafts we can infer that the developing T cells are not self-reactive for either of the two MHC antigens. The only cells that could present self-peptide:MHC^b complexes to thymocytes, and thus induce tolerance to MHC^b, are the bone marrow derived cells. The dendritic cells and macrophages are therefore assumed to have a crucial role in negative selection.

In addition, both the thymocytes themselves and thymic epithelial cells also have the ability to cause the deletion of self-reactive cells. Such reactions may normally be of secondary significance compared to the dominant role of bone marrow derived cells in negative selection. In patients undergoing bone marrow transplantation from an unrelated donor, however, where all the thymic macrophages and dendritic cells are of donor type, negative selection mediated by thymic epithelial cells can assume a special importance in maintaining tolerance to the recipient's own antigens.

Bone marrow transplant from $MHC^{a \times b} F_1$ mouse into MHC^a recipient

$MHC^{a \times b} F_1$ MHC^b

bone marrow

MHC^a

Skin graft from MHC^b mouse onto ($MHC^{a \times b} \rightarrow MHC^a$) bone marrow chimera

$MHC^{a \times b} F_1$ MHC^b

skin graft

$MHC^{a \times b}$ MHC^a chimera

($MHC^{a \times b} \rightarrow MHC^a$) chimeric mouse tolerates MHC^b skin graft

Fig. 7.35 Bone marrow derived cells mediate negative selection in the thymus. When $MHC^{a \times b}$ F_1 bone marrow is injected into an irradiated MHC^a mouse, the T cells mature on thymic epithelium expressing only MHC^a molecules. Nevertheless, the chimeric mice are tolerant to skin grafts expressing MHC^b molecules (provided that these grafts do not present skin-specific peptides that differ between strains a and b). This implies that the T cells whose receptors recognize self antigens presented by MHC^b have been eliminated in the thymus. Because the transplanted $MHC^{a \times b}$ F_1 bone marrow cells are the only source of MHC^b molecules in the thymus, bone marrow derived cells must be able to induce negative selection.

7-25 The specificity and/or the strength of signals for negative and positive selection must differ.

We have described some of the experiments that contributed to the large body of evidence that T cells are selected for both self MHC restriction and self tolerance by self-MHC:self-peptide complexes expressed on stromal cells in the thymus. We now turn to the central question posed by positive and negative selection: how can engagement of the receptor by self-MHC:self-peptide complexes lead both to further maturation of thymocytes during positive selection and to cell death during negative selection? The answers to these questions are still not known for certain, but two possible mechanisms have been suggested. We will briefly describe each, before going on to discuss some recent experiments that bear on the mechanism of positive selection.

There are two issues to be resolved. First, the interactions that lead to positive selection must include more receptor specificities than those that lead to negative selection. Otherwise, all the cells that were positively selected in the thymic cortex would be eliminated by negative selection, and no T cells would ever leave the thymus (Fig. 7.36). Second, the consequences of the interactions that lead to positive and negative selection must differ: cells that recognize self-peptide:self-MHC complexes on cortical epithelial cells are induced to mature, whereas those whose receptors might confer strong and potentially damaging autoreactivity are induced to die.

Fig. 7.36 The specificity or affinity of positive selection must differ from that of negative selection. Immature T cells are positively selected in such a way that only those thymocytes whose receptors can engage the peptide:MHC complexes on thymic epithelium mature, giving rise to a population of thymocytes restricted for self MHC. Negative selection removes those thymocytes whose receptors can be activated by self peptides complexed with self-MHC molecules, giving a self-tolerant population of thymocytes. If the specificity and avidity of positive and negative selection were the same (left panels), all the T cells that survive positive selection would be deleted during negative selection. Only if the specificity and avidity of negative selection are different from those of positive selection (right panels) can thymocytes mature into T cells.

Two main hypotheses have been proposed to account for these differences between positive and negative selection. The first is the **avidity hypothesis**. This states that the outcome of MHC:peptide binding by thymocyte T-cell receptors depends on the strength of the signal delivered by the receptor and co-receptor on binding, and that this will, in turn, depend upon both the affinity of the T-cell receptor for the MHC:peptide complex and the density of the complex on a thymic cortical epithelial cell. Thymocytes that are signaled weakly are rescued from apoptosis and are thus positively selected, whereas thymocytes that are signaled strongly are driven to apoptosis and are thus negatively selected. Because more complexes are likely to bind weakly than strongly, this will result in the positive selection of a larger repertoire of cells than are negatively selected.

Alternatively, the delivery of incomplete activating signals by self peptides could account for positive selection: we will call this the **qualitative signaling hypothesis**. Under this hypothesis, it is the nature of the signal delivered by the receptor, not just the number of receptors engaged, that distinguishes positive from negative selection. According to the avidity hypothesis, the same MHC:peptide complex could drive positive or negative selection of the same receptor, depending on its density on the cell surface. This could not occur under the qualitative signaling hypothesis, because it proposes that the signals leading to positive and negative selection are qualitatively different.

So-called **antagonist peptides** have been used to try to distinguish between these hypotheses. These are known as antagonist peptides because they inhibit the response of mature T cells to their normal stimulatory, or **agonist**, peptide. On binding to the antigen receptor of a mature T cell, antagonist peptide:MHC complexes generate some, but not all, of the intracellular signaling events that are associated with full agonist-driven T-cell activation (see Section 6-14). Recognition of antagonist peptides by thymocytes has in many cases been shown to induce positive selection, whereas recognition of agonist peptides induces negative selection (Fig. 7.37). Thus the differences between the ways in which agonist and antagonist peptides interact with the receptor and signal to the cell are likely to be relevant to how positive selection works.

The experiments shown in Fig. 7.37 used a T-cell receptor of known specificity whose behavior *in vivo* with different variants of its peptide antigen had been characterized. The affinities of agonist and antagonist peptides for the receptor were found to be quite similar when measured using an affinity sensor (see Appendix I, Section A-30), but it was found that complexes of MHC class I molecules with agonist peptides induced dimerization of the T-cell receptors, whereas antagonist peptides did not. This could mean that *in vivo* agonist peptides induce the receptor clustering required for generating signals that lead to activation (see Section 6-2) and, during thymocyte development, to deletion. Antagonist peptides, in contrast, seem to bind to the T-cell receptor but fail to induce receptor clustering, and therefore deliver a qualitatively different signal. During thymocyte development this would be a survival signal to the cell. Because the agonist and antagonist peptides bind the T-cell receptor with similar affinity, but only the antagonist induces positive selection, this implies that the signals delivered by the agonist peptides that cause deletion and those delivered by the antagonist peptides that mediate positive selection are fundamentally different, suggesting that the qualitative signaling hypothesis of T-cell selection is correct. While only one group has reported a dimerization of the TCR on interaction with agonist ligands, there is more consensus that a conformational change of some kind occurs in the T-cell receptor on binding its ligand. Binding of an adaptor protein, Nck, to the cytoplasmic tail of the CD3ζ chain only occurs after binding of the T-cell receptor to its ligand and is not dependent on the phosphorylation of the

Fig. 7.37 The differences between negative and positive selection may be due to differences in the aggregation of T-cell receptors upon ligand binding. Agonist, antagonist, and null peptides can be identified for a particular T-cell receptor by assaying the responses of mature T-cell clones. Their effects on mature T cells *in vivo* can be tested in mice made transgenic for this T-cell receptor (left-hand panels). Using thymic lobe organ cultures from mice that have also been genetically engineered to express only the MHC class I molecule recognized by the receptor, it is possible to test for the effects of these peptides on thymocyte development (right-hand panels). Binding to an agonist peptide (top panels) induces the organized aggregation of T-cell receptors on the cell surface and effective signaling through the T-cell receptor. Agonist peptides trigger the full activation of mature T cells; however, if they are encountered as self peptides by developing thymocytes they induce apoptosis and hence negative selection. Antagonist peptides (center panels) bind the T-cell receptor but fail to induce T-cell receptor aggregation. These peptides inhibit mature T cells but can drive the positive selection of developing thymocytes. Irrelevant peptides fail to engage the T-cell receptor at all and are ignored by mature T cells and developing thymocytes. If only irrelevant peptides are presented, the thymocyte is not positively selected and it dies by neglect.

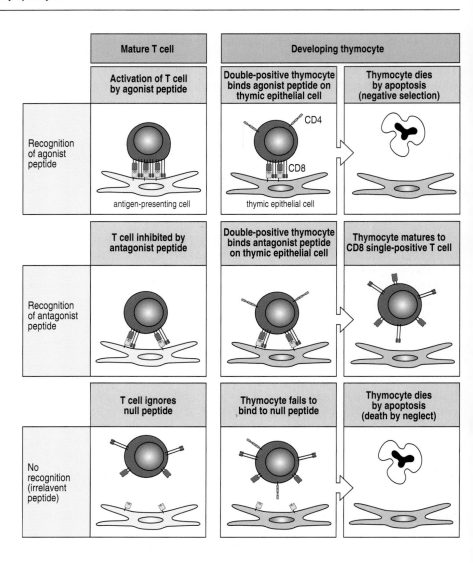

CD3ζ chain. Instead, it appears to depend on a conformational change in the receptor itself allowing Nck to bind and to develop the full array of signals from the receptor. In the absence of Nck binding, a different pattern of intracellular signals will be generated and this may constitute the qualitative difference in signaling that would allow the discrimination between positive and negative selection.

Summary.

Initially, random receptor gene segment rearrangements and junctional diversity create a broad repertoire of antigen receptors. Only some of these will not be dangerously self-reactive and yet be useful to the immune system. Cells meeting these criteria are selected, a process that begins as soon as immature lymphocytes express antigen receptors. Lymphocyte development involves both negative and positive selection. Negative selection includes deletion from the repertoire, receptor editing, and anergy. Positive selection is best defined for T cells; as we will discuss in the next part of this chapter, B cells can also be positively selected as they mature to populate the periphery. For developing T cells, recognition of self-MHC:self-peptide complexes on thymic cortical epithelial cells provides an as yet poorly defined positive survival signal. T-cell receptors capable of responding to foreign peptides presented by self MHC molecules are thus selected from a primary repertoire that has an inherent specificity for all the different MHC molecules in the population. Positive selection also ensures the functional matching of receptor, co-receptor, and the class of MHC molecule recognized. The paradox that recognition of self-MHC:self-peptide ligands by the T-cell receptor can lead to two opposing effects, namely positive and negative selection, remains unsolved. Its solution will come from a full understanding of the ligand–receptor interactions, the signal transduction mechanisms, and the physiology of each step of the process.

Survival and maturation of lymphocytes in peripheral lymphoid tissues.

Once lymphocytes have left the central lymphoid tissues, they are carried in the blood to the peripheral lymphoid tissues. These tissues have a highly organized architecture, with distinct areas of B cells and T cells. Their organization is determined by interactions between the lymphocytes and the other cell types that make up the lymphoid tissues. The survival and maturation of lymphocytes reaching the peripheral lymphoid tissue in turn depends upon further interactions with their self ligands as well as neighboring cells in the tissue. Before considering the factors governing the survival and maturation of newly formed lymphocytes in the periphery, we therefore look briefly at the organization and development of these tissues and the signals that guide lymphocytes to their correct locations within them. Normally a lymphocyte will leave peripheral lymphoid tissue and recirculate via lymph and blood (see Section 1-4), continually reentering lymphoid tissues until either antigen is encountered or the lymphocyte dies. On encountering antigen, the lymphocyte stops recirculating, proliferates and differentiates, as will be described in Chapters 8–10. When a lymphocyte dies, its place is then taken by a newly formed lymphocyte; this enables a turnover of the receptor repertoire and ensures that lymphocyte numbers remain constant.

7-26 Lymphocytes are found in particular locations in peripheral lymphoid tissues.

As we saw in Chapter 1, the various peripheral lymphoid organs are organized roughly along the same lines, with distinct areas of B cells and T cells. Besides lymphocytes, peripheral lymphoid tissues also contain macrophages and dendritic cells, as well as nonleukocyte stromal cells. The lymphoid tissue of the spleen is the white pulp, whose overall design is illustrated in Fig. 1.9. Each area of white pulp is demarcated by a marginal sinus, a vascular network that branches from the central arteriole. The **marginal zone** of the white pulp, the outer border of which is the edge of the marginal sinus, is a highly organized region whose function is poorly understood. It has few T cells but is rich in macrophages and contains a unique population of B cells, the **marginal zone B cells**, which do not recirculate. Pathogens reaching the bloodstream are efficiently trapped in the marginal zone by the macrophages, and it could be that marginal zone B cells are uniquely adapted to provide the first responses to such pathogens, as will be discussed further below.

Within the white pulp are clearly separated areas of T cells and B cells. T cells are clustered around the central arteriole, with the globular B-cell areas or follicles located farther out. Some follicles contain germinal centers, areas in which B cells involved in an adaptive immune response are proliferating and undergoing somatic hypermutation (see Section 4-9). In follicles with germinal centers, the resting B cells that are not part of the immune response are pushed outward to make up the **mantle zone** around the proliferating lymphocytes. The antigen-driven production of germinal centers will be described in detail when we consider B-cell responses in Chapter 9.

B cells and T cells are not the only cells in their respective areas. The B-cell zone contains a network of **follicular dendritic cells** (**FDCs**), which are mainly concentrated in the area of the follicle most distant from the central arteriole. Follicular dendritic cells have long processes, from which they get their name, and they are in contact with B cells. They differ, however, from the dendritic cells we have encountered previously (see Section 1-6) in that they are not leukocytes and are not derived from bone marrow precursors; in addition, they are not phagocytic and do not express MHC class II proteins. Follicular dendritic cells seem to be specialized to capture antigen in the form of immune complexes—complexes of antigen, antibody, and complement. The immune complexes are not internalized but remain intact on the follicular dendritic cell surface, where the antigen can be recognized by B cells. Follicular dendritic cells are also important in the development of B-cell follicles, as will be described in the next section. Beyond this, their functions are not entirely clear.

T-cell zones contain a network of bone marrow derived dendritic cells, sometimes known as **interdigitating dendritic cells** from the way their processes interweave among the T cells. There are two subtypes of these dendritic cells, distinguished by characteristic cell-surface proteins. The so-called **lymphoid dendritic cells** express the α chain of CD8, whereas the **myeloid dendritic cells** express not CD8 but CD11b:CD18, an integrin that is also expressed by macrophages. Both types of dendritic cell seem to derive from a common myeloid precursor. Whether they subsequently represent two separate lineages of dendritic cells with discrete functions, two different developmental stages within the same lineage, or two alternative fates for a dendritic cell depending on environmental stimuli is not known, and is an area of active research.

Lymph nodes have a very similar architecture to that of the spleen (see Fig. 1.8). B-cell follicles with a similar structure and composition to those in the spleen are located just under the outer capsule. T-cell zones surround the follicles in the paracortical areas. Unlike the spleen, lymph nodes have no marginal sinus surrounding the lymphocyte areas and thus there is no marginal zone. Also unlike the spleen, lymph nodes collect lymph, which enters in the subcapsular space.

Lymphoid tissues are also associated with epithelial surfaces that provide physical barriers against infection. Peyer's patches are lymph node-like structures that are interspersed at intervals just beneath the gut epithelium (see Fig. 1.10). They comprise B-cell follicles located immediately under specialized areas, or 'domes,' of epithelium known as follicular-associated epithelium, with T-cell zones that lie more deeply. Follicular-associated epithelium is composed of cells that lack the typical brush border. Instead, these so-called M (for multifold) cells are adapted to channel antigens and pathogens from the gut lumen to the Peyer's patch. Peyer's patches and similar tissue present in the tonsils provide specialized sites where B cells can become committed to synthesizing IgA. The mucosal epithelial surfaces lining the mouth and the intestine, respiratory tract, and reproductive tract have their own specialized immune systems called collectively the mucosal-associated lymphoid tissues (MALT) (see Section 1-3). The epithelial cells of these surfaces as well as the skin are interspersed with a dense network of dendritic cells, which in the skin are called Langerhans' cells. The stromal cells of the MALT, and in particular the gut-associated lymphoid tissues (GALT), a part of the overall MALT, secrete the cytokine TGF-β, which has been shown to induce IgA secretion in culture. In addition, as discussed in Section 7-16, during fetal development, waves of γ:δ T cells with specific γ- and δ-gene rearrangements leave the thymus and migrate to these epithelial barriers.

7-27 The development and organization of peripheral lymphoid tissues is controlled by tumor necrosis factor family molecules, and the homing of lymphocytes is mediated by chemokines.

Newly formed lymphocytes enter the spleen via the blood, exiting first in the marginal sinus, from which they migrate to the appropriate areas of the white pulp. Lymphocytes that survive their passage through the spleen most probably leave via venous sinuses in the red pulp. In lymph nodes, lymphocytes enter from the blood through the walls of specialized blood vessels, the high endothelial venules (HEVs), which are located within the T-cell zones. Naive B cells migrate through the HEVs in the T-cell area and come to rest in the follicle where, unless they encounter their specific antigen and become activated, they remain for about a day. B cells and T cells leave in the lymph via the efferent lymphatic, which returns them eventually to the blood.

Once lymphocytes enter the spleen or lymph node, how do they find their way to their respective zones? They are directed there mainly by responses to chemokines; B and T cells have different sets of receptors that respond to chemokines differentially secreted in the T and B zones. This answer then begs the question of how these zones develop in the first place and how they come to secrete specific chemokines. Surprisingly, members of the tumor necrosis factor (TNF)/TNF receptor (TNFR) family, which were originally thought to be involved in inflammation and cell death, have a critical role in the development and maintenance of normal lymphoid architecture. This has been best demonstrated in a series of knockout mice in which either the ligand or its receptor has been inactivated (Fig. 7.38). These knockouts have complicated phenotypes, which is partly due to the fact that individual TNF-family proteins can bind to multiple receptors and, conversely, many receptors can bind more than one protein. In addition, it seems clear that there is some overlapping function or cooperation between TNF-family proteins. Nonetheless, some general conclusions can be drawn.

Fig. 7.38 Members of the TNF family and their receptors have important roles in lymphoid development and in determining the architecture of the secondary lymphoid organs. These roles have been deduced mainly from the study of knockout mice deficient in one or more TNF family members (ligands) or receptors. Some receptors bind more than one ligand, and some ligands bind more than one receptor, complicating the effects of their deletion. The defects are organized here with respect to the two main receptors, TNFR-I and the LT-β receptor, along with a relatively newly recognized receptor, the herpes virus entry mediator (HVEM), which may also be involved in lymphoid organization. (Note that receptors are named for the first ligand known to bind them.) In some cases, the loss of ligands that bind the same receptor leads to a different phenotype in each case. This is due to the ability of the ligand to bind another receptor, and is indicated in the figure. In addition, the LT-α protein chain contributes to two distinct ligands, LT-α3 and LTα2β1, each of which has a distinct receptor. In general, signaling through the LT-β receptor is required for lymph node and follicular dendritic cell development and normal splenic architecture, whereas signaling through the TNFR-I receptor is also required for follicular dendritic cells and normal splenic architecture but not for lymph node development.

Receptor	Ligands	Effects seen in knockout (KO) mice				
		Spleen	Peripheral lymph node	Mesenteric lymph node	Peyer's patch	Follicular dendritic cells
TNFR-I	TNF-α LT-α3	Distorted architecture	Present in TNF-α KO Absent in LT-α KO owing to lack of LT-β signals	Present	Reduced	Absent
LT-β receptor	TNF-α LT-α2/β1 LIGHT	Distorted No marginal zones	Absent	Present in LT-β KO Absent in LT-β receptor KO	Absent	Absent
HVEM	LT-α3 LIGHT	Although both LT-α and LIGHT can bind HVEM, there is no known role for HVEM signaling in organogenesis				

Lymph node development depends on the expression of a subset of TNF-family proteins known as the lymphotoxin (LT) proteins. Interestingly, not all lymph nodes are dependent on signals from the same family members. LT-α_3, a soluble homotrimer of the LT-α chain, supports the development of cervical and mesenteric lymph nodes, and possibly lumbar and sacral lymph nodes. All these lymph nodes drain mucosal sites. LT-α_3 probably exerts its effects by binding to TNFR-I and possibly also to another TNFR-family member called HVEM. The membrane-bound heterotrimer comprising LT-α and the distinct protein chain LT-β (LT-α_2:β_1) binds only to the LT-β receptor and supports the development of all the other lymph nodes. In addition, Peyer's patches do not form in the absence of the membrane-bound LT-α_2:β_1 heterotrimer. These effects are not reversible in adult animals and, in fact, it can be shown that there are certain critical developmental periods during which the absence or inhibition of these LT-family proteins will prevent the development of lymph nodes and Peyer's patches irrevocably.

The spleen develops in all mice deficient in TNF or TNFR family members that have been studied. However, its architecture is very abnormal in many of these mutant mice (see Fig. 7.38). LT (most probably the membrane-bound heterotrimer) is required for the normal segregation of T-cell and B-cell zones. TNF-α, binding to the TNFR-I, also contributes to the organization of the white pulp: when TNF-α signals are disrupted, B cells surround T-cell zones in a ring rather than in discrete follicles. In addition, the marginal zones are not well defined when TNF-α or its receptor is absent. Perhaps most importantly, follicular dendritic cells are not found in mice that lack TNF-α or TNFR-I. These mice, which do have lymph nodes and Peyer's patches, because they express LT family members, nonetheless lack follicular dendritic cells in those lymph nodes and Peyer's patches. Similarly, mice that cannot form or signal via membrane-bound LT-α_2:β_1 also lack normal follicular dendritic cells in spleen and any residual lymph nodes. Unlike the situation in lymph node development, which is irreversible, the disorganized lymphoid architecture in the spleen is reversible when the missing TNF family member is restored. B cells are the likely source for the membrane-bound LT because normal B cells can restore follicular dendritic cells and follicles when transferred to RAG-deficient recipients (which lack lymphocytes). A similar role for B cells in the development of the M cells that lie over Peyer's patches was recently discovered. In this case it seems that signals independent of LT-α are required, because B cells deficient in LT-α will still restore the development of M cells in Peyer's patches.

The precise location of B cells, T cells, macrophages, and dendritic cells in peripheral lymphoid tissue is controlled by chemoattractant cytokines, or chemokines, which are produced by both stromal cells and bone marrow derived cells (Fig. 7.39). B cells are attracted to the follicles by CXCL13 (B-lymphocyte chemokine, BLC), for which B cells constitutively express the receptor, CXCR5. The most likely source of CXCL13 is the follicular dendritic cell, possibly along with other follicular stromal cells. B cells are, in turn, the source of LT that is required for the development of follicular dendritic cells. This reciprocal dependence of B cells and follicular dendritic cells illustrates the complex web of interactions that organizes secondary lymphoid tissues. T cells can also express CXCR5, although at a lower level, and this may explain how T cells are able to enter B-cell follicles, which they do on activation, to participate in the formation of the germinal center.

Two chemokines, CCL19 (MIP-3β) and CCL21 (secondary lymphoid chemokine, SLC), account for T-cell localization to the T zones. They both bind to the receptor CCR7, which is present on T cells; mice that lack CCR7 do not form normal T zones and have markedly impaired primary immune responses. CCL21 is produced by stromal cells of the T zone in spleen, and by

| Stromal cells and high endothelial venules (HEV) secrete the chemokine CCL21 (SLC) | Dendritic cells express a receptor for CCL21 and migrate into the developing lymph node | Dendritic cells secrete CCL21 and CCL19 (MIP-3β), which attract T cells to the developing lymph node | B cells are initially attracted into the developing lymph node by the same chemokines | B cells induce follicular dendritic cells, which in turn secrete the chemokine CXCL13 (BLC) to attract more B cells |

Fig. 7.39 The organization of a lymphoid organ is orchestrated by chemokines. The cellular organization of a lymphoid organ is initiated by stromal cells and by vascular endothelial cells, which express the chemokine CCL21 (first panel). Dendritic cells express a receptor for CCL21 and are attracted by it to the site of the developing lymph node (second panel). There the dendritic cells also secrete CCL21, augmenting the expression by stromal cells and vascular endothelial cells. The dendritic cells also express a second chemokine, CCL19, and the combination of CCL21 and CCL19 attracts T cells to the developing lymph node (third panel).

The same combination of chemokines also attracts B cells into the developing lymph node (fourth panel). The B cells are able to either induce the differentiation of follicular dendritic cells or direct their recruitment into the lymph node. Once present, the follicular dendritic cells secrete a chemokine, CXCL13, which is a chemoattractant for B cells. The production of CXCL13 drives the organization of B cells into discrete B-cell areas (follicles) around the follicular dendritic cells and contributes to the further recruitment of B cells from the circulation into the lymph node (fifth panel).

the endothelial cells of HEVs in lymph nodes and Peyer's patches. Another source of CCL19 and CCL21 is the interdigitating dendritic cells, which are also prominent in the T zones. Indeed, dendritic cells themselves express CCR7 and will localize to T zones even in RAG-deficient mice, which lack lymphocytes. Thus, the T zone might be organized first through the attraction of dendritic cells and T cells by CCL21 produced by stromal cells. This organization would then be reinforced by CCL21 and CCL19 secreted by resident mature dendritic cells, which in turn attract more T cells and dendritic cells.

B cells—particularly activated ones—also express CCR7 but at lower levels than do T cells or dendritic cells. This may account for their characteristic migration pattern, which is first through the T zone (where they may linger if activated) and then to the follicle. Although the cellular organization of T-cell and B-cell areas in lymph nodes and Peyer's patches has been less well studied, it seems likely that it is controlled by similar, if not identical, chemokines and receptors.

7-28 The further development and homeostasis of peripheral lymphocytes is determined via cytokines and by signals that lymphocytes continually receive through their antigen receptors.

When newly formed lymphocytes reach the peripheral lymphoid tissues, they are not fully qualified to enter the pool of long-lived naive cells. As a population, these cells have been purged of autoreactivity in the central lymphoid organs; however, this was only effective for autoantigens that are expressed in or could reach these organs. Therefore, one step that newly emigrated lymphocytes must undergo is **peripheral tolerance**, or the process of eliminating or inactivating self-reactive cells that encounter autoantigens for the first time in the periphery, as described in the next section. In addition, B cells that leave the bone marrow are still immature; even after peripheral tolerance is complete, only a fraction of these immature cells are destined to complete development and enter the long-lived pool.

Moreover, lymphocytes in the periphery can also receive positive signals that are thought to control the further differentiation of immature B cells as well as their survival. Similarly, the survival of mature T cells depends on interactions with positively selecting ligands encountered in the periphery. These further selective processes—both negative and positive—will be described in the next four sections.

7-29 Lymphocytes that encounter sufficient quantities of self antigens for the first time in the periphery are eliminated or inactivated.

Not all potential self antigens are expressed in central lymphoid organs. Some, like the thyroid product thyroglobulin, are tissue specific and/or are compartmentalized such that there is little if any available in the circulation. Lymphocytes that do encounter self antigens *de novo* in the periphery can have three fates, much like those that recognize such antigens in central lymphoid organs: deletion, anergy, or survival (also known as 'ignorance').

Mature B cells that encounter a strongly cross-linking antigen in the periphery will undergo clonal deletion. This was elegantly shown in studies of B cells expressing immunoglobulin specific for H-2K^b MHC class I molecules. These cells are deleted even when, in transgenic animals, the expression of the H-2K^b molecule is restricted to the liver by use of a liver-specific gene promoter. B cells that encounter strongly cross-linking antigens in the periphery undergo apoptosis directly, unlike their counterparts in the bone marrow, which attempt further receptor rearrangements instead. The different outcomes may be due to the fact that the B cells in the periphery are more mature and can no longer rearrange their light-chain loci. However, stromal signals may be important; some experiments suggest that stromal cells in the spleen instruct B cells to respond in a different way to signals delivered through the antigen receptor compared with the stromal cells of the bone marrow.

As with immature B cells, mature B cells that encounter and bind an abundant soluble antigen become anergized. This was demonstrated in mice by placing the HEL transgene under the control of an inducible promoter that can be regulated by changes in the diet. It is thus possible to induce the production of lysozyme at any time and thereby study its effects on HEL-specific B cells at different stages of maturation. These experiments have shown that both mature and immature B cells are inactivated when they are chronically exposed to soluble antigen.

The situation is similar for T cells. Again, our understanding of the fates of autoreactive T cells in the periphery comes mainly from the study of T-cell receptor transgenic mice. In some cases, T cells reacting to self antigens in the periphery are eliminated, though this may follow a brief period of activation and cell division known as **activation-induced cell death**. In other cases, these cells may be rendered anergic. When studied *in vitro*, these anergic T cells prove refractory to signals given through the T-cell receptor.

Thus, the outcomes of peripheral negative selection are analogous to those of immature lymphocytes reacting to autoantigens in central lymphoid organs. This creates a problem because mature lymphocytes need to be activated under certain circumstances to generate productive immune responses to pathogenic microbes. The solution is that, in the absence of signals from the innate immune system, which induces inflammatory cytokines and the expression of co-stimulatory molecules, even mature lymphocytes interpret an antigen-receptor signal as a negative one. This was recently demonstrated *in vivo* for T cells. It was shown that, in the absence of inflammation, dendritic cells present self antigens. The consequences for a T cell of recognizing this self antigen on quiescent dendritic cells are either activation-induced cell death or anergy. Thus, when the innate immune system is not activated, antigens presented by dendritic cells may lead to T-cell tolerance rather than activation. The fate of mature B cells is also determined by the context of the signal, although in this case the direct effects of the innate immune system are also integrated with the presence or absence of activated helper T cells, which in turn depends on thymic and peripheral tolerance.

7-30   Most immature B cells arriving in the spleen are short-lived and require cytokines and positive signals through the B-cell receptor for maturation and survival.

When B cells emerge from bone marrow into the periphery, they are still functionally immature, expressing high levels of sIgM but little sIgD. Most of these immature cells will not survive to become fully mature B cells bearing low levels of sIgM and high levels of sIgD. Fig. 7.40 shows the possible fates of newly produced B cells that enter the periphery.

The daily output of new B cells is roughly 5–10% of the total B-lymphocyte population in the steady-state peripheral pool. Although the size of this pool is not easy to measure, it seems to remain constant in unimmunized animals, and the stream of new B cells must be balanced by the death of an equal number of peripheral B cells. The great majority of peripheral B cells (about 90%) are long-lived, however, and only 1–2% of these die each day. Most of the B cells that die are in the short-lived immature peripheral B-cell population, of which more than 50% die every 3 days. Thus most B cells have a life-span of

Fig. 7.40 Proposed population dynamics of conventional B cells. B cells are produced as receptor-positive immature B cells in the bone marrow. The most avidly self-reactive B cells are removed at this stage. B cells then migrate to the periphery, where they enter the secondary lymphoid tissues. It is estimated that $10–20 \times 10^6$ B cells are produced by the bone marrow and exported each day in a mouse, and an equal number are lost from the periphery. There seem to be two classes of peripheral B cell: long-lived B cells and short-lived B cells. The short-lived B cells are, by definition, recently formed B cells. Most of the turnover of short-lived B cells might result from B cells that fail to enter lymphoid follicles. In some cases this is a consequence of being rendered anergic by binding to soluble self antigen; for the remaining immature B cells, entry into lymphoid follicles is thought to entail some form of positive selection. Thus the remainder of the short-lived B cells fail to join the long-lived pool because they are not positively selected. About 90% of all peripheral B cells are relatively long-lived mature B cells that seem to have undergone positive selection in the periphery. These mature naive B cells recirculate through peripheral lymphoid tissues and have a half-life of 6–8 weeks in mice. Memory B cells, which have been activated previously by antigen and T cells, are thought to have a longer life.

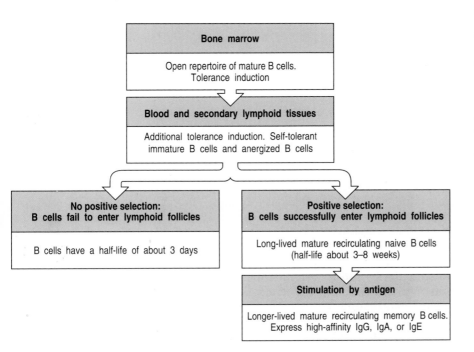

only a few days once they leave the bone marrow and enter the periphery; only a small number of newly produced B cells survive to become part of the pool of relatively long-lived peripheral B cells.

The failure of most B cells to survive for more than a few days in the periphery seems to be due to competition between peripheral B cells for access to the follicles in the peripheral lymphoid tissues. The follicles seem to provide essential survival and possibly maturation signals for naive B cells. If newly produced immature B cells do not enter a follicle, their passage through the periphery is halted and they die. The limited number of lymphoid follicles cannot accommodate the very large numbers of naive B cells poured out into the periphery each day and so there is continual competition for entry. In addition, competition for a factor called BAFF has an important role, as will be discussed further in the next section.

The population dynamics indicate that competition for follicular entry favors mature B cells that are already established in the relatively long-lived and stable peripheral B-cell pool. Why this should be is not entirely clear. Mature B cells have undergone phenotypic changes that might make their access to the follicles easier; for example, they express the receptor, CXCR5, for the chemoattractant CXCL13, expressed by follicular dendritic cells. They also have increased expression of the B-cell co-receptor component CR2 (CD21), which affects the signaling capacity of the B cell.

What determines the fate of an immature B cell? Is its survival simply a matter of chance, or are survival and further development determined by positive selection involving the specificity of its antigen receptor, as in the positive selection of T cells in the thymus? Several experiments indicate that signaling through the B-cell receptor has a positive role in the maturation and continued recirculation of peripheral B cells. A clever method of inactivating the B-cell receptor in mature B cells by conditional gene deletion has demonstrated that continuous expression of the B-cell receptor is required for B-cell survival. Mice that lack the tyrosine kinase Syk, which is involved in signaling from the B-cell receptor (see Section 6-10), fail to develop mature B cells although they do have immature B cells. Thus, a Syk-transduced signal may be required for final B-cell maturation or for the survival of mature B cells. Although each B-cell receptor has a unique specificity, such signaling need not depend on antigen-specific interactions; the receptor could, for example, be responsible for 'tonic' signaling, in which a weak but significant signal is generated by the assembly of the receptor complex and infrequently triggers some or all of the downstream signaling events.

7-31 The specificity of the B-cell receptor is important in determining the differentiation and survival of B cells in the periphery.

Although tonic signaling through the B-cell receptor may be important, evidence is accumulating that receptor specificity has an important role in shaping the peripheral B-cell pools that derive from immature B cells that reach the spleen. This is most clearly shown in the role of the B-cell receptor and antigen in the selection of two subsets of B cells that do not reside in B-cell follicles: so-called **B-1** or **CD5$^+$ B cells** and 'marginal zone' B cells. B-1 B cells are a minority subset of B cells comprising about 5% of all B cells in mice and humans, and are the major population in rabbits. The B cells belonging to this subset were first identified by surface expression of the protein CD5 and are also characterized by high levels of sIgM with little sIgD, even when mature. These cells appear first during fetal development (Fig. 7.41); they are therefore termed B-1 cells because their development precedes that of the conventional B cells whose development has been discussed up to now and which are sometimes termed **B-2 cells**.

Property	B-1 cells	Conventional B-2 cells	Marginal zone B cells
When first produced	Fetus	After birth	After birth
N-regions in VDJ junctions	Few	Extensive	Yes
V-region repertoire	Restricted	Diverse	Partly restricted
Primary location	Body cavities (peritoneal, pleural)	Secondary lymphoid organs	Spleen
Mode of renewal	Self-renewing	Replaced from bone marrow	Long-lived
Spontaneous production of immunoglobulin	High	Low	Low
Isotypes secreted	IgM >> IgG	IgG > IgM	IgM > IgG
Response to carbohydrate antigen	Yes	Maybe	Yes
Response to protein antigen	Maybe	Yes	Yes
Requirement for T-cell help	No	Yes	Sometimes
Somatic hypermutation	Low–none	High	?
Memory development	Little or none	Yes	?

Fig. 7.41 A comparison of the properties of B-1 cells, conventional B cells (B-2 cells), and marginal zone B cells. B-1 cells can develop in unusual sites in the fetus, such as the omentum, in addition to the liver. B-1 cells predominate in the young animal although they probably can be produced throughout life. Being produced mainly during fetal and neonatal life, their rearranged variable-region sequences contain few N-nucleotides. In contrast, marginal zone B cells accumulate after birth and do not reach peak levels in the mouse until 8 weeks of age. B-1 cells are best thought of as a partly activated self-renewing pool of lymphocytes that are selected by ubiquitous self and foreign antigens. Because of this selection, and possibly because the cells are produced early in life, the B-1 cells have a restricted repertoire of variable regions and antigen-binding specificities. Marginal zone B cells also have a restricted repertoire that may be selected by a set of antigens similar to those that select B-1 cells. B-1 cells seem to be the major population of B cells in certain body cavities, most probably because of exposure at these sites to antigens that drive B-1 cell proliferation. Marginal zone B cells remain in the marginal zone of the spleen and are not thought to recirculate. Partial activation of B-1 cells leads to the secretion of mainly IgM antibody; B-1 cells contribute much of the IgM that circulates in the blood. The limited diversity of both the B-1 and marginal zone B-cell repertoire and the propensity of these cells to react with common bacterial carbohydrate antigens suggest that they carry out a more primitive, less adaptive, immune response than conventional B cells (B-2 cells). In this regard they are comparable to γ:δ T cells.

There is great debate about the origin of B-1 cells. It is clear that their antigen specificity affects the fate of B-1 cells and/or their precursors, in that certain autoantigens and environmental antigens drive the expansion and maintenance of B-1 cells in the periphery. Interestingly, although there are some B-1 cells in the spleen and blood, they are greatly enriched in the peritoneal and pleural cavity fluid. At these sites they may encounter the relevant selecting antigens as well as other signals, including IL-10, that promote their survival. Some of the antigens that drive B-1 expansion, such as phosphatidylcholine, are encountered on the surface of bacteria that colonize the gut.

Although B-1 cells are selected by environmental antigens and autoantigens, it is not yet clear whether they arise as a distinct lineage from a unique precursor cell, or instead differentiate to the B-1 phenotype from a precursor cell that could also give rise to B-2 cells. In the mouse, fetal liver produces mainly B-1 cells, whereas adult bone marrow generates predominantly B-2 cells, and this has been interpreted as support for the unique precursor hypothesis. However, the weight of evidence favors the idea that commitment to the B-1 or B-2 subset is due to a selection step rather than being a distinct lineage difference such as that between γ:δ and α:β T cells. It is, however, difficult to rule out the idea that such cells are precommitted but survive only if their receptor specificity matches the predetermined fate.

Marginal zone B cells, so called because they reside in the marginal sinus of the white pulp, are another unique subset of B cells. They seem to be resting mature B cells, yet they have a different set of surface proteins from the major follicular population of B cells. For example, they express lower levels of CD23, a C-type lectin, and high levels of both the MHC class I-like molecule CD1 (see Section 5-18) and the receptors for the C3 fragment of complement, CD21/35. Marginal zone B cells have restricted antigen specificities, biased toward common environmental and even self antigens, and may be adapted to provide a quick response if such antigens enter the bloodstream. They may not require T-cell help to become activated. Both functionally and phenotypically, marginal zone B cells resemble B-1 cells; recent experiments suggest they are positively selected by certain self antigens, much as B-1 cells are. However, they are distinct both in location and in surface protein expression; for example, marginal zone B cells do not have high levels of CD5.

The functions of B-1 cells and marginal zone B cells are being clarified. Their locations suggest a role for B-1 cells in defending the body cavities, and for marginal zone B cells in defense against pathogens that penetrate the bloodstream. The restricted repertoire of receptors of both cell types seems to equip them for a function in the early, nonadaptive phase of an immune response (see Section 2-29). Indeed, the V gene segments that are used to encode the receptors of B-1 and marginal zone B cells might have evolved by natural selection to recognize common bacterial antigens, thus allowing them to contribute to the very early phases of the adaptive immune response. In practice, it is found that B-1 cells make little contribution to adaptive immune responses to most protein antigens but contribute strongly to some antibody responses against carbohydrate antigens. Moreover, a large proportion of the IgM that normally circulates in the blood of unimmunized mice derives from B-1 cells. The existence of these so-called 'natural antibodies,' which are highly cross-reactive and bind with low affinity to both microbial and self antigens, supports the view that B-1 cells are partly activated, because they are selected for self-renewal by ubiquitous self and environmental antigens.

Whereas positive selection in the periphery has a clear role in the development and maintenance of marginal zone and B-1 cells, the situation is less clear for the majority follicular B cells. Even among long-lived peripheral B cells, studies in mice reveal a broad distribution of life-span. One part of this population is composed of relatively long-lived mature naive B cells with a half-life of 1–2 months. We know that some of the short-lived peripheral B cells fail to survive because they have bound soluble self antigen and become anergic (see Section 7-17), leading to their exclusion from the lymphoid follicles. We have seen that most immature B cells reaching the spleen do not survive for long there. Evidence is accumulating that the B-cell receptor repertoire of surviving mature B cells is enriched for certain antigen specificities compared with the immature population, strongly favoring the idea that there is positive selection of a subset of these immature B cells for further maturation and long-term survival. However, the extent to which the recruitment of immature B cells into the long-lived pool of recirculating mature B cells is ligand-mediated and governed by receptor specificity is not as clear as for B-1 or marginal zone B cells.

The nature of other signals required for the maintenance of follicular B cells is not fully known. They might obtain a variety of survival signals from their normal environment, the B-cell follicle, through which they recirculate. One receptor–ligand pair from the TNF family, BAFF-R/BAFF, has recently been shown to have an important role in follicular B-cell survival, because mutants lacking BAFF-R have mainly immature B cells and few long-lived peripheral B cells. Interestingly, BAFF is secreted by myeloid cells that are mainly not in B-cell follicles. Peripheral B cells also include B cells that are very long-lived. These include the memory B cells that differentiate from mature B cells after their first encounter with antigen (see Section 1-13). Memory B cells persist for extended periods after antigenic stimulation and may require intermittent follicular signals for their survival; we will return to B-cell memory in Chapter 10.

The continual production and loss of new B cells ensures that the receptor repertoire is broadly maintained to meet new antigenic challenges. In contrast, the persistence of memory cells—the progeny of cells that have been activated—ensures that those cells proved to recognize pathogens are retained to combat reinfection.

7-32 The life-span of T cells in the periphery is determined by cytokines as well as ongoing contact with self-peptide:self-MHC complexes similar to those that initially selected them.

When T cells have expressed their receptors and co-receptors, and matured within the thymus for a further week or so, they emigrate to the periphery. Unlike B cells emigrating from bone marrow, only small numbers of T cells are exported from the thymus, roughly $1–2 \times 10^6$ per day in the mouse. Mature naive CD8 and CD4 T cells outside the thymus are sustained by repeated contact with MHC:self-peptide complexes similar or identical to those that originally positively selected them. This was shown by a transfer of T cells from their normal environment to recipients that lacked MHC molecules, or lacked the 'correct' MHC molecules that originally selected the T cells. The T cells did not survive long in such environments, whereas T cells transferred into recipients that had the correct MHC molecules survived. Contact with the appropriate self-peptide:self-MHC complex leads to infrequent division of mature naive T cells, which are maintained in the peripheral lymphoid organs; this slow increase in T-cell numbers must be balanced by a slow loss of T cells, such that the number of T cells remains roughly constant. Most probably, this loss involves the daughters of such dividing naive cells.

Where do the CD4 and CD8 T cells encounter their positively selecting ligands in the periphery? Current evidence favors molecules on lymphoid dendritic cells in T-cell zones (see Section 7-26). These cells are similar to the dendritic cells that migrate to the lymph nodes from peripheral sites (see Section 1-6) but lack sufficient co-stimulatory potential to induce full T-cell activation. However, the study of peripheral positive selection is in its infancy, and a clear picture has yet to emerge.

Memory T cells also persist, like memory B cells, after immunization. Paradoxically, their turnover is faster than that of the naive T cells, although expanded clones of memory cells are maintained at a relatively constant size by balanced proliferation and cell death. Unlike the naive cells, memory T cells do not seem to require continual stimulation by self-peptide:self-MHC ligands for this turnover to take place. Memory T cells transferred into mice that lack both MHC class I and MHC class II molecules are able to survive and to proliferate; these cells seem to depend on cytokine stimulation by IL-7 and IL-15 and the presence of the transcription factor lung Kruppel-like factor (LKLF) rather than on antigenic stimulation. However, in at least one study, memory cells that have survived for long periods in the absence of MHC molecules seem to be nonfunctional. Emerging evidence indicates that the survival and function of memory T cells may be controlled by a combination of cytokines—IL-7 in particular—and T-cell receptor signals. Memory T and B cells consist of clones of normal long-lived lymphocytes. Tumors of lymphocyte origin represent abnormally growing and surviving clones, which we consider in the next sections.

Multiple
Myeloma

7-33 B-cell tumors often occupy the same site as their normal counterparts.

Tumors retain many of the characteristics of the cell type from which they arose, especially when the tumor is relatively differentiated and slow growing. This is clearly illustrated by B-cell tumors. Tumors corresponding to essentially all stages of B-cell development have been found in humans, from the earliest stages to the myelomas that represent malignant outgrowths of plasma cells (Fig. 7.42).

Furthermore, each type of tumor retains its characteristic homing properties. Thus, a tumor that resembles mature, germinal center or memory cells homes to follicles in lymph nodes and spleen, giving rise to a **follicular center cell lymphoma**, whereas a tumor of plasma cells usually disperses to many different sites in the bone marrow much as normal plasma cells do, from which comes the clinical name of **multiple myeloma** (tumor of bone marrow). These similarities mean that it is often possible to use tumor cells, which are available in large quantities, to study the cell-surface molecules and signaling pathways responsible for homing and other cellular functions.

Fig. 7.42 B-cell tumors represent clonal outgrowths of B cells at various stages of development. Each type of tumor cell has a normal B-cell equivalent, homes to similar sites, and has behavior similar to that cell. Thus, myeloma cells look much like the plasma cells from which they derive, they secrete immunoglobulin, and they are found predominantly in the bone marrow. The most enigmatic of B-cell tumors is Hodgkin's disease, which consists of two cell phenotypes: a lymphoid cell and a large, odd-looking cell known as a Reed–Sternberg (RS) cell. The RS cell seems to derive from a germinal center B cell that has a decreased expression of surface immunoglobulin, possibly owing to somatic mutation. Chronic lymphocytic leukemia (CLL) was previously thought to derive from the B-1 lineage because it expresses CD5. However, recent gene expression profile studies of CLL suggest that it resembles an activated or memory B cell. Many lymphomas and myelomas can go through a preliminary, less aggressive, lymphoproliferative phase, and some mild lympho-proliferations seem to be benign.

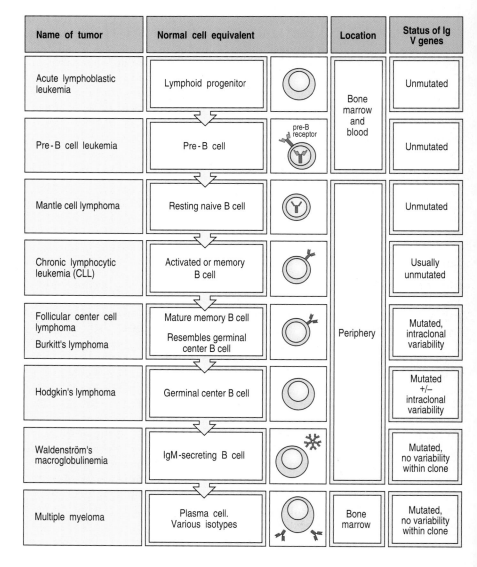

Name of tumor	Normal cell equivalent		Location	Status of Ig V genes
Acute lymphoblastic leukemia	Lymphoid progenitor		Bone marrow and blood	Unmutated
Pre-B cell leukemia	Pre-B cell	pre-B receptor		Unmutated
Mantle cell lymphoma	Resting naive B cell			Unmutated
Chronic lymphocytic leukemia (CLL)	Activated or memory B cell			Usually unmutated
Follicular center cell lymphoma / Burkitt's lymphoma	Mature memory B cell / Resembles germinal center B cell		Periphery	Mutated, intraclonal variability
Hodgkin's lymphoma	Germinal center B cell			Mutated +/- intraclonal variability
Waldenström's macroglobulinemia	IgM-secreting B cell			Mutated, no variability within clone
Multiple myeloma	Plasma cell. Various isotypes		Bone marrow	Mutated, no variability within clone

The general conclusion that a tumor represents the clonal outgrowth of a single transformed cell is very clearly illustrated by tumors of B-lineage cells. All the cells in a B-cell tumor have identical immunoglobulin gene rearrangements, decisively documenting their origin from one cell. This is useful for clinical diagnosis, because tumor cells can be detected by sensitive assays for these homogeneous rearrangements (Fig. 7.43). Indeed, the presence of rearrangements at the B-cell receptor loci is highly indicative of a tumor's B cell origin, just as rearrangements at the T-cell receptor loci are indicative of T-cell origin. This approach has proved useful in typing acute lymphoblastic leukemia, a common malignancy of childhood. Most of these have rearrangements of the heavy-chain but not the light-chain loci, indicating their origin from a pre-B cell and consistent with their relatively undifferentiated phenotype. Some of these have rearranged light chains as well and may have arisen from a slightly more developed precursor. A few lymphoblastic leukemias have rearrangements at the T-cell receptor loci and thus are not of B-cell origin.

Similarly, gene rearrangement status has recently enabled the origin of a class of tumors known as **Hodgkin's disease** to be settled. The bizarre-looking cell that is characteristic of Hodgkin's disease, known as a **Reed–Sternberg (RS) cell**, was previously thought to be of T-cell or dendritic cell origin. DNA analysis has now shown that these cells have rearranged immunoglobulin genes, classifying them as outgrowths of a single B cell. How the originally transformed B cell changes morphology to become an RS cell is not known. Curiously, in Hodgkin's disease, RS cells are sometimes a minority population; the more numerous surrounding cells are usually polyclonal T and B cells that may be reacting to the RS cells or to a soluble factor they secrete. One of the reasons that the origin of RS cells was unclear is that in nearly all cases they lack surface immunoglobulin. We now know that in many cases the reason for loss of surface immunoglobulin is a somatic mutation that inactivates one of the immunoglobulin V-region genes.

Whether the immunoglobulin genes in a B-cell tumor contain somatic mutations also provides important information on its origin (see Fig. 7.42); in particular, if the genes are mutated this suggests that the cell of origin had passed through a germinal center reaction. Pre-B cell leukemias and most **chronic lymphocytic leukemias (CLL)** have no mutations. By contrast, follicular

Fig. 7.43 Clonal analysis of B-cell and T-cell tumors. DNA analysis of tumor cells by Southern blotting techniques can detect and monitor lymphoid malignancy. Left panel: B-cell tumor analysis. In a sample from a healthy person (left lane), immunoglobulin genes are in the germline configuration in non-B cells, so a digest of their DNA with a suitable restriction endonuclease yields a single germline DNA fragment when probed with an immunoglobulin heavy-chain J-region probe (J_H). Normal B cells present in this sample make many different rearrangements to J_H, producing a spectrum of 'bands' each so faint that it is undetectable. By contrast, in samples from patients with B-cell malignancies (patient 1 and patient 2), where a single cell has given rise to all the tumor cells in the sample, two extra bands are seen with the J_H probe. These bands are characteristic of each patient's tumor and result from the rearrangement of both alleles of the J_H gene in the original tumor cells. The intensity of the bands compared with that of the germline band gives an indication of the abundance of tumor cells in the sample. After antitumor treatment (see patient 1), the intensity of the tumor-specific bands can be seen to diminish. Right panel: the unique rearrangement events in each T cell can be used similarly to identify tumors of T cells by Southern blotting. The probe used in this case was for the T-cell receptor β-chain constant regions ($C_\beta 1$ and $C_\beta 2$). DNA from a placenta (P), a tissue in which the T-cell receptor genes are not rearranged, shows one prominent band for each region. DNA from peripheral blood lymphocytes from two patients suffering from T-cell tumors (T_1 and T_2) gives additional bands that correspond to specific rearrangements (arrowed) that are present in a large number of cells (the tumor). As with B cells, no bands deriving from rearranged genes in normal T cells also present in the patients' samples can be seen, because no one rearranged band is present at sufficient concentration to be detected in this assay. Left panel: photograph courtesy of T.J. Vulliamy and L. Luzzatto. Right panel: photograph courtesy of T. Diss.

lymphoma or **Burkitt's lymphoma**, arising from germinal center B cells, express mutated V genes. If the V genes from several different lymphoma lines of these types from the same patient are sequenced, minor variations (intraclonal variations) are seen because somatic hypermutation continues in the tumor cells. Later-stage B-cell tumors such as multiple myelomas contain mutated genes but do not display intraclonal variation; this is because by this stage in B-cell development somatic hypermutation has ceased. Some caution is needed in generalizing from the somatic mutation status of immunoglobulin genes because it is not entirely clear that mutation is restricted to germinal centers, and it is certainly true that some memory cells can pass through a germinal center reaction and not acquire any somatic mutations.

Recently, techniques referred to as microarray-based gene expression analysis have allowed the comprehensive description of genes expressed in tumor cells and in normal cells and thereby have provided greater insights into how tumors relate to normal tissues (see Appendix I, Section A-35). These approaches are much more powerful than those used previously and permit more precise classification and insight into the biology of tumor cells. Such insights may in turn lead to the discovery of therapeutic targets. This work has confirmed previous classifications based on homing patterns and has even allowed the further subdivision of tumor types, such as diffuse non-Hodgkin's lymphoma, into groups that resemble in this case either activated B cells or germinal center B cells. These molecularly based subdivisions have prognostic significance in that tumors that resemble germinal center cells respond much better to therapy. The analysis of CLL by gene expression profiling is particularly revealing. Because these tumors express CD5 and typically lack somatic mutations, they were thought for many years to arise from a B-1 cell precursor (see Section 7-31). However, gene expression analysis revealed little resemblance to normal CD5 B cells and instead suggested a relationship to a resting B cell, possibly a memory-type B cell. This would agree with the fact that some CLLs do have somatic mutations. Indeed, the mutated and unmutated CLLs share expression of nearly all genes. Yet the mutated CLLs do express a unique subset of genes, and this is probably responsible for the fact that they have a particularly benign prognosis. Expansions and variations on this molecular approach to classifying tumors of the immune system will no doubt lead to a further understanding of tumors as well as better prognosis and therapy.

7-34 A range of tumors of immune system cells throws light on different stages of T-cell development.

Tumors of T-lineage cells have been identified but, unlike B-cell tumors, few that correspond to intermediate stages in T-cell development have been identified in humans. Instead, the tumors resemble either mature T cells or, in **acute lymphoblastic leukemia**, the earliest type of lymphoid progenitor (Fig. 7.44). One possible reason for the rarity of tumors corresponding to intermediate stages is that immature T cells are programmed to die unless rescued within a very narrow time window by positive selection (see Section 7-20). Thymocytes might simply not linger long enough at the intermediate stages of their development to provide an opportunity for malignant transformation. Thus, only cells that are already transformed at earlier stages, or that do not become transformed until the T cell has matured, are ever seen as tumors.

T-Cell Lymphoma

As with B cells, the behavior of mature T-cell tumors has provided insight into different aspects of T-cell biology, and vice versa. For example, **cutaneous T-cell lymphomas**, which home to the skin and proliferate slowly, are clonal outgrowths of a CD4 T cell that, when activated, homes to the skin. A tumor

Disease	Cell		Characteristic cell-surface markers	Location
	Stem cell		CD34	Bone marrow
Common acute lymphoblastic leukemia (C-ALL or B-ALL)	Lymphoid progenitor		CD10 CD19 CD20	
Thymoma	Thymic stromal cell or epithelial cell		Cytokeratins	Thymus
Acute lymphoblastic leukemia (T-ALL)	Thymocyte		CD1	
Sézary syndrome Adult T-cell leukemia Mycosis fungoides Chronic lymphocytic leukemia (CLL) T prolymphocytic leukemia (TPLL)	T cell		CD3/TCR CD4 or CD8	Periphery

Fig. 7.44 T-cell tumors represent monoclonal outgrowths of normal cell populations. Each distinct T-cell tumor has a normal equivalent and retains many of the properties of the cell from which it develops. However, tumors of T cells lack the intermediates in the T-cell developmental pathway. Some of these tumors represent a massive outgrowth of a rare cell type. For example, acute lymphoblastic leukemia is derived from the lymphoid progenitor cell. One T-cell-related tumor is also included. Thymomas derive from thymic stromal or epithelial cells. Some characteristic cell-surface markers for each stage are also shown. For example, CD10 (common acute lymphoblastic leukemia antigen or CALLA) is used as a marker for common acute lymphoblastic leukemia. Note that T-cell chronic lymphocytic leukemia (CLL) cells express CD8, whereas the other T-cell tumors listed express CD4. Adult T-cell leukemia is caused by the retrovirus HTLV-1.

of thymic stroma, called a **thymoma**, is frequently present in certain types of autoimmune disease, and removal of these tumors often ameliorates the disease. The reasons for this are not yet known.

7-35 Malignant lymphocyte tumors frequently carry chromosomal translocations that join immunoglobulin loci to genes that regulate cell growth.

The unregulated accumulation of cells of a single clone, which is the most striking characteristic of tumors, is caused by mutations that release the founder cell from the normal restraints on its growth or prevent its normal programmed death. In B-cell tumors the disruption of normal cellular homeostatic controls is often associated with an aberrant immunoglobulin gene rearrangement, in which one of the immunoglobulin loci is joined to a gene on another chromosome. This genetic fusion with another chromosome is known as a **translocation**, and in B-cell tumors translocations are found that disrupt the expression and function of genes important for controlling cell growth. Cellular genes that cause cancer when their function or expression is disrupted are termed **oncogenes**.

Translocations give rise to chromosomal abnormalities that are visible microscopically in metaphase. Characteristic translocations are seen in different B-cell tumors and reflect the involvement of a particular oncogene in each tumor type. Characteristic translocations that involve the T-cell receptor loci are also seen in T-cell tumors. Immunoglobulin and T-cell receptor loci are sites at which double-stranded DNA breaks occur during gene rearrangement, and during isotype switching and somatic hypermutation in

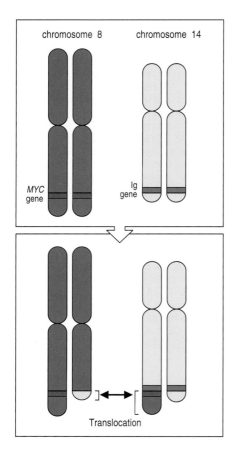

Fig. 7.45 Specific chromosomal rearrangements are found in some lymphoid tumors. If a chromosomal rearrangement joins one of the immunoglobulin genes to a cellular oncogene, it can result in the aberrant expression of the oncogene under the control of the immunoglobulin regulatory sequences. Such chromosomal rearrangements are frequently associated with B-cell tumors. In the example shown, from Burkitt's lymphoma, the translocation of the oncogene *MYC* from chromosome 8 to the immunoglobulin heavy-chain locus on chromosome 14 results in the deregulated expression of *MYC* and the unregulated growth of the B cell. The immunoglobulin gene on the normal chromosome 14 is usually productively rearranged, and the tumors that result from such translocations generally have a mature B-cell phenotype and express immunoglobulin.

B cells, so it is not surprising that they are especially likely to be sites of chromosomal translocation.

The analysis of chromosomal abnormalities has revealed much about the regulation of B-cell growth and the disruption of growth control in tumor cells. In Burkitt's lymphoma cells, the *MYC* oncogene on chromosome 8 is recombined with an immunoglobulin locus by translocations that involve either chromosome 14 (heavy chain) (Fig. 7.45), chromosome 2 (κ light chain), or chromosome 22 (λ light chain). The Myc protein is known to be involved in the control of the cell cycle in normal cells. The translocation deregulates expression of the Myc protein, which leads to an increased proliferation of B cells, although other mutations elsewhere in the genome are also needed before a B-cell tumor results.

Other B-cell tumors, particularly follicular lymphomas, carry a chromosomal translocation of immunoglobulin genes to the oncogene *bcl-2*, increasing the production of Bcl-2 protein. The Bcl-2 protein prevents apoptosis in B-lineage cells, so its abnormal expression allows some B cells to survive and accumulate beyond their normal life-span. During this time, further genetic changes can occur that lead to malignant transformation. Proof that Bcl-2 rearrangement and consequent overexpression can promote lymphoma comes from mice that carry a constitutively overexpressed *bcl-2* transgene. These mice tend to develop B-cell lymphomas in later life. Similarly, the gene *bcl-6* is commonly rearranged in diffuse large B-cell lymphomas and is thought to have a causative role in the transformation of these cells.

Summary.

Lymphocytes that survive the selective processes that operate in the central lymphoid organs are exported to the peripheral lymphoid organs. Here, their fate is still controlled by their antigen receptors. In the absence of encounter with their specific foreign antigen, naive lymphocytes require at least weak engagement of their antigen receptors for long-term survival. The evidence for such receptor-mediated survival signals is clearest for T cells, but they also seem to be needed for B-1 cells and marginal zone B cells, in which case they may promote differentiation, expansion, and survival, and most probably also for B-2 cells, in which case they promote survival without expansion. Although ligands that select B cells are known in a few cases for B-1 and marginal zone B cells, in general the ligands involved are unknown.

The organization of the peripheral lymphoid tissues and the homing of B and T cells to distinct areas are controlled by TNF-family proteins and chemokines. Large numbers of immature B cells leave the bone marrow daily. Most of these emigrants die soon after their arrival in the periphery, thus keeping the number of circulating B cells fairly constant. A small number acquire the signs of maturity and become longer-lived naive B cells. The lymphoid follicle, through which B cells must circulate to survive, seems to provide signals for maturation and survival. T cells leave the thymus as fully mature cells and in smaller numbers than B cells. They are generally long-lived and are thought to be slowly self-renewing in the peripheral lymphoid tissues, being maintained by repeated contacts with self-peptide:self-MHC complexes that can be recognized by the T-cell receptor but that do not cause T-cell activation. Memory cell clones are long-lived and may not require as much contact with selecting ligands for survival and function. Memory T cells require IL-7 and/or IL-15 for survival. The distinct minority subpopulations of lymphocytes, such as the B-1 cells, marginal zone B cells, γ:δ T cells, and the double-negative T cells with α:β receptors of very limited diversity, have different developmental histories and functional properties from conventional B-2 cells and α:β T cells, and are likely to be regulated independently of these majority B-cell and T-cell populations.

Very rarely, an individual B cell or T cell undergoes mutation and gives rise to a leukemia or lymphoma. The properties of the different lymphoid tumors reflect the developmental stage of the cell from which the tumor derives. All lymphoid tumors except those derived from very early uncommitted cells have characteristic gene rearrangements that allow their placement in the B or T lineage. These rearrangements are frequently accompanied by chromosomal translocations, often between a locus involved in generating the antigen receptor and a cellular proto-oncogene. Detailed and extensive gene expression analysis of these tumors is revealing their origins as well as the key genes involved in malignant transformation. Such studies are already aiding in diagnosis and are likely to lead to specific therapies.

Summary to Chapter 7.

In this chapter we have learned about the formation of the B-cell and T-cell lineages from a primitive lymphoid progenitor. The somatic gene rearrangements that generate the highly diverse repertoire of antigen receptors—immunoglobulin for B cells and the T-cell receptor for T cells—occur in the early stages of the development of T cells and B cells from a common lymphoid progenitor. Mammalian B-cell development takes place in fetal liver and, after birth, in the bone marrow; T cells also originate in the bone marrow but undergo most of their development in the thymus. B-cell specific and T-cell specific transcription factors and other proteins ensure that the immunoglobulin genes are rearranged in developing B cells and the T-cell receptor genes in developing T cells, but much of the somatic recombination machinery, including the RAG proteins that are an essential part of the V(D)J recombinase, is common to both. Gene rearrangement proceeds successively at each gene locus, beginning with loci that contain D genes. The cell is only allowed to proceed to the next stage of development if the rearrangement has been successful and has produced an in-frame sequence that can be translated into a protein chain. Cells that do not generate successful rearrangements for both receptor chains die by apoptosis. The course of B-cell development is summarized in Fig. 7.46, and that of $\alpha{:}\beta$ T cells in Fig. 7.47.

Once a functional antigen receptor has appeared on the cell surface, the newly minted lymphocyte is ready for stringent tests of its potential usefulness on the one hand and its autoreactivity on the other. Positive selection selects potentially useful cells for survival, whereas negative selection removes self-reactive cells from the lymphocyte repertoire, rendering it tolerant to the antigens of the body. Tolerance is enforced at different stages throughout the development of both B and T cells, and positive selection likewise seems to represent a continuous process. Positive selection is particularly essential for T cells, because it ensures that only cells bearing T-cell receptors that can recognize antigen in combination with self MHC molecules will continue to mature. It occurs in the thymus, in thymocytes that have just started to produce a T-cell receptor and are still expressing both of the co-receptors CD4 and CD8. Although signals through co-receptors are clearly important, precisely how the thymocyte matches up the specificity of its T-cell receptor, the specificity of the co-receptor for MHC molecules, and the appropriate differentiated cellular function is not completely resolved. For B cells, positive selection seems to occur at the final transition from immature to mature B cells, which occurs in peripheral lymphoid tissues. How it is effected is not known at present.

Occasionally, B cells and T cells undergo malignant transformation, giving rise to tumors that have escaped normal growth controls while retaining most features of the parent cell, including its characteristic homing pattern. These tumors frequently carry translocations involving the antigen-receptor loci and other genes that are intimately involved in lymphocyte growth regulation

Fig. 7.46 A summary of the development of human conventional B-lineage cells. The state of the immunoglobulin genes, the expression of some essential intracellular proteins, and the expression of some cell-surface molecules are shown for successive stages of B-2-cell development. Note that because the immunoglobulin genes undergo further changes during antigen-driven development, such as isotype switch and somatic hypermutation (see Chapter 4), these are chronicled throughout development. The antigen-dependent stages are described in more detail in Chapter 9.

B cells		Heavy-chain genes	Light-chain genes	Intra-cellular proteins	Surface marker proteins
Stem cell		Germline	Germline		CD34 CD45 AA4.1
Early pro-B cell		D–J rearranged	Germline	RAG-1 RAG-2 TdT λ5, VpreB	CD34 CD45R AA4.1, IL-7R MHC class II CD10, CD19 CD38
Late pro-B cell		V–DJ rearranged	Germline	TdT λ5, VpreB	CD45R AA4.1, IL-7R MHC class II CD10, CD19 CD38, CD20 CD40
Large pre-B cell	pre-B receptor	VDJ rearranged	Germline	λ5, VpreB	CD45R AA4.1, IL-7R MHC class II pre-B-R CD19, CD38 CD20, CD40
Small pre-B cell	cytoplasmic μ	VDJ rearranged	V–J rearrangement	μ RAG-1 RAG-2	CD45R AA4.1 MHC class II CD19, CD38 CD20, CD40
Immature B cell	IgM	VDJ rearranged. μ heavy chain produced in membrane form	VJ rearranged		CD45R AA4.1 MHC class II IgM CD19, CD20 CD40
Mature naive B cell	IgD IgM	VDJ rearranged. μ chain produced in membrane form. Alternative splicing yields μ + δ mRNA			CD45R MHC class II IgM, IgD CD19, CD20 CD21, CD40
Lympho-blast	IgM	Alternative splicing yields secreted μ chains		Ig	CD45R MHC class II CD19, CD20 CD21, CD40
Memory B cell	IgG	Isotype switch to Cγ, Cα, or Cε. Somatic hypermutation	Somatic hypermutation		CD45R MHC class II IgG, IgA CD19, CD20 CD21, CD40
Plasma blast and Plasma cell	IgG	Alternative splicing yields both membrane and secreted Ig	VJ rearranged	Ig	CD135 Plasma cell antigen-1 CD38

ANTIGEN INDEPENDENT

ANTIGEN DEPENDENT

TERMINAL DIFFERENTIATION

BONE MARROW

PERIPHERY

T cells		β-chain gene rearrangements	α-chain gene rearrangements	Intra-cellular proteins	Surface marker proteins	
Stem cell		Germline	Germline		CD34?	**BONE MARROW**
Early double-negative thymocyte		D–J rearranged	Germline	RAG-1 RAG-2 TdT Lck ZAP-70	CD2 HSA CD44hi	**THYMUS**
Late double-negative thymocyte		V–DJ rearranged	Germline	RAG-1 RAG-2 TdT Lck ZAP-70	CD25 CD44lo HSA	
Early double-positive thymocyte	pre-T receptor		V–J rearranged	RAG-1 RAG-2	PTα CD4 CD8 HSA	
Late double-positive thymocyte	T-cell receptor			Lck ZAP-70	CD69 CD4 CD8 HSA	
Naive CD4 T cell				Lck ZAP-70 LKLF	CD4 CD62L CD45RA CD5	**PERIPHERY**
Memory CD4 T cell				Lck ZAP-70	CD4 CD45RO CD44	
Effector CD4 T cell				Type 1: IL-2 IFN-γ Type 2: IL-5 IL-4 IL-10	CD4 CD45RO CD44hi Fas FasL (type 1)	
Naive CD8 T cell					CD8 CD45RA	
Memory CD8 T cell					CD8 CD45RO CD44	
Effector CD8 T cell				IFN-γ granzyme perforin	FasL Fas CD8 CD44hi	

Left margin labels: ANTIGEN INDEPENDENT; ANTIGEN DEPENDENT; TERMINAL DIFFERENTIATION; ANTIGEN DEPENDENT; TERMINAL DIFFERENTIATION

Fig. 7.47 A summary of the development of human α:β T cells. The state of the T-cell receptor genes, the expression of some essential intracellular proteins, and the expression of some cell-surface molecules are shown for successive stages of α:β T-cell development. Note that since the T-cell receptor genes do not undergo further changes during antigen-driven development, only the phases during which they are actively undergoing rearrangement in the thymus are indicated. The antigen-dependent phases of CD4 and CD8 cells are depicted separately, and are detailed in Chapter 8.

or cell death; thus these translocations have been a goldmine of information about the genes and proteins that regulate lymphocyte homeostasis. Most recently, gene expression analysis has proved to be an even more powerful and comprehensive way to gain insight into the origins of lymphocyte tumors, as well as many tumors of nonlymphoid origin.

Chapter 7 questions.

7.1   What are the two major goals of lymphocyte development?

7.2   Discuss the ordered steps of receptor rearrangement in B and T cells, drawing the parallels between the two cell types.

7.3   Lymphocyte development is notable for huge cell losses at several steps. What are the major reasons that lymphocytes die without (a) progressing beyond the pre-T/B stage; (b) after reaching the immature stage of expressing a complete TCR/BCR? Cover both T and B cells.

7.4   What is the function of the pre-T/B cell receptor?

7.5   Discuss the process of positive selection of T cells in the thymus. (a) Where does it take place? (b) What are the ligands? (c) When (at what stage) during T-cell development does positive selection occur? (d) How does the cell 'know' which co-receptor—CD4 or CD8—to express?

7.6   (a) What families of molecules are critical for the proper organization of peripheral lymphoid tissues? (b) Name one that is important for organizing the B-cell zone and discuss how it works, and (c) name one that is important for organizing the T-cell zone.

7.7   There are three main subsets of B cells: follicular, marginal zone and B-1. Compare and contrast their development and functions, covering at least five different categories.

7.8   What does the presence or absence of somatic hypermutations in immunoglobulin V regions of B-lineage tumors tell us about the origin of the neoplastic cells?

General references.

Casali, P., and Silberstein, L.E.S. (eds): *Immunoglobulin Gene Expression in Development and Disease.* New York, New York Academy of Sciences, 1995.

Loffert, D., Schaal, S., Ehlich, A., Hardy, R.R., Zou, Y.R., Muller, W., and Rajewsky, K.: **Early B-cell development in the mouse—insights from mutations introduced by gene targeting.** *Immunol. Rev.* 1994, **137**:135–153.

Melchers, F., ten Boekel, E., Seidl, T., Kong, X.C., Yamagami, T., Onishi, K., Shimizu, T., Rolink, A.G., and Andersson, J.: **Repertoire selection by pre-B-cell receptors and B-cell receptors, and genetic control of B-cell development from immature to mature B cells.** *Immunol. Rev.* 2000, **175**:33–46.

Starr, T.K., Jameson, S.C., and Hogquist, K.A.: **Positive and negative selection of T cells.** *Annu. Rev. Immunol.* 2003, **21**:139–176.

von Boehmer, H.: **The developmental biology of T lymphocytes.** *Annu. Rev. Immunol.* 1993, **6**:309–326.

Section references.

7-1   Lymphocyte development occurs in specialized environments and is regulated by signals from the environment along with the somatic rearrangement of the antigen-receptor genes.

Akashi, K., Kondo, M., Cheshier, S., Shizuru, J., Gandy, K., Domen, J., Mebius, R., Traver, D., and Weissman, I.L.: **Lymphoid development from stem cells and the common lymphocyte progenitors.** *Cold Spring Harbor Symp. Quant. Biol.* 1999, **64**:1–12.

van Ewijk, W., Hollander, G., Terhorst, C., and Wang, B.: **Stepwise development of thymic microenvironments *in vivo* is regulated by thymocyte subsets.** *Development* 2000, **127**:1583–1591.

Funk, P.E., Kincade, P.W., and Witte, P.L.: **Native associations of early hematopoietic stem-cells and stromal cells isolated in bone-marrow cell aggregates.** *Blood* 1994, **83**:361–369.

7-2   B cells develop in the bone marrow with the help of stromal cells and achieve maturity in peripheral lymphoid organs.

Jacobsen, K., Kravitz, J., Kincade, P.W., and Osmond, D.G.: **Adhesion receptors on bone-marrow stromal cells—*in vivo* expression of vascular cell adhesion molecule-1 by reticular cells and sinusoidal endothelium in normal and γ-irradiated mice.** *Blood* 1996, **87**:73–82.

Nagasawa, T., Hirota, S., Tachibana, V., Takakura, N., Nishikawa, S., Kitamura, Y., Yoshida, V., Kikutani, H., and Kishimoto, T.: **Defects of B-cell lymphopoiesis and bone-marrow myelopoiesis in mice lacking the CXC chemokine PBSF/SDF-1.** *Nature* 1996, **382**:635–638.

7-3   Stages in B-cell development are distinguished by the expression of immunoglobulin chains and particular cell-surface proteins.

Allman, D., Li, J., and Hardy, R.R.: **Commitment to the B lymphoid lineage occurs before DH-JH recombination.** *J. Exp. Med.* 1999, **189**:735–740.

Allman, D., Lindsley, R.C., DeMuth, W., Rudd, K., Shinton, S.A., and Hardy, R.R.: **Resolution of three nonproliferative immature splenic B cell subsets reveals multiple selection points during peripheral B cell maturation.** *J. Immunol.* 2001, **167**:6834–6840.

Hardy, R.R., Carmack, C.E., Shinton, S.A., Kemp, J.D., and Hayakawa, K.: **Resolution and characterization of pro-B and pre-pro-B cell stages in normal mouse bone marrow.** *J. Exp. Med.* 1991, **173**:1213–1225.

Osmond, D.G., Rolink, A., and Melchers, F.: **Murine B lymphopoiesis: towards a unified model.** *Immunol. Today* 1998, **19**:65–68.

7-4   T cells also originate in the bone marrow, but all the important events in their development occur in the thymus.

Anderson, G., Moore, N.C., Owen, J.J.T., and Jenkinson, E.J.: **Cellular interactions in thymocyte development.** *Annu. Rev. Immunol.* 1996, **14**:73–99.

Carlyle, J.R., and Zúñiga-Pflücker, J.C.: **Requirement for the thymus in alpha-beta T lymphocyte lineage commitment.** *Immunity* 1998, **9**:187–197.

Cordier, A.C., and Haumont, S.M.: **Development of thymus, parathyroids, and ultimobranchial bodies in NMRI and *nude* mice.** *Am. J. Anat.* 1980, **157**:227–263.

Nehls, M., Kyewski, B., Messerle, M., Waldschütz, R., Schüddekopf, K., Smith, A.J.H., and Boehm, T.: **Two genetically separable steps in the differentiation of thymic epithelium.** *Science* 1996, **272**:886–889.

Zúñiga-Pflücker, J.C., and Lenardo, M.J.: **Regulation of thymocyte development from immature progenitors.** *Curr. Opin. Immunol.* 1996, **8**:215–224.

7-5   T-cell precursors proliferate extensively in the thymus but most die there.

Shortman, K., Egerton, M., Spangrude, G.J., and Scollay, R.: **The generation and fate of thymocytes.** *Semin. Immunol.* 1990, **2**:3–12.

Surh, C.D., and Sprent, J.: **T-cell apoptosis detected *in situ* during positive and negative selection in the thymus.** *Nature* 1994, **372**:100–103.

7-6   Successive stages in the development of thymocytes are marked by changes in cell-surface molecules.

Borowski, C., Martin, C., Gounari, F., Haughn, L., Aifantis, I., Grassi, F., and von Boehmer, H.: **On the brink of becoming a T cell.** *Curr. Opin. Immunol.* 2002, **14**:200–206.

Saint-Ruf, C., Ungewiss, K., Groetrrup, M., Bruno, L., Fehling, H.J., and von Boehmer, H.: **Analysis and expression of a cloned pre-T-cell receptor gene.** *Science* 1994, **266**:1208–1212.

Shortman, K., and Wu, L.: **Early T lymphocyte progenitors.** *Annu. Rev. Immunol.* 1996, **14**:29–47.

7-7   Thymocytes at different developmental stages are found in distinct parts of the thymus.

Bleul, C.C., and Boehm, T.: **Chemokines define distinct microenvironments in the developing thymus.** *Eur. J. Immunol.* 2000, **30**:3371–3379.

Picker, L.J., and Siegelman, M.H.: Lymphoid tissues and organs, in Paul, W.E. (ed): *Fundamental Immunology*, 3rd edn. New York, Raven Press, 1993.

7-8   B cells undergo a programmed series of gene rearrangements in the bone marrow.

Ehrlich, A., and Kuppers, R.: **Analysis of immunoglobulin gene rearrangements in single B cells.** *Curr. Opin. Immunol.* 1995, **7**:281–284.

Ten-Boekel, E., Melchers, F., and Rolink, A.: **The status of Ig loci rearrangements in single cells from different stages of B-cell development.** *Int. Immunol.* 1995, **7**:1013–1019.

7-9   Successful rearrangement of heavy-chain immunoglobulin gene segments leads to the formation of a pre-B-cell receptor that halts further V_H to DJ_H rearrangement and triggers the cell to divide.

Grawunder, U., Leu, T.M.J., Schatz, D.G., Werner, A., Rolink, A.G., Melchers, F., and Winkler, T.H.: **Down-regulation of Rag1 and Rag2 gene expression in pre-B cells after functional immunoglobulin heavy-chain rearrangement.** *Immunity* 1995, **3**:601–608.

Loffert, D., Ehlich, A., Muller, W., and Rajewsky, K.: **Surrogate light-chain expression is required to establish immunoglobulin heavy-chain allelic exclusion during early B-cell development.** *Immunity* 1996, **4**:133–144.

Melchers, F., ten Boekel, E., Yamagami, T., Andersson, J., and Rolink, A.: **The roles of preB and B cell receptors in the stepwise allelic exclusion of mouse IgH and L chain gene loci.** *Semin. Immunol.* 1999, **11**:307–317.

7-10   Rearrangement at the immunoglobulin light-chain locus leads to cell-surface expression of the B-cell receptor.

Arakawa, H., Shimizu, T., and Takeda, S.: **Reevaluation of the probabilities for productive rearrangements on the κ-loci and λ-loci.** *Int. Immunol.* 1996, **8**:91–99.

Gorman, J.R., van der Stoep, N., Monroe, R., Cogne, M., Davidson, L., and Alt, F.W.: **The Igκ 3′ enhancer influences the ratio of Igκ versus Igλ B lymphocytes.** *Immunity* 1996, **5**:241–252.

Takeda, S., Sonoda, E., and Arakawa, H.: **The κ–λ ratio of immature B cells.** *Immunol. Today* 1996, **17**:200–201.

7-11   The expression of proteins regulating immunoglobulin gene rearrangement and function is developmentally programmed.

Hesslein, D.G., and Schatz, D.G.: **Factors and forces controlling V(D)J recombination.** *Adv. Immunol.* 2001, **78**:169–232.

Kee, B.L., and Murre, C.: **Transcription factor regulation of B lineage commitment.** *Curr. Opin. Immunol.* 2001, **13**:180–185.

Sleckman, B.P., Gorman, J.R., and Alt, F.W.: **Accessibility control of antigen receptor variable region gene assembly—role of *cis*-acting elements.** *Annu. Rev. Immunol.* 1996, **14**:459–481.

7-12   T cells in the thymus undergo a series of gene segment rearrangements similar to those of B cells.

Lauzurica, P., and Krangel, M.S.: **Temporal and lineage-specific control of T-cell receptor α/δ gene rearrangement by T-cell receptor α and δ enhancers.** *J. Exp. Med.* 1994, **179**:1913–1921.

Livak, F., Petrie, H.T., Crispe, I.N., and Schatz, D.G.: **In-frame TCR δ gene rearrangements play a critical role in the αβ/γδ T cell lineage decision.** *Immunity* 1995, **2**:617–627.

Sleckman, B.P., Bassing, C.H., Bardon, C.G., Okada, A., Khor, B., Bories, J.C., Monroe, R., and Alt, F.W.: **Accessibility control of variable region gene assembly during T-cell development.** *Immunol. Rev.* 1998, **165**:121–130.

7-13   Successful rearrangement at the β-chain locus and synthesis of a β chain leads to the production of a pre-T-cell receptor that triggers cell proliferation and cessation of β-chain gene rearrangement.

von Boehmer, H., Aifantis, I., Azogui, O., Feinberg, J., Saint-Ruf, C., Zober, C., Garcia, C., and Buer, J.: **Crucial function of the pre-T-cell receptor (TCR) in TCR beta selection, TCR beta allelic exclusion and alpha beta versus gamma delta lineage commitment.** *Immunol. Rev.* 1998, **165**:111–119.

Dudley, E.C., Petrie, H.T., Shah, L.M., Owen, M.J., and Hayday, A.C.: **T-cell receptor β chain gene rearrangement and selection during thymocyte development in adult mice.** *Immunity* 1994, **1**:83–93.

Philpott, K.I., Viney, J.L., Kay, G., Rastan, S., Gardiner, E.M., Chae, S., Hayday, A.C., and Owen, M.J.: **Lymphoid development in mice congenitally lacking T cell receptor α β-expressing cells.** *Science* 1992, **256**:1448–1453.

7-14   T-cell α-chain genes undergo successive rearrangements until positive selection or cell death intervenes.

Hardardottir, F., Baron, J.L., and Janeway, C.A., Jr.: **T cells with two functional antigen-specific receptors.** *Proc. Natl. Acad. Sci. USA* 1995, **92**:354–358.

Marrack, P., and Kappler, J.: **Positive selection of thymocytes bearing alpha beta T cell receptors.** *Curr. Opin. Immunol.* 1997, **9**:250–255.

Padovan, E., Casorati, G., Dellabona, P., Meyer, S., Brockhaus, M., and Lanzavecchia, A.: **Expression of two T-cell receptor α chains: dual receptor T cells.** *Science* 1993, **262**:422–424.

Petrie, H.T., Livak, F., Schatz, D.G., Strasser, A., Crispe, I.N., and Shortman, K.: **Multiple rearrangements in T-cell receptor α-chain genes maximize the production of useful thymocytes.** *J. Exp. Med.* 1993, **178**:615–622.

7-15   T cells with α:β or γ:δ receptors arise from a common progenitor.

Fehling, H.J., Gilfillan, S., and Ceredig, R.: **Alpha beta/gamma delta lineage commitment in the thymus of normal and genetically manipulated mice.** *Adv. Immunol.* 1999, **71**:1–76.

Hayday, A.C., Barber, D.F., Douglas, N., and Hoffman, E.S.: **Signals involved in gamma/delta T cell versus alpha/beta T cell lineage commitment.** *Semin. Immunol.* 1999, **11**:239–249.

Hayes, S.M., and Love, P.E.: **Distinct structure and signaling potential of the gamma delta TCR complex.** *Immunity* 2002, **16**:827–838.

Kang, J., Coles, M., Cado, D., and Raulet, D.H.: **The developmental fate of T cells is critically influenced by TCRγδ expression.** *Immunity* 1998, **8**:427–438.

Kang, J., and Raulet, D.H.: **Events that regulate differentiation of α βTCR⁺ and γ δTCR⁺ T cells from a common precursor.** *Semin. Immunol.* 1997, **9**:171–179.

7-16   T cells expressing particular γ- and δ-chain V regions arise in an ordered sequence early in life.

Dunon, D., Courtois, D., Vainio, O., Six, A., Chen, C.H., Cooper, M.D., Dangy J.P., and Imhof, B.A.: **Ontogeny of the immune system: γδ and αβ T cells migrate from thymus to the periphery in alternating waves.** *J. Exp. Med.* 1997, **186**:977–988.

Havran, W.L., and Boismenu, R.: **Activation and function of γδ T cells.** *Curr. Opin. Immunol.* 1994, **6**:442–446.

7-17   Immature B cells that bind self antigens undergo further receptor rearrangement, die, or are inactivated.

Casellas, R., Shih, T.A., Kleinewietfeld, M., Rakonjac, J., Nemazee, D., Rajewsky, K., and Nussenzweig, M.C.: **Contribution of receptor editing to the antibody repertoire.** *Science* 2001, **291**:1541–1544.

Chen, C., Nagy, Z., Radic, M.Z., Hardy, R.R., Huszar, D., Camper, S.A., and Weigert, M.: **The site and stage of anti-DNA B-cell deletion.** *Nature* 1995, **373**:252–255.

Cornall, R.J., Goodnow, C.C., and Cyster, J.G.: **The regulation of self-reactive B cells.** *Curr. Opin. Immunol.* 1995, **7**:804–811.

Melamed, D., Benschop, R.J., Cambier, J.C., and Nemazee, D.: **Developmental regulation of B lymphocyte immune tolerance compartmentalizes clonal selection from receptor selection.** *Cell* 1998, **92**:173–182.

Prak, E.L., and Weigert, M.: **Light-chain replacement—a new model for antibody gene rearrangement.** *J. Exp. Med.* 1995, **182**:541–548.

Tiegs, S.L., Russell, D.M., and Nemazee, D.: **Receptor editing in self-reactive bone marrow B cells.** *J. Exp. Med.* 1993, **177**:1009–1020.

7-18   The MHC type of the thymic stroma selects a repertoire of mature T cells that can recognize foreign antigens presented by the same MHC type.

Fink, P.J., and Bevan, M.J.: **H-2 antigens of the thymus determine lymphocyte specificity.** *J. Exp. Med.* 1978, **148**:766–775.

Zinkernagel, R.M., Callahan, G.N., Klein, J., and Dennert, G.: **Cytotoxic T cells learn specificity for self H-2 during differentiation in the thymus.** *Nature* 1978, **271**:251–253.

7-19   Only thymocytes whose receptors interact with self-MHC:self-peptide complexes can survive and mature.

Hogquist, K.A., Tomlinson, A.J., Kieper, W.C., McGargill, M.A., Hart, M.C., Naylor, S., and Jameson, S.C.: **Identification of a naturally occurring ligand for thymic positive selection.** *Immunity* 1997, **6**:389–399.

Huessman, M., Scott, B., Kisielow, P., and von Boehmer, H.: **Kinetics and efficacy of positive selection in the thymus of normal and T-cell receptor transgenic mice.** *Cell* 1991, **66**:533–562.

Stefanski, H.E., Mayerova, D., Jameson, S.C., and Hogquist, K.A.: **A low affinity TCR ligand restores positive selection of CD8+ T cells in vivo.** *J. Immunol.* 2001, **166**:6602–6607.

7-20 Positive selection acts on a repertoire of receptors with inherent specificity for MHC molecules.

Merkenschlager, M., Graf, D., Lovatt, M., Bommhardt, U., Zamoyska, R., and Fisher, A.G.: **How many thymocytes audition for selection?** *J. Exp. Med.* 1997, **186**:1149–1158.

Zerrahn, J., Held, W., and Raulet, D.H.: **The MHC reactivity of the T cell repertoire prior to positive and negative selection.** *Cell* 1997, **88**:627–636.

7-21 Positive selection coordinates the expression of CD4 or CD8 with the specificity of the T-cell receptor and the potential effector functions of the T cell.

Basson, M.A., Bommhardt, U., Cole, M.S., Tso, J.Y., and Zamoyska, R.: **CD3 ligation on immature thymocytes generates antagonist-like signals appropriate for CD8 lineage commitment, independently of T cell receptor specificity.** *J. Exp. Med.* 1998, **187**:1249–1260.

von Boehmer, H., Kisielow, P., Lishi, H., Scott, B., Borgulya, P., and Teh, H.S.: **The expression of CD4 and CD8 accessory molecules on mature T cells is not random but correlates with the specificity of the αβ receptor for antigen.** *Immunol. Rev.* 1989, **109**:143–151.

Bommhardt, U., Cole, M.S., Tso, J.Y., and Zamoyska, R.: **Signals through CD8 or CD4 can induce commitment to the CD4 lineage in the thymus.** *Eur. J. Immunol.* 1997, **27**:1152–1163.

Germain, R.N.: **T-cell development and the CD4-CD8 lineage decision.** *Nat. Rev. Immunol.* 2002, **2**:309–322.

Lundberg, K., Heath, W., Kontgen, F., Carbone, F.R., and Shortman, K.: **Intermediate steps in positive selection: differentiation of CD4$^+$8^{int} TCR^{int} thymocytes into CD4$^-$8$^+$TCR^{hi} thymocytes.** *J. Exp. Med.* 1995, **181**:1643–1651.

Singer, A., Bosselut, R., and Bhandoola, A.: **Signals involved in CD4/CD8 lineage commitment: current concepts and potential mechanisms.** *Semin. Immunol.* 1999, **11**:273–281.

7-22 Thymic cortical epithelial cells mediate positive selection of developing thymocytes.

Cosgrove, D., Chan, S.H., Waltzinger, C., Benoist, C., and Mathis, D.: **The thymic compartment responsible for positive selection of CD4$^+$ T cells.** *Int. Immunol.* 1992, **4**:707–710.

Ernst, B.B., Surh, C.D., and Sprent, J.: **Bone marrow-derived cells fail to induce positive selection in thymus reaggregation cultures.** *J. Exp. Med.* 1996, **183**:1235–1240.

Fowlkes, B.J., and Schweighoffer, E.: **Positive selection of T cells.** *Curr. Opin. Immunol.* 1995, **7**:188–195.

7-23 T cells that react strongly with ubiquitous self antigens are deleted in the thymus.

Kishimoto, H., and Sprent, J.: **Negative selection in the thymus includes semimature T cells.** *J. Exp. Med.* 1997, **185**:263–271.

Zal, T., Volkmann, A., and Stockinger, B.: **Mechanisms of tolerance induction in major histocompatibility complex class II-restricted T cell specific for a blood-borne self antigen.** *J. Exp. Med.* 1994, **180**:2089–2099.

7-24 Negative selection is driven most efficiently by bone marrow derived antigen-presenting cells.

Matzinger, P., and Guerder, S.: **Does T cell tolerance require a dedicated antigen-presenting cell?** *Nature* 1989, **338**:74–76.

Sprent, J., and Webb, S.R.: **Intrathymic and extrathymic clonal deletion of T cells.** *Curr. Opin. Immunol.* 1995, **7**:196–205.

Webb, S.R., and Sprent, J.: **Tolerogenicity of thymic epithelium.** *Eur. J. Immunol.* 1990, **20**:2525–2528.

7-25 The specificity and/or the strength of signals for negative and positive selection must differ.

Alberola-Ila, J., Hogquist, K.A., Swan, K.A., Bevan, M.J., and Perlmutter, R.M.: **Positive and negative selection invoke distinct signaling pathways.** *J. Exp. Med.* 1996, **184**:9–18.

Ashton-Rickardt, P.G., Bandeira, A., Delaney, J.R., Van Kaer, L., Pircher, H.P., Zinkernagel, R.M., and Tonegawa, S.: **Evidence for a differential avidity model of T-cell selection in the thymus.** *Cell* 1994, **76**:651–663.

Bommhardt, U., Basson, M.A., Krummrei, U., and Zamoyska, R.: **Activation of the extracellular signal-related kinase/mitogen-activated protein kinase pathway discriminates CD4 versus CD8 lineage commitment in the thymus.** *J. Immunol.* 1999, **163**:715–722.

Bommhardt, U., Scheuring, Y., Bickel, C., Zamoyska, R., and Hunig, T.: **MEK activity regulates negative selection of immature CD4$^+$CD8$^+$ thymocytes.** *J. Immunol.* 2000, **164**:2326–2337.

Hogquist, K.A., Jameson, S.C., Heath, W.R., Howard, J.L., Bevan, M.J., and Carbone, F.R.: **T-cell receptor antagonist peptides induce positive selection.** *Cell* 1994, **76**:17–27.

7-26 Lymphocytes are found in particular locations in peripheral lymphoid tissues.

Liu, Y.J.: **Sites of B lymphocyte selection, activation, and tolerance in spleen.** *J. Exp. Med.* 1997, **186**:625–629.

Loder, F., Mutschler, B., Ray, R.J., Paige, C.J., Sideras, P., Torres, R., Lamers, M.C., and Carsetti, R.: **B cell development in the spleen takes place in discrete steps and is determined by the quality of B cell receptor-derived signals.** *J. Exp. Med.* 1999, **190**:75–89.

Mebius, R.E.: **Organogenesis of lymphoid tissues.** *Nat. Rev. Immunol.* 2003, **3**:292–303.

7-27 The development and organization of peripheral lymphoid tissues is controlled by tumor necrosis factor family molecules, and the homing of lymphocytes is mediated by chemokines.

Ansel, K.M., and Cyster, J.G.: **Chemokines in lymphopoiesis and lymphoid organ development.** *Curr. Opin. Immunol.* 2001, **13**:172–179.

Cyster, J.G.: **Chemokines and cell migration in secondary lymphoid organs.** *Science* 1999, **286**:2098–2102.

Cyster, J.G.: **Leukocyte migration: scent of the T zone.** *Curr. Biol.* 2000, **10**:R30–R33.

Cyster, J.G., Ansel, K.M., Reif, K., Ekland, E.H., Hyman, P.L., Tang, H.L., Luther, S.A., and Ngo, V.N.: **Follicular stromal cells and lymphocyte homing to follicles.** *Immunol. Rev.* 2000, **176**:181–193.

Douni, E., Akassoglou, K., Alexopoulou, L., Georgopoulos, S., Haralambous, S., Hill, S., Kassiotis, G., Kontoyiannis, D., Pasparakis, M., Plows, D., Probert, L., and Kollias, G.: **Transgenic and knockout analysis of the role of TNF in immune regulation and disease pathogenesis.** *J. Inflamm.* 1996, **47**:27–38.

Fu, Y.X., and Chaplin, D.D.: **Development and maturation of secondary lymphoid tissues.** *Annu. Rev. Immunol.* 1999, **17**:399–433.

Mariathasan, S., Matsumoto, M., Baranyay, F., Nahm, M.H., Kanagawa, O., and Chaplin, D.D.: **Absence of lymph nodes in lymphotoxin-α (LTα)-deficient mice is due to abnormal organ development, not defective lymphocyte migration.** *J. Inflamm.* 1995, **45**:72–78.

7-28 The further development and homeostasis of peripheral lymphocytes is determined via cytokines and by signals that lymphocytes continually receive through their antigen receptors.

Cyster, J.G., Hartley, S.B., and Goodnow, C.C.: **Competition for follicular niches excludes self-reactive cells from the recirculating B-cell repertoire.** *Nature* 1994, **371**:389–395.

Lam, K.P., Kuhn, R., and Rajewsky, K.: *In vivo* **ablation of surface immunoglobulin on mature B cells by inducible gene targeting results in rapid cell death.** *Cell* 1997, **90**:1073–1083.

7-29   Lymphocytes that encounter sufficient quantities of self antigens for the first time in the periphery are eliminated or inactivated.

Arnold, B.: **Levels of peripheral T cell tolerance.** *Transpl. Immunol.* 2002, **10**:109–114.

Goodnow, C.C., Crosbie, J., Jorgensen, H., Brink, R.A., and Basten, A.: **Induction of self-tolerance in mature peripheral B lymphocytes.** *Nature* 1989, **342**:385–391.

Russell, D.M., Dembic, Z., Morahan, G., Miller, J.F.A.P., Burki, K., and Nemazee, D.: **Peripheral deletion of self-reactive B cells.** *Nature* 1991, **354**:308–311.

Steinman, R.M., and Nussenzweig, M.C.: **Avoiding horror autotoxicus: the importance of dendritic cells in peripheral T cell tolerance.** *Proc. Natl. Acad. Sci. USA* 2002, **99**:351–358.

7-30   Most immature B cells arriving in the spleen are short-lived and require cytokines and positive signals through the B-cell receptor for maturation and survival.

Allman, D.M., Ferguson, S.E., Lentz, V.M., and Cancro, M.P.: **Peripheral B cell maturation. II. Heat-stable antigen**[hi] **splenic B cells are an immature developmental intermediate in the production of long-lived marrow-derived B cells.** *J. Immunol.* 1993, **151**:4431–4444.

Harless, S.M., Lentz, V.M., Sah, A.P., Hsu, B.L., Clise-Dwyer, K., Hilbert, D.M., Hayes, C.E., and Cancro, M.P.: **Competition for BLyS-mediated signaling through Bcmd/BR3 regulates peripheral B lymphocyte numbers.** *Curr. Biol.* 2001, **11**:1986–1989.

Levine, M.H., Haberman, A.M., Sant'Angelo, D.B., Hannum, L.G., Cancro, M.P., Janeway, C.A., Jr., and Shlomchik, M.J.: **A B-cell receptor-specific selection step governs immature to mature B cell differentiation.** *Proc. Natl. Acad. Sci. USA* 2000, **97**:2743–2748.

Rolink, A.G., Tschopp, J., Schneider, P., and Melchers, F.: **BAFF is a survival and maturation factor for mouse B cells.** *Eur. J. Immunol.* 2002, **32**:2004–2010.

7-31   The specificity of the B-cell receptor is important in determining the differentiation and survival of B cells in the periphery.

Clarke, S.H., and Arnold, L.W.: **B-1 cell development: evidence for an uncommitted immunoglobulin (Ig)M**[+] **B cell precursor in B-1 cell differentiation.** *J. Exp. Med.* 1998, **187**:1325–1334.

Hardy, R.R., and Hayakawa, K.: **A developmental switch in B lymphopoiesis.** *Proc. Natl. Acad. Sci. USA* 1991, **88**:11550–11554.

Hayakawa, K., Asano, M., Shinton, S.A., Gui, M., Allman, D., Stewart, C.L., Silver, J., and Hardy, R.R.: **Positive selection of natural autoreactive B cells.** *Science*

1999, **285**:113–116.

Martin, F., and Kearney, J.F.: **Marginal-zone B cells.** *Nat. Rev. Immunol.* 2002, **2**:323–335.

7-32   The life-span of T cells in the periphery is determined by cytokines as well as ongoing contact with self-peptide:self-MHC complexes similar to those that initially selected them.

Freitas, A.A., and Rocha, B.: **Peripheral T cell survival.** *Curr. Opin. Immunol.* 1999, **11**:152–156.

Judge, A.D., Zhang, X., Fujii, H., Surh, C.D., and Sprent, J.: **Interleukin 15 controls both proliferation and survival of a subset of memory-phenotype CD8**[+] **T cells.** *J. Exp. Med.* 2002, **196**:935–946.

Kassiotis, G., Garcia, S., Simpson, E., and Stockinger, B.: **Impairment of immunological memory in the absence of MHC despite survival of memory T cells.** *Nature Immunol.* 2002, **3**:244–250.

Ku, C.C., Murakami, M., Sakamoto, A., Kappler, J., and Marrack, P.: **Control of homeostasis of CD8+ memory T cells by opposing cytokines.** *Science* 2000, **288**:675–678.

Murali-Krishna, K., Lau, L.L., Sambhara, S., Lemonnier, F., Altman, J., and Ahmed, R.: **Persistence of memory CD8 T cells in MHC class I-deficient mice.** *Science* 1999, **286**:1377–1381.

Seddon, B., Tomlinson, P., and Zamoyska, R.: **IL-7 and T cell receptor signals regulate homeostasis of CD4 memory cells.** *Nat. Immunol.* 2003, **4**:680–686.

7-33   B-cell tumors often occupy the same site as their normal counterparts.

Alizadeh, A.A., and Staudt, L.M.: **Genomic-scale gene expression profiling of normal and malignant immune cells.** *Curr. Opin. Immunol.* 2000, **12**:219–225.

Cotran, R.S., Kumar, V., and Robbins, S.L.: *Diseases of White Cells, Lymph Nodes, and Spleen. Pathologic Basis of Disease*, 5th edn, 629–672. Philadelphia, W.B. Saunders, 1994.

7-34   A range of tumors of immune system cells throws light on different stages of T-cell development.

Hwang, L.Y., and Baer, R.J.: **The role of chromosome translocations in T cell acute leukemia.** *Curr. Opin. Immunol.* 1995, **7**:659–664.

Rabbitts, T.H.: **Chromosomal translocations in human cancer.** *Nature* 1994, **372**:143–149.

7-35   Malignant lymphocyte tumors frequently carry chromosomal translocations that join immunoglobulin loci to genes that regulate cell growth.

Cory, S.: **Regulation of lymphocyte survival by the Bcl-2 gene family.** *Annu. Rev. Immunol.* 1995, **13**:513–543.

Rabbitts, T.H.: **Chromosomal translocations in human cancer.** *Nature* 1994, **372**:143–149.

Yang, E., and Korsmeyer, S.J.: **Molecular thanatopsis—a discourse on the Bcl-2 family and cell death.** *Blood* 1996, **88**:386–401.

T Cell-Mediated Immunity

Once they have completed their development in the thymus, T cells enter the bloodstream and are carried by the circulation. On reaching a peripheral lymphoid organ they leave the blood again to migrate through the lymphoid tissue, returning to the bloodstream to recirculate between blood and peripheral lymphoid tissue. Mature recirculating T cells that have not yet encountered their specific antigens are known as **naive T cells**. During this seemingly endless recirculation, the naive T cells receive periodic survival signals from encounter with self-peptide:self-MHC complexes and also through their IL-7 receptors. To participate in an adaptive immune response, a naive T cell must first encounter its specific antigen, and then be induced to proliferate and differentiate into cells that can contribute to the removal of the antigen. We will term these latter cells **armed effector T cells** because they act very rapidly when they encounter their specific antigen on other cells. The cells on which armed effector T cells act will be referred to as their **target cells**.

In this chapter we will see how naive T cells are activated to produce armed effector T cells the first time they encounter their specific antigen in the form of a peptide:MHC complex on the surface of an activated **antigen-presenting cell** (APC). The most important antigen-presenting cells are the highly specialized **dendritic cells**, whose only known function is to ingest and present antigen. Tissue dendritic cells ingest antigen at sites of infection and are activated as part of the innate immune response. This induces their migration to local lymphoid tissue and their maturation into cells that are highly effective at presenting antigen to recirculating T cells. These mature dendritic cells are distinguished by surface molecules, known as **co-stimulatory molecules**, that synergize with antigen in the activation of naive T cells. **Macrophages**, which we described in Chapter 2 as phagocytic cells that provide a first line of defense against infection, can also be activated to express co-stimulatory and MHC class II molecules. This enables them to act as antigen-presenting cells, although they are less powerful than dendritic cells at activating naive T cells. B cells can also serve as antigen-presenting cells in some circumstances. Once a T-cell response has been initiated, macrophages and B cells that have taken up specific antigen also become targets for armed effector T cells. Dendritic cells, macrophages, and B cells are often known as professional antigen-presenting cells.

As we learned in Chapter 5, effector T cells fall into three functional classes that detect peptide antigens derived from different types of pathogen. Peptides from intracellular pathogens that multiply in the cytoplasm are carried to the cell surface by MHC class I molecules and presented to CD8

T cells. These differentiate into **cytotoxic T cells** that kill infected target cells. Peptide antigens from pathogens multiplying in intracellular vesicles, and those derived from ingested extracellular bacteria and toxins, are carried to the cell surface by MHC class II molecules and presented to CD4 T cells. These can differentiate into two types of effector T cell, called T_H1 and T_H2. Pathogens that accumulate in large numbers inside macrophage and dendritic cell vesicles tend to stimulate the differentiation of T_H1 cells, whereas extracellular antigens tend to stimulate the production of T_H2 cells. T_H1 cells activate the microbicidal properties of macrophages and induce B cells to make IgG antibodies that are very effective at opsonizing extracellular pathogens for ingestion by phagocytic cells. Both T_H2 and T_H1 cells can initiate the humoral immune response by activating naive antigen-specific B cells to produce IgM antibodies. The T_H2 cells can subsequently stimulate the production of different isotypes, including IgA and IgE, as well as neutralizing and/or weakly opsonizing subtypes of IgG. Fig. 8.1 shows the involvement of the different effector T cells in the immune responses to different classes of pathogens.

The activation of naive T cells in response to antigen, and their subsequent proliferation and differentiation into armed effector cells, constitutes a **primary cell-mediated immune response**. At the same time as providing armed effector T cells, this response generates immunological memory, which gives protection from subsequent challenge by the same pathogen. The generation of memory T cells, long-lived cells that give an accelerated response to antigen, is much less well understood than the generation of effector T cells and will be dealt with in Chapter 10. Memory T cells differ in several ways from naive T cells, but like naive T cells they are quiescent and require activation by antigen-presenting cells with co-stimulatory activity to regenerate effector T cells.

Armed effector T cells differ in many ways from their naive precursors, and these changes equip them to respond quickly and efficiently when they encounter specific antigen on target cells. In the last two sections of this chapter we will describe the specialized mechanisms of T cell-mediated cytotoxicity and of macrophage activation by armed effector T cells, the major components of **cell-mediated immunity**. We will only touch on the activation of B cells by helper T cells until Chapter 9, where the humoral or antibody-mediated immune response is discussed.

Fig. 8.1 The role of effector T cells in cell-mediated and humoral immune responses to representative pathogens. Cell-mediated immune responses are directed principally at intracellular pathogens. They involve the destruction of infected cells by cytotoxic T cells, or the destruction of intracellular pathogens by macrophages activated by T_H1 cells. Both T_H2 and T_H1 cells can also contribute to humoral immunity by inducing the production of antibodies. T_H1 cells induce strongly opsonizing antibody isotypes, whereas T_H2 cells initiate the humoral response by activating naive B cells to secrete IgM, and induce the production of other antibody isotypes including weakly opsonizing antibodies such as IgG1 and IgG3 (mouse) and IgG2 and IgG4 (human) as well as IgA and IgE (mouse and human). All types of antibody contribute to humoral immunity, which is directed principally at extracellular pathogens. Note, however, that both cell-mediated and humoral immunity are involved in many infections, such as the response to *Pneumocystis carinii*, which requires antibody for ingestion by phagocytes and macrophage activation for effective destruction of the ingested pathogen.

	Cell-mediated immunity		Humoral immunity
Typical pathogens	Vaccinia virus Influenza virus Rabies virus *Listeria*	*Mycobacterium tuberculosis* *Mycobacterium leprae* *Leishmania donovani* *Pneumocystis carinii*	*Clostridium tetani* *Staphylococcus aureus* *Streptococcus pneumoniae* Polio virus *Pneumocystis carinii* *Trichinella spiralis*
Location	Cytosol	Macrophage vesicles	Extracellular fluid
Effector T cell	Cytotoxic CD8 T cell	T_H1 cell	T_H1 and T_H2 cells
Antigen recognition	Peptide:MHC class I complex on infected cell	Peptide:MHC class II complex on infected macrophage	Peptide:MHC class II complex on antigen-specific B cell
Effector action	Killing of infected cell	Activation of infected macrophages	Activation of specific B cell to make antibody

The production of armed effector T cells.

For activation, a naive T cell must recognize a foreign peptide bound to a self MHC molecule. But this is not, on its own, sufficient for activation. That requires the simultaneous delivery of a **co-stimulatory signal** by a specialized antigen-presenting cell. Only dendritic cells, macrophages, and B cells are able to express both classes of MHC molecule as well as the co-stimulatory cell-surface molecules that drive the clonal expansion of naive T cells and their differentiation into armed effector T cells.

The most potent activators of naive T cells are mature dendritic cells, and these are thought to initiate most, if not all, T-cell responses *in vivo.* As we will describe in this part of the chapter, immature dendritic cells in the tissues take up antigen at sites of infection and are activated to travel to local lymphoid tissues. Here they mature into cells that express high levels of co-stimulatory molecules and the adhesion molecules that mediate interactions with the naive T cells continually recirculating through these tissues. The activation and clonal expansion of a naive T cell on initial encounter with antigen on the surface of an antigen-presenting cell is often called **priming**, to distinguish it from the responses of armed effector T cells to antigen on their target cells and from the responses of primed memory T cells.

8-1   T-cell responses are initiated in peripheral lymphoid organs by activated antigen-presenting cells.

Adaptive immune responses are not initiated in the tissues where a pathogen first establishes a focus of infection but in the peripheral lymphoid tissues through which naive T cells are continually migrating. Pathogens and their products are transported to lymphoid tissue by the lymph that drains the infected tissue, or, more rarely, by the blood. Pathogens infecting mucosal surfaces accumulate in the Peyer's patches of the gut or the tonsils; those that enter the blood are trapped in the spleen; and those infecting other sites are trapped in the lymph nodes directly downstream of the site of infection (see Section 1-3). All lymphoid organs contain mature dendritic cells that have captured antigen at the site of infection.

The delivery of antigen from a site of infection to downstream lymphoid tissue and its subsequent presentation to naive T cells is actively aided by the innate immune response. As discussed in Chapter 2, this is rapidly triggered at the site of infection by nonclonal receptors that recognize molecular patterns that are associated with pathogens but not with host cells. One of the induced responses of innate immunity is an inflammatory reaction that increases the entry of plasma into the infected tissues and the consequent drainage of these tissue fluids into the lymph. Another is the induced maturation of tissue dendritic cells that have been taking up particulate and soluble antigens at the site of infection (Fig. 8.2). These cells are activated through receptors that signal the presence of pathogen components or by cytokines produced during the inflammatory response. The dendritic cells respond by migrating to the lymph node and expressing the co-stimulatory molecules that are required, in addition to antigen, for the activation of naive T cells. Macrophages, which are phagocytic cells found in tissues and scattered throughout lymphoid tissue, and B cells, which bind pathogen components, may be similarly induced through the same non-antigen-specific receptors to express co-stimulatory molecules and act as antigen-presenting cells. Thus the innate immune response to infection hastens the transport of antigens to the local lymphoid tissue and enables those cells that have taken up antigen to present it effectively to the naive T cells that migrate through this tissue.

Fig. 8.2 Immature dendritic cells ingest antigen in the tissues.

Immature dendritic cells in the tissues have a very dendritic morphology, with many long processes, as shown in the top panels. On the left, the tissue is stained for MHC class II molecules in green and for a lysosomal protein in red. The cell bodies of these immature dendritic cells are difficult to distinguish in this figure, but you can see that the cell contains many endocytic vesicles that stain both for MHC class II molecules and for the lysosomal protein; when these two colors overlap they give rise to a yellow fluorescence. On the right, in the scanning electron micrograph, you can see the many long processes, or dendrites, from which the cell gets its name. These immature cells are activated and leave the tissues to migrate through the lymphatics to secondary lymphoid tissues. During this migration their morphology changes, as shown in the middle panels. The dendritic cells also stop phagocytosing antigen, and in the left panel you can see that the staining for lysosomal proteins is beginning to be distinct from that for MHC class II molecules. The dendritic cell now has many folds of membrane, as shown in the photo on the right, which gave these cells their original name of 'veil' cells. Finally, in the lymph nodes (bottom panels), they become mature dendritic cells that express high levels of peptide:MHC complexes and co-stimulatory molecules, and are very good at stimulating naive CD4 and naive CD8 T cells. Here the cells do not phagocytose and again the red staining of lysosomal proteins is quite distinct from the green-stained MHC class II molecules displayed at high density on many dendritic processes. The micrograph on the left shows the typical morphology of a mature dendritic cell. Fluorescent micrographs courtesy of I. Mellman, P. Pierre, and S. Turley. Scanning electron micrographs courtesy of K. Dittmar.

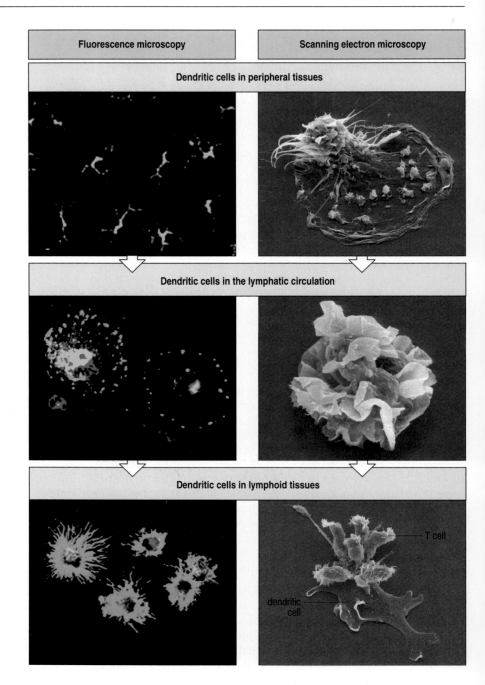

The distribution of dendritic cells, macrophages, and B cells in a lymph node is shown schematically in Fig. 8.3. Dendritic cells are present mainly in the T-cell areas. They are named after their fingerlike processes, which form a network of branches among the T cells. By the time they arrive in the lymph nodes, dendritic cells have lost their ability to capture new antigen. They are, however, able to present the antigens they ingested at the site of infection, and in their mature activated form they are the most potent antigen-presenting cells for naive T cells.

Macrophages are found in many areas of the lymph node, especially in the marginal sinus, where the afferent lymph enters the lymphoid tissue, and in the medullary cords, where the efferent lymph collects before flowing into the blood. Here they can actively ingest microbes and particulate antigens and so prevent them from entering the blood. Because most pathogens are particulate, macrophages in the T-cell areas may stimulate immune responses to many sources of infection.

Finally, the B cells, which recirculate through the lymphoid tissues and concentrate in the lymphoid follicles, are particularly efficient at taking up soluble antigens such as bacterial toxins by the specific binding of antigen to the B-cell surface immunoglobulin. The antigen:receptor complex is internalized by receptor-mediated phagocytosis, and degraded fragments of the antigen can return to the B-cell surface complexed with MHC class II molecules. Antigen-specific B cells can thus activate naive CD4 T cells if the B cells are also induced to express co-stimulatory molecules. B cells are, however, very inefficient at initiating adaptive immune responses. This is because only those with the appropriate receptor specificity can internalize and present a particular antigen at high density, and these will be very scarce. Thus, the probability of their encountering a naive T cell specific for the same antigen is very low.

The antigen-presenting function of dendritic cells, macrophages, and B cells will be discussed in more detail in Sections 8-6 to 8-8. Only these three cell types express the specialized co-stimulatory molecules required to activate naive T cells; furthermore, all of these cell types express these molecules only when suitably activated in the context of a response to infection. Dendritic cells can take up, process, and present a wide variety of pathogens and antigens, and seem to be the most important activators of naive T cells; in contrast, macrophages and B cells specialize in processing and presenting antigens from ingested pathogens and soluble antigens, respectively, and are also the targets of subsequent actions of armed effector CD4 T cells.

8-2   Naive T cells sample the MHC:peptide complexes on the surface of antigen-presenting cells as they migrate through peripheral lymphoid tissue.

Naive T cells enter lymphoid tissue by crossing the walls of specialized venules known as **high endothelial venules** (**HEVs**). They circulate continuously from the bloodstream to the lymphoid organs and back to the blood, making contact with many thousands of antigen-presenting cells in the lymphoid tissues every day. These contacts allow the naive T cells to sample MHC:peptide complexes on the surface of these antigen-presenting cells, which is important for two reasons. One is that it seems to reinforce the positive selection for self-peptide:self-MHC recognition that occurred during T-cell development. As discussed in Chapter 7, T-cell receptors are selected for their ability to interact with self-MHC:self-peptide complexes. In this way, a repertoire of mature T cells is selected that can be activated by nonself peptides bound to the same MHC molecules. Recent experiments show that T-cell survival in the periphery also depends on contact with self-MHC:self-peptide ligands (see Section 7-32), and that these signals are delivered effectively through interactions with such complexes on dendritic cells. Thus, as naive T cells migrate through peripheral lymphoid tissue, they receive survival signals through their interactions with dendritic cells. At the same time, the sampling of MHC:peptide ligands ensures that each T cell has a high probability of encountering antigens derived from pathogens at any site of infection. This is crucial for the initiation of an adaptive immune response, as only one naive T cell in 10^4–10^6 is likely to be specific for a particular antigen, and adaptive immunity depends on the activation and expansion of these rare cells (Fig. 8.4). The T cells that do not encounter their specific antigen eventually reach the medulla of the lymph node, from whence they are carried by the efferent lymphatics back to the blood to continue recirculating through other

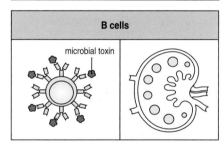

Fig. 8.3 Antigen-presenting cells are distributed differentially in the lymph node. Dendritic cells are found throughout the cortex of the lymph node in the T-cell areas. Macrophages are distributed throughout but are found mainly in the marginal sinus, where the afferent lymph collects before percolating through the lymphoid tissue, and also in the medullary cords, where the efferent lymph collects before passing via the efferent lymphatics into the blood. B cells are found mainly in the follicles. The three types of antigen-presenting cell are thought to be adapted to present different types of pathogen or products of pathogens, but mature dendritic cells are by far the strongest activators of naive T cells.

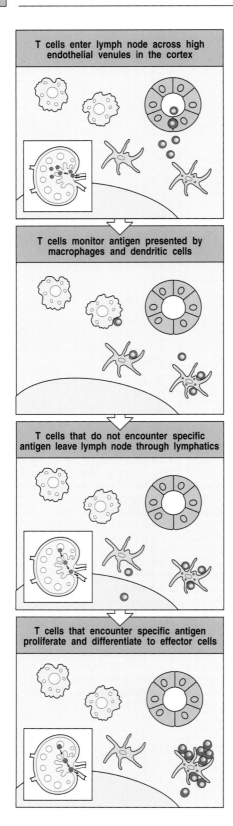

T cells enter lymph node across high endothelial venules in the cortex

T cells monitor antigen presented by macrophages and dendritic cells

T cells that do not encounter specific antigen leave lymph node through lymphatics

T cells that encounter specific antigen proliferate and differentiate to effector cells

Fig. 8.4 Naive T cells encounter antigen during their recirculation through peripheral lymphoid organs. Naive T cells recirculate through peripheral lymphoid organs, such as the lymph node shown here, entering through specialized regions of vascular endothelium called high endothelial venules. On leaving the blood vessel, the T cells enter the deep cortex of the lymph node, where they encounter mature dendritic cells. Those T cells shown in green do not encounter their specific antigen. They receive a survival signal through their interaction with self-MHC:self-peptide complexes and IL-7, and leave the lymph node through the lymphatics to return to the circulation. T cells shown in blue encounter their specific antigen on the surface of an antigen-presenting cell and are activated to proliferate and to differentiate into armed effector T cells. These antigen-specific armed effector T cells, now increased 100–1000-fold in number, also leave the lymph node via the efferent lymphatics and enter the circulation.

lymphoid organs. Naive T cells that recognize their specific antigen on the surface of a dendritic cell cease to migrate, and embark on the generation of armed effector cells, which takes several days. At the end of this period the armed effector T cells leave the lymphoid organ and reenter the bloodstream to migrate to sites of infection.

8-3 Lymphocyte migration, activation, and effector function depend on cell–cell interactions mediated by cell-adhesion molecules.

The migration of naive T cells through the lymph nodes, and their initial interactions with antigen-presenting cells, depend on lymphocytes binding to high endothelial venules through interactions that are not antigen-specific. Similar interactions eventually guide the effector T cells into the peripheral tissues and have an important role in their interaction with target cells. Binding of T cells to high endothelial venules is controlled by an array of adhesion molecules on the surface of the T lymphocyte that recognize a complementary array of adhesion molecules on the surface of the venule. The main classes of adhesion molecule involved in lymphocyte interactions are the selectins, the integrins, members of the immunoglobulin superfamily, and some mucin-like molecules. We have already encountered members of the first three classes in the recruitment of neutrophils and monocytes to sites of infection during an innate immune response (see Section 2-22). Most adhesion molecules have fairly broad roles in the generation of immune responses. Many that are involved in lymphocyte migration and the interactions of armed effector T cells with their targets are also involved in interactions of other leukocytes with endothelium. Adhesion molecules are also important in getting lymphocytes together in adaptive immune responses that involve T-cell–B-cell interactions, and we will describe these in Chapter 10, where we present an integrated view of the immune response.

The selectins (Fig. 8.5) are particularly important for leukocyte homing to particular tissues and can be expressed either on leukocytes (**L-selectin**, CD62L) or on vascular endothelium (**P-selectin**, CD62P, and **E-selectin**, CD62E). L-selectin is expressed on naive T cells and guides their exit from the blood into peripheral lymphoid tissues. P-selectin and E-selectin are expressed on the vascular endothelium at sites of infection and serve to recruit effector cells into the tissues at these sites (see Sections 2-22 and 2-23). Selectins are cell-surface molecules with a common core structure, distinguished from each other by the presence of different lectin-like domains in their extracellular portion (see Fig. 2.42). The lectin domains bind to particular sugar groups, and each selectin binds to a cell-surface carbohydrate. L-selectin binds to the carbohydrate moiety, sulfated sialyl-Lewis^x, of mucin-like molecules called **vascular addressins**, which are expressed on the surface of vascular endothelial cells. Two of these addressins, **CD34** and

GlyCAM-1, are expressed as sulfated sialyl-Lewis^x molecules on high endothelial venules in lymph nodes. A third, **MAdCAM-1**, is expressed on endothelium in mucosa, and guides lymphocyte entry into mucosal lymphoid tissue such as those of the gut.

The interaction between L-selectin and the vascular addressins is responsible for the specific homing of naive T cells to lymphoid organs but does not, on its own, enable the cell to cross the endothelial barrier into the lymphoid tissue. For this, proteins from two other families—the integrins and the immunoglobulin superfamily—are required. These proteins also have a crucial role in the subsequent interactions of lymphocytes with antigen-presenting cells and later with their target cells.

The integrins comprise a large family of cell-surface proteins that mediate adhesion between cells, and between cells and the extracellular matrix, in normal development as well as in immune and inflammatory responses. Integrins bind tightly to their ligands after receiving signals that induce a change in their conformation. For example, as we saw in Chapter 2, signaling by chemokines activates integrins on leukocytes to bind tightly to the vascular surface during the migration of leukocytes into sites of inflammation. Chemokines similarly activate T-cell integrins during the migration of T lymphocytes into lymphoid organs and in the migration of activated T lymphocytes to sites of infection.

The migration of naive T cells into lymphoid tissues is mediated by the chemokine **CCL21**, also known as **SLC** (secondary lymphoid tissue chemokine). This is expressed by high vascular endothelial cells, stromal cells, and dendritic cells in lymphoid tissue, and binds to the CCR7 chemokine receptor on naive T cells. This interaction stimulates the receptor-associated Gα_i G protein, which in turn, by a mechanism not yet fully worked out, rapidly increases both the affinity of integrin binding and the mobility of integrin in the T-cell membrane so that an increased number of integrin molecules can migrate into the area of cell–cell contact. The combination of these changes in integrin affinity and avidity arrest the T cell's progress through the blood and enable it to enter the lymphoid tissue. Similar interactions with chemokines produced at sites of inflammation direct effector T-cell migration into the tissues; this will be discussed in more detail in Chapter 10. Chemokines are not the only molecules able to stimulate increased integrin affinity; later in this chapter we will see how signaling through the T-cell receptor also triggers T-cell integrins to adhere tightly to their ligands on antigen-presenting cells and on the target cells that bear specific peptide:MHC complexes.

The integrins were introduced in Chapter 2, so we will just review their most important characteristics here. An integrin molecule consists of a large α chain that pairs noncovalently with a smaller β chain. There are several

Fig. 8.5 L-selectin and the mucin-like vascular addressins direct naive lymphocyte homing to lymphoid tissues. L-selectin is expressed on naive T cells, which bind to sulfated sialyl-Lewis^x moieties on the vascular addressins CD34 and GlyCAM-1 on high endothelial venules in order to enter lymph nodes. The relative importance of CD34 and GlyCAM-1 in this interaction is unclear. GlyCAM-1 is expressed exclusively on high endothelial venules but has no transmembrane region and it is unclear how it is attached to the membrane; CD34 has a transmembrane anchor and is expressed in appropriately glycosylated form only on high endothelial venule cells, although it is found in other forms on other endothelial cells. The addressin MAdCAM-1 is expressed on mucosal endothelium and guides entry into mucosal lymphoid tissue. The icon shown represents mouse MAdCAM-1, which contains an IgA-like domain closest to the cell membrane; human MAdCAM-1 has an elongated mucin-like domain and lacks the IgA-like domain. L-selectin recognizes the carbohydrate moieties on the vascular addressins.

Fig. 8.6 Integrins are important in T-lymphocyte adhesion. Integrins are heterodimeric proteins containing a β chain, which defines the class of integrin, and an α chain, which defines the different integrins within a class. The α chain is larger than the β chain and contains binding sites for divalent cations that may be important in signaling. LFA-1 is a β$_2$ integrin that is expressed on all T cells and indeed on all leukocytes. It binds ICAMs and is important in the adhesive interactions that mediate cell migration and in the interactions of T cells with antigen-presenting or target cells; the level of its expression is increased on armed effector T cells. Lymphocyte Peyer's patch adhesion molecule, LPAM-1 (integrin α$_4$:β$_7$), is expressed by a subset of naive T cells and contributes to mucosal homing by supporting adhesive interactions with MAdCAM-1. VLA-4 is a β$_1$ integrin that increases its expression after T-cell activation. It binds to VCAM-1 on activated endothelium and, as we will discuss further in Chapter 10, is important for recruiting armed effector T cells into sites of infection.

Leukocyte
Adhesion Deficiency

subfamilies of integrins, broadly defined by their common β chains. We will be concerned chiefly with the **leukocyte integrins**, which have a common β$_2$ chain with distinct α chains (Fig. 8.6). All T cells express a β$_2$ integrin known as **lymphocyte function-associated antigen-1** (**LFA-1**). This leukocyte integrin is also found on macrophages and neutrophils, and is involved in their recruitment to sites of infection (see Section 2-22). LFA-1 has a similar role in the migration of both naive and effector T cells out of the blood. In addition, it is thought to be the most important adhesion molecule for T-cell activation, because antibodies against LFA-1 effectively inhibit the activation of both naive and armed effector T cells.

Despite this, however, T-cell responses can be normal in patients lacking the β$_2$ integrin chain and hence all integrins that contain β$_2$, including LFA-1. This is probably because T cells also express other adhesion molecules, including CD2 and β$_1$ integrins, that may be able to compensate for the absence of LFA-1. Expression of the β$_1$ integrins increases significantly at a late stage in T-cell activation, and they are thus often called **VLAs**, for **very late activation antigens**; we will see in Chapter 10 that they are important in directing armed effector T cells to their inflamed target tissues.

Many cell-adhesion molecules are members of the immunoglobulin superfamily, which also includes the antigen receptors of T and B cells, the co-receptors CD4, CD8, and CD19, and the invariant domains of MHC molecules. At least five adhesion molecules of the immunoglobulin superfamily are especially important in T-cell activation (Fig. 8.7). Three very similar **intercellular adhesion molecules** (**ICAMs**)—**ICAM-1**, **ICAM-2**, and **ICAM-3**—all bind to the T-cell integrin LFA-1. ICAM-1 and ICAM-2 are expressed on endothelium as well as on antigen-presenting cells; binding to these molecules enables lymphocytes to migrate through blood vessel walls. ICAM-3 is expressed only on leukocytes and is thought to have an important role in adhesion between

Fig. 8.7 Immunoglobulin superfamily adhesion molecules involved in leukocyte interactions. Adhesion molecules of the immunoglobulin superfamily bind to adhesion molecules of various types, including integrins (LFA-1 and VLA-4), other immunoglobulin superfamily members (the CD2–CD58 (LFA-3) interaction) and lectins (DC-SIGN). These interactions have a role in lymphocyte migration, homing, and cell–cell interactions; most of the molecules listed here have been introduced in Fig. 2.42.

Immunoglobulin superfamily	Name	Tissue distribution	Ligand
Various roles in cell adhesion. Ligands for integrins	CD2 (LFA-2)	T cells	CD58 (LFA-3)
	ICAM-1 (CD54)	Activated vessels, lymphocytes, dendritic cells	LFA-1, Mac1
	ICAM-2 (CD102)	Resting vessels	LFA-1
	ICAM-3 (CD50)	Naive T cells	DC-SIGN, LFA-1
	LFA-3 (CD58)	Lymphocytes, antigen-presenting cells	CD2
	VCAM-1 (CD106)	Activated endothelium	VLA-4

T cells and antigen-presenting cells, particularly dendritic cells. In addition to binding LFA-1, ICAM-3 binds with high affinity to a recently discovered lectin called **DC-SIGN**, which is found only on dendritic cells. The two remaining immunoglobulin superfamily adhesion molecules, **CD58** (formerly known as LFA-3) on the antigen-presenting cell and CD2 on the T cell, bind to each other; this interaction synergizes with that of ICAM-1 or ICAM-2 with LFA-1.

8-4   The initial interaction of T cells with antigen-presenting cells is mediated by cell-adhesion molecules.

As they migrate through the cortical region of the lymph node, naive T cells bind transiently to each antigen-presenting cell that they encounter. Antigen-presenting cells, and dendritic cells in particular, bind naive T cells very efficiently through interactions between LFA-1, ICAM-3, and CD2 on the T cell, and ICAM-1, ICAM-2, DC-SIGN, and CD58 on the antigen-presenting cell (Fig. 8.8). The binding of ICAM-3 to DC-SIGN is unique to the interaction between dendritic cells and T cells, whereas the other molecules synergize in the binding of lymphocytes to all three types of antigen-presenting cell. Perhaps because of this synergy, the precise role of each adhesion molecule has been difficult to distinguish. People lacking LFA-1 can have normal T-cell responses, and this also seems to be true for genetically engineered mice lacking CD2. It would not be surprising if there were enough redundancy in the molecules mediating T-cell adhesive interactions to enable immune responses to occur in the absence of any one of them; such molecular redundancy has been observed in other complex biological processes.

The transient binding of naive T cells to antigen-presenting cells is crucial in providing time for T cells to sample large numbers of MHC molecules on each antigen-presenting cell for the presence of a specific peptide. In those rare cases in which a naive T cell recognizes its peptide:MHC ligand, signaling through the T-cell receptor induces a conformational change in LFA-1, which greatly increases its affinity for ICAM-1 and ICAM-2. This conformational change is the same as that induced by signaling through chemokine receptors during the migration of leukocytes to sites of infection (see Section 2-21), although its mechanism is not known. The change in LFA-1 stabilizes the association between the antigen-specific T cell and the antigen-presenting cell (Fig. 8.9). The association can persist for several days, during which time the naive T cell proliferates and its progeny, which also adhere to the antigen-presenting cell, differentiate into armed effector T cells.

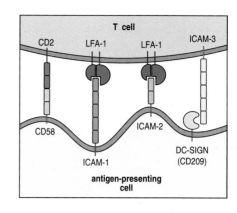

Fig. 8.8 Cell-surface molecules of the immunoglobulin superfamily are important in the interactions of lymphocytes with antigen-presenting cells. In the initial encounter of T cells with antigen-presenting cells, CD2 binding to CD58 on the antigen-presenting cell synergizes with LFA-1 binding to ICAM-1 and ICAM-2. One interaction that seems to be exclusive to the interaction of naive T cells with dendritic cells is that between ICAM-3 on the naive T cell and DC-SIGN (CD209), a C-type lectin that is specific to dendritic cells and binds ICAM-3 with high affinity. LFA-1 is the $\alpha_L{:}\beta_2$ integrin heterodimer CD11a:CD18. ICAM-1, -2, and -3 are also known as CD54, CD102, and CD50, respectively.

Fig. 8.9 Transient adhesive interactions between T cells and antigen-presenting cells are stabilized by specific antigen recognition. When a T cell binds to its specific ligand on an antigen-presenting cell, intracellular signaling through the T-cell receptor (TCR) induces a conformational change in LFA-1 that causes it to bind with higher affinity to ICAMs on the antigen-presenting cell. The T cell shown here is a CD4 T cell.

Specific signal and co-stimulator

APC

MHC class II

antigen

T-cell receptor

CD4

T cell

Activates T cell

Fig. 8.10 Activation of naive T cells requires two independent signals delivered by the same antigen-presenting cell. Binding of the foreign peptide:self-MHC complex by the T-cell receptor and, in this example, a CD4 co-receptor, transmits a signal (arrow 1) to the T cell that antigen has been encountered. Activation of naive T cells requires a second signal (arrow 2), the co-stimulatory signal, to be delivered by the same antigen-presenting cell.

Most T-cell encounters with antigen-presenting cells do not, however, result in the recognition of an antigen; instead, they deliver a survival signal. In these encounters, the T cells must be able to separate efficiently from the antigen-presenting cells so that they can continue to migrate through the lymph node, eventually leaving via the efferent lymphatic vessels to reenter the blood and continue circulating. Dissociation, like stable binding, may also involve signaling between the T cell and the antigen-presenting cells, but little is known of its mechanism.

8-5   Both specific antigen and co-stimulatory signals provided by the same antigen-presenting cell are required for the clonal expansion of naive T cells.

We saw in Chapter 6 that armed effector T cells are triggered into action when their antigen-specific receptors and either the CD4 or CD8 co-receptors bind to peptide:MHC complexes. By contrast, ligation of the T-cell receptor and co-receptor does not, on its own, stimulate naive T cells to proliferate and differentiate into armed effector T cells. The antigen-specific clonal expansion of naive T cells requires a second, or co-stimulatory, signal (Fig. 8.10), which must be delivered by the same antigen-presenting cell on which the T cell recognizes its antigen. CD8 T cells seem to require a stronger co-stimulatory signal than CD4 T cells and, as we will see later, their clonal expansion is aided by CD4 cells interacting with the same antigen-presenting cell.

The best-characterized co-stimulatory molecules are the structurally related glycoproteins **B7.1** (CD80) and **B7.2** (CD86). We will call them the **B7 molecules** from here on, as functional differences between the two have yet to be defined. The B7 molecules are homodimeric members of the immunoglobulin superfamily that are found exclusively on the surfaces of cells that stimulate T-cell proliferation. Their role in co-stimulation has been demonstrated by transfecting fibroblasts that express a T-cell ligand with genes encoding B7 molecules and showing that the fibroblasts could then stimulate the clonal expansion of naive T cells. The receptor for B7 molecules on the T cell is **CD28**, yet another member of the immunoglobulin superfamily (Fig. 8.11). Ligation of CD28 by B7 molecules or by anti-CD28 antibodies is absolutely required for the clonal expansion of naive T cells, whereas anti-B7 antibodies, which inhibit the binding of B7 molecules to CD28, inhibit T-cell responses. Although other molecules have been reported to co-stimulate naive T cells, so far only the B7 molecules have been shown definitively to provide co-stimulatory signals for naive T cells in normal immune responses.

Once a naive T cell is activated it expresses a number of proteins that contribute to sustaining or modifying the co-stimulatory signal that drives clonal expansion and differentiation. One such protein is **CD40 ligand** (CD154), so called because it binds to **CD40** on antigen-presenting cells. Binding of CD40 by CD40 ligand transmits activating signals to the T cell and also activates the antigen-presenting cell to express B7 molecules, thus stimulating further T-cell proliferation. CD40 and CD40 ligand belong to the tumor necrosis factor (TNF)

T cell

CD4

TCR/CD3 complex

CD28

B7.1 or B7.2

APC   MHC class II

Fig. 8.11 The principal co-stimulatory molecules expressed on antigen-presenting cells are B7 molecules, which bind the T-cell protein CD28. Binding of the T-cell receptor:CD3 complex (TCR:CD3) and its co-receptor CD4 to the peptide:MHC class II complex on the antigen-presenting cell (APC) delivers a signal (arrow 1) that can induce the clonal expansion of T cells only when the co-stimulatory signal (arrow 2) is given by binding of CD28 to B7 molecules. Both CD28 and B7 molecules are members of the immunoglobulin superfamily. B7.1 (CD80) and B7.2 (CD86) are homodimers, each of whose chains has one immunoglobulin V-like domain and one C-like domain. CD28 is a disulfide-linked homodimer in which each chain has one V-like domain.

family of receptors and ligands, which, as we will describe later in this chapter, have a central role in the effector function of fully differentiated T cells. Their earlier role in sustaining the development of a T-cell response is demonstrated in mice lacking CD40 ligand; when these mice are immunized, the clonal expansion of responding T cells is curtailed at an early stage. Another pair of TNF family molecules that seem to contribute to the co-stimulation of T cells are the T-cell molecule **4-1BB** (CD137) and its ligand **4-1BBL**, which is expressed on activated dendritic cells, macrophages, and B cells. As with CD40 ligand and CD40, the effects of this receptor–ligand interaction are bidirectional, with both the T cell and the antigen-presenting cell receiving activating signals; this process is sometimes referred to as the T-cell:antigen-presenting cell dialogue.

CD28-related proteins are also induced on activated T cells and serve to modify the co-stimulatory signal as the T-cell response develops. One is **CTLA-4** (CD152), an additional receptor for B7 molecules. CTLA-4 closely resembles CD28 in sequence, and the two proteins are encoded by closely linked genes. However, CTLA-4 binds B7 molecules about 20 times more avidly than does CD28 and delivers an inhibitory signal to the activated T cell (Fig. 8.12). This makes the activated progeny of a naive T cell less sensitive to stimulation by the antigen-presenting cell and limits production of the autocrine T-cell growth factor IL-2. Thus, binding of CTLA-4 to B7 molecules is essential for limiting the proliferative response of activated T cells to antigen and B7. This was confirmed by producing mice with a disrupted CTLA-4 gene; such mice develop a fatal disorder characterized by a massive overgrowth of lymphocytes.

A third CD28-related protein is induced on activated T cells and can enhance T-cell responses; this inducible co-stimulator, or **ICOS**, binds a ligand known as **LICOS**, the ligand of ICOS, which is distinct from B7.1 and B7.2. LICOS is produced on activated dendritic cells, monocytes, and B cells, but its contribution to immune responses has not yet been clearly defined. Although it resembles CD28 in driving T-cell growth, it differs from CD28 in not inducing IL-2; instead it induces the cytokine IL-10, which inhibits the differentiation of T_H1 cells.

Fig. 8.12 T-cell activation through the T-cell receptor and CD28 leads to the increased expression of CTLA-4, an inhibitory receptor for B7 molecules. Naive T cells express CD28, which delivers a co-stimulatory signal on binding B7 molecules (left panel), thereby driving the activation and expansion of T cells that encounter specific antigen presented by a B7-positive antigen-presenting cell. Once activated, T cells express increased levels of CTLA-4 (CD152; right panel). CTLA-4 has a higher affinity for B7 molecules than does CD28 and thus binds most or all of the B7 molecules, effectively shutting down the proliferative phase of the response.

Thus, antigen-presenting cells engage in a co-stimulatory dialogue with naive T cells that recognize the antigens they display. This involves the delivery and receipt of signals through several different molecules, but seems to be initiated through the binding of B7 molecules to CD28 on the T cell. Antigen-presenting cells are activated to express B7 molecules on detecting the presence of infection through receptors of the innate immune system. There is therefore a requirement for the simultaneous delivery of antigen-specific and co-stimulatory signals by one cell in the activation of naive T cells. This means that only activated antigen-presenting cells, principally the dendritic cells that migrate into lymphoid tissue after being activated by binding and ingesting pathogens, can initiate T-cell responses. This is important because not all potentially self-reactive T cells are deleted in the thymus; peptides derived from proteins made only in specialized cells in peripheral tissues might not be encountered during negative selection of thymocytes. Self-tolerance could be broken if naive autoreactive T cells could recognize self antigens on tissue cells and then be co-stimulated by an antigen-presenting cell, either locally or at a distant site. Thus, the requirement that the same cell present both the specific antigen and the co-stimulatory signal is important in preventing destructive immune responses to self tissues. Indeed, antigen binding to the T-cell receptor in the absence of co-stimulation not only fails to activate the cell, it instead leads to a state called **anergy**, in which the T cell becomes refractory to activation by specific antigen even when the antigen is subsequently presented to it by a professional antigen-presenting cell (Fig. 8.13).

Fig. 8.13 The requirement for one cell to deliver both the antigen-specific signal and the co-stimulatory signal is crucial in preventing immune responses to self antigens. In the upper panels, a T cell recognizes a viral peptide on the surface of an antigen-presenting dendritic cell (DC) and is activated to proliferate and differentiate into an effector cell capable of eliminating any virus-infected cell. In contrast, naive T cells that recognize antigen on cells that cannot provide co-stimulation become anergic, as when a T cell recognizes a self antigen expressed by an uninfected epithelial cell (lower panels). This T cell does not differentiate into an armed effector cell, and cannot even be activated by a subsequent encounter with a professional antigen-presenting cell bearing the same antigen.

Now that we have discussed the molecular interactions that allow naive T cells to adhere transiently to antigen-presenting cells and scan their MHC:peptide complexes, and also the adhesion and co-stimulatory molecules that contribute to T-cell activation once a specific antigen is encountered, we will look more closely at the properties of the three types of antigen-presenting cell. Dendritic cells, macrophages, and B cells differ in their selectivity of antigen uptake, their antigen-processing properties, and their co-stimulatory and migratory behavior, and thus have distinctive functions in initiating T-cell responses.

8-6   Dendritic cells specialize in ingesting antigen and activating naive T cells.

The only known function of dendritic cells is to present antigen to T cells, and the mature dendritic cells found in peripheral lymphoid tissues are by far the most potent stimulators of naive T cells. This ability is not shared, however, by the immature dendritic cells found under most surface epithelia and in most solid organs such as the heart and kidneys. Dendritic cells can arise from both myeloid and lymphoid progenitors within the bone marrow, and emerge from the bone marrow to migrate via the blood to peripheral tissues. There they have an immature phenotype that is associated with low levels of MHC proteins, and they lack co-stimulatory B7 molecules (Fig 8.14, top panel). They are not yet equipped to stimulate naive T cells. However, they share with their close relatives, the macrophages, the ability to recognize and ingest pathogens through receptors that recognize features common to microbial surfaces, and they are very active in taking up antigens by phagocytosis using receptors such as the lectin DEC 205. Other extracellular antigens are taken up nonspecifically by **macropinocytosis**, in which large volumes of surrounding fluid are engulfed.

Typical of immature dendritic cells are the **Langerhans' cells** of the skin. These are actively phagocytic and contain large granules, known as Birbeck granules, which may be a type of phagosome. An infection triggers the migration of Langerhans'cells to the regional lymph nodes (Fig. 8.15). Here they rapidly lose the ability to take up and process antigen but synthesize new MHC molecules that present peptides of pathogens at a high level. On arriving in the regional lymph node they also express B7 molecules, which can co-stimulate naive T cells, and also large numbers of adhesion molecules, which enable them to interact with antigen-specific T cells. In this way the Langerhans' cells capture antigens from invading pathogens and differentiate into mature dendritic cells that are uniquely fitted for presenting these antigens and activating naive T cells.

Fig. 8.14 Dendritic cells mature through at least two definable stages to become potent antigen-presenting cells in peripheral lymphoid tissue. Dendritic cells originate from bone marrow progenitors and migrate via the blood to peripheral tissues and organs, where they are highly phagocytic via receptors such as DEC 205 and are actively macropinocytic but do not express co-stimulatory molecules (top panel). At sites of infection they pick up antigen and are induced to migrate via the afferent lymphatic vessels to the regional lymph node (see Fig. 8.15). Here they are powerful activators of naive T cells but are no longer phagocytic. Dendritic cells in lymphoid tissue express B7.1, B7.2, and high levels of MHC class I and class II molecules, as well as high levels of the adhesion molecules ICAM-1, ICAM-2, LFA-1, and CD58 (center panel). They also express high levels of the dendritic-cell-specific adhesion molecule DC-SIGN, which binds ICAM-3 with high affinity. Dendritic cells also secrete DC-CK (CCL18), secreted chemokine with high DC-CK (CCL18), secreted chemokine affinity. The photograph shows a mature dendritic cell. Photograph courtesy of J. Barker.

Fig. 8.15 Langerhans' cells can take up antigen in the skin, migrate to the peripheral lymphoid organs, and present foreign antigens to T cells. Langerhans' cells can ingest antigen by several means, but have no co-stimulatory activity. In the presence of infection, they take up antigen locally in the skin and then migrate to the lymph nodes. There they differentiate into dendritic cells that can no longer ingest antigen but now have co-stimulatory activity.

Immature dendritic cells persist in the peripheral tissues for variable lengths of time. When an infection occurs, they are stimulated to migrate via the lymphatics to the local lymphoid tissues, where they have a completely different phenotype. The dendritic cells in lymphoid tissue are no longer able to engulf antigens by phagocytosis or by macropinocytosis. However, they now express very high levels of long-lived MHC class I and MHC class II molecules; this enables them to stably present peptides from proteins acquired from the infecting pathogens. They also express very high levels of adhesion molecules, including DC-SIGN, as well as high levels of B7 molecules (see Fig. 8.14, center panel). They also secrete a chemokine that specifically attracts naive T cells; this chemokine, called DC-CK (CCL18), is expressed only in dendritic cells in lymphoid tissues. These properties help to explain the dendritic cell's ability to stimulate strong naive T-cell responses.

Although activated mature dendritic cells will also present some self peptides, the T-cell receptor repertoire has been purged in the thymus of receptors that recognize self peptides presented by dendritic cells (see Chapter 7), and thus T-cell responses against ubiquitous self antigens are avoided. In addition, tissue dendritic cells reaching the end of their life-span in body tissues without having been activated by infection also travel via the lymphatics to local lymphoid tissue. Because they do not express the appropriate co-stimulatory molecules, these cells induce tolerance to any self antigens that they display which are derived from the peripheral tissues.

The signals that activate tissue dendritic cells to migrate and mature after taking up antigen are clearly of key importance in determining whether an adaptive immune response will be initiated. These signals can be generated through direct interactions with pathogens or by stimulation by cytokines, but in both cases they are thought to be a consequence of the recognition of invading pathogens by nonclonotypic receptors of the innate immune system. The best-understood example is the response to Gram-negative bacteria, whose cell walls contain lipopolysaccharide (LPS). Receptors that recognize

LPS are found on dendritic cells and macrophages, and these associate with the Toll-like signaling receptor TLR-4, which then activates the transcription factor NFκB (see Sections 2-8 and 6-17). Signaling through this pathway induces the expression of B7 molecules and of cytokines such as TNF-α, which stimulate the migration of tissue dendritic cells. Thus, an immature tissue dendritic cell that binds and internalizes Gram-negative bacteria is induced to migrate to local lymphoid tissue and to present bacterial-derived peptide antigens to naive T cells. Other members of the TLR family are expressed on tissue dendritic cells and are thought to be involved in detecting and signaling the presence of other classes of pathogen (see Fig. 2.12). Other types of receptor that can bind pathogens, such as receptors for complement, or phagocytic receptors such as the mannose receptor, are also expressed on dendritic cells and may contribute to their activation.

Pathogens that have evolved to escape recognition by phagocytic receptors are taken up by tissue dendritic cells through the process of macropinocytosis. Intracellular degradation of the pathogen produces peptides that can subsequently be presented to naive T cells and is thought to reveal components that trigger activation of the dendritic cell. Bacterial DNA containing unmethylated CpG dinucleotide motifs induces the rapid activation of dendritic cells. This probably occurs after recognition of the DNA by a receptor called TLR-9, which is present in intracellular vesicles. Exposure to bacterial DNA activates NFκB and mitogen-activated protein kinase (MAP kinase) signaling pathways, leading to the production of cytokines such as IL-6, IL-12, IL-18, and interferon (IFN)-α and IFN-γ. In turn, these cytokines augment the expression of the co-stimulatory molecules. Heat-shock proteins are another internal bacterial constituent that can activate the antigen-presenting function of dendritic cells. Some viruses are thought to be recognized inside the dendritic cell, as a consequence of the production of double-stranded RNA in the course of their replication. As discussed in Section 2-26, viral infection also induces the production of IFN-α and IFN-β by infected cells. IFN-α and IFN-β can further activate dendritic cells to express increased levels of co-stimulatory molecules.

Dendritic cells are likely to be particularly important in stimulating T-cell responses to viruses, which fail to induce co-stimulatory activity in other types of antigen-presenting cell. Viruses may infect dendritic cells by binding to any of several molecules on the cell surface, or after being engulfed but not destroyed by immature dendritic cells. Such viruses synthesize their proteins by using the dendritic cell's own protein synthesis machinery, leading to the surface expression of viral peptides bound to MHC class I molecules just as in other types of infected cell. Viral peptides will also be presented on both MHC class I and MHC class II molecules as a result of ingesting viral particles by phagocytic receptors such as the mannose receptor, which can recognize many viruses, or through macropinocytosis. The mechanism by which peptides generated by degradation of viral proteins in the endosomal pathway can be presented by MHC class I molecules is not known; nor, in fact, is it known whether there is only one such mechanism. Nevertheless, it is clear that extracellular proteins taken up by dendritic cells can give rise to peptides presented by MHC class I molecules, leading to the mechanism known as **cross-priming**. In this way, viruses that are not able to infect dendritic cells are still able to stimulate effective immune responses. Thus, any virus infection can lead to the activation of virus-specific naive CD8 T cells, generating cytotoxic CD8 effector T cells that can kill infected cells. In addition, viral peptides presented on the dendritic cell's MHC class II molecules will activate CD4 T cells that can stimulate the production of antibodies as well as the production of IFN-γ and members of the TNF family of cytokines.

Dendritic cells are believed to present antigens from fungal as well as viral and bacterial pathogens. Indeed, they are thought to initiate immune responses to a wide range of pathogens, and to be able to distinguish between different classes of pathogen. This is reflected in the synthesis of different effector molecules by the activated dendritic cells, which in turn influence the differentiation of the responding T cells into different subclasses, which is discussed further in Section 10-5. In addition to pathogen-associated antigens, dendritic cells are known to present alloantigens deriving from a transplanted organ, which form the basis for graft rejection (see Chapter 13), and are thought to present protein antigens from environmental sources that trigger allergic reactions upon inhalation (see Chapter 12). In principle, any nonself antigen will be immunogenic if it is taken up and subsequently presented by an activated dendritic cell. The normal physiology of dendritic cells is to migrate, and this is increased by stimuli such as transplantation, which activate the linings of the lymphatics; this is why dendritic cells are so potent at stimulating allograft reactions.

8-7 Macrophages are scavenger cells that can be induced by pathogens to present foreign antigens to naive T cells.

As we learned in Chapter 2, many of the microorganisms that enter the body are engulfed and destroyed by phagocytes, which provide an innate, antigen-nonspecific first line of defense against infection. Microorganisms that are destroyed by phagocytes without additional help from T cells do not cause disease and do not require an adaptive immune response. Pathogens, by definition, have developed mechanisms to avoid elimination by innate immunity, and the targeting and removal of such pathogens is the function of the adaptive immune response. Mononuclear phagocytes or macrophages that have bound and ingested microorganisms, but have failed to destroy them, contribute to the adaptive immune response by acting as antigen-presenting cells. As we will see later in this chapter and in Chapter 10, the adaptive immune response is in turn able to stimulate the microbicidal and phagocytic capacities of these cells.

Resting macrophages have few or no MHC class II molecules on their surface and do not express B7 molecules. The expression of both MHC class II and B7 molecules is induced by the ingestion of microorganisms and recognition of their foreign molecular patterns. Macrophages, like tissue dendritic cells, have a variety of receptors that recognize microbial surface components, including the mannose receptor, the scavenger receptor, complement receptors, and several Toll-like receptors (see Chapter 2). These receptors function in innate immune defense mediated by macrophages; they are involved in the ingestion of microorganisms by phagocytosis and in signaling for the secretion of pro-inflammatory cytokines, which recruit and activate more phagocytes. The phagocytic receptors can function similarly to those on tissue dendritic cells and thus allow the macrophage to function as an antigen-presenting cell. Once bound, microorganisms are engulfed and degraded in the endosomes and lysosomes, generating peptides that can be presented by MHC class II molecules. At the same time, the receptors recognizing these microorganisms transmit a signal that leads to the expression of MHC class II molecules and B7 molecules.

Thus, the induction of co-stimulatory activity by common microbial constituents occurs in both dendritic cells and macrophages. This is believed to allow the immune system to distinguish antigens borne by infectious agents from antigens associated with innocuous proteins, including self proteins. Indeed, many foreign proteins do not induce an immune response when injected on their own, presumably because they fail to induce co-stimulatory

Fig. 8.16 Microbial substances can induce co-stimulatory activity in macrophages. If protein antigens are taken up and presented by macrophages in the absence of bacterial components that induce co-stimulatory activity in the macrophage, T cells specific for the antigen will become anergic (refractory to activation). Almost all microbes can induce the expression of co-stimulators by antigen-presenting cells, and macrophages presenting peptide antigens derived by degradation of such bacteria can activate naive T cells. When bacteria are mixed with protein antigens, the protein antigens are rendered immunogenic because the bacteria induce co-stimulatory B7 molecules in the antigen-presenting cells. Such added bacteria act as adjuvants (see Appendix I, Section A-4).

activity in antigen-presenting cells. When such protein antigens are mixed with bacteria, however, they become immunogenic, because the bacteria induce the essential co-stimulatory activity in cells that ingest the protein (Fig. 8.16). Bacteria used in this way are known as **adjuvants** (see Appendix I, Section A-4). We will see in Chapter 13 how self tissue proteins mixed with bacterial adjuvants can induce autoimmune diseases, illustrating the crucial importance of the regulation of co-stimulatory activity in the discrimination of self from nonself.

As macrophages continuously scavenge dead or dying cells, which are rich sources of self antigens, it is particularly important that they should not activate T cells in the absence of microbial infection. The Kupffer cells of the liver sinusoids and the macrophages of the splenic red pulp, in particular, remove large numbers of dying cells from the blood daily. Kupffer cells express little MHC class II and no TLR-4, the Toll-like receptor on human cells that signals the presence of LPS. Thus, although they generate large amounts of self peptides in their endosomes and lysosomes, these macrophages are not likely to elicit an autoimmune response.

8-8   B cells are highly efficient at presenting antigens that bind to their surface immunoglobulin.

Macrophages cannot take up soluble antigens efficiently, whereas immature dendritic cells can take up large amounts of antigen from extracellular fluid by nonspecific macropinocytosis. B cells, by contrast, are uniquely adapted to bind specific soluble molecules through their cell-surface immunoglobulin. B cells internalize the antigens bound by their surface immunoglobulin receptors and then display peptide fragments of antigen as peptide:MHC class II complexes. Because this mechanism of antigen uptake is highly efficient and B cells constitutively express high levels of MHC class II molecules,

Fig. 8.17 B cells can use their surface immunoglobulin to present specific antigen very efficiently to T cells.
Surface immunoglobulin allows B cells to bind and internalize specific antigen very efficiently, especially if the antigen is present as a soluble protein, as most toxins are. The internalized antigen is processed in intracellular vesicles where it binds to MHC class II molecules. The vesicles are transported to the cell surface where the MHC class II:foreign-peptide complexes can be recognized by T cells. When the protein antigen is not specific for the B-cell receptor, its internalization is inefficient and only a few fragments of such proteins are subsequently presented at the B-cell surface (not shown).

Antigen-specific B cell binds antigen	Specific antigen efficiently internalized by receptor-mediated endocytosis	High density of specific antigen fragments presented

high levels of specific peptide:self-MHC class II complexes are generated at the B-cell surface (Fig. 8.17). This pathway of antigen presentation allows B cells to be targeted by antigen-specific CD4 T cells, which drive their differentiation, as we will see in Chapter 9. In circumstances in which the presenting B cells are induced to express co-stimulatory activity they can also activate naive T cells.

B cells do not constitutively express co-stimulatory activity but, as with dendritic cells and macrophages, they can be induced by various microbial constituents to express B7 molecules, especially B7.2. In fact, B7.1 was first identified as a molecule expressed on B cells activated by microbial LPS. These observations help to explain why it is essential to co-inject bacterial adjuvants to produce an immune response to soluble proteins such as ovalbumin, hen egg-white lysozyme, and cytochrome *c*, which may require B cells as antigen-presenting cells.

The requirement for induced co-stimulatory activity also helps to explain why, although B cells present soluble proteins efficiently, they are unlikely to initiate responses to soluble self proteins in the absence of infection. In the absence of co-stimulation, antigen not only fails to activate naive T cells but causes them to become anergic or unresponsive (see Fig. 8.13). This provides an additional safeguard to the mechanisms discussed in Chapter 7 whereby potentially self-reactive T and B cells are eliminated or inactivated as they develop in the thymus and bone marrow.

Although much of what we know about the immune system in general, and about T-cell responses in particular, has been learned from the study of immune responses to soluble protein immunogens presented by B cells, it is not clear how important B cells are in priming naive T cells in natural immune responses. Soluble protein antigens are not abundant during natural infections; most natural antigens, such as bacteria and viruses, are particulate, whereas soluble bacterial toxins act by binding to cell surfaces and so are present only at low concentrations in solution. Some natural immunogens enter the body as soluble molecules: examples are insect toxins, anticoagulants injected by blood-sucking insects, snake venoms, and many allergens. However, tissue dendritic cells could also be responsible for activating naive T cells that recognize these antigens. Although tissue dendritic cells could not concentrate these antigens in the same way as antigen-specific B cells, they may be more likely to encounter a naive T cell with the appropriate antigen specificity than the limited number of B cells able to bind and concentrate a particular antigen. The chances of a B cell's encountering a T cell that can recognize the peptide antigens it displays is greatly increased once a naive T cell has been detained in lymphoid tissue by finding its antigen on the surface of a dendritic cell.

	Dendritic cells	Macrophages	B cells
Antigen uptake	+++ Macropinocytosis and phagocytosis by tissue dendritic cells Viral infection	Phagocytosis +++	Antigen-specific receptor (Ig) ++++
MHC expression	Low on tissue dendritic cells High on dendritic cells in lymphoid tissues	Inducible by bacteria and cytokines – to +++	Constitutive Increases on activation +++ to ++++
Co-stimulator delivery	Constitutive by mature, nonphagocytic lymphoid dendritic cells ++++	Inducible – to +++	Inducible – to +++
Antigen presented	Peptides Viral antigens Allergens	Particulate antigens Intracellular and extracellular pathogens	Soluble antigens Toxins Viruses
Location	Ubiquitous throughout the body	Lymphoid tissue Connective tissue Body cavities	Lymphoid tissue Peripheral blood

Fig. 8.18 The properties of the various antigen-presenting cells. Dendritic cells, macrophages, and B cells are the main cell types involved in the presentation of foreign antigens to naive T cells. These cells vary in their means of antigen uptake, MHC class II expression, co-stimulator expression, the type of antigen they present effectively, their locations in the body, and their surface adhesion molecules (not shown).

T-cell responses can thus be primed by three distinct types of antigen-presenting cell. Dendritic cells are optimally equipped to present a wide variety of antigens to naive T cells, whereas macrophages stimulate T-cell responses to the pathogens they take up but are unable to eliminate, and B cells specialize in presenting fragments of the antigen to which their surface immunoglobulin binds. The three types of antigen-presenting cell are compared in Fig. 8.18. In each of these cell types, as we saw in Chapter 2, the expression of co-stimulatory activity is controlled so as to provoke responses against pathogens while avoiding immunization against self.

8-9   Activated T cells synthesize the T-cell growth factor interleukin-2 and its receptor.

Naive T cells can live for many years by dividing infrequently and equally infrequently undergoing apoptosis. They are found as small resting cells with condensed chromatin and scanty cytoplasm and synthesize little RNA or protein. On activation, they must reenter the cell cycle and divide rapidly to produce the large numbers of progeny that will differentiate into armed effector T cells. Their proliferation and differentiation are driven by the cytokine **interleukin-2** (**IL-2**), which is produced by the activated T cell itself.

The initial encounter with specific antigen in the presence of a co-stimulatory signal triggers entry of the T cell into the G_1 phase of the cell cycle; at the same time, it also induces the synthesis of IL-2 along with the α chain of the IL-2 receptor (also known as **CD25**). The IL-2 receptor has three chains: α, β, and γ (Fig. 8.19). Resting T cells express a form of this receptor composed of β and γ chains that binds IL-2 with moderate affinity, allowing resting T cells to respond to very high concentrations of IL-2. Association of the α chain

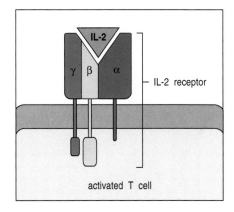

Fig. 8.19 High-affinity IL-2 receptors are three-chain structures that are present only on activated T cells. On resting T cells, the β and γ chains are expressed constitutively. They bind IL-2 with moderate affinity. Activation of T cells induces the synthesis of the α chain and the formation of the high-affinity heterotrimeric receptor. The β and γ chains show similarities in amino-acid sequence to cell-surface receptors for growth hormone and prolactin, both of which also regulate cell growth and differentiation.

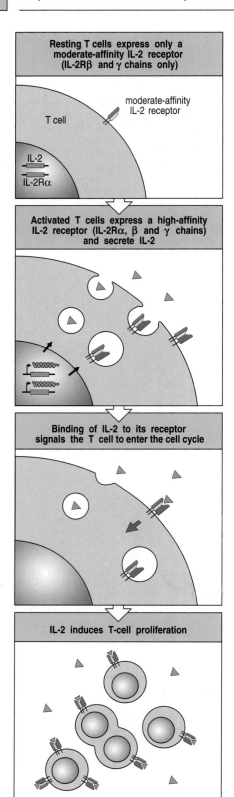

Resting T cells express only a moderate-affinity IL-2 receptor (IL-2Rβ and γ chains only)

moderate-affinity IL-2 receptor

T cell

IL-2

IL-2Rα

Activated T cells express a high-affinity IL-2 receptor (IL-2Rα, β and γ chains) and secrete IL-2

Binding of IL-2 to its receptor signals the T cell to enter the cell cycle

IL-2 induces T-cell proliferation

Fig. 8.20 Activated T cells secrete and respond to IL-2. Activation of naive T cells induces the expression and secretion of IL-2 and the expression of high-affinity IL-2 receptors. IL-2 binds to the high-affinity IL-2 receptors to promote T-cell growth in an autocrine fashion.

with the β and γ heterodimer creates a receptor with a much higher affinity for IL-2, allowing the cell to respond to very low concentrations of IL-2. Binding of IL-2 to the high-affinity receptor then triggers progression through the rest of the cell cycle (Fig. 8.20). T cells activated in this way can divide two or three times a day for several days, allowing one cell to give rise to a clone of thousands of cells that all bear the same receptor for antigen. IL-2 is a survival factor for these cells, and the removal of IL-2 from activated T cells results in their death; it also promotes the differentiation of these activated cells into armed effector T cells.

8-10 The co-stimulatory signal is necessary for the synthesis and secretion of IL-2.

Antigen recognition by the T-cell receptor induces the synthesis of several transcription factors (see Chapter 6). One of these, **NFAT (nuclear factor of activated T cells)**, binds to the promoter region of the IL-2 gene and is needed to activate its transcription. IL-2 gene transcription on its own, however, does not lead to the production of IL-2; this additionally requires ligation of CD28 by the co-stimulatory molecule B7. One effect of signaling through CD28 is thought to be the stabilization of IL-2 mRNA. Cytokine mRNAs are very short-lived because of an 'instability' sequence in their 3′ untranslated region. This instability prevents sustained cytokine production and release, and enables cytokine activity to be tightly regulated. The stabilization of IL-2 mRNA increases IL-2 synthesis 20–30-fold. A second effect of CD28 ligation is to activate transcription factors (AP-1 and NFκB) that increase the transcription of IL-2 mRNA about threefold. These two effects together increase IL-2 protein production as much as 100-fold. When a T cell recognizes specific antigen in the absence of co-stimulation through its CD28 molecule, little IL-2 is produced and the T cell does not proliferate. Thus, the most important function of the co-stimulatory signal is to promote the synthesis of IL-2.

The central importance of IL-2 in initiating adaptive immune responses is well illustrated by the drugs that are most commonly used to suppress undesirable immune responses such as transplant rejection. The immunosuppressive drugs cyclosporin A and FK506 (tacrolimus) inhibit IL-2 production by disrupting signaling through the T-cell receptor, whereas rapamycin (sirolimus) inhibits signaling through the IL-2 receptor. Cyclosporin A and rapamycin act synergistically to inhibit immune responses by preventing the IL-2-driven clonal expansion of T cells. The mode of action of these drugs will be considered in detail in Chapter 14.

8-11 Antigen recognition in the absence of co-stimulation leads to the inactivation of peripheral T cells.

Antigen recognition in the absence of co-stimulation inactivates naive T cells, inducing a state known as anergy. The most important change in anergic T cells is their inability to produce IL-2. This prevents them from proliferating and differentiating into effector cells when they encounter antigen, even if the antigen is subsequently presented by antigen-presenting cells that express co-stimulatory molecules. This helps to ensure the tolerance of T cells to self tissue antigens. Although anergy has only been demonstrated

Fig. 8.21 T-cell tolerance to antigens expressed on tissue cells results from antigen recognition in the absence of co-stimulation. An antigen-presenting cell (APC) will neither activate nor inactivate a T cell if the appropriate antigen is not present on the APC surface, even if it expresses a co-stimulatory molecule and can deliver signal 2 (left panel). However, when a T cell recognizes antigen in the absence of co-stimulatory molecules, it receives signal 1 alone and is inactivated (right panel). This allows self antigens expressed on tissue cells to induce tolerance in the peripheral T-cell population.

formally *in vitro*, there is sufficiently compelling evidence from studies *in vivo* showing peripheral tolerance to various antigens to assume that it happens in this setting as well.

As we saw in Section 7-23, any protein synthesized by all cells will be presented by antigen-presenting cells in the thymus and will induce clonal deletion of the T cells reactive to these ubiquitous self proteins. However, many proteins have specialized functions and are made only by the cells of certain tissues. Because MHC class I molecules present only peptides derived from proteins synthesized within the cell, such tissue-specific self peptides will not be displayed on the MHC molecules of thymic cells, and T cells recognizing them are unlikely to be deleted in the thymus. An important factor in avoiding autoimmune responses to such tissue-specific proteins is the absence of co-stimulatory activity on tissue cells. Naive T cells recognizing self peptides on tissue cells are not activated; instead, they are induced to enter a state of anergy (Fig. 8.21).

Although the deletion of potentially autoreactive T cells is readily understood as a simple way to maintain self tolerance, the retention of anergic T cells specific for tissue antigens is less easy to understand. It would seem more economical and efficient to eliminate such cells; indeed, binding of the T-cell receptor on peripheral T cells in the absence of co-stimulators can lead to programmed cell death as well as to anergy. Nevertheless, some T cells persist in an anergic state *in vivo*. One possible explanation for this is that such anergic T cells have a role in preventing responses by naive, nonanergic T cells to foreign antigens that mimic self-peptide:self-MHC complexes. The persisting anergic T cells could recognize and bind to such peptide:MHC complexes on antigen-presenting cells without responding, and thus could compete with naive, potentially autoreactive cells of the same specificity. In this way, anergic T cells could serve to prevent the accidental activation of autoreactive T cells by infectious agents, thus actively contributing to tolerance.

8-12 Proliferating T cells differentiate into armed effector T cells that do not require co-stimulation to act.

Late in the proliferative phase of the T-cell response induced by IL-2, after 4–5 days of rapid growth, activated T cells differentiate into armed effector T cells that can synthesize all the effector molecules required for their specialized functions as helper or cytotoxic T cells. In addition, all classes of armed effector T cells have undergone changes that distinguish them from naive T cells.

Stimulation of naive T cell	Proliferating T cell	Active effector T cells kill virus-infected target cells
RECOGNITION	PROLIFERATION · DIFFERENTIATION	EFFECTOR FUNCTION

Fig. 8.22 Armed effector T cells can respond to their target cells without co-stimulation. A naive T cell that recognizes antigen on the surface of an antigen-presenting cell and receives the required two signals (arrows 1 and 2, left panel) becomes activated, and both secretes and responds to IL-2. IL-2-driven clonal expansion (center panel) is followed by the differentiation of the T cells to armed effector cell status. Once the cells have differentiated into effector T cells, any encounter with specific antigen triggers their effector actions without the need for co-stimulation. Thus, as illustrated here, a cytotoxic T cell can kill targets that express only the peptide:MHC ligand and not co-stimulatory signals (right panel).

One of the most important is in their activation requirements: once a T cell has differentiated into an armed effector cell, encounter with its specific antigen results in immune attack without the need for co-stimulation (Fig. 8.22).

This applies to all classes of armed effector T cells. Its importance is particularly easy to understand for cytotoxic CD8 T cells, which must be able to act on any cell infected with a virus, whether or not the infected cell can express co-stimulatory molecules. However, it is also important for the effector function of CD4 cells, as armed effector CD4 T cells must be able to activate B cells and macrophages that have taken up antigen even if these cells are not expressing co-stimulatory molecules.

Changes are also seen in the cell-adhesion molecules expressed by armed effector T cells. They express higher levels of LFA-1 and CD2 but lose cell-surface L-selectin and therefore cease to recirculate through lymph nodes. Instead, they express the integrin VLA-4, which allows them to bind to vascular endothelium bearing the molecule **VCAM-1**, which is expressed at sites of inflammation. This allows the armed effector T cells to enter sites of infection and put their armory of effector proteins to good use. These changes in the T-cell surface are summarized in Fig. 8.23.

Fig. 8.23 Activation of T cells changes the expression of several cell-surface molecules. The example here is a CD4 T cell. Resting naive T cells express L-selectin, through which they home to lymph nodes, with relatively low levels of other adhesion molecules such as CD2 and LFA-1. Upon activation, expression of L-selectin ceases and, instead, increased amounts of the integrin LFA-1 are produced, which is activated to bind its ligands ICAM-1 and ICAM-2. A newly expressed integrin called VLA-4, which acts as a homing receptor for vascular endothelium at sites of inflammation, ensures that activated T cells enter peripheral tissues where they may encounter sites of infection. Activated T cells also have a higher density of the adhesion molecule CD2 on their surface, increasing the avidity of the interaction with potential target cells, and a higher density of the adhesion molecule CD44. Finally, the isoform of CD45 expressed changes, by alternative splicing of the RNA transcript of the CD45 gene, so that activated T cells express the CD45RO isoform, which associates with the T-cell receptor and CD4. This change makes the T cell more sensitive to stimulation by lower concentrations of peptide:MHC complexes.

	Cell-surface molecules								
CD4 T cell	L-selectin	VLA-4	LFA-1	CD2	CD4	T-cell receptor	CD44	CD45RA	CD45RO
Resting	+	–	+	+	+	+	+	+	–
Activated	–	+	++	++	+	+	++	–	+

8-13 The differentiation of CD4 T cells into T$_H$1 or T$_H$2 cells determines whether humoral or cell-mediated immunity will predominate.

Naive CD8 T cells emerging from the thymus are already predestined to become cytotoxic cells, even though they are not yet expressing any of the differentiated functions of armed effector cells. The case of CD4 T cells, however, is more complex. Naive CD4 T cells can differentiate upon activation into either T$_H$1 or T$_H$2 cells, which differ in the cytokines that they produce and therefore in their function. The decision on which fate the progeny of a naive CD4 T cell will follow is made during the clonal expansion that takes place after the first encounter with antigen (Fig. 8.24).

The factors that determine whether a proliferating CD4 T cell *in vivo* will differentiate into a T$_H$1 or a T$_H$2 cell are not fully understood. The cytokines elicited by infectious agents (principally IFN-γ, IL-12, and IL-4), the co-stimulators used to drive the response, and the nature of the peptide:MHC ligand all have an effect. In particular, because the decision to differentiate into T$_H$1 versus T$_H$2 cells occurs early in the immune response, the cytokines produced in response to pathogens by cells of the innate immune system have an important role in shaping the subsequent adaptive response; we will learn more about this in Chapter 10.

The consequences of inducing T$_H$1 versus T$_H$2 cells are profound: the selective production of T$_H$1 cells leads to cell-mediated immunity and the production of opsonizing antibody classes (predominantly IgG), whereas the production of predominantly T$_H$2 cells provides humoral immunity, especially IgM, IgA, and IgE. A striking example of the difference this can make to the outcome of infection is seen in leprosy, a disease caused by infection with *Mycobacterium leprae*. *M. leprae*, like *M. tuberculosis*, grows in macrophage vesicles, and effective host defense requires macrophage activation by T$_H$1 cells. In patients with tuberculoid leprosy, in which T$_H$1 cells are preferentially induced, few live bacteria are found, little antibody is produced, and, although skin and peripheral nerves are damaged by the inflammatory responses associated with macrophage activation, the disease progresses slowly and the patient usually survives. However, when T$_H$2 cells are preferentially induced, the main response is humoral, the antibodies produced cannot reach the intracellular bacteria, and the patients develop lepromatous leprosy, in which *M. leprae* grows abundantly in macrophages, causing gross tissue destruction that is eventually fatal.

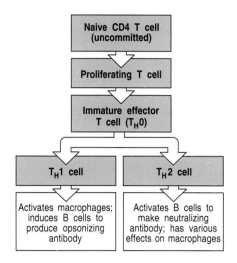

Fig. 8.24 The stages of activation of CD4 T cells. Naive CD4 T cells first respond to their specific peptide:MHC class II complexes by making IL-2 and proliferating. These cells then differentiate into a cell type known as T$_H$0, which has some of the effector functions characteristic of both T$_H$1 and T$_H$2 cells. The T$_H$0 cell has the potential to become either a T$_H$1 cell or a T$_H$2 cell.

Lepromatous Leprosy

8-14 Naive CD8 T cells can be activated in different ways to become armed cytotoxic effector cells.

Naive CD8 T cells differentiate into cytotoxic cells, and perhaps because the effector actions of these cells are so destructive, naive CD8 T cells require more co-stimulatory activity to drive them to become armed effector cells than do naive CD4 T cells. This requirement can be met in two ways. The simplest is activation by mature dendritic cells, which have high intrinsic co-stimulatory activity. These cells can directly stimulate CD8 T cells to synthesize the IL-2 that drives their own proliferation and differentiation (Fig. 8.25). This has been exploited to generate cytotoxic T-cell responses against tumors, as we will see in Chapter 14.

Cytotoxic T-cell responses to some viruses and tissue grafts, however, seem to require the presence of CD4 T cells during the priming of the naive CD8 T cell. In these responses, both the naive CD8 T cell and the CD4 T cell must recognize related antigens on the surface of the same antigen-presenting cell. In this case, it is thought that the actions of the CD4 T cell may be needed to compensate for inadequate co-stimulation of naive CD8 T cells by the infected antigen-presenting cell. This compensatory effect is currently thought

Fig. 8.25 Naive CD8 T cells can be activated directly by potent antigen-presenting cells. Naive CD8 T cells that encounter peptide:MHC class I complexes on the surface of dendritic cells, which express high levels of co-stimulatory molecules (left panel), are activated to produce IL-2 (right panel) and proliferate in response to it, eventually differentiating into armed cytotoxic CD8 T cells (not shown).

Dendritic cells express high levels of B7 and can activate naive CD8 T cells

Activated CD8 T cell makes IL-2, driving its own proliferation and differentiation

APC stimulates effector CD4 T cell, which in turn activates the APC

Activated APC expresses CD40 and 4-IBBL, which co-stimulates naive CD8 T cell

Fig. 8.26 Some CD8 T-cell responses require CD4 T cells. CD8 T cells recognizing antigen on weakly co-stimulatory cells may become activated only in the presence of CD4 T cells bound to the same antigen-presenting cell. This happens mainly by an effector CD4 T cell recognizing antigen on the antigen-presenting cell and being triggered to induce increased levels of co-stimulatory activity on the antigen-presenting cell, which in turn activates the CD8 T cell to make its own IL-2.

to occur by the recruitment of an armed effector CD4 T cell that activates the antigen-presenting cell to express higher levels of co-stimulatory activity. We have seen that this is one of the actions of CD40 ligand, which is expressed once T cells have been activated. Binding of CD40 ligand on the CD4 T cell to CD40 on the antigen-presenting cell induces B7 expression and enables the antigen-presenting cell to co-stimulate the CD8 T cell directly (Fig. 8.26).

Summary.

The crucial first step in adaptive immunity is the activation of naive antigen-specific T cells by antigen-presenting cells. This occurs in the lymphoid tissues and organs through which naive T cells are constantly passing. The most distinctive feature of antigen-presenting cells is the expression of co-stimulatory molecules, of which the B7.1 and B7.2 molecules are the best characterized. Naive T cells will respond to antigen only when one cell presents both a specific antigen to the T-cell receptor and a B7 molecule to CD28, the receptor for B7 on the T cell. The three cell types that can serve as antigen-presenting cells are dendritic cells, macrophages, and B cells. Each of these cells has a distinct function in eliciting immune responses. Tissue dendritic cells take up antigens by phagocytosis and macropinocytosis and are stimulated by infection to migrate to the local lymphoid tissue, where they differentiate into mature dendritic cells expressing co-stimulatory activity. They are the most potent activators of naive T cells. Macrophages efficiently ingest particulate antigens such as bacteria and are induced by infectious agents to express MHC class II molecules and co-stimulatory activity. The unique ability of B cells to bind and internalize soluble protein antigens via their receptors may be important in activating T cells to this class of antigen, provided that co-stimulatory molecules are also induced on the B cell. In all three types of antigen-presenting cell, the expression of co-stimulatory molecules is activated in response to signals from receptors that also function in innate immunity to signal the presence of infectious agents (see Chapter 2).

The activation of T cells by antigen-presenting cells leads to their proliferation and the differentiation of their progeny into armed effector T cells. This depends on the production of cytokines, in particular the T-cell growth factor IL-2, which binds to a high-affinity receptor on the activated T cell. T cells whose antigen receptors are ligated in the absence of co-stimulatory signals fail to make IL-2 and instead become anergic or die. This dual requirement for both receptor ligation and co-stimulation by the same antigen-presenting cell helps to prevent naive T cells from responding to self antigens on tissue cells, which lack co-stimulatory activity.

Proliferating T cells develop into armed effector T cells, the critical event in most adaptive immune responses. Once an expanded clone of T cells achieves effector function, its progeny can act on any target cell that displays antigen on its surface. Effector T cells have a variety of functions. The most important are the killing of infected cells by CD8 cytotoxic T cells and the activation of macrophages by T_H1 cells, which together make up cell-mediated immunity, and the activation of B cells by both T_H2 and T_H1 cells to produce different classes of antibody, thus driving the humoral immune response.

General properties of armed effector T cells.

All T-cell effector functions involve the interaction of an armed effector T cell with a target cell displaying specific antigen. The effector proteins released by these T cells are focused on the appropriate target cell by mechanisms that are activated by recognition of antigen on the target cell. The focusing mechanism is common to all types of effector T cells, whereas their effector actions depend on the array of membrane and secreted proteins that they express or release upon receptor ligation. The different types of effector T cell are specialized to deal with different types of pathogen, and the effector molecules that they are programmed to produce cause distinct and appropriate effects on the target cell (Fig. 8.27).

Fig. 8.27 There are three classes of effector T cell, specialized to deal with three classes of pathogen. CD8 cytotoxic cells (left panels) kill target cells that display peptide fragments of cytosolic pathogens, most notably viruses, bound to MHC class I molecules at the cell surface. T_H1 cells (middle panels) and T_H2 cells (right panels) both express the CD4 co-receptor and recognize fragments of antigens degraded within intracellular vesicles, displayed at the cell surface by MHC class II molecules. T_H1 cells activate macrophages, enabling them to destroy intracellular microorganisms more efficiently. They can also activate B cells to produce strongly opsonizing antibodies belonging to certain IgG subclasses (IgG1 and IgG3 in humans, and their homologs IgG2a and IgG2b in the mouse). T_H2 cells, in contrast, drive B cells to differentiate and produce immunoglobulins of all other types, and are responsible for initiating B-cell responses by activating naive B cells to proliferate and secrete IgM. The various types of immunoglobulin together make up the effector molecules of the humoral immune response.

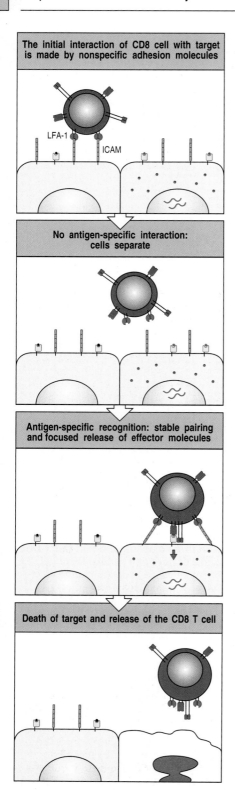

The initial interaction of CD8 cell with target is made by nonspecific adhesion molecules

LFA-1

ICAM

No antigen-specific interaction: cells separate

Antigen-specific recognition: stable pairing and focused release of effector molecules

Death of target and release of the CD8 T cell

Fig. 8.28 Interactions of T cells with their targets initially involve nonspecific adhesion molecules. The major initial interaction is between LFA-1 on the T cell, illustrated here as a cytotoxic CD8 T cell, and ICAM-1 or ICAM-2 on the target cell (top panel). This binding allows the T cell to remain in contact with the target cell and to scan its surface for the presence of specific peptide:MHC complexes. If the target cell does not carry the specific antigen, the T cell disengages (second panel) and can scan other potential targets until it finds the specific antigen (third panel). Signaling through the T-cell receptor increases the strength of the adhesive interactions, prolonging the contact between the two cells and stimulating the T cell to deliver its effector molecules. The T cell then disengages (bottom panel).

8-15 Effector T-cell interactions with target cells are initiated by antigen-nonspecific cell-adhesion molecules.

Once an effector T cell has completed its differentiation in the lymphoid tissue, it must find target cells that are displaying the MHC:peptide complex that it recognizes. Some T_H2 cells encounter their B-cell targets without leaving the lymphoid tissue, as we discuss further in Chapter 9. However, most of the armed effector T cells emigrate from their site of activation in lymphoid tissues and enter the blood via the thoracic duct. Because of the cell-surface changes that have occurred during differentiation, they can now migrate into tissues, particularly at sites of infection. They are guided to these sites by changes in the adhesion molecules expressed on the endothelium of the local blood vessels as a result of infection, and by local chemotactic factors, as we will see in Chapter 10.

The initial binding of an effector T cell to its target, like that of a naive T cell to an antigen-presenting cell, is an antigen-nonspecific interaction mediated by LFA-1 and CD2. The level of LFA-1 and of CD2 is two to fourfold higher on armed effector T cells than on naive T cells, and so armed effector T cells can bind efficiently to target cells that have lower levels of ICAMs and CD58 on their surface than do the antigen-presenting cells. This interaction is normally transient unless recognition of antigen on the target cell through the T-cell receptor triggers an increase in the affinity of the T-cell's LFA-1 for its ligands on the target cell. The T cell then binds more tightly to its target and remains bound for long enough to release its effector molecules. Armed CD4 effector T cells, which activate macrophages or induce B cells to secrete antibody, must maintain contact with their targets for relatively long periods. Cytotoxic T cells, by contrast, can be observed under the microscope attaching to and dissociating from successive targets relatively rapidly as they kill them (Fig. 8.28). Killing of the target, or some local change in the T cell, allows the effector T cell to detach and address new targets. How armed CD4 effector T cells disengage from their antigen-negative targets is not known, although current evidence suggests that CD4 binding directly to MHC class II molecules on target cells that are not displaying specific antigen signals the cell to detach.

8-16 Binding of the T-cell receptor complex directs the release of effector molecules and focuses them on the target cell.

When binding to their specific antigenic peptide:self-MHC complexes or to self-peptide:self-MHC complexes, the T-cell receptors and their associated co-receptors cluster at the site of cell–cell contact, forming what is called the supramolecular adhesion complex, or SMAC. Clustering of the T-cell receptors then signals a reorientation of the cytoskeleton that polarizes the effector cell so as to focus the release of effector molecules at the site of contact with the target cell. This is illustrated for a cytotoxic T cell in Fig. 8.29. Polarization starts with the local reorganization of the cortical actin cytoskeleton at the site

Collision and nonspecific adhesion

cytotoxic T cell | target cell
GA
MTOC

Specific recognition redistributes cytoskeleton and cytoplasmic components of T cell

Release of granules at site of cell contact

a

b

c

Fig. 8.29 The polarization of T cells during specific antigen recognition allows effector molecules to be focused on the antigen-bearing target cell. The example illustrated here is a CD8 cytotoxic T cell. Cytotoxic T cells contain specialized lysosomes called lytic granules (shown in red in the left panels), which contain cytotoxic proteins. Initial binding to a target cell through adhesion molecules does not have any effect on the location of the lytic granules. Binding of the T-cell receptor causes the T cell to become polarized: reorganization within the cortical actin cytoskeleton at the site of contact aligns the microtubule-organizing center (MTOC), which in turn aligns the secretory apparatus, including the Golgi apparatus (GA), towards the target cell. Proteins stored in lytic granules derived from the Golgi are then directed specifically onto the target cell. The photomicrograph in panel a shows an unbound, isolated cytotoxic T cell. The microtubule cytoskeleton is stained in green and the lytic granules in red. Note how the lytic granules are dispersed throughout the T cell. Panel b depicts a cytotoxic T cell bound to a (larger) target cell. The lytic granules are now clustered at the site of cell–cell contact in the bound T cell. The electron micrograph in panel c shows the release of granules from a cytotoxic T cell. Panels a and b courtesy of G. Griffiths. Panel c courtesy of E. Podack.

of contact; this in turn leads to the reorientation of the microtubule-organizing center (MTOC), the center from which the microtubule cytoskeleton is produced, and of the Golgi apparatus (GA), through which most proteins destined for secretion travel. In the cytotoxic T cell, the cytoskeletal reorientation focuses exocytosis of the preformed lytic granules at the site of contact with its target cell.

The polarization of a T cell also focuses the secretion of soluble effector molecules whose synthesis is induced *de novo* by ligation of the T-cell receptor. For example, the secreted cytokine IL-4, which is the principal effector molecule of T_H2 cells, is confined and concentrated at the site of contact with the target cell (see Fig. 9.6). Other cell-surface molecules are oriented at the immunological synapse, the site of contact between the T cell and its target. For example, the enhanced binding of LFA-1 to ICAM-1 creates a molecular seal that surrounds the T-cell receptor and its co-receptor, focusing on the antigenic peptide: self-MHC complex, which also clusters in this site (Fig. 8.30).

Fig. 8.30 The area of contact between an armed effector T cell and its contact forms an 'immunological synapse.' Confocal fluorescence micrograph of the area of contact between a CD4 T cell and a B cell (as viewed through one of the cells). This region of contact, called the supramolecular adhesion complex, or SMAC, is organized into two distinct regions, the outer, or peripheral, SMAC (pSMAC) and the inner, or central, SMAC (cSMAC). The outer red ring shown here is made up of LFA-1 on the T cell and its counter-receptors on the target cell, whereas molecules that cluster in the center of the ring (bright green) include the T-cell receptor complex, bound to its peptide:MHC complex, the co-receptor CD4, and CD28. Photograph courtesy of A. Kupfer.

Outer ring (red) pSMAC	Inner circle (green) cSMAC
LFA-1:ICAM-1	TCR, CD4, CD28 MHC:peptide

The central zone, in which the antigen receptor and co-receptors cluster, is referred to as the central SMAC, or cSMAC; the outer zone in which adhesion molecules cluster is known as the peripheral SMAC, or pSMAC.

Thus, the antigen-specific T-cell receptor controls the delivery of effector signals in three ways: it induces the stable binding of effector cells to their specific target cells to create a tightly held, narrow space in which effector molecules can be concentrated; it focuses their delivery at the site of contact by inducing a reorientation of the secretory apparatus of the effector cell; and it triggers their synthesis and/or release. All these receptor-coordinated mechanisms contribute to the selective action of effector molecules on the target cell bearing specific antigen. In this way, effector T-cell activity is highly selective for those target cells that display specific peptide:MHC complexes, although the effector molecules themselves are not antigen-specific.

8-17 The effector functions of T cells are determined by the array of effector molecules that they produce.

The effector molecules produced by armed effector T cells fall into two broad classes: **cytotoxins**, which are stored in specialized lytic granules and released by cytotoxic CD8 T cells (see Fig. 8.29), and **cytokines** and related membrane-associated proteins, which are synthesized *de novo* by all effector T cells. The cytotoxins are the principal effector molecules of cytotoxic T cells and will be discussed further in Section 8-22. Their release, in particular, must be tightly regulated because they are not specific: they can penetrate the lipid bilayer and trigger an intrinsic death program in any cell. By contrast, cytokines and membrane-associated proteins act by binding to specific receptors on the target cell. CD4 effector T cells act mainly through the production of cytokines and membrane-associated proteins, and their actions are therefore directed at cells bearing MHC class II molecules and expressing receptors for these proteins.

The effector actions and main effector molecules of all three functional classes of effector T cell are summarized in Fig. 8.31. The cytokines are a diverse group of proteins and we will review them briefly before discussing the T-cell cytokines and their contributions to the effector actions of cytotoxic CD8 T cells, T_H1 cells, and T_H2 cells. As we will see, soluble cytokines and membrane-associated molecules often act in combination to mediate the effects of T cells on their target cells.

The membrane-associated effector molecules, which we will discuss further in Section 8-20, are all structurally related to **tumor necrosis factor (TNF)**, and their receptors on target cells are members of the **TNF receptor (TNFR)** family. All three classes of effector T cell express one or more members of the TNF family upon recognizing their specific antigen on the target cell. The membrane-bound TNF-family member CD40 ligand is particularly important for CD4 T-cell effector function; it is induced on T_H1 and T_H2 cells, and delivers activating signals to B cells and macrophages through the TNFR-family protein CD40. TNF-α is made by T_H1 cells, some T_H2 cells, and by cytotoxic T cells in soluble and membrane-associated forms, and can also deliver activating signals to macrophages. Some members of the TNF family can stimulate death by apoptosis. Thus **Fas ligand** (CD178), the principal membrane-associated TNF-related molecule expressed by cytotoxic T cells, can trigger death by apoptosis in target cells bearing the receptor protein **Fas** (CD95); some T_H1 cells also express Fas ligand and can kill Fas-bearing cells with which they interact. Death by this mechanism seems to be important for removing activated Fas-bearing lymphocytes; if it fails, a lymphoproliferative disease associated with severe autoimmunity results.

Autoimmune Lymphoproliferative Syndrome (ALPS)

CD8 T cells: peptide + MHC class I		CD4 T cells: peptide + MHC class II			
Cytotoxic (killer) T cells		**T$_H$1 cells**		**T$_H$2 cells**	

Cytotoxic effector molecules	Others	Macrophage-activating effector molecules	Others	B-cell-activating effector molecules	Others
Perforin Granzymes Granulysin Fas ligand	IFN-γ TNF-β TNF-α	IFN-γ GM-CSF TNF-α CD40 ligand Fas ligand	IL-3 TNF-β (IL-2) CXCL2 (GROβ)	IL-4 IL-5 IL-15 CD40 ligand	IL-3 GM-CSF IL-10 TGF-β CCL11 (eotaxin) CCL17 (TARC)

Fig. 8.31 The three main types of armed effector T cell produce distinct sets of effector molecules. CD8 T cells are predominantly killer T cells that recognize pathogen-derived peptides bound to MHC class I molecules. They release perforin (which creates holes in the target cell membrane), granzymes (which are pro-proteases that are activated intracellularly to trigger apoptosis), and often the cytokine IFN-γ. A membrane-bound effector molecule expressed on CD8 T cells is the Fas ligand (CD178). When this binds to Fas (CD95) on a target cell it activates apoptosis in the Fas-bearing cell. CD4 T cells recognize peptides bound to MHC class II molecules and are of two functional types: T$_H$1 and T$_H$2. T$_H$1 cells are specialized to activate macrophages that are infected by or have ingested pathogens; they secrete IFN-γ to activate the infected cell, as well as other effector molecules. They can also express membrane-bound CD40 ligand and/or Fas ligand. These are both members of the TNF family of proteins, but CD40 ligand triggers the activation of the target cell, whereas Fas ligand triggers the death of Fas-expressing cells, so their pattern of expression has a strong influence on their function. T$_H$2 cells are specialized for B-cell activation; they secrete the B-cell growth factors IL-4, IL-5, IL-9, and IL-13. The principal membrane-bound effector molecule expressed by T$_H$2 cells is CD40 ligand, which binds to CD40 on the B cell and induces B-cell proliferation and isotype switching (see Chapter 9).

8-18 Cytokines can act locally or at a distance.

Cytokines are small soluble proteins secreted by one cell that can alter the behavior or properties of the cell itself or of another cell. They are released by many cells in addition to those of the immune system. We have already discussed the cytokines released by phagocytic cells in Chapter 2, where we dealt with the inflammatory reactions that are important in innate immunity. Here we are concerned mainly with the cytokines that mediate the effector functions of T cells. Cytokines produced by lymphocytes are often called **lymphokines**, but this nomenclature can be confusing because some lymphokines are also secreted by nonlymphoid cells; we will therefore use the generic term 'cytokine' for all of them. Most cytokines produced by T cells are given the name **interleukin** (**IL**) followed by a number: we have encountered several interleukins already in this chapter. The cytokines produced by T cells are shown in Fig. 8.32, and a more comprehensive list of cytokines of immunological interest is in Appendix III.

Most cytokines have a multitude of different biological effects when tested at high concentration in biological assays *in vitro*, but targeted disruption of the genes for cytokines and cytokine receptors in gene-knockout mice (see Appendix I, Section A-47) has helped to clarify their physiological roles.

The main cytokine released by CD8 effector T cells is IFN-γ, which can block viral replication or even lead to the elimination of virus from infected cells without killing them. T$_H$1 cells and T$_H$2 cells release different, but overlapping, sets of cytokines, which define their distinct actions in immunity. T$_H$2 cells secrete IL-4, IL-5, IL-9, and IL-13, as well as having CD40 ligand on their surface, all of which activate B cells, and IL-10, which inhibits macrophage activation. T$_H$1 cells secrete IFN-γ, which is the main macrophage-activating

Cytokine	T-cell source	Effects on					Effect of gene knockout
		B cells	T cells	Macrophages	Hematopoietic cells	Other somatic cells	
Interleukin-2 (IL-2)	Naive, T$_H$1, some CD8	Stimulates growth and J-chain synthesis	Growth	–	Stimulates NK cell growth	–	↓ T-cell responses IBD
Interferon-γ (IFN-γ)	T$_H$1, CTL	Differentiation IgG2a synthesis (mouse)	Inhibits T$_H$2 cell growth	Activation, ↑ MHC class I and class II	Activates NK cells	Antiviral ↑ MHC class I and class II	Susceptible to mycobacteria, some viruses
Lymphotoxin (LT, TNF-β)	T$_H$1, some CTL	Inhibits	Kills	Activates, induces NO production	Activates neutrophils	Kills fibroblasts and tumor cells	Absence of lymph nodes Disorganized spleen
Interleukin-4 (IL-4)	T$_H$2	Activation, growth IgG1, IgE ↑ MHC class II induction	Growth, survival	Inhibits macrophage activation	↑Growth of mast cells	–	No T$_H$2
Interleukin-5 (IL-5)	T$_H$2	Mouse: Differentiation IgA synthesis	–	–	↑ Eosinophil growth and differentiation	–	Reduced eosinophilia
Interleukin-10 (IL-10)	T$_H$2, (human: some T$_H$1)	↑ MHC class II	Inhibits T$_H$1	Inhibits cytokine release	Co-stimulates mast cell growth		IBD
Interleukin-3 (IL-3)	T$_H$1, T$_H$2, some CTL	–	–	–	Growth factor for progenitor hematopoietic cells (multi-CSF)	–	–
Tumor necrosis factor-α (TNF-α)	T$_H$1, some T$_H$2, some CTL	–	–	Activates, induces NO production		Activates microvascular endothelium	Resistance to Gram –ve sepsis
Granulocyte-macrophage colony-stimulating factor (GM-CSF)	T$_H$1, some T$_H$2, some CTL	Differentiation	Inhibits growth ?	Activation Differentiation to dendritic cells	↑ Production of granulocytes and macrophages (myelopoiesis) and dendritic cells	–	–
Transforming growth factor-β (TGF-β)	CD4 T cells	Inhibits growth IgA switch factor	Inhibits growth, promotes survival	Inhibits activation	Activates neutrophils	Inhibits/ stimulates cell growth	Death at ~10 weeks

Fig. 8.32 The nomenclature and functions of well-defined T-cell cytokines. The major actions are noted in boxes. Each cytokine has multiple activities on different cell types. The mixture of cytokines secreted by a given cell type produces many effects through what is called a 'cytokine network.' Major activities of effector cytokines are highlighted in red. ↑, increase; ↓, decrease; CTL, cytotoxic lymphocyte; NK, natural killer cell; CSF, colony-stimulating factor; IBD, inflammatory bowel disease; NO, nitric oxide.

cytokine, and lymphotoxin (also called LT-α or TNF-β), which activates macrophages, inhibits B cells and is directly cytotoxic for some cells. The T$_H$0 cells from which both of these functional classes derive (see Fig. 8.24) also secrete cytokines, including IL-2, IL-4, and IFN-γ, and may as a result have a distinctive effector function.

We have already discussed in Section 8-16 how the T-cell receptor can orchestrate the polarized release of these cytokines so that they are concentrated at the site of contact with the target cell. Furthermore, most of the soluble cytokines have local actions that synergize with those of the membrane-bound effector molecules. The effect of all these molecules is therefore combinatorial, and, because the membrane-bound effectors can bind only to receptors on an interacting cell, this is another mechanism by which selective effects of cytokines are focused on the target cell. The effects of some cytokines are further confined to target cells by tight regulation of their synthesis: as we will see later, the synthesis of cytokines such as IL-2, IL-4, and IFN-γ is controlled, so that their secretion by T cells does not continue after the interaction with a target cell ends.

Some cytokines, however, have more distant effects. IL-3 and GM-CSF (see Fig. 8.32) are released by both types of CD4 effector T cell and act on bone marrow cells to stimulate the production of macrophages and granulocytes, both of which are important nonspecific effector cells in both humoral and cell-mediated immunity. IL-3 and GM-CSF also stimulate the production of dendritic cells from bone marrow precursors. IL-5, produced by T$_H$2 cells, can increase the production of eosinophils, which contribute to the late phase of allergic reactions, in which the predominant cell activated is a T$_H$2 cell (see Chapter 12). Whether a given cytokine effect is local or more distant is likely to reflect the amounts released, the degree to which this release is focused on the target cell, and the stability of the cytokine *in vivo* but, for most of the cytokines, in particular those with more distant effects, these factors are not yet known.

8-19 Cytokines and their receptors fall into distinct families of structurally related proteins.

Cytokines can be grouped by structure into families—the hematopoietins, the interferons, and the TNF family (see Fig. 2.38)—and their receptors can likewise be grouped (Fig. 8.33). We have already encountered members of all of these families in Chapter 2 and have given an overview of the chemokine family there (see Section 2-21). We will focus here on the receptors for the hematopoietins, the TNF family, and IFN-γ on account of their role in T-cell effector function. Members of the TNF family act as trimers, most of which are membrane-bound and so are quite distinct in their properties from the other cytokines. Nevertheless, they share some important properties with the soluble T-cell cytokines, because they are also synthesized *de novo* upon antigen recognition by T cells and affect the behavior of the target cell.

Fig. 8.33 Cytokine receptors belong to superfamilies of receptor proteins, each with a distinctive structure. Many cytokine receptors are members of the hematopoietin-receptor superfamily, named after the first of its members to be defined. This large superfamily, also known as the class I cytokine receptors, is divided into three subsets on the basis of differences in sequence and structure. A smaller number of receptors fall into the class II cytokine receptor superfamily; many of these are receptors for interferons or interferon-like cytokines. Other superfamilies of cytokine receptors are the tumor necrosis factor receptor (TNFR) family, and the chemokine receptor family, the latter belonging to the very large family of G-protein-coupled receptors. Each family member is a variant with a distinct specificity, performing a particular function on the cell that expresses it. In the hematopoietin receptor family, the α chain often defines the ligand specificity of the receptor, whereas the β or γ chain confers the intracellular signaling function. For the TNFR family, the ligands act as trimers and may be associated with the cell membrane rather than being secreted. Of the receptors listed here, some have been mentioned already in this book, some will occur in later chapters, and some are important examples from other biological systems. The diagrams indicate the representations of these receptors that you will encounter throughout this book.

Class I cytokine receptor (hematopoietin-receptor family)	α β	Receptors for erythropoietin, growth hormone, and IL-13
		Receptors for IL-3, IL-5, and GM-CSF share a common chain, CD131 or β$_c$ (common beta chain)
		Receptors for IL-2, IL-4, IL-7, IL-9 and IL-15 share a common chain CD132 or γ$_c$ (common gamma chain). IL-2 receptor also has a third chain, a high-affinity subunit IL-2Rα (CD25)
Class II cytokine receptor		Interferon-α, -β, and -γ receptor, IL-10 receptor
TNF-receptor family		Tumor necrosis factor (TNF) receptors I and II CD40, Fas (Apo 1, CD95), CD30, CD27, nerve growth factor receptor
Chemokine-receptor family		CCR1–10, CXCR1–5, XCR1, CX3CR1

Many of the soluble cytokines made by effector T cells are members of the hematopoietin family. These cytokines and their receptors can be further divided into subfamilies characterized by functional similarities and genetic linkage. For instance, IL-3, IL-4, IL-5, IL-13, and GM-CSF are related structurally, their genes are closely linked in the genome, and all are major cytokines produced by T_H2 cells. In addition, they bind to closely related receptors, which form the family of class I cytokine receptors. The IL-3, IL-5, and GM-CSF receptors share a common β chain. Another subgroup of class I cytokine receptors is defined by their use of the γ chain of the IL-2 receptor. This chain is shared by receptors for the cytokines IL-2, IL-4, IL-7, IL-9, and IL-15 and is now called the **common γ chain** ($γ_c$). More distantly related, the receptor for IFN-γ is a member of a small family of cytokine receptors with some similarities to the hematopoietin receptor family. These so-called class II cytokine receptors include the receptor for IFN-α and IFN-β, and the IL-10 receptor. Overall, the structural, functional, and genetic relations between the cytokines and their receptors suggest that they may have diversified in parallel during the evolution of increasingly specialized effector functions.

These specific functional effects depend on intracellular signaling events that are triggered by the cytokines binding to their specific receptors. The hematopoietin and interferon receptors all signal through a similar pathway, which is described in Chapter 6. The key signaling molecules of this pathway are members of the Janus family of cytoplasmic tyrosine kinases (JAKs) and their targets, the signal transducing activators of transcription (STATs), which enter the nucleus to activate specific genes. As the JAKs and STATs are present as families of related molecules, different members may be activated to achieve different effects.

8-20 The TNF family of cytokines are trimeric proteins that are usually associated with the cell surface.

TNF-α is made by T cells in soluble and membrane-associated forms, both of which are made up of three identical protein chains (a homotrimer; see Fig. 2.38). TNF-β (LT-α) can be produced as a secreted homotrimer but is usually linked to the cell surface by forming heterotrimers with a third, membrane-associated, member of this family called LT-β. The receptors for these molecules, TNFR-I and TNFR-II, form homotrimers when bound to either TNF-α or LT. The trimeric structure is characteristic of all members of the TNF family, and the ligand-induced trimerization of their receptors seems to be the critical event in initiating signaling.

Most effector T cells express members of the TNF protein family as cell-surface molecules. The most important TNF-family proteins in T-cell effector function are TNF-α, TNF-β, Fas ligand, and CD40 ligand, the latter two always being cell-surface associated. These molecules all bind receptors that are members of the TNFR family; TNFR-I and TNFR-II can each interact with either TNF-α or TNF-β, whereas Fas ligand and CD40 ligand bind respectively to the transmembrane protein Fas and to the transmembrane protein CD40 on target cells

Fas is expressed on many cells but is especially prominent on activated lymphocytes. Activation of Fas by the Fas ligand has profound consequences for the cell as Fas contains a 'death domain' in its cytoplasmic tail, which can initiate an activation cascade of cellular proteases called caspases that leads to apoptotic cell death (see Fig. 6.23). Fas is important in maintaining lymphocyte homeostasis, as can be seen from the effects of mutations in the Fas or Fas ligand genes. Mice and humans with a mutant form of Fas develop a lymphoproliferative disease associated with severe autoimmunity. A mutation in the gene encoding the Fas ligand in another mouse strain creates a nearly identical phenotype. These mutant phenotypes represent the best-characterized examples of generalized autoimmunity caused by single-gene defects. Other TNFR-family members, including TNFR-I, are also associated with death domains and can also induce programmed cell death. Thus, TNF-α and TNF-β can induce programmed cell death by binding to TNFR-I.

The cytoplasmic tail of CD40 lacks a death domain; instead, it seems to be linked downstream to proteins called **TRAFs** (TNF-receptor-associated factors). CD40 is involved in macrophage and B-cell activation; the ligation of CD40 on B cells promotes growth and isotype switching, whereas CD40 ligation on macrophages induces them to secrete TNF-α and to become receptive to much lower concentrations of IFN-γ. Deficiency in CD40 ligand expression is associated with immunodeficiency, as we will learn in Chapters 9 and 11.

Hyper IgM
Immunodeficiency

Summary.

Interactions between armed effector T cells and their targets are initiated by transient nonspecific adhesion between the cells. T-cell effector functions are elicited only when peptide:MHC complexes on the surface of the target cell are recognized by the receptor on an armed effector T cell. This recognition event triggers the armed effector T cell to adhere more strongly to the antigen-bearing target cell and to release its effector molecules directly at the target cell, leading to the activation or death of the target. The consequences of antigen recognition by an armed effector T cell are determined largely by the set of effector molecules that it produces on binding a specific target cell. CD8 cytotoxic T cells store preformed cytotoxins in specialized lytic granules whose release can be tightly focused at the site of contact with the infected target cell. Cytokines, and one or more members of the TNF family of membrane-associated effector proteins, are synthesized *de novo* by all three types of effector T cell. T_H2 cells express B-cell-activating effector molecules, whereas T_H1 cells express effector molecules that activate macrophages. CD8 T cells express membrane-associated Fas ligand, which induces programmed cell death in cells bearing Fas; they also release IFN-γ. Membrane-associated effector molecules can deliver signals only to an interacting cell bearing the appropriate receptor, whereas soluble cytokines can act on cytokine receptors expressed locally on the target cell, or on hematopoietic cells at a distance. The actions of cytokines and membrane-associated effector molecules through their specific receptors, together with the effects of cytotoxins released by CD8 cells, account for most of the effector functions of T cells.

T cell-mediated cytotoxicity.

All viruses, and some bacteria, multiply in the cytoplasm of infected cells; indeed, a virus is a highly sophisticated parasite that has no biosynthetic or metabolic apparatus of its own and, in consequence, can replicate only inside cells. Although susceptible to antibody before they enter cells (see Chapter 9), once they are inside cells these pathogens are not accessible to antibodies and can be eliminated only by the destruction or modification of the infected cells on which they depend. This role in host defense is fulfilled by cytotoxic CD8 T cells. The crucial role of cytotoxic T cells in limiting such infections is seen in the increased susceptibility of animals artificially depleted of these T cells, or of mice or humans that lack the MHC class I molecules that present antigen to CD8 T cells. The elimination of infected cells without the destruction of healthy tissue requires the cytotoxic mechanisms of CD8 T cells to be both powerful and accurately targeted.

8-21   Cytotoxic T cells can induce target cells to undergo programmed cell death.

Fig. 8.34 Cytotoxic CD8 T cells can induce apoptosis in target cells. Specific recognition of peptide:MHC complexes on a target cell (top panels) by a cytotoxic CD8 T cell (CTL) leads to the death of the target cell by apoptosis. Cytotoxic T cells can recycle to kill multiple targets. Each killing requires the same series of steps, including receptor binding and directed release of cytotoxic proteins stored in lytic granules. The process of apoptosis is shown in the micrographs (bottom panels), where panel a shows a healthy cell with a normal nucleus. Early in apoptosis (panel b) the chromatin becomes condensed (red) and, although the cell sheds membrane vesicles, the integrity of the cell membrane is retained, in contrast to the necrotic cell in the upper part of the same field. In late stages of apoptosis (panel c), the cell nucleus (middle cell) is very condensed, no mitochondria are visible, and the cell has lost much of its cytoplasm and membrane through the shedding of vesicles. Photographs (× 3500) courtesy of R. Windsor and E. Hirst.

Cells can die in either of two ways. Physical or chemical injury, such as the deprivation of oxygen that occurs in heart muscle during a heart attack or membrane damage with antibody and complement, leads to cell disintegration or **necrosis**. The dead or necrotic tissue is taken up and degraded by phagocytic cells, which eventually clear the damaged tissue and heal the wound. The other form of cell death is known as **programmed cell death** or **apoptosis**. Apoptosis is a normal cellular response that is crucial in the tissue remodeling that occurs during development and metamorphosis in all multi-cellular animals. As we saw in Chapter 7, most thymocytes die an apoptotic death when they fail positive selection or, much less often, are negatively selected as a result of recognizing self antigens. Early changes seen in apoptosis are nuclear blebbing, alteration in cell morphology, and, eventually, fragmentation of the DNA. The cell then destroys itself from within, shrinking by shedding membrane-bound vesicles, and degrading itself until little is left. A hallmark of this type of cell death is the fragmentation of nuclear DNA into 200-base-pair (bp) pieces through the activation of endogenous nucleases that cleave the DNA between nucleosomes, each of which contains about 200 bp of DNA.

Cytotoxic T cells kill their targets by programming them to undergo apoptosis (Fig. 8.34). When cytotoxic T cells are mixed with target cells and rapidly brought into contact by centrifugation, they can program antigen-specific target cells to die within 5 minutes, although death can take hours to become

| CTL recognizes and binds virus-infected cell | CTL programs target for death, inducing DNA fragmentation | CTL migrates to new target | Target cell dies by apoptosis |

fully evident. The rapidity of this response reflects the release of preformed effector molecules, which activate an endogenous apoptotic pathway within the target cell.

As well as killing the host cell, the apoptotic mechanism may also act directly on cytosolic pathogens. For example, the nucleases that are activated in apoptosis to destroy cellular DNA can also degrade viral DNA. This prevents the assembly of virions and thus the release of infectious virus, which could otherwise infect nearby cells. Other enzymes activated in the course of apoptosis may destroy nonviral cytosolic pathogens. Apoptosis is therefore preferable to necrosis as a means of killing infected cells; in cells dying by necrosis, intact pathogens are released from the dead cell and these can continue to infect healthy cells, or can parasitize the macrophages that ingest them.

8-22   Cytotoxic effector proteins that trigger apoptosis are contained in the granules of CD8 cytotoxic T cells.

The principal mechanism of cytotoxic T cell action is the calcium-dependent release of specialized **lytic granules** upon recognition of antigen on the surface of a target cell. These granules are modified lysosomes that contain at least three distinct classes of cytotoxic effector protein that are expressed selectively in cytotoxic T cells (Fig. 8.35). Such proteins are stored in the lytic granules in an active form, but conditions within the granules prevent them from functioning until after their release. One of these cytotoxic proteins, known as **perforin**, polymerizes in target-cell membranes to form transmembrane pores. Another class of cytotoxic proteins comprises at least three proteases called **granzymes**, which belong to the same family of enzymes— the serine proteases—as the digestive enzymes trypsin and chymotrypsin. The third cytotoxic protein, **granulysin**, is able to induce apoptosis in target cells and also has antimicrobial action. Granules that store perforin, granzymes, and granulysin can be seen in armed CD8 cytotoxic effector cells in tissue lesions.

When purified granules from cytotoxic T cells are added to target cells *in vitro*, they lyse the cells by creating pores in the lipid bilayer. The pores consist of polymers of perforin, which is a major constituent of these granules. Perforin monomers bind to phosphorylcholine on the target-cell membrane in a Ca^{2+}-dependent fashion, and then polymerize to form a pore similar to that formed by polymerized complement component C9, a protein related to perforin. This pore is lipophilic on the outside with a hydrophilic central channel of diameter 16 nm (Fig. 8.36) through which water and salts pass rapidly into the cell. With the integrity of the cell membrane destroyed, the cells die rapidly.

Both perforin and granzymes are required for effective cell killing. Their separate roles have been investigated in experiments that rely on similarities between the lytic granules of CD8 T cells and the granules of mast cells. The release of mast-cell granules occurs on cross-linking of a cell-surface receptor for IgE, just as the release of lytic granules from T cells occurs upon aggregating the T-cell receptor. The mechanism of signaling for granule release is thought to be the same or similar in both cases, because both the IgE receptor and the T-cell receptor have ITAM motifs in their cytoplasmic domains, and their cross-linking leads to tyrosine phosphorylation of the ITAMs (see Chapter 6). When a mast-cell line is transfected with the genes for perforin or a granzyme, the gene products are stored in mast-cell granules, and when the cell is activated these granules are released. When transfected with the gene for perforin alone, mast cells can kill other cells, but large numbers of transfected cells are needed as killing is very inefficient. By contrast,

Protein in lytic granules of cytotoxic T cells	Actions on target cells
Perforin	Polymerizes to form a pore in target membrane
Granzymes	Serine proteases, which activate apoptosis once in the cytoplasm of the target cell
Granulysin	Induces apoptosis

Fig. 8.35 Cytotoxic effector proteins released by cytotoxic T cells.

Fig. 8.36 Perforin released from the lytic granules of cytotoxic T cells can insert into the target cell membrane to form pores. Perforin molecules, as well as several other effector molecules, are contained in the granules of cytotoxic T cells (panel a). When a CD8 cytotoxic T cell recognizes its target, the granule contents are released onto the target cell (panel b, bottom right quadrant). The perforin molecules released from the granules polymerize in the membrane of the target cell to form pores. The structure of these pores is best seen when purified perforin is added to synthetic lipid vesicles (panel c: pores are seen both end on, as circles, and sideways on, arrow). The pores span the target cell membrane (panel d). G, granule; N, nucleus; M, mitochondrion; Go, Golgi apparatus. Photographs courtesy of E. Podack.

mast cells transfected with the gene for granzyme B alone are unable to kill other cells. However, when perforin-transfected mast cells are also transfected with the gene encoding granzyme B, the cells or their purified granules become as effective at killing targets as granules from cytotoxic cells. This suggests that perforin makes pores through which the granzymes can move into the target cell. However, it seems that granzyme B does not simply diffuse from the extracellular space through the perforin pore; rather, it seems first to bind to a cell-surface molecule, the mannose-6-phosphate receptor. This is normally involved in targeting molecules to the lysosomal compartment of cells but seems to be vital in rendering cells susceptible to killing by cytotoxic T cells. Although the exact mechanism is not yet defined, the role of perforin seems to be to mediate the release of the bound granzyme into the cytosol of the target cell.

The granzymes are proteases, so although they can trigger apoptosis in the target cell, they cannot cleave DNA. Granzyme B cleaves and activates the ubiquitous cellular enzyme caspase-3, which is a cysteine protease that cuts after aspartic acid residues (hence the name caspase). Caspase-3 activates a caspase proteolytic cascade, which eventually activates the caspase-activated deoxyribonuclease (CAD) by cleaving an inhibitory protein (ICAD) that binds to and inactivates CAD. This nuclease is believed to be the enzyme that finally degrades the DNA.

Cells undergoing programmed cell death are rapidly ingested by phagocytic cells, which recognize a change in the cell membrane: phosphatidylserine, which is normally found only in the inner leaflet of the membrane, replaces phosphatidylcholine as the predominant phospholipid in the outer leaflet. The ingested cell is broken down and completely digested by the phagocyte without the induction of co-stimulatory proteins. Thus, apoptosis is normally an immunologically 'quiet' process; that is, apoptotic cells do not normally contribute to or stimulate immune responses.

The importance of perforin in cytotoxicity is well illustrated in mice that have had their perforin gene knocked out. They are severely defective in their ability to mount a cytotoxic T-cell response to many, but not all, viruses. Mice defective in the granzyme B gene have a less profound defect, probably because there are several enzymes feeding into the caspase cascade.

8-23 Activated CD8 T cells and some CD4 effector T cells express Fas ligand, which can also activate apoptosis.

The release of granule contents accounts for most of the cytotoxic activity of CD8 effector T cells, as shown by the loss of most killing activity in perforin knockout mice. This granule-mediated killing is strictly calcium-dependent, yet some cytotoxic actions of CD8 T cells survive calcium depletion. Moreover, some CD4 T cells can also kill other cells, yet do not contain granules and make neither perforin nor granzymes. These observations imply that there must be a second perforin-independent mechanism of cytotoxicity. This involves the binding of Fas in the target-cell membrane by the Fas ligand, which is present in the membranes of activated cytotoxic T cells, T_H1 cells, and some T_H2 cells. Ligation of Fas leads to the activation of caspases, which induce apoptosis in the target cell (see Fig. 6.24). As discussed in Section 8-20, the lymphoproliferative and autoimmune disorders seen in mice and humans with mutations in genes for either Fas or Fas ligand imply that this pathway of killing is very important in regulating peripheral immune responses. Fas is expressed on activated lymphocytes, and Fas–Fas ligand interactions are important in terminating lymphocyte growth after the removal of the initiating pathogen.

8-24 Cytotoxic T cells are selective and serial killers of targets expressing specific antigen.

When cytotoxic T cells are offered a mixture of equal amounts of two target cells, one bearing specific antigen and the other not, they kill only the target cell bearing the specific antigen. The 'innocent bystander' cells and the cytotoxic T cells themselves are not killed. The cytotoxic T cells are probably not killed because release of the cytotoxic effector molecules is highly polarized. As we saw in Fig. 8.29, cytotoxic T cells orient their Golgi apparatus and microtubule-organizing center to focus secretion on the point of contact with a target cell. Granule movement toward the point of contact is shown in Fig. 8.37. Cytotoxic T cells attached to several different target cells reorient their

Fig. 8.37 Effector molecules are released from T-cell granules in a highly polar fashion. The granules of cytotoxic T cells can be labeled with fluorescent dyes, allowing them to be seen under the microscope, and their movements can be followed by time-lapse photography. Here we show a series of pictures taken during the interaction of a cytotoxic T cell with a target cell, which is eventually killed. In the top panel, at time 0, the T cell (upper right) has just made contact with a target cell (diagonally below). At this time, the granules of the T cell, labeled with a red fluorescent dye, are distant from the point of contact. In the second panel, after 1 minute has elapsed, the granules have begun to move towards the target cell, a move that has essentially been completed in the third panel, after 4 minutes. After 40 minutes, in the last panel, the granule contents have been released into the space between the T cell and the target, which has begun to undergo apoptosis (note the fragmented nucleus). The T cell will now disengage from the target cell and can recognize and kill other targets. Photographs courtesy of G. Griffiths.

Time = 0

After 1 minute

After 4 minutes

After 40 minutes

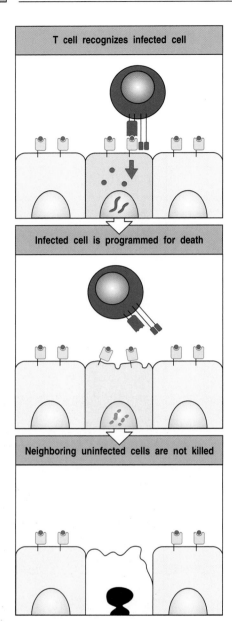

Fig. 8.38 Cytotoxic T cells kill target cells bearing specific antigen while sparing neighboring uninfected cells. All the cells in a tissue are susceptible to lysis by the cytotoxic proteins of armed effector CD8 T cells, but only infected cells are killed. Specific recognition by the T-cell receptor identifies which target cell to kill, and the polarized release of granules (not shown) ensures that neighboring cells are spared.

secretory apparatus toward each cell in turn and kill them one by one, strongly suggesting that the mechanism whereby cytotoxic mediators are released allows attack at only one point of contact at any one time. The narrowly focused action of cytotoxic CD8 T cells allows them to kill single infected cells in a tissue without creating widespread tissue damage (Fig. 8.38) and is of crucial importance in tissues where cell regeneration does not occur, as in neurons of the central nervous system, or is very limited, as in the pancreatic islets.

Cytotoxic T cells can kill their targets rapidly because they store preformed cytotoxic proteins in forms that are inactive in the environment of the lytic granule. Cytotoxic proteins are synthesized and loaded into the lytic granules during the first encounter of a naive cytotoxic precursor T cell with its specific antigen. Ligation of the T-cell receptor similarly induces *de novo* synthesis of perforin and granzymes in armed effector CD8 T cells, so that the supply of lytic granules is replenished. This makes it possible for a single CD8 T cell to kill a series of targets in succession.

8-25   Cytotoxic T cells also act by releasing cytokines.

Inducing apoptosis in target cells is the main way in which cytotoxic CD8 T cells eliminate infection. However, most cytotoxic CD8 T cells also release the cytokines IFN-γ, TNF-α, and TNF-β, which contribute to host defense in several ways. IFN-γ inhibits viral replication directly, and also induces the increased expression of MHC class I and other molecules involved in peptide loading of the newly synthesized MHC class I proteins in infected cells. This increases the chance that infected cells will be recognized as target cells for cytotoxic attack. IFN-γ also activates macrophages, recruiting them to sites of infection both as effector cells and as antigen-presenting cells. IFN-γ also lowers the tryptophan concentration in cells with an IFN-γ receptor and thus can kill intracellular pathogens by starvation. TNF-α or TNF-β can synergize with IFN-γ in macrophage activation and in killing some target cells through their interaction with TNFR-I. Thus, armed effector cytotoxic CD8 T cells act in a variety of ways to limit the spread of cytosolic pathogens. The relative importance of each of these mechanisms is being rapidly determined through gene-knockout technology.

Summary.

Armed effector cytotoxic CD8 T cells are essential in host defense against pathogens that live in the cytosol, the commonest of which are viruses. These cytotoxic T cells can kill any cell harboring such pathogens by recognizing foreign peptides that are transported to the cell surface bound to MHC class I molecules. Cytotoxic CD8 T cells perform their killing function by releasing two types of preformed cytotoxic protein: the granzymes, which seem able to induce apoptosis in any type of target cell, and the pore-forming protein perforin, which punches holes in the target cell membrane through which the granzymes can enter. These properties allow the cytotoxic T cell to attack and destroy virtually any cell that is infected with a cytosolic pathogen. A membrane-bound molecule, the Fas ligand, expressed by CD8 and some CD4 T cells, can also induce apoptosis by binding to Fas expressed by some target cells. Cytotoxic CD8 T cells also produce IFN-γ, which inhibits viral replication and is an important inducer of MHC class I molecule expression and macrophage activation. Cytotoxic T cells kill infected targets with great precision, sparing adjacent normal cells. This precision is crucial in minimizing tissue damage while allowing the eradication of infected cells.

Macrophage activation by armed CD4 T$_H$1 cells.

Some microorganisms such as mycobacteria, the causative agents of tuberculosis and leprosy, are intracellular pathogens that grow primarily in the phagosomes of macrophages. There they are shielded from the effects of both antibodies and cytotoxic T cells. These microbes maintain themselves in the usually hostile environment of the phagocyte by inhibiting the fusion of lysosomes to the phagosomes in which they grow, or by preventing the acidification of these vesicles that is required to activate lysosomal proteases. Such microorganisms can be eliminated when the macrophage is activated by a T$_H$1 cell. Armed T$_H$1 cells act by synthesizing membrane-associated proteins and a range of soluble cytokines whose local and distant actions coordinate the immune response to these intracellular pathogens. Armed T$_H$1 effector cells also activate macrophages to kill recently ingested pathogens, and can activate B cells to secrete a limited but highly effective set of immunoglobulin isotypes, as described in the next chapter.

8-26   Armed T$_H$1 cells have a central role in macrophage activation.

Several important pathogens live within macrophages, whereas many others are ingested by macrophages from the extracellular fluid. In many cases the macrophage is able to destroy such pathogens without the need for T-cell activation, as we have seen in Chapter 2, but in several clinically important infections CD4 T cells are needed to provide activating signals for macrophages. The induction of antimicrobial mechanisms in macrophages is known as **macrophage activation** and is the principal effector action of T$_H$1 cells. Among the extracellular pathogens that are killed when macrophages are activated is *Pneumocystis carinii*; this microorganism is a common cause of death in people with AIDS, because of their deficiency of CD4 T cells. Macrophage activation can be measured by the ability of activated macrophages to damage a broad spectrum of microbes as well as certain tumor cells. This ability to act on extracellular targets extends to healthy tissue cells, which means that macrophages must normally be maintained in an unactivated state.

Macrophages require two signals for activation. One of these is provided by IFN-γ; the other can be provided in a variety of ways and sensitizes the macrophage to respond to IFN-γ. Armed effector T$_H$1 cells can deliver both signals. IFN-γ is the most characteristic cytokine produced by armed T$_H$1 cells on interacting with their specific target cells, whereas the CD40 ligand expressed by the T$_H$1 cell delivers the sensitizing signal by contacting CD40 on the macrophage (Fig. 8.39). CD8 T cells are also an important source of IFN-γ and can activate macrophages presenting antigens derived from cytosolic proteins; mice lacking MHC class I molecules, and thus having no CD8 T cells, show increased susceptibility to some parasitic infections. Macrophages can also be made more sensitive to IFN-γ by very small amounts of bacterial LPS, and this latter pathway may be particularly important when CD8 T cells are the primary source of the IFN-γ. It is also possible that membrane-associated TNF-α or TNF-β can substitute for CD40 ligand in macrophage activation. These cell-associated molecules apparently stimulate the macrophage to secrete TNF-α, and antibody against TNF-α can inhibit macrophage activation. T$_H$2 cells are inefficient macrophage activators because they produce IL-10, a cytokine that can deactivate macrophages, and they also do not produce IFN-γ. They do express CD40 ligand, however, and can deliver the contact-dependent signal required to activate macrophages to respond to IFN-γ.

Fig. 8.39 T$_H$1 cells activate macrophages to become highly microbicidal. When an armed effector T$_H$1 cell specific for a bacterial peptide contacts an infected macrophage, the T cell is induced to secrete the macrophage-activating factor IFN-γ and to express CD40 ligand. Together these newly synthesized T$_H$1 proteins activate the macrophage.

8-27 The production of cytokines and membrane-associated molecules by armed CD4 T$_H$1 cells requires new RNA and protein synthesis.

Within minutes of the recognition of specific antigen by armed effector cytotoxic CD8 T cells, directed exocytosis of preformed perforins and granzymes programs the target cell to die by apoptosis. In contrast, when armed T$_H$1 cells encounter their specific ligand, they must synthesize *de novo* the cytokines and cell-surface molecules that mediate their effects. This process requires hours rather than minutes, so T$_H$1 cells must adhere to their target cells for far longer than cytotoxic T cells.

Recognition of its target by a T$_H$1 cell rapidly induces the transcription of cytokine genes and new protein synthesis begins within an hour of receptor triggering. The newly synthesized cytokines are then delivered directly through microvesicles of the constitutive secretory pathway to the site of contact between the T-cell membrane and the macrophage. It is thought that the newly synthesized cell-surface CD40 ligand is also expressed in this polarized fashion. This means that, although all macrophages have receptors for IFN-γ, the macrophage actually displaying antigen to the armed T$_H$1 cell is far more likely to become activated by it than are neighboring uninfected macrophages.

8-28 Activation of macrophages by armed T$_H$1 cells promotes microbial killing and must be tightly regulated to avoid tissue damage.

T$_H$1 cells activate infected macrophages through cell contact and the focal secretion of IFN-γ. This generates a series of biochemical responses that convert the macrophage into a potent antimicrobial effector cell (Fig. 8.40). Activated macrophages fuse their lysosomes more efficiently to phagosomes, exposing intracellular or recently ingested microbes to a variety of microbicidal lysosomal enzymes. Activated macrophages also make oxygen radicals and nitric oxide (NO), both of which have potent antimicrobial activity, as well as synthesizing antimicrobial peptides and proteases that can be released to attack extracellular parasites.

Additional changes in the activated macrophage help to amplify the immune response. The number of MHC class II molecules, B7 molecules, CD40 molecules, and TNF receptors on the macrophage surface increases, making the cell more effective at presenting antigen to fresh T cells, and more responsive to CD40 ligand and to TNF-α. TNF-α produced by the activated macrophage can synergize with IFN-γ produced by armed T$_H$1 cells in macrophage activation, particularly in the induction of the reactive nitrogen metabolite NO, which has broad antimicrobial activity. The NO is produced by the enzyme **inducible NO synthase (iNOS)**, and mice that have had the gene for iNOS knocked out are highly susceptible to infection by several intracellular pathogens. Activated macrophages also secrete IL-12, which directs the differentiation of activated naive CD4 T cells into T$_H$1 effector cells, as we will learn in Chapter 10. These and many other surface and secreted molecules of activated macrophages are instrumental in the effector actions of macrophages in cell-mediated responses, and they are also important effectors in humoral immune responses, which we will discuss in Chapter 9, and in recruiting other immune cells to sites of infection, a function to which we will return in Chapter 10.

Because activated macrophages are extremely effective in destroying pathogens, one may ask why macrophages are not simply maintained in a state of constant activation. Besides the fact that macrophages consume huge quantities of energy to maintain the activated state, macrophage activation *in*

Fig. 8.40 Activated macrophages undergo changes that greatly increase their antimicrobial effectiveness and amplify the immune response. Activated macrophages increase their expression of CD40 and of TNF receptors, and are stimulated to secrete TNF-α. This autocrine stimulus synergizes with IFN-γ secreted by T$_H$1 cells to increase the antimicrobial action of the macrophage, in particular by inducing the production of nitric oxide (NO) and superoxide ions (O$_2$). The macrophage also upregulates its B7 molecules in response to binding to CD40 ligand on the T cell, and increases its expression of MHC class II molecules, thus allowing further activation of resting CD4 T cells.

vivo is usually associated with localized tissue destruction that apparently results from the release of antimicrobial mediators such as oxygen radicals, NO, and proteases, which are toxic to host cells as well as to pathogens. The ability of activated macrophages to release toxic mediators is important in host defense because it enables them to attack large extracellular pathogens that they cannot ingest, such as parasitic worms. However, this can be achieved only at the expense of tissue damage. Tight regulation of the activity of macrophages by T_H1 cells thus allows the specific and effective deployment of this potent means of host defense while minimizing local tissue damage and energy consumption.

Macrophage activation is mediated by mechanisms that control IFN-γ synthesis by activated effector T cells. This seems to be achieved by regulating the half-life of the mRNA encoding IFN-γ. IFN-γ mRNA, like that encoding a variety of other cytokines, contains a sequence $(AUUUA)_n$ in its 3′ untranslated region that greatly reduces its half-life, and this serves to limit the period of cytokine production. Activation of the T cell seems to induce the production of a new protein that promotes cytokine mRNA degradation: treatment of activated effector T cells with the protein synthesis inhibitor cycloheximide greatly increases the level of cytokine mRNA. The rapid destruction of cytokine mRNA, together with the focal delivery of IFN-γ at the point of contact between the activated T_H1 cell and its macrophage target, thus limits the action of the effector T cell to the infected macrophage. We will see in Chapter 9 that the same mechanisms direct and limit T-cell help to B cells. In addition, macrophage activation itself is markedly inhibited by cytokines such as transforming growth factor-β (TGF-β), and IL-10. Because several of these inhibitory cytokines are produced by T_H2 cells, the induction of CD4 T cells belonging to the T_H2 subset is an important pathway for controlling the effector functions of activated macrophages.

8-29 T_H1 cells coordinate the host response to intracellular pathogens.

The activation of macrophages by armed T_H1 cells expressing CD40 ligand and secreting IFN-γ is central to the host response to pathogens that proliferate in macrophage vesicles. In mice whose IFN-γ gene or CD40 ligand gene has been destroyed by targeted gene disruption, production of antimicrobial agents by macrophages is impaired, and the animals succumb to sublethal doses of *Mycobacterium* and *Leishmania* species. Macrophage activation is also crucial in controlling vaccinia virus. Mice lacking TNF receptors are also more susceptible to these pathogens. However, although IFN-γ and CD40 ligand are probably the most important effector molecules synthesized by T_H1 cells, the immune response to pathogens that proliferate in macrophage vesicles is complex, and other cytokines secreted by T_H1 cells may also be crucial in coordinating these responses (Fig. 8.41). For example, macrophages that are chronically infected with intracellular bacteria may lose the ability to become activated. Such cells could provide a reservoir of infection that is shielded from immune attack. Activated T_H1 cells can also express Fas ligand and thus kill a limited range of target cells that express Fas, including macrophages, thereby destroying these infected cells.

Whereas some intravesicular bacteria pose a hazard by incapacitating chronically infected macrophages, others, including some mycobacteria and *Listeria monocytogenes*, can escape from cell vesicles and enter the cytoplasm, where they are not susceptible to macrophage activation. Their presence can, however, be detected by cytotoxic CD8 T cells, which can release them by killing the cell. The pathogens released when macrophages are killed either by T_H1 cells or by cytotoxic CD8 T cells can be taken up by freshly recruited macrophages still capable of activation to antimicrobial activity.

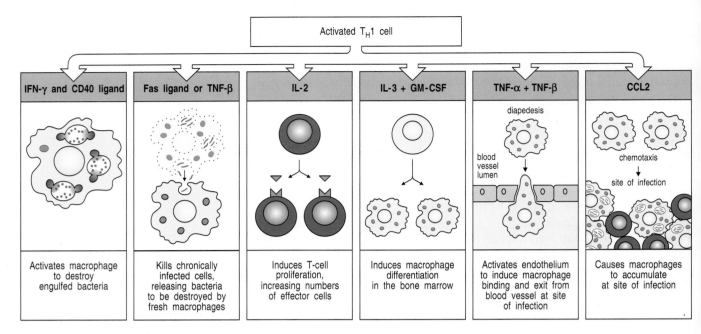

Fig. 8.41 The immune response to intracellular bacteria is coordinated by activated T_H1 cells. The activation of T_H1 cells by infected macrophages results in the synthesis of cytokines that both activate the macrophage and coordinate the immune response to intracellular pathogens. IFN-γ and CD40 ligand synergize in activating the macrophage, which allows it to kill engulfed pathogens. Chronically infected macrophages lose the ability to kill intracellular bacteria, and Fas ligand or TNF-β produced by the T_H1 cell can kill these macrophages, releasing the engulfed bacteria, which are taken up and killed by fresh macrophages. In this way, IFN-γ and TNF-β synergize in the removal of intracellular bacteria. IL-2 produced by T_H1 cells induces T-cell proliferation and potentiates the release of other cytokines. IL-3 and GM-CSF stimulate the production of new macrophages by acting on hematopoietic stem cells in the bone marrow. New macrophages are recruited to the site of infection by the action of TNF-α, TNF-β, and other cytokines on vascular endothelium, which signal macrophages to leave the bloodstream and enter the tissues. A chemokine with macrophage chemotactic activity (CCL2) signals macrophages to migrate into sites of infection and accumulate there. Thus, the T_H1 cell coordinates a macrophage response that is highly effective in destroying intracellular infectious agents.

Another very important function of T_H1 cells is the recruitment of phagocytic cells to sites of infection. T_H1 cells recruit macrophages by two mechanisms. First, they make the hematopoietic growth factors IL-3 and GM-CSF, which stimulate the production of new phagocytic cells in the bone marrow. Second, TNF-α and TNF-β, which are secreted by T_H1 cells at sites of infection, change the surface properties of endothelial cells so that phagocytes adhere to them. Chemokines such as the macrophage chemotactic protein CCL2, which is produced by T_H1 cells in the inflammatory response, serve to direct the migration of these phagocytic cells through the vascular endothelium and to the site of the infection (see Section 2-21).

When microbes effectively resist the microbicidal effects of activated macrophages, chronic infection with inflammation can develop. Often, this has a characteristic pattern, consisting of a central area of macrophages surrounded by activated lymphocytes. This pathological pattern is called a **granuloma** (Fig. 8.42). Giant cells consisting of fused macrophages can form in the center of these granulomas. A granuloma serves to 'wall off' pathogens that resist destruction. T_H2 cells seem to participate in granulomas along with T_H1 cells, perhaps by regulating their activity and preventing widespread tissue damage. In tuberculosis, the center of the large granulomas can become isolated and the cells there die, probably from a combination of lack of oxygen and the cytotoxic effects of activated macrophages. As the dead tissue in the center resembles cheese, this process is called **caseation necrosis**. Thus, the activation of T_H1 cells can cause significant pathology. Their

Fig. 8.42 Granulomas form when an intracellular pathogen or its constituents cannot be totally eliminated. When mycobacteria (red) resist the effects of macrophage activation, a characteristic localized inflammatory response called a granuloma develops. This consists of a central core of infected macrophages. The core may include multinucleated giant cells, which are fused macrophages, surrounded by large macrophages often called epithelioid cells, but in granulomas caused by mycobacteria the core usually becomes necrotic. Mycobacteria can persist in the cells of the granuloma. The central core is surrounded by T cells, many of which are CD4-positive. The exact mechanisms by which this balance is achieved, and how it breaks down, are unknown. Granulomas, as seen in the bottom panel, also form in the lungs and elsewhere in a disease known as sarcoidosis, which may be caused by inapparent mycobacterial infection. Photograph courtesy of J. Orrell.

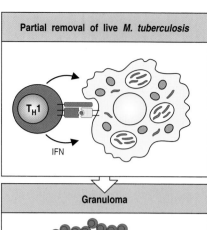

Partial removal of live *M. tuberculosis*

Granuloma

— mycobacteria
— multi-nucleated giant cell
— epithelioid cell
— T cells

nonactivation, however, leads to the more serious consequence of death from disseminated infection, which is now seen frequently in patients with AIDS and concomitant mycobacterial infection.

Summary.

CD4 T cells that can activate macrophages have a critical role in host defense against those intracellular and extracellular pathogens that resist killing after being engulfed by macrophages. Macrophages are activated by membrane-bound signals delivered by activated T_H1 cells and by the potent macrophage-activating cytokine IFN-γ, which is secreted by activated T cells. Once activated, the macrophage can kill intracellular and ingested bacteria. Activated macrophages can also cause local tissue damage, and this explains why their activity is strictly regulated by antigen-specific T cells. T_H1 cells produce a range of cytokines, chemokines, and surface molecules that not only activate infected macrophages but also kill chronically infected senescent macrophages, stimulate the production of new macrophages in bone marrow, and recruit fresh macrophages to sites of infection. Thus, T_H1 cells control and coordinate host defense against certain intracellular pathogens. It is likely that the absence of this function explains the preponderance of infections with intracellular pathogens in adult AIDS patients.

Summary to Chapter 8.

An adaptive immune response is initiated when naive T cells encounter specific antigen on the surface of an antigen-presenting cell that also expresses the co-stimulatory molecules B7.1 and B7.2. In most cases, these first encounters with antigen are thought to occur with a dendritic cell that has taken up antigen at a site of infection, migrated to local lymphoid tissue, and matured to become a potent activator of naive T cells. The activated T cells produce IL-2, which drives them to proliferate and differentiate into armed effector T cells. All T-cell effector functions involve cell–cell interactions. When armed effector T cells recognize specific antigen on target cells, they release mediators that act directly on the target cell, altering its behavior. The triggering of armed effector T cells by peptide:MHC complexes is independent of co-stimulation, so that any infected target cell can be activated or destroyed by an armed effector T cell. CD8 cytotoxic T cells kill target cells infected with cytosolic pathogens, removing sites of pathogen replication. CD4 T_H1 cells activate macrophages to kill intracellular parasites. CD4 T cells are also essential in the activation of B cells to secrete the antibodies that mediate humoral immune responses directed against extracellular pathogens, as we shall see in Chapter 9. Thus, effector T cells control virtually all known effector mechanisms of the adaptive immune response.

Chapter 8 questions.

8.1   T-cell activation requires that the naive T cell find and interact with an antigen-presenting cell. (a) What different molecules are involved in these processes? (b) What consequences would you expect if these molecules were deficient in an individual? (c) What scope do these molecules offer for the design of anti-inflammatory or immunosuppressive drugs?

8.2   In some particle-physics experiments, coincidence detection—the simultaneous measurement of the same event by two separate detectors—is used to discriminate real events from spurious fluctuations in the detector systems. How do the requirements for T-cell activation follow the same principle in: (a) the recognition of pathogens? (b) the prevention of autoimmune reactions?

8.3   T-cell effector functions are primarily mediated by secreted products. (a) To what extent is this true for (i) CD4 cells and (ii) CD8 T cells? (b) What are the roles of T-cell membrane effector molecules in the immune response?

General references.

Dustin, M.L.: **Coordination of T cell activation and migration through formation of the immunological synapse.** *Ann. N.Y. Acad. Sci.* 2003, **987:** 51–59.

Ihle, J.N.: **Cytokine receptor signaling.** *Nature* 1995, **377:**591–594.

Janeway, C.A., and Bottomly, K.: **Signals and signs for lymphocyte responses.** *Cell* 1994, **76:**275–285.

Lanzavecchia, A., and Sallusto, F.: **Antigen decoding by T lymphocytes: from synapses to fate determination.** *Nat. Immunol.* 2001, **2:** 487–492.

McBride, J.M., and Fathman, C.G.: **A complicated relationship: fulfilling the interactive needs of the T lymphocyte and the dendritic cell.** *Pharmacogenomics J.* 2002, **2:** 367–376.

Mosmann, T.R., Li, L., Hengartner, H., Kagi, D., Fu, W., and Sad, S.: **Differentiation and functions of T cell subsets.** *Ciba Found. Symp.* 1997, **204:** 148–154; discussion 154–158.

Snyder, J.E., and Mosmann, T.R.: **How to 'spot' a real killer.** *Trends Immunol.* 2003, **24:** 231–232.

Springer, T.A.: **Traffic signals for lymphocyte recirculation and leukocyte emigration: the multistep paradigm.** *Cell* 1994, **76:**301–314.

Tseng, S.Y., and Dustin, M.L.: **T-cell activation: a multidimensional signaling network.** *Curr. Opin. Cell Biol.* 2002, **14:** 575–580.

Section references.

8-1   **T-cell responses are initiated in peripheral lymphoid organs by activated antigen-presenting cells.**

Caux, C., Ait-Yahia, S., Chemin, K., de Bouteiller, O., Dieu-Nosjean, M.C., Homey, B., Massacrier, C., Vanbervliet, B., Zlotnik, A., and Vicari, A.: **Dendritic cell biology and regulation of dendritic cell trafficking by chemokines.** *Springer Semin. Immunopathol.* 2000, **22:**345–369.

Dupuis, M., Denis-Mize, K., LaBarbara, A., Peters, W., Charo, I.F., McDonald, D.M., and Ott, G.: **Immunization with the adjuvant MF59 induces macrophage trafficking and apoptosis.** *Eur. J. Immunol.* 2001, **31:**2910–2918.

Itano, A.A., and Jenkins, M.K.: **Antigen presentation to naive CD4 T cells in the lymph node.** *Nat. Immunol.* 2003, **4:**733–739.

Picker, L.J., and Butcher, E.C.: **Physiological and molecular mechanisms of lymphocyte homing.** *Annu. Rev. Immunol.* 1993, **10:**561–591.

Steptoe, R.J., Li, W., Fu, F., O'Connell, P.J., and Thomson, A.W.: **Trafficking of APC from liver allografts of Flt3L-treated donors: augmentation of potent allostimulatory cells in recipient lymphoid tissue is associated with a switch from tolerance to rejection.** *Transpl. Immunol.* 1999, **7:**51–57.

Yoshino, M., Yamazaki, H., Nakano, H., Kakiuchi, T., Ryoke, K., Kunisada, T., and

Hayashi, S.: **Distinct antigen trafficking from skin in the steady and active states.** *Int. Immunol.* 2003, **15**:773–779.

8-2 Naive T cells sample the MHC:peptide complexes on the surface of antigen-presenting cells as they migrate through peripheral lymphoid tissue.

Miller, M.J., Wei, S.H., Cahalan, M.D., and Parker, I.: **Autonomous T cell trafficking examined in vivo with intravital two-photon microscopy.** *Proc. Natl. Acad. Sci. USA* 2003, **100**:2604–2609.

Miller, M.J., Wei, S.H., Parker, I., and Cahalan, M.D.: **Two-photon imaging of lymphocyte motility and antigen response in intact lymph node.** *Science* 2002, **296**:1869–1873.

Schlienger, K., Craighead, N., Lee, K.P., Levine, B.L., and June, C.H.: **Efficient priming of protein antigen-specific human CD4+ T cells by monocyte-derived dendritic cells.** *Blood* 2000, **96**:3490–3498.

Thery, C., and Amigorena, S.: **The cell biology of antigen presentation in dendritic cells.** *Curr. Opin. Immunol.* 2001, **13**:45–51.

8-3 Lymphocyte migration, activation, and effector function depend on cell–cell interactions mediated by cell-adhesion molecules.

Hogg, N., Henderson, R., Leitinger, B., McDowall, A., Porter, J., and Stanley, P.: **Mechanisms contributing to the activity of integrins on leukocytes.** *Immunol. Rev.* 2002, **186**:164–171.

Iwata, S., Kobayashi, H., Miyake-Nishijima, R., Sasaki, T., Souta-Kuribara, A., Nori, M., Hosono, O., Kawasaki, H., Tanaka, H., and Morimoto, C.: **Distinctive signaling pathways through CD82 and beta1 integrins in human T cells.** *Eur. J. Immunol.* 2002, **32**:1328–1337.

Kunkel, E.J., Campbell, D.J., and Butcher, E.C.: **Chemokines in lymphocyte trafficking and intestinal immunity.** *Microcirculation* 2003, **10**:313–323.

Laudanna, C., Kim, J.Y., Constantin, G., and Butcher, E.: **Rapid leukocyte integrin activation by chemokines.** *Immunol. Rev.* 2002, **186**:37–46.

Lo, C.G., Lu, T.T., and Cyster, J.G.: **Integrin-dependence of lymphocyte entry into the splenic white pulp.** *J. Exp. Med.* 2003, **197**:353–361.

Madri, J.A., and Graesser, D.: **Cell migration in the immune system: the evolving inter-related roles of adhesion molecules and proteinases.** *Dev. Immunol.* 2000, **7**:103–116.

Picker, L.J.: **Control of lymphocyte homing.** *Curr. Opin. Immunol.* 1994, **6**:394–406.

Yusuf-Makagiansar, H., Anderson, M.E., Yakovleva, T.V., Murray, J.S., and Siahaan, T.J.: **Inhibition of LFA-1/ICAM-1 and VLA-4/VCAM-1 as a therapeutic approach to inflammation and autoimmune diseases.** *Med. Res. Rev.* 2002, **22**:146–167.

8-4 The initial interaction of T cells with antigen-presenting cells is mediated by cell-adhesion molecules.

Bromley, S.K., Burack, W.R., Johnson, K.G., Somersalo, K., Sims, T.N., Sumen, C., Davis, M.M., Shaw, A.S., Allen, P.M., and Dustin, M.L.: **The immunological synapse.** *Annu. Rev. Immunol.* 2001, **19**:375–396.

Friedl, P., and Brocker, E.B.: **TCR triggering on the move: diversity of T-cell interactions with antigen-presenting cells.** *Immunol. Rev.* 2002, **186**:83–89.

Gunzer, M., Schafer, A., Borgmann, S., Grabbe, S., Zanker, K.S., Brocker, E.B., Kampgen, E., and Friedl, P.: **Antigen presentation in extracellular matrix: interactions of T cells with dendritic cells are dynamic, short lived, and sequential.** *Immunity* 2000, **13**:323–332.

Montoya, M.C., Sancho, D., Vicente-Manzanares, M., and Sanchez-Madrid, F.: **Cell adhesion and polarity during immune interactions.** *Immunol. Rev.* 2002, **186**:68–82.

Wang, J., and Eck, M.J.: **Assembling atomic resolution views of the immunological synapse.** *Curr. Opin. Immunol.* 2003, **15**:286–293.

8-5 Both specific antigen and co-stimulatory signals provided by the same antigen-presenting cell are required for the clonal expansion of naive T cells.

Bour-Jordan, H., and Bluestone, J.A.: **CD28 function: a balance of costimulatory and regulatory signals.** *J. Clin. Immunol.* 2002, **22**:1–7.

Gonzalo, J.A., Delaney, T., Corcoran, J., Goodearl, A., Gutierrez-Ramos, J.C., and Coyle, A.J.: **Cutting edge: the related molecules CD28 and inducible costimulator deliver both unique and complementary signals required for optimal T cell activation.** *J. Immunol.* 2001, **166**:1–5.

Wang, S., Zhu, G., Chapoval, A.I., Dong, H., Tamada, K., Ni, J., and Chen, L.: **Costimulation of T cells by B7-H2, a B7-like molecule that binds ICOS.** *Blood* 2000, **96**:2808–2813.

8-6 Dendritic cells specialize in ingesting antigen and activating naive T cells.

Belz, G.T., Carbone, F.R., and Heath, W.R.: **Cross-presentation of antigens by dendritic cells.** *Crit. Rev. Immunol.* 2002, **22**:439–448.

Gatti, E., and Pierre, P.: **Understanding the cell biology of antigen presentation: the dendritic cell contribution.** *Curr. Opin. Cell Biol.* 2003, **15**:468–473.

Guermonprez, P., Valladeau, J., Zitvogel, L., Thery, C., and Amigorena, S.: **Antigen presentation and T cell stimulation by dendritic cells.** *Annu. Rev. Immunol.* 2002, **20**:621–667.

8-7 Macrophages are scavenger cells that can be induced by pathogens to present foreign antigens to naive T cells.

Barker, R.N., Erwig, L.P., Hill, K.S., Devine, A., Pearce, W.P., and Rees, A.J.: **Antigen presentation by macrophages is enhanced by the uptake of necrotic, but not apoptotic, cells.** *Clin. Exp. Immunol.* 2002, **127**:220–225.

Underhill, D.M., Bassetti, M., Rudensky, A., and Aderem, A.: **Dynamic interactions of macrophages with T cells during antigen presentation.** *J. Exp. Med.* 1999, **190**:1909–1914.

Zhu, F.G., Reich, C.F., and Pisetsky, D.S.: **The role of the macrophage scavenger receptor in immune stimulation by bacterial DNA and synthetic oligonucleotides.** *Immunology* 2001, **103**:226–234.

8-8 B cells are highly efficient at presenting antigens that bind to their surface immunoglobulin.

Guermonprez, P., England, P., Bedouelle, H., and Leclerc, C.: **The rate of dissociation between antibody and antigen determines the efficiency of antibody-mediated antigen presentation to T cells.** *J. Immunol.* 1998, **161**:4542–4548.

Lanzavecchia, A.: **Receptor-mediated antigen uptake and its effect on antigen presentation to class II-restricted T lymphocytes.** *Annu. Rev. Immunol.* 1993, **8**:773–793.

Shirota, H., Sano, K., Hirasawa, N., Terui, T., Ohuchi, K., Hattori, T., and Tamura, G.: **B cells capturing antigen conjugated with CpG oligodeoxynucleotides induce Th1 cells by elaborating IL-12.** *J. Immunol.* 2002, **169**:787–794.

Zaliauskiene, L., Kang, S., Sparks, K., Zinn, K.R., Schwiebert, L.M., Weaver, C.T., and Collawn, J.F.: **Enhancement of MHC class II-restricted responses by receptor-mediated uptake of peptide antigens.** *J. Immunol.* 2002, **169**:2337–2345.

8-9 Activated T cells synthesize the T-cell growth factor interleukin-2 and its receptor.

&

8-10 The co-stimulatory signal is necessary for the synthesis and secretion of IL-2.

Appleman, L.J., Berezovskaya, A., Grass, I., and Boussiotis, V.A.: **CD28 costimulation mediates T cell expansion via IL-2-independent and IL-2-dependent regulation of cell cycle progression.** *J. Immunol.* 2000, **164**:144–151.

Chang, J.T., Segal, B.M., and Shevach, E.M.: **Role of costimulation in the induction of the IL-12/IL-12 receptor pathway and the development of autoimmunity.** *J. Immunol.* 2000, **164**:100–106.

Gaffen, S.L.: **Signaling domains of the interleukin 2 receptor.** *Cytokine* 2001, **14**:63–77.

Michel, F., Attal-Bonnefoy, G., Mangino, G., Mise-Omata, S., and Acuto, O.: **CD28 as a molecular amplifier extending TCR ligation and signaling capabilities.** *Immunity* 2001, **15**:935–945.

Zhou, X.Y., Yashiro-Ohtani, Y., Nakahira, M., Park, W.R., Abe, R., Hamaoka, T., Naramura, M., Gu, H., and Fujiwara, H.: **Molecular mechanisms underlying differential contribution of CD28 versus non-CD28 costimulatory molecules to IL-2 promoter activation.** *J. Immunol.* 2002, **168**:3847–3854.

8-11 Antigen recognition in the absence of co-stimulation leads to the inactivation of peripheral T cells.

Schwartz, R.H.: **T cell anergy.** *Annu. Rev. Immunol.* 2003, **21**:305–334.

Vanhove, B., Laflamme, G., Coulon, F., Mougin, M., Vusio, P., Haspot, F., Tiollier, J., and Soulillou, J.P.: **Selective blockade of CD28 and not CTLA-4 with a single-chain Fv-alpha1-antitrypsin fusion antibody.** *Blood* 2003, **102**:564–570.

Wekerle, T., Blaha, P., Langer, F., Schmid, M., and Muehlbacher, F.: **Tolerance through bone marrow transplantation with costimulation blockade.** *Transpl. Immunol.* 2002, **9**:125–133.

8-12 Proliferating T cells differentiate into armed effector T cells that do not require co-stimulation to act.

Gudmundsdottir, H., Wells, A.D., and Turka, L.A.: **Dynamics and requirements of T cell clonal expansion *in vivo* at the single-cell level: effector function is linked to proliferative capacity.** *J. Immunol.* 1999, **162**:5212–5223.

London, C.A., Lodge, M.P., and Abbas, A.K.: **Functional responses and co-stimulator dependence of memory CD4+ T cells.** *J. Immunol.* 2000, **164**:265–272.

Schweitzer, A.N., and Sharpe, A.H.: **Studies using antigen-presenting cells lacking expression of both B7-1 (CD80) and B7-2 (CD86) show distinct requirements for B7 molecules during priming versus restimulation of Th2 but not Th1 cytokine production.** *J. Immunol.* 1998, **161**:2762–2771.

8-13 The differentiation of CD4 T cells into T$_H$1 or T$_H$2 cells determines whether humoral or cell-mediated immunity will predominate.

Ansel, K.M., Lee, D.U., and Rao, A.: **An epigenetic view of helper T cell differentiation.** *Nat. Immunol.* 2003, **4**:616–623.

Farrar, J.D., Ouyang, W., Lohning, M., Assenmacher, M., Radbruch, A., Kanagawa, O., and Murphy, K.M.: **An instructive component in T helper cell type 2 (Th2) development mediated by GATA-3.** *J. Exp. Med.* 2001, **193**:643–650.

Holzer, U., Kwok, W.W., Nepom, G.T., and Buckner, J.H.: **Differential antigen sensitivity and costimulatory requirements in human Th1 and Th2 antigen-specific CD4+ cells with similar TCR avidity.** *J. Immunol.* 2003, **170**:1218–1223.

Murphy, K.M., and Reiner, S.L.: **The lineage decisions of helper T cells.** *Nat. Rev. Immunol.* 2002, **2**:933–944.

Nath, I., Vemuri, N., Reddi, A.L., Jain, S., Brooks, P., Colston, M.J., Misra, R.S., and Ramesh, V.: **The effect of antigen presenting cells on the cytokine profiles of stable and reactional lepromatous leprosy patients.** *Immunol. Lett.* 2000, **75**:69–76.

Szabo, S.J., Sullivan, B.M., Peng, S.L., and Glimcher, L.H.: **Molecular mechanisms regulating Th1 immune responses.** *Annu. Rev. Immunol.* 2003, **21**:713–758.

Zhou, M., and Ouyang, W.: **The function role of GATA-3 in Th1 and Th2 differentiation.** *Immunol. Res.* 2003, **28**:25–37.

8-14 Naive CD8 T cells can be activated in different ways to become armed cytotoxic effector cells.

Andreasen, S.O., Christensen, J.E., Marker, O., and Thomsen, A.R.: **Role of CD40 ligand and CD28 in induction and maintenance of antiviral CD8+ effector T cell responses.** *J. Immunol.* 2000, **164**:3689–3697.

Blazevic, V., Trubey, C.M., and Shearer, G.M.: **Analysis of the costimulatory requirements for generating human virus-specific in vitro T helper and effector responses.** *J. Clin. Immunol.* 2001, **21**:293–302.

Croft, M.: **Co-stimulatory members of the TNFR family: keys to effective T-cell immunity?** *Nat. Rev. Immunol.* 2003, **3**:609–620.

Liang, L., and Sha, W.C.: **The right place at the right time: novel B7 family**

members regulate effector T cell responses. *Curr. Opin. Immunol.* 2002, **14**:384–390.

Seder, R.A., and Ahmed, R.: **Similarities and differences in CD4+ and CD8+ effector and memory T cell generation.** *Nat. Immunol.* 2003, **4**:835–842.

Weninger, W., Manjunath, N., and von Andrian, U.H.: **Migration and differentiation of CD8+ T cells.** *Immunol. Rev.* 2002, **186**:221–233.

8-15 Effector T-cell interactions with target cells are initiated by antigen-nonspecific cell-adhesion molecules.

Dustin, M.L.: **Role of adhesion molecules in activation signaling in T lymphocytes.** *J. Clin. Immunol.* 2001, **21**:258–263.

van der Merwe, P.A., and Davis, S.J.: **Molecular interactions mediating T cell antigen recognition.** *Annu. Rev. Immunol.* 2003, **21**:659–684.

8-16 Binding of the T-cell receptor complex directs the release of effector molecules and focuses them on the target cell.

Bossi, G., Trambas, C., Booth, S., Clark, R., Stinchcombe, J., and Griffiths, G.M.: **The secretory synapse: the secrets of a serial killer.** *Immunol. Rev.* 2002, **189**:152–160.

Dustin, M.L.: **Coordination of T cell activation and migration through formation of the immunological synapse.** *Ann. N.Y. Acad. Sci.* 2003, **987**:51–59.

Montoya, M.C., Sancho, D., Vicente-Manzanares, M., and Sanchez-Madrid, F.: **Cell adhesion and polarity during immune interactions.** *Immunol. Rev.* 2002, **186**:68–82.

Trambas, C.M., and Griffiths, G.M.: **Delivering the kiss of death.** *Nat. Immunol.* 2003, **4**:399–403.

8-17 The effector functions of T cells are determined by the array of effector molecules that they produce.

&

8-18 Cytokines can act locally or at a distance.

Guidotti, L.G., and Chisari, F.V.: **Cytokine-mediated control of viral infections.** *Virology* 2000, **273**:221–227.

Harty, J.T., Tvinnereim, A.R., and White, D.W.: **CD8+ T cell effector mechanisms in resistance to infection.** *Annu. Rev. Immunol.* 2000, **18**:275–308.

Santana, M.A., and Rosenstein, Y.: **What it takes to become an effector T cell: the process, the cells involved, and the mechanisms.** *J. Cell Physiol.* 2003, **195**:392–401.

8-19 Cytokines and their receptors fall into distinct families of structurally related proteins.

Basler, C.F., and Garcia-Sastre, A.: **Viruses and the type I interferon antiviral system: induction and evasion.** *Int. Rev. Immunol.* 2002, **21**:305–337.

Boulay, J.L., O'Shea, J.J., and Paul, W.E.: **Molecular phylogeny within type I cytokines and their cognate receptors.** *Immunity* 2003, **19**:159–163.

Collette, Y., Gilles, A., Pontarotti, P., and Olive, D.: **A co-evolution perspective of the TNFSF and TNFRSF families in the immune system.** *Trends Immunol.* 2003, **24**:387–394.

Proudfoot, A.E.: **Chemokine receptors: multifaceted therapeutic targets.** *Nat. Rev. Immunol.* 2002, **2**:106–115.

Taniguchi, T., and Takaoka, A.: **The interferon-alpha/beta system in antiviral responses: a multimodal machinery of gene regulation by the IRF family of transcription factors.** *Curr. Opin. Immunol.* 2002, **14**:111–116.

Wong, M.M., and Fish, E.N.: **Chemokines: attractive mediators of the immune response.** *Semin. Immunol.* 2003, **15**:5–14.

8-20 The TNF family of cytokines are trimeric proteins that are usually associated with the cell surface.

Hehlgans, T., and Mannel, D.N.: **The TNF-TNF receptor system.** *Biol. Chem.* 2002, **383**:1581–1585.

Locksley, R.M., Killeen, N., and Lenardo, M.J.: **The TNF and TNF receptor** superfamilies: integrating mammalian biology. *Cell* 2001, **104**:487–501.

Screaton, G., and Xu, X.N.: **T cell life and death signalling via TNF-receptor family members.** *Curr. Opin. Immunol.* 2000, **12**:316–322.

Theill, L.E., Boyle, W.J., and Penninger, J.M.: **RANK-L and RANK: T cells, bone loss, and mammalian evolution.** *Annu. Rev. Immunol.* 2002, **20**:795–823.

Zhou, T., Mountz, J.D., and Kimberly, R.P.: **Immunobiology of tumor necrosis factor receptor superfamily.** *Immunol. Res.* 2002, **26**:323–336.

8-21   Cytotoxic T cells can induce target cells to undergo programmed cell death.

Barry, M., and Bleackley, R.C.: **Cytotoxic T lymphocytes: all roads lead to death.** *Nat. Rev. Immunol.* 2002, **2**:401–409.

Russell, J.H., and Ley, T.J.: **Lymphocyte-mediated cytotoxicity.** *Annu. Rev. Immunol.* 2002, **20**:323–370.

Zimmermann, K.C., and Green, D.R.: **How cells die: apoptosis pathways.** *J. Allergy Clin. Immunol.* 2001, **108**:S99–S103.

8-22   Cytotoxic effector proteins that trigger apoptosis are contained in the granules of CD8 cytotoxic T cells.

Barry, M., Heibein, J.A., Pinkoski, M.J., Lee, S.F., Moyer, R.W., Green, D.R., and Bleackley, R.C.: **Granzyme B short-circuits the need for caspase 8 activity during granule-mediated cytotoxic T-lymphocyte killing by directly cleaving Bid.** *Mol. Cell Biol.* 2000, **20**:3781–3794.

Lieberman, J.: **The ABCs of granule-mediated cytotoxicity: new weapons in the arsenal.** *Nat. Rev. Immunol.* 2003, **3**:361–370.

Smyth, M.J., Kelly, J.M., Sutton, V.R., Davis, J.E., Browne, K.A., Sayers, T.J., and Trapani, J.A.: **Unlocking the secrets of cytotoxic granule proteins.** *J. Leukoc. Biol.* 2001, **70**:18–29.

8-23   Activated CD8 T cells and some CD4 effector T cells express Fas ligand, which can also activate apoptosis.

Green, D.R., Droin, N., and Pinkoski, M.: **Activation-induced cell death in T cells.** *Immunol. Rev.* 2003, **193**:70–81.

Greil, R., Anether, G., Johrer, K., and Tinhofer, I.: **Tracking death dealing by Fas and TRAIL in lymphatic neoplastic disorders: pathways, targets, and therapeutic tools.** *J. Leukoc. Biol.* 2003, **74**:311–330.

Medana, I.M., Gallimore, A., Oxenius, A., Martinic, M.M., Wekerle, H., and Neumann, H.: **MHC class I-restricted killing of neurons by virus-specific CD8+ T lymphocytes is effected through the Fas/FasL, but not the perforin pathway.** *Eur. J. Immunol.* 2000, **30**:3623–3633.

Wallin, R.P., Screpanti, V., Michaelsson, J., Grandien, A., and Ljunggren, H.G.: **Regulation of perforin-independent NK cell-mediated cytotoxicity.** *Eur. J. Immunol.* 2003, **33**:2727–2735.

8-24   Cytotoxic T cells are selective and serial killers of targets expressing specific antigen.

Bossi, G., Trambas, C., Booth, S., Clark, R., Stinchcombe, J., and Griffiths, G.M.: **The secretory synapse: the secrets of a serial killer.** *Immunol. Rev.* 2002, **189**:152–160.

Stinchcombe, J.C., Bossi, G., Booth, S., and Griffiths, G.M.: **The immunological synapse of CTL contains a secretory domain and membrane bridges.** *Immunity* 2001, **15**:751–761.

Trambas, C.M., and Griffiths, G.M.: **Delivering the kiss of death.** *Nat. Immunol.* 2003, **4**:399–403.

8-25   Cytotoxic T cells also act by releasing cytokines.

Amel-Kashipaz, M.R., Huggins, M.L., Lanyon, P., Robins, A., Todd, I., and Powell, R.J.: **Quantitative and qualitative analysis of the balance between type 1 and type 2 cytokine-producing CD8– and CD8+ T cells in systemic lupus erythematosus.** *J. Autoimmun.* 2001, **17**:155–163.

Kemp, R.A., and Ronchese, F.: **Tumor-specific Tc1, but not Tc2, cells deliver protective antitumor immunity.** *J. Immunol.* 2001, **167**:6497–6502.

Prezzi, C., Casciaro, M.A., Francavilla, V., Schiaffella, E., Finocchi, L., Chircu, L.V., Bruno, G., Sette, A., Abrignani, S., and Barnaba, V.: **Virus-specific CD8+ T cells with type 1 or type 2 cytokine profile are related to different disease activity in chronic hepatitis C virus infection.** *Eur. J. Immunol.* 2001, **31**:894–906.

Woodland, D.L., and Dutton, R.W.: **Heterogeneity of CD4+ and CD8+ T cells.** *Curr. Opin. Immunol.* 2003, **15**:336–342.

8-26   Armed T_H1 cells have a central role in macrophage activation.

Monney, L., Sabatos, C.A., Gaglia, J.L., Ryu, A., Waldner, H., Chernova, T., Manning, S., Greenfield, E.A., Coyle, A.J., Sobel, R.A., Freeman, G.J., and Kuchroo, V.K.: **Th1-specific cell surface protein Tim-3 regulates macrophage activation and severity of an autoimmune disease.** *Nature* 2002, **415**:536–541.

Munoz Fernandez, M.A., Fernandez, M.A., and Fresno, M.: **Synergism between tumor necrosis factor-α and interferon-γ on macrophage activation for the killing of intracellular *Trypanosoma cruzi* through a nitric oxide-dependent mechanism.** *Eur. J. Immunol.* 1992, **22**:301–307.

Stout, R., and Bottomly, K.: **Antigen-specific activation of effector macrophages by interferon-γ producing (T_H1) T-cell clones: failure of IL-4 producing (T_H2) T-cell clones to activate effector functions in macrophages.** *J. Immunol.* 1989, **142**:760–765.

8-27   The production of cytokines and membrane-associated molecules by armed CD4 T_H1 cells requires new RNA and protein synthesis.

Shaw, G., and Kamen, R.: **A conserved AU sequence from the 3′ untranslated region of GM-CSF mRNA mediates selective mRNA degradation.** *Cell* 1986, **46**:659–667.

8-28   Activation of macrophages by armed T_H1 cells promotes microbial killing and must be tightly regulated to avoid tissue damage.

Duffield, J.S.: **The inflammatory macrophage: a story of Jekyll and Hyde.** *Clin. Sci. (Lond.)* 2003, **104**:27–38.

James, D.G.: **A clinicopathological classification of granulomatous disorders.** *Postgrad. Med. J.* 2000, **76**:457–465.

Labow, R.S., Meek, E., and Santerre, J.P.: **Model systems to assess the destructive potential of human neutrophils and monocyte-derived macrophages during the acute and chronic phases of inflammation.** *J. Biomed. Mater. Res.* 2001, **54**:189–197.

Wigginton, J.E., and Kirschner, D.: **A model to predict cell-mediated immune regulatory mechanisms during human infection with *Mycobacterium tuberculosis*.** *J. Immunol.* 2001, **166**:1951–1967.

8-29 T_H1 cells coordinate the host response to intracellular pathogens.

Alexander, J., Satoskar, A.R., and Russell, D.G.: **Leishmania species: models of intracellular parasitism.** *J. Cell Sci.* 1999, **112**:2993–3002.

Berberich, C., Ramirez-Pineda, J.R., Hambrecht, C., Alber, G., Skeiky, Y.A., and Moll, H.: **Dendritic cell (DC)-based protection against an intracellular pathogen is dependent upon DC-derived IL-12 and can be induced by molecularly defined antigens.** *J. Immunol.* 2003, **170**:3171–3179.

Biedermann, T., Zimmermann, S., Himmelrich, H., Gumy, A., Egeter, O., Sakrauski, A.K., Seegmuller, I., Voigt, H., Launois, P., Levine, A.D., Wagner, H., Heeg, K., Louis, J.A., and Rocken, M.: **IL-4 instructs TH1 responses and resistance to Leishmania major in susceptible BALB/c mice.** *Nat. Immunol.* 2001, **2**:1054–1060.

Koguchi, Y., and Kawakami, K.: **Cryptococcal infection and Th1-Th2 cytokine balance.** *Int. Rev. Immunol.* 2002, **21**:423–438.

Neighbors, M., Xu, X., Barrat, F.J., Ruuls, S.R., Churakova, T., Debets, R., Bazan, J.F., Kastelein, R.A., Abrams, J.S., and O'Garra, A.: **A critical role for interleukin 18 in primary and memory effector responses to *Listeria monocytogenes* that extends beyond its effects on Interferon gamma production.** *J. Exp. Med.* 2001, **194**:343–354.

The Humoral Immune Response

9

Many of the bacteria that cause infectious disease in humans multiply in the extracellular spaces of the body, and most intracellular pathogens spread by moving from cell to cell through the extracellular fluids. The extracellular spaces are protected by the **humoral immune response**, in which antibodies produced by B cells cause the destruction of extracellular microorganisms and prevent the spread of intracellular infections. The activation of B cells and their differentiation into antibody-secreting plasma cells (Fig. 9.1) and memory B cells is triggered by antigen and usually requires helper T cells. The term 'helper T cell' is often used to mean a cell from the T_H2 class of CD4 T cells (see Chapter 8), but a subset of T_H1 cells can also help in B-cell activation. In this chapter we therefore use the term **helper T cell** to mean any armed effector CD4 T cell that can activate a B cell. Helper T cells also control isotype switching and have a role in initiating the somatic hypermutation of antibody V-region genes, molecular processes that were described in Chapter 4.

Antibodies contribute to immunity in three main ways (see Fig. 9.1). To enter cells, viruses and intracellular bacteria bind to specific molecules on the target cell surface. Antibodies that bind to the pathogen can prevent this and are said to **neutralize** the pathogen. Neutralization by antibodies is also important in preventing bacterial toxins from entering cells. Antibodies protect against bacteria that multiply outside cells mainly by facilitating uptake of the pathogen by phagocytic cells that are specialized to destroy ingested bacteria. Coating the surface of a pathogen to enhance phagocytosis is called **opsonization**. Antibodies do this in either of two ways. In the first, bound

Fig. 9.1 The humoral immune response is mediated by antibody molecules that are secreted by plasma cells. Antigen that binds to the B-cell antigen receptor signals B cells and is, at the same time, internalized and processed into peptides that activate armed helper T cells. Signals from the bound antigen and from the helper T cell induce the B cell to proliferate and differentiate into plasma cells secreting specific antibody (top two panels). These antibodies protect the host from infection in three main ways. First, they can inhibit the toxic effects or infectivity of pathogens by binding to them: this is termed neutralization (bottom left panel). Second, by coating the pathogens they can enable accessory cells that recognize the Fc portions of arrays of antibodies to ingest and kill the pathogen, a process called opsonization (bottom center panel). Third, antibodies can trigger the activation of the complement system. Complement proteins can strongly enhance opsonization, and can directly kill certain bacterial cells (bottom right panel).

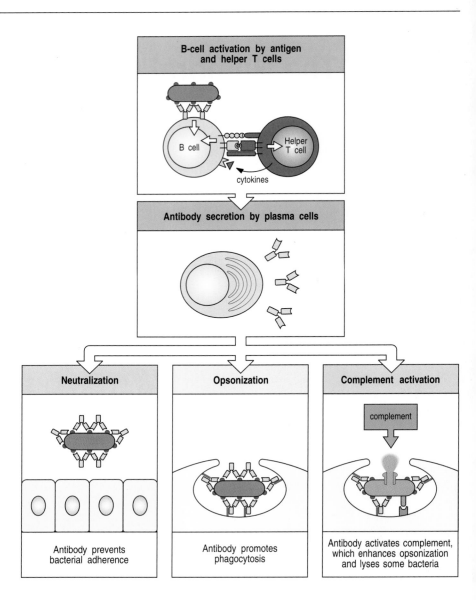

antibodies coating the pathogen are recognized by Fc receptors on phagocytic cells that bind to the antibody C-region (see Section 4-19). Alternatively, antibodies binding to the surface of a pathogen can activate the proteins of the complement system, which was described in Chapter 2. **Complement activation** results in complement proteins being bound to the pathogen surface, and these opsonize the pathogen by binding complement receptors on phagocytes. Other complement components recruit phagocytic cells to the site of infection, and the terminal components of complement can lyse certain microorganisms directly by forming pores in their membranes. Which effector mechanisms are engaged in a particular response is determined by the isotype or class of the antibodies produced.

In the first part of this chapter we describe the interactions of B cells with helper T cells that lead to the production of antibodies, the affinity maturation of this antibody response, the isotype switching that confers functional diversity, and the generation of memory B cells that provide long-lasting immunity to reinfection. In the rest of the chapter we discuss in detail the mechanisms whereby antibodies contain and eliminate infections.

B-cell activation by armed helper T cells.

The surface immunoglobulin that serves as the **B-cell antigen receptor** (**BCR**) has two roles in B-cell activation. First, like the antigen receptor on T cells, it transmits signals directly to the cell's interior when it binds antigen (see Section 6-1). Second, the B-cell antigen receptor delivers the antigen to intracellular sites where it is degraded and returned to the B-cell surface as peptides bound to MHC class II molecules (see Chapter 5). The peptide:MHC class II complex can be recognized by antigen-specific armed helper T cells, stimulating them to make proteins that, in turn, cause the B cell to proliferate and its progeny to differentiate into antibody-secreting cells and into memory B cells (the latter will be described in more detail in Chapter 10). Some microbial antigens can activate B cells directly in the absence of T-cell help. The ability of B cells to respond directly to these antigens provides a rapid response to many important pathogens. However, somatic hypermutation and switching to certain immunoglobulin isotypes depend on the interaction of antigen-stimulated B cells with helper T cells and other cells in the peripheral lymphoid organs. Antibodies induced by microbial antigens alone are therefore less variable and less functionally versatile than those induced with T-cell help.

9-1 The humoral immune response is initiated when B cells that bind antigen are signaled by helper T cells or by certain microbial antigens alone.

It is a general rule in adaptive immunity that naive antigen-specific lymphocytes are difficult to activate by antigen alone. Naive T cells require a co-stimulatory signal from professional antigen-presenting cells; naive B cells require accessory signals that can come either from an armed helper T cell or, in some cases, directly from microbial constituents.

Antibody responses to protein antigens require antigen-specific T-cell help. B cells can receive help from armed helper T cells when antigen bound by surface immunoglobulin is internalized and returned to the cell surface as peptides bound to MHC class II molecules. Armed helper T cells that recognize the peptide:MHC complex then deliver activating signals to the B cell. Thus, protein antigens binding to B cells both provide a specific signal to the B cell by cross-linking its antigen receptors and allow the B cell to attract antigen-specific T-cell help. These antigens are unable to induce antibody responses in animals or humans who lack T cells, and they are therefore known as **thymus-dependent** or **TD antigens** (Fig. 9.2, top two panels).

Fig. 9.2 A second signal is required for B-cell activation by either thymus-dependent or thymus-independent antigens. The first signal required for B-cell activation is delivered through its antigen receptor (top panel). For thymus-dependent antigens, the second signal is delivered by a helper T cell that recognizes degraded fragments of the antigen as peptides bound to MHC class II molecules on the B-cell surface (center panel); the interaction between CD40 ligand (CD40L, also called CD154) on the T cell and CD40 on the B cell contributes an essential part of this second signal. For thymus-independent antigens, the second signal can be delivered by the antigen itself (bottom panel), either through direct binding of a part of the antigen to a receptor of the innate immune system, such as a Toll-like receptor (green), or simply by extensive cross-linking of the membrane IgM by a polymeric antigen (not shown).

The **B-cell co-receptor** complex of CD19:CD21:CD81 (see Section 6-9) can greatly enhance B-cell responsiveness to antigen. CD21 (also known as complement receptor 2, CR2) is a receptor for the complement fragment C3dg (see Section 2-16). When mice are immunized with hen egg lysozyme coupled to three linked molecules of the complement fragment C3dg, the dose of modified lysozyme needed to induce antibody in the absence of added adjuvant is up to 10,000 times smaller than that needed for unmodified hen egg lysozyme. It is not yet known whether binding of CD21 enhances B-cell responsiveness by increasing B-cell signaling, by inducing co-stimulatory molecules on the B cell, or by increasing the receptor-mediated uptake of antigen. As we will see later in this chapter, antibodies already bound to antigens can activate the complement system, thus coating the antigen with C3dg and producing a more potent antigen, which in turn leads to more efficient B-cell activation and antibody production.

Although armed peptide-specific helper T cells are required for B-cell responses to protein antigens, many microbial constituents, such as bacterial polysaccharides, can induce antibody production in the absence of helper T cells. These microbial antigens are known as **thymus-independent** or **TI antigens** because they induce antibody responses in individuals who have no T lymphocytes. The second signal required to activate antibody production to TI antigens is either provided directly by recognition of a common microbial constituent (see Fig. 9.2, bottom panel) or by massive cross-linking of B-cell receptors, which would occur when a B cell binds repeating epitopes on the bacterial cell. Thymus-independent antibody responses provide some protection against extracellular bacteria, and we will return to them later.

9-2   Armed helper T cells activate B cells that recognize the same antigen.

Armed helper T cells activate B cells to proliferate and differentiate when they recognize the appropriate peptide:MHC class II complex on the B-cell surface (Fig. 9.3). T-cell dependent antibody responses require the activation of B cells by helper T cells that respond to the same antigen; this is called **linked recognition**. This means that before B cells can be induced to make antibody against an infecting pathogen, a CD4 T cell specific for peptides from this pathogen must first be activated to produce appropriately armed helper T cells. This presumably occurs when the T cell interacts with an antigen-

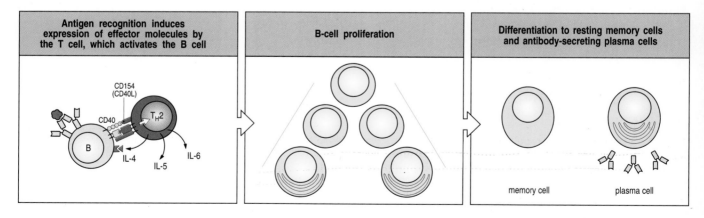

Fig. 9.3 Armed helper T cells stimulate the proliferation and then the differentiation of antigen-binding B cells. The specific interaction of an antigen-binding B cell with an armed helper T cell leads to the expression of the B-cell stimulatory molecule CD40 ligand (CD154) on the helper T-cell surface and to the secretion of the B-cell stimulatory cytokines IL-4, IL-5, and IL-6, which drive the proliferation and differentiation of the B cell into antibody-secreting plasma cells. An activated B cell can alternatively become a memory cell.

Fig. 9.4 B cells and helper T cells must recognize epitopes of the same molecular complex in order to interact. An epitope on a viral coat protein is recognized by the surface immunoglobulin on a B cell, and the virus is internalized and degraded. Peptides derived from viral proteins, including internal proteins, are returned to the B-cell surface bound to MHC class II molecules (see Chapter 5). Here, these complexes are recognized by helper T cells, which help to activate the B cells to produce antibody against the coat protein.

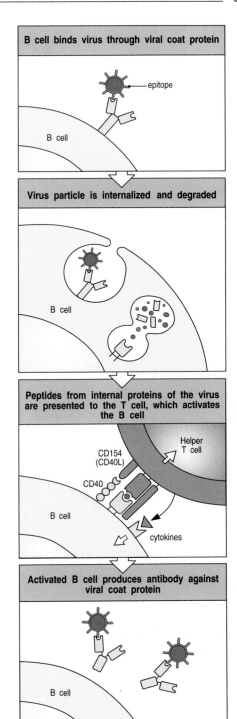

presenting dendritic cell or macrophage (see Section 8-1). Although the epitope recognized by the armed helper T cell must be linked to that recognized by the B cell, the two cells need not recognize identical epitopes. Indeed, we saw in Chapter 5 that T cells can recognize peptides derived from the core region of proteins that are quite distinct from the surface epitopes on the same protein recognized by B cells. For more complex natural antigens, such as viruses, the T cell and the B cell might not even recognize the same protein. It is, however, crucial that the peptide recognized by the T cell be physically associated with the antigen recognized by the B cell, which can thus produce the appropriate peptide after internalization of the antigen bound to its B-cell receptors.

For example, by recognizing an epitope on a viral protein coat, a B cell can internalize a complete virus particle. After internalization, the virus particle is degraded and peptides from internal viral proteins as well as coat proteins can be displayed by MHC class II molecules on the B-cell surface. Helper T cells that have been primed earlier in an infection by macrophages or dendritic cells presenting these internal peptides can then activate the B cell to make antibodies that recognize the coat protein (Fig. 9.4).

The specific activation of the B cell by a T cell sensitized to the same antigen or pathogen depends on the ability of the antigen-specific B cell to concentrate the appropriate peptide on its surface MHC class II molecules. B cells that bind a particular antigen are up to 10,000 times more efficient at displaying peptide fragments of that antigen on their MHC class II molecules than are B cells that do not bind the antigen. Armed helper T cells will therefore help only those B cells whose receptors bind an antigen containing the peptide that they recognize.

The requirement for linked recognition has important consequences for the regulation and manipulation of the humoral immune response. One is that linked recognition helps to ensure self tolerance, because an autoimmune response requires the simultaneous presence of a self-reactive T cell as well as the self-reactive B cell, as will be described in Chapter 13. Another important application of linked recognition is in the design of vaccines, such as that used to immunize infants against *Haemophilus influenzae* type b. This bacterial pathogen can infect the covering of the brain, called the meninges, causing meningitis. Protective immunity to this pathogen is mediated by antibodies against its capsular polysaccharide. Although adults make very effective thymus-independent responses to these polysaccharide antigens, such responses are weak in the immature immune system of the infant. To make an effective vaccine for use in infants, therefore, the polysaccharide is linked chemically to tetanus toxoid, a foreign protein against which infants are routinely and successfully vaccinated (see Chapter 14). B cells that bind the polysaccharide component of the vaccine can be activated by helper T cells specific for peptides of the linked toxoid (Fig. 9.5).

Linked recognition was originally discovered through studies of the production of antibodies against haptens (see Appendix I, Section A-1). Haptens are small chemical groups that cannot elicit antibody responses on their own

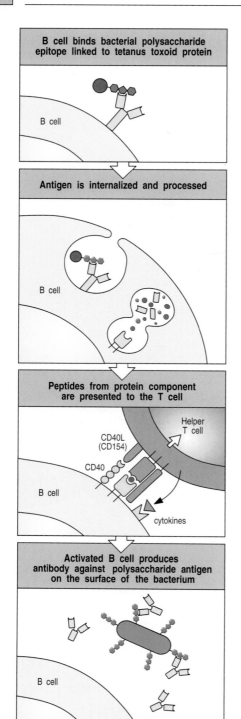

B cell binds bacterial polysaccharide epitope linked to tetanus toxoid protein

B cell

Antigen is internalized and processed

B cell

Peptides from protein component are presented to the T cell

Helper T cell

CD40L (CD154)

CD40

B cell

cytokines

Activated B cell produces antibody against polysaccharide antigen on the surface of the bacterium

B cell

Fig. 9.5 Protein antigens attached to polysaccharide antigens allow T cells to help polysaccharide-specific B cells. The vaccine against *Haemophilus influenzae* type b is a conjugate of bacterial polysaccharide and the tetanus toxoid protein. The B cell recognizes and binds the polysaccharide, internalizes and degrades the whole conjugate and then displays toxoid-derived peptides on surface MHC class II molecules. Helper T cells generated in response to earlier vaccination against the toxoid recognize the complex on the B-cell surface and activate the B cell to produce anti-polysaccharide antibody. This antibody can then protect against infection with *H. influenzae* type b.

because they cannot cross-link B-cell receptors and they cannot recruit T-cell help. When coupled to a carrier protein, however, they become immunogenic, because the protein will carry multiple hapten groups that can now cross-link B-cell receptors. In addition, T-cell dependent responses are possible because T cells can be primed to respond to peptides derived from the protein. Coupling of a hapten to a protein is responsible for the allergic responses shown by many people to the antibiotic penicillin, which reacts with host proteins to form a coupled hapten that can stimulate an antibody response, as we will learn in Chapter 12.

9-3   Antigenic peptides bound to self MHC class II molecules trigger armed helper T cells to make membrane-bound and secreted molecules that can activate a B cell.

Recognition of peptide:MHC class II complexes on B cells triggers armed helper T cells to synthesize both cell-bound and secreted effector molecules that synergize in activating the B cell. One particularly important T-cell effector molecule is a membrane-bound molecule of the tumor necrosis factor (TNF) family known as **CD40 ligand** (**CD40L**, now called **CD154**) because it binds to the B-cell surface molecule **CD40**. CD40 is a member of the TNF-receptor family of cytokine receptors (see Section 8-20); however, it does not contain a 'death domain.' It is involved in directing all phases of the B-cell response and is also important in the activation of dendritic cells and macrophages, as described in Chapter 8. Binding of CD40 by CD40 ligand helps to drive the resting B cell into the cell cycle and is essential for B-cell responses to thymus-dependent antigens. It also causes the B cell to increase expression of co-stimulatory molecules, especially those of the B7 family. These in turn provide important signals that sustain T-cell growth and differentiation, thus enhancing the mutual T cell–B cell interaction.

B cells are stimulated to proliferate *in vitro* when they are exposed to a mixture of artificially synthesized CD40 ligand and the cytokine interleukin-4 (IL-4). IL-4 is made by T_H2 cells when they recognize their specific ligand on the B-cell surface, and IL-4 and CD40 ligand are thought to synergize in driving the clonal expansion that precedes antibody production *in vivo*. IL-4 is secreted in a polar fashion by the T_H2 cell and is focused at the site of contact with the B cell (Fig. 9.6) so that it acts selectively on the antigen-specific target B cell. The combination of B-cell receptor and CD40 ligation, along with IL-4 and other signals derived from direct T-cell contact, leads to B-cell proliferation. Some of these additional contact signals have recently been elucidated. They involve other TNF/TNF-receptor family members, including **CD30** and **CD30 ligand** (now called CD153) and 41BB and 41BB ligand, as well as additional homologs of B7 and CD28, including **B7-RP** and ICOS (inducible co-stimulator). After several rounds of proliferation, B cells can differentiate into antibody-secreting plasma cells. Two additional cytokines, IL-5 and IL-6, both secreted by helper T cells, contribute to these later stages of B-cell activation.

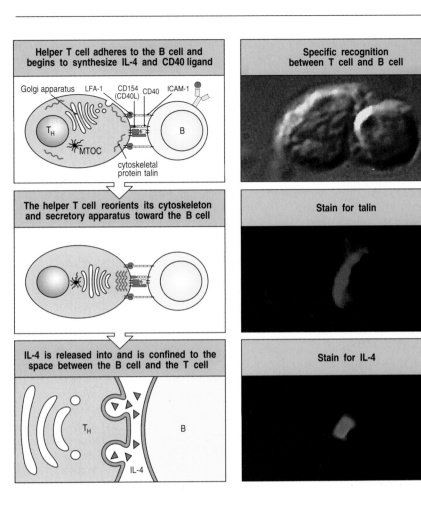

Helper T cell adheres to the B cell and begins to synthesize IL-4 and CD40 ligand

Golgi apparatus LFA-1 CD154 (CD40L) CD40 ICAM-1
T_H   MTOC   cytoskeletal protein talin   B

The helper T cell reorients its cytoskeleton and secretory apparatus toward the B cell

IL-4 is released into and is confined to the space between the B cell and the T cell

T_H   B   IL-4

Specific recognition between T cell and B cell

Stain for talin

Stain for IL-4

Fig. 9.6 When an armed helper T cell encounters an antigen-binding B cell, it becomes polarized and secretes IL-4 and other cytokines as well as the cell-associated TNF family member CD40 ligand at the point of cell–cell contact. On binding antigen on the B cell through its T-cell receptor, the helper T cell is induced to express CD40 ligand, which binds to CD40 on the B cell. As shown in the top left panel, the tight junction formed between the cells upon antigen-specific binding seems to be sealed by a ring of adhesion molecules, with LFA-1 on the T cell interacting with ICAM-1 on the B cell (see Fig. 8.30). The cytoskeleton becomes polarized, as revealed by the relocation of the cytoskeletal protein talin (stained red in right center panel), to the point of cell–cell contact, and the secretory apparatus (the Golgi apparatus) is reoriented by the cytoskeleton toward the point of contact with the B cell. As shown in the bottom panels, cytokines are released at the point of contact. The bottom right panel shows IL-4 (stained green) confined to the space between the B cell and the helper T cell. MTOC, microtubule-organizing center. Photographs courtesy of A. Kupfer.

9-4   Isotype switching in thymus-dependent responses requires expression of CD40 ligand by the helper T cell and is directed by cytokines.

Antibodies are remarkable not only for the diversity of their antigen-binding sites but also for their versatility as effector molecules. The specificity of an antibody response is determined by the antigen-binding site, which consists of the two variable V domains, V_H and V_L; however, the effector action of the antibody is determined by the isotype of its heavy-chain C-region (see Section 4-19). A given heavy-chain V domain can become associated with the C-region of any isotype through the process of isotype switching (see Section 4-18). We will see later in this chapter how antibodies of each isotype contribute to the elimination of pathogens. The DNA rearrangements that underlie isotype switching and confer this functional diversity on the humoral immune response are directed by cytokines, especially those released by armed effector CD4 T cells.

All naive B cells express cell-surface IgM and IgD, yet IgM makes up less than 10% of the immunoglobulin found in plasma, where the most abundant isotype is IgG. Much of the antibody in plasma has therefore been produced by B cells that have undergone isotype switching. Little IgD antibody is produced at any time, so the early stages of the antibody response are dominated by IgM antibodies. Later, IgG and IgA are the predominant isotypes, with IgE contributing a small but biologically important part of the response. The overall predominance of IgG is also due in part to its longer lifetime in the plasma (see Fig. 4.17).

Isotype switching is markedly reduced in individuals who lack functional CD40 ligand, which is necessary for productive interactions between B cells and helper T cells; such individuals do make IgM antibodies in response to thymus-dependent antigens, indicating that CD40L–CD40 interactions are most important for a sustained immune response that includes isotype switching. Individuals lacking CD40 ligand have abnormally high levels of IgM in their plasma, which has given rise to the name **hyper IgM immunodeficiency** for this condition. Many of these antibodies may be induced by thymus-independent antigens expressed by the pathogens that chronically infect these patients, who suffer from severe humoral immunodeficiency, as we will see in Chapter 11. Thymus-independent responses can include IgG. It seems in this case that BAFF (see Section 7-30), another molecule in the TNF family that is expressed by macrophages and dendritic cells, can provide the necessary signal to promote isotype switching in the absence of CD40 ligand.

Most of what is known about the regulation of isotype switching by helper T cells has come from experiments *in vitro* in which mouse B cells are given various nonspecific stimuli, such as bacterial lipopolysaccharide (LPS), along with purified cytokines. These experiments show that different cytokines preferentially induce switching to different isotypes. In the mouse, IL-4 preferentially induces switching to IgG1 and IgE, whereas transforming growth factor (TGF)-β induces switching to IgG2b and IgA. T_H2 cells make both of these cytokines, and also make IL-5, which promotes IgA secretion by cells that have already undergone switching. Although T_H1 cells are relatively poor initiators of antibody responses, they participate in isotype switching by releasing interferon (IFN)-γ, which preferentially induces switching to IgG2a and IgG3. The role of cytokines in directing B cells to make the different antibody isotypes is summarized in Fig. 9.7. Such a directed mechanism is supported by the observation that individual B cells frequently undergo switching to the same C gene on both chromosomes, even though the antibody heavy chain is being expressed from only one of the chromosomes.

Cytokines induce isotype switching in part by stimulating the formation and splicing of mRNA transcribed from the switch recombination sites that lie 5′ to each heavy-chain C gene (see Fig. 4.21). When activated B cells are exposed to IL-4, for example, transcription from a site upstream of the switch regions of $C_{\gamma 1}$ and C_ε can be detected a day or two before switching occurs (Fig. 9.8). Recent findings suggest that the production of a spliced switch transcript has a role in directing switching, but the mechanism is not yet clear. Interestingly, each of the cytokines that induce switching seems to induce transcription

Hyper IgM
Immunodeficiency

Fig. 9.7 Different cytokines induce switching to different isotypes. The individual cytokines induce (violet) or inhibit (red) the production of certain isotypes. Much of the inhibitory effect is probably the result of directed switching to a different isotype. These data are drawn from experiments with mouse cells.

		Role of cytokines in regulating Ig isotype expression					
Cytokines	IgM	IgG3	IgG1	IgG2b	IgG2a	IgE	IgA
IL-4	Inhibits	Inhibits	Induces		Inhibits	Induces	
IL-5							Augments production
IFN-γ	Inhibits	Induces	Inhibits		Induces	Inhibits	
TGF-β	Inhibits	Inhibits		Induces			Induces

Fig. 9.8 Isotype switching is preceded by transcriptional activation of heavy-chain C-region genes. Resting naive B cells transcribe the μ and δ genes at a low rate, giving rise to surface IgM and IgD. Bacterial lipopolysaccharide (LPS), which can activate B cells independently of antigen, induces IgM secretion. In the presence of IL-4, however, $C_{\gamma1}$ and C_{ε} are transcribed at a low rate, presaging switches to IgG1 and IgE production. The transcripts originate before the 5′ end of the region to which switching occurs, and do not code for protein. Similarly, TGF-β gives rise to $C_{\gamma2b}$ and C_{α} transcripts and drives switching to IgG2b and IgA. It is not known what determines which of the two transcriptionally activated heavy-chain C genes undergoes switching. Arrows indicate transcription. The figure shows isotype switching in the mouse.

from the switch regions of two different heavy-chain C genes, promoting specific recombination to one or other of these genes only. Thus, helper T cells regulate both the production of antibody by B cells as well as the isotype that determines the effector function of the antibody.

9-5   Antigen-binding B cells are trapped in the T-cell zone of secondary lymphoid tissues and are activated by encounter with armed helper T cells.

One of the most puzzling features of the antibody response is how an antigen-specific B cell manages to encounter a helper T cell with an appropriate antigen specificity. This question arises because the frequency of naive lymphocytes specific for any given antigen is estimated to be between 1 in 10,000 and 1 in 1,000,000. Thus, the chance of an encounter between a T lymphocyte and a B lymphocyte that recognize the same antigen should be between 1 in 10^8 and 1 in 10^{12}. Achieving such an encounter is a far more difficult challenge than getting effector T cells activated, because, in the latter case, only one of the two cells involved has specific receptors. Moreover, T cells and B cells mostly occupy quite distinct zones in peripheral lymphoid tissue (see Fig. 1.8). As in naive T-cell activation (see Chapter 8), the answer seems to lie in the antigen-specific trapping of migrating lymphocytes.

When an antigen is introduced into an animal, it is captured and processed by professional antigen-presenting cells, especially the dendritic cells that migrate from the tissues into the T-cell zones of local lymph nodes. Recirculating naive T cells pass by such cells continuously and those rare T cells whose receptors bind peptides derived from the antigen are trapped very efficiently. This trapping clearly involves the specific antigen receptor on the T cell, although it is stabilized by the activation of adhesion molecules and chemokines, as we learned in Sections 8-3 and 8-4. Ingenious experiments using mice transgenic for rearranged immunoglobulin genes show that, in the presence of the appropriate antigen, B cells with antigen-specific receptors are also trapped at the border of the T-cell and B-cell zones of lymphoid tissue by a similar mechanism. On encountering antigen, migrating antigen-binding B cells are arrested by the activation of adhesion molecules and the engagement of chemokine receptors such as CCR7, a receptor for CCL19 and CCL21.

Initial trapping of B cells at the border of the T-cell zones provides an elegant solution to the problem posed at the beginning of this section. T cells are themselves trapped and activated to helper status at the same sites, and when B cells migrate into lymph nodes through high endothelial venules they first enter these same T-cell zones. Most of the B cells move quickly through the T-cell zone into the B-cell zone (the primary follicle), but those B cells that have bound antigen are trapped. B cells that are already in follicles or in the marginal zone most probably also migrate to the border between T zone and B zone on antigen encounter. Thus, antigen-binding B cells are selectively trapped in precisely the correct location to maximize their chance of encountering a helper T cell that can activate them. B cells receive key signals from T cells and enter the cell cycle. However, after this initial encounter B cells migrate from this site to continue their proliferation and differentiation. In the spleen they move to the border of the T zone and red pulp (specifically called the marginal sinus bridging channels because at these areas the marginal sinus connects to the red pulp). Here they establish a **primary focus** of clonal expansion (Fig. 9.9). In lymph nodes the analogous site is the medullary cords where lymph drains out of the node.

In this focus, both types of lymphocyte proliferate for several days to constitute the first phase of the primary humoral immune response. Some of the proliferating B cells differentiate into antibody-synthesizing **plasmablasts**. These are cells that have begun to secrete antibody yet are still dividing and still express many of the characteristics of activated B cells that allow their interaction with T cells. After a few more days the plasmablasts stop dividing

Fig. 9.9 Meeting of antigen-binding B and T cells at the border between the T-cell and B-cell zones in the spleen. Upon entry into the spleen through the marginal sinus, T cells and B cells home to different regions, as described in Chapter 7. Antigen-specific T cells remain in the T-cell zone, where they might encounter antigen on the surface of an antigen-presenting cell such as a dendritic cell (left panel). B cells that encounter antigen migrate to the border of the B-cell zone and the T-cell zone, and thus can interact with antigen-specific armed helper T cells. This interaction gives rise to initial proliferation (center panel). After that, the antigen-specific lymphocytes migrate to the border of the T-cell zone and the red pulp, where they continue to proliferate and the B cells differentiate into plasmablasts, forming a so-called 'primary focus' (right panel). In lymph nodes, the equivalent structures are the medullary cords.

Property						
	Intrinsic			Inducible		
B-lineage cell	Surface Ig	Surface MHC class II	High-rate Ig secretion	Growth	Somatic hyper-mutation	Isotype switch
Resting B cell	High	Yes	No	Yes	Yes	Yes
Plasmablast	High	Yes	Yes	Yes	Unknown	Yes
Plasma cell	Low	No	Yes	No	No	No

Fig. 9.10 Plasma cells secrete antibody at a high rate but can no longer respond to antigen or helper T cells. Resting naive B cells carry surface immunoglobulin (usually IgM and IgD) and MHC class II molecules on their surface. Their V genes do not carry somatic mutations. They can take up antigen and present it to helper T cells, which then induce the B cells to proliferate, switch isotype, and undergo somatic hypermutation; however, B cells do not secrete significant amounts of antibody. Plasmablasts have an intermediate phenotype. They do secrete antibody, but retain substantial surface immunoglobulin and MHC class II molecules and so can continue to take up and present antigen to T cells. Plasma cells are terminally differentiated B cells that secrete antibodies. They can no longer interact with helper T cells because they have very low levels of surface immunoglobulin and lack MHC class II molecules, although they have usually already undergone isotype switching and somatic hypermutation. Plasma cells have also lost the ability to change isotype or to undergo further somatic hypermutation.

and either die or differentiate further into plasma cells. The differentiation of a B cell into a plasma cell is accompanied by many morphological changes that reflect its commitment to the production of large amounts of secreted antibody. The properties of resting B cells, plasmablasts, and plasma cells are compared in Fig. 9.10. Plasmablasts and plasma cells have abundant cytoplasm dominated by multiple layers of rough endoplasmic reticulum (see Fig. 1.19). The nucleus shows a characteristic pattern of peripheral chromatin condensation, a prominent perinuclear Golgi apparatus is visible, and the cisternae of the endoplasmic reticulum are rich in immunoglobulin, which in a plasma cell makes up 10–20% of all the protein synthesized. Although plasmablasts still express B7 co-stimulatory molecules and MHC class II molecules, plasma cells do not. Thus, plasma cells can no longer present antigen to helper T cells, although these T cells may still provide important signals for plasma-cell differentiation and survival, such as IL-6 and CD40L. Plasmablasts express surface immunoglobulin but it is expressed on plasma cells only at low levels. Nonetheless, these low levels of surface immunoglobulin may be physiologically important, because recent evidence suggests that the survival of plasma cells may be determined in part by their ability to continue to bind antigen. Plasma cells have a range of life-spans. Some survive for only days to a few weeks after their final differentiation, whereas others are very long-lived and account for the persistence of antibody responses.

9-6 The second phase of the primary B-cell immune response occurs when activated B cells migrate to follicles and proliferate to form germinal centers.

There is another fate for some of the B cells and T cells that proliferate early in the immune response. Some of these cells migrate into a **primary lymphoid follicle** (Fig. 9.11) where they continue to proliferate and ultimately form a **germinal center** (Fig. 9.12). It is unclear whether these cells that seed the germinal center come from cells initially activated at the T zone–B zone border and/or from cells that arise later in the primary focus, which in the spleen is at the T zone–red pulp border. Germinal centers are composed mainly of proliferating B cells, but antigen-specific T cells make up about 10% of germinal center lymphocytes and provide indispensable help to the B cells. The germinal center is essentially an island of cell division that sets up amid a sea of resting B cells in the primary follicles; germinal center B cells displace the resting

B cells develop in the bone marrow

stem cell
pro-B
pre-B
B
B
B
stromal cell

Mature B cells travel to the lymph node via the bloodstream and leave via the efferent lymph

primary lymphoid follicle
secondary lymphoid follicle
high endothelial venule
germinal center
T-cell area
medullary cords
B cell
blood vessels
efferent lymphatic vessel

B cells that encounter antigen at the T-cell/B-cell border become activated. They form primary foci in the medullary cords. Some cells then migrate to the primary follicle, forming a germinal center

HEV

Plasma cells migrate to the medullary cords or leave via the efferent lymphatics

Plasma cells migrate to the bone marrow

Fig. 9.11 Activated B cells form germinal centers in lymphoid follicles. Some B cells activated at the T-cell/B-cell border migrate to form a germinal center within a primary follicle. Germinal centers are sites of rapid B-cell proliferation and differentiation. Follicles in which germinal centers have formed are known as secondary follicles. Within the germinal center, B cells begin their differentiation into either antibody-secreting plasma cells or memory B cells. Plasma cells leave the germinal center and migrate to the medullary cords or leave the lymph node altogether via the efferent lymphatics and migrate to the bone marrow. Memory B cells continue to recirculate through the B-cell zones of secondary lymphoid tissue (not shown) and some may preferentially reside in the splenic marginal zone as described in Chapter 7.

B cells toward the periphery of the follicle, forming a **mantle zone** of resting cells around the center. Primary follicles contain resting B cells clustered around a dense network of processes extending from a specialized cell type, the **follicular dendritic cell** (**FDC**). Follicular dendritic cells attract both naive and activated B cells into the follicles by secreting the chemokine CXCL13 (see Section 7-30).

The early events in the primary focus lead to the prompt secretion of specific antibody that serves as immediate protection to the infected individual. In contrast, the germinal center reaction provides for a more effective later response, should the pathogen establish a chronic infection or the host become reinfected. To this end, B cells undergo several important modifications in the germinal center. These include **somatic hypermutation** (see Chapter 4), which alters the V-regions of immunoglobulin genes, **affinity maturation**, which selects for survival of B cells with high affinity for the antigen, and **isotype switching** (see Sections 9-4 and 4-18), which allows these selected B cells to express a variety of effector functions in the form of antibodies of different isotypes. The selected B cells will differentiate either into memory B cells, the function of which will be described in Chapter 10, or into plasma cells, which will begin to secrete higher-affinity and isotype-switched antibody during the latter part of the primary immune response.

The germinal center is a site of intense cell proliferation, with B cells dividing every 6–8 hours. Initially, these rapidly proliferating B cells markedly reduce their expression of surface immunoglobulin, particularly of IgD. These B cells are termed **centroblasts**. As time goes on, some B cells reduce their rate of division and begin to express higher levels of surface immunoglobulin. These are termed **centrocytes** and they presumably arise from centroblasts. The centroblasts at first proliferate in the **dark zone** of the germinal center (see Fig. 9.12), so called because the proliferating cells are densely packed. With further development, B cells begin to fill the **light zone** of the germinal center, an area of the follicle that is more richly supplied with follicular dendritic cells and less densely packed with cells. It was thought originally that only the centroblasts in the dark zone proliferated, whereas centrocytes in the light zone did not divide. Indeed, this may be true in chronic germinal centers found in inflamed tonsils that have been surgically removed. However, in newly forming germinal centers in mice, proliferation can occur in both light and dark zones, and proliferative cells in the dark zone can express moderate amounts of immunoglobulin on their surface. Follicular dendritic cells, which originally were most prominent in the light zone, seem to react to germinal center formation and their dendritic processes become more evident throughout the germinal center as it develops. The result is that a mature germinal center at day 15 after immunization more closely resembles a light zone, with few of the classic dark zone characteristics. This view of germinal center evolution may help to explain how B cells with high affinity for the stimulating antigen are selected, as we now discuss.

Schematic representation of a germinal center	Light micrograph of germinal center (high power)	Germinal center stained to show T cells, follicular dendritic cells, and proliferating B cells
		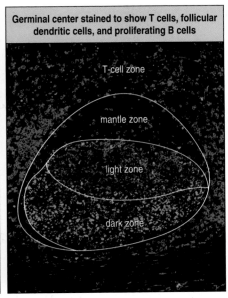

Fig. 9.12 Germinal centers are formed when activated B cells enter lymphoid follicles. The germinal center is a specialized microenvironment in which B-cell proliferation, somatic hypermutation, and selection for antigen binding all occur. Closely packed centroblasts form the so-called 'dark zone' of the germinal center, as can be seen in the lower part of the photomicrograph in the center, which shows a high-power view of a section through a human tonsillar germinal center. The photomicrograph on the right shows a lower-power view of a tonsillar germinal center; B cells are found in the dark zone, light zone, and mantle zone. Proliferating cells are stained green for Ki67, an antigen expressed in nuclei of dividing cells, revealing the centroblasts in the dark zone. The dense network of follicular dendritic cells, stained red, mainly occupies the light zone. Cells in the light zone are also proliferating, though to a lesser degree in most germinal centers. Small recirculating B cells occupy the mantle zone at the edge of the B-cell follicle. Large masses of CD4 T cells, stained blue, can be seen in the T-cell zones, which separate the follicles. There are also significant numbers of T cells in the light zone of the germinal center; CD4 staining in the dark zone is mainly associated with CD4-positive phagocytes. Photographs courtesy of I. MacLennan.

9-7 Germinal center B cells undergo V-region somatic hypermutation, and cells with mutations that improve affinity for antigen are selected.

The process of somatic hypermutation, as one of the four mechanisms that create immunoglobulin diversity, was described in Chapter 4. Here we describe the signals that initiate hypermutation and the biological consequences of mutation for those cells. Somatic hypermutation is normally restricted to B cells that are proliferating in germinal centers. This was first shown by FACS sorting of germinal center B cells (see Appendix I, Section A-22) and sequencing of the V genes of cell lines derived from them; later, it was shown more directly by sequencing the V genes that were amplified by PCR of DNA isolated from germinal center B cells that had been micro-dissected from histologic sections. However, studies *in vitro* have shown that B cells can be induced to undergo hypermutation outside germinal centers when their B-cell receptors are cross-linked and they receive help, including cytokines and stimulation by CD40L, from activated T cells.

Unlike the other mechanisms of immunoglobulin diversification (see Section 4-6), which generate B cells with radically differing B-cell receptors, somatic hypermutation has the potential to create a series of related B cells that differ subtly in their specificity and affinity for antigen. This is because somatic hypermutation generally involves individual point mutations that change only a single amino acid. Immunoglobulin V-region genes accumulate mutations at a rate of about one base pair change per 10^3 base pairs per cell division. The mutation rates of all other somatic cell DNA are much lower: around one base pair change per 10^{10} base pairs per cell division. These mutations also affect some DNA flanking the rearranged V gene, but they generally do not extend into the C-region exons. Thus, random point mutations are somehow targeted to the rearranged V genes in a B cell. Because each of the expressed heavy-chain and light-chain V-region genes is encoded by about 360 base pairs, and about three out of every four base changes results in an altered amino acid, every second B cell will acquire a mutation in its receptor at each division.

The point mutations accumulate in a stepwise manner as the descendents of an individual B cell (B-cell clones) expand in the germinal center. Mutations can affect the ability of a B cell to bind antigen and thus will affect the fate of the B cell in the germinal center, as diagrammed in Fig. 9.13. Most mutations have a negative impact on the ability of the B-cell receptor to bind the original antigen. For example, some mutations abolish receptor function altogether by introducing a stop codon that prevents proper translation; other deleterious mutations alter framework region amino acids that are essential for correct immunoglobulin folding (see Chapter 3); and still others alter amino acids in the complementarity-determining regions that are responsible for contacting antigen. These deleterious mutations are disastrous for the cells that harbor them; these cells are eliminated by apoptosis either because they can no longer make a B-cell receptor or because they cannot compete with sibling cells that bind antigen more strongly. Deleterious mutation is evidently a frequent event, because germinal centers are filled with apoptotic B cells that are quickly engulfed by macrophages, resulting in **tingible body macrophages**, which contain dark-staining nuclear debris in their cytoplasm and are a long-recognized histologic feature of germinal centers.

Less frequently, mutations improve the affinity of a B-cell receptor for antigen. Cells that harbor these mutations are efficiently selected and expanded. Whether this is due to the prevention of cell death and/or an enhancement of cell division is still unclear. In either case it is clear that selection is incremental. After each round of mutation, B cells begin to express the new receptor, and it determines the cell's fate, whether favorable or unfavorable. If favorable, the cell undergoes another round of division and mutation, and the expression and selection process is repeated. In this way the affinity and specificity of positively selected B cells are continually refined during the germinal center response.

The fact that both centroblasts and centrocytes proliferate and can express immunoglobulin explains how mutation and positive selection can take place simultaneously throughout the germinal center without the need for migration back and forth between the dark and light zones.

Evidence of positive and negative selection is seen in the pattern of somatic hypermutations in V-regions of B cells that have survived passage through the germinal center (see Section 4-9). The existence of negative selection is shown by the relative scarcity of amino acid replacements in the framework regions, reflecting the loss of cells that had mutated any one of the many residues that are critical for immunoglobulin V-region folding. Negative selection is an important force in the germinal center, most probably eliminating more than one in every two cells. Were it not for substantial negative selection, B cells dividing three to four times per day in a single germinal center would quickly create enough progeny to overwhelm the entire organism; more than a billion cells could be created in 10 days in a single germinal center. Instead, a germinal center actually contains a few thousand B cells at its peak.

The mark of positive selection, in contrast, is an accumulation of numerous amino acid replacements in the complementarity-determining regions (see Fig. 4.9). The consequence of these cycles of proliferation, mutation, and selection, all of which happen within the germinal center, is that the average affinity of the population of responding B cells for its antigen increases over time, largely explaining the observed phenomenon of affinity maturation of the antibody response. The selection process can be quite stringent: although 50–100 B cells may seed the germinal center, most of them leave no progeny, and by the time the germinal center reaches maximum size, it is typically composed of the descendants of only one or a few B cells.

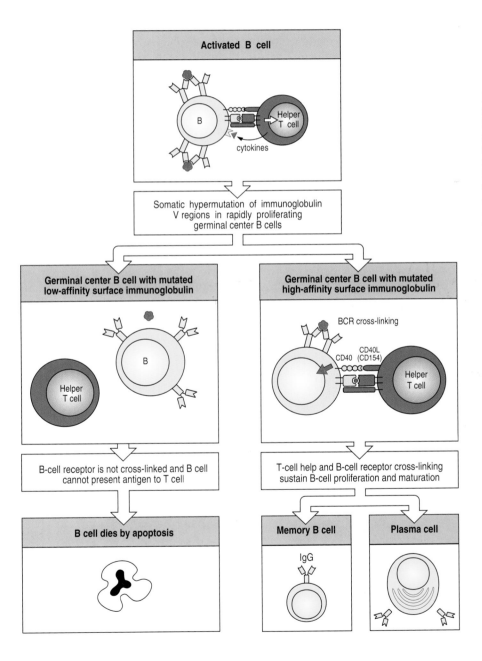

Fig. 9.13 Activated B cells undergo rounds of mutation and selection for higher-affinity mutants in the germinal center, resulting in high-affinity antibody-secreting plasma cells and high-affinity memory B cells. B cells are first activated outside follicles by the combination of antigen and T cells (top panel). They migrate to germinal centers (not shown), where the remaining events occur. Somatic hypermutation can result in amino acid replacements in immunoglobulin V regions that affect the fate of the B cell. Mutations that result in a B-cell receptor (BCR) of lower affinity for the antigen (left panels) will prevent the B cell from being activated as efficiently, because both B-cell receptor cross-linking and the ability of the B cell to present peptide antigen to T cells are reduced. This results in the B cell dying by apoptosis. In this way, low-affinity cells are purged from the germinal center. Most mutations are either negative or neutral (not shown) and thus the germinal center is a site of massive B-cell death as well as of proliferation. Some mutations, however, will improve the ability of the B-cell receptor to bind antigen. This increases the B cell's chance of interacting with T cells, and thus of proliferating and surviving (right panels). Surviving cells undergo repeated cycles of mutation and selection during which some of the progeny B cells undergo differentiation to either memory B cells or plasma cells (bottom right panels) and leave the germinal center. The signals that control these differentiation decisions are unknown.

9-8   Ligation of the B-cell receptor and CD40, together with direct contact with T cells, are all required to sustain germinal center B cells.

Germinal center B cells are inherently prone to dying, and to survive they must receive specific signals. It was originally discovered *in vitro* that germinal center B cells could be kept alive by simultaneously cross-linking their B-cell receptors and ligating their cell-surface CD40. *In vivo* these signals are delivered by antigen and T cells, respectively. Additional signals are also required for survival, which are delivered by direct contact with T cells. The nature of these signals is still obscure but might include ICOS and B7-RP as well as additional members of the TNF/TNF-receptor family.

The source of antigen in the germinal center has been a matter of some controversy. Antigen can be trapped and stored for long periods in the form of immune complexes on follicular dendritic cells (Figs 9.14 and 9.15) and it was therefore assumed that this was the antigen that sustained germinal center B-cell proliferation. Although this may be true under certain circumstances, there is now evidence that antigen on follicular dendritic cells is not required to sustain a normal germinal center response. Indeed, the role of the antigen depot on these cells is unknown, although one role could be to maintain long-lived plasma cells. Where, then, does the antigen that sustains the germinal center come from? Under normal circumstances it is most likely that live pathogens will continue to provide antigens until they are eliminated by the immune response, after which the germinal center decays. Immunizations with protein antigens are usually given in a form that slowly releases the antigen over time, which mimics the situation with live pathogens. Indeed, it is difficult to stimulate germinal center formation by immunization without either a live replicating pathogen or a sustained release of antigen in adjuvant (see Appendix I, Section A-4).

How the various signals that maintain the germinal center exert their effects on B cells is not completely understood. The combined signals from the B-cell receptor and CD40 seem to increase the expression of a protein called Bcl-X_L, a relative of Bcl-2, which promotes B-cell survival (see Chapter 6). There may be many other signals yet to be discovered that promote B-cell differentiation.

Fig. 9.14 Immune complexes bind to the surface of follicular dendritic cells. Radiolabeled antigen localizes to, and persists in, lymphoid follicles of draining lymph nodes (see light micrograph and the schematic representation below, showing a germinal center in a lymph node). Radiolabeled antigen has been injected 3 days previously and its localization in the germinal center is shown by the intense dark staining. The antigen is in the form of antigen:antibody:complement complexes bound to Fc and complement receptors on the surface of the follicular dendritic cell. These complexes are not internalized, as depicted schematically for immune complexes bound to both Fc and CR3 receptors in the right panel and insert. Antigen can persist in this form for long periods. Photograph courtesy of J. Tew.

Fig. 9.15 Immune complexes bound to follicular dendritic cells form iccosomes, which are released and can be taken up by B cells in the germinal center. Follicular dendritic cells have a prominent cell body and many dendritic processes. Immune complexes, bound to complement and Fc receptors on the follicular dendritic cell surface, become clustered, forming prominent 'beads' along the dendrites. An intermediate form of follicular dendritic cell is shown (left panel) with both straight filiform dendrites and those that are becoming beaded. These beads are shed from the cell as iccosomes (immune complex-coated bodies), which can bind (center panel) and be taken up by B cells in the germinal center (right panel). In the center and right panels, the iccosome has been formed with immune complexes containing horseradish peroxidase, which is electron-dense and therefore appears dark in the transmission electron micrographs. Photographs courtesy of A.K. Szakal.

9-9 Surviving germinal center B cells differentiate into either plasma cells or memory cells.

The purpose of the germinal center reaction is to enhance the later part of the primary immune response. Some germinal center cells differentiate first into plasmablasts and then into plasma cells. These plasma cells migrate to the bone marrow, where a subset of them live for a long period. Plasma cells obtain signals from bone marrow stromal cells that are essential for their survival. These long-lived plasma cells provide a source of long-lasting high-affinity antibody.

Other germinal center B cells differentiate into **memory B cells**. Memory B cells are long-lived descendants of cells that were once stimulated by antigen and had proliferated in the germinal center. These cells divide very slowly if at all; they express surface immunoglobulin but secrete no antibody, or do so only at a low rate. Because the precursors of memory B cells once participated in a germinal center reaction, memory B cells inherit the genetic changes that occurred in germinal center cells, including somatic mutations and the gene rearrangements that result in an isotype switch (see Sections 4-9 and 4-18). The signals that control which differentiation path a B cell takes, and even whether at any given point the B cell continues to divide instead of differentiating, are still being investigated. We will discuss the existence and features of memory B cells in Chapter 10.

9-10 B-cell responses to bacterial antigens with intrinsic ability to activate B cells do not require T-cell help.

Although antibody responses to most protein antigens are dependent on helper T cells, humans and mice with T-cell deficiencies nevertheless make antibodies against many bacterial antigens. This is because the special properties of some bacterial polysaccharides, polymeric proteins, and lipopolysaccharides enable them to stimulate naive B cells in the absence of T-cell help. These antigens are known as thymus-independent antigens (TI antigens) because they stimulate strong antibody responses in athymic individuals. The nonprotein bacterial products cannot elicit classical T-cell responses, yet they induce antibody responses in normal individuals. Although responses to TI antigens can occur in mice that lack all T cells and natural killer (NK) cells, if such cells are activated during the course of a physiologic immune response (for example by other protein antigens or via the innate immune system) they can affect the TI immune response. In particular, cytokines secreted by T cells, NK T cells or NK cells (see Section 10-5) can affect the isotype of the antibody secreted. NK T cells are particularly intriguing as cells that might influence the TI response to nonprotein antigens because the T-cell receptors on these cells recognize certain polysaccharides bound to unconventional MHC class I or class I-like molecules such as CD1.

Thymus-independent antigens fall into two classes which activate B cells by two different mechanisms. **TI-1 antigens** possess an intrinsic activity that can directly induce B-cell division. At high concentration these molecules cause the proliferation and differentiation of most B cells regardless of their antigen specificity; this is known as **polyclonal activation** (Fig. 9.16, top two panels). TI-1 antigens are thus often called **B-cell mitogens**, a mitogen being a substance that induces cells to undergo mitosis. An example of a B-cell mitogen and TI-1 antigen is LPS, which binds to LPS-binding protein and CD14 (see Chapter 2), which then associates with the activating receptor TLR-4 on B cells. LPS activates B cells only at doses at least 100 times those needed to activate dendritic cells. Thus, when B cells are exposed to concentrations of TI-1 antigens that are 10^3–10^5 times lower than those used for polyclonal activation, only those B cells whose B-cell receptors also specifically bind the TI-1 molecules become activated. At these low antigen concentrations, sufficient amounts of TI-1 for B-cell activation can only be concentrated on the B-cell surface with the aid of this specific binding (Fig. 9.16, bottom two panels).

It is likely that, as with any pathogen antigen, concentrations of TI-1 antigens are low during the early stages of infections *in vivo*; thus, only antigen-specific B cells are likely to be activated and these will produce antibodies specific for the TI-1 antigen that may in turn neutralize the toxic effects of these molecules. Such responses have an important role in defense against several extracellular pathogens, as they arise earlier than thymus-dependent responses because they do not require prior priming and clonal expansion of helper T cells. However, TI-1 antigens are inefficient inducers of affinity maturation and memory B cells, both of which require antigen-specific T-cell help. Thymus-independent responses include isotype switching to certain isotypes, such as IgG3 in the mouse. This is probably the result of help from dendritic cells, which provide secreted cytokines and membrane-bound signals to nearby proliferating plasmablasts as they respond to TI antigens. One important factor provided by dendritic cells is BAFF, which promotes switching (see Section 9-4).

High concentration of TI-1 antigen

Polyclonal B-cell activation; nonspecific antibody response

Low concentration of TI-1 antigen

TI-1 antigen-specific antibody response

Fig. 9.16 Thymus-independent type 1 antigens (TI-1 antigens) are polyclonal B-cell activators at high concentrations, whereas at low concentrations they induce an antigen-specific antibody response. At high concentration, the signal delivered by the B-cell-activating moiety of TI-1 antigens is sufficient to induce proliferation and antibody secretion by B cells in the absence of specific antigen binding to surface immunoglobulin. Thus, all B cells respond (top panels). At low concentration, only B cells specific for the TI-1 antigen bind enough of it to focus its B-cell activating properties onto the B cell; this gives a specific antibody response to epitopes on the TI-1 antigen (lower panels).

9-11   B-cell responses to bacterial polysaccharides do not require peptide-specific T-cell help.

The second class of thymus-independent antigens consists of molecules such as bacterial capsular polysaccharides that have highly repetitive structures. These thymus-independent antigens, called **TI-2 antigens**, contain no intrinsic B-cell-stimulating activity. Whereas TI-1 antigens can activate both immature and mature B cells, TI-2 antigens can activate only mature B cells; immature B cells, as we saw in Chapter 7, are inactivated by repetitive epitopes. This might be why infants do not make antibodies against polysaccharide antigens efficiently: most of their B cells are immature. Responses to several TI-2 antigens are made prominently by B-1 cells (also known as CD5 B cells), which comprise an autonomously replicating subpopulation of B cells, and by marginal zone B cells, another unique subset of nonrecirculating B cells that line the border of the splenic white pulp (see Sections 7-26 and 7-31). Although B-1 cells arise early in development, young children do not make a fully effective response to carbohydrate antigens until about 5 years of age. In contrast, marginal zone B cells are rare at birth and accumulate with age; they might therefore be responsible for most physiological TI-2 responses, which also increase with age.

TI-2 antigens most probably act by simultaneously cross-linking a critical number of B-cell receptors of mature B cells specific for the antigen (Fig. 9.17,

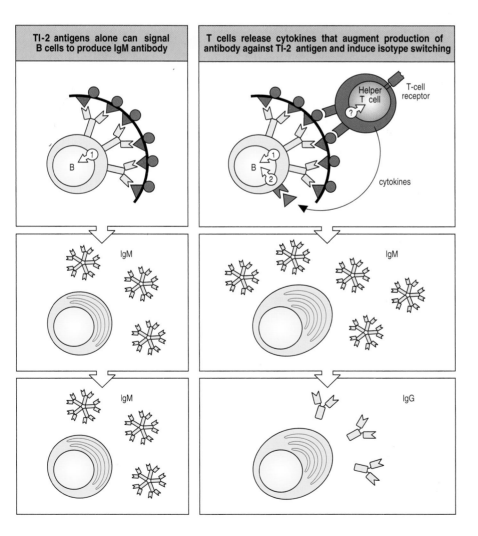

Fig. 9.17 B-cell activation by thymus-independent type 2 antigens (TI-2 antigens) requires, or is greatly enhanced by, cytokines. Multiple cross-linking of the B-cell receptor by TI-2 antigens can lead to IgM antibody production (left panels), but there is evidence that helper T cells greatly augment these responses and lead to isotype switching as well (right panels). It is not clear how T cells are activated in this case, because polysaccharide antigens cannot produce peptide fragments that might be recognized by T cells on the B-cell surface. One possibility is that a component of the antigen binds to a cell-surface molecule common to all helper T cells, as shown in the figure. Another possibility (not shown) is that certain γ:δ T cells or CD4 CD8 double-negative α:β T cells can provide help, as some of these cells have T-cell receptors that recognize certain polysaccharides bound to unconventional MHC molecules such as CD1.

left panels). Excessive receptor cross-linking, however, renders mature B cells unresponsive or anergic, just as it does immature B cells. Thus, the density of TI-2 antigen epitopes presented to the B cell is critical: if it is too low, receptor cross-linking is insufficient to activate the cell; if too high, the B cell becomes anergic.

B-cell responses to TI-2 antigens provide a prompt and specific response to an important class of pathogen. Many common extracellular bacterial pathogens are surrounded by a polysaccharide capsule that enables them to resist ingestion by phagocytes. The bacteria not only escape direct destruction by phagocytes but also avoid stimulating T-cell responses through the presentation of bacterial peptides by macrophages. Antibody that is produced rapidly in response to this polysaccharide capsule without the help of peptide-specific T cells can coat these bacteria, promoting their ingestion and destruction by phagocytes and NK cells by mechanisms that we will describe in Sections 9-20 and 9-21. Both IgM and IgG antibodies are induced by TI-2 antigens (Fig. 9.17, right panels) and are likely to be an important part of the humoral immune response in many bacterial infections. We mentioned earlier the importance of antibodies to the capsular polysaccharide of *Haemophilus influenzae* type b, a TI-2 antigen, in protective immunity to this bacterium. A further example of the importance of TI-2 responses can be seen in patients with an immunodeficiency disease known as the **Wiskott–Aldrich syndrome**. These patients can respond, although poorly, to protein antigens but fail to make antibody against polysaccharide antigens and are highly susceptible to infection with encapsulated bacteria. Thus, the TI responses are important components of the humoral immune response to nonprotein antigens that do not engage peptide-specific T-cell help; the distinguishing features of thymus-dependent, TI-1, and TI-2 antibody responses are summarized in Fig. 9.18.

Wiskott–Aldrich Syndrome

	TD antigen	TI-1 antigen	TI-2 antigen
Antibody response in infants	Yes	Yes	No
Antibody production in congenitally athymic individual	No	Yes	Yes
Antibody response in absence of all T cells	No	Yes	No
Primes T cells	Yes	No	No
Polyclonal B-cell activation	No	Yes	No
Requires repeating epitopes	No	No	Yes
Examples of antigen	Diphtheria toxin Viral hemagglutinin Purified protein derivative (PPD) of *Mycobacterium tuberculosis*	Bacterial lipopolysaccharide *Brucella abortus*	Pneumococcal polysaccharide *Salmonella* polymerized flagellin Dextran Hapten-conjugated Ficoll (polysucrose)

Fig. 9.18 Properties of different classes of antigen that elicit antibody responses.

Summary.

B-cell activation by many antigens, especially oligomeric proteins, requires both binding of the antigen by the B-cell surface immunoglobulin—the B-cell receptor—and interaction of the B cell with antigen-specific helper T cells. Helper T cells recognize peptide fragments derived from the antigen internalized by the B cell and displayed by the B cells as peptide:MHC class II complexes. Helper T cells stimulate the B cell through the binding of CD40 ligand on the T cell to CD40 on the B cell, through the interaction of other TNF–TNF-receptor family ligand pairs, and by the directed release of cytokines. Activated B cells also provide signals to T cells, for example via B7-family molecules, that promote their continued activation. The initial interaction occurs at the border of the T-cell and B-cell areas of secondary lymphoid tissue, where both antigen-specific helper T cells and antigen-specific B cells are trapped as a consequence of binding antigen. This initial interaction is quickly followed by the migration of antigen-specific B and T cells to the T-zone:red pulp border, where there are marginal sinus-bridging channels in which further proliferation and plasmablast differentiation happens. Finally, further interactions between T cells and B cells continue after migration into the B-cell zone or follicle, and the formation of a germinal center.

Helper T cells induce a phase of vigorous B-cell proliferation and direct the differentiation of the clonally expanded progeny of naive B cells into either antibody-secreting plasma cells or memory B cells. During the differentiation of activated B cells, the antibody isotype can change in response to cytokines released by helper T cells, and the antigen-binding properties of the antibody can change by somatic hypermutation of V-region genes. Somatic hypermutation and selection for high-affinity binding occur in the germinal centers. Helper T cells control these processes by selectively activating cells that have retained their specificity for the antigen and by inducing proliferation and differentiation into plasma cells and memory B cells. Some nonprotein antigens stimulate B cells in the absence of linked recognition by peptide-specific helper T cells. These thymus-independent antigens induce only limited isotype switching and do not induce memory B cells. However, responses to these antigens have a crucial role in host defense against pathogens whose surface antigens cannot elicit peptide-specific T-cell responses.

The distribution and functions of immunoglobulin isotypes.

Extracellular pathogens can find their way to most sites in the body, and antibodies must be equally widely distributed to combat them. Most classes of antibody are distributed by diffusion from their site of synthesis, but specialized transport mechanisms are required to deliver antibodies to epithelial surfaces lining the lumina of organs such as those of the lung and intestine. The distribution of antibodies is determined by their isotype, which can limit their diffusion or enable them to engage specific transporters that deliver them across epithelia. In this part of the chapter we describe the mechanisms by which antibodies of different isotypes are directed to the compartments of the body in which their particular effector functions are appropriate, and discuss the protective functions of antibodies that result solely from their binding to pathogens. In the last part of the chapter we discuss the effector cells and molecules that are specifically engaged by different isotypes.

9-12 Antibodies of different isotype operate in distinct places and have distinct effector functions.

Pathogens most commonly enter the body across the epithelial barriers of the mucosa lining the respiratory, digestive, and urogenital tracts, or through damaged skin. Less often, insects, wounds, or hypodermic needles introduce microorganisms directly into the blood. The body's mucosal surfaces, tissues, and blood are all protected by antibodies from such infections; these antibodies serve to neutralize the pathogen or promote its elimination before it can establish a significant infection. Antibodies of different isotypes are adapted to function in different compartments of the body. Because a given V-region can become associated with any C-region through isotype switching (see Section 4-18), the progeny of a single B cell can produce antibodies that share the same specificity yet provide all of the protective functions appropriate for each body compartment.

The first antibodies to be produced in a humoral immune response are always IgM, because IgM can be expressed without isotype switching (see Fig. 4.20). These early IgM antibodies are produced before B cells have undergone somatic hypermutation and therefore tend to be of low affinity. However, IgM molecules form pentamers whose ten antigen-binding sites can bind simultaneously to multivalent antigens such as bacterial capsular polysaccharides. This compensates for the relatively low affinity of the IgM monomers by multipoint binding that confers high overall avidity. As a result of the large size of the pentamers, IgM is mainly found in the blood and, to a smaller extent, the lymph. The pentameric structure of IgM makes it especially effective in activating the complement system, as we will see in the last part of this chapter. Infection of the bloodstream has serious consequences unless it is controlled quickly, and the rapid production of IgM and its efficient activation of the complement system are important in controlling such infections. Some IgM is produced in secondary and subsequent responses, and also after somatic hypermutation, although other isotypes dominate the later phases of the antibody response. IgM is also produced by B-1 cells that reside in the peritoneal cavity and the pleural spaces. As discussed in Chapter 7 (Section 7-31), these cells are naturally activated and secrete antibodies against environmental pathogens, thus providing in these body cavities a preformed repertoire of IgM antibodies that can recognize invading pathogens.

Antibodies of the other isotypes—IgG, IgA, and IgE—are smaller, and diffuse easily out of the blood into the tissues. Although IgA can form dimers, as we saw in Chapter 4, IgG and IgE are always monomeric. The affinity of the individual antigen-binding sites for their antigen is therefore critical for the effectiveness of these antibodies, and most of the B cells expressing these isotypes have been selected for increased affinity of antigen-binding in germinal centers. IgG is the principal isotype in the blood and extracellular fluid, whereas IgA is the principal isotype in secretions, the most important being those of the epithelium lining the intestinal and respiratory tracts. IgG efficiently opsonizes pathogens for engulfment by phagocytes and activates the complement system, but IgA is a less potent opsonin and a weak activator of complement. This difference is not surprising because IgG operates mainly in the body tissues, where accessory cells and molecules are available, whereas IgA operates mainly on epithelial surfaces where complement and phagocytes are not normally present, and therefore IgA functions chiefly as a neutralizing antibody.

Finally, IgE antibody is present only at very low levels in blood or extracellular fluid but is bound avidly by receptors on mast cells that are found just beneath the skin and mucosa, and along blood vessels in connective tissue.

Functional activity	IgM	IgD	IgG1	IgG2	IgG3	IgG4	IgA	IgE
Neutralization	+	−	++	++	++	++	++	−
Opsonization	+	−	+++	*	++	+	+	−
Sensitization for killing by NK cells	−	−	++	−	++	−	−	−
Sensitization of mast cells	−	−	+	−	+	−	−	+++
Activates complement system	+++	−	++	+	+++	−	+	−

Distribution	IgM	IgD	IgG1	IgG2	IgG3	IgG4	IgA	IgE
Transport across epithelium	+	−	−	−	−	−	+++ (dimer)	−
Transport across placenta	−	−	+++	+	++	+/−	−	−
Diffusion into extravascular sites	+/−	−	+++	+++	+++	+++	++ (monomer)	+
Mean serum level (mg ml^{-1})	1.5	0.04	9	3	1	0.5	2.1	3×10^{-5}

Fig. 9.19 Each human immunoglobulin isotype has specialized functions and a unique distribution. The major effector functions of each isotype (+++) are shaded in dark red, whereas lesser functions (++) are shown in dark pink, and very minor functions (+) in pale pink. The distributions are marked similarly, with actual average levels in serum being shown in the bottom row. *IgG2 can act as an opsonin in the presence of an Fc receptor of the appropriate allotype, found in about 50% of white people.

Antigen binding to this cell-associated IgE triggers mast cells to release powerful chemical mediators that induce reactions, such as coughing, sneezing, and vomiting, that in turn can expel infectious agents, as will be discussed later in this chapter when we describe the receptors that bind immunoglobulin C-regions and engage effector functions. The distribution and main functions of antibodies of the different isotypes are summarized in Fig. 9.19.

9-13 Transport proteins that bind to the Fc regions of antibodies carry particular isotypes across epithelial barriers.

IgA-secreting plasma cells are found predominantly in the lamina propria, which lies immediately below the basement membrane of many surface epithelia. From there the IgA antibodies can be transported across the epithelium to its external surface, for example to the lumen of the gut or the bronchi. IgA antibody synthesized in the lamina propria is secreted as a dimeric IgA molecule associated with a single J chain (see Fig. 4.23). This polymeric form of IgA binds specifically to the poly-Ig receptor, which is present on the basolateral surfaces of the overlying epithelial cells (Fig. 9.20). When the poly-Ig receptor has bound a molecule of dimeric IgA, the complex is internalized and carried through the cytoplasm of the epithelial cell in a transport vesicle to its luminal surface. This process is called **transcytosis**. At the apical or luminal surface of the epithelial cell, the poly-Ig receptor is cleaved enzymatically, releasing the extracellular portion of the receptor still

Fig. 9.20 Transcytosis of IgA antibody across epithelia is mediated by the poly-Ig receptor, a specialized transport protein. Most IgA antibody is synthesized in plasma cells lying just beneath epithelial basement membranes of the gut, the respiratory epithelia, the tear and salivary glands, and the lactating mammary gland. The IgA dimer bound to a J chain diffuses across the basement membrane and is bound by the poly-Ig receptor on the basolateral surface of the epithelial cell. The bound complex undergoes transcytosis in which it is transported in a vesicle across the cell to the apical surface, where the poly-Ig receptor is cleaved to leave the extracellular IgA-binding component bound to the IgA molecule as the so-called secretory component. Carbohydrate on the secretory component binds to mucins in mucus and holds the IgA at the epithelial surface (not shown). The residual piece of the poly-Ig receptor is nonfunctional and is degraded. In this way, IgA is transported across epithelia into the lumens of several organs that are in contact with the external environment.

| Binding of IgA to receptor on basolateral face of epithelial cell | Endocytosis | Transport to apical face of epithelial cell | Release of IgA dimer at apical face of epithelial cell |

attached to the Fc region of the dimeric IgA. This fragment of receptor, called the **secretory component**, may help to protect the IgA dimer from proteolytic cleavage. The IgA is then held at the mucosal surface, being bound to mucins in mucus by the carbohydrate of the secretory component. The secretory component binds to the same regions on the Fc portion of IgA as the Fcα receptor I, thus blocking the binding of secretory IgA to this receptor (see Section 9-19). Some molecules of dimeric IgA diffuse from the lamina propria into the extracellular spaces of the tissues, draining into the bloodstream before being excreted into the gut via the bile. It is therefore not surprising that patients with obstructive jaundice, a condition in which bile is not excreted, show a marked increase in dimeric IgA in the plasma.

The principal sites of IgA synthesis and secretion are the gut, the respiratory epithelium, the lactating breast, and various other exocrine glands such as the salivary and tear glands. It is believed that the primary functional role of IgA antibodies is to protect epithelial surfaces from infectious agents, just as IgG antibodies protect the extracellular spaces of the internal tissues. IgA antibodies prevent the attachment of bacteria or toxins to epithelial cells and the absorption of foreign substances, and provide the first line of defense against a wide variety of pathogens. Newborn infants are especially vulnerable to infection, having had no prior exposure to the microbes in the environment they enter at birth. IgA antibodies are secreted in breast milk and are thereby transferred to the gut of the newborn infant, where they provide protection from newly encountered bacteria until the infant can synthesize its own protective antibody.

IgA is not the only protective antibody that a mother passes on to her baby. Maternal IgG is transported across the placenta directly into the bloodstream of the fetus during intrauterine life; human babies at birth have as high a level of plasma IgG as their mothers, and with the same range of antigen specificities. The selective transport of IgG from mother to fetus is due to an IgG transport protein in the placenta, FcRn, which is closely related in structure to

Fig. 9.21 FcRn binds to the Fc portion of IgG. The structure of a molecule of FcRn (blue and green) is shown bound to one chain of the Fc portion of IgG (red), at the interface of the Cγ2 and Cγ3 domains, with the Cγ2 region at the top. The β_2-microglobulin component of the FcRn is green. The dark-blue structure attached to the Fc portion of IgG is a carbohydrate chain, reflecting glycosylation. FcRn transports IgG molecules across the placenta in humans and also across the gut in rats and mice. It also has a role in maintaining the levels of IgG in adults. Although only one molecule of FcRn is shown binding to the Fc portion, it is thought that it takes two molecules of FcRn to capture one molecule of IgG. Courtesy of P. Björkman.

MHC class I molecules. Despite this similarity, FcRn binds IgG quite differently from the binding of peptide to MHC class I molecules, because its peptide-binding groove is occluded. It binds to the Fc portion of IgG molecules (Fig. 9.21). Two molecules of FcRn bind one molecule of IgG, bearing it across the placenta. In some rodents, FcRn also delivers IgG to the circulation of the neonate from the gut lumen. Maternal IgG is ingested by the newborn animal in its mother's milk and colostrum, the protein-rich fluid secreted by the early postnatal mammary gland. In this case, FcRn transports the IgG from the lumen of the neonatal gut into the blood and tissues. Interestingly, FcRn is also found in adults in the gut and liver and on endothelial cells. Its function in adults is to maintain the levels of IgG in plasma, which it does by binding antibody, endocytosing it, and recycling it to the blood, thus preventing its excretion.

By means of these specialized transport systems, mammals are supplied from birth with antibodies against pathogens common in their environments. As they mature and make their own antibodies of all isotypes, these are distributed selectively to different sites in the body (Fig. 9.22). Thus, throughout life, isotype switching and the distribution of isotypes through the body provide effective protection against infection in extracellular spaces.

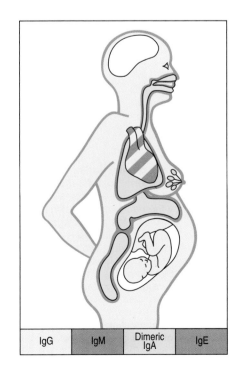

Fig. 9.22 Immunoglobulin isotypes are selectively distributed in the body. IgG and IgM predominate in plasma, whereas IgG and monomeric IgA are the major isotypes in extracellular fluid within the body. Dimeric IgA predominates in secretions across epithelia, including breast milk. The fetus receives IgG from the mother by transplacental transport. IgE is found mainly associated with mast cells just beneath epithelial surfaces (especially of the respiratory tract, gastrointestinal tract, and skin). The brain is normally devoid of immunoglobulin.

9-14   High-affinity IgG and IgA antibodies can neutralize bacterial toxins.

Many bacteria cause disease by secreting proteins called toxins, which damage or disrupt the function of the host's cells (Fig. 9.23). To have an effect, a toxin must interact specifically with a molecule that serves as a receptor on the surface of the target cell. In many toxins the receptor-binding domain is on one polypeptide chain but the toxic function is carried by a second chain. Antibodies that bind to the receptor-binding site on the toxin molecule can prevent the toxin from binding to the cell and thus protect the cell from attack (Fig. 9.24). Antibodies that act in this way to neutralize toxins are referred to as **neutralizing antibodies**.

Most toxins are active at nanomolar concentrations: a single molecule of diphtheria toxin can kill a cell. To neutralize toxins, therefore, antibodies must be able to diffuse into the tissues and bind the toxin rapidly and with high affinity. The ability of IgG antibodies to diffuse easily throughout the extracellular fluid and their high affinity make these the principal neutralizing antibodies for toxins found in tissues. IgA antibodies similarly neutralize toxins at the mucosal surfaces of the body.

Diphtheria and tetanus toxins are two bacterial toxins in which the toxic and receptor-binding functions are on separate protein chains. It is therefore possible to immunize individuals, usually as infants, with modified toxin

Toxic Shock
Syndrome

Fig. 9.23 Many common diseases are caused by bacterial toxins. These toxins are all exotoxins—proteins secreted by the bacteria. High-affinity IgG and IgA antibodies protect against these toxins. Bacteria also have nonsecreted endotoxins, such as lipopolysaccharide, which are released when the bacterium dies. The endotoxins are also important in the pathogenesis of disease, but there the host response is more complex because the innate immune system has receptors for some of these (see Chapters 2 and 10).

Disease	Organism	Toxin	Effects *in vivo*
Tetanus	*Clostridium tetani*	Tetanus toxin	Blocks inhibitory neuron action, leading to chronic muscle contraction
Diphtheria	*Corynebacterium diphtheriae*	Diphtheria toxin	Inhibits protein synthesis, leading to epithelial cell damage and myocarditis
Gas gangrene	*Clostridium perfringens*	Clostridial toxin	Phospholipase activation, leading to cell death
Cholera	*Vibrio cholerae*	Cholera toxin	Activates adenylate cyclase, elevates cAMP in cells, leading to changes in intestinal epithelial cells that cause loss of water and electrolytes
Anthrax	*Bacillus anthracis*	Anthrax toxic complex	Increases vascular permeability, leading to edema, hemorrhage, and circulatory collapse
Botulism	*Clostridium botulinum*	Botulinum toxin	Blocks release of acetylcholine, leading to paralysis
Whooping cough	*Bordetella pertussis*	Pertussis toxin	ADP-ribosylation of G proteins, leading to lymphoproliferation
		Tracheal cytotoxin	Inhibits cilia and causes epithelial cell loss
Scarlet fever	*Streptococcus pyogenes*	Erythrogenic toxin	Vasodilation, leading to scarlet fever rash
		Leukocidin Streptolysins	Kill phagocytes, allowing bacterial survival
Food poisoning	*Staphylococcus aureus*	Staphylococcal enterotoxin	Acts on intestinal neurons to induce vomiting. Also a potent T-cell mitogen (SE superantigen)
Toxic-shock syndrome	*Staphylococcus aureus*	Toxic-shock syndrome toxin	Causes hypotension and skin loss. Also a potent T-cell mitogen (TSST-1 superantigen)

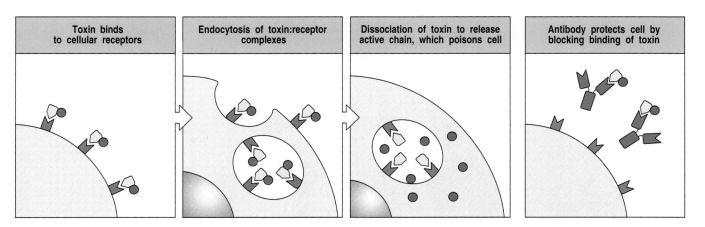

Fig. 9.24 Neutralization of toxins by IgG antibodies protects cells from their damaging action. Many bacteria (as well as venomous insects and snakes) cause their damaging effects by elaborating toxic proteins (see Fig. 9.23). These toxins are usually composed of several distinct moieties. One part of the toxin molecule binds a cellular receptor, which enables the molecule to be internalized. Another part of the toxin molecule then enters the cytoplasm and poisons the cell. Antibodies that inhibit toxin binding can prevent, or neutralize, these effects.

molecules in which the toxic chain has been denatured. These modified toxins, called toxoids, lack toxic activity but retain the receptor-binding site. Thus, immunization with the toxoid induces neutralizing antibodies that protect against the native toxin.

For some insect or animal venoms that are so toxic that a single exposure can cause severe tissue damage or death, the adaptive immune response is too slow to be protective. Exposure to these venoms is a rare event and protective vaccines have not been developed for use in humans. Instead, neutralizing antibodies are generated by immunizing other species, such as horses, with insect and snake venoms to produce anti-venom antibodies (antivenins). These antivenins are injected into exposed individuals to protect them against the toxic effects of the venom. Transfer of antibodies in this way is known as **passive immunization** (see Appendix I, Section A-37).

9-15 High-affinity IgG and IgA antibodies can inhibit the infectivity of viruses.

Animal viruses infect cells by binding to a particular cell-surface receptor, often a cell-type-specific protein that determines which cells they can infect. The **hemagglutinin** of influenza virus, for example, binds to terminal sialic acid residues on the carbohydrates of glycoproteins present on epithelial cells of the respiratory tract. It is known as hemagglutinin because it recognizes and binds to similar sialic acid residues on chicken red blood cells and agglutinates these red blood cells. Antibodies against the hemagglutinin can prevent infection by the influenza virus. Such antibodies are called virus-neutralizing antibodies and, as with the neutralization of toxins, high-affinity IgA and IgG antibodies are particularly important.

Many antibodies that neutralize viruses do so by directly blocking viral binding to surface receptors (Fig. 9.25). However, viruses are sometimes successfully neutralized when only a single molecule of antibody is bound to a virus particle that has many receptor-binding proteins on its surface. In these cases, the antibody must cause some change in the virus that disrupts its structure and either prevents it from interacting with its receptors or interferes with the fusion of the virus membrane with the cell surface after the virus has engaged its surface receptor.

| Virus binds to receptors on cell surface | Receptor-mediated endocytosis of virus | Acidification of endosome after endocytosis triggers fusion of virus with cell and entry of viral DNA | Antibody blocks binding to virus receptor and can also block fusion event |

Fig. 9.25 Viral infection of cells can be blocked by neutralizing antibodies. For a virus to multiply within a cell, it must introduce its genes into the cell. The first step in entry is usually the binding of the virus to a receptor on the cell surface. For enveloped viruses, as shown in the figure, entry into the cytoplasm requires fusion of the viral envelope and the cell membrane. For some viruses this fusion event takes place on the cell surface (not shown); for others it can occur only within the more acidic environment of endosomes, as shown here. Nonenveloped viruses must also bind to receptors on cell surfaces but they enter the cytoplasm by disrupting endosomes. Antibodies bound to viral surface proteins neutralize the virus, inhibiting either its initial binding to the cell or its subsequent entry.

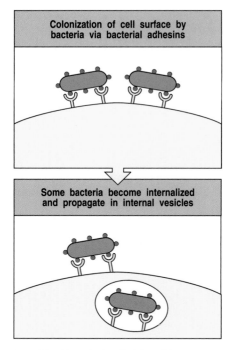

| Colonization of cell surface by bacteria via bacterial adhesins |

| Some bacteria become internalized and propagate in internal vesicles |

9-16   Antibodies can block the adherence of bacteria to host cells.

Many bacteria have cell-surface molecules called adhesins that enable them to bind to the surface of host cells. This adherence is critical to the ability of these bacteria to cause disease, whether they subsequently enter the cell, as do *Salmonella* species, or remain attached to the cell surface as extracellular pathogens (Fig. 9.26). *Neisseria gonorrhoeae*, the causative agent of the sexually transmitted disease gonorrhea, has a cell-surface protein known as pilin, which enables the bacterium to adhere to the epithelial cells of the urinary and reproductive tracts and is essential to its infectivity. Antibodies against pilin can inhibit this adhesive reaction and prevent infection.

IgA antibodies secreted onto the mucosal surfaces of the intestinal, respiratory, and reproductive tracts are particularly important in preventing infection by inhibiting the adhesion of bacteria, viruses, or other pathogens to the epithelial cells lining these surfaces. The adhesion of bacteria to cells within tissues can also contribute to pathogenesis, and IgG antibodies against adhesins can protect from damage much as IgA antibodies protect at mucosal surfaces.

| Antibodies against adhesins block colonization and uptake |

Fig. 9.26 Antibodies can prevent the attachment of bacteria to cell surfaces. Many bacterial infections require an interaction between the bacterium and a cell-surface receptor. This is particularly true for infections of mucosal surfaces. The attachment process involves very specific molecular interactions between bacterial adhesins and their receptors on host cells; antibodies against bacterial adhesins can block such infections.

9-17   Antibody:antigen complexes activate the classical pathway of complement by binding to C1q.

Another way in which antibodies can protect against infection is by activation of the cascade of complement proteins. We described these proteins in Chapter 2 because they can also be activated on pathogen surfaces in the absence of antibody, as part of the innate immune response. Complement activation proceeds via a series of proteolytic cleavage reactions, in which inactive components present in plasma are cleaved to form proteolytic enzymes that attach covalently to the pathogen surface. All known pathways of complement activation converge to generate the same set of effector actions: the pathogen surface or immune complex is coated with covalently attached fragments (principally C3b) that act as opsonins to promote uptake and removal by phagocytes. At the same time, small peptides with inflammatory and chemotactic activity are released (principally C5a) so that phagocytes are recruited to the site. In addition, the terminal complement components can form a membrane-attack complex that damages some bacteria.

Antibodies initiate complement activation by a pathway known as the classical pathway because it was the first pathway of complement activation to be discovered. The full details of this pathway, and of the other two known pathways of complement activation, are given in Chapter 2, but we will describe here how antibody is able to initiate the classical pathway after binding to pathogen, or after forming immune complexes.

The first component of the classical pathway of complement activation is C1, which is a complex of three proteins called C1q, C1r, and C1s. Two molecules each of C1r and C1s are bound to each molecule of C1q (see Fig. 2.21). Complement activation is initiated when antibodies attached to the surface of a pathogen bind C1q. C1q can be bound by either IgM or IgG antibodies but, because of the structural requirements of binding to C1q, neither of these antibody isotypes can activate complement in solution; the cascade is initiated only when the antibodies are bound to multiple sites on a cell surface, normally that of a pathogen.

The C1q molecule has six globular heads joined to a common stem by long, filamentous domains that resemble collagen molecules; the whole C1q complex has been likened to a bunch of six tulips held together by the stems. Each globular head can bind to one Fc domain, and binding of two or more globular heads activates the C1q molecule. In plasma the pentameric IgM molecule has a planar conformation that does not bind C1q (Fig. 9.27, left panel); however, binding to the surface of a pathogen deforms the IgM pentamer so that it looks like a staple (Fig. 9.27, right panel), and this distortion

IgM planar conformation

IgM 'staple' conformation

Fig. 9.27 The two conformations of IgM. The left panel shows the planar conformation of soluble IgM; the right panel shows the 'staple' conformation of IgM bound to a bacterial flagellum. Photographs (× 760,000) courtesy of K.H. Roux.

Fig. 9.28 The classical pathway of complement activation is initiated by the binding of C1q to antibody on a surface such as a bacterial surface. In the left panels one molecule of IgM, bent into the 'staple' conformation by binding several identical epitopes on a pathogen surface, allows the globular heads of C1q to bind to its Fc pieces on the surface of the pathogen. In the right panels, multiple molecules of IgG bound on the surface of a pathogen allow the binding of a single molecule of C1q to two or more Fc pieces. In both cases, the binding of C1q activates the associated C1r, which becomes an active enzyme that cleaves the pro-enzyme C1s, generating a serine protease that initiates the classical complement cascade (not illustrated).

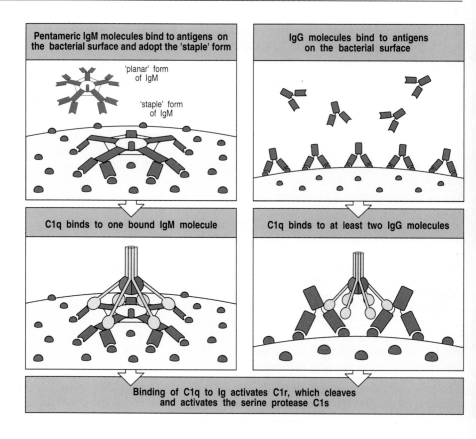

exposes binding sites for the C1q heads. Although C1q binds with low affinity to some subclasses of IgG in solution, the binding energy required for C1q activation is achieved only when a single molecule of C1q can bind two or more IgG molecules that are held within 30–40 nm of each other as a result of binding antigen. This requires that multiple molecules of IgG be bound to a single pathogen. For this reason, IgM is much more efficient than IgG in activating complement. The binding of C1q to a single bound IgM molecule, or to two or more bound IgG molecules (Fig. 9.28), leads to the activation of an enzymatic activity in C1r, triggering the complement cascade. This translates antibody binding into the activation of the complement cascade, which, as we learned in Chapter 2, can also be triggered by the direct binding of C1q to the pathogen surface.

9-18   Complement receptors are important in the removal of immune complexes from the circulation.

Many small soluble antigens form antibody:antigen complexes known as **immune complexes** that contain too few molecules of IgG to be readily bound to the Fcγ receptors that we will discuss in the next part of the chapter. These antigens include toxins bound by neutralizing antibodies and debris from dead microorganisms. Such immune complexes are found after most infections and are removed from the circulation through the action of complement. The soluble immune complexes trigger their own removal by activating complement, again through the binding of C1q, leading to the covalent binding of the activated components C4b and C3b to the complex, which is then cleared from the circulation by the binding of C4b and C3b to complement receptor 1 (CR1) on the surface of erythrocytes. The erythrocytes transport the bound complexes of antigen, antibody, and complement to the liver and spleen. Here, macrophages bearing CR1 and Fc receptors

Fig. 9.29 Erythrocyte CR1 helps to clear immune complexes from the circulation. CR1 on the erythrocyte surface has an important role in the clearance of immune complexes from the circulation. Immune complexes bind to CR1 on erythrocytes, which transport them to the liver and spleen, where they are removed by macrophages expressing receptors for both Fc and bound complement components.

Small antigen:antibody complexes form in the circulation and activate complement

C1q

Many molecules of C3b are bound covalently to the complex

C3b

C4b2b3b

Bound C3b binds to the receptor CR1 on erythrocyte surfaces

CR1

In the spleen and liver, phagocytic cells remove the immune complexes

FcR

remove the complexes from the erythrocyte surface without destroying the cell, and then degrade them (Fig. 9.29). Even larger aggregates of particulate antigen and antibody can be made soluble upon activation of the classical complement pathway and the consequent binding of C3b to the aggregates; these can then be removed by binding to complement receptors.

Immune complexes that are not removed tend to deposit in the basement membranes of small blood vessels, most notably those of the renal glomerulus, where the blood is filtered to form urine. Immune complexes that pass through the basement membrane of the glomerulus bind to the complement receptor CR1 on the renal podocytes, cells that lie beneath the basement membrane. The functional significance of these receptors in the kidney is unknown; however, they have an important role in the pathology of some autoimmune diseases.

In the autoimmune disease systemic lupus erythematosus, which we will describe in Chapter 13, excessive levels of circulating immune complexes cause huge deposits of antigen, antibody, and complement on the podocytes, damaging the glomerulus; kidney failure is the principal danger in this disease. Immune complexes can also be a cause of pathology in patients with deficiencies in the early components of complement. Such patients do not clear immune complexes effectively and they also suffer tissue damage, especially in the kidneys, in a similar way.

Summary.

The T-cell dependent antibody response begins with IgM secretion but quickly progresses to the production of additional isotypes. Each isotype is specialized both in its localization in the body and in the functions it can perform. IgM antibodies are found mainly in blood; they are pentameric in structure. IgM is specialized to activate complement efficiently upon binding antigen and to compensate for the low affinity of a typical IgM antigen-binding site. IgG antibodies are usually of higher affinity and are found in blood and in extracellular fluid, where they can neutralize toxins, viruses, and bacteria, opsonize them for phagocytosis, and activate the complement system. IgA antibodies are synthesized as monomers, which enter blood and extracellular fluids, or as dimeric molecules in the lamina propria of various epithelial tissues. IgA dimers are selectively transported across the epithelial layer into sites such as the lumen of the gut, where they neutralize toxins and viruses and block the entry of bacteria across the intestinal epithelium. Most IgE antibody is bound to the surface of mast cells that reside mainly just below body surfaces; antigen binding to this IgE triggers local defense reactions. Antibodies can defend the body against extracellular pathogens and their toxic products in several ways. The simplest is by direct interactions with pathogens or their products, for example by binding to the active sites of toxins and neutralizing them or by blocking their ability to bind to host cells through specific receptors. When antibodies of the appropriate isotype bind to antigens, they can activate the classical pathway of complement, which leads to the elimination of the pathogen by the various mechanisms described in Chapter 2. Soluble immune complexes of antigen and antibody also fix complement and are cleared from the circulation via complement receptors on red blood cells.

Systemic Lupus Erythematosus

The destruction of antibody-coated pathogens via Fc receptors.

The ability of high-affinity antibodies to neutralize toxins, viruses, or bacteria can protect against infection but does not, on its own, solve the problem of how to remove the pathogens and their products from the body. Moreover, many pathogens cannot be neutralized by antibody and must be destroyed by other means. Many pathogen-specific antibodies do not bind to neutralizing targets on pathogen surfaces and thus need to be linked to other effector mechanisms to play their part in host defense. We have already seen how the binding of antibody to antigen can activate complement. Another important defense mechanism is the activation of a variety of **accessory effector cells** bearing receptors called **Fc receptors** because they are specific for the Fc portion of antibodies. These receptors facilitate the phagocytosis of neutralized microorganisms and resistant extracellular pathogens by macrophages, dendritic cells and neutrophils. Other nonphagocytic cells—NK cells, eosinophils, basophils, and mast cells (see Fig. 1.4)—are triggered to secrete stored mediators when their Fc receptors are engaged. These mechanisms maximize the effectiveness of all antibodies regardless of where they bind. Fc receptor-bearing cells are activated when their Fc receptors are aggregated by binding to the multiple Fc regions of antibody molecules coating a pathogen. They can also be activated by soluble mediators; these include products of the complement cascade, which can itself be activated by antibody.

9-19   The Fc receptors of accessory cells are signaling receptors specific for immunoglobulins of different isotypes.

The Fc receptors are a family of cell-surface molecules that bind the Fc portion of immunoglobulins. Each member of the family recognizes immunoglobulin of one isotype or a few closely related isotypes through a recognition domain on the α chain of the Fc receptor. Most Fc receptors are themselves members of the immunoglobulin gene superfamily. Different cell types bear Fc receptors for antibodies of different isotypes, and the isotype of the antibody thus determines which types of cell will be engaged in a given response. The different Fc receptors, the cells that express them, and their isotype specificities are shown in Fig. 9.30.

Most Fc receptors function as part of a multisubunit complex. Only the α chain is required for specific recognition; the other chains are required for transport to the cell surface and for signal transduction when an Fc region is bound. Some Fcγ receptors, the Fcα receptor I, and the high-affinity receptor for IgE use a γ chain for signaling; the γ chain, which is closely related to the ζ chain of the T-cell receptor complex, associates noncovalently with the Fc-binding α chain. The human FcγRII-A is a single-chain receptor in which the cytoplasmic domain of the α chain replaces the function of the γ chain. FcγRII-B1 and FcγRII-B2 are also single-chain receptors but function as inhibitory receptors because they contain an ITIM that engages the inositol 5'-phosphatase SHIP (see Section 6-16). Although the most prominent function of Fc receptors is the activation of accessory cells to attack pathogens, they can also contribute in other ways to immune responses. For example, the FcγRII-B receptor negatively regulates B cells, mast cells, macrophages, and neutrophils by adjusting the threshold at which immune complexes will activate these cells. Fc receptors expressed by dendritic cells enable them to ingest antigen:antibody complexes and to present antigenic peptides to T cells.

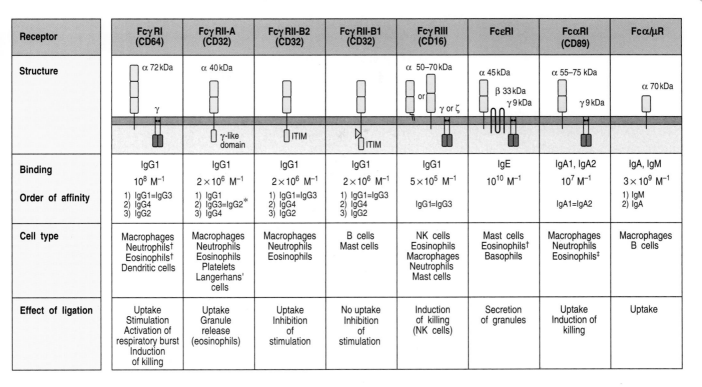

Receptor	Fcγ RI (CD64)	Fcγ RII-A (CD32)	Fcγ RII-B2 (CD32)	Fcγ RII-B1 (CD32)	Fcγ RIII (CD16)	FcεRI	FcαRI (CD89)	Fcα/μR
Structure	α 72 kDa γ	α 40 kDa γ-like domain	ITIM	ITIM	α 50–70 kDa or γ or ζ	α 45 kDa β 33 kDa γ 9 kDa	α 55–75 kDa γ 9 kDa	α 70 kDa
Binding Order of affinity	IgG1 10^8 M^{-1} 1) IgG1=IgG3 2) IgG4 3) IgG2	IgG1 2×10^6 M^{-1} 1) IgG1 2) IgG3=IgG2* 3) IgG4	IgG1 2×10^6 M^{-1} 1) IgG1=IgG3 2) IgG4 3) IgG2	IgG1 2×10^6 M^{-1} 1) IgG1=IgG3 2) IgG4 3) IgG2	IgG1 5×10^5 M^{-1} IgG1=IgG3	IgE 10^{10} M^{-1}	IgA1, IgA2 10^7 M^{-1} IgA1=IgA2	IgA, IgM 3×10^9 M^{-1} 1) IgM 2) IgA
Cell type	Macrophages Neutrophils† Eosinophils† Dendritic cells	Macrophages Neutrophils Eosinophils Platelets Langerhans' cells	Macrophages Neutrophils Eosinophils	B cells Mast cells	NK cells Eosinophils Macrophages Neutrophils Mast cells	Mast cells Eosinophils† Basophils	Macrophages Neutrophils Eosinophils‡	Macrophages B cells
Effect of ligation	Uptake Stimulation Activation of respiratory burst Induction of killing	Uptake Granule release (eosinophils)	Uptake Inhibition of stimulation	No uptake Inhibition of stimulation	Induction of killing (NK cells)	Secretion of granules	Uptake Induction of killing	Uptake

Fig. 9.30 Distinct receptors for the Fc region of the different immunoglobulin isotypes are expressed on different accessory cells. The subunit structure and binding properties of these receptors and the cell types expressing them are shown. The exact chain composition of any receptor can vary from one cell type to another. For example, FcγRIII in neutrophils is expressed as a molecule with a glycosylphosphatidylinositol membrane anchor, without γ chains, whereas in NK cells it is a transmembrane molecule associated with γ chains as shown. The FcγRII-B1 differs from the FcγRII-B2 by the presence of an additional exon in the intracellular region. This exon prevents the FcγRII-B1 from being internalized upon cross-linking. The binding affinities are taken from data on human receptors. *Only some allotypes of FcγRII-A bind IgG2. †In these cases Fc receptor expression is inducible rather than constitutive. ‡In eosinophils, the molecular weight of CD89α chain is 70–100 kDa.

9-20 Fc receptors on phagocytes are activated by antibodies bound to the surface of pathogens and enable the phagocytes to ingest and destroy pathogens.

Phagocytes are activated by IgG antibodies, especially IgG1 and IgG3, that bind to specific Fcγ receptors on the phagocyte surface (see Fig. 9.30). Because phagocyte activation can initiate an inflammatory response and cause tissue damage, it is essential that the Fc receptors on phagocytes are able to distinguish antibody molecules bound to a pathogen from the much larger number of free antibody molecules that are not bound to anything. This distinction is made possible by the aggregation or multimerization of antibodies that occurs when they bind to multimeric antigens or to multi-valent antigenic particles such as viruses and bacteria. Fc receptors on the surface of a cell bind antibody-coated particles with higher avidity than immunoglobulin monomers, and this is the principal mechanism by which bound antibodies are distinguished from free immunoglobulin (Fig. 9.31). The result is that Fc receptors enable cells to detect pathogens through bound antibody molecules. Thus, specific antibody together with Fc receptors gives to phagocytic cells that lack intrinsic specificity the ability to identify and remove pathogens and their products from the extracellular spaces.

The most important Fc-bearing cells in humoral immune responses are the phagocytic cells of the monocytic and myelocytic lineages, particularly macrophages and neutrophils (see Chapter 2). Many bacteria are directly

Free immunoglobulin does not cross-link Fc receptors

bacterium

Fc receptors

macrophage

No activation of macrophage, no destruction of bacterium

Aggregation of immunoglobulin on bacterial surface allows cross-linking of Fc receptors

Activation of macrophage, leading to phagocytosis and destruction of bacterium

Fig. 9.31 Bound antibody is distinguishable from free immunoglobulin by its state of aggregation. Free immunoglobulin molecules bind most Fc receptors with very low affinity and cannot cross-link Fc receptors. Antigen-bound immunoglobulin, however, binds to Fc receptors with high avidity because several antibody molecules that are bound to the same surface bind to multiple Fc receptors on the surface of the accessory cell. This Fc receptor cross-linking sends a signal to activate the cell bearing it. With Fc receptors that have ITIMs, the result is inhibition.

recognized, ingested, and destroyed by phagocytes, and these bacteria are not pathogenic in normal individuals (see Chapter 2). Bacterial pathogens, however, often have polysaccharide capsules that allow them to resist direct engulfment by phagocytes. However, these bacteria become susceptible to phagocytosis when they are coated with antibody and complement that engages the Fcγ or Fcα receptors and CR1 on phagocytic cells, triggering bacterial uptake (Fig. 9.32). Phagocytosis by binding to complement receptors is particularly important early in the immune response, before isotype-switched antibodies have been made. Capsular polysaccharides belong to the TI-2 class of thymus-independent antigens (see Section 9-11) and can therefore stimulate the early production of IgM antibodies. IgM is very effective at activating the complement system. IgM binding to encapsulated bacteria thus triggers the opsonization of these bacteria by complement and their prompt ingestion and destruction by phagocytes bearing complement receptors. Recently, an Fc receptor for IgM has been discovered, suggesting that IgM may promote phagocytosis directly *in vivo*.

Both the internalization and destruction of microorganisms are greatly enhanced by interactions between the molecules coating an opsonized microorganism and their receptors on the phagocyte surface. When an antibody-coated pathogen binds to Fcγ receptors on the surface of a phagocyte, for example, the cell surface extends around the surface of the particle

| Bacterium is coated with complement and IgG antibody | When C3b binds to CR1 and antibody binds to Fc receptor, bacteria are phagocytosed | Macrophage membranes fuse, creating a membrane-bounded vesicle, the phagosome | Lysosomes fuse with these vesicles, delivering enzymes that degrade the bacterium |

bacterium

C3b

Fc receptors

CR1

macrophage

lysosome

Fig. 9.32 Fc and complement receptors on phagocytes trigger the uptake and degradation of antibody-coated bacteria. Many bacteria resist phagocytosis by macrophages and neutrophils. Antibodies bound to these bacteria, however, enable them to be ingested and degraded through the interaction of the multiple Fc domains arrayed on the bacterial surface with Fc receptors on the phagocyte surface. Antibody coating also induces activation of the complement system and the binding of complement components to the bacterial surface. These can interact with complement receptors (for example CR1) on the phagocyte. Fc receptors and complement receptors synergize in inducing phagocytosis. Bacteria coated with IgG antibody and complement are therefore more readily ingested than those coated with IgG alone. Binding of Fc and complement receptors signals the phagocyte to increase the rate of phagocytosis, to fuse lysosomes with phagosomes, and to increase its bactericidal activity.

Fig. 9.33 Eosinophils attacking a schistosome larva in the presence of serum from an infected patient. Large parasites, such as worms, cannot be ingested by phagocytes; however, when the worm is coated with antibody, especially IgE, eosinophils can attack it through their binding to the high-affinity FcεRI. Similar attacks can be mounted by other Fc receptor-bearing cells on various large targets. These cells release the toxic contents of their granules directly onto the target, a process known as exocytosis. Photograph courtesy of A. Butterworth.

through successive binding of Fcγ receptors to the antibody Fc regions bound to the pathogen surface. This is an active process triggered by the stimulation of Fcγ receptors. Endocytosis leads to enclosure of the particle in an acidified cytoplasmic vesicle called a phagosome. The phagosome then fuses with one or more lysosomes to generate a phagolysosome, releasing the lysosomal enzymes into the phagosome interior, where they destroy the bacterium (see Fig. 9.32). The process of bacterial destruction in the phagolysosome was described in detail in Section 2-3.

Some particles are too large for a phagocyte to ingest; parasitic worms are one example. In this case the phagocyte attaches to the surface of the antibody-coated parasite via its Fcγ, Fcα, or Fcε receptors, and the lysosomes fuse with the attached surface membrane. This reaction discharges the contents of the lysosome onto the surface of the parasite, damaging it directly in the extracellular space. Thus, Fcγ and Fcα receptors can trigger the internalization of external particles by phagocytosis or the externalization of internal vesicles by exocytosis. Whereas the principal phagocytes in the destruction of bacteria are macrophages and neutrophils, large parasites such as helminths are more usually attacked by eosinophils (Fig. 9.33). Cross-linking of IgE bound to the high-affinity FcεRI usually results in exocytosis. We will see in the next three sections that NK cells and mast cells also release mediators stored in their vesicles when their Fc receptors are aggregated.

9-21 Fc receptors activate NK cells to destroy antibody-coated targets.

Infected cells are usually destroyed by T cells that are activated by foreign peptides bound to cell-surface MHC molecules. However, virus-infected cells can also signal the presence of intracellular infection by expressing on their surfaces viral proteins that can be recognized by antibodies. Cells bound by such antibodies can then be killed by a specialized non-T, non-B lymphoid cell called a **natural killer cell** (**NK cell**), which we met in Chapter 2. NK cells are large lymphoid cells with prominent intracellular granules; they make up a small fraction of peripheral blood lymphoid cells. They bear no known antigen-specific receptors but are able to recognize and kill a limited range of abnormal cells. They were first discovered because of their ability to kill some tumor cells, but are now known to have an important role in innate immunity.

The destruction of antibody-coated target cells by NK cells is called **antibody-dependent cell-mediated cytotoxicity** (**ADCC**) and is triggered when antibody bound to the surface of a cell interacts with Fc receptors on the NK cell (Fig. 9.34). NK cells express the receptor FcγRIII (CD16), which recognizes the IgG1 and IgG3 subclasses. The mechanism of attack is exactly analogous to that of cytotoxic T cells, involving the release of cytoplasmic granules containing perforin and granzymes (see Section 8-22). The importance of ADCC in defense against infection with bacteria or viruses has not yet been fully established. However, ADCC represents yet another mechanism by which, through engaging an Fc receptor, antibodies can direct an antigen-specific attack by an effector cell that itself lacks specificity for antigen.

| Antibody binds antigens on the surface of target cells | Fc receptors on NK cells recognize bound antibody | Cross-linking of Fc receptors signals the NK cell to kill the target cell | Target cell dies by apoptosis |

Fig. 9.34 Antibody-coated target cells can be killed by NK cells in antibody-dependent cell-mediated cytotoxicity (ADCC). NK cells (see Chapter 2) are large granular non-T, non-B lymphoid cells that have FcγRIII (CD16) on their surface. When these cells encounter cells coated with IgG antibody, they rapidly kill the target cell. The importance of ADCC in host defense or tissue damage is still controversial.

9-22   Mast cells, basophils, and activated eosinophils bind IgE antibody via the high-affinity Fcε receptor.

When pathogens cross epithelial barriers and establish a local focus of infection, the host must mobilize its defenses and direct them to the site of pathogen growth. One mechanism by which this is achieved is to activate a specialized cell type known as a **mast cell**. Mast cells are large cells containing distinctive cytoplasmic granules that contain a mixture of chemical mediators, including histamine, that act rapidly to make local blood vessels more permeable. Mast cells have a distinctive appearance after staining with the dye toluidine blue that makes them readily identifiable in tissues (see Fig. 1.4). They are found in particularly high concentrations in vascularized connective tissues just beneath body epithelial surfaces, including the submucosal tissues of the gastrointestinal and respiratory tracts and the dermis that lies just below the surface of the skin.

Mast cells can be activated to release their granules, and to secrete lipid inflammatory mediators and cytokines, via antibody bound to Fc receptors specific for IgE (FcεRI) and IgG (FcγRIII). We have seen earlier that most Fc receptors bind stably to the Fc region of antibodies only when these are bound to antigen. By contrast, FcεRI binds monomeric IgE antibodies with a very high affinity, measured at approximately 10^{10} M^{-1}. Thus, even at the low levels of IgE found circulating in normal individuals, a substantial portion of the total IgE is bound to the FcεRI on mast cells and on the analogous circulating basophilic granulocytes or **basophils**. Eosinophils can also express Fc receptors, but express FcεRI only when activated and recruited to an inflammatory site.

Although mast cells are usually stably associated with bound IgE, they are not activated simply by the binding of monomeric antigens to this IgE. Mast-cell activation occurs only when the bound IgE is cross-linked by multivalent antigen. This signal activates the mast cell to release the contents of its granules, which occurs in seconds (Fig. 9.35), to synthesize and release lipid mediators such as prostaglandin D_2 and leukotriene C4, and to secrete cytokines such as TNF-α, thereby initiating a local inflammatory response. Degranulation releases the stored histamine, causing a local increase in

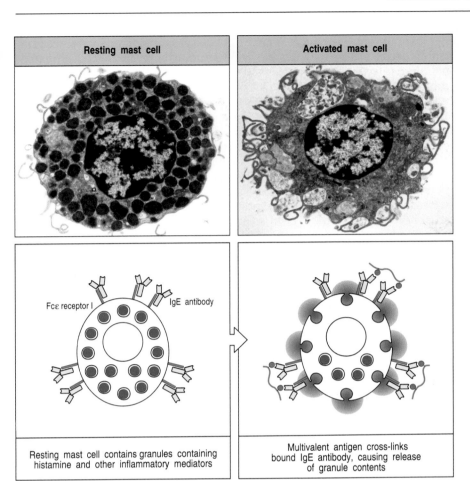

Resting mast cell	Activated mast cell

Fcε receptor I   IgE antibody

Resting mast cell contains granules containing histamine and other inflammatory mediators	Multivalent antigen cross-links bound IgE antibody, causing release of granule contents

Fig. 9.35 IgE antibody cross-linking on mast-cell surfaces leads to a rapid release of inflammatory mediators. Mast cells are large cells found in connective tissue that can be distinguished by secretory granules containing many inflammatory mediators. They bind stably to monomeric IgE antibodies through the very high-affinity Fcε receptor I. Antigen cross-linking of the bound IgE antibody molecules triggers rapid degranulation, releasing inflammatory mediators into the surrounding tissue. These mediators trigger local inflammation, which recruits cells and proteins required for host defense to sites of infection. These cells are also triggered during allergic reactions when allergens bind to IgE on mast cells. Photographs courtesy of A.M. Dvorak.

blood flow and vascular permeability that quickly leads to an accumulation of fluid and blood proteins, including antibodies, in the surrounding tissue. Shortly afterwards there is an influx of blood-borne cells such as polymorphonuclear leukocytes and, later, macrophages, eosinophils, and effector lymphocytes. This influx can last from a few minutes to a few hours and produces an inflammatory response at the site of infection. Thus, mast cells are part of the front-line host defenses against pathogens that enter the body across epithelial barriers.

9-23 IgE-mediated activation of accessory cells has an important role in resistance to parasite infection.

Mast cells are thought to serve at least three important functions in host defense. First, their location near body surfaces allows them to recruit both specific and nonspecific effector elements to sites where infectious agents are most likely to enter the internal milieu. Second, they increase the flow of lymph from sites of antigen deposition to the regional lymph nodes, where naive lymphocytes are first activated. Third, their ability to trigger muscular contraction can contribute to the physical expulsion of pathogens from the lungs or the gut. Mast cells respond rapidly to the binding of antigen to surface-bound IgE antibodies, and their activation leads to the recruitment and activation of basophils and eosinophils, which contribute further to the IgE-mediated response. There is increasing evidence that such IgE-mediated responses are crucial to defense against parasite infestation.

A role for mast cells in the clearance of parasites is suggested by the accumulation of mast cells in the intestine, known as **mastocytosis**, that accompanies helminth infection, and by observations in W/W^V mutant mice, which have a profound mast-cell deficiency caused by mutation of the gene c-*kit*. These mutant mice show impaired clearance of the intestinal nematodes *Trichinella spiralis* and *Strongyloides* species. Clearance of *Strongyloides* is even more impaired in W/W^V mice that lack IL-3 and that therefore, besides lacking mast cells, fail to produce basophils. Thus, both mast cells and basophils seem to contribute to defense against these helminth parasites. Other evidence also points to the importance of IgE antibodies and eosinophils in defense against parasites. Infections by certain classes of parasite, particularly helminths, are strongly associated with the production of IgE antibodies and the presence of an abnormally large number of eosinophils (**eosinophilia**) in blood and tissues. Furthermore, experiments in mice show that depletion of eosinophils by using polyclonal anti-eosinophil antisera increases the severity of infection by the parasitic helminth *Schistosoma mansoni*. Eosinophils seem to be directly responsible for helminth destruction; examination of infected tissues shows degranulated eosinophils adhering to helminths, and experiments *in vitro* have shown that eosinophils can kill *S. mansoni* in the presence of specific IgE (see Fig. 9.33), IgG, or IgA anti-schistosome antibodies.

The role of IgE, mast cells, basophils, and eosinophils can also be seen in resistance to the feeding of blood-sucking ixodid ticks. Normal skin at the site of a tick bite shows degranulated mast cells and an accumulation of basophils and eosinophils that are degranulated, an indicator of recent activation. Resistance to subsequent feeding by these ticks develops after the first exposure, suggesting a specific immunological mechanism. Mast-cell deficient mice show no such acquired resistance to tick species, and in guinea pigs the depletion of either basophils or eosinophils by specific polyclonal antibodies also reduces resistance to tick feeding. Finally, recent experiments have shown that resistance to ticks in mice is mediated by specific IgE antibody.

Thus, many clinical studies and experiments support a role for this system of IgE binding to the high-affinity FcεRI in host resistance to pathogens that enter across epithelia. We will see later, in Chapter 12, that the same system accounts for many of the symptoms in allergic diseases such as asthma and hay fever, and in the life-threatening response known as systemic anaphylaxis.

Summary.

Antibody-coated pathogens are recognized by effector cells through Fc receptors that bind to an array of constant regions (Fc portions) provided by the pathogen-bound antibodies. Binding activates the cell and triggers destruction of the pathogen, through either phagocytosis, granule release, or both. Fc receptors comprise a family of proteins, each of which recognizes immunoglobulins of particular isotypes. Fc receptors on macrophages and neutrophils recognize the constant regions of IgG or IgA antibodies bound to a pathogen and trigger the engulfment and destruction of bacteria coated with IgG or IgA. Binding to the Fc receptor also induces the production of microbicidal agents in the intracellular vesicles of the phagocyte. Eosinophils are important in the elimination of parasites too large to be engulfed: they bear Fc receptors specific for the constant region of IgG, as well as high-affinity receptors for IgE; aggregation of these receptors triggers the release of toxic substances onto the surface of the parasite. NK cells, tissue mast cells, and blood basophils also release their granule contents when their Fc receptors are engaged. The high-affinity receptor for IgE is expressed constitutively by mast cells and basophils, and is induced in activated eosinophils. It differs from other Fc receptors in that it can bind free monomeric antibody, thus enabling an immediate response to pathogens at their site of first entry into the tissues. When IgE bound to the surface of a mast cell is aggregated by binding to antigen, it triggers the release of histamine and many other mediators that increase the blood flow to sites of infection; it thereby recruits antibodies and effector cells to these sites. Mast cells are found principally below epithelial surfaces of the skin and beneath the basement membrane of the digestive and respiratory tracts. Their activation by innocuous substances is responsible for many of the symptoms of acute allergic reactions, as will be described in Chapter 12.

Summary to Chapter 9.

The humoral immune response to infection involves the production of antibody by plasma cells derived from B lymphocytes, the binding of this antibody to the pathogen, and the elimination of the pathogen by phagocytic cells and molecules of the humoral immune system. The production of antibody usually requires the action of helper T cells specific for a peptide fragment of the antigen recognized by the B cell. The B cell then proliferates and differentiates, first at the T zone–B zone boundary in secondary lymphoid tissues, then at the T zone–red pulp border, and finally in the germinal center, where somatic hypermutation diversifies the B-cell receptors expressed by a clone of B cells. The B cells that bind antigen most avidly are selected for further differentiation by the continual requirement for contact with antigen and the requirement to present antigen-derived peptides to germinal center helper T cells. These events allow the affinity of antibodies to increase over the course of an immune response, especially in repeated responses to the same antigen. Helper T cells also direct isotype switching, leading to the production of antibody of various isotypes that can be distributed to various body compartments.

IgM is produced naturally by B-1 cells, as well as early in the response of conventional or B-2 cells. IgM has a major role in protecting against infection in the bloodstream, whereas isotypes secreted later, such as IgG, diffuse into the tissues. Certain pathogens that have highly repeating antigenic determinants and express mitogens that intrinsically stimulate B cells can elicit IgM and some IgG independently of T-cell help. Such antigens are called TI antigens, and the antibody elicited by these antigens can provide an early protective immune response. Multimeric IgA is produced in the lamina propria and transported across epithelial surfaces, whereas IgE is made in small amounts and binds avidly to the surface of mast cells. Antibodies that bind with high affinity to critical sites on toxins, viruses, and bacteria can neutralize them. However, pathogens and their products are destroyed and removed from the body largely through uptake into phagocytes and degradation inside these cells. Antibodies that coat pathogens bind to Fc receptors on phagocytes, which are thereby triggered to engulf and destroy the pathogen. Binding of antibody C-regions to Fc receptors on other cells leads to the exocytosis of stored mediators; this is particularly important in parasite infections, in which Fcε-expressing mast cells and activated eosinophils are triggered by the binding of antigen to IgE antibody to release inflammatory mediators directly onto parasite surfaces. Antibodies can also initiate the destruction of pathogens by activating the complement system. Complement components can opsonize pathogens for uptake by phagocytes, recruit phagocytes to sites of infection, and directly destroy pathogens by creating pores in their cell membrane. Receptors for complement components and Fc receptors often synergize in activating the uptake and destruction of pathogens and immune complexes. Thus, the humoral immune response is targeted to the infecting pathogen through the production of specific antibody; however, the effector actions of that antibody are determined by its isotype and are the same for all pathogens bound by antibody of a particular isotype.

Chapter 9 questions.

9.1 *(a) Why have multiple isotypes of immunoglobulin evolved? (b) Describe unique roles for IgM, IgG, IgA, and IgE.*

9.2 *Compare and contrast the thymus-dependent and thymus-independent humoral immune responses in terms of: requirements for stimulation, isotype, site in the spleen, affinity, and memory cell formation.*

9.3 *(a) What is somatic hypermutation? (b) Where does it occur? (c) Discuss two main functions or results of somatic hypermutation.*

9.4 *Compare and contrast plasma cells, plasmablasts and memory B cells in terms of: proliferation, antibody secretion, life-span, and location in the body.*

9.5 *Most of the effector functions of antibodies require accessory cells or molecules. (a) Which function does not? (b) Why is this important and what site(s) of the body require this for protection?*

9.6 *(a) What are the two main categories of effector functions that do require accessory cells and molecules? (b) Discuss one aspect in which they are similar or provide overlapping functions and one aspect in which they are different.*

General references.

Liu, Y.J., Zhang, J., Lane, P.J., Chan, E.Y., and MacLennan, I.C.: **Sites of specific B cell activation in primary and secondary responses to T cell-dependent and T cell-independent antigens.** *Eur. J. Immunol.* 1991, **21**:2951–2962.

Metzger, H. (ed): *Fc Receptors and the Action of Antibodies*, 1st edn. Washington, DC, American Society for Microbiology, 1990.

Rajewsky, K.: **Clonal selection and learning in the antibody system.** *Nature* 1996, **381**:751–758.

Section references.

9-1 The humoral immune response is initiated when B cells that bind antigen are signaled by helper T cells or by certain microbial antigens alone.

Gulbranson-Judge, A., and MacLennan, I.: **Sequential antigen-specific growth of T cells in the T zones and follicles in response to pigeon cytochrome c.** *Eur. J. Immunol.* 1996, **26**:1830–1837.

O'Rourke, L., Tooze, R., and Fearon, D.T.: **Co-receptors of B lymphocytes.** *Curr. Opin. Immunol.* 1997, **9**:324–329.

9-2 Armed helper T cells activate B cells that recognize the same antigen.

Lanzavecchia, A.: **Receptor-mediated antigen uptake and its effect on antigen presentation to class II-restricted T lymphocytes.** *Annu. Rev. Immunol.* 1990, **8**:773–793.

MacLennan, I.C.M., Gulbranson-Judge, A., Toellner, K.M., Casamayor-Palleja, M., Chan, E., Sze, D.M.Y., Luther, S.A., and Orbea, H.A.: **The changing preference of T and B cells for partners as T-dependent antibody responses develop.** *Immunol. Rev.* 1997, **156**:53–66.

Parker, D.C.: **T cell-dependent B-cell activation.** *Annu. Rev. Immunol.* 1993, **11**:331–340.

9-3 Antigenic peptides bound to self MHC class II molecules trigger armed helper T cells to make membrane-bound and secreted molecules that can activate a B cell.

Jaiswal, A.I., and Croft, M.: **CD40 ligand induction on T cell subsets by peptide-presenting B cells.** *J. Immunol.* 1997, **159**:2282–2291.

Lane, P., Traunecker, A., Hubele, S., Inui, S., Lanzavecchia, A., and Gray, D.: **Activated human T cells express a ligand for the human B cell-associated antigen CD40 which participates in T cell-dependent activation of B lymphocytes.** *Eur. J. Immunol.* 1992, **22**:2573–2578.

Mackay, F., and Browning, J.L.: **BAFF: a fundamental survival factor for B cells.** *Nat. Rev. Immunol.* 2002, **2**:465–475.

Noelle, R.J., Roy, M., Shepherd, D.M., Stamenkovic, I., Ledbetter, J.A., and Aruffo, A.: **A 39-kDa protein on activated helper T cells binds CD40 and transduces the signal for cognate activation of B cells.** *Proc. Natl. Acad. Sci. USA* 1992, **89**:6550–6554.

Shanebeck, K.D., Maliszewski, C.R., Kennedy, M.K., Picha, K.S., Smith, C.A., Goodwin, R.G., and Grabstein, K.H.: **Regulation of murine B cell growth and differentiation by CD30 ligand.** *Eur. J. Immunol.* 1995, **25**:2147–2153.

Sharpe, A.H., and Freeman, G.J.: **The B7-CD28 superfamily.** *Nat. Rev. Immunol.* 2002, **2**:116–126.

Valle, A., Zuber, C.E., Defrance, T., Djossou, O., De, R.M., and Banchereau, J.: **Activation of human B lymphocytes through CD40 and interleukin 4.** *Eur. J. Immunol.* 1989, **19**:1463–1467.

Yoshinaga, S.K., Whoriskey, J.S., Khare, S.D., Sarmiento, U., Guo, J., Horan, T., Shih, G., Zhang, M., Coccia, M.A., Kohno, T., Tafuri-Bladt, A., Brankow, D., Campbell, P., Chang, D., Chiu, L., Dai, T., Duncan, G., Elliott, G.S., Hui, A., McCabe, S.M., Scully, S., Shahinian, A., Shaklee, C.L., Van, G., Mak, T.W. *et al.*: **T-cell co-stimulation through B7RP-1 and ICOS.** *Nature* 1999, **402**:827–832.

9-4 Isotype switching in thymus-dependent responses requires expression of CD40 ligand by the helper T cell and is directed by cytokines.

Francke, U., and Ochs, H.D.: **The CD40 ligand, gp39, is defective in activated T cells from patients with X-linked hyper-IgM syndrome.** *Cell* 1993, **72**:291–300.

Jumper, M., Splawski, J., Lipsky, P., and Meek, K.: **Ligation of CD40 induces sterile transcripts of multiple Ig H chain isotypes in human B cells.** *J. Immunol.* 1994, **152**:438–445.

Litinskiy, M.B., Nardelli, B., Hilbert, D.M., He, B., Schaffer, A., Casali, P., and Cerutti, A.: **DCs induce CD40-independent immunoglobulin class switching through BLyS and APRIL.** *Nat. Immunol.* 2002, **3**:822–829.

Snapper, C.M., Kehry, M.R., Castle, B.E., and Mond, J.J.: **Multivalent, but not divalent, antigen receptor cross-linkers synergize with CD40 ligand for induction of Ig synthesis and class switching in normal murine B cells.** *J. Immunol.* 1995, **154**:1177–1187.

Snapper, C.M., and Paul, W.E.: **Interferon γ and B cell stimulatory factor-1 reciprocally regulate Ig isotype production.** *Science* 1987, **236**:944–947.

Stavnezer, J.: **Immunoglobulin class switching.** *Curr. Opin. Immunol.* 1996, **8**:199–205.

9-5 Antigen-binding B cells are trapped in the T-cell zone of secondary lymphoid tissues and are activated by encounter with armed helper T cells.

Garside, P., Ingulli, E., Merica, R.R., Johnson, J.G., Noelle, R.J., and Jenkins, M.K.: **Visualization of specific B and T lymphocyte interactions in the lymph node.** *Science* 1998, **281**:96–99.

Jacob, J., Kassir, R., and Kelsoe, G.: **In situ studies of the primary immune response to (4-hydroxy-3-nitrophenyl)acetyl. I. The architecture and dynamics of responding cell population.** *J. Exp. Med.* 1991, **173**:1165–1175.

Pape, K.A., Kouskoff, V., Nemazee, D., Tang, H.L., Cyster, J.G., Tze, L.E., Hippen, K.L., Behrens, T.W., and Jenkins, M.K.: **Visualization of the genesis and fate of isotype-switched B cells during a primary immune response.** *J. Exp. Med.* 2003, **197**:1677–1687.

9-6 The second phase of the primary B-cell immune response occurs when activated B cells migrate to follicles and proliferate to form germinal centers.

Brachtel, E.F., Washiyama, M., Johnson, G.D., Tenner-Racz, K., Racz, P., and MacLennan, I.C.: **Differences in the germinal centres of palatine tonsils and lymph nodes.** *Scand. J. Immunol.* 1996, **43**:239–247.

Camacho, S.A., Kosco-Vilbois, M.H., and Berek, C.: **The dynamic structure of the germinal center.** *Immunol. Today* 1998, **19**:511–514.

Jacob, J., and Kelsoe, G.: **In situ studies of the primary immune response to (4-hydroxy-3-nitrophenyl)acetyl. II. A common clonal origin for periarteriolar lymphoid sheath-associated foci and germinal centers.** *J. Exp. Med.* 1992, **176**:679–687.

Jacob, J., Przylepa, J., Miller, C., and Kelsoe, G.: **In situ studies of the primary immune response to (4-hydroxy-3-nitrophenyl)acetyl. III. The kinetics of V region mutation and selection in germinal center B cells.** *J. Exp. Med.* 1993, **178**:1293–1307.

Kelsoe, G.: **The germinal center: a crucible for lymphocyte selection.** *Semin. Immunol.* 1996, **8**:179–184.

MacLennan, I.C.M.: **Germinal centers.** *Annu. Rev. Immunol.* 1994, **12**:117–139.

9-7 Germinal center B cells undergo V-region somatic hypermutation, and cells with mutations that improve affinity for antigen are selected.

Clarke, S.H., Huppi, K., Ruezinsky, D., Staudt, L., Gerhard, W., and Weigert, M.: **Inter- and intraclonal diversity in the antibody response to influenza hemagglutinin.** *J. Exp. Med.* 1985, **161**:687–704.

Jacob, J., Kelsoe, G., Rajewsky, K., and Weiss, U.: **Intraclonal generation of antibody mutants in germinal centres.** *Nature* 1991, **354**:389–392.

Shlomchik, M.J., Litwin, S., and Weigert, M.: **The influence of somatic mutation on clonal expansion.** *Prog. Immunol. Proc. 7th Int. Cong. Immunol.* 1990, **7**:415–423.

Ziegner, M., Steinhauser, G., and Berek, C.: **Development of antibody diversity in single germinal centers: selective expansion of high-affinity variants.** *Eur. J. Immunol.* 1994, **24**:2393–2400.

9-8 Ligation of the B-cell receptor and CD40, together with direct contact with T cells, are all required to sustain germinal center B cells.

Han, S., Hathcock, K., Zheng, B., Kepler, T.B., Hodes, R., and Kelsoe, G.: **Cellular interaction in germinal centers. Roles of CD40 ligand and B7–2 in established germinal centers.** *J. Immunol.* 1995, **155**:556–567.

Hannum, L.G., Haberman, A.M., Anderson, S.M., and Shlomchik, M.J.: **Germinal center initiation, variable gene region hypermutation, and mutant B cell selection without detectable immune complexes on follicular dendritic cells.** *J. Exp. Med.* 2000, **192**:931–942.

Humphrey, J.H., Grennan, D., and Sundaram, V.: **The origin of follicular dendritic cells in the mouse and the mechanism of trapping of immune complexes on them.** *Eur. J. Immunol.* 1984, **14**:859–864.

Liu, Y.J., Joshua, D.E., Williams, G.T., Smith, C.A., Gordon, J., and MacLennan, I.C.M.: **Mechanism of antigen-driven selection in germinal centres.** *Nature* 1989, **342**:929–931.

Wang, Z., Karras, J.G., Howard, R.G., and Rothstein, T.L.: **Induction of bcl-x by CD40 engagement rescues sIg-induced apoptosis in murine B cells.** *J. Immunol.* 1995, **155**:3722–3725.

9-9 Surviving germinal center B cells differentiate into either plasma cells or memory cells.

Coico, R.F., Bhogal, B.S., and Thorbecke, G.J.: **Relationship of germinal centers in lymphoid tissue to immunologic memory. IV. Transfer of B cell memory with lymph node cells fractionated according to their receptors for peanut agglutinin.** *J. Immunol.* 1983, **131**:2254–2257.

Koni, P.A., Sacca, R., Lawton, P., Browning, J.L., Ruddle, N.H., and Flavell, R.A.: **Distinct roles in lymphoid organogenesis for lymphotoxins alpha and beta revealed in lymphotoxin beta-deficient mice.** *Immunity* 1997, **6**:491–500.

Matsumoto, M., Lo, S.F., Carruthers, C.J.L., Min, J., Mariathasan, S., Huang, G., Plas, D.R., Martin, S.M., Geha, R.S., Nahm, M.H., and Chaplin, D.D.: **Affinity maturation without germinal centres in lymphotoxin-α-deficient mice.** *Nature* 1996, **382**:462–466.

Tew, J.G., DiLosa, R.M., Burton, G.F., Kosco, M.H., Kupp, L.I., Masuda, A., and Szakal, A.K.: **Germinal centers and antibody production in bone marrow.** *Immunol. Rev.* 1992, **126**:99–112.

9-10 B-cell responses to bacterial antigens with intrinsic ability to activate B cells do not require T-cell help.

Anderson, J., Coutinho, A., Lernhardt, W., and Melchers, F.: **Clonal growth and maturation to immunoglobulin secretion in vitro of every growth-inducible B lymphocyte.** *Cell* 1977, **10**:27–34.

Dubois, B., Vanbervliet, B., Fayette, J., Massacrier, C., Kooten, C.V., Briere, F., Banchereau, J., and Caux, C.: **Dendritic cells enhance growth and differentiation of CD40-activated B lymphocytes.** *J. Exp. Med.* 1997, **185**:941–952.

Garcia De Vinuesa, C., Gulbranson-Judge, A., Khan, M., O'Leary, P., Cascalho, M., Wabl, M., Klaus, G.G., Owen, M.J., and MacLennan, I.C.: **Dendritic cells associated with plasmablast survival.** *Eur. J. Immunol.* 1999, **29**:3712–3721.

9-11 B-cell responses to bacterial polysaccharides do not require peptide-specific T-cell help.

Mond, J.J., Lees, A., and Snapper, C.M.: **T cell-independent antigens type 2.** *Annu. Rev. Immunol.* 1995, **13**:655–692.

9-12 Antibodies of different isotype operate in distinct places and have distinct effector functions.

Clark, M.R.: **IgG effector mechanisms.** *Chem. Immunol.* 1997, **65**:88–110.

Herrod, H.G.: **IgG subclass deficiency.** *Allergy Proc.* 1992, **13**:299–302.

Janeway, C.A., Rosen, F.S., Merler, E., and Alper, C.A.: *The Gamma Globulins,*

2nd edn. Boston, Little Brown and Co., 1967.

Ward, E.S., and Ghetie, V.: **The effector functions of immunoglobulins: implications for therapy.** *Ther. Immunol.* 1995, **2**:77–94.

9-13   Transport proteins that bind to the Fc regions of antibodies carry particular isotypes across epithelial barriers.

Burmeister, W.P., Gastinel, L.N., Simister, N.E., Blum, M.L., and Bjorkman, P.J.: **Crystal structure at 2.2 Å resolution of the MHC-related neonatal Fc receptor.** *Nature* 1994, **372**:336–343.

Corthesy, B., and Kraehenbuhl, J.P.: **Antibody-mediated protection of mucosal surfaces.** *Curr. Top. Microbiol. Immunol.* 1999, **236**:93–111.

Ghetie, V., and Ward, E.S.: **Multiple roles for the major histocompatibility complex class I-related receptor FcRn.** *Annu. Rev. Immunol.* 2000, **18**:739–766.

Lamm, M.E.: **Current concepts in mucosal immunity. IV. How epithelial transport of IgA antibodies relates to host defense.** *Am. J. Physiol.* 1998, **274**:G614-G617.

Mostov, K.E.: **Transepithelial transport of immunoglobulins.** *Annu. Rev. Immunol.* 1994, **12**:63–84.

Simister, N.E., and Mostov, K.E.: **An Fc receptor structurally related to MHC class I antigens.** *Nature* 1989, **337**:184–187.

9-14   High-affinity IgG and IgA antibodies can neutralize bacterial toxins.

Robbins, F.C., and Robbins, J.B.: **Current status and prospects for some improved and new bacterial vaccines.** *Am. J. Pub. Health* 1986, **7**:105–125.

9-15   High-affinity IgG and IgA antibodies can inhibit the infectivity of viruses.

Mandel, B.: **Neutralization of polio virus: a hypothesis to explain the mechanism and the one hit character of the neutralization reaction.** *Virology* 1976, **69**:500–510.

Possee, R.D., Schild, G.C., and Dimmock, N.J.: **Studies on the mechanism of neutralization of influenza virus by antibody: evidence that neutralizing antibody (anti-haemagglutinin) inactivates influenza virus *in vivo* by inhibiting virion transcriptase activity.** *J. Gen. Virol.* 1982, **58**:373–386.

Roost, H.P., Bachmann, M.F., Haag, A., Kalinke, U., Pliska, V., Hengartner, H., and Zinkernagel, R.M.: **Early high-affinity neutralizing anti-viral IgG responses without further overall improvements of affinity.** *Proc. Natl. Acad. Sci. USA* 1995, **92**:1257–1261.

9-16   Antibodies can block the adherence of bacteria to host cells.

Fischetti, V.A., and Bessen, D.: Effect of mucosal antibodies to M protein in colonization by group A streptococci, in Switalski, L., Hook, M., and Beachery, E. (eds): *Molecular Mechanisms of Microbial Adhesion.* New York, Springer, 1989.

9-17   Antibody:antigen complexes activate the classical pathway of complement by binding to C1q.

Cooper, N.R.: **The classical complement pathway. Activation and regulation of the first complement component.** *Adv. Immunol.* 1985, **37**:151–216.

Perkins, S.J., and Nealis, A.S.: **The quaternary structure in solution of human complement subcomponent $C1r_2C1s_2$.** *Biochem. J.* 1989, **263**:463–469.

9-18   Complement receptors are important in the removal of immune complexes from the circulation.

Nash, J.T., Taylor, P.R., Botto, M., Norsworthy, P.J., Davies, K.A., and Walport, Schifferli, J.A., and Taylor, J.P.: **Physiologic and pathologic aspects of circulating immune complexes.** *Kidney Int.* 1989, **35**:993–1003.

Schifferli, J.A., Ng, Y.C., and Peters, D.K.: **The role of complement and its receptor in the elimination of immune complexes.** *N. Engl. J. Med.* 1986, **315**:488–495.

Nash, J.T., Taylor, P.R., Botto, M., Norsworthy, P.J., Davies, K.A., Walport, M.J.: **Immune complex processing in C1q-deficient mice.** *Clin. Exp. Immunol.* 2001, **123**:196–202.

Walport, M.J., Davies, K.A., and Botto, M.: **C1q and systemic lupus erythematosus.** *Immunobiology* 1998, **199**:265–285.

9-19   The Fc receptors of accessory cells are signaling receptors specific for immunoglobulins of different isotypes.

Kinet, J.P., and Launay, P.: **Fc alpha/microR: single member or first born in the family?** *Nat. Immunol.* 2000, **1**:371–372.

Ravetch, J.V., and Bolland, S.: **IgG Fc receptors.** *Annu. Rev. Immunol.* 2001, **19**:275–290.

Ravetch, J.V., and Clynes, R.A.: **Divergent roles for Fc receptors and complement *in vivo*.** *Annu. Rev. Immunol.* 1998, **16**:421–432.

Shibuya, A., Sakamoto, N., Shimizu, Y., Shibuya, K., Osawa, M., Hiroyama, T., Eyre, H.J., Sutherland, G.R., Endo, Y., Fujita, T., Miyabayashi, T., Sakano, S., Tsuji, T., Nakayama, E., Phillips, J.H., Lanier, L.L., and Nakauchi, H.: **Fc alpha/mu receptor mediates endocytosis of IgM-coated microbes.** *Nat. Immunol.* 2000, **1**:441–446.

9-20   Fc receptors on phagocytes are activated by antibodies bound to the surface of pathogens and enable the phagocytes to ingest and destroy pathogens.

Gounni, A.S., Lamkhioued, B., Ochiai, K., Tanaka, Y., Delaporte, E., Capron, A., Kinet, J.P., and Capron, M.: **High-affinity IgE receptor on eosinophils is involved in defence against parasites.** *Nature* 1994, **367**:183–186.

Karakawa, W.W., Sutton, A., Schneerson, R., Karpas, A., and Vann, W.F.: **Capsular antibodies induce type-specific phagocytosis of capsulated *Staphylococcus aureus* by human polymorphonuclear leukocytes.** *Infect. Immun.* 1986, **56**:1090–1095.

9-21   Fc receptors activate NK cells to destroy antibody-coated targets.

Lanier, L.L., and Phillips, J.H.: **Evidence for three types of human cytotoxic lymphocyte.** *Immunol. Today* 1986, **7**:132.

Leibson, P.J.: **Signal transduction during natural killer cell activation: inside the mind of a killer.** *Immunity* 1997, **6**:655–661.

Takai, T.: **Multiple loss of effector cell functions in FcR gamma-deficient mice.** *Int. Rev. Immunol.* 1996, **13**:369–381.

9-22   Mast cells, basophils, and activated eosinophils bind IgE antibody via the high-affinity Fcε receptor.

Beaven, M.A., and Metzger, H.: **Signal transduction by Fc receptors: the FcεRI case.** *Immunol. Today* 1993, **14**:222–226.

Kalesnikoff, J., Huber, M., Lam, V., Damen, J.E., Zhang, J., Siraganian, R.P., and Krystal, G.: **Monomeric IgE stimulates signaling pathways in mast cells that lead to cytokine production and cell survival.** *Immunity* 2001, **14**:801–811.

Sutton, B.J., and Gould, H.J.: **The human IgE network.** *Nature* 1993, **366**:421–428.

9-23   IgE-mediated activation of accessory cells has an important role in resistance to parasite infection.

Capron, A., and Dessaint, J.P.: **Immunologic aspects of schistosomiasis.** *Annu. Rev. Med.* 1992, **43**:209–218.

Grencis, R.K., Else, K.J., Huntley, J.F., and Nishikawa, S.I.: **The *in vivo* role of stem cell factor (c-kit ligand) on mastocytosis and host protective immunity to the intestinal nematode *Trichinella spiralis* in mice.** *Parasite Immunol.* 1993, **15**:55–59.

Kasugai, T., Tei, H., Okada, M., Hirota, S., Morimoto, M., Yamada, M., Nakama, A., Arizono, N., and Kitamura, Y.: **Infection with *Nippostrongylus brasiliensis* induces invasion of mast cell precursors from peripheral blood to small intestine.** *Blood* 1995, **85**:1334–1340.

Ushio, H., Watanabe, N., Kiso, Y., Higuchi, S., and Matsuda, H.: **Protective immunity and mast cell and eosinophil responses in mice infested with larval *Haemaphysalis longicornis* ticks.** *Parasite Immunol.* 1993, **15**:209–214.

Adaptive Immunity to Infection

Throughout this book we have examined various individual mechanisms by which both the innate and the adaptive immune responses function to protect the individual from invading microorganisms. In this chapter we consider how the cells and molecules of the immune system work as an integrated defense system to eliminate or control an infectious agent and how the adaptive immune system provides long-lasting protective immunity. This is the first of several chapters that consider how the immune system functions as a whole in health and disease. Subsequent chapters examine how failures of immune defense and unwanted immune responses occur, and how the immune response can be manipulated to benefit the individual.

In the first part of this chapter we briefly consider the diversity of pathogens the immune system can encounter and outline the general course of an infection. The mechanisms of innate immunity, which we discussed in detail in Chapter 2, are brought into play in the earliest phases of the infection and may succeed in repelling it. Pathogens, however, have developed strategies that allow them, at least on occasion, to elude or overcome the mechanisms of innate immune defense and to establish a focus of infection from which they can spread. In these circumstances, the innate immune response sets the scene for the induction of an adaptive immune response, the focus of the second part of the chapter. Several days are required for the clonal expansion and differentiation of naive lymphocytes into effector T cells and antibody-secreting B cells that, in most cases, effectively target the pathogen for elimination (Fig. 10.1). During this period, specific immunological memory is also established. This ensures a rapid reinduction of antigen-specific antibody and armed effector T cells on subsequent encounters with the same pathogen, thus providing long-lasting protection against reinfection.

Innate immunity is an essential prerequisite for the adaptive immune response, because the antigen-specific lymphocytes of the adaptive immune response are activated by co-stimulatory molecules that are induced on cells of the innate immune system during their interaction with microorganisms. The cytokines produced during these early phases also have an important role in stimulating the subsequent adaptive immune response and shaping its development. We have already described the generation and function of armed effector T cells and antibodies in Chapters 8 and 9. In this chapter we discuss how the different phases of host defense are orchestrated in space and time, and how changes in specialized cell-surface molecules and chemokines guide lymphocytes to the appropriate site of action at different stages of the adaptive immune response.

The most frequent sites of encounter between the body and microorganisms and other antigens are the mucosal surfaces. A mucosal immune system lines the airways, gastrointestinal tract, and urogenital system, and is the most extensive compartment of the immune system. The third part of the chapter describes the functions and properties of the adaptive immune responses

Fig. 10.1 The course of a typical acute infection that is cleared by an adaptive immune reaction. 1. The level of infectious agent increases as the pathogen replicates. 2. When numbers of the pathogen exceed the threshold dose of antigen required for an adaptive response, the response is initiated; the pathogen continues to grow, retarded only by responses of the innate immune system. At this stage, immunological memory also starts to be induced. 3. After 4–7 days, effector cells and molecules of the adaptive response start to clear the infection. 4. When the infection is cleared and the dose of antigen falls below the response threshold, the response ceases, but antibody, residual effector cells, and also immunological memory provide lasting protection against reinfection in most cases.

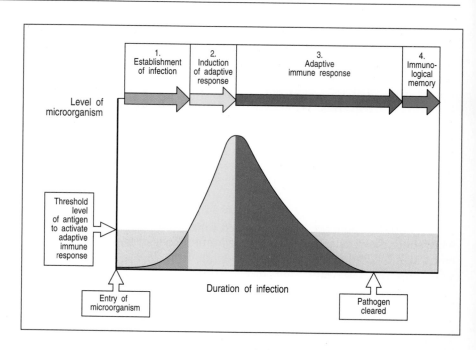

mounted by the mucosal immune system. These not only protect the body from infection but are also designed to stop the immune system from responding inappropriately to the many environmental antigens and potential allergens with which the mucosal lymphoid tissues come into contact, most particularly the foods we eat every day.

We then return to immunological memory, which provides long-lasting and sometimes lifelong protection against reinfection by many pathogens. Memory responses differ in several ways from primary responses. We discuss the reasons for this, and what is known of how immunological memory is maintained.

Infectious agents and how they cause disease.

Infectious disease can be devastating, and sometimes fatal, to the host. In this part of the chapter we briefly examine the stages of infection, and the various types of infectious agent.

10-1   The course of an infection can be divided into several distinct phases.

The process of infection can be broken down into stages, each of which can be blocked by different defense mechanisms. In the first stage a new host is exposed to infectious particles shed by an infected individual or present in the environment. The number, route, mode of transmission, and stability of an infectious agent outside the host determine its infectivity. Some pathogens, such as anthrax, are spread by spores that are highly resistant to heat and drying, whereas others, such as the human immunodeficiency virus (HIV), are spread only by the exchange of bodily fluids or tissues because they are unable to survive as infectious agents outside the body.

The first contact with a new host occurs through an epithelial surface. This may be the skin or the internal mucosal surfaces of the respiratory, gastrointestinal, or urogenital tracts. After making contact, an infectious agent must establish a focus of infection. This involves adhering to the epithelial surface and then colonizing it, or penetrating it to replicate in the tissues (Fig. 10.2, left-hand panels). Wounds and insect and tick bites that breach the epidermal barrier help some pathogens to get through the skin. Many microorganisms are repelled or kept in check at this stage by innate immunity, as discussed in Chapter 2. These innate immune responses use a variety of germline-encoded receptors to discriminate between foreign microbial and self host-cell surfaces, or between infected and normal cells. They are not as effective as adaptive immune responses, which can afford to be more powerful on account of their antigen specificity. However, they can prevent an infection from being established or, failing that, contain it and prevent the spread of the pathogen into the bloodstream while an adaptive immune response develops.

Only when a microorganism has successfully established a site of infection in the host does disease occur. With the possible exception of lung infections, in which primary infection can cause life-threatening disease, little damage will be caused unless the agent is able to spread from the original site of infection or can secrete toxins that can spread to other parts of the body. Extracellular pathogens spread by direct extension of the focus of infection through the lymphatics or the bloodstream. Usually, spread by the bloodstream occurs only after the lymphatic system has been overwhelmed by the burden of infectious agent. Obligate intracellular pathogens must spread from cell to cell; they do so either by direct transmission from one cell to the next or by release into the extracellular fluid and reinfection of both adjacent and distant cells.

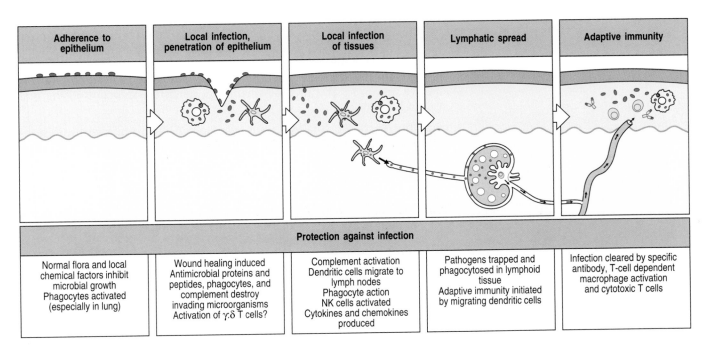

Adherence to epithelium	Local infection, penetration of epithelium	Local infection of tissues	Lymphatic spread	Adaptive immunity
Protection against infection				
Normal flora and local chemical factors inhibit microbial growth Phagocytes activated (especially in lung)	Wound healing induced Antimicrobial proteins and peptides, phagocytes, and complement destroy invading microorganisms Activation of γ:δ T cells?	Complement activation Dendritic cells migrate to lymph nodes Phagocyte action NK cells activated Cytokines and chemokines produced	Pathogens trapped and phagocytosed in lymphoid tissue Adaptive immunity initiated by migrating dendritic cells	Infection cleared by specific antibody, T-cell dependent macrophage activation and cytotoxic T cells

Fig. 10.2 Infections and the responses to them can be divided into a series of stages. These are illustrated here for an infectious microorganism (red) entering across an epithelium, the commonest route of entry. The microorganism must first adhere to epithelial cells and then cross the epithelium. A local nonadaptive response helps to contain the infection and delivers antigen to local lymph nodes, leading to adaptive immunity and clearance of the infection. The role of γ:δ T cells is uncertain, as indicated by the question mark.

Some of the bacteria that cause gastroenteritis exert their effects without spreading into the tissues. They establish a site of infection on the epithelial surface in the lumen of the gut and cause no direct pathology themselves, but secrete toxins that cause damage either *in situ* or after crossing the epithelial barrier and entering the circulation.

Most infectious agents show a significant degree of host specificity, causing disease only in one or a few related species. What determines host specificity for every agent is not known, but the requirement for attachment to a particular cell-surface molecule is one critical factor. As other interactions with host cells are also commonly needed to support replication, most pathogens have a limited host range. The molecular mechanisms of host specificity comprise an area of research known as molecular pathogenesis, which falls outside the scope of this book.

Although most microorganisms are repelled by innate host defenses, an initial infection, once established, generally leads to perceptible disease followed by an effective host adaptive immune response. This is initiated in the local lymphoid tissue, in response to antigens presented by dendritic cells activated during the course of the innate immune response (Fig. 10.2, third and fourth panels). Antigen-specific effector T cells and antibody-secreting B cells are generated by clonal expansion and differentiation over the course of several days, during which time the induced responses of innate immunity continue to function. Eventually, antigen-specific T cells and then antibodies are released into the blood and recruited to the site of infection (Fig. 10.2, last panel). A cure involves the clearance of extracellular infectious particles by antibodies and the clearance of intracellular residues of infection through the actions of effector T cells.

After many types of infection there is little or no residual pathology following an effective primary response. In some cases, however, the infection or the response to it causes significant tissue damage. In yet other cases, such as infection with cytomegalovirus or *Mycobacterium tuberculosis*, the infection is contained but not eliminated, and can persist in a latent form. If the adaptive immune response is later weakened, as it is in acquired immune deficiency syndrome (AIDS), these diseases reappear as virulent systemic infections. We will focus on the strategies used by certain pathogens to evade or subvert adaptive immunity and thereby establish a persistent infection in the first part of Chapter 11.

In addition to clearing the infectious agent, an effective adaptive immune response prevents reinfection. For some infectious agents, this protection is essentially absolute, whereas for others infection is reduced or attenuated upon reexposure.

10-2   Infectious diseases are caused by diverse living agents that replicate in their hosts.

The agents that cause disease fall into five groups: viruses, bacteria, fungi, protozoa, and helminths (worms). Protozoa and worms are usually grouped together as parasites, and are the subject of the discipline of parasitology, whereas viruses, bacteria, and fungi are the subject of microbiology. In Fig. 10.3, the classes of microorganisms and parasites that cause disease are listed, with typical examples of each. The remarkable variety of these pathogens has caused the natural selection of two crucial features of adaptive immunity. First, the advantage of being able to recognize a wide range of different pathogens has driven the development of receptors on B and T cells of equal or greater diversity. Second, the distinct habitats and life cycles of pathogens have to be countered by a range of distinct effector mechanisms. The characteristic features of each pathogen are its mode of transmission,

Some common causes of disease in humans			
Viruses	DNA viruses	Adenoviruses	Human adenoviruses (eg, types 3, 4, and 7)
		Herpesviruses	Herpes simplex, varicella zoster, Epstein–Barr virus, cytomegalovirus, HHV8
		Poxviruses	Variola, vaccinia virus
		Parvoviruses	Human parvovirus
		Papovaviruses	Papilloma virus
		Hepadnaviruses	Hepatitis B virus
	RNA viruses	Orthomyxoviruses	Influenza virus
		Paramyxoviruses	Mumps, measles, respiratory syncytial virus
		Coronaviruses	Cold viruses, SARS
		Picornaviruses	Polio, coxsackie, hepatitis A, rhinovirus
		Reoviruses	Rotavirus, reovirus
		Togaviruses	Rubella, arthropod-borne encephalitis
		Flaviviruses	Arthropod-borne viruses (yellow fever, dengue fever)
		Arenaviruses	Lymphocytic choriomeningitis, Lassa fever
		Rhabdoviruses	Rabies
		Retroviruses	Human T-cell leukemia virus, HIV
Bacteria	Gram +ve cocci	Staphylococci	*Staphylococcus aureus*
		Streptococci	*Streptococcus pneumoniae, Strep. pyogenes*
	Gram −ve cocci	Neisseriae	*Neisseria gonorrhoeae, N. meningitidis*
	Gram +ve bacilli		*Corynebacterium diphtheriae, Bacillus anthracis, Listeria monocytogenes*
	Gram −ve bacilli		*Salmonella typhi, Shigella flexneri, Campylobacter jejuni, Vibrio cholerae, Yersinia pestis, Pseudomonas aeruginosa, Brucella melitensis, Haemophilus influenzae, Legionella pneumophilus, Bordetella pertussis*
	Firmicutes	Clostridia	*Clostridium tetani, C. botulinum, C. perfringens*
	Spirochetes	Spirochetes	*Treponema pallidum, Borrelia burgdorferi, Leptospira interrogans*
	Actinobacteria	Mycobacteria	*Mycobacterium tuberculosis, M. leprae, M. avium*
	Protobacteria	Rickettsias	*Rickettsia prowazekii*
	Chlamydiae	Chlamydias	*Chlamydia trachomatis*
	Mollicutes	Mycoplasmas	*Mycoplasma pneumoniae*
Fungi	Ascomycetes		*Candida albicans, Cryptococcus neoformans, Aspergillus fumigatus, Histoplasma capsulatum, Coccidioides immitis, Pneumocystis carinii*
Protozoa			*Entamoeba histolytica, Giardia intestinalis, Leishmania donovani, Plasmodium falciparum, Trypanosoma brucei, Toxoplasma gondii, Cryptosporidium parvum*
Worms	Nematodes	Intestinal	*Trichuris trichura, Trichinella spiralis, Enterobius vermicularis, Ascaris lumbricoides, Ancylostoma duodenale, Strongyloides stercoralis*
		Tissues	*Onchocerca volvulus, Loa loa, Dracuncula medinensis*
	Flukes	Blood, liver	*Schistosoma mansoni, Clonorchis sinensis*

Fig. 10.3 A variety of microorganisms can cause disease. Pathogenic organisms are of five main types: viruses, bacteria, fungi, protozoa, and worms. Some common pathogens in each group are listed.

its mechanism of replication, its pathogenesis—the means by which it causes disease—and the response it elicits. We focus here on the immune responses to these pathogens.

Infectious agents can grow in various body compartments, as shown schematically in Fig. 10.4. We have already seen that two major compartments can be defined—intracellular and extracellular. Obligate intracellular pathogens must invade host cells to replicate, whereas facultative intracellular pathogens, such as mycobacteria, can replicate either intracellularly or outside the cell. Intracellular pathogens must either be prevented from entering cells or be detected and eliminated once they have done so. They can be subdivided further into those that replicate free in the cell, such as viruses and certain bacteria (for example, *Chlamydia*, *Rickettsia*, and *Listeria*), and those, such as the mycobacteria, that replicate in intracellular vesicles. Viruses can be prevented from entering cells by neutralizing antibodies, whose production relies on helper T cells (see Section 9-15), while once inside cells they are dealt with by virus-specific cytotoxic T cells, which recognize and kill the infected cell (see Section 8-21). Intravesicular pathogens, in contrast, infect mainly macrophages and can be eliminated with the aid of pathogen-specific T_H1 cells, which activate infected macrophages to destroy the pathogen (see Section 8-26).

Many microorganisms live and replicate in the extracellular spaces, either within the body or on the surface of epithelia. Extracellular bacteria are usually susceptible to killing by phagocytes and thus pathogenic species have developed means of resisting engulfment. Encapsulated Gram-positive cocci such as the streptococci and staphylococci, for example, grow in extracellular spaces and resist phagocytosis by means of their polysaccharide capsule. This means that an infection in a previously unexposed host is not immediately eliminated by tissue phagocytes. However, opsonization by complement or specific antibody, or both, can overcome this, allowing the bacteria to be killed by phagocytes. Thus, these extracellular bacteria are cleared by means of the humoral immune response (see Chapter 9).

Fig. 10.4 Pathogens can be found in various compartments of the body, where they must be combated by different host defense mechanisms. Virtually all pathogens have an extracellular phase in which they are vulnerable to antibody-mediated effector mechanisms. However, intracellular phases are not accessible to antibody, and these are attacked by T cells.

	Extracellular		Intracellular	
	Interstitial spaces, blood, lymph	**Epithelial surfaces**	**Cytoplasmic**	**Vesicular**
Site of infection				
Organisms	Viruses Bacteria Protozoa Fungi Worms	*Neisseria gonorrhoeae* *Mycoplasma* spp. *Streptococcus pneumoniae* *Vibrio cholerae* *Escherichia coli* *Helicobacter pylori* *Candida albicans* Worms	Viruses *Chlamydia* spp. *Rickettsia* spp. *Listeria monocytogenes* Protozoa	*Mycobacterium* spp. *Salmonella typhimurium* *Yersinia pestis* *Listeria* spp. *Legionella pneumophila* *Cryptococcus neoformans* *Histoplasma* *Leishmania* spp. *Trypanosoma* spp.
Protective immunity	Antibodies Complement Phagocytosis Neutralization	Antibodies, especially IgA Antimicrobial peptides	Cytotoxic T cells NK cells	T-cell and NK-cell dependent macrophage activation

	Direct mechanisms of tissue damage by pathogens			Indirect mechanisms of tissue damage by pathogens		
	Exotoxin production	Endotoxin	Direct cytopathic effect	Immune complexes	Anti-host antibody	Cell-mediated immunity
Pathogenic mechanism						
Infectious agent	*Streptococcus pyogenes* *Staphylococcus aureus* *Corynebacterium diphtheriae* *Clostridium tetani* *Vibrio cholerae*	*Escherichia coli* *Haemophilus influenzae* *Salmonella typhi* *Shigella* *Pseudomonas aeruginosa* *Yersinia pestis*	Variola Varicella-zoster Hepatitis B virus Polio virus Measles virus Influenza virus Herpes simplex virus Human herpes virus 8 (HHV8)	Hepatitis B virus Malaria *Streptococcus pyogenes* *Treponema pallidum* Most acute infections	*Streptococcus pyogenes* *Mycoplasma pneumoniae*	*Mycobacterium tuberculosis* *Mycobacterium leprae* Lymphocytic choriomeningitis virus *Borrelia burgdorferi* *Schistosoma mansoni* Herpes simplex virus
Disease	Tonsilitis, scarlet fever Boils, toxic shock syndrome, food poisoning Diphtheria Tetanus Cholera	Gram-negative sepsis Meningitis, pneumonia Typhoid Bacillary dysentery Wound infection Plague	Smallpox Chickenpox, shingles Hepatitis Poliomyelitis Measles, subacute sclerosing panencephalitis Influenza Cold sores Kaposi's sarcoma	Kidney disease Vascular deposits Glomerulonephritis Kidney damage in secondary syphilis Transient renal deposits	Rheumatic fever Hemolytic anemia	Tuberculosis Tuberculoid leprosy Aseptic meningitis Lyme arthritis Schistosomiasis Herpes stromal keratitis

Fig. 10.5 Pathogens can damage tissues in a variety of different ways. The mechanisms of damage, representative infectious agents, and the common names of the diseases associated with each are shown. Exotoxins are released by microorganisms and act at the surface of host cells, for example by binding to receptors. Endotoxins, which are intrinsic components of microbial structure, trigger phagocytes to release cytokines that produce local or systemic symptoms. Many pathogens are cytopathic, directly damaging the cells they infect. Finally, adaptive immune response to the pathogen can generate antigen:antibody complexes that can activate neutrophils and macrophages, antibodies that can cross-react with host tissues, or T cells that kill infected cells. All of these have some potential to damage the host's tissues. In addition, neutrophils, the most abundant cells early in infection, release many proteins and small-molecule inflammatory mediators that both control infection and cause tissue damage (see Fig. 2.6).

Different infectious agents cause markedly different diseases, reflecting the diverse ways in which they damage tissues (Fig. 10.5). Many extracellular pathogens cause disease by releasing specific toxic products or protein toxins (see Fig. 9.23). These are counteracted by neutralizing antibodies (see Section 9-14). Intracellular infectious agents frequently cause disease by damaging the cells that house them. The specific killing of virus-infected cells by cytotoxic T cells thus not only prevents virus spread but removes damaged cells. The immune response to the infectious agent can itself be a major cause of pathology in several diseases (see Fig. 10.5). The damage caused by a particular infectious agent also depends on the site in which it grows; *Streptococcus pneumoniae* in the lung causes pneumonia, whereas in the blood it causes a rapidly fatal systemic illness, pneumococcal sepsis.

As we learned in Chapter 2, for a pathogen to invade the body, it must first bind to or cross an epithelium. When the infection is due to intestinal pathogens such as *Salmonella typhi*, the causal agent of typhoid fever, or *Vibrio cholerae*, which causes cholera, the adaptive immune response occurs in the specialized mucosal immune system associated with the gastrointestinal tract, as described later in this chapter. As a means of entry, some intestinal pathogens even target the M cells that lie over the Peyer's patches and are specialized to transport antigens and pathogens across the intestinal epithelium.

Many pathogens cannot be entirely eliminated by the immune response. But neither are most pathogens universally lethal. Those pathogens that have persisted for many thousands of years in the human population are highly evolved to exploit their human hosts; such pathogens cannot alter their pathogenicity without upsetting the compromise they have achieved with the human immune system. Rapidly killing every host it infects is no better for the long-term survival of a pathogen than being wiped out by the immune response before the pathogen has had time to infect another individual. In short, we have learned to live with our enemies, and they with us. However, we must be on the alert at all times for new pathogens and new threats to health. The human immunodeficiency virus that causes AIDS serves as a warning that we remain constantly vulnerable to the emergence of new infectious agents.

Summary.

The mammalian body is susceptible to infection by many pathogens, which must first make contact with the host and then establish a focus of infection so as to cause disease. To establish an infection, the pathogen must first colonize the skin or the internal mucosal surfaces of the respiratory, gastrointestinal, or urogenital tracts and then overcome or bypass the innate immune defenses associated with the epithelia and the phagocytes in the underlying tissues. If the pathogen succeeds in doing this, it will provoke an adaptive immune response that will take effect after several days and will usually clear the infection. Pathogens differ greatly in their lifestyles and means of pathogenesis, requiring an equally diverse set of defensive responses from the host immune system.

The course of the adaptive response to infection.

It is not known how many infections are dealt with solely by the nonadaptive mechanisms of innate immunity discussed in Chapter 2; this is because such infections are eliminated early and produce little in the way of symptoms or pathology. Moreover, deficiencies in nonadaptive defenses are rare, so it has seldom been possible to study their consequences. Innate immunity does, however, seem to be essential for effective host defense, as shown by the progression of infection in mice that lack components of innate immunity but have an intact adaptive immune system (Fig. 10.6). Adaptive immunity is also essential, as shown by the immunodeficiency syndromes associated with failure of one or the other arm of the adaptive immune response (see Chapter 11). Adaptive immunity is triggered when an infection eludes or overwhelms the innate defense mechanisms and generates a threshold dose of antigen (see Fig. 10.1). This antigen then initiates an adaptive immune response, which becomes effective only after several days, the time required for antigen-specific T cells and B cells to locate their specific foreign antigen, to proliferate, and to differentiate into armed effector cells. In the earlier chapters of this

Fig. 10.6 The time course of infection in normal and immunodeficient mice and humans. The red curve shows the rapid growth of microorganisms in the absence of innate immunity, when macrophages (MAC) and polymorphonuclear leukocytes (PMN) are lacking. The green curve shows the course of infection in mice and humans that have innate immunity but have no T or B lymphocytes and so lack adaptive immunity. The yellow curve shows the normal course of an infection in immunocompetent mice or humans.

book we discussed the cells and molecules that mediate the adaptive immune response, and the interactions between them. We are now ready to see how each cell type is recruited in turn in the course of a primary adaptive immune response to a pathogen, and how the effector lymphocytes and antibodies that are generated in response to antigen are dispersed to their sites of action. These clear the infection and protect against reinfection in the short term. A primary adaptive response also establishes a state of long-lasting protective immunity that is ultimately mediated by long-lived resting memory cells, to which we return in the last part of this chapter.

10-3 The nonspecific responses of innate immunity are necessary for an adaptive immune response to be initiated.

The establishment of a focus of infection in tissues and the response of the innate immune system to it produce changes in the immediate environment of the infection. In a bacterial infection, the first thing that usually happens is that the infected tissue becomes inflamed. As we learned in Chapter 2, this is initially the result of the activation of the resident macrophages by bacterial components such as lipopolysaccharide (LPS) acting through Toll-like receptors on the macrophage. The cytokines and chemokines secreted by the activated macrophages, especially the cytokine tumor necrosis factor-α (TNF-α), induce numerous changes in the endothelial cells of nearby blood capillaries, a process known as endothelial cell activation. Inflammation can also result from the activation of complement, resulting in the production of the anaphylatoxins C3a and C5a, which are able to activate vascular endothelium. In a primary infection, complement is activated mainly via the alternative and MBL pathways. Activation of the vascular endothelium causes the release of Weibel–Palade bodies from within the endothelial cells, which deliver the cell adhesion molecule P-selectin to the endothelial cell surface. Activation also induces the transcription and translation of RNA encoding E-selectin, which then appears on the endothelial cell surface.

These two selectins cause leukocytes, including neutrophils and monocytes, to adhere to and roll on the endothelial surface. The cytokines also induce the production of the adhesion molecule VCAM-1 on endothelial cells. By binding to adhesion molecules on neutrophils and monocytes, VCAM-1 strengthens their interaction with endothelial cells and aids their entry in large numbers into the infected tissue to form an inflammatory focus (see Fig. 2.44). As monocytes mature into tissue macrophages and become activated in their turn, more and more inflammatory cells are attracted into the infected tissue and the inflammatory response is maintained and reinforced. The inflammatory response can be thought of as putting up a flag on the endothelial cells to signal the presence of infection, but as yet the response is entirely nonspecific for the pathogen's antigens.

A second crucial effect of infection is the activation of potential professional antigen-presenting cells—the dendritic cells—that reside in most tissues. These take up antigen in the infected tissues and, like macrophages, they are activated through innate immune receptors that respond to common constituents of pathogens. For example, a combination of LPS and LPS-binding protein (LBP) binding to the cell-surface receptors CD14 and the Toll-like receptor TLR-4 induces dendritic cells to mature into potent antigen-presenting cells. Activated dendritic cells increase their synthesis of MHC class II molecules and, most importantly, begin to express the co-stimulatory molecules B7.1 (CD80) and B7-2 (CD86) on their surface. As described in Chapter 8, these antigen-presenting cells are carried away from the infected tissue in lymph, along with their antigen cargo, to enter peripheral lymphoid tissues, in which they can initiate the adaptive immune response. They arrive in large numbers at the draining lymph nodes, or other nearby lymphoid tissue, attracted by the chemokines CCL19, CCL20, and CCL21, which are produced by the lymph-node stroma and high endothelial venules.

Once dendritic cells arrive in the lymphoid tissues, they seem to have reached their final destination. They eventually die in these tissues, but before this their role is to activate antigen-specific naive T lymphocytes. Naive lymphocytes are continually passing through the lymph nodes, which they enter from the blood across the walls of high endothelial venules, as we describe below. Those naive T cells that are able to recognize antigen on the surface of dendritic cells are activated and both divide and mature into effector cells that reenter the circulation. When there is a local infection, the changes induced by inflammation in the walls of nearby venules, as we will see later, induce these effector T cells to leave the blood vessel and migrate to the site of infection.

Thus, the local release of cytokines and chemokines at the site of infection has far-reaching consequences. As well as recruiting neutrophils and macrophages, which are not specific for antigen, the changes induced in the blood vessel walls also enable newly activated effector T lymphocytes to enter infected tissue.

10-4 An adaptive immune response is initiated when circulating T cells encounter their corresponding antigen in draining lymphoid tissues and become activated.

The importance of the peripheral lymphoid organs in the initiation of adaptive immune responses was first shown by ingenious experiments in which a skin flap was isolated from the body wall so that it had a blood circulation but no lymphatic drainage. Antigen placed in the flap of skin did not elicit a T-cell response, showing that T cells do not become sensitized in the infected tissue itself. We now know that naive T lymphocytes are activated in the peripheral lymphoid organs by antigens brought there by dendritic cells. The immune response to pathogens that enter through the skin rather than across mucosal surfaces is generally believed to occur in the lymph nodes, which are sites of intersection of two pathways of circulation, those of the lymph and the blood (see Fig. 1.8).

As described in Chapter 8, immature dendritic cells in tissues take up antigens and are stimulated by infection to migrate to draining lymph nodes. Antigens introduced directly into the bloodstream are picked up by antigen-presenting cells in the spleen, and lymphocytes are activated in the splenic white pulp (see Fig. 1.9). The trapping of antigen by antigen-presenting cells that migrate to these lymphoid tissues, and the continuous recirculation of naive T cells through these tissues, ensure that rare antigen-specific T cells will encounter their specific antigen on an antigen-presenting cell surface. The unique architecture of the peripheral lymphoid organs virtually guarantees contact of foreign antigen with specific T-cell receptors in the lymph nodes and spleen or in mucosa-associated lymphoid tissues (MALT) (see Fig. 1.10).

Naive T cells enter the lymphoid organs in essentially the same way as described in Chapter 2 for the entry of phagocytes into sites of infection, except that selectin is expressed on the T cell rather than the endothelium. L-selectin on naive T cells binds to sulfated carbohydrates on proteins such as the vascular addressins GlyCAM-1 and CD34. CD34 is expressed on endothelial cells in many tissues but is properly glycosylated for L-selectin binding only on the high endothelial venule cells of lymph nodes (Fig. 10.7). Binding of L-selectin causes the lymphocyte to roll on the endothelial surface, and although the interaction is too weak to promote extravasation, it is critical for the lymphocyte to home selectively to the lymphoid organs, because it is essential for the

| Circulating lymphocyte enters the high endothelial venule in the lymph node | Binding of L-selectin to GlyCAM-1 and CD34 allows rolling interaction | LFA-1 is activated by chemokines bound to extracellular matrix | Activated LFA-1 binds tightly to ICAM-1 | Lymphocyte migrates into the lymph node by diapedesis |

Fig. 10.7 Lymphocytes in the blood enter lymphoid tissue by crossing the walls of high endothelial venules. The first step is the binding of L-selectin on the lymphocyte to sulfated carbohydrates of GlyCAM-1 and CD34 on the high endothelial cells. Local chemokines activate LFA-1 on the lymphocyte and cause it to bind tightly to ICAM-1 on the endothelial cell, allowing migration across the endothelium. For the lymphocyte to cross the high endothelial barrier successfully, migration has to lead to the activation of matrix metalloproteinases, as with the migration of neutrophils out of the blood (see Fig. 2.44).

initiation of the stronger interactions that follow between the T cell and the high endothelium, which are mediated by molecules with a relatively broad tissue distribution.

Chemokines produced by the cells of the lymph node are also important for initiating strong adhesion. These chemokines bind to proteoglycan molecules in the extracellular matrix and high endothelial venule cell walls, and are recognized by receptors on the naive T cell (see Section 8-3). Stimulation by these locally bound chemokines activates the adhesion molecule LFA-1 on the T cell, increasing its affinity for ICAM-2, which is expressed constitutively on all endothelial cells, and ICAM-1, which, in the absence of inflammation, is expressed only on the high endothelial venule cells of peripheral lymphoid tissues. The binding of LFA-1 to its ligands ICAM-1 and ICAM-2 has a major role in T-cell adhesion to and migration through the wall of the venule into the lymph node (see Fig. 10.7).

T cells that have arrived in the T-cell zone via the high endothelial venules scan the surface of the antigen-presenting dendritic cells for specific peptide:MHC complexes. If they do not recognize antigen, they eventually leave the lymph node via an efferent lymphatic vessel. This returns them to the blood so that they can recirculate through other lymph nodes. Rarely, a naive T cell recognizes its specific peptide:MHC complex on the surface of a dendritic cell. This signals the activation of LFA-1, causing the T cell to adhere strongly to the dendritic cell and cease migrating. Binding to the peptide:MHC complexes and co-stimulatory molecules on the dendritic cell surface stimulate the naive T cell to proliferate and differentiate, resulting in the production of an expanded population of armed, antigen-specific effector T cells (see Fig. 8.4). The efficiency with which T cells screen each antigen-presenting cell in lymph nodes is very high, as can be seen by the rapid trapping of antigen-specific T cells in a single lymph node containing antigen: all of the antigen-specific T cells in a sheep were trapped in one lymph node within 48 hours of antigen deposition (Fig. 10.8).

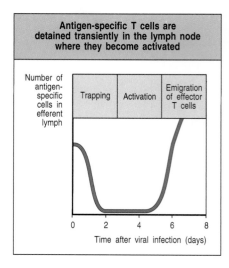

Antigen-specific T cells are detained transiently in the lymph node where they become activated

Fig. 10.8 Trapping and activation of antigen-specific naive T cells in lymphoid tissue. Naive T cells entering the lymph node from the blood encounter many antigen-presenting dendritic cells in the lymph node cortex. Most T cells will not recognize their specific antigen in the cortex and leave via the efferent lymphatics to reenter the blood. T cells that do recognize their specific antigen bind stably to the dendritic cell and are activated through their T-cell receptors, resulting in the production of armed effector T cells. Lymphocyte recirculation and recognition is so effective that all the specific naive T cells in the peripheral circulation can be trapped by antigen in one node within 2 days. By 5 days after the arrival of antigen, activated effector T cells are leaving the lymph node in large numbers via the efferent lymphatics.

10-5 Cytokines made in the early phases of an infection influence the functional differentiation of CD4 T cells.

The differentiation of naive CD4 T cells into the two major classes of CD4 effector T cell occurs during the initial response of these cells to antigen in the peripheral lymphoid tissues. This step, at which a naive CD4 T cell becomes either an armed T_H1 cell or an armed T_H2 cell, has an impact on the outcome of an adaptive immune response, determining the relative amounts of the different types of T cell produced and thus the extent of macrophage activation and which isotypes of antibody will predominate.

The mechanisms that control this step in CD4 T-cell differentiation are not yet fully defined; however, it is clear that it can be profoundly influenced by cytokines present during the initial proliferative phase of T-cell activation. Experiments *in vitro* have shown that naive CD4 T cells initially stimulated in the presence of IL-12 and interferon (IFN)-γ tend to develop into T_H1 cells (Fig. 10.9, left panels), in part because IFN-γ inhibits the proliferation of T_H2

Fig. 10.9 The differentiation of naive CD4 T cells into different subclasses of effector T cells is influenced by cytokines elicited by the pathogen. Many pathogens, especially intracellular bacteria and viruses, activate dendritic cells and NK cells to produce IL-12 and IFN-γ, which cause proliferating CD4 T cells to differentiate into T_H1 cells. IL-4 can inhibit these responses. IL-4, which can be produced by various cells, is made in response to parasitic worms and other pathogens and acts on proliferating CD4 T cells to cause them to become T_H2 cells. The mechanisms by which these cytokines induce the selective differentiation of CD4 T cells is now largely worked out. Selective induction of transcription factors induced by cytokine binding to cytokine receptors leads to the activation of these two different fates.

cells. Because IL-12, produced by dendritic cells and macrophages, and IFN-γ, produced by NK cells and CD8 T cells, predominate in the early phase of the response to viruses and to some intracellular bacteria, such as *Listeria* (see Section 2-27), CD4 T-cell responses in these infections tend to be dominated by T_H1 cells.

Signals that stimulate dendritic cells to release IL-12 include the chemokines CCL3 (MIP-1α), CCL4 (MIP-1β), and CCL5 (RANTES). These can be produced by many activated cell types, including macrophages, dendritic cells, and endothelial cells. They bind to the receptors CCR5 and CCR1 on dendritic cells, promoting the production of IL-12, and attract T_H1 cells, which also bear these receptors. Production of IL-12 by dendritic cells is also stimulated by IFN-γ and prostaglandin E2 derived from sites of tissue inflammation, or by the binding of Toll-like receptors on the dendritic cell surface by ligands such as LPS.

The importance of the ligation of Toll-like receptors in driving dendritic cells to produce IL-12 has been shown in mice lacking myeloid differentiation factor 88 (MyD88), a component of an intracellular signaling pathway activated by the ligation of some Toll-like receptors. Mice deficient in MyD88 do not survive a challenge with *Toxoplasma gondii*, a protozoan pathogen that can survive inside macrophage vesicles and that normally elicits a strong T_H1 response. Dendritic and other cells from the animals lacking MyD88 failed to produce IL-12 in response to parasite antigens and failed to mount a T_H1 response (Fig. 10.10).

By contrast, CD4 T cells activated in the presence of IL-4, especially when IL-6 is also present, tend to differentiate into T_H2 cells (see Fig. 10.9, right panels). This is because IL-4 and IL-6 promote the differentiation of T_H2 cells, and IL-4 or IL-10, either alone or in combination, also inhibit the generation of T_H1 cells. Although several types of lymphocyte and leukocyte can secrete IL-4, the source of the IL-4 that initiates the primary T_H2 response is not yet entirely clear. Mast cells are potent producers of IL-4 after stimulation and have been found to migrate to peripheral lymphoid organs, making them a possible candidate for an early source of IL-4.

The differential capacity of pathogens to interact with dendritic cells, macrophages, and NK cells can therefore influence the overall balance of cytokines present early in the immune response, and thus determine the balance

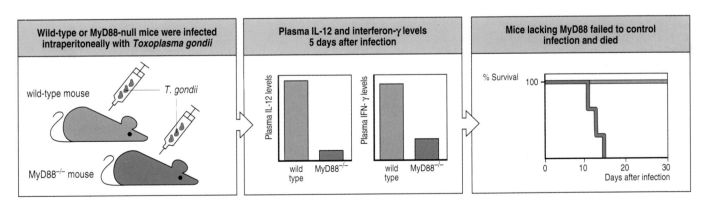

Fig. 10.10 Infection may trigger T_H1 polarization through Toll-like receptor signaling pathways. The adaptor protein MyD88 is a key component of Toll-like receptor signaling. Wild-type mice and mice deficient in MyD88 were infected intraperitoneally with the protozoan parasite *Toxoplasma gondii*. Five days after infection, mice lacking MyD88 showed a severe reduction in the amount of IL-12 in plasma compared with wild-type mice (middle panels), and dendritic cells from the spleens of these animals failed to produce IL-12 on stimulation with antigens from *T. gondii*. The mice lacking MyD88 also failed to produce a large IFN-γ response (middle panel) and a T_H1 response to the infection, and died at about 2 weeks after infection (right panel). In contrast, wild-type mice produced a strong IL-12, IFN-γ, and T_H1 response, controlled the infection and survived.

of T_H1 and T_H2 cells in any immune response (Fig. 10.11). Some pathogens may even have evolved to interact with the innate immune system so as to generate responses that are beneficial to them rather than to the host.

	T_H1 cells		T_H2 cells	
	Molecule	Cellular expression	Molecule	Cellular expression
Toll-like receptor (ligand)	TLR2 (bacterial peptidoglycan) TLR4 (LPS) TLR5 (flagellin) TLR9 (unmethylated DNA)	Receptor: dendritic cells		
Cytokine	IL-12 IL-27	Monocytes, macrophages and dendritic cells	IL-4	NK T cells, mast cell
	IFN-γ TNF-α LT	T_H1 lymphocytes, NK cells, macrophages	IL-4 IL-13 IL-5 IL-9 IL-10	T_H2 lymphocytes
Signaling molecule (downstream from)	Stat-4 (IL-12) Stat-1 (IFN-γ) T-bet (Stat-1)	T_H1 lymphocytes	Stat-6 (IL-4, IL-13) GATA3 (Stat-6) c-Maf (TCR signaling)	T_H2 lymphocytes
Chemokine (receptor)	CCL3, CCL4, CCL5 (CCR5, CCR1)	Chemokines: activated macrophages, dendritic cells, endothelial cells Receptors: dendritic cells	CCL2 (CCR2)	Chemokine: monocytes / dendritic cells Receptor: dendritic cells
	CCL3, CCL4, CCL5 (CCR5, CCR1) CXCL10 (CXCR3)	Chemokines: dendritic cells, T_H1 lymphocytes Receptors: T_H1 lymphocytes	CCL17, CCL22 (CCR4)	Chemokines: epithelial cells, macrophages, T_H2 lymphocytes Receptors: T_H2 lymphocytes
			CCL1 (CCR8)	Chemokine: T_H2 lymphocytes, endothelial cells, macrophages Receptor: T_H2 lymphocyte, vascular smooth muscle
			CCL5, CCL7, CCL11, CCL13, CCL24, CCL26 (CCR3)	Chemokine: epithelial cells, macrophages, T_H2 lymphocytes Receptor: Basophils, eosinophils, mast cells, epithelial cells
Other (receptor)			Prostaglandin D2 (CRTH2)	PGD2: mast cells Receptor: T_H2 lymphocytes, eosinophils

Fig. 10.11 The molecular programs of T_H1 and T_H2 responses. The figure shows the molecules that are associated with the polarization of a T-cell response to become dominated by either T_H1 or T_H2. T_H1 responses are promoted by antigen presentation by dendritic cells mainly in the context of dendritic cell co-stimulation by the products of infection. In contrast, T_H2 responses seem to be the 'default' response to antigen presentation by dendritic cells to naive T cells. An array of cytokines, chemokines, and their receptors are characteristic of either T_H1 or T_H2 responses. The activation of specific signaling pathways in T cells destined for a T_H1 or T_H2 fate leads to the production of either T_H1 or T_H2 cytokines and shuts down the pathway to synthesis of the cytokines that promote the development of the reciprocal subset of T_H cells.

10-6   Distinct subsets of T cells can regulate the growth and effector functions of other T-cell subsets.

The two subsets of CD4 T cells—T_H1 and T_H2—have very different functions: T_H2 cells are the most effective activators of B cells, especially in primary responses, whereas T_H1 cells are crucial for activating macrophages and are also involved in directing the production of certain antibody isotypes. T_H1 cells also produce IL-2, which is required for the proliferation of CD8 T cells, and IFN-γ, which augments CD8 T-cell function by upregulating MHC class I molecules on their target cells. It is also clear that the two CD4 T-cell subsets can regulate each other; once one subset becomes dominant, it is often hard to shift the response to the other subset. One reason for this is that cytokines from one type of CD4 T cell inhibit the activation of the other. Thus, IL-10, a product of T_H2 cells, can inhibit the development of T_H1 cells by blocking activation by the antigen-presenting cell, whereas IFN-γ, a product of T_H1 cells, can prevent the activation of T_H2 cells (Fig. 10.12). If a particular CD4 T-cell subset is activated first or preferentially in a response, it can suppress the development of the other subset. The overall effect is that certain responses are dominated by either a T_H2 or a T_H1 response. However, under many circumstances *in vivo* there is a mixed T_H1 and T_H2 response.

One class of CD4 T cells that might regulate T_H1 versus T_H2 development is the so-called **NK T cells** (see Section 2-29). These express the cell-surface marker NK1.1 normally associated with NK cells, but have an $\alpha{:}\beta$ T-cell receptor. This is, however, nearly invariant; in fact, essentially the same receptor seems to be used in the NK T cells of mice and their counterparts in humans. In mice, the invariant α chain is composed of the gene segments $V\alpha_{14}J\alpha_{28}$, and the human α chain uses the equivalent gene segments, $V\alpha_{24}J\alpha_Q$. Many NK T cells express CD4—others lack CD4 and CD8—but the development of the NK T cells, unlike that of other CD4 T cells, does not depend on the expression of MHC class II molecules. Instead, they recognize an MHC class IB molecule,

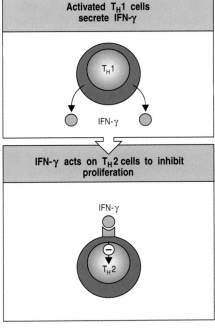

Fig. 10.12 The two subsets of CD4 T cells each produce cytokines that can negatively regulate the other subset. T_H2 cells make IL-10, which acts on macrophages to inhibit T_H1 activation, perhaps by blocking macrophage IL-12 synthesis, and TGF-β, which acts directly on the T_H1 cells to inhibit their growth (left panels). T_H1 cells make IFN-γ, which blocks the growth of T_H2 cells (right panels). These effects allow either subset to dominate a response by suppressing the outgrowth of cells of the other subset.

CD1, which is not encoded within the MHC (see Section 5-18). In mice there are two CD1 genes (CD1.1 and CD1.2), whereas in humans there are five (CD1a–e), of which only CD1d is homologous to the murine CD1.1 and CD1.2. CD1 molecules are expressed by thymocytes, antigen-presenting cells, and intestinal epithelium. Lymphocytes such as NK T cells are known as innate-like lymphocytes (ILLs) (see Section 2-29).

Although the exact function of CD1 molecules is not well defined, CD1b is known to present a bacterial lipid, mycolic acid, to α:β T cells, whereas other CD1 molecules are recognized by γ:δ T cells. The activation of NK T cells is thought to depend on the expression of CD1 molecules induced in response to infection; whether all NK T cells recognize a specific antigen presented by these CD1 molecules is not known, but some at least are able to recognize glycolipid antigens presented by CD1d. Upon activation, these NK T cells secrete very large amounts of IL-4 and IFN-γ. Deficits in NK T cells are associated with autoimmune disease, such as diabetes, and implicate the NK T cells as immune regulators.

The interplay of cytokines is important in human disease, but it has been explored at present mainly in mouse models, where polarized responses are easier to study. For example, when BALB/c mice are experimentally infected with the protozoan parasite *Leishmania*, their CD4 T cells fail to differentiate into T_H1 effector cells; instead, the mice preferentially make T_H2 cells in response to this pathogen. These T_H2 cells are unable to activate macrophages to inhibit leishmanial growth, resulting in susceptibility to disease. By contrast, C57BL/6 mice respond by producing T_H1 cells that protect the host by activating infected macrophages to kill the *Leishmania*. The preferential activation of T_H2 rather than T_H1 cells in BALB/c mice can be reversed if IL-4 is blocked in the first days of infection by injecting anti-IL-4 antibody, but this treatment is ineffective after a week or so of infection.

Because cytokines seem to regulate the balance between T_H1 and T_H2 cells, one might expect that it would be possible to shift this balance by administering appropriate cytokines. IL-2 and IFN-γ have been used to stimulate cell-mediated immunity in diseases such as lepromatous leprosy and can cause both a local resolution of the lesion and a systemic change in T-cell responses.

CD8 T cells are also able to regulate the immune response by producing cytokines. It has become clear recently that effector CD8 T cells can, in addition to their familiar cytolytic function, also respond to antigen by secreting cytokines typical of either T_H1 or T_H2 cells. Such CD8 T cells, called T_C1 or T_C2 by analogy to the T_H subsets, seem to be responsible for the development of leprosy in its lepromatous rather than its tuberculoid form, which we will discuss in detail in Chapter 11. Patients with the less destructive tuberculoid leprosy make T_C1 cells whose cytokines induce T_H1 cells, which can activate macrophages to rid the body of its burden of leprosy bacilli. Patients with lepromatous leprosy have CD8 T cells that suppress the T_H1 response by making IL-10 and transforming growth factor (TGF)-β. Thus, the suppression of CD4 T cells by CD8 T cells that has been observed in various situations can be explained by their expression of different sets of cytokines.

10-7 The nature and amount of antigenic peptide can also affect the differentiation of CD4 T cells.

Another factor that influences the differentiation of CD4 T cells into distinct effector subsets is the amount and exact sequence of the antigenic peptide that initiates the response. Large amounts of peptide that achieve a high density on the surface of antigen-presenting cells tend to stimulate T_H1-cell

Fig. 10.13 The nature and amount of ligand presented to a CD4 T cell during primary stimulation can determine its functional phenotype. CD4 T cells presented with low levels of a ligand that binds the T-cell receptor poorly differentiate preferentially into T_H2 cells making IL-4 and IL-5. Such T cells are most active in stimulating naive B cells to differentiate into plasma cells and make antibody. T cells presented with a high density of a ligand that strongly binds the T-cell receptor differentiate into T_H1 cells that secrete IL-2, lymphotoxin (LT; formerly known as TNF-β), and IFN-γ, and are most effective in activating macrophages.

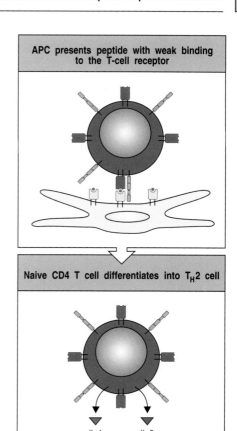

responses, whereas low-density presentation tends to elicit T_H2-cell responses. Moreover, peptides that interact strongly with the T-cell receptor tend to stimulate T_H1-like responses, whereas peptides that bind weakly tend to stimulate T_H2-like responses (Fig. 10.13).

This difference could be very important in several circumstances. For instance, allergy is caused by the production of IgE antibody, which, as we learned in Chapter 9, requires high levels of IL-4 but does not occur in the presence of IFN-γ, a potent inhibitor of IL-4-driven class switching to IgE. Antigens that elicit IgE-mediated allergy are generally delivered in minute doses, and they elicit T_H2 cells that make IL-4 and no IFN-γ. It is also relevant that allergens do not elicit any of the known innate immune responses, which produce cytokines that tend to bias CD4 T-cell differentiation toward T_H1 cells. Finally, allergens are delivered to humans in minute doses across a thin mucosa, such as that of the lung. Something about this route of sensitization allows even potent generators of T_H1 responses such as *Leishmania major* to induce T_H2 responses.

Most protein antigens that elicit CD4 T-cell responses stimulate the production of both T_H1 and T_H2 cells. This reflects the presence in most proteins of several different peptide sequences that can bind to MHC class II molecules and be presented to CD4 T cells. Some of these peptides are likely to bind to MHC class II molecules with high affinity, and consequently will be present at high density on the antigen-presenting cell, whereas others are likely to bind MHC class II molecules with low affinity and be present only at low density. Naive T cells specific for peptide antigens that have high affinity for MHC molecules are therefore likely to encounter a high density of their ligand, whereas others might only encounter a low density, and these differences could affect the subsequent response of the T cell. Indeed, it can be shown experimentally that some peptides in a protein tend to elicit the production of T_H2 cells, whereas other peptides tend to elicit T_H1 cells.

10-8   Armed effector T cells are guided to sites of infection by chemokines and newly expressed adhesion molecules.

The full activation of naive T cells takes 4–5 days and is accompanied by marked changes in the homing behavior of these cells. Armed effector cytotoxic CD8 T cells must travel from the lymph node, or other peripheral lymphoid tissue in which they have been activated, to attack and destroy infected cells. Armed effector CD4 T_H1 cells must also leave the lymphoid tissues to activate macrophages at the site of infection. Most of the antigen-specific armed effector T cells cease production of L-selectin, which mediates homing to the lymph nodes, whereas the expression of other adhesion molecules is increased (Fig. 10.14). One important change is a marked increase in the expression of the integrin $\alpha_4:\beta_1$, also known as VLA-4. This binds to the VCAM-1 molecule that is induced on activated endothelial cell surfaces and initiates the extravasation of the effector T cells. Thus, if the innate immune response

Fig. 10.14 Armed effector T cells change their surface molecules, allowing them to home to sites of infection. Naive T cells home to lymph nodes through the binding of L-selectin to sulfated carbohydrates displayed by various proteins, such as CD34 and GlyCAM-1, on the high endothelial venule (HEV, top panel). If they encounter antigen and differentiate into armed effector T cells, many lose expression of L-selectin, leave the lymph node about 4–5 days later, and now express the integrin VLA-4 and increased levels of LFA-1. These bind to VCAM-1 and ICAM-1, respectively, on peripheral vascular endothelium at sites of inflammation (bottom panel). On differentiating into effector cells, T cells also alter their splicing of the mRNA encoding the cell-surface molecule CD45. The CD45RO isoform expressed by effector T cells lacks one or more exons that encode extracellular domains present in the CD45RA isoform expressed by naive T cells, and somehow makes effector T cells more sensitive to stimulation by specific antigen.

has already activated the endothelium at the site of infection, as described in Section 10-3, effector T cells will rapidly be recruited. At the early stage of the immune response, only a few of the effector T cells that enter the infected tissues will be expected to be specific for pathogen, because any effector T cell specific for any antigen will also be able to enter. However, specificity of the reaction is maintained, because only those effector T cells that recognize pathogen antigens will carry out their function, destroying infected cells or specifically activating pathogen-loaded macrophages. By the peak of an adaptive immune response, most of the recruited T cells will be specific for the infecting pathogen, because after several days of clonal expansion and differentiation these cells predominate in numbers.

Differential expression of adhesion molecules can direct different subsets of armed effector T cells to specific sites. As we discuss later in this chapter, the peripheral immune system is compartmentalized such that different populations of lymphocytes migrate through different lymphoid compartments and—after activation—through the different tissues they serve. The selective expression of different homing receptors that bind to tissue-specific 'addressins' is the mechanism by which this is achieved.

Not all infections trigger innate immune responses that activate local endothelial cells, and it is not so clear how armed effector T cells are guided to the sites of infection in these cases. However, activated T cells seem to enter all tissues in very small numbers, perhaps via adhesive interactions such as the binding of P-selectin to P-selectin glycolipid-1, and could thus encounter their antigens even in the absence of a previous inflammatory response.

Effector T cells that recognize pathogen antigens in the tissues produce cytokines such as TNF-α, which activates endothelial cells to express E-selectin, VCAM-1, and ICAM-1, and chemokines such as CCL5 (see Fig. 2.41), which can then act on effector T cells to activate their adhesion molecules. The increased levels of VCAM-1 and ICAM-1 on endothelial cells bind VLA-4 and LFA-1, respectively, on armed effector T cells, recruiting more of these cells into tissues that contain the antigen. At the same time, monocytes and polymorphonuclear leukocytes are recruited to these sites by adhesion to E-selectin. TNF-α and IFN-γ released by the activated T cells also act synergistically to change the shape of endothelial cells, allowing increased blood flow, increased vascular permeability, and increased emigration of leukocytes, fluid, and protein into a site of infection.

Thus, one or a few specific effector T cells encountering antigen in a tissue can initiate a potent local inflammatory response that recruits both a greater number of specific armed effector cells and many more nonspecific inflammatory cells to that site. By contrast, effector T cells that enter the tissues but do not recognize their antigen are rapidly lost. They either enter afferent lymph in the tissues and return to the bloodstream, or undergo apoptosis.

Most of the T cells in the afferent lymph that drains tissues are memory or effector T cells, which characteristically express the CD45RO isoform of the cell-surface molecule CD45 and lack L-selectin. Effector T cells and memory T cells have similar phenotypes, as we discuss later, and both seem to be committed to migration through potential sites of infection. As well as allowing effector T cells to clear all sites of infection, this pattern of migration allows them to contribute, along with memory cells, to protecting the host against reinfection with the same pathogen (see Sections 10-11 and 10-12).

10-9   Antibody responses develop in lymphoid tissues under the direction of armed helper T cells.

Migration out of lymphoid tissues is clearly important for the effector actions of antigen-specific CD8 cytotoxic T cells and armed T_H1 cells. However, the most important functions of helper CD4 T cells, predominantly T_H2 cells, depend on their interactions with B cells, and these interactions occur in the lymphoid tissues themselves. B cells specific for a protein antigen cannot be activated to proliferate, form germinal centers, or differentiate into plasma cells until they encounter a helper T cell that is specific for one of the peptides derived from that antigen. Humoral immune responses to protein antigens thus cannot occur until after antigen-specific helper T cells have been generated.

One of the most interesting questions in immunology is how two antigen-specific lymphocytes—the naive antigen-binding B cell and the armed helper T cell—find one another to initiate a T-cell dependent antibody response. As we learned in Chapter 9, the likely answer lies in the migratory path of B cells through the lymphoid tissues and the presence of armed helper T cells on that path (Fig. 10.15).

Fig. 10.15 The specialized regions of peripheral lymphoid tissue provide an environment where antigen-specific naive B cells can interact with armed helper T cells specific for the same antigen. The initial encounter of antigen-specific naive B cells with the appropriate helper T cells occurs in the T-cell areas in lymphoid tissue and stimulates the proliferation of B cells in contact with the helper T cells to form a primary focus, as shown in the first three panels. This also results in some isotype switching in the antigen-specific B cells. Some of the activated B-cell blasts then migrate to medullary cords, where they divide, differentiate into plasma cells, and secrete antibody for a few days (third panel). Other B-cell blasts migrate into primary lymphoid follicles, where they proliferate rapidly to form a germinal center under the influence of antigen and of helper T cells (fourth panel). The germinal center is the site of somatic hypermutation and selection of high-affinity B cells that are able to bind antigen better than lower-affinity cells and thus survive either because they are protected from apoptotic signals delivered by T cells or/and they are more capable of presenting antigen to T cells and thereby receiving positive signals such as IL-4 and CD40 ligand (fifth panel). FDC, follicular dendritic cell.

If B cells binding their specific antigen in the T-cell zone of peripheral lymphoid organs receive specific signals from armed helper T cells, they proliferate in the T-cell areas (see Fig. 10.15, second panel). In the absence of T-cell signals, these antigen-stimulated B cells die within 24 hours of arriving in the T-cell zone.

About 5 days after primary immunization, primary foci of proliferating B cells appear in the T-cell areas, which correlates with the time needed for helper T cells to differentiate. Some of the B cells activated in the primary focus may migrate to the medullary cords of the lymph node, or to those parts of the red pulp that are next to the T-cell zones of the spleen, where they become plasma cells and secrete specific antibody for a few days (see Fig. 10.15, third panel). Others migrate to the follicle (see Fig. 10.15, fourth panel), where they proliferate further, forming a germinal center in which they undergo somatic hypermutation (see Sections 4-9 and 9-7). The antibodies secreted by B cells differentiating early in the response not only provide early protection; they may also be important in trapping antigen in the form of antigen:antibody complexes on the surface of the local follicular dendritic cells. The antigen:antibody complexes, which become coated with fragments of C3, are held by complement fragment receptors (CR1, CR2, and CR3) as well as by a non-phagocytic Fc receptor on the follicular dendritic cells. Antigen can be retained in lymphoid follicles in this form for very long periods. The function of this antigen is unclear, but it may regulate the long-term antibody response.

The proliferation, somatic hypermutation, and selection that occur in the germinal centers during a primary antibody response have been described in Chapter 9. The adhesion and chemokine molecules that govern the migratory behavior of B cells are likely to be very important to this process but, as yet, little is known of their nature or of the ligands to which they bind. The chemokine/receptor pair CXCL13/CXCR5, which controls B-cell migration into the follicle, may be important, particularly for B cells homing to the germinal center. Another chemokine receptor, CCR7, which is strongly expressed on T cells and weakly expressed on B cells, may be involved in temporarily directing B cells to the interface with the T-cell zone. The ligands for CCR7 are CCL19 (MIP-3β) and CCL21 (SLE), which are highly expressed in the T zone (see Section 7-27) and could attract B cells that have an increased expression of CCR7.

10-10 Antibody responses are sustained in medullary cords and bone marrow.

The B cells activated in primary foci migrate either to adjacent follicles or to local extrafollicular sites of proliferation. B cells grow exponentially in these sites for 2–3 days and undergo six or seven cell divisions before the progeny come out of the cell cycle and form antibody-producing plasma cells *in situ* (Fig. 10.16, upper panel). Most of these plasma cells have a life-span of 2–4

Fig. 10.16 Plasma cells are dispersed in medullary cords and bone marrow. In these sites they secrete antibody at high rates directly into the blood for distribution to the rest of the body. In the upper micrograph, plasma cells in lymph node medullary cords are stained green (with fluorescein anti-IgA) if they are secreting IgA, and red (with rhodamine anti-IgG) if they are secreting IgG. The plasma cells in these local extrafollicular sites are short lived (2–4 days). The lymphatic sinuses are outlined by green granular staining selective for IgA. In the lower micrograph, longer-lived plasma cells (3 weeks to 3 months or more) in the bone marrow are revealed with antibodies specific for light chains (fluorescein anti-λ and rhodamine anti-κ stain). Plasma cells secreting immunoglobulins containing λ light chains show on this micrograph as yellow. Those secreting immunoglobulins containing κ light chains stain red. Photographs courtesy of P. Brandtzaeg.

days, after which they undergo apoptosis. About 10% of plasma cells in these extrafollicular sites live longer; their origin and ultimate fate are unknown. The B cells that migrate to the primary follicles to form germinal centers undergo isotype switching and affinity maturation before either becoming memory cells or leaving the germinal center to become relatively long-lived antibody-producing cells (see Sections 9-7 to 9-9).

These B cells leave germinal centers as plasmablasts (pre-plasma cells). Plasmablasts originating in the follicles of Peyer's patches and mesenteric lymph nodes migrate via lymph to the blood and then enter the lamina propria of the gut and other epithelial surfaces. Those originating in peripheral lymph node or splenic follicles migrate to the bone marrow (see Fig. 10.16, lower panel). In these distant sites of antibody production, the plasmablasts differentiate into plasma cells that have a life-span of months to years. These are thought to provide the antibody that can last in the blood for years after an initial immune response. Whether this supply of plasma cells is replenished by the continual but occasional differentiation of memory cells is not yet known. Studies of responses to nonreplicating antigens show that germinal centers are present for only 3–4 weeks after initial antigen exposure. However, small numbers of B cells continue to proliferate in the follicles for months. These may be the precursors of antigen-specific plasma cells in the mucosa and bone marrow throughout the subsequent months and years.

10-11 The effector mechanisms used to clear an infection depend on the infectious agent.

A primary adaptive immune response usually serves to clear the primary infection from the body and in most cases provides protection against reinfection with the same pathogen. However, as we will discuss further in Chapter 11, some pathogens evade complete clearance and persist for the life of the host, for example *Leishmania, Toxoplasma*, and herpes viruses. Figure 10.17 summarizes the different types of infection in humans and the ways in which they can be eliminated or held in check by a primary adaptive immune response. It also indicates the mechanisms involved in immunity to reinfection, or protective immunity, against these pathogens. Inducing protective immunity is the goal of vaccine development, and to achieve this it is necessary to induce an adaptive immune response that has both the antigen specificity and the appropriate functional elements to combat the particular pathogen concerned.

Protective immunity consists of two components—immune reactants, such as antibody or effector T cells generated in the initial infection or by vaccination, and long-lived immunological memory (Fig. 10.18), which we consider in the last part of this chapter. The type of antibody or effector T cell that offers protection depends on the infectious strategy and lifestyle of the pathogen. In many cases the most efficient protective immunity is mediated by neutralizing antibody that can prevent pathogens from establishing an infection. Effective immunity against polio virus, for example, requires preexisting antibody, because the virus rapidly infects motor neurons and destroys them unless it is immediately neutralized by antibody and prevented from spreading within the body. Specific IgA on epithelial surfaces can also neutralize the virus before it enters the body. Thus, protective immunity can involve effector mechanisms (IgA in this case) that do not operate in the elimination of the primary infection (see Fig. 10.17).

Preformed reactants can also allow the immune system to respond more rapidly and efficiently to a second exposure to a pathogen. Thus, when opsonizing antibodies such as IgG1 are present (see Section 9-12), opsonization and phagocytosis of pathogens will be more efficient. If specific IgE is present, then pathogens will also be able to activate mast cells, rapidly initiating an inflammatory response through the release of histamine and leukotrienes.

Infectious agent	Disease	Humoral immunity				Cell-mediated immunity	
		IgM	IgG	IgE	IgA	CD4 T cells (macrophages)	CD8 killer T cells
Viruses							
Variola	Smallpox						
Varicella zoster	Chickenpox						
Epstein–Barr virus	Mononucleosis						
Influenza virus	Influenza						
Mumps virus	Mumps						
Measles virus	Measles						
Polio virus	Poliomyelitis						
Human immunodeficiency virus	AIDS						
Bacteria							
Staphylococcus aureus	Boils						
Streptococcus pyogenes	Tonsilitis						
Streptococcus pneumoniae	Pneumonia						
Neisseria gonorrhoeae	Gonorrhea						
Neisseria meningitidis	Meningitis						
Corynebacterium diphtheriae	Diphtheria						
Clostridium tetani	Tetanus						
Treponema pallidum	Syphilis			Transient			
Borrelia burgdorferi	Lyme disease			Transient			
Salmonella typhi	Typhoid						
Vibrio cholerae	Cholera						
Legionella pneumophila	Legionnaire's disease						
Rickettsia prowazekii	Typhus						
Chlamydia trachomatis	Trachoma						
Mycobacteria	Tuberculosis, leprosy						
Fungi — *Candida albicans*	Candidiasis						
Protozoa							
Plasmodium spp.	Malaria						
Toxoplasma gondii	Toxoplasmosis						
Trypanosoma spp.	Trypanosomiasis						
Leishmania spp.	Leishmaniasis						
Worms — Schistosome	Schistosomiasis						

Fig. 10.17 Different effector mechanisms are used to clear primary infections with different pathogens and to protect against subsequent reinfection. The pathogens are listed in order of increasing complexity, and the defense mechanisms used to clear a primary infection are identified by the red shading of the boxes where these are known. Yellow shading indicates a role in protective immunity. Paler shades indicate less well established mechanisms. Much has to be learned about such host–pathogen interactions. It is clear that classes of pathogens elicit similar protective immune responses, reflecting similarities in their lifestyles.

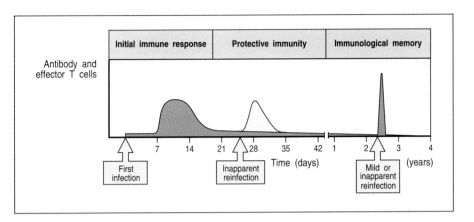

Fig. 10.18 Protective immunity consists of preformed immune reactants and immunological memory. Antibody levels and effector T-cell activity gradually decline after an infection is cleared. An early reinfection is rapidly cleared by these immune reactants. There are few symptoms but levels of immune reactants increase. Reinfection at later times leads to rapid increases in antibody and effector T cells owing to immunological memory, and infection can be mild or even inapparent.

10-12 Resolution of an infection is accompanied by the death of most of the effector cells and the generation of memory cells.

When an infection is effectively repelled by the adaptive immune system, two things occur. The actions of effector cells remove the specific stimulus that originally recruited them. In the absence of this stimulus, they then undergo 'death by neglect,' removing themselves by apoptosis. The dying cells are rapidly cleared by phagocytes and other cells, which recognize the membrane lipid phosphatidylserine. This lipid is normally found only on the inner surface of the plasma membrane, but in apoptotic cells it rapidly redistributes to the outer surface, where it can be recognized by specific receptors on many cells. Thus, not only does the ending of infection lead to the removal of the pathogen, it also leads to the loss of most of the pathogen-specific effector cells.

However, some of the effector cells are retained, and these provide the raw material for memory T-cell and B-cell responses. These are crucially important to the operation of the adaptive immune system. The memory T cells, which we consider at the end of this chapter, are retained virtually forever. However, the mechanisms underlying the decision to induce apoptosis in most effector cells and to retain only a few are not known. It seems likely that the answer will lie in the cytokines produced by the environment, by the T cells themselves, or by the affinity of the receptors retained as memory cells.

Summary.

The adaptive immune response is required for effective protection of the host against pathogenic microorganisms. The response of the innate immune system to pathogens helps to initiate the adaptive immune response, as interactions with these pathogens lead to the production of cytokines and the activation of dendritic cells to activated antigen-presenting cell status. The antigens of the pathogen are transported to local lymphoid organs by these migrating antigen-presenting cells and are presented to antigen-specific naive T cells that continuously recirculate through the lymphoid organs. T-cell priming and the differentiation of armed effector T cells occur here on the surface of antigen-loaded dendritic cells, and the armed effector T cells either leave the lymphoid organ to effect cell-mediated immunity in sites of infection in the tissues or remain in the lymphoid organ to participate in humoral immunity by activating antigen-binding B cells. CD8 T cells have an important role in protective immunity, especially in protecting the host against infection by viruses and intracellular infections by *Listeria* and other micro-bial pathogens that have special means for entering the host cell's cytoplasm. Ideally, the adaptive immune response eliminates the infectious agent and provides the host with a state of protective immunity against reinfection with the same pathogen.

The mucosal immune system.

The immune system can be viewed as an organ that is distributed through-out the body to defend against pathogens wherever these may enter or spread. Within the immune system, a series of anatomically distinct com-partments can be distinguished, each of which is specially adapted to gener-ate a response to pathogens present in a particular set of body tissues. The previous part of this chapter illustrated the general principles underlying the initiation of an adaptive immune response in the compartment comprising the peripheral lymph nodes and spleen. This is the compartment that re-sponds to antigens that have entered the tissues or spread into the blood. A second compartment of the adaptive immune system of equal size to this, and located near the surfaces where most pathogens invade, is the mucosal immune system (commonly described by the acronym MALT). Two further distinct compartments are those of the body cavities (peritoneum and pleura) and the skin. Immune responses initiated within each compartment remain largely confined to that compartment. Compartmentalization of the immune response is achieved by the programming of naive T cells during ex-posure to antigen in the peripheral lymphoid tissues of each compartment. Effector T cells express a repertoire of adhesion molecules and chemokine re-ceptors that confer tissue-specific homing properties that confine them to the compartment in which they first met antigen as naive cells. The tissues of the compartment that are surveyed and protected by the T cells express tissue-specific ligands for the T-cell adhesion molecules and chemokines that are bound by their own 'police force' of T cells. We will illustrate the con-cept of compartmentalization of the immune system by considering the mu-cosal immune system. The mucosal surfaces of the body are particularly vulnerable to infection. They are thin and permeable barriers to the interior of the body because of their physiological activities in gas exchange (the lungs), food absorption (the gut), sensory activities (eyes, nose, mouth, and throat), and reproduction (uterus and vagina). The necessity for permeabil-ity of the surface lining these sites creates obvious vulnerability to infection, and it is not surprising that the vast majority of infectious agents invade the human body by these routes.

A second important point to bear in mind when considering the immunobi-ology of mucosal surfaces is that the gut acts as a portal of entry to a vast array of foreign antigens in the form of food. The immune system has evolved mechanisms to avoid a vigorous immune response to food antigens on the one hand and, on the other, to detect and kill pathogenic organisms gaining entry through the gut. To complicate matters further, most of the gut is heav-ily colonized by approximately 10^{14} commensal microorganisms, which live in symbiosis with their host. These bacteria are beneficial to their host in many ways. They provide protection against pathogenic bacteria by occupy-ing the ecological niches for bacteria in the gut. They also serve a nutritional role in their host by synthesizing vitamin K and some of the components of the vitamin B complex. However, in certain circumstances they can also cause disease, as we will see later.

10-13 Mucosa-associated lymphoid tissue is located in anatomically defined microcompartments throughout the gut.

The mucosa-associated peripheral lymphoid tissues lining the gut are known as **gut-associated lymphoid tissue** or **GALT**. The tonsils and adenoids form a ring, known as Waldeyer's ring, at the back of the mouth at the entrance of the gut and airways. They consist of large aggregates of mucosal lymphoid tissue, which often become extremely enlarged in childhood because of recurrent infections, and which in the past were victims of a vogue for surgical removal. A reduced IgA response to oral polio vaccination has been seen in individuals who have had their tonsils and adenoids removed, which illustrates the importance of this subcompartment of the mucosal immune system.

The other principal sites within the gut mucosal immune system for the induction of immune responses are the Peyer's patches of the small intestine, the appendix (which is another frequent victim of the surgeon's knife), and solitary lymphoid follicles of the large intestine and rectum. **Peyer's patches** are an extremely important site for the induction of immune responses in the small intestine and have a distinctive appearance, forming dome-like structures extending into the lumen of the intestine (see Fig. 1.10). The overlying layer of follicle-associated epithelium of the Peyer's patches contains specialized epithelial cells. These have microfolds on their luminal surface, instead of the microvilli present on the absorptive epithelial cells of the intestine, and are known as **multifenestrated** or **microfold cells** (**M cells**). They are much less prominent than the absorptive gut epithelial cells, known as enterocytes, and form a membrane overlying the lymphoid tissue within the Peyer's patch. M cells lack a thick surface glycocalyx and do not secrete mucus. Hence, they are adapted to interact directly with molecules and particles within the lumen of the gut.

M cells take up molecules and particles from the gut lumen by endocytosis or phagocytosis (Fig. 10.19). This material is then transported through the interior of the cell in vesicles to the basal cell membrane, where it is released into the extracellular space. This process is known as **transcytosis**. At their basal surface, the cell membrane of M cells is extensively folded around underlying lymphocytes and antigen-presenting cells, which take up the transported material released from the M cells and process it for antigen presentation.

Because M cells are much more accessible than enterocytes to particles within the gut, a number of pathogens target M cells to gain access to the subepithelial space, even though such pathogens then find themselves in the heart of the adaptive immune system of the intestine, the Peyer's patches. We consider some of these pathogens in Section 10-19.

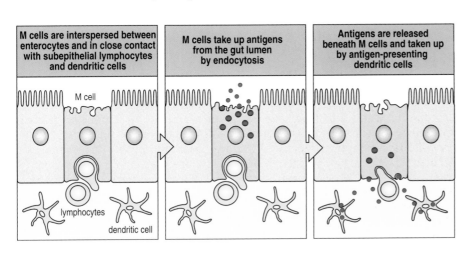

| M cells are interspersed between enterocytes and in close contact with subepithelial lymphocytes and dendritic cells | M cells take up antigens from the gut lumen by endocytosis | Antigens are released beneath M cells and taken up by antigen-presenting dendritic cells |

Fig. 10.19 M cells take up antigens from the lumen of the gut by endocytosis. The cell membrane at the base of these cells is folded around lymphocytes and dendritic cells within the Peyer's patches. Antigens are transported through M cells by the process of transcytosis and delivered directly to antigen-presenting cells and lymphocytes of the mucosal immune system.

10-14 The trafficking of lymphocytes within different compartments of the immune system is controlled by tissue-specific adhesion and chemokine interactions.

In addition to the organized lymphoid tissue in which induction of immune responses occurs within the mucosal immune system, small foci of lymphocytes and plasma cells are scattered widely throughout the lamina propria of the gut wall. These represent the effector cells of the gut mucosal immune system. The life history of these cells is as follows. As naive lymphocytes, they emerge from the primary lymphoid organs of bone marrow and thymus to enter the inductive peripheral lymphoid tissue of the mucosal immune system, the Peyer's patches, via the bloodstream. This migration is controlled by the chemokines CCL21 and CCL19 released from peripheral lymphoid tissues ligating the receptor CCR7 on the naive lymphocytes. These naive lymphocytes may encounter foreign antigens presented within the Peyer's patches, and become activated to effector status. Activation includes a reprogramming step that alters the migratory behavior of these effector cells and directs them to extralymphoid sites.

Leaving the Peyer's patches, the activated lymphocytes are carried via the lymphatics draining the intestines, pass through mesenteric lymph nodes, and eventually end up in the thoracic duct, from where they circulate in the blood throughout the entire body (Fig. 10.20). They reenter the mucosal tissues from the small blood vessels lining the gut wall and other sites of MALT, such as the respiratory or reproductive mucosa, and the lactating breast. T lymphocytes that migrate to the lamina propria of the gut express both L-selectin and the $\alpha_4{:}\beta_7$ integrin, which bind to separate sites on the gut vascular addressin MAdCAM-1, carried on endothelial cells lining blood vessels within the gut wall (Fig. 10.21). T cells that home to the epithelium of the gut express instead an integrin called $\alpha_e{:}\beta_7$ and bind to the E-cadherin expressed

Fig. 10.20 Anatomy of mucosal immune responses. The left panel shows the afferent immune response. Antigen from pathogenic microorganisms is presented beneath mucosal surfaces to naive lymphocytes within organized mucosal lymphoid tissue, for example Peyer's patches. Activated lymphocytes leave this tissue via draining lymph nodes and reenter the circulation through the thoracic duct. The right panel shows the efferent immune response, in which primed lymphocytes reenter mucosal tissues throughout the body from the circulation, thereby disseminating a mucosal immune response.

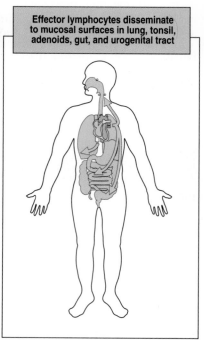

Lymphocytes and lymph return to blood via mesenteric lymph nodes and thoracic duct

Naive lymphocytes enter mucosal tissue from blood

Effector lymphocytes disseminate to mucosal surfaces in lung, tonsil, adenoids, gut, and urogenital tract

Antigens from infectious agents taken into submucosal lymphoid tissues

Fig. 10.21 Effector T cells home to the gut by combinations of relatively specific interactions involving adhesion molecules and chemokines. Left panel: a gut-homing lymphocyte adheres to the vascular endothelium of an intestinal blood vessel by the binding of lymphocyte L-selectin and $\alpha_4{:}\beta_7$ integrin to MAdCAM-1 expressed on the endothelial surface. Right panel: having migrated across the endothelium, further binding of the T cell to intestinal epithelial cells is mediated by CCR9 (T cell)–CCL25 (epithelial cell) interactions in the small intestine, or CCR10–CCL28 interactions in the large intestine. A further interaction between the T-cell integrin $\alpha_e{:}\beta_7$ and epithelial E-cadherin strengthens T-cell localization to the intestinal epithelium.

on epithelial cells. In addition to tissue-specific adhesion of lymphocytes, there is also tissue-specific expression of the chemokines that lure T cells to specific organs. In the gut, the chemokine CCL25 (TECK) is expressed by the epithelium of the small intestine and is a ligand for the chemokine receptor CCR9, expressed on gut-homing T cells. Even within the intestine there seems to be regional specialization of chemokine expression. The colon and salivary glands express CCL28 (MEC, mucosal epithelial chemokine) which is a ligand for the CCR10 on gut- and skin-homing lymphocytes (we explain below why skin-homing lymphocytes do not migrate to the gut in response to CCL28).

In this way an immune response that may be started by foreign antigens presented in a limited number of Peyer's patches is disseminated throughout the mucosa of the body. This pathway of lymphocyte trafficking is distinct from and parallel to that of lymphocytes in the rest of the peripheral lymphoid system (see Fig. 1.11).

T lymphocytes that home to the skin express an adhesion molecule named cutaneous lymphocyte antigen (CLA) (Fig. 10.22). This is a glycosylated isoform of P-selectin glycolipid-1, and binds to E-selectin on cutaneous vascular

Fig. 10.22 Skin-homing T cells use specific combinations of integrins and chemokines to home to the skin. Left panel: a skin-homing lymphocyte binds to the endothelium lining a cutaneous blood vessel by interactions between cutaneous lymphocyte antigen (CLA) and constitutively expressed E-selectin on the endothelial cells. The adhesion is strengthened by an interaction between lymphocyte chemokine receptor CCR4 and the endothelial chemokine CCL17. Right panel: once through the endothelium, keratinocytes of the epidermis anchor the effector T lymphocyte by the chemokine CCL27 that they produce, which binds to the receptor CCR10 on lymphocytes.

endothelium. CLA-expressing T lymphocytes also produce the chemokine receptor CCR4. This binds the chemokine CCL17 (TARC), which is present at high levels on the endothelium of cutaneous vessels. The interaction of CLA with E-selectin causes the T lymphocyte to roll against the wall of the vessel, and further interaction between T lymphocyte CCR4 and endothelial CCL17 is thought to cause the arrest and adhesion of lymphocytes to the wall. In addition to CCR4, skin-homing T lymphocytes carry the chemokine receptor CCR10 (GPR-2), which ligates the chemokine CCL27 (CTACK) expressed by the epithelial cells of the skin, the keratinocytes. As both skin- and gut-homing lymphocytes express the same chemokine receptor, CCR10, why do they not both home promiscuously to either of these organs? The explanation probably lies in the monogamy of their adhesion mechanisms. CLA-positive skin-homing cells do not bind to MAdCAM-1, and $\alpha_4{:}\beta_7$ integrin-positive gut-homing lymphocytes do not bind to E-selectin.

10-15 The mucosal immune system contains a distinctive repertoire of lymphocytes.

The distinctiveness of the mucosal immune system from the rest of the peripheral lymphoid system is further underlined by the different lymphocyte repertoires in the different compartments. The T cells of the gut can be divided into two types. One type (designated type a) bears the conventional $\alpha{:}\beta$ T-cell receptors in conjunction with either CD4 or CD8, and participates in conventional T-cell responses to foreign antigens, as discussed in earlier chapters. The second class, designated type b, is made up of T cells with unusual surface phenotypes such as TCR$\gamma{:}\delta$ CD4 CD8 double-negative, TCR$\gamma{:}\delta$ CD8$\alpha{:}\alpha$ and TCR$\alpha{:}\beta$ CD8$\alpha{:}\alpha$. The receptors of these T cells do not bind the normal MHC:peptide ligands, but instead bind to a number of different ligands, including MHC class IB molecules. T cells are abundant in the gut mucosa as intraepithelial lymphocytes, interspersed between the epithelial cells that line the gut, and have a restricted repertoire of T-cell receptor specificities. There are as many as 10–20 intraepithelial lymphocytes for every 100 epithelial cells in the small intestine in humans and these are about 50% type a and 50% type b. The T-cell receptor gene rearrangements in type a intraepithelial lymphocytes are shared with those of the effector T cells in the lamina propria of the gut and with thoracic duct T cells. This shows that these cells originate from naive T cells primed with antigen in the Peyer's patches and circulate as described in Section 10-14.

Unlike these conventional type a intraepithelial T cells, many of the type b intraepithelial lymphocytes do not undergo positive and negative selection in the thymus (see Chapter 7) and can be found in athymic mice. They express receptors with sequences that have undergone no or minimal divergence from their germline-encoded sequences and can be classified in phylogenetic terms as being at the interface between innate and adaptive immunity.

T cells bearing a $\gamma{:}\delta$ receptor are especially abundant in the gut mucosa compared with other lymphoid tissues. One subset of these $\gamma{:}\delta$ T cells in humans, which expresses a T-cell receptor that uses the Vδ_1 gene segment, carries an activating C-type lectin NK receptor, NKG2D. This binds to two MHC-like molecules—MIC-A and MIC-B—that are expressed on intestinal epithelial cells in response to cellular injury and stress. The injured cells may then be recognized and killed by this subset of $\gamma{:}\delta$ T cells (Fig. 10.23). This illustrates one of the key roles of T cells, which is to patrol and survey the body, destroying cells that express an abnormal phenotype as a result of stress or infection.

The Vδ_1-containing receptor on these T cells may also have a role in allowing them to survey tissues for injured cells. Some human T cells expressing this receptor bind to CD1c, one of the isotypes of the CD1 family of MHC class I-like

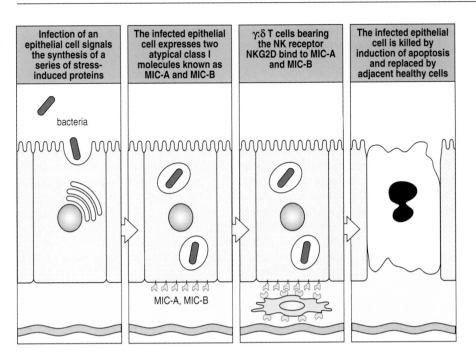

Infection of an epithelial cell signals the synthesis of a series of stress-induced proteins	The infected epithelial cell expresses two atypical class I molecules known as MIC-A and MIC-B	γ:δ T cells bearing the NK receptor NKG2D bind to MIC-A and MIC-B	The infected epithelial cell is killed by induction of apoptosis and replaced by adjacent healthy cells

Fig. 10.23 T cells of the mucosal immune system bearing γ:δ T-cell receptors and an activating NK receptor recognize and kill injured enterocytes. Infection or other injury to enterocytes, the epithelial cells lining the lumen of the gut, stimulates a stress response, which causes expression on the cell surface of two atypical MHC class IB molecules, known as MIC-A and MIC-B. Intraepithelial T cells carrying the NK receptor NKG2D bind MIC-A and MIC-B and induce apoptosis in the injured enterocytes. The dying enterocyte is removed from the epithelium and the local tissue injury is repaired.

molecules that we encountered in Section 10-6. This protein, which shows increased expression on activated monocytes and dendritic cells, presents endogenous lipid and glycolipid antigens to some types of T cell. In response to antigen presentation by CD1c, these T cells secrete IFN-γ, which may be important in polarizing the response of conventional T cells bearing α:β receptors toward a T_H1 response.

A second group of specialized mucosal T cells, so far characterized only in mice, express α:β T-cell receptors together with a CD8 α:α homodimer, instead of the normal CD8 α:β heterodimer that characterizes MHC class I-restricted cytotoxic T cells. These cells can be found in the gut of mice lacking conventional MHC class I molecules, which shows that their development is not dependent on positive selection in the thymus by peptides bound to classical MHC class I molecules. They are, however, absent from mice lacking expression of β_2-microglobulin, which is necessary for the expression of MHC class IB molecules. The ligand recognized by these T cells in mice has been identified as the nonpolymorphic MHC class IB molecule known as Qa-2. These cells are likely to represent a further class of T cells that have a major role in maintaining the integrity of the gut mucosa by recognizing and destroying injured mucosal cells.

About 70% of all intraepithelial lymphocytes are CD8 positive and the large majority of these express the CD8 α:α homodimer. It has been discovered that this CD8 α:α homodimer binds to a nonclassical MHC class I molecule that does not present antigenic peptides, named thymus leukemia antigen (TL). The TL antigen is expressed almost exclusively by intestinal epithelial cells. The interaction of TL with the CD8α:α homodimer seems to modulate the activity of the intraepithelial T cells, reducing their direct cytotoxic activity and increasing their production of cytokines. This discovery further underlines the role of intraepithelial lymphocytes in controlling the repair of damaged mucosal epithelium.

10-16 Secretory IgA is the antibody isotype associated with the mucosal immune system.

The dominant antibody isotype of the mucosal immune system is IgA. This class of antibody is found in humans in two isotypic forms, IgA1 and IgA2. The expression of IgA differs between the two main compartments in which it is found—blood and mucosal secretions. In the blood IgA is found mainly as a monomer, and the ratio of IgA1 to IgA2 is about 4:1. In mucosal secretions IgA is almost exclusively produced as a dimer, and the ratio of IgA1 to IgA2 is about 3:2. Several common intestinal pathogens possess proteolytic enzymes that can digest IgA1, whereas IgA2 is much more resistant to digestion. The higher proportion of plasma cells secreting IgA2 in the gut lamina propria may therefore be the consequence of selective pressure by pathogens against individuals with low IgA2 levels in the gut. The mechanism of isotype switching to IgA was discussed in Section 9-4. The localization of IgA-secreting plasma cells to mucosal tissues is achieved by similar mechanisms to the localization of effector T lymphocytes that we considered in Section 10-14. The B-cell precursors of IgA-secreting plasma cells express the mucosal homing integrin $\alpha_4:\beta_7$ and the chemokine receptor CCR9.

There are special mechanisms for the secretion of polymeric IgA and IgM antibody into the gut lumen (see Section 9-13). Both these antibodies are synthesized throughout the gut by plasma cells located in the lamina propria and are transported into the gut by immature epithelial cells located at the base of the intestinal crypts. These express the polymeric immunoglobulin receptor (poly-Ig receptor) on their basolateral surfaces. This receptor binds polymeric IgA or IgM and transports the antibody by transcytosis to the luminal surface of the gut. Upon reaching the luminal surface of the enterocyte, the antibody is released into the secretions by proteolytic cleavage of the extracellular domain of the polymeric Ig receptor. The cleaved extracellular domain of the polymeric Ig receptor is known as secretory component (frequently abbreviated to SC) and remains associated with polymeric IgA and IgM (see Fig. 9.20). Secretory component serves several physiological roles, including acting as 'glue' to bind secreted IgA and IgM to the mucus layer on the luminal surface of the epithelial layer of the gut, where they can bind to and neutralize gut pathogens and their toxic products (Fig. 10.24). SC also protects these antibodies against proteolytic cleavage. Some SC released into gut mucosal secretions is not bound to antibody; this SC may have a direct innate antibacterial role by binding directly to certain bacteria or bacterial toxins, including fimbrial proteins of *Escherichia coli* and *Clostridium difficile* toxin.

Fig. 10.24 The major antibody isotype present in the lumen of the gut is secretory polymeric IgA. This is synthesized by plasma cells in the lamina propria and transported into the lumen of the gut through epithelial cells at the base of the crypts. Polymeric IgA binds to the mucus layer overlying the gut epithelium and acts as an antigen-specific barrier to pathogens and toxins in the gut lumen.

Polymeric IgA is transported into the gut lumen through epithelial cells at the base of the crypts

Polymeric IgA binds to the mucus layer overlying the gut epithelium

IgA in the gut neutralizes pathogens and their toxins

bacterial toxin

Intestinal mucosal IgA has an important role in the symbiotic relationship between an individual and their gut commensal bacteria, helping to restrict these organisms to the gut lumen. The IgA repertoire in the gut includes antibodies specific for antigens expressed by commensal bacteria; these antibody specificities are not found in serum except in pathological circumstances, when commensal bacteria invade the bloodstream (see Section 10-18). These IgA antibodies are produced locally in the gut by lymphocytes of the B-1 subset (see Section 7-31). B-1 cells are present in mice that lack organized follicular lymphoid tissues and also in mice that are deficient in T lymphocytes: that is, they are T-cell independent and can arise from B-1 cells that are not organized into follicular structures. This mechanism for IgA production may offer a glimpse into the evolutionary history of specific antibody responses.

10-17 Most antigens presented to the mucosal immune system induce tolerance.

We are continuously exposed to a huge array of foreign antigens in the form of food, but these do not normally induce an adaptive immune response. For example, IgA antibodies with high affinity for food antigens do not normally develop. This lack of response occurs despite the fact that the repertoire of lymphocyte antigen receptors has not been negatively selected to remove those specific for food antigens. This is because, like any other foreign antigen, food antigens do not have a role in the central mechanisms of lymphocyte tolerance to self, which are established in the thymus and bone marrow (see Chapter 7).

The feeding of foreign antigens leads typically to a state of specific and active unresponsiveness, a phenomenon known as **oral tolerance**. Thus, no antibody response follows the feeding of a foreign protein such as ovalbumin, although a strong antibody response to this protein can be induced by injecting it subcutaneously, especially if an adjuvant is given as well. However, the feeding of ovalbumin is followed by a prolonged period during which the administration of ovalbumin by injection, even in the presence of adjuvant, elicits no antibody response. This suppression is antigen-specific, because antibody responses to other injected antigens are not affected. These experiments show that there are antigen-specific mechanisms for suppressing peripheral immune responses to antigens delivered by mouth. The mechanisms of oral tolerance are partly understood but, before considering them, we first discuss the contrasting immune responses that are seen in response to bacterial infections of the gut.

10-18 The mucosal immune system can mount an immune response to the normal bacterial flora of the gut.

We each harbor more than 400 species of commensal bacteria, which are present in largest numbers in the colon and ileum. Despite the fact that these bacteria collectively weigh about 1 kg and outnumber us by approximately 10^{14} to 1 (or 10 to 1 in terms of numbers of cells, because there are about 10^{13} cells in the human body), for most of the time we cohabit with our intestinal bacterial flora in a happy symbiotic relationship.

One protective activity of our normal gut flora is to compete with pathogenic bacteria for space and nutrients, preventing their colonization of the gut. This activity is dramatically illustrated by one of the adverse effects of antibiotics. Taking an antibiotic kills large numbers of commensal gut bacteria and thereby offers an ecological niche to bacteria that would not otherwise be able to compete successfully with the normal flora and grow in the gut. One

Fig. 10.25 Treatment with antibiotics causes massive death of the commensal bacteria that normally colonize the colon. This allows pathogenic bacteria to proliferate and occupy an ecological niche that is normally occupied by harmless commensal bacteria. *Clostridium difficile* is an example of a pathogen that produces toxins that can cause severe bloody diarrhea in patients treated with antibiotics.

| The colon is colonized by large numbers of commensal bacteria | Antibiotics kill many of these commensal bacteria | *Clostridium difficile* gains a foothold and produces toxins that cause mucosal injury | Neutrophils and red blood cells leak into gut between injured epithelial cells |

example of a bacterium that grows in the antibiotic-treated gut and can cause a severe infection is *Clostridium difficile*; this produces two toxins, which can cause severe bloody diarrhea associated with mucosal injury (Fig. 10.25).

There are some circumstances in which the normal bacterial inhabitants of the gut cause disease, for example after breakdown of the integrity of the mucosa lining the gut. This can occur after poor blood flow in the gut, or after endotoxemia. In these circumstances, normally innocuous gut bacteria, such as nonpathogenic *Escherichia coli*, can cross the mucosa, invade the bloodstream, and cause fatal systemic infection (see Section 2-24). This illustrates the vital importance of the mucosal surfaces as a barrier to infection. The normal gut flora also become an important cause of systemic infection in patients with immunodeficiency. This illustrates the role of the adaptive immune system in defending the body against the resident gut bacteria, but also shows that this response does not eliminate them from the lumen of the gut, but rather causes a state resembling symbiosis.

The scale of the normal immune response to gut bacteria is illustrated by the study of animals delivered by Cesarean section into a sterile environment in which there is no colonization of the gut by microorganisms. These are known as **germ-free** or **gnotobiotic** animals: they have marked reductions in the size of all peripheral lymphoid organs and reduced levels of antibodies of all isotypes.

10-19 Enteric pathogens cause a local inflammatory response and the development of protective immunity.

In spite of the array of innate immune mechanisms in the gut, and stiff competition from the indigenous flora, the gut is a frequent site of infection by pathogenic microorganisms. These include many species of viruses, pathogenic enteric bacteria including *Salmonella*, *Yersinia*, *Shigella*, and *Listeria*, and protozoa such as *Entamoeba histolytica* and *Cryptosporidium*. These pathogens cause disease in many different ways, but certain common features of infection are crucial to understanding how they stimulate an immune response by the host in contrast to the immunological tolerance shown to the foreign antigens in food.

The most important consequence of infection in the gut, as elsewhere in the body, is the development of an inflammatory response. The release of cytokines and chemokines in this response is key to the induction of an adaptive immune response. The inflammatory mediators stimulate the maturation of dendritic cells and other antigen-presenting cells so that they express co-stimulatory molecules.

The first step in the induction of an inflammatory response to intestinal infection is the detection of the presence of pathogenic organisms. The environment outside the body is rich in microorganisms, in complete contrast to the normally sterile interior. Reflecting this, innate immune mechanisms for sensing bacterial infection are different at epithelial surfaces compared with the interior of the body. As we learned in Section 2-5, cells of myeloid origin, patrolling the sterile interior of the body, carry on their surfaces pattern-recognition receptors such as lectins and Toll-like receptors that can bind and signal the presence of extracellular bacteria. By contrast, epithelial surfaces are constantly exposed to environmental bacteria and, in the case of the gut epithelium, are inundated by the commensal organisms of the gut. To establish an infection through the intestine, potential pathogens have to cross the physical barrier of the epithelium. They can achieve this by invasion of M cells, intracellular invasion of epithelial cells, or through breaches in the epithelial lining of the gut (Fig. 10.26).

Gut epithelial cells do not act as passive victims of infection. They express intracellular receptors that detect bacterial invasion. Two such receptors belong to a family of proteins that are structurally similar to disease-resistance proteins in plants: they contain two structural domains known as NBS (nucleotide-binding site) and LRR (leucine-rich repeat). One of these receptors, Nod1 (also known as CARD4, so named because it contains a caspase-recruitment domain in addition to an NBS and LRR domain), is found in many cell types. It signals the presence of intracellular endotoxin and has been shown to mediate a response to intracellular infection by the gut pathogen *Shigella flexneri*, which causes bacillary dysentery (Fig. 10.27). A second member of the family, Nod2, is largely restricted to monocytes. Nod2 has also been shown to bind intracellular endotoxin, and genetic variants of this protein cause increased susceptibility to the development of the inflammatory bowel disease, Crohn's disease (see Section 12-18). Oligomerization of Nod1 or Nod2 allows them to bind the protein kinase RICK (also known as Rip2 and CARDIAK) through that protein's caspase-recruitment domain, leading to the activation of the NFκB pathway (see Section 6-17).

Salmonellae enter and kill M cells and then infect macrophages and epithelial cells

Gut lumen

M cell

TLR-5

Salmonellae invade the luminal surface of epithelial cells

Salmonellae enter dendrites of dendritic cells that are sampling the gut luminal contents

Fig. 10.26 *Salmonella typhimurium*, an important cause of food poisoning, can penetrate the gut epithelial layer by three routes. In the first route (left panel), *S. typhimurium* adheres to and enters M cells, which it then kills by causing apoptosis. Having penetrated the epithelium, it infects macrophages and gut epithelial cells. Epithelial cells express TLR-5 on their basal membrane; this binds flagellin on the salmonella, activating an inflammatory response via the NFκB pathway. Salmonella can also invade gut epithelial cells directly by adherence of their fimbriae to the luminal epithelial surface (middle panel). In the third route of entry, dendritic cells sampling the gut lumen protrude dendrites between epithelial cells. These effectively breach the epithelial layer and can be infected by salmonellae in the lumen (right panel).

| Shigellae penetrate gut epithelium through M cells | Shigellae invade basal surface of epithelial cells and spread to other epithelial cells | Shigella LPS binds and oligomerizes Nod1, activating the NFκB pathway | Activated epithelium secretes CXCL8, recruiting neutrophils |

Fig. 10.27 *Shigella flexneri*, a cause of bacterial dysentery, infects intestinal epithelial cells, triggering activation of the NFκB pathway. *Shigella flexneri* binds to M cells and is translocated beneath the gut epithelium (first panel). The bacteria infect intestinal epithelial cells from their basal surface and are released into the cytoplasm (second panel). The lipopolysaccharide (LPS) on the shigellae binds to and oligomerizes the protein Nod1; oligomerized Nod1 binds the protein kinase RICK, which triggers activation of the NFκB pathway, leading to transcription of chemokines and cytokines (third panel). Activated epithelial cells release the chemokine CXCL8 (IL-8), which acts as a neutrophil chemoattractant (fourth panel). IκK, IκB kinase; IκB, inhibitor of NFκB.

Epithelial cells also have molecules on their surface that can detect infection. These are of two types. The first are polarized in distribution, expressed on the basal surface of the cell, and only accessible to organisms that have penetrated beneath the epithelium, for example by trafficking through M cells. An example of this type of receptor is TLR-5, which binds bacterial flagellin and signals via the NFκB pathway to synthesize and release inflammatory mediators. Mutant mice that lack this receptor show increased susceptibility to salmonella infection. The second group of molecules found on epithelial cell surfaces comprises receptors such as TLR-4, which are expressed at a significant level only on the luminal surface in the presence of inflammation, in which context they may augment host defense.

Epithelial cells that have sensed bacteria and activated the NFκB pathway release cytokines and chemokines. These include the chemokine CXCL8 (IL-8), which is a potent neutrophil chemoattractant, and CC chemokines, including CCL2, CCL3, CCL4, and CCL5, which are chemoattractants for monocytes, eosinophils, and T lymphocytes (see Fig. 2.41). In this way, the onset of infection triggers an influx of inflammatory cells and lymphocytes, leading to the induction of an immune response to the antigens of the infectious agent. Injury and stress to the enterocytes lining the gut may also stimulate the expression of nonclassical MHC molecules, such as MIC-A and MIC-B (see Section 10-15). These act as ligands to the receptors on γ:δ T cells at the base of the crypts, which kill the infected mucosal cell, thereby promoting repair and recovery of the injured mucosa (see Fig. 10.23).

Several pathogens directly exploit the M cell as a means of invasion. Some viruses are transported through the M cell by transcytosis and from the subepithelial space are able to establish systemic infection. For example, from this site polio virus and retroviruses enter intestinal neuronal cells and spread to the central nervous system. HIV, which we will discuss in detail in Chapter 11, may use a similar route into the lymphoid tissue of the rectal mucosa, where it first encounters and infects macrophages.

Many of the most important enteric bacteria that cause infections in humans gain entry to the body through M cells. Invasion by this route delivers bacteria straight to the lymphoid system of the host. Depending on the pathogenicity of the organism and the strength of the host adaptive immune response, infections that breach the gut mucosa may be cleared with little tissue injury, or cause a local inflammatory response, or invade the bloodstream or lymphatics and result in a systemic infection. Bacteria that specifically target M cells include *Salmonella typhi*, the causative agent of typhoid, and *S. typhimurium*, a major cause of bacterial food poisoning (see Fig. 10.26). These bacteria cause a brisk local and systemic inflammatory response associated with the induction of T_H1-type T-cell responses and antibody responses of the IgG and IgA classes.

10-20 Infection by *Helicobacter pylori* causes a chronic inflammatory response, which can cause peptic ulcers, carcinoma of the stomach, and unusual lymphoid tumors.

There is one exceptional bacterial infection of the stomach, in which the inflammatory and immune response to the organism causes the disease instead of clearing the infection. *Helicobacter pylori*, which infects many millions of people around the world, adheres to the mucosa of the stomach and causes a local inflammatory response, with the release of the chemokine CXCL8 and the influx of leukocytes. There is no overt disease in most people infected, but up to 5% make one of two very different responses to the infection. In some, there is excessive release of the hormone gastrin, which stimulates acid production and the development of peptic ulcers. In others, chronic inflammation has the opposite effect, leading to atrophy of the stomach, which is associated with reduced acid production and an increased risk of carcinoma of the stomach (Fig. 10.28). Rarely, lymphomas known as MALT lymphomas, because of their origin from the mucosa-associated lymphoid tissue, arise from the B lymphocytes that accumulate in the chronic inflammatory lymphoid infiltrates of the stomach. These are extraordinary tumors because some of them, despite being monoclonal proliferations with a transformed phenotype, are still dependent for survival and growth on antigenic or other inflammatory stimulation by *H. pylori*. These tumors may regress if the *H. pylori* infection is effectively eliminated by antibiotics alone.

Fig. 10.28 *Helicobacter pylori* infects the stomachs of many millions of people. In some, it stimulates the G cells of the stomach to secrete gastrin, which leads to excess acid production by the stomach, causing peptic ulceration. In others, it causes chronic inflammation of the mucosa, leading to atrophy and loss of acid production. The chronic inflammation of the stomach wall in these individuals can lead to the development of gastric carcinoma.

10-21 In the absence of inflammatory stimuli, the normal response of the mucosal immune system to foreign antigens is tolerance.

We have seen that there are two opposing outcomes of exposure to foreign antigens entering through the mucosa of the gut. Tolerance to food antigens contrasts with a vigorous antibody and T-cell response after exposure to pathogens. The essential difference between antigenic challenge by food and that by pathogens is that the pathogens cause inflammation whereas food does not. Both the antigens within food and the antigens within pathogens are presented by antigen-presenting cells to T lymphocytes, but the contexts in which these two sources of antigen are presented are quite different.

Three different responses that T cells can make to peptides derived from foods and other antigens delivered via the mucosa may account for the phenomenon of oral tolerance. The first is the deletion of antigen-specific T cells by the induction of apoptosis, which has been found to occur in experimental animals in response to the oral intake of very large, and probably nonphysiological, doses of antigen. This is probably not the most important mechanism of oral tolerance, although it may contribute.

The second response is anergy, in which T cells presented with peptide in the absence of co-stimulatory signals become refractory to further stimulation with antigen (see Section 8-11). The development of anergy in response to a food antigen was demonstrated by feeding ovalbumin to mice that had large numbers of T cells carrying a transgenically expressed T-cell receptor for an ovalbumin peptide epitope (see Appendix I, Section A-46). After feeding of ovalbumin, T cells bearing the transgenic T-cell receptor could still be detected, but these were totally refractory to further stimulation by ovalbumin *in vitro* and *in vivo*, even when ovalbumin was injected systemically together with an adjuvant (Fig. 10.29).

The third response involves the development of regulatory T cells, which can actively suppress antigen-specific responses after rechallenge with antigen. One subset of T cells has been described that produces IL-4, IL-10, and TGF-β on stimulation with antigen. These cells have been called T_H3 cells. A similar population secretes TGF-β in an IL-10-dependent manner and has been named T_R1 (T regulatory 1 cells). This pattern of cytokine secretion in response to antigen-specific stimulation inhibits the development of T_H1 responses and is associated with low levels of antibody and a virtual absence of inflammatory T-cell responses. These and other regulatory T cells will be discussed in more detail in Chapter 13 in the context of autoimmunity. The γ:δ T cells that are abundant throughout the mucosal immune system may also have a role in oral tolerance, because tolerance seems to be reduced in mice lacking this subset of T lymphocytes.

	Mice fed	
	Ovalbumin	Control
Number of ovalbumin-specific CD4 T cells	Low	High
Response to ovalbumin	–	+++

Fig. 10.29 T-cell anergy following feeding of antigen. Mice were injected with CD4 T cells bearing a transgenic receptor specific for an ovalbumin peptide. Two days later they were fed with ovalbumin or a control protein; 4 days later they were injected with the relevant ovalbumin peptide with adjuvant, and 8 days later the draining lymph node was harvested. The number of ovalbumin-specific transgenic T cells in this was measured and the cells' proliferative response was assessed to stimulation by ovalbumin peptide *in vitro*. Mice fed with ovalbumin demonstrated a small reduction, compared with control-fed mice, in the number of transgenic T cells recovered, showing some deletion of T cells by orally fed antigen. However, many transgenic T cells remained in the ovalbumin-fed mice and these were refractory to stimulation by antigen *in vitro*, compared with the control-fed mice, which showed vigorous proliferative responses. These transgenic T cells had become anergic after oral intake of antigen.

Antigen-specific suppression is a form of oral tolerance that can be transferred experimentally to recipient animals by lymphocytes derived from animals that have been fed with antigen. When an animal that has been injected with such lymphocytes is exposed to the same antigen for the first time, these regulatory cells respond to the antigen and inhibit the responses of naive T cells in the recipient animal. This contrasts with anergic T cells, which cannot transfer oral tolerance after transfer to a naive animal.

To understand the phenomenon of oral tolerance, it is essential to understand how antigens delivered orally are presented to T cells. Two routes of antigen presentation of soluble food antigens have been characterized that may induce T-cell responses favoring tolerance rather than immune activation. The first is presentation of soluble food antigens by the professional antigen-presenting cells of the gut and other peripheral lymphoid organs. In the absence of inflammatory stimuli, antigen presentation by dendritic cells favors the induction of tolerance rather than T-cell activation. Dendritic cells in Peyer's patches have been shown to express IL-10 and IL-4, in contrast to dendritic cells in peripheral lymph nodes, which express IFN-γ and IL-12. However, this heterogeneity of cytokine responses does not fully explain tolerance to food antigens. These antigens may be detected in the bloodstream after feeding and there is evidence that the induction of tolerance to food antigens takes place in lymph nodes and spleen as well as in the mucosal lymphoid system.

The second possible route of presentation of food antigens is by the enterocytes of the gut. These express MHC class I and MHC class II molecules in the absence of co-stimulatory molecules, and thus may induce anergy when they present antigens to intraepithelial lymphocytes.

We will discuss each of these mechanisms of tolerance further in Chapter 13, where we consider how the loss of tolerance to self tissues may contribute to the development of autoimmune disease. As we will see in Chapter 14, one of the strategies for treating allergy and autoimmune disease is to attempt to manipulate the nature of the antigen-specific response to stimulate T cells with the properties of such regulatory T cells.

Summary.

The immune system can be divided into a series of functional anatomical compartments, of which the two most important are the peripheral lymphoid system made up of the conventionally studied spleen and lymph nodes, and the mucosal lymphoid system. Specific homing mechanisms for lymphocytes to each of these compartments serve to maintain a separate population of lymphocytes in each. The mucosal surfaces of the body are highly vulnerable to infection and possess a complex array of innate and adaptive mechanisms of immunity. The adaptive immune system of the mucosa-associated lymphoid tissues differs from that of the rest of the peripheral lymphoid system in several respects. The types and distribution of T cells differ, with significantly greater numbers of γ:δ T cells in the gut mucosa compared with peripheral lymph nodes and blood. The major antibody type secreted across the epithelial cells lining mucosal surfaces is secretory polymeric IgA. The mucosal lymphoid system is exposed to a vast array of foreign antigens from foods, from the commensal bacteria of the gut, and from pathogenic microorganisms and parasites. No immune response can normally be detected to food antigens. Indeed, soluble antigens taken by mouth may induce antigen-specific tolerance or antigen-specific suppression. In contrast, pathogenic microorganisms induce strong protective T_H1 responses. It is an important challenge to understand these contrasting specific immune responses. The key distinction between tolerance and the development of powerful protective adaptive immune responses is the context in which peptide antigen is presented to T lymphocytes in the mucosal immune system. In the absence of inflammation, presentation of peptides to T cells by MHC molecules on antigen-presenting cells occurs in the absence of co-stimulation. By contrast, pathogenic microorganisms induce inflammatory responses in the tissues, which stimulate the maturation and expression of co-stimulatory molecules on antigen-presenting cells. This form of antigen presentation to T cells favors the development of a protective T_H1 response.

Immunological memory.

Having considered how an appropriate primary immune response is mounted to pathogens in both the peripheral lymphoid system and the mucosa-associated lymphoid tissues, we now turn to immunological memory, which is a feature of both compartments. Perhaps the most important consequence of an adaptive immune response is the establishment of a state of immunological memory. **Immunological memory** is the ability of the immune system to respond more rapidly and effectively to pathogens that have been encountered previously, and reflects the preexistence of a clonally expanded population of antigen-specific lymphocytes. Memory responses, which are called secondary, tertiary, and so on, depending on the number of exposures to antigen, also differ qualitatively from primary responses. This is particularly clear in the antibody response, in which the characteristics of antibodies produced in secondary and subsequent responses are distinct from those produced in the primary response to the same antigen. Memory T-cell responses can also be distinguished qualitatively from the responses of naive or effector T cells. The principal focus of this section is the altered character of memory responses, although we also discuss emerging explanations of how immunological memory persists after exposure to antigen.

10-22 Immunological memory is long-lived after infection or vaccination.

Most children in developed countries are now vaccinated against measles virus; before vaccination was widespread, most were naturally exposed to this virus and suffered from an acute, unpleasant, and potentially dangerous viral illness. Whether through vaccination or infection, children exposed to the virus acquire long-term protection from measles. The same is true of many other acute infectious diseases: this state of protection is a consequence of immunological memory.

The basis of immunological memory has been hard to explore experimentally. Although the phenomenon was first recorded by the ancient Greeks and has been exploited routinely in vaccination programs for over 200 years, it is just now becoming clear that memory reflects a small but persistent population of specialized **memory cells** that is independent of the continued persistence of the original antigen that induced them. This mechanism of maintaining memory is consistent with the finding that only individuals who were themselves previously exposed to a given infectious agent are immune, and that memory is not dependent on repeated exposure to infection as a result of contacts with other infected individuals. This was established by observations made of populations on remote islands, where a virus such as measles can cause an epidemic, infecting all people living on the island at that time, after which the virus disappears for many years. On reintroduction from outside the island, the virus does not affect the original population but causes disease in those people born since the first epidemic. This means that immunological memory need not be maintained by repeated exposure to infectious virus.

Instead, it is most likely that memory is sustained by long-lived antigen-specific lymphocytes that were induced by the original exposure and that persist until a second encounter with the pathogen. Although most of the memory cells are in a resting state, careful studies have shown that a small percentage are dividing at any one time. What stimulates this infrequent cell division is unclear. However, cytokines such as those produced either constitutively or during the course of antigen-specific immune responses directed at non-cross-reactive antigens could be responsible. IL-7 helps to maintain memory T cells generally, and IL-15 has been shown to maintain memory CD8 T cells. Regardless of cell division, the number of memory cells for a given antigen is highly regulated, remaining practically constant during the memory phase. Naive T cells require contact with self MHC molecules for their long-term survival in the periphery. It seems that memory T cells do not have this requirement, instead depending on IL-7 and IL-15 for survival. However, it was recently discovered that memory T cells surviving after transfer to MHC-deficient hosts have some defects in typical T-cell memory functions, indicating that stimulation by self-MHC:self-peptide complexes may be required for their optimal function.

Immunological memory can be measured experimentally in various ways. Adoptive transfer assays (see Appendix I, Section A-42) of lymphocytes from animals immunized with simple, nonliving antigens have been favored for such studies, as the antigen cannot proliferate. In these experiments, the existence of memory cells is measured purely in terms of the transfer of specific responsiveness from an immunized, or 'primed,' animal to a nonimmunized recipient. After antigen administration, animals that received memory cells have a faster and more robust response than controls that did not receive cells or that received cells from nonimmune donors.

When an animal is first immunized with a protein antigen, functional helper T-cell memory against that antigen appears abruptly and is at its maximal level after 5 days or so. Functional antigen-specific B-cell memory appears some days later, because B-cell activation cannot begin until armed helper T cells are available, and B cells must then enter a phase of proliferation and selection in lymphoid tissue. By 1 month after immunization, memory B cells are present at their maximal levels. These levels are then maintained with little alteration for the lifetime of the animal. It is important to recognize in these experiments that functional memory can include both the precursors to memory cells and the memory cells themselves. These precursors are probably activated T and B cells, some of whose progeny will later differentiate into memory cells. Thus, precursors to memory can appear shortly after immunization, even though resting memory-type lymphocytes may not yet have developed. In the following sections we look in more detail at the changes that occur in lymphocytes after antigen priming that lead to the development of resting memory lymphocytes, and discuss the mechanisms that might account for these changes.

10-23 Both clonal expansion and clonal differentiation contribute to immunological memory in B cells.

Immunological memory in B cells can be examined by isolating B cells from immunized mice and restimulating them with antigen in the presence of armed helper T cells specific for the same antigen. The response of these primed B cells can be compared with the primary B-cell response seen on isolating B cells from unimmunized mice and stimulating them with antigen in the same way (Fig. 10.30). By these means it is possible to show that antigen-specific memory B cells differ both quantitatively and qualitatively from naive B cells. B cells that can respond to antigen increase in frequency by up to 100-fold after priming (see Fig. 10.30) and produce antibody of higher

Fig. 10.30 The generation of secondary antibody responses from memory B cells is distinct from the generation of the primary antibody response. These responses can be studied and compared by isolating B cells from immunized and unimmunized donor mice, and stimulating them in culture in the presence of armed antigen-specific effector T cells. The primary response usually consists of antibody molecules made by plasma cells derived from a relatively large number of different precursor B cells. The antibodies are of relatively low affinity, with few somatic mutations. The secondary response derives from far fewer high-affinity precursor B cells, which have undergone significant clonal expansion. Their receptors and antibodies are of high affinity for the antigen and show extensive somatic mutation. Thus, there is usually only a 10–100-fold increase in the frequency of activatable B cells after priming; however, the quality of the antibody response is altered radically, such that these precursors induce a far more intense and effective response.

	Source of B cells	
	Unimmunized donor Primary response	Immunized donor Secondary response
Frequency of specific B cells	$1{:}10^4 - 1{:}10^5$	$1{:}10^2 - 1{:}10^3$
Isotype of antibody produced	IgM > IgG	IgG, IgA
Affinity of antibody	Low	High
Somatic hypermutation	Low	High

average affinity than unprimed B lymphocytes; the affinity of that antibody continues to increase during the ongoing secondary and subsequent antibody responses (Fig. 10.31). The secondary antibody response is characterized in its first few days by the production of small amounts of IgM antibody and larger amounts of IgG antibody, with some IgA and IgE. These antibodies are produced by memory B cells that have already switched from IgM to these more mature isotypes and express IgG, IgA, or IgE on their surface, as well as a somewhat higher level of MHC class II molecules and B7.1 (CD80) than is characteristic of naive B cells. Increased affinity for antigen and increased levels of MHC class II and co-stimulatory molecules facilitate antigen uptake and presentation, and allow memory B cells to initiate their critical interactions with armed helper T cells at lower doses of antigen. Unlike memory T cells, which can enter nonlymphoid tissues as a result of changes in cell-surface molecules that affect migration and homing, it is thought that memory B cells continue to recirculate through the same secondary lymphoid compartments that contain naive B cells, principally the follicles of the spleen, lymph nodes, and Peyer's patches. Some memory B cells can also be found in splenic marginal zones (Fig. 1.9), although it is not clear whether these represent a distinct subset of memory B cells.

The distinction between primary and secondary antibody responses is most clearly seen in those cases in which the primary response is dominated by antibodies that are closely related to each other and show little if any somatic hypermutation. This occurs in inbred mouse strains in response to certain haptens that are recognized by a limited set of naive B cells. The antibodies produced are encoded by the same V_H and V_L genes in all animals of the strain, suggesting that these variable regions have been selected during evolution for recognition of determinants on pathogens that happen to cross-react with some haptens. As a result of the uniformity of these primary responses, changes in the antibody molecules produced in secondary responses to the same antigens are easy to observe. These differences include

Fig. 10.31 Both the affinity and the amount of antibody increase with repeated immunization. The upper panel shows the increase in the level of antibody with time after primary, followed by secondary and tertiary, immunization; the lower panel shows the increase in the affinity of the antibodies. The increase in affinity (affinity maturation) is seen largely in IgG antibody (as well as in IgA and IgE, which are not shown) coming from mature B cells that have undergone isotype switching and somatic hypermutation to yield higher-affinity antibodies. Although some affinity maturation occurs in the primary antibody response, most arises in later responses to repeated antigen injections. Note that these graphs are on a logarithmic scale.

not only numerous somatic hypermutations in antibodies containing the dominant V regions but also the addition of antibodies containing V_H and V_L gene segments not detected in the primary response. These are thought to derive from B cells that were activated at low frequency during the primary response, and thus were not detected, and which differentiated into memory B cells.

10-24 Repeated immunization leads to increasing affinity of antibody owing to somatic hypermutation and selection by antigen in germinal centers.

Upon reexposure to the same antigen, a secondary immune response will ensue. In some ways this resembles the primary immune response, with the initial proliferation of B cells and T cells at the interface between the T-cell and B-cell zones. The secondary response is characterized by early and vigorous generation of plasma cells, thus accounting for early profuse IgG production. Some B cells that have not yet undergone terminal differentiation can migrate into the follicle and become **germinal center B cells**. There, these B cells enter a second proliferative phase, during which the DNA encoding their immunoglobulin V domains again undergoes somatic hypermutation before the B cells differentiate into antibody-secreting plasma cells (see Section 9-7).

The antibodies produced by plasma cells in the primary and early secondary response are important in driving affinity maturation in the secondary response. In secondary and subsequent immune responses, any persisting antibodies produced by the B cells that differentiated in the primary response are immediately available to bind the newly introduced antigen. Some of these antibodies divert antigen to phagocytes for degradation and disposal (see Section 9-20). If there is sufficient preexisting antibody to clear or inactivate the pathogen, it is possible that no immune response will ensue. However, if there is a trace excess of antigen, B cells whose receptors bind the antigen with sufficient avidity to compete with the preexisting antibody will take up the uncomplexed antigen and process it into peptide fragments that bind to MHC class II molecules. These foreign peptide:self-MHC class II complexes are presented to armed helper T cells surrounding and infiltrating the germinal centers (see Section 9-2). Contact between the B cells presenting antigenic peptides and armed helper T cells specific for the same peptide leads to an exchange of activating signals and the rapid proliferation of both activated antigen-specific B cells and helper T cells. Thus, only the higher-affinity memory B cells are efficiently stimulated in the secondary immune response. In this way the affinity of the antibody produced rises progressively, because only B cells with high-affinity antigen receptors can bind antigen efficiently and be driven to proliferate by antigen-specific helper T cells (Fig. 10.32).

Fig. 10.32 The mechanism of affinity maturation in an antibody response. At the beginning of a primary response, B cells with receptors of a wide variety of affinities (K_A), most of which will bind antigen with low affinity, take up antigen, present it to helper T cells, and become activated to produce antibody of varying and relatively low affinity (top panel). These antibodies then bind and clear antigen, so that only those B cells with receptors of the highest affinity can continue to capture antigen and interact effectively with helper T cells. Such B cells will therefore be selected to undergo further expansion and clonal differentiation, and the antibodies they produce will dominate a secondary response (middle panel). These higher-affinity antibodies will in turn compete for antigen and select for the activation of B cells bearing receptors of still higher affinity in the tertiary response (bottom panel).

10-25 Memory T cells are increased in frequency and have distinct activation requirements and cell-surface proteins that distinguish them from armed effector T cells.

Because the T-cell receptor does not undergo isotype switching or somatic hypermutation, it is not as easy to identify a memory T cell unequivocally as it is a memory B cell. After immunization, the number of T cells reactive to a given antigen increases markedly as effector T cells are produced, and then falls back to persist at a level significantly (100–1000-fold) above the initial frequency for the rest of the animal's or person's life (Fig. 10.33). These persisting cells are designated memory T cells (Fig. 10.34). They carry cell-surface proteins more characteristic of armed effector cells than of naive T cells but are long-lived cells with distinctive cell-surface proteins, responses to stimuli, and expression of genes that control cell survival. In B cells, the distinction between effector and memory cells is more obvious and has been recognized for some time. This is because effector B cells, as we saw in Chapter 9, are terminally differentiated plasma cells that have already been activated to secrete antibody until they die.

A major problem in experiments aimed at establishing the existence of memory T cells is that most assays for T-cell effector function take several days, during which the putative memory T cells are reinduced to effector cell status. Thus, these assays do not distinguish preexisting effector cells from memory T cells. This problem does not apply to cytotoxic T cells, however, because cytotoxic effector T cells can program a target cell for lysis in 5 minutes. Memory CD8 T cells need to be reactivated to become cytotoxic, but they can do so without undergoing DNA synthesis, as shown by studies carried out in the presence of mitotic inhibitors. Recently it has become possible to track particular clones of antigen-specific CD8 T cells by staining them with tetrameric MHC:peptide complexes (see Appendix I, Section A-28). It has been found that the number of antigen-specific CD8 T cells increases markedly during an infection, and then decreases by up to 100-fold; nevertheless, this final level is distinctly higher than before priming. These cells continue to express some markers characteristic of activated cells, such as CD44, but stop expressing other activation markers, such as CD69. In addition they express more Bcl-2, a protein that promotes cell survival and may be responsible for the long half-life of memory CD8 cells. The proteins that are differentially expressed among naive, effector, and memory T cells are summarized in Fig. 10.35. Memory cells are more sensitive to restimulation by antigen than are naive cells, and more quickly and more vigorously produce cytokines such as IFN-γ in response to such stimulation.

The issue is more difficult to address for CD4 T-cell responses, in part because their responses are smaller than those of CD8 T cells and also because until recently there was a lack of peptide:MHC class II reagents such as the peptide:MHC class I tetramers that can be used to reveal antigen-specific T cells. Nonetheless, the transfer and priming of naive T cells carrying T-cell receptor transgenes that give the T cells a known MHC:peptide specificity has made it possible to visualize memory CD4 T cells. They appear as a long-lived population of cells that share some surface characteristics of activated

Fig.10.33 Generation of memory T cells after a virus infection. After an infection, in this case a reactivation of latent cytomegalovirus (CMV), the number of T cells specific for viral antigen increases dramatically and then falls back to give a sustained low level of memory T cells. The top panel shows the numbers of T cells (orange); the bottom panel shows the course of the virus infection (blue), as estimated by the amount of viral DNA in the blood. Data courtesy of G. Aubert.

effector T cells but are distinct from effector T cells in that they require additional restimulation before acting on target cells. Changes in three cell-surface proteins—L-selectin, CD44, and CD45—are particularly significant after exposure to antigen. L-selectin is lost on most memory CD4 T cells, whereas CD44 levels are increased on all memory T cells; these changes contribute to directing the migration of memory T cells from the blood into the tissues rather than directly into lymphoid tissues. The isoform of CD45 changes because of alternative splicing of exons that encode the extracellular domain of CD45, leading to isoforms that are smaller and more readily associated with the T-cell receptor and facilitate antigen recognition (see Fig. 10.35). These changes are characteristic of cells that have been activated to become armed effector T cells (see Section 8-12), yet some of the cells on which these changes have occurred have many characteristics of resting CD4 T cells, suggesting that they represent memory CD4 T cells. Only after reexposure to antigen on an antigen-presenting cell do they achieve armed effector T-cell status and acquire all the characteristics of armed T_H2 or T_H1 cells, secreting IL-4 and IL-5, or IFN-γ, respectively.

It therefore seems reasonable to designate these cells as memory CD4 T cells, and to surmise that naive CD4 T cells can differentiate into armed effector T cells or into memory T cells that can later be activated to effector status. Recent experiments show that both CD4 and CD8 T cells can differentiate into two types of memory cell (Fig. 10.36), with distinct activation characteristics. One type are called **effector memory cells** because they can rapidly mature into effector T cells and secrete large amounts of IFN-γ, IL-4, and IL-5 early after restimulation. These cells lack the chemokine receptor CCR7 but express high levels of β_1 and β_2 integrins, as well as receptors for inflammatory chemokines. This profile suggests that these effector memory cells are specialized for quickly entering inflamed tissues. The other type are called **central memory cells**. They express CCR7 and would therefore be expected to recirculate more easily to the T-cell zones of peripheral lymphoid tissues, as do naive T cells. These central memory cells are very sensitive to T-cell receptor cross-linking and rapidly express CD40 ligand in response to it; however, they take longer to differentiate into effector cells and thus do not secrete as much cytokine as effector memory cells do early after restimulation.

As with memory CD8 T cells, the field is currently being revolutionized by the direct staining of CD4 T cells with peptide:MHC class II oligomers (see Appendix I, Section A-28). This technique allows one not only to identify antigen-specific CD4 T cells but also, by using intracellular cytokine staining (see Appendix I, Section A-27), to determine whether they are T_H1 or T_H2 cells. These improvements in the identification and phenotyping of CD4 T cells will rapidly increase our knowledge of these hitherto mysterious cells and could contribute valuable information on naive, memory, and effector CD4 T cells.

10-26 In immune individuals, secondary and subsequent responses are mediated mainly by memory lymphocytes.

In the normal course of an infection, a pathogen first proliferates to a level sufficient to elicit an adaptive immune response and then stimulates the production of antibodies and effector T cells that eliminate the pathogen from the body. Most of the armed effector T cells then die, and antibody levels gradually decline after the pathogen is eliminated, because the antigens that elicited the response are no longer present at the level needed to sustain it. We can think of this as feedback inhibition of the response. Memory T and B cells remain, however, and maintain a heightened ability to mount a response to a recurrence of infection with the same pathogen.

Fig. 10.34 Encounter with antigen generates effector T cells and long-lived memory T cells. On priming with antigen, a naive T cell divides and differentiates. Most of the progeny are relatively short-lived effector cells. However, some become long-lived memory T cells, which are sustained by cytokines. The continued function, but not survival, of memory T cells also requires contact with MHC molecules.

Fig. 10.35 Expression of many cell-surface molecules alters when naive T cells become memory T cells. The changes include increases in molecules that control the adhesion of the T cell to antigen-presenting cells and endothelial cells; molecules such as chemokine receptors that affect migration to sites of inflammation; factors and receptors that promote survival of memory cells; and proteins that are involved in effector functions, such as granzyme B. Some changes also increase the sensitivity of the memory T cell to antigen stimulation. Many of these changes are also seen on cells that have been activated to become armed effector T cells, but some changes, such as expression of CD25 and CD69, are specific to effector cells, whereas others, such as expression of the survival factor Bcl-2, are limited to long-lived memory cells. The chart represents a general picture that applies to both CD4 and CD8 T cells in mice and humans, but some details that may differ between these sets of cells have been omitted for simplicity.

Molecule	Naive	Effector	Memory	Comments
CD44	+	+++	+++	Cell adhesion molecule
CD45RO	+	+++	+++	Modulates T-cell receptor signaling
CD45RA	+++	+	+++	Modulates T-cell receptor signaling
CD62L	+++	–	Some +++	Receptor for homing to lymph node
CCR7	+++	+/–	Some +++	Chemokine receptor for homing to lymph node
CD69	–	+++	–	Early activation antigen
Bcl-2	++	+/–	+++	Promotes cell survival
Interferon-γ	–	+++	+++	Effector cytokine; mRNA present and protein made on activation
Granzyme B	–	+++	+/–	Effector molecule in cell killing
FasL	–	+++	+	Effector molecule in cell killing
CD122	+/–	++	++	Part of receptor for IL-15 and IL-2
CD25	–	++	–	Part of receptor for IL-2
CD127	++	–	+++	Part of receptor for IL-7
Ly6C	+	+++	+++	GPI-linked protein
CXCR4	+	+	++	Receptor for chemokine CXCL12; controls tissue migration
CCR5	+	++	Some +++	Receptor for chemokines CCL3 and CCL4; tissue migration

The antibody and memory lymphocytes remaining in an immunized individual also largely prevent the activation of naive B and T cells by the same antigen. The suppression of naive lymphocyte activation can be shown by passively transferring antibody or memory T cells to naive recipients; when the recipient is thus immunized, naive lymphocytes do not respond to the original antigen, but responses to other antigens are unaffected. This has been put to practical use to prevent the response of Rh⁻ mothers to their Rh⁺ children; if anti-Rh antibody is given to the mother before she reacts to her child's red blood cells, her response will be inhibited. The mechanism of this suppression is likely to involve the antibody-mediated clearance and destruction of the child's red blood cells, thus preventing naive B cells and T cells from mounting an immune response. Memory B-cell responses are not inhibited by antibody against the antigen, so the Rh⁻ mothers at risk must be identified and treated before a response has occurred. Memory B cells are much more sensitive, because of their high affinity and alterations in their B-cell receptor signaling requirements, to smaller amounts of antigen that cannot be efficiently cleared by

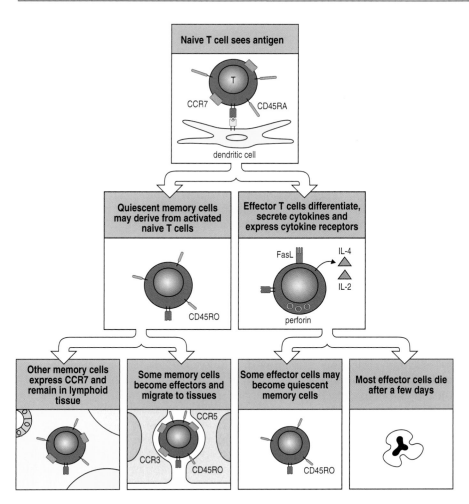

Fig. 10.36 T cells can differentiate into different types of memory cell. Quiescent memory cells bearing the characteristic CD45RO surface protein can arise from activated effector cells (right half of diagram) or directly from activated naive T cells (left half of diagram). Two types of memory T cell can derive from quiescent memory cells. One type matures rapidly into effector T cells after restimulation and secretes large amounts of IFN-γ, IL-4, and IL-5. They do not express the receptor CCR7, but express receptors (CCR3 and CCR5) for inflammatory chemokines. The other type of memory T cell expresses CCR7 and remains in peripheral lymphoid tissues after restimulation.

the passive anti-Rh antibody. The ability of memory B cells to be activated to produce antibody, even when exposed to preexisting antibody, also allows secondary antibody responses to occur in individuals who are already immune.

Adoptive transfer of immune T cells (see Appendix I, Section A-42) to naive syngeneic mice also prevents the activation of naive T cells by antigen. This has been shown most clearly for cytotoxic T cells. It is possible that, once re-activated, the memory CD8 T cells regain cytotoxic activity sufficiently rapidly to kill the antigen-presenting cells that are required to activate naive CD8 T cells, thereby inhibiting the latter's activation.

These mechanisms might also explain the phenomenon known as **original antigenic sin**. This term was coined to describe the tendency of people to make antibodies only against epitopes expressed on the first influenza virus variant to which they are exposed, even in subsequent infections with variants that bear additional, highly immunogenic, epitopes (Fig. 10.37). Antibodies against the original virus will tend to suppress responses of naive B cells specific for the new epitopes. This might benefit the host by using only those B cells that can respond most rapidly and effectively to the virus. This pattern is broken only if the person is exposed to an influenza virus that lacks all epitopes seen in the original infection, because now no preexisting antibodies bind the virus and naive B cells are able to respond.

Summary.

Protective immunity against reinfection is one of the most important consequences of adaptive immunity operating through the clonal selection of lymphocytes. Protective immunity depends not only on preformed antibody and armed effector T cells but most importantly on the establishment of a population of lymphocytes that mediate long-lived immunological memory. The capacity of these cells to respond rapidly to restimulation with the same antigen can be transferred to naive recipients by primed B and T cells. The precise changes that distinguish naive, effector, and memory lymphocytes are now being characterized and, with the advent of receptor-specific reagents, the relative contributions of clonal expansion and differentiation to the memory phenotype are rapidly being clarified. Memory B cells can also be distinguished by changes in their immunoglobulin genes because of isotype switching and somatic hypermutation, and secondary and subsequent immune responses are characterized by antibodies with increasing affinity for the antigen.

Summary to Chapter 10.

Vertebrates resist infection by pathogenic microorganisms in several ways. The innate defenses can act immediately and may succeed in repelling the infection, but if not they are followed by a series of induced early responses that help to contain the infection as adaptive immunity develops. These first two phases of the immune response rely on recognizing the presence of infection by using the nonclonotypic receptors of the innate immune system. They are covered in detail in Chapter 2 but are summarized in Fig. 10.38. Specialized subsets of T cells and B cells, which can be viewed as intermediates between innate and adaptive immunity, are referred to as innate-like lymphocytes. These include NK T cells, which can bias the CD4 T-cell response towards a T_H1 or a T_H2 phenotype, and a subset of γ:δ T cells, particularly common in the gut, that secrete IFN-γ and therefore promote a T_H1 response. Both these subsets recognize CD1 molecules rather than MHC antigens. The mucosal immune system functions as a separate compartment of the peripheral immune system and has a distinctive anatomy and repertoire of lymphocytes. The gut-associated lymphoid tissue shows a remarkable ability to discriminate between different types of foreign antigens, responding differently to food antigens, innocuous

Fig. 10.37 When individuals who have already been infected with one variant of influenza virus are infected with a second variant they make antibodies only against epitopes that were present on the initial virus.
A child infected for the first time with an influenza virus at 2 years of age makes a response to all epitopes (left panel). At age 5 years, the same child exposed to a variant influenza virus responds preferentially to those epitopes shared with the original virus, and makes a smaller than normal response to new epitopes on the virus (middle panel). Even at age 20 years, this commitment to respond to epitopes shared with the original virus, and the subnormal response to new epitopes, is retained (right panel). This phenomenon is called 'original antigenic sin.'

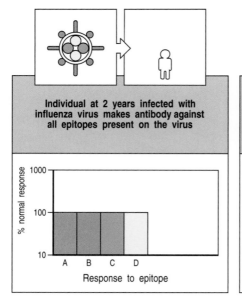

Individual at 2 years infected with influenza virus makes antibody against all epitopes present on the virus

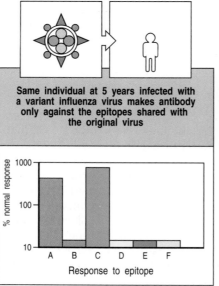

Same individual at 5 years infected with a variant influenza virus makes antibody only against the epitopes shared with the original virus

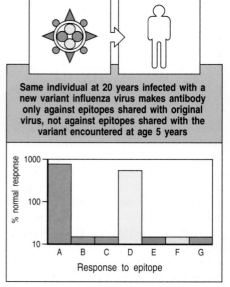

Same individual at 20 years infected with a new variant influenza virus makes antibody only against epitopes shared with original virus, not against epitopes shared with the variant encountered at age 5 years

Phases of the immune response		
Immediate (0–4 hours)	**Early (4–96 hours)**	**Late (96–100 hours)**
Nonspecific Innate No memory No specific T cells	Nonspecific + specific Inducible No memory No specific T cells	Specific Inducible Memory Specific T cells

	Immediate (0–4 hours)	**Early (4–96 hours)**	**Late (96–100 hours)**
Barrier functions	Skin, epithelia	Local inflammation (C5a) Local TNF-α	IgA antibody in luminal spaces IgE antibody on mast cells Local inflammation
Response to extracellular pathogens	Phagocytes Alternative and MBL complement pathway	Mannan-binding lectin C-reactive protein Thymus independent B-cell antibody Complement	IgG antibody and Fc receptor- bearing cells IgG, IgM antibody + classical complement pathway
Response to intracellular bacteria	Macrophages	Activated NK- dependent macrophage activation IL-1, IL-6, TNF-α, IL-12	T-cell activation of macrophages by IFN-γ
Response to virus-infected cells	Natural killer (NK) cells	Interferon-α and -β IL-12-activated NK cells	Cytotoxic T cells IFN-γ

Fig. 10.38 The components of the three phases of the immune response against different classes of microorganisms. The mechanisms of innate immunity that operate in the first two phases of the immune response have been covered in Chapter 2, and thymus-independent B-cell responses are covered in Chapter 9. The early phases contribute to the initiation of adaptive immunity, and they influence the functional character of the antigen-specific effector T cells and antibodies that appear on the scene in the late phase of the response. There are striking similarities in the effector mechanisms at each phase of the response; the main change is in the recognition structures used.

gut flora, and pathogens, with only the latter provoking inflammation and a protective adaptive immune response. An adaptive immune response is mounted in the specialized lymphoid tissue that serves the particular site of infection and takes several days to develop, because T and B lymphocytes must encounter their specific antigen, proliferate, and differentiate into effector cells. T-cell dependent B-cell responses cannot be initiated until antigen-specific T cells have had a chance to proliferate and differentiate. Once an adaptive immune response has occurred, the antibodies and effector T cells are dispersed via the circulation and recruited into the infected tissues; the infection is usually controlled and the pathogen is contained or eliminated. The final effector mechanisms used to clear an infection depend on the type of infectious agent, and in most cases they are the same as those employed in the early phases of immune defense; only the recognition mechanism changes and is more selective (see Fig. 10.38). An effective adaptive immune response leads to a state of protective immunity. This state consists of the presence of effector cells and molecules produced in the initial response, and of immunological memory. Immunological memory is manifested as a heightened ability to respond to pathogens that have previously been encountered and successfully eliminated. It is a property of memory T and B lymphocytes, which can transfer immune memory to naive recipients. The precise mechanism of the maintenance of immunological memory, which is arguably the crucial feature of adaptive immunity, seems to be due to the presence of certain cytokines and to homeostatic interactions with self-MHC:self-peptide complexes. The artificial induction of protective immunity, which includes immunological memory, by vaccination is the most outstanding accomplishment of immunology in the field of medicine. The understanding of how this is accomplished is now catching up with its practical success. However, as we will see in Chapter 11, many pathogens do not induce protective immunity that completely eliminates the pathogen, so we will need to learn what prevents this before we can prepare effective vaccines against these pathogens.

Chapter 10 questions.

10.1   *Communication is critical in any large empire. (a) How is the body alerted to an invasion by microbes, and (b) how does it ensure that its responses reach the site of infection?*

10.2   *Describe how the immune system is organized anatomically into different compartments.*

10.3   *We are exposed to foreign antigens in large quantities in the food that we eat. (a) Why don't we mount immune responses against these food antigens? (b) How does the immune system distinguish between food antigens and the antigens of invading bacteria that it must fight?*

10.4   *Memory immune responses differ from primary immune responses in a number of important properties. (a) Name three ways in which they differ, and (b) describe the underlying mechanism(s) involved in each case.*

10.5   *(a) Discuss the roles of cytokine signals and signals received through the T-cell receptor in the survival and function of memory T cells. (b) Compare and contrast their requirements and responses to such signals with those of naive T cells.*

General references.

Brandtzaeg, P., Farstad, I.N., Johansen, F.E., Morton, H.C., Norderhaug, I.N., and Yamanaka, T.: **The B-cell system of human mucosae and exocrine glands.** *Immunol. Rev.* 1999, **171**:45–87.

Campbell, N., Yio, X.Y., So, L.P., Li, Y., and Mayer, L.: **The intestinal epithelial cell: processing and presentation of antigen to the mucosal immune system.** *Immunol. Rev.* 1999, **172**:315–324.

Hayday, A., and Viney, J.L.: **The ins and outs of body surface immunology.** *Science* 2000, **290**:97–100.

Section references.

10-1   The course of an infection can be divided into several distinct phases.
&

10-2   Infectious diseases are caused by diverse living agents that replicate in their hosts.

Mandell, G., Bennett, J., and Dolin, R. (eds): *Principles and Practice of Infectious Diseases*, 5th edn. New York, Churchill Livingstone, 2000.

10-3   The nonspecific responses of innate immunity are necessary for an adaptive immune response to be initiated.

Fearon, D.T., and Carroll, M.C.: **Regulation of B lymphocyte responses to foreign and self-antigens by the CD19/CD21 complex.** *Annu. Rev. Immunol.* 2000, **18**:393–422.

Fearon, D.T., and Locksley, R.M.: **The instructive role of innate immunity in the acquired immune response.** *Science* 1996, **272**:50–53.

Janeway, C.A., Jr.: **The immune system evolved to discriminate infectious nonself from noninfectious self.** *Immunol. Today* 1992, **13**:11–16.

Medzhitov, R., and Janeway, C., Jr.: **Innate immunity.** *N. Engl. J. Med.* 2000, **343**:338–344.

10-4   An adaptive immune response is initiated when circulating T cells encounter their corresponding antigen in draining lymphoid tissues and become activated.

Finger, E.B., Purl, K.D., Alon, R., Lawrence, M.B., von Andrian, U.H., and Springer, T.A.: **Adhesion through L-selectin requires a threshold hydrodynamic shear.** *Nature* 1996, **379**:266–269.

Roake, J.A., Rao, A.S., Morris, P.J., Larson, C.P., Hankins, D.F., and Austyn, J.M.: **Dendritic cell loss from nonlymphoid tissues after systemic administration of lipopolysaccharide, tumor necrosis factor, and interleukin-1.** *J. Exp. Med.* 1995, **181**:2237–2247.

Shaw, S., Ebnet, K., Kaldjian, E.P., and Anderson, A.O.: **Orchestrated information transfer underlying leukocyte:endothelial interactions.** *Annu. Rev. Immunol.* 1996, **14**:155–177.

10-5   Cytokines made in the early phases of an infection influence the functional differentiation of CD4 T cells.

Bendelac, A., Rivera, M.N., Park, S.H., and Roark, J.H.: **Mouse CD1-specific NK1 T cells: development, specificity, and function.** *Annu. Rev. Immunol.* 1997, **15**:535–562.

Finkelman, F.D., Shea-Donohue, T., Goldhill, J., Sullivan, C.A., Morris, S.C., Madden, K.B., Gauser, W.C., and Urban, J.F., Jr.: **Cytokine regulation of host defense against parasitic intestinal nematodes.** *Annu. Rev. Immunol.* 1997, **15**:505–533.

Hsieh, C.S., Macatonia, S.E., Tripp, C.S., Wolf, S.F., O'Garra, A., and Murphy, K.M.: **Development of T_H1 CD4+ T cells through IL-12 produced by Listeria-induced macrophages.** *Science* 1993, **260**:547–549.

Moser, M., and Murphy, K.M.: **Dendritic cell regulation of T$_H$1–T$_H$2 development**. *Nat. Immunol.* 2000, **1**:199–205.

10-6   Distinct subsets of T cells can regulate the growth and effector functions of other T-cell subsets.

Croft, M., Carter, L., Swain, S.L., and Dutton, R.W.: **Generation of polarized antigen-specific CD8 effector populations: reciprocal action of interleukin-4 and IL-12 in promoting type 2 versus type 1 cytokine profiles.** *J. Exp. Med.* 1994, **180**:1715–1728.

Nakamura, T., Kamogawa, Y., Bottomly, K., and Flavell, R.A.: **Polarization of IL-4- and IFN-γ-producing CD4$^+$ T cells following activation of naive CD4$^+$ T cells.** *J. Immunol.* 1997, **158**:1085–1094.

Seder, R.A., and Paul, W.E.: **Acquisition of lymphokine producing phenotype by CD4$^+$ T cells.** *Annu. Rev. Immunol.* 1994, **12**:635–673.

10-7   The nature and amount of antigenic peptide can also affect the differentiation of CD4 T cells.

Constant, S.L., and Bottomly, K.: **Induction of Th1 and Th2 CD4$^+$ T cell responses: the alternative approaches.** *Annu. Rev. Immunol.* 1997, **15**:297–322.

Wang, L.F., Lin, J.Y., Hsieh, K.H., and Lin, R.H.: **Epicutaneous exposure of protein antigen induces a predominant T$_H$2-like response with high IgE production in mice.** *J. Immunol.* 1996, **156**:4079–4082.

Wang, R., Abrams, S.I., Loh, D.Y., Hsieh, C.S., Murphy, K.M., and Russell, J.H.: **Separation of CD4$^+$ functional responses by peptide dose in Th1 and Th2 subsets expressing the same transgenic antigen receptor.** *Cell. Immunol.* 1993, **148**:357–370.

10-8   Armed effector T cells are guided to sites of infection by chemokines and newly expressed adhesion molecules.

MacKay, C.R., Marston, W., and Dudler, L.: **Altered patterns of T-cell migration through lymph nodes and skin following antigen challenge.** *Eur. J. Immunol.* 1992, **22**:2205–2210.

Romanic, A.M., Graesser, D., Baron, J.L., Visintin, I., Janeway, C.A., Jr., and Madri, J.A.: **T cell adhesion to endothelial cells and extracellular matrix is modulated upon transendothelial cell migration.** *Lab. Invest.* 1997, **76**:11–23.

Sallusto, F., Kremmer, E., Palermo, B., Hoy, A., Ponath, P., Qin, S., Forster, R., Lipp, M., and Lanzavecchia, A.: **Switch in chemokine receptor expression upon TCR stimulation reveals novel homing potential for recently activated T cells.** *Eur. J. Immunol.* 1999, **29**:2037–2045.

10-9   Antibody responses develop in lymphoid tissues under the direction of armed helper T cells.

Jacob, J., Kassir, R., and Kelsoe, G.: *In situ* **studies of the primary immune response to (4-hydroxy-3-nitrophenyl)acetyl. I. The architecture and dynamics of responding cell populations.** *J. Exp. Med.* 1991, **173**:1165–1175.

Kelsoe, G., and Zheng, B.: **Sites of B-cell activation** *in vivo. Curr. Opin. Immunol.* 1993, **5**:418–422.

Liu, Y.J., Zhang, J., Lane, P.J., Chan, E.Y., and MacLennan, I.C.: **Sites of specific B cell activation in primary and secondary responses to T cell-dependent and T cell-independent antigens.** *Eur. J. Immunol.* 1991, **21**:2951–2962.

MacLennan, I.C.M.: **Germinal centres.** *Annu. Rev. Immunol.* 1994, **12**:117–139.

10-10   Antibody responses are sustained in medullary cords and bone marrow.

Benner, R., Hijmans, W., and Haaijman, J.J.: **The bone marrow: the major source of serum immunoglobulins, but still a neglected site of antibody formation.** *Clin. Exp. Immunol.* 1981, **46**:1–8.

Manz, R.A., Thiel, A., and Radbruch, A.: **Lifetime of plasma cells in the bone marrow.** *Nature* 1997, **388**:133–134.

Slifka, M.K., Antia, R., Whitmire, J.K., and Ahmed, R.: **Humoral immunity due to long-lived plasma cells.** *Immunity* 1998, **8**:363–372.

Takahashi, Y., Dutta, P.R., Cerasoli, D.M., and Kelsoe, G.: *In situ* **studies of the primary immune response to (4-hydroxy-3-nitrophenyl)acetyl. V. Affinity maturation develops in two stages of clonal selection.** *J. Exp. Med.* 1998, **187**:885–895.

10-11   The effector mechanisms used to clear an infection depend on the infectious agent.

Mims, C.A.: *The Pathogenesis of Infectious Disease*, 3rd edn. London, Academic Press, 1987.

10-12   Resolution of an infection is accompanied by the death of most of the effector cells and the generation of memory cells.

Murali-Krishna, K., Altman, J.D., Suresh, M., Sourdive, D.J., Zajac, A.J., Miller, J.D., Slansky, J., and Ahmed, R.: **Counting antigen-specific CD8 T cells: a reevaluation of bystander activation during viral infection.** *Immunity* 1998, **8**:177–187.

Webb, S., Hutchinson, J., Hayden, K., and Sprent, J.: **Expansion/deletion of mature T cells exposed to endogenous superantigens** *in vivo. J. Immunol.* 1994, **152**:586–597.

10-13   Mucosa-associated lymphoid tissue is located in anatomically defined microcompartments throughout the gut.

Finke, D., and Kraehenbuhl, J.P.: **Formation of Peyer's patches.** *Curr. Opin. Genet. Dev.* 2001, **11**:561–567.

Hein, W.R.: **Organization of mucosal lymphoid tissue.** *Curr. Top. Microbiol. Immunol.* 1999, **236**:1–15.

Mowat, A.M., and Viney, J.L.: **The anatomical basis of intestinal immunity.** *Immunol. Rev.* 1997, **156**:145–166.

Nagler-Anderson, C.: **Man the barrier! Strategic defences in the intestinal mucosa.** *Nat. Rev. Immunol.* 2001, **1**:59–67.

Neutra, M.R., Mantis, N.J., and Kraehenbuhl, J.P.: **Collaboration of epithelial cells with organized mucosal lymphoid tissues.** *Nat. Immunol.* 2001, **2**:1004–1009.

Niedergang, F., and Kraehenbuhl, J.P.: **Much ado about M cells.** *Trends Cell Biol.* 2000, **10**:137–141.

10-14   The trafficking of lymphocytes within different compartments of the immune system is controlled by tissue-specific adhesion and chemokine interactions.

Homey, B., Alenius, H., Muller, A., Soto, H., Bowman, E.P., Yuan, W., McEvoy, L., Lauerma, A.I., Assmann, T., Bunemann, E., *et al.*: **CCL27–CCR10 interactions regulate T cell-mediated skin inflammation.** *Nat. Med.* 2002, **8**:157–165.

Hudak, S., Hagen, M., Liu, Y., Catron, D., Oldham, E., McEvoy, L.M., and Bowman, E.P.: **Immune surveillance and effector functions of CCR10$^+$ skin homing T cells.** *J. Immunol.* 2002, **169**:1189–1196.

Kunkel, E.J., and Butcher, E.C.: **Chemokines and the tissue-specific migration of lymphocytes.** *Immunity* 2002, **16**:1–4.

10-15   The mucosal immune system contains a distinctive repertoire of lymphocytes.

Bendelac, A., Bonneville, M., and Kearney, J.F.: **Autoreactivity by design: innate B and T lymphocytes.** *Nat. Rev. Immunol.* 2001, **1**:177–186.

Guy-Grand, D., and Vassalli, P.: **Gut intraepithelial lymphocyte development.** *Curr. Opin. Immunol.* 2002, **14**:255–259.

Hayday, A.C.: **γ δ cells: a right time and a right place for a conserved third way of protection.** *Annu. Rev. Immunol.* 2000, **18**:975–1026.

Hayday, A.C., Theodoridis, E., Ramsburg, E., and Shires, J.: **Intraepithelial lymphocytes: exploring the Third Way in immunology.** *Nat. Immunol.* 2001, **2**:997–1003.

Leishman, A.J., Naidenko, O.V., Attinger, A., Koning, F., Lena, C.J., Xiong, Y.,

Chang, H.C., Reinherz, E., Kronenberg, M., and Cheroutre, H.: **T cell responses modulated through interaction between CD8αα and the nonclassical MHC class I molecule, TL.** *Science* 2001, **294**:1936–1939.

Porcelli, S.A., and Modlin, R.L.: **The CD1 system: antigen-presenting molecules for T cell recognition of lipids and glycolipids.** *Annu. Rev. Immunol.* 1999, **17**:297–329.

Roberts, S.J., Smith, A.L., West, A.B., Wen, L., Findly, R.C., Owen, M.J., and Hayday, A.C.: **T-cell αβ+ and γδ+ deficient mice display abnormal but distinct phenotypes toward a natural, widespread infection of the intestinal epithelium.** *Proc. Natl. Acad. Sci. USA* 1996, **93**:11774–11779.

10-16 Secretory IgA is the antibody isotype associated with the mucosal immune system.

Corthesy, B., and Kraehenbuhl, J.P.: **Antibody-mediated protection of mucosal surfaces.** *Curr. Top. Microbiol. Immunol.* 1999, **236**:93–111.

Macpherson, A.J., Gatto, D., Sainsbury, E., Harriman, G.R., Hengartner, H., and Zinkernagel, R.M.: **A primitive T cell-independent mechanism of intestinal mucosal IgA responses to commensal bacteria.** *Science* 2000, **288**:2222–2226.

Mostov, K.E.: **Transepithelial transport of immunoglobulins.** *Annu. Rev. Immunol.* 1994, **12**:63–84.

Phalipon, A., Cardona, A., Kraehenbuhl, J.P., Edelman, L., Sansonetti, P.J., and Corthesy, B.: **Secretory component: a new role in secretory IgA-mediated immune exclusion *in vivo*.** *Immunity* 2002, **17**:107–115.

Phalipon, A., and Corthesy, B.: **Novel functions of the polymeric Ig receptor: well beyond transport of immunoglobulins.** *Trends Immunol.* 2003, **24**:55–58.

10-17 Most antigens presented to the mucosal immune system induce tolerance.

Strobel, S., and Mowat, A.M.: **Immune responses to dietary antigens: oral tolerance.** *Immunol. Today* 1998, **19**:173–181.

10-18 The mucosal immune system can mount an immune response to the normal bacterial flora of the gut.

Berg, R.D.: **Bacterial translocation from the gastrointestinal tract.** *Adv. Exp. Med. Biol.* 1999, **473**:11–30.

Berg, R.D.: **The indigenous gastrointestinal microflora.** *Trends Microbiol.* 1996, **4**:430–435.

Bos, N.A., Kimura, H., Meeuwsen, C.G., De Visser, H., Hazenberg, M.P., Wostmann, B.S., Pleasants, J.R., Benner, R., and Marcus, D.M.: **Serum immunoglobulin levels and naturally occurring antibodies against carbohydrate antigens in germ-free BALB/c mice fed chemically defined ultrafiltered diet.** *Eur. J. Immunol.* 1989, **19**:2335–2339.

Kelly, C.P., and LaMont, J.T.: ***Clostridium difficile* infection.** *Annu. Rev. Med.* 1998, **49**:375–390.

Pothoulakis, C., and LaMont, J.T.: **Microbes and microbial toxins: paradigms for microbial–mucosal interactions. II. The integrated response of the intestine to *Clostridium difficile* toxins.** *Am. J. Physiol. Gastrointest. Liver Physiol.* 2001, **280**:G178–G183.

10-19 Enteric pathogens cause a local inflammatory response and the development of protective immunity.

Cario, E., Brown, D., McKee, M., Lynch-Devaney, K., Gerken, G., and Podolsky, D.K.: **Commensal-associated molecular patterns induce selective toll-like receptor-trafficking from apical membrane to cytoplasmic compartments in polarized intestinal epithelium.** *Am. J. Pathol.* 2002, **160**:165–173.

Gewirtz, A.T., and Madara, J.L.: **Periscope, up! Monitoring microbes in the intestine.** *Nat. Immunol.* 2001, **2**:288–290.

Gewirtz, A.T., Navas, T.A., Lyons, S., Godowski, P.J., and Madara, J.L.: **Cutting edge: bacterial flagellin activates basolaterally expressed TLR5 to induce epithelial proinflammatory gene expression.** *J. Immunol.* 2001, **167**:1882–1885.

Girardin, S.E., Sansonetti, P.J., and Philpott, D.J.: **Intracellular vs extracellular recognition of pathogens—common concepts in mammals and flies.** *Trends Microbiol.* 2002, **10**:193–199.

Holmes, K.V., Tresnan, D.B., and Zelus, B.D.: **Virus–receptor interactions in the enteric tract. Virus–receptor interactions.** *Adv. Exp. Med. Biol.* 1997, **412**:125–133.

Inohara, N., Ogura, Y., and Nunez, G.: **Nods: a family of cytosolic proteins that regulate the host response to pathogens.** *Curr. Opin. Microbiol.* 2002, **5**:76–80.

Philpott, D.J., Girardin, S.E., and Sansonetti, P.J.: **Innate immune responses of epithelial cells following infection with bacterial pathogens.** *Curr. Opin. Immunol.* 2001, **13**:410–416.

Rescigno, M., Urbano, M., Valzasina, B., Francolini, M., Rotta, G., Bonasio, R., Granucci, F., Kraehenbuhl, J.P., and Ricciardi-Castagnoli, P.: **Dendritic cells express tight junction proteins and penetrate gut epithelial monolayers to sample bacteria.** *Nat. Immunol.* 2001, **2**:361–367.

Sansonetti, P.: **Host–pathogen interactions: the seduction of molecular cross talk.** *Gut* 2002, 50 Suppl 3: III2–III8.

Sansonetti, P.J.: **Microbes and microbial toxins: paradigms for microbial–mucosal interactions. III. Shigellosis: from symptoms to molecular pathogenesis.** *Am. J. Physiol. Gastrointest. Liver Physiol.* 2001, **280**:G319–G323.

Spies, T.: **Induction of T cell alertness by bacterial colonization of intestinal epithelium.** *Proc. Natl. Acad. Sci. USA* 2002, **99**:2584–2586.

10-20 Infection by *Helicobacter pylori* causes a chronic inflammatory response, which can cause peptic ulcers, carcinoma of the stomach, and unusual lymphoid tumors.

Blaser, M.J.: ***Helicobacter pylori* and gastric diseases.** *Br. Med. J.* 1998, **316**:1507–1510.

Isaacson, P.G.: **Gastric MALT lymphoma: from concept to cure.** *Ann. Oncol.* 1999, **10**:637–645.

Peek, R.M., Jr.: **Intoxicated cells and stomach ulcers.** *Nat. Genet.* 2003, **33**:328–330.

Stolte, M., Bayerdorffer, E., Morgner, A., Alpen, B., Wundisch, T., Thiede, C., and Neubauer, A.: ***Helicobacter* and gastric MALT lymphoma.** *Gut* 2002, **50 Suppl** 3:III19–III24.

10-21 In the absence of inflammatory stimuli, the normal response of the mucosal immune system to foreign antigens is tolerance.

Bilsborough, J., and Viney, J.L.: **Getting to the guts of immune regulation.** *Immunology* 2002, **106**:139–143.

Czerkinsky, C., Anjuere, F., McGhee, J.R., George-Chandy, A., Holmgren, J., Kieny, M.P., Fujiyashi, K., Mestecky, J.F., Pierrefite-Carle, V., Rask, C., and Sun, J.B.: **Mucosal immunity and tolerance: relevance to vaccine development.** *Immunol. Rev.* 1999, **170**:197–222.

Levings, M.K., and Roncarolo, M.G.: **T-regulatory 1 cells: a novel subset of CD4 T cells with immunoregulatory properties.** *J. Allergy Clin. Immunol.* 2000, **106**:S109-S112.

MacDonald, T.T.: **Effector and regulatory lymphoid cells and cytokines in mucosal sites.** *Curr. Top. Microbiol. Immunol.* 1999, **236**:113–135.

Neurath, M.F., Finotto, S., and Glimcher, L.H.: **The role of Th1/Th2 polarization in mucosal immunity.** *Nat. Med.* 2002, **8**:567–573.

Van Houten, N., and Blake, S.F.: **Direct measurement of anergy of antigen-specific T cells following oral tolerance induction.** *J. Immunol.* 1996, **157**:1337–1341.

Weiner, H.L.: **The mucosal milieu creates tolerogenic dendritic cells and T_R1 and T_H3 regulatory cells.** *Nat. Immunol.* 2001, **2**:671–672.

10-22 Immunological memory is long-lived after infection or vaccination.

Black, F.L., and Rosen, L.: **Patterns of measles antibodies in residents of Tahiti and their stability in the absence of re-exposure.** *J. Immunol.* 1962, **88**:725–731.

Hammarlund, E., Lewis, M.W., Hansen, S.G., Strelow, L.I., Nelson, J.A., Sexton, G.J., Hanifin, J.M., and Slifka, M.K.: **Duration of antiviral immunity after smallpox vaccination.** *Nat. Med.* 2003, **9**:1131–1137.

Kassiotis, G., Garcia, S., Simpson, E., and Stockinger, B.: **Impairment of immunological memory in the absence of MHC despite survival of memory**

T cells. *Nat. Immunol.* 2002, **3**:244–250.

Ku, C.C., Murakami, M., Sakamoto, A., Kappler, J., and Marrack, P.: **Control of homeostasis of CD8⁺ memory T cells by opposing cytokines.** *Science* 2000, **288**:675–678.

Murali-Krishna, K., Lau, L.L., Sambhara, S., Lemonnier, F., Altman, J., and Ahmed, R.: **Persistence of memory CD8 T cells in MHC class I-deficient mice.** *Science* 1999, **286**:1377–1381.

Seddon, B., Tomlinson, P., and Zamoyska, R.: **Interleukin 7 and T cell receptor signals regulate homeostasis of CD4 memory cells.** *Nat. Immunol.* 2003, **4**:680–686.

10-23   Both clonal expansion and clonal differentiation contribute to immunological memory in B cells.

Berek, C., and Milstein, C.: **Mutation drift and repertoire shift in the maturation of the immune response.** *Immunol. Rev.* 1987, **96**:23–41.

Cumano, A., and Rajewsky, K.: **Clonal recruitment and somatic mutation in the generation of immunological memory to the hapten NP.** *EMBO J.* 1986, **5**:2459–2468.

Klein, U., Tu, Y., Stolovitzky, G.A., Keller, J.L., Haddad, J., Jr., Miljkovic, V., Cattoretti, G., Califano, A., and Dalla-Favera, R.: **Transcriptional analysis of the B cell germinal center reaction.** *Proc. Natl. Acad. Sci. USA* 2003, **100**:2639–2644.

Tarlinton, D.: **Germinal centers: form and function.** *Curr. Opin. Immunol.* 1998, **10**:245–251.

10-24   Repeated immunization leads to increasing affinity of antibody owing to somatic hypermutation and selection by antigen in germinal centers.

Berek, C., Jarvis, J.M., and Milstein, C.: **Activation of memory and virgin B cell clones in hyperimmune animals.** *Eur. J. Immunol.* 1987, **17**:1121–1129.

Liu, Y.J., Zhang, J., Lane, P.J., Chan, E.Y., and MacLennan, I.C.: **Sites of specific B cell activation in primary and secondary responses to T cell-dependent and T cell-independent antigens.** *Eur. J. Immunol.* 1991, **21**:2951–2962.

Siskind, G.W., Dunn, P., and Walker, J.G.: **Studies on the control of antibody synthesis: II. Effect of antigen dose and of suppression by passive antibody on the affinity of antibody synthesized.** *J. Exp. Med.* 1968, **127**:55–66.

10-25   Memory T cells are increased in frequency and have distinct activation requirements and cell-surface proteins that distinguish them from armed effector T cells.

Bradley, L.M., Atkins, G.G., and Swain, S.L.: **Long-term CD4⁺ memory T cells from the spleen lack MEL-14, the lymph node homing receptor.** *J. Immunol.* 1992, **148**:324–331.

Kaech, S.M., Hemby, S., Kersh, E., and Ahmed, R.: **Molecular and functional profiling of memory CD8 T cell differentiation.** *Cell* 2002, **111**:837–851.

Rogers, P.R., Dubey, C., and Swain, S.L.: **Qualitative changes accompany memory T cell generation: faster, more effective responses at lower doses of antigen.** *J. Immunol.* 2000, **164**:2338–2346.

Sallusto, F., Lenig, D., Forster, R., Lipp, M., and Lanzavecchia, A.: **Two subsets of memory T lymphocytes with distinct homing potentials and effector functions.** *Nature* 1999, **401**:708–712.

Wherry, E.J., Teichgraber, V., Becker, T.C., Masopust, D., Kaech, S.M., Antia, R., von Andrian, U.H., and Ahmed, R.: **Lineage relationship and protective immunity of memory CD8 T cell subsets.** *Nat. Immunol.* 2003, **4**:225–234.

10-26   In immune individuals, secondary and subsequent responses are mediated mainly by memory lymphocytes.

Fazekas de St Groth, B., and Webster, R.G.: **Disquisitions on original antigenic sin. I. Evidence in man.** *J. Exp. Med.* 1966, **140**:2893–2898.

Fridman, W.H.: **Regulation of B cell activation and antigen presentation by Fc receptors.** *Curr. Opin. Immunol.* 1993, **5**:355–360.

Pollack, W., Gorman, J.G., Freda, V.J., Ascari, W.Q., Allen, A.E., and Baker, W.J.: **Results of clinical trials of RhoGAm in women.** *Transfusion* 1968, **8**:151–153.

PART V

THE IMMUNE SYSTEM IN HEALTH AND DISEASE

Failures of Host Defense Mechanisms

In the normal course of an infection, the infectious agent triggers an innate immune response that causes symptoms. The foreign antigens of the infectious agent, enhanced by signals from the innate immune response, induce an adaptive immune response that clears the infection and establishes a state of protective immunity. This does not always happen, however, and in this chapter we examine three circumstances in which there are failures of host defense against infection: avoidance or subversion of a normal immune response by the pathogen; inherited failures of defense because of gene defects; and the acquired immune deficiency syndrome (AIDS), a generalized susceptibility to infection that is itself due to the failure of the host to control and eliminate the human immunodeficiency virus (HIV).

The propagation of a pathogen depends on its ability to replicate in a host and to spread to new hosts. Common pathogens must therefore grow without activating too vigorous an immune response and, conversely, must not kill the host too quickly. The most successful pathogens persist either because they do not elicit an immune response, or because they evade the response once it has occurred. Over millions of years of coevolution with their hosts, pathogens have developed various strategies for avoiding destruction by the immune system, and we have encountered some of them in earlier chapters. In the first part of this chapter we examine these in more detail, and discuss some that have not yet been mentioned.

In the second part of the chapter we turn to the **immunodeficiency diseases**, in which host defense fails. In most of these diseases, a defective gene results in the elimination of one or more components of the immune system, leading to heightened susceptibility to infection with particular classes of pathogen. Immunodeficiency diseases caused by defects in T- or B-lymphocyte development, phagocyte function, and components of the complement system have all been discovered. Finally, we consider how the persistent infection of immune system cells by the human immunodeficiency virus, HIV, leads to the acquired immune deficiency syndrome, AIDS. The analysis of all these diseases has already made an important contribution to our understanding of host defense mechanisms and, in the longer term, might help to provide new methods of controlling or preventing infectious diseases, including AIDS.

Pathogens have evolved various means of evading or subverting normal host defenses.

Just as vertebrates have developed many different defenses against pathogens, so pathogens have evolved elaborate strategies to evade these defenses. Many pathogens use one or more of these strategies to evade the immune system. At the end of this chapter we will see how HIV succeeds in defeating the immune response by using several of them in combination.

11-1 Antigenic variation allows pathogens to escape from immunity.

One way in which an infectious agent can evade immune surveillance is by altering its antigens; this is particularly important for extracellular pathogens, against which the principal defense is the production of antibody against their surface structures. There are three ways in which **antigenic variation** can occur. First, many infectious agents exist in a wide variety of antigenic types. There are, for example, 84 known types of *Streptococcus pneumoniae*, an important cause of bacterial pneumonia. Each type differs from the others in the structure of its polysaccharide capsule. The different types are distinguished by serological tests and so are often known as **serotypes**. Infection with one serotype of such an organism can lead to type-specific immunity, which protects against reinfection with that type but not with a different serotype. Thus, from the point of view of the adaptive immune system, each serotype of *S. pneumoniae* represents a distinct organism. The result is that essentially the same pathogen can cause disease many times in the same individual (Fig. 11.1).

Fig. 11.1 Host defense against *Streptococcus pneumoniae* is type specific. The different strains of *S. pneumoniae* have antigenically distinct capsular polysaccharides. The capsule prevents effective phagocytosis until the bacterium is opsonized by specific antibody and complement, allowing phagocytes to destroy it. Antibody against one type of *S. pneumoniae* does not cross-react with the other types, so an individual immune to one type has no protective immunity to a subsequent infection with a different type. An individual must generate a new adaptive immune response each time he or she is infected with a different type of *S. pneumoniae*.

Streptococcus pneumoniae

There are many types of *S. pneumoniae*, which differ in their capsular polysaccharides

| Individual infected with one type of *S. pneumoniae* | Response clears infection | Subsequent infection with a different type of *S. pneumoniae* is unaffected by response to first type | New response clears infection |

A second, more dynamic, mechanism of antigenic variation is seen in the influenza virus. At any one time, a single virus type is responsible for most infections throughout the world. The human population gradually develops protective immunity to this virus type, chiefly by directing neutralizing antibody against the major surface protein of the influenza virus, its hemagglutinin. Because the virus is rapidly cleared from individual hosts, its survival depends on the presence of a large pool of unprotected individuals among whom it spreads very readily. The virus might therefore be in danger of running out of potential hosts if it had not evolved two distinct ways of changing its antigenic type (Fig. 11.2).

The first of these, **antigenic drift**, is caused by point mutations in the genes encoding hemagglutinin and a second surface protein, neuraminidase. Every 2–3 years a variant arises with mutations that allow the virus to evade neutralization by antibodies in the population; other mutations affect epitopes that are recognized by T cells and, in particular, CD8 T cells, so that cells infected with the mutant virus also escape destruction. Individuals who were previously infected with, and hence are immune to, the old variant are thus susceptible to the new variant. This causes an epidemic that is relatively mild because there is still some cross-reaction with antibodies and T cells produced against the previous variant of the virus, and therefore most of the population have some level of immunity (see Section 10-26).

Major influenza pandemics resulting in widespread and often fatal disease occur as the result of the second process, which is termed **antigenic shift**. This happens when there is reassortment of the segmented RNA genome of

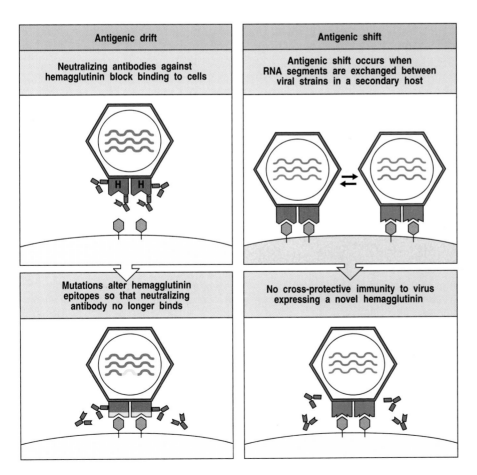

Fig. 11.2 Two types of variation allow repeated infection with type A influenza virus. Neutralizing antibody that mediates protective immunity is directed at the viral surface protein hemagglutinin (H), which is responsible for viral binding to and entry into cells. Antigenic drift (left panels) involves the emergence of point mutants that alter the binding sites for protective antibodies on the hemagglutinin. When this happens, the new virus can grow in a host that is immune to the previous strain of virus. However, as T cells and some antibodies can still recognize epitopes that have not been altered, the new variants cause only mild disease in previously infected individuals. Antigenic shift (right panels) is a rare event involving reassortment of the segmented RNA viral genomes of two different influenza viruses, probably in a bird. These antigen-shifted viruses have large changes in their hemagglutinin molecule and therefore T cells and antibodies produced in earlier infections are not protective. These shifted strains cause severe infection that spreads widely, causing the influenza pandemics that occur every 10–50 years. (There are eight RNA molecules in each viral genome but for simplicity only three are shown.)

the influenza virus and related animal influenza viruses in an animal host, leading to major changes in the hemagglutinin protein on the viral surface. The resulting virus is recognized poorly, if at all, by antibodies and by T cells directed against the previous variant, so that most people are highly susceptible to the new virus, and severe infection results.

The third mechanism of antigenic variation involves programmed rearrangements in the DNA of the pathogen. The most striking example occurs in African trypanosomes, where changes in the major surface antigen occur repeatedly within a single infected host. Trypanosomes are insect-borne protozoa that replicate in the extracellular tissue spaces of the body and cause sleeping sickness in humans. The trypanosome is coated with a single type of glycoprotein, the variant-specific glycoprotein (VSG), which elicits a potent protective antibody response that rapidly clears most of the parasites. The trypanosome genome, however, contains about 1000 VSG genes, each encoding a protein with distinct antigenic properties. Only one of these is expressed at any one time by being placed into an active 'expression site' in the genome. The VSG gene expressed can be changed by gene rearrangement that places a new VSG gene into the expression site (Fig. 11.3). So, by having their own system of gene rearrangement that can change the VSG protein produced, trypanosomes keep one step ahead of an immune system capable of generating many distinct antibodies by gene rearrangement. A few trypanosomes with such changed surface glycoproteins thus evade the antibodies made by the host, and these soon grow and cause a recurrence of disease (see Fig. 11.3, bottom panel). Antibodies are then made against the new VSG, and the whole cycle repeats. This chronic cycle of antigen clearance leads to immune-complex damage and inflammation, and eventually to neurological damage, finally resulting in coma. This gives African trypanosomiasis its common name of sleeping sickness. These cycles of evasive action make trypanosome infections very difficult for the immune system to defeat, and they are a major health problem in Africa. Malaria is another major disease caused by a protozoan parasite that varies its antigens to evade elimination by the immune system.

Antigenic variation also occurs in bacteria: DNA rearrangements help to account for the success of two important bacterial pathogens—*Salmonella typhimurium*, a common cause of salmonella food poisoning, and *Neisseria gonorrhoeae*, which causes gonorrhea, a major sexually transmitted disease and an increasing public health problem in the United States. *S. typhimurium* regularly alternates its surface flagellin protein by inverting a segment of its DNA containing the promoter for one flagellin gene. This turns off expression of the gene and allows the expression of a second flagellin gene, which

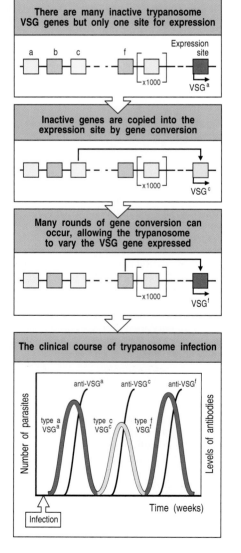

Fig. 11.3 Antigenic variation in trypanosomes allows them to escape immune surveillance. The surface of a trypanosome is covered with a variant-specific glycoprotein (VSG). Each trypanosome has about 1000 genes encoding different VSGs, but only the gene in a specific expression site within the telomere at one end of the chromosome is active. Although several genetic mechanisms have been observed for changing the VSG gene expressed, the usual mechanism is gene conversion. An inactive gene, which is not at the telomere, is copied and transposed into the telomeric expression site, where it becomes active. When an individual is first infected, antibodies are raised against the VSG initially expressed by the trypanosome population. A small number of trypanosomes spontaneously switch their VSG gene to a new type, and while the host antibody eliminates the initial variant, the new variant is unaffected. As the new variant grows, the whole sequence of events is repeated.

encodes an antigenically distinct protein. *N. gonorrhoeae* has several variable antigens, the most striking of which is the pilin protein, which, like the variable surface glycoproteins of the African trypanosome, is encoded by several variant genes, only one of which is active at any given time. Silent versions of the gene from time to time replace the active version downstream of the pilin promoter. All of these mechanisms help the pathogen to evade an otherwise specific and effective immune response.

11-2   Some viruses persist *in vivo* by ceasing to replicate until immunity wanes.

Viruses usually betray their presence to the immune system once they have entered cells by directing the synthesis of viral proteins, fragments of which are displayed on the surface MHC molecules of the infected cell, where they are detected by T lymphocytes. To replicate, a virus must make viral proteins, and rapidly replicating viruses that produce acute viral illnesses are therefore readily detected by T cells, which normally control them. Some viruses, however, can enter a state known as **latency** in which the virus is not being replicated. In the latent state, the virus does not cause disease but, because there are no viral peptides to flag its presence, the virus cannot be eliminated. Such latent infections can be reactivated and this results in recurrent illness.

Herpes viruses often enter latency. Herpes simplex virus, the cause of cold sores, infects epithelia and spreads to sensory neurons serving the area of infection. After an effective immune response controls the epithelial infection, the virus persists in a latent state in the sensory neurons. Factors such as sunlight, bacterial infection, or hormonal changes reactivate the virus, which then travels down the axons of the sensory neuron and reinfects the epithelial tissues (Fig. 11.4). At this point, the immune response again becomes active and controls the local infection by killing the epithelial cells, producing a new sore. This cycle can be repeated many times. There are two reasons why the sensory neuron remains infected: first, the virus is quiescent in the nerve and therefore few viral proteins are produced, generating few virus-derived peptides to present on MHC class I molecules; second, neurons carry very low levels of MHC class I molecules, which makes it harder for CD8 T cells to recognize infected neurons and attack them. This low level of MHC class I expression might be beneficial, as it reduces the risk that neurons, which do not regenerate, or regenerate only very slowly, will be attacked inappropriately by CD8 T cells. It also makes neurons unusually vulnerable to persistent infections. Another example of this is provided by herpes zoster (varicella zoster), the virus that causes chickenpox. This virus remains latent in one or a few dorsal root ganglia after the acute illness is over and can be reactivated by stress or immunosuppression to spread down the nerve and reinfect the skin. The reinfection causes the reappearance of the classic rash of varicella in the area of skin served by the infected dorsal root, a disease commonly called shingles. Herpes simplex reactivation is frequent, but herpes zoster usually reactivates only once in a lifetime in an immunocompetent host.

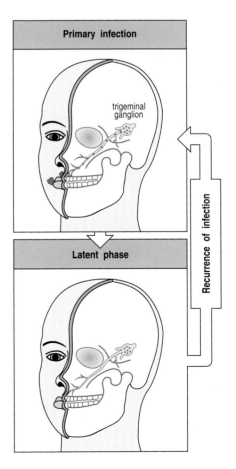

Fig. 11.4 Persistence and reactivation of herpes simplex virus infection. The initial infection in the skin is cleared by an effective immune response, but residual infection persists in sensory neurons such as those of the trigeminal ganglion, whose axons innervate the lips. When the virus is reactivated, usually by some environmental stress and/or alteration in immune status, the skin in the area served by the nerve is reinfected from virus in the ganglion and a new cold sore results. This process can be repeated many times.

The Epstein–Barr virus (EBV), yet another herpes virus, enters latency in B cells after a primary infection that often passes without being diagnosed. In a minority of infected individuals, the initial acute infection of B cells is more severe, causing a disease known as infectious mononucleosis or glandular fever. EBV infects B cells by binding to CR2 (CD21), a component of the B-cell co-receptor complex. The infection causes most of the infected cells to proliferate and produce virus, leading in turn to the proliferation of antigen-specific T cells and the excess of mononuclear white cells in the blood that gives the disease its name. The infection is controlled eventually by specific CD8 T cells, which kill the infected proliferating B cells. A fraction of B lymphocytes become latently infected, however, and EBV remains quiescent in these cells. Latently infected cells express a viral protein, EBNA-1, which is needed to maintain the viral genome, but EBNA-1 interacts with the proteasome (see Section 5-3) to prevent its own degradation into peptides that would elicit a T-cell response.

Latently infected B cells can be isolated by taking B cells from individuals who have apparently cleared their EBV infection and placing them in tissue culture: in the absence of T cells, the latently infected cells that have retained the EBV genome become transformed into so-called immortal cell lines, the equivalent of tumorigenesis *in vitro*. Infected B cells sometimes undergo malignant transformation *in vivo*, giving rise to a B-cell lymphoma called Burkitt's lymphoma (see Section 7-33). This is a rare event, and it seems likely that a crucial part of this process is a failure of T-cell surveillance. Further support for this hypothesis comes from the increased risk of EBV-associated B-cell lymphomas developing in patients with acquired and inherited immunodeficiencies of T-cell function (see Sections 11-15 and 11-28).

11-3 Some pathogens resist destruction by host defense mechanisms or exploit them for their own purposes.

Some pathogens induce a normal immune response but have evolved specialized mechanisms for resisting its effects. For instance, some bacteria that are engulfed in the normal way by macrophages have evolved means of avoiding destruction by these phagocytes; indeed, they use macrophages as their primary host. *Mycobacterium tuberculosis*, for example, is taken up by macrophages but prevents the fusion of the phagosome with the lysosome, protecting itself from the bactericidal actions of the lysosomal contents.

Other microorganisms, such as *Listeria monocytogenes*, escape from the phagosome into the cytoplasm of the macrophage, where they can multiply readily. They then spread to adjacent cells in tissues without emerging from the cell into the extracellular environment. They do this by hijacking the host cytoskeletal protein actin, which assembles into filaments at the rear of the bacterium. The actin filaments drive the bacteria forward into vacuolar projections to adjacent cells; these vacuoles are then lysed by the *Listeria*, releasing the bacteria directly into the cytoplasm of the adjacent cell. In this way they avoid attack by antibodies. Cells infected with *L. monocytogenes* are, however, susceptible to killing by cytotoxic T cells. The protozoan parasite *Toxoplasma gondii* can apparently generate its own vesicle, which isolates it from the rest of the cell because it does not fuse with any cellular vesicle. This might actually enable *T. gondii* to avoid making peptides derived from its proteins accessible for loading onto MHC molecules, and thus remain invisible to the immune system.

Two prominent spirochetal infections, **Lyme disease** and **syphilis**, avoid elimination by antibodies through less well understood mechanisms and establish a persistent and extremely damaging infection in tissues. Lyme disease is caused by the spirochete bacterium *Borrelia burgdorferi*, whereas syphilis, the more widespread and much the better understood of the two diseases, is caused by *Treponema pallidum*. *T. pallidum* is believed to avoid recognition by antibodies by coating its surface with host molecules until it has invaded tissues such as the central nervous system, where it is less easily reached by antibodies.

Finally, many viruses have evolved mechanisms to subvert various arms of the immune system. These range from capturing cellular genes for cytokines or cytokine receptors, to synthesizing complement-regulatory molecules, inhibiting MHC class I synthesis or assembly, or producing decoy proteins that mimic so-called TIR domains that we learned about in Section 6-17. This is one of the most rapidly expanding areas of research into host–pathogen relationships. Examples of how members of the herpes and poxvirus families subvert host responses are shown in Fig. 11.5.

Viral strategy	Specific mechanism	Result	Virus examples
Inhibition of humoral immunity	Virally encoded Fc receptor	Blocks effector functions of antibodies bound to infected cells	Herpes simplex Cytomegalovirus
	Virally encoded complement receptor	Blocks complement-mediated effector pathways	Herpes simplex
	Virally encoded complement control protein	Inhibits complement activation by infected cell	Vaccinia
Inhibition of inflammatory response	Virally encoded chemokine receptor homolog, eg, β-chemokine receptor	Sensitizes infected cells to effects of β-chemokine; advantage to virus unknown	Cytomegalovirus
	Virally encoded soluble cytokine receptor, eg, IL-1 receptor homolog, TNF receptor homolog, interferon-γ receptor homolog	Blocks effects of cytokines by inhibiting their interaction with host receptors	Vaccinia Rabbit myxoma virus
	Viral inhibition of adhesion molecule expression, eg, LFA-3 ICAM-1	Blocks adhesion of lymphocytes to infected cells	Epstein–Barr virus
	Protection from NFκB activation by short sequences that mimic TLRs	Blocks inflammatory responses elicited by IL-1 or bacterial pathogens	Vaccinia
Blocking of antigen processing and presentation	Inhibition of MHC class I expression	Impairs recognition of infected cells by cytotoxic T cells	Herpes simplex Cytomegalovirus
	Inhibition of peptide transport by TAP	Blocks peptide association with MHC class I	Herpes simplex
Immunosuppression of host	Virally encoded cytokine homolog of IL-10	Inhibits T$_H$1 lymphocytes Reduces interferon-γ production	Epstein–Barr virus

Fig. 11.5 Mechanisms of subversion of the host immune system by viruses of the herpes and pox families.

11-4   Immunosuppression or inappropriate immune responses can contribute to persistent disease.

Toxic Shock
Syndrome

Many pathogens suppress immune responses in general. For example, staphylococci produce toxins, such as the **staphylococcal enterotoxins** and **toxic shock syndrome toxin-1**, that act as superantigens. Superantigens are proteins that bind the antigen receptors of very large numbers of T cells (see Section 5-15), stimulating them to produce cytokines that cause significant suppression of all immune responses. The details of this suppression are not understood. The stimulated T cells proliferate and then rapidly undergo apoptosis, leaving a generalized immunosuppression together with the deletion of certain families of peripheral T cells.

Many other pathogens cause mild or transient immunosuppression during acute infection. These forms of suppressed immunity are poorly understood but important, as they often make the host susceptible to secondary infections by common environmental microorganisms. A crucially important example of immune suppression follows trauma, burns, or even major surgery. The burned patient has a clearly diminished capability to respond to infection, and generalized infection is a common cause of death in these patients. The reasons for this are also not fully understood.

Measles virus infection, in spite of the widespread availability of an effective vaccine, still accounts for 10% of the global mortality of children under 5 years old and is the eighth leading cause of death worldwide. Malnourished children are the main victims and the cause of death is usually secondary bacterial infection, particularly pneumonia caused by measles-induced immunosuppression. The immunosuppression that follows measles infection can last for several months and is associated with reduced T- and B-cell function. There is reduced or absent delayed-type hypersensitivity and, during this period of acquired immunodeficiency, children have markedly increased susceptibility to mycobacterial infection, reflecting the important role of macrophage activation by T_H1 cells in host defense against mycobacteria. An important mechanism for measles-induced immunosuppression is the infection of dendritic cells by measles virus. Infected dendritic cells cause unresponsiveness of T lymphocytes by mechanisms that are not yet understood, and it seems likely that this is the proximate cause of the immunosuppression induced by measles virus.

Acquired Immune
Deficiency Syndrome
(AIDS)

The most extreme case of immune suppression caused by a pathogen is the acquired immune deficiency syndrome caused by infection with HIV. The ultimate cause of death in AIDS is usually infection with an **opportunistic pathogen**, a term used to describe a microorganism that is present in the environment but does not usually cause disease because it is well controlled by normal host defenses. HIV infection leads to a gradual loss of immune competence, allowing infection with organisms that are not normally pathogenic. We return to this topic in the last part of this chapter.

Lepromatous
Leprosy

Leprosy, which we discussed in Section 8-13, is a more complex case, in which the causal bacterium, *Mycobacterium leprae*, is associated either with the suppression of cell-mediated immunity or with a strong cell-mediated antibacterial response. This leads to two major forms of the disease—lepromatous and tuberculoid leprosy. In **lepromatous leprosy**, cell-mediated immunity is profoundly depressed, *M. leprae*-infected cells are present in great profusion, and cellular immune responses to many antigens are suppressed. This leads to a phenotypic state in such patients called **anergy**, here meaning the absence of delayed-type hypersensitivity to a wide range of antigens unrelated to *M. leprae*. In **tuberculoid leprosy**, by contrast, there is potent cell-mediated immunity with macrophage activation, which controls but does not eradicate infection. Few viable microorganisms are found in tissues, the patients usually survive, and most of the symptoms and pathology are caused by the inflammatory response to these persistent microorganisms (Fig. 11.6). The difference between the two forms of disease might lie in a difference in the ratio of T_H1 to T_H2 cells, and this is thought to be caused by cytokines produced by CD8 T cells, as we learned in Section 10-6.

Infection with *Mycobacterium leprae* can result in different clinical forms of leprosy
There are two polar forms, tuberculoid and lepromatous leprosy, but several intermediate forms also exist

Tuberculoid leprosy	Lepromatous leprosy
Organisms present at low to undetectable levels	Organisms show florid growth in macrophages
Low infectivity	High infectivity
Granulomas and local inflammation. Peripheral nerve damage	Disseminated infection. Bone, cartilage, and diffuse nerve damage
Normal serum immunoglobulin levels	Hypergammaglobulinemia
Normal T-cell responsiveness. Specific response to *M. leprae* antigens	Low or absent T-cell responsiveness. No response to *M. leprae* antigens

Cytokine patterns in leprosy lesions

Fig. 11.6 T-cell and macrophage responses to *Mycobacterium leprae* are sharply different in the two polar forms of leprosy. Infection with *M. leprae*, which stain as small dark red dots in the photographs, can lead to two very different forms of disease. In tuberculoid leprosy (left), growth of the organism is well controlled by T_H1-like cells that activate infected macrophages. The tuberculoid lesion contains granulomas and is inflamed, but the inflammation is local and causes only local effects, such as peripheral nerve damage. In lepromatous leprosy (right), infection is widely disseminated and the bacilli grow uncontrolled in macrophages; in the late stages of disease there is major damage to connective tissues and to the peripheral nervous system. There are several intermediate stages between these two polar forms. The cytokine patterns in the two polar forms of the disease are sharply different, as shown by the analysis of RNA isolated from lesions of four patients with lepromatous leprosy and four patients with tuberculoid leprosy (Northern blot, lower panel). Cytokines typically produced by T_H2 cells (IL-4, IL-5, and IL-10) dominate in the lepromatous form, whereas cytokines produced by T_H1 cells (IL-2, IFN-γ, and TNF-β) dominate in the tuberculoid form. It therefore seems that T_H1-like cells predominate in tuberculoid leprosy, and T_H2-like cells in lepromatous leprosy. IFN-γ would be expected to activate macrophages, enhancing killing of *M. leprae*, whereas IL-4 can actually inhibit the induction of bactericidal activity in macrophages. High levels of IL-4 would also explain the hypergammaglobulinemia observed in lepromatous leprosy. The determining factors in the initial induction of T_H1- or T_H2-like cells are suspected to be so-called T_C1 or T_C2 cells, by analogy with T_H1 and T_H2 cells. The mechanism for the anergy or generalized loss of effective cell-mediated immunity in lepromatous leprosy is not understood. Photographs courtesy of G. Kaplan; cytokine patterns courtesy of R.L. Modlin.

11-5 Immune responses can contribute directly to pathogenesis.

Tuberculoid leprosy is just one example of an infection in which the pathology is caused largely by the immune response. This is true to some degree in most infections; for example, the fever that accompanies a bacterial infection is caused by the release of cytokines by macrophages. One medically important example of immunopathology is the wheezy broncheolitis caused by **respiratory syncytial virus** (**RSV**) infection. Broncheolitis caused by RSV is the major cause of admission of young children to hospital in the Western world, with as many as 90,000 admissions and 4500 deaths each year in the United States alone. The first indication that the immune response to the virus might have a role in the pathogenesis of this disease came from the observation that young infants vaccinated with an alum-precipitated killed virus preparation suffered a worse disease than children who did not receive this vaccine. This occurred because the vaccine failed to induce neutralizing antibodies but succeeded in producing T_H2 cells. On infection, the T_H2 cells released interleukin (IL)-3, IL-4, and IL-5, which induced bronchospasm, increased secretion of mucus, and tissue eosinophilia. Mice can be infected with RSV and develop a disease similar to that seen in humans.

Another example of a pathogenic immune response is the response to the eggs of the schistosome. Schistosomes are parasitic worms that lay eggs in the hepatic portal vein. Some of the eggs reach the intestine and are shed in the feces, spreading the infection; others lodge in the portal circulation of the liver, where they elicit a potent immune response leading to chronic inflammation, hepatic fibrosis, and eventually liver failure. This process reflects the excessive activation of T_H1 cells and can be modulated by T_H2 cells, IL-4, or CD8 T cells, which can also act by producing IL-4.

Summary.

Infectious agents can cause recurrent or persistent disease by avoiding normal host defense mechanisms or by subverting them to promote their own replication. There are many different ways of evading or subverting the immune response. Antigenic variation, latency, resistance to immune effector mechanisms, and suppression of the immune response all contribute to persistent and medically important infections. In some cases the immune response is part of the problem: some pathogens use immune activation to spread infection, and others would not cause disease if it were not for the immune response. Each of these mechanisms teaches us something about the nature of the immune response and its weaknesses, and each requires a different medical approach to prevent or to treat infection.

Immunodeficiency diseases.

Immunodeficiencies occur when one or more components of the immune system is defective. The immunodeficiencies are classified as primary or secondary. Primary immunodeficiencies are caused by mutations affecting any of a large number of genes that control the expression and activities of immune responses. Most primary immunodeficiencies present in the clinic as recurrent or overwhelming infections in very young children, although milder inherited abnormalities may not show clinical symptoms until later in life. By contrast, secondary immunodeficiencies are acquired as a consequence of other diseases, or are secondary to environmental factors such as starvation, or are an adverse consequence of medical intervention.

By examining which infections accompany a particular inherited or acquired immunodeficiency, we can see which components of the immune system are important in the response to particular infectious agents. The inherited immunodeficiency diseases also reveal how interactions between different cell types contribute to the immune response and to the development of T and B lymphocytes. Finally, these inherited diseases can lead us to the defective gene, often revealing new information about the molecular basis of immune processes and providing the necessary information for diagnosis, for genetic counseling, and eventually for gene therapy.

11-6   A history of repeated infections suggests a diagnosis of immunodeficiency.

Patients with immune deficiency are usually detected clinically by a history of recurrent infection with the same or similar pathogens. The type of infection is a guide to which part of the immune system is deficient. Recurrent infection by **pyogenic**, or pus-forming, bacteria suggests a defect in antibody, complement, or phagocyte function, reflecting the role of these parts of the immune system in host defense against such infections. By contrast, a history of persistent fungal skin infection, cutaneous candidiasis, or recurrent viral infections is more suggestive of a defect in host defense mediated by T lymphocytes.

To determine the competence of the immune system in patients with possible immunodeficiency, a battery of tests is usually conducted (Fig. 11.7); these focus with increasing precision as the nature of the defect is narrowed down to a single element. The presence of the various cell types in blood is determined by routine hematology, often followed by FACS analysis (see

Evaluation of the cellular components of the human immune system			
	B cells	T cells	Phagocytes
Normal numbers ($\times 10^9$ per liter of blood)	Approximately 0.3	Total 1.0–2.5 CD4 0.5–1.6 CD8 0.3–0.9	Monocytes 0.15–0.60 Polymorphonuclear leukocytes Neutrophils 3.00–5.50 Eosinophils 0.05–0.25 Basophils 0.02
Measurement of function *in vivo*	Serum Ig levels Specific antibody levels	Skin test	—
Measurement of function *in vitro*	Induced antibody production in response to pokeweed mitogen	T-cell proliferation in response to phytohemagglutinin or to tetanus toxoid	Phagocytosis Nitro blue tetrazolium uptake Intracellular killing of bacteria
Specific defects	See Fig. 11.8	See Fig. 11.8	See Fig. 11.8

Evaluation of the humoral components of the human immune system				
	Immunoglobulins			Complement
Component	IgG	IgM	IgA	IgE	
Normal levels in adults	600–1400 mg dl^{-1}	40–345 mg dl^{-1}	60–380 mg dl^{-1}	0–200 IU ml^{-1}	CH$_{50}$ of 125–300 IU ml^{-1}

Fig. 11.7 Evaluation of immune competence.

Appendix I, Section A-22) of lymphocyte subsets, and the measurement of serum immunoglobulins. The phagocytic competence of freshly isolated polymorphonuclear leukocytes and monocytes is tested, and the efficiency of the complement system is determined by testing the dilution of serum required for the lysis of 50% of antibody-coated red blood cells (this is denoted the CH_{50}).

In general, if such tests reveal a defect in one of these broad compartments of immune function, more specialized testing is then needed to determine the precise nature of the defect. Tests of lymphocyte function are often valuable, starting with the ability of polyclonal mitogens to induce T-cell proliferation and B-cell secretion of immunoglobulin in tissue culture (see Appendix I, Section A-31). These tests can eventually pinpoint the cellular defect in immunodeficiency.

11-7   Inherited immunodeficiency diseases are caused by recessive gene defects.

Before the advent of highly effective antibiotic therapy, it is likely that most individuals with inherited immune defects died in infancy or early childhood because of their susceptibility to particular classes of pathogen (Fig. 11.8). Such cases would not have been easy to identify, as many normal infants also died of infection. Thus, although many inherited immunodeficiency diseases have now been identified, the first immunodeficiency disease was not described until 1952. Most of the gene defects that cause these inherited immunodeficiencies are recessive and, for this reason, many of the known immunodeficiencies are caused by mutations in genes on the X chromosome. Recessive defects cause disease only when both chromosomes are defective. However, as males have only one X chromosome, all males who inherit an X chromosome carrying a defective gene will manifest disease, whereas female carriers, having two X chromosomes, are usually healthy. Immunodeficiency diseases that affect various steps in B- and T-lymphocyte development have been described, as have defects in surface molecules that are important for T- or B-cell function. Defects in phagocytic cells, in complement, in cytokines, in cytokine receptors, and in molecules that mediate effector responses also occur (see Fig. 11.8). Thus, immunodeficiency can be caused by defects in either the adaptive or the innate immune system. Individual examples of these diseases will be described in later sections.

More recently, the use of gene knockout techniques in mice has allowed the creation of many immunodeficient states that are adding rapidly to our knowledge of the contribution of individual molecules to normal immune function. Nevertheless, human immunodeficiency disease is still the best source of insight into normal pathways of host defense against infectious diseases in humans. For example, a deficiency of antibody, of complement, or of phagocytic function each increases the risk of infection by certain pyogenic bacteria. This shows that the normal pathway of host defense against such bacteria is the binding of antibody followed by fixation of complement, which allows the opsonized bacteria to be taken up by phagocytic cells. Breaking any one of the links in this chain of events leading to bacterial killing causes a similar immunodeficient state.

The study of immunodeficiency also teaches us about the redundancy of mechanisms of host defense against infectious disease. The first two people to be discovered with a hereditary deficiency of complement were healthy immunologists. This teaches us two lessons. The first is that there are multiple protective immune mechanisms against infection; for example, although there is abundant evidence that complement deficiency increases susceptibility to pyogenic infection, not every human with complement deficiency

Name of deficiency syndrome	Specific abnormality	Immune defect	Susceptibility
Severe combined immune deficiency	ADA deficiency	No T or B cells	General
	PNP deficiency	No T or B cells	General
	X-linked *scid*, γ_c chain deficiency	No T cells	General
	Autosomal *scid* DNA repair defect	No T or B cells	General
DiGeorge's syndrome	Thymic aplasia	Variable numbers of T and B cells	General
MHC class I deficiency	TAP mutations	No CD8 T cells	Chronic lung and skin inflammation
MHC class II deficiency	Lack of expression of MHC class II	No CD4 T cells	General
Wiskott–Aldrich syndrome	X-linked; defective WASP gene	Defective anti-polysaccharide antibody and impaired T-cell activation responses	Encapsulated extracellular bacteria
X-linked agamma-globulinemia	Loss of Btk tyrosine kinase	No B cells	Extracellular bacteria, viruses
X-linked hyper IgM syndrome	Defective CD40 ligand	No isotype switching	Extracellular bacteria *Pneumocystis carinii* *Cryptosporidium parvum*
Common variable immunodeficiency	Unknown; MHC-linked	Defective IgA and IgG production	Extracellular bacteria
Selective IgA	Unknown; MHC-linked	No IgA synthesis	Respiratory infections
Phagocyte deficiencies	Many different	Loss of phagocyte function	Extracellular bacteria and fungi
Complement deficiencies	Many different	Loss of specific complement components	Extracellular bacteria especially *Neisseria* spp.
Natural killer (NK) cell defect	Unknown	Loss of NK function	Herpes viruses
X-linked lympho-proliferative syndrome	SH2D1A mutant	Inability to control B cell growth	EBV-driven B cell tumors
Ataxia telangiectasia	Gene with PI 3-kinase homology	T cells reduced	Respiratory infections
Bloom's syndrome	Defective DNA helicase	T cells reduced Reduced antibody levels	Respiratory infections

Fig. 11.8 Human immunodeficiency syndromes. The specific gene defect, the consequence for the immune system, and the resulting disease susceptibilities are listed for some common and some rare human immunodeficiency syndromes. ADA, adenosine deaminase; PNP, purine nucleotide phosphorylase; TAP, transporters associated with antigen processing; WASP, Wiskott–Aldrich syndrome protein; EBV, Epstein–Barr virus; NK, natural killer.

See various cases in
Case Studies in Immunology

suffers from recurrent infections. The second lesson concerns the phenomenon of **ascertainment artifact**. When an unusual observation is made in a patient with disease, there is a temptation to seek a causal link; however, no one would suggest that complement deficiency causes a genetic predisposition to becoming an immunologist. Complement deficiency was discovered in immunologists because they used their own blood in their experiments. If a particular measurement is made only in a highly selected group of patients with a particular disease, it is inevitable that the only abnormal results will be discovered in patients with that disease. This is an ascertainment artifact and emphasizes the importance of studying appropriate controls.

11-8   The main effect of low levels of antibody is an inability to clear extracellular bacteria.

Pyogenic bacteria have polysaccharide capsules that are not directly recognized by the receptors on macrophages and neutrophils that stimulate phagocytosis. They therefore escape immediate elimination by the innate immune response and are successful extracellular pathogens. Normal individuals can clear infections by such bacteria because antibody and complement opsonize the bacteria, making it possible for phagocytes to ingest and destroy them. The principal effect of deficiencies in antibody production is therefore a failure to control this class of bacterial infection. In addition, susceptibility to some viral infections, most notably those caused by enteroviruses, is also increased, because of the importance of antibodies in neutralizing infectious viruses that enter the body through the gut (see Chapter 10).

The first description of an immunodeficiency disease was Ogden C. Bruton's account, in 1952, of the failure of a male child to produce antibody. Because this defect is inherited in an X-linked fashion and is characterized by the absence of immunoglobulin in the serum, it was called **Bruton's X-linked agammaglobulinemia** (**XLA**). The absence of antibody can be detected using immunoelectrophoresis (Fig. 11.9). Since then, many more diseases of antibody production have been described, most of them the consequence of failures in the development or activation of B lymphocytes. Infants with these diseases are usually identified as a result of recurrent infections with pyogenic bacteria such as *Streptococcus pneumoniae*.

The defective gene in XLA is now known to encode a protein tyrosine kinase called Btk (Bruton's tyrosine kinase) which is a member of the recently described family of Tec kinases (see Section 6-11). This protein is expressed in neutrophils as well as in B cells, although only B cells are defective in these patients, in whom B-cell maturation is largely arrested at the pre-B-cell stage. Thus, it is likely that Btk is required to couple the pre-B-cell receptor (which

Fig. 11.9 Immunoelectrophoresis reveals the absence of several distinct immunoglobulin isotypes in serum from a patient with X-linked agammaglobulinemia (XLA). Serum samples from a normal control and from a patient with recurrent bacterial infection caused by the absence of antibody production, as reflected in an absence of gamma globulins, are separated by electrophoresis on an agar-coated slide. Antiserum raised against whole normal human serum and containing antibodies against many of its different proteins is put in a trough down the middle; each antibody forms an arc of precipitation with the protein it recognizes. The position of each arc is determined by the electrophoretic mobility of the serum protein; immunoglobulins migrate to the gamma globulin region of the gel. The absence of immunoglobulins in a patient who has X-linked agammaglobulinemia is shown in the panel at the bottom, where several arcs are missing from the patient's serum (upper set). These are IgA, IgM, and several subclasses of IgG, each recognized in normal serum (lower set) by antibodies in the antiserum against human serum proteins. Bottom panel from the collection of the late C.A. Janeway Sr.

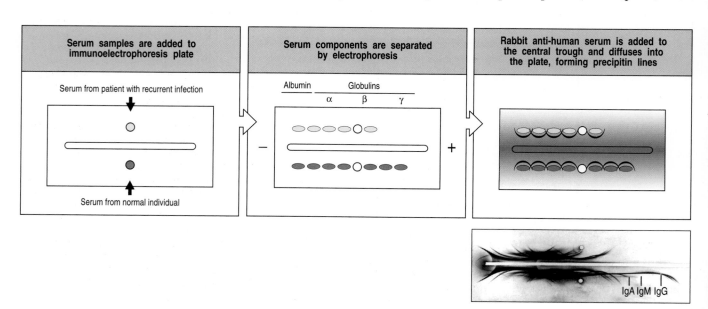

consists of heavy chains, surrogate light chains, and Igα and Igβ) to nuclear events that lead to pre-B-cell growth and differentiation (see Section 7-9). In patients with Btk deficiencies, some B cells mature despite the defect in the signaling kinase, suggesting that signals transmitted by these kinases are not absolutely required.

Because the gene responsible for XLA is found on the X chromosome, it is possible to identify female carriers by analyzing X-chromosome inactivation in their B cells. During development, female cells randomly inactivate one of their two X chromosomes. Because the product of a normal *btk* gene is required for normal B-lymphocyte development, only cells in which the normal allele of *btk* is active can develop into mature B cells. Thus, in female carriers of mutant *btk* genes, all B cells have the normal X chromosome as the active X. By contrast, the active X chromosomes in the T cells and macrophages of carriers are an equal mixture of the normal and *btk* mutant X chromosomes. This fact allowed female carriers of XLA to be identified even before the nature of *btk* was known. Nonrandom X inactivation only in B cells also demonstrates conclusively that the *btk* gene is required for normal B-cell development but not for the development of other cell types, and that Btk must act within B cells rather than on stromal cells or other cells required for B-cell development (Fig. 11.10).

X-linked Agammaglobulinemia

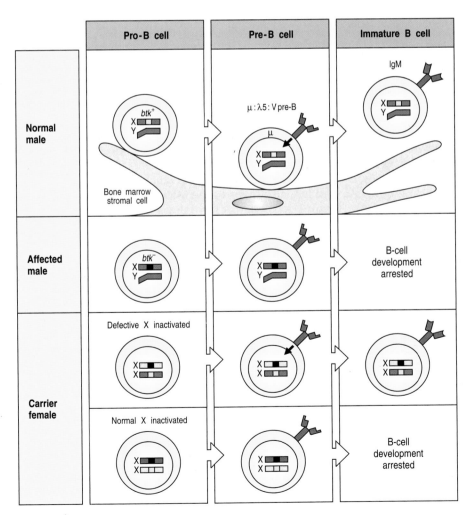

Fig. 11.10 The product of the *btk* gene is important for B-cell development. In X-linked agammaglobulinemia (XLA), a protein tyrosine kinase of the Tec family called Btk, encoded on the X chromosome, is defective. In normal individuals, B-cell development proceeds through a stage in which the pre-B-cell receptor consisting of μ:λ5: V pre-B transduces a signal via Btk, triggering further B-cell development. In males with XLA, no signal can be transduced and, although the pre-B-cell receptor is expressed, the B cells develop no further. In female mammals, including humans, one of the two X chromosomes in each cell is permanently inactivated early in development. Because the choice of which chromosome to inactivate is random, half of the pre-B cells in a carrier female will have inactivated the chromosome with the wild-type *btk*, meaning that they can express only the defective *btk* gene and cannot develop further. Therefore, in the carrier, mature B cells always have the nondefective X chromosome active. This is in sharp contrast to all other cell types, which have the nondefective X chromosome active in only half of their cells. Nonrandom X-chromosome inactivation in a particular cell lineage is a clear indication that the product of the X-linked gene is required for the development of cells of that lineage. It is also sometimes possible to identify the stage at which the gene product is required, by detecting the point in development at which X-chromosome inactivation develops bias. Using this kind of analysis, one can identify carriers of X-linked traits such as XLA without needing to know the nature of the mutant gene.

Fig. 11.11 Immunoglobulin levels in newborn infants fall to low levels at about 6 months of age. Babies are born with high levels of IgG, which is actively transported across the placenta from the mother during gestation. After birth, the production of IgM starts almost immediately; the production of IgG, however, does not begin for about 6 months, during which time the total level of IgG falls as the maternally acquired IgG is catabolized. Thus, IgG levels are low from about the age of 3 months to 1 year, which can lead to susceptibility to disease.

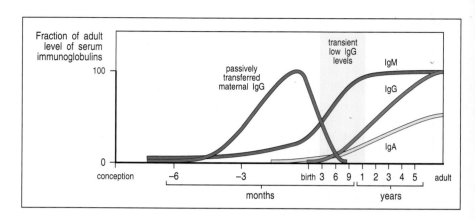

The commonest humoral immune defect is the transient deficiency in immunoglobulin production that occurs in the first 6–12 months of life. The newborn infant has initial antibody levels comparable to those of the mother, because of the transplacental transport of maternal IgG (see Section 9-13). As the transferred IgG is catabolized, antibody levels gradually decrease until the infant begins to produce useful amounts of its own IgG at about 6 months of age (Fig. 11.11). Thus, IgG levels are quite low between the ages of 3 months and 1 year when active IgG antibody responses are poor. In some infants this can lead to a period of heightened susceptibility to infection. This is especially true for premature babies, who begin with lower levels of maternal IgG and also reach immune competence later after birth.

The most common inherited form of immunoglobulin deficiency in populations of European origin is **selective IgA deficiency**, which is seen in about 1 person in 800. Although no obvious disease susceptibility is associated with selective IgA defects, they are commoner in people with chronic lung disease than in the general population. Lack of IgA might thus result in a predisposition to lung infections with various pathogens and is consistent with the role of IgA in defense at the body's surfaces. The genetic basis of this defect is unknown, but some data suggest that a gene of unidentified function mapping in the class III region of the MHC could be involved. A related syndrome called **common variable immunodeficiency**, in which there is usually a deficiency in IgM, IgG, and IgA, also maps to the MHC region. In familial cases, common variable immunodeficiency or IgA deficiency can be seen in different family members, and conversion from one phenotype to the other can occur over time.

People with pure B-cell defects resist many pathogens successfully. However, effective defense against a subset of extracellular pyogenic bacteria, including staphylococci and streptococci, requires the opsonization of these bacteria with specific antibody. In people with B-cell defects, these infections can be suppressed with antibiotics and monthly infusions of human immunoglobulin collected from a large pool of donors. Because there are antibodies against many pathogens in this pooled immunoglobulin, it serves as a fairly successful shield against infection.

11-9 T-cell defects can also result in low antibody levels.

Patients with **hyper IgM syndrome** have normal B- and T-cell development and high serum levels of IgM, but make very limited IgM antibody responses against T-cell dependent antigens and produce immunoglobulin isotypes other than IgM and IgD only in trace amounts. This makes them highly susceptible to infection with extracellular pathogens. Two types of hyper IgM syndrome have been distinguished that illustrate two different pathways that are essential for normal isotype-switch recombination and somatic hypermutation in B cells.

The commonest variant of hyper IgM syndrome is **X-linked hyper IgM syndrome**, which is caused by mutations in the gene for CD40 ligand (CD154). CD40 ligand is normally expressed on activated T cells, which therefore can engage the CD40 molecule on B cells. In cases of CD40 ligand deficiency, the B cells do not have their CD40 engaged although the B cells themselves are normal. We learned in Chapter 9 that CD40 ligand is critical in the T-cell dependent activation of B-cell proliferation, and these patients illustrate that CD40 ligand is also essential for the induction of the isotype switch and the formation of germinal centers (Fig. 11.12). There are also defects in cell-mediated immunity in these individuals. For example, they are susceptible to infection with the opportunistic lung pathogen *Pneumocystis carinii*, which is normally killed by activated macrophages. The susceptibility is thought to be due, at least in part, to the inability of the T cells to deliver an activating signal to infected macrophages by engaging the CD40 expressed on these cells (see Section 8-29). A defect in T-cell activation could also contribute to the profound immunodeficiency suffered by these patients, as studies on mice that lack CD40 ligand have revealed a failure of antigen-specific T cells to expand in response to primary immunization with antigen. A very similar syndrome has been identified in patients with mutations in two other genes. The first is the *CD40* gene, in which mutations have been found in several patients with a recessive variant of hyper IgM syndrome. The second mutated gene was found in a rare group of patients with a developmental disorder that includes hyper IgM syndrome, called **hypohydrotic ectodermal dysplasia with immunodeficiency**, in which patients lack sweat glands and have abnormal hair and tooth development. In this disease, also known as **NEMO deficiency**, mutations were found in the gene for a zinc-finger domain-containing protein named NEMO (NFκB essential modulator, also known as IKKγ), which is an essential component of the intracellular signaling pathway leading to activation of the transcription factor NFκB. These discoveries show that mutations in the pathway triggered by CD40 ligand on T cells binding to CD40, its receptor on B cells, and leading to NFκB activation by downstream signaling by CD40, all result in closely similar immunodeficiency syndromes.

The second type of hyper IgM syndrome is caused by an intrinsic defect in B cells and is associated with a milder form of immunodeficiency in which patients show increased susceptibility to severe bacterial infections but do not suffer from opportunistic infections such as *Pneumocystis carinii*. This syndrome is caused by mutations in the gene encoding an enzyme called **activation-induced cytidine deaminase** (AID; see Section 4-9). The B cells in these patients show two abnormalities: they fail to switch antibody isotype and also have severely reduced somatic hypermutation. The consequence is that immature B cells accumulate in abnormal germinal centers, causing enlargement of the lymph nodes and spleen. Activation-induced cytidine deaminase is expressed only in B cells that have been activated to isotype switch by ligation of CD40 or by stimulation with bacterial lipopolysaccharide or the appropriate cytokines. The degree of immunodeficiency associated with hyper IgM syndrome caused by **AID deficiency** is less than that associated with CD40 ligand, CD40, or NEMO deficiency. This is because AID deficiency only causes the failure of normal antibody responses, whereas deficiency of the latter proteins is associated with B- and T-cell defects.

These diseases illustrate the fact that the study of immunodeficiency can both lead us to new genes and help us to determine the roles of known genes in normal immune-system function.

Hyper IgM Immunodeficiency

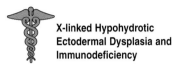

X-linked Hypohydrotic Ectodermal Dysplasia and Immunodeficiency

Activation-induced Cytidine Deaminase (AID) Deficiency

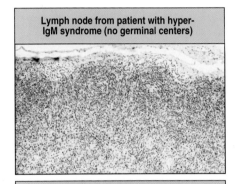

Lymph node from patient with hyper-IgM syndrome (no germinal centers)

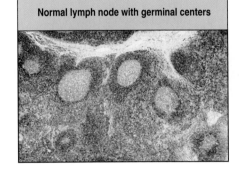

Normal lymph node with germinal centers

Fig. 11.12 Patients with X-linked hyper IgM syndrome are unable to activate their B cells fully. Lymphoid tissues in patients with hyper IgM syndrome are devoid of germinal centers (top panel), unlike a normal lymph node (bottom panel). B-cell activation by T cells is required both for isotype switching and for the formation of germinal centers, where extensive B-cell proliferation takes place. Photographs courtesy of R. Geha and A. Perez-Atayde.

Deficiency of the C8
Complement Component

11-10 Defects in complement components cause defective humoral immune function.

Not surprisingly, the spectrum of infections associated with complement deficiencies overlaps substantially with that seen in patients with deficiencies in antibody production. Defects in the activation of C3, and in C3 itself, are associated with a wide range of pyogenic infections, emphasizing the important role of C3 as an opsonin, promoting the phagocytosis of bacteria (Fig. 11.13). In contrast, defects in the membrane-attack components of complement (C5–C9) have more limited effects and result exclusively in susceptibility to *Neisseria* species. This indicates that host defense against these bacteria, which are capable of intracellular survival, is mediated by extracellular lysis by the membrane-attack complex of complement. Accurate data from large population studies in Japan, where endemic *N. meningitidis* infection is rare, show that the risk each year of infection with this organism is approximately 1 in 2,000,000 to a normal person. This compares with a risk of 1 in 200 in the same population to a person with inherited deficiency of one of the membrane-attack complex proteins—a 10,000-fold increase in risk compared with a person with normal complement activity. The early components of the classical complement pathway are particularly important for the elimination of immune complexes and apoptotic cells, which can cause significant pathology in autoimmune diseases such as systemic lupus erythematosus. This aspect of inherited complement deficiency is discussed in Chapter 13.

Another set of diseases are caused by defects in complement control proteins (see Section 2-19). People lacking decay-accelerating factor (DAF) and CD59, which protect a person's own cell surfaces from complement activation, destroy their own red blood cells. This results in the disease paroxysmal nocturnal hemoglobinuria, as we learned in Chapter 2. A more striking consequence

Fig. 11.13 Defects in complement components are associated with susceptibility to certain infections and accumulation of immune complexes. Defects in the early components of the alternative pathway and in C3 lead to susceptibility to extracellular pathogens, particularly pyogenic bacteria. Defects in the early components of the classical pathway predominantly affect the processing of immune complexes and clearance of apoptotic cells, leading to immune-complex disease. Deficiency of mannose-binding lectin (MBL), the recognition molecule of the mannose-binding lectin pathway, is associated with bacterial infections, mainly in early childhood. Finally, defects in the membrane-attack components are associated only with susceptibility to strains of *Neisseria* species, the causative agents of meningitis and gonorrhea, implying that the effector pathway is important chiefly in defense against these organisms.

of the loss of a regulatory protein is seen in patients with C1-inhibitor defects. C1 inhibitor irreversibly inhibits the activity of several serine proteinase enzymes. These include two enzymes that participate in the contact activation system of blood clotting, factor XIIa (activated Hageman factor) and kallikrein, in addition to the two enzymes that together initiate the classical pathway of complement, C1r and C1s. Deficiency of C1 inhibitor leads to a failure to regulate these two pathways. Their unregulated activity results in the excessive production of vasoactive mediators that cause fluid accumulation in the tissues and epiglottal swelling that can lead to suffocation. These mediators are bradykinin, produced by the cleavage of high molecular weight kininogen by kallikrein and the C2 kinin, produced by the activity of C1s on C2a. This syndrome is called **hereditary angioneurotic edema**.

Hereditary
Angioneurotic Edema

11-11 Defects in phagocytic cells permit widespread bacterial infections.

Deficiencies in phagocyte numbers or function can be associated with severe immunodeficiency; indeed a total absence of neutrophils is incompatible with survival in the normal environment. Inherited deficiencies of neutrophils (**neutropenias**) are classified as **severe congenital neutropenia** or as **cyclic neutropenia**. In severe congenital neutropenia, which can be inherited as a dominant or recessive trait, the neutrophil count is persistently extremely low, at less than 0.2×10^9 per liter, and patients depend on successful bone marrow transplantation for survival. Cyclic neutropenia is a dominantly inherited disease in which neutrophil numbers fluctuate from near normal to very low or none, with an approximate cycle time of 21 days. Other bone marrow derived cells—monocytes, platelets, lymphocytes, and reticulocytes—undergo smaller fluctuations in numbers with the same periodicity. Surprisingly, it transpires that mutations in neutrophil elastase cause cyclic neutropenia and also cause a significant fraction of the dominant variant of severe congenital neutropenia. The mutations in the neutrophil elastase seem to lead to the production of dysfunctional proteins that have a dominant-negative effect. It seems likely that the mutant neutrophil elastase may be resistant to serine proteinase inhibitors and/or be targeted to the wrong intracellular compartment. This can lead to the expression of a toxic intracellular protein that blocks neutrophil maturation. How the mutant elastase causes a 21-day cycle in neutropenia and the effects on other bone marrow cell types is still a mystery.

Defects in the recruitment of phagocytic cells to extravascular sites of infection can cause serious immunodeficiency. Leukocytes reach such sites by emigrating from blood vessels in a tightly regulated process consisting of three stages. The first is the rolling adherence of leukocytes to endothelial cells, through the binding of a fucosylated tetrasaccharide ligand known as sialyl-Lewis^x to E-selectin and P-selectin. Sialyl-Lewis^x is expressed on monocytes and neutrophils, whereas E-selectin and P-selectin are expressed on endothelium activated by mediators from the site of infection. The second stage is the tight adherence of the leukocytes to the endothelium through the binding of leukocyte β_2 integrins such as CD11b:CD18 (Mac-1:CR3) to counter-receptors on endothelial cells. The third and final stage is the transmigration of leukocytes through the endothelium along gradients of chemotactic molecules originating from the site of tissue injury. Neutrophil recruitment is illustrated in Fig. 2.44 and described in more detail in Section 2-22.

Deficiencies in the molecules involved in each of these stages can prevent neutrophils and macrophages from reaching sites of infection to ingest and destroy bacteria. Reduced rolling adhesion has been described in patients with a lack of sialyl-Lewis^x caused by a deficiency in a putative GDP-fucose transporter that participates in fucosylation during sialyl-Lewis^x biosynthesis.

Fig. 11.14 Defects in phagocytic cells are associated with persistence of bacterial infection. Defects in the leukocyte integrins with a common β$_2$ subunit (CD18) or defects in the selectin ligand, sialyl-Lewis^x, prevent phagocytic cell adhesion and migration to sites of infection (leukocyte adhesion deficiency). The respiratory burst is defective in chronic granulomatous disease, glucose-6-phosphate dehydrogenase (G6PD) deficiency, and myeloperoxidase deficiency. In chronic granulomatous disease, infections persist because macrophage activation is defective, leading to chronic stimulation of CD4 T cells and hence to granulomas. Vesicle fusion in phagocytes is defective in Chediak–Higashi syndrome. These diseases illustrate the critical role of phagocytes in removing and killing pathogenic bacteria.

Type of defect / name of syndrome	Associated infectious or other diseases
Leukocyte adhesion deficiency	Widespread pyogenic bacterial infections
Chronic granulomatous disease	Intracellular and extracellular infection, granulomas
G6PD deficiency	Defective respiratory burst, chronic infection
Myeloperoxidase deficiency	Defective intracellular killing, chronic infection
Chediak–Higashi syndrome	Intracellular and extracellular infection, granulomas

Leukocyte
Adhesion Deficiency

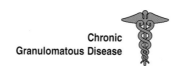

Chronic
Granulomatous Disease

Similarly, deficiencies in the leukocyte integrin common β$_2$ subunit CD18 have been identified and these prevent leukocyte migration to sites of infection by abolishing the leukocyte's ability to adhere tightly to the endothelium, causing the **leukocyte adhesion deficiency** syndrome. A third genetic defect, preventing neutrophil migration, was identified in the *Rac2* gene. The Rac2 protein is a member of the Rho family of GTPases, which regulate neutrophil activation and cytoskeletal function. All these deficiencies lead to infections that are resistant to antibiotic treatment and that persist despite an apparently effective cellular and humoral adaptive immune response. Acquired deficiency of neutrophils (neutropenia) associated with chemotherapy, malignancy, or aplastic anemia is also associated with a similar spectrum of severe pyogenic bacterial infections.

Most of the other known defects in phagocytic cells affect their ability to kill intracellular and/or ingest extracellular bacteria (Fig. 11.14). In **chronic granulomatous disease**, phagocytes cannot produce the superoxide radical, and their antibacterial activity is thereby seriously impaired. Several different genetic defects, affecting any one of the four constituent proteins of the NADPH oxidase system, can cause this. Patients with this disease have chronic bacterial infections, which in some cases lead to the formation of granulomas. Deficiencies in the enzymes glucose-6-phosphate dehydrogenase and myeloperoxidase also impair intracellular killing and lead to a similar, although less severe, phenotype. Finally, in **Chediak–Higashi syndrome**, a complex syndrome characterized by partial albinism, abnormal platelet function, and severe immunodeficiency, a defect in a gene encoding a protein involved in intracellular vesicle formation causes a failure to fuse lysosomes properly with phagosomes; the phagocytes in these patients have enlarged granules and impaired intracellular killing ability.

11-12 Defects in T-cell function result in severe combined immunodeficiencies.

Although patients with B-cell defects can deal with many pathogens adequately, patients with defects in T-cell development are highly susceptible to a broad range of infectious agents. This demonstrates the central role of T cells in adaptive immune responses to virtually all antigens. Because such patients make neither specific T-cell dependent antibody responses nor cell-mediated immune responses, and thus cannot develop immunological memory, they are said to suffer from **severe combined immunodeficiency** (**SCID**).

Several different defects can lead to the SCID phenotype. In X-linked SCID, which is the commonest form of SCID, T cells fail to develop because of a mutation in the common γ chain of several cytokine receptors, including those for the interleukins IL-2, IL-4, IL-7, IL-9, and IL-15. We examine this defect further in Section 11-13. The commonest forms of autosomally inherited SCID are due to **adenosine deaminase** (**ADA**) **deficiency** and **purine nucleotide phosphorylase** (**PNP**) **deficiency**. These enzyme defects affect purine degradation, and both result in an accumulation of nucleotide metabolites that are particularly toxic to developing T cells. B cells are also somewhat compromised in these patients, more so in ADA than in PNP deficiency.

One class of people with SCID lack expression of all MHC class II molecules on their cells, and therefore have an **MHC class II deficiency**. Because the thymus in such individuals lacks MHC class II molecules, CD4 T cells cannot be positively selected and therefore few develop. The antigen-presenting cells in these individuals also lack MHC class II molecules and so the few CD4 T cells that do develop cannot be stimulated by antigen. In these individuals, MHC class I expression is normal and CD8 T cells develop normally. However, such people suffer from SCID, illustrating the central importance of CD4 T cells in adaptive immunity to most pathogens. The syndrome is caused not by mutations in the MHC genes themselves but by mutations in one of several different genes encoding gene-regulatory proteins that are required for the transcriptional activation of MHC class II promoters. Four complementing gene defects (known as groups A, B, C, and D) have been defined in patients who fail to express MHC class II molecules, which implies that at least four different genes are required for normal MHC class II gene expression. One of these, named the *MHC class II transactivator*, or *CIITA*, is the gene mutated in group A. The genes mutated in groups B, C, and D are named *RFXANK*, *RFX5*, and *RFXAP*. These genes encode three proteins that are components of a multimeric complex, RFX, involved in controlling transcription; this complex binds a sequence named an X-box, present in the promoter of all MHC class II genes.

In contrast, a more limited immunodeficiency, associated with chronic respiratory bacterial infections and skin ulceration with vasculitis, has been observed in a small number of patients showing almost complete absence of cell-surface MHC class I molecules, known as **MHC class I deficiency**. Affected individuals have normal levels of mRNA encoding MHC class I molecules and normal production of MHC class I proteins, but very few of these proteins reach the cell surface. The defect was shown to be similar to that in the *TAP* mutant cells mentioned in Section 5-2 and, indeed, affected patients have been found to have mutations in the *TAP1* or *TAP2* genes that encode the two subunits of the peptide transporter. The absence of MHC class I molecules at the cell surface leads to a lack of CD8 T cells expressing the α:β T cell receptor, but these patients do have CD8 T cells that bear the γ:δ receptor. It is surprising that they are not abnormally susceptible to viral infections, given the key role of MHC class I presentation and cytotoxic CD8 α:β T cells in the control of viral infections. However, there is evidence for TAP-independent pathways of antigen presentation of certain peptides by MHC class I molecules. The clinical phenotype of TAP1- and TAP2-deficient patients illustrates that these pathways may be sufficient to allow the control of viral infections.

Another set of defects leading to SCID are those that cause failures of DNA rearrangement in developing lymphocytes. For example, defects in either the *RAG-1* or *RAG-2* gene result in the arrest of lymphocyte development because

X-linked Severe Combined Immunodeficiency

Adenosine Deaminase Deficiency

MHC Class II Deficiency

MHC Class I Deficiency

Omenn
Syndrome

of a failure to rearrange the antigen receptor genes. Thus, there is a complete lack of T and B cells in mice with genetically engineered defects in the *RAG* genes, and in patients with autosomally inherited forms of SCID who lack a functional RAG protein. There are other patients with mutations in either the *RAG-1* or *RAG-2* gene who can nonetheless make a small amount of functional RAG protein, allowing a small amount of V(D)J recombination. They suffer from a distinctive and severe disease called **Omenn's syndrome**, which, in addition to increased susceptibility to multiple opportunistic infections, has clinical features very similar to graft-versus-host disease (see Section 13-38), with rashes, eosinophilia, diarrhea, and enlargement of the lymph nodes. Normal or increased numbers of T cells, all of which are activated, are found in these unfortunate children. A possible explanation for this phenotype is that very low levels of *RAG* activity allow some limited T-cell receptor gene recombination. However, no B cells are found and it may be that B cells have more stringent requirements for *RAG* activity. The T cells that are produced in these patients show an abnormal and highly restricted receptor repertoire, both in the thymus and in the periphery, where they have undergone clonal expansion and activation. The clinical features strongly suggest that these peripheral T cells are autoreactive and responsible for the graft-versus-host phenotype.

Another group of patients with autosomal SCID have a phenotype very similar to that of a mutant mouse strain called *scid*; *scid* mice suffer from an abnormal sensitivity to ionizing radiation as well as from severe combined immunodeficiency. They produce very few mature B and T cells, because there is a failure of DNA rearrangement in their developing lymphocytes; only rare VJ or VDJ joints are seen and most of these are abnormal. The underlying defect in *scid* mice has now been shown to be in the enzyme DNA-dependent protein kinase (DNA-PK$_{CS}$), which binds to the DNA hairpin structures that form at the end of the double-stranded breaks that occur during the process of antigen receptor gene rearrangement. Mutations in a protein called Artemis, which is functionally related to DNA-PK$_{CS}$, are found in some people with autosomal SCID. Artemis is an exonuclease that forms a complex with, and is activated by, DNA-PK$_{CS}$. The normal role of the Artemis:DNA-PK$_{CS}$ complex is to open the hairpin structures to allow the formation of the VDJ joints, to complete the process of VDJ recombination (see Section 4-5).

Other defects in DNA repair and metabolizing enzymes are associated with a combination of immunodeficiency, increased sensitivity to the damaging effects of ionizing radiation, and cancer development. One example is **Bloom's syndrome**, a disease caused by mutations in a DNA helicase enzyme, which unwinds DNA. Another is **ataxia telangiectasia (AT)**, in which the underlying defect is in a protein called ATM, which contains a kinase domain thought to be involved in intracellular signaling in response to DNA damage. Because repair of double-strand DNA breaks and lymphocyte division are central to the function of the adaptive immune system, it is not surprising that defects such as these are associated with the development of immunodeficiency. Defective repair of DNA breaks also causes increased susceptibility to cancer, in both lymphoid and other tissues.

In a final example of a severe combined immunodeficiency—**DiGeorge's syndrome**—the thymic epithelium fails to develop normally. The genetic abnormality underlying this complex developmental disorder is a hemizygous deletion in chromosome 22q11. The deletion varies between 1.5 and 5 megabases in extent, with the smallest deletion that causes the syndrome containing approximately 24 genes. The relevant gene within this interval is *TBX1*, which encodes a transcription factor, T-box 1. DiGeorge's syndrome is caused by the deletion of a single copy of this gene. Without the proper inductive environment T cells cannot mature, and both T-cell dependent antibody production and cell-mediated immunity are absent. Patients with this syndrome have some serum immunoglobulin and variable numbers of B and T cells.

A second disorder of thymic development, associated with SCID and absent expression of body hair, is found in mice; the mutant strain is descriptively named ***nude***. A small number of people have been described with the same phenotype. This syndrome is caused by mutations in a gene named winged-helix-nude (*WHN*). It encodes a transcription factor normally expressed in skin and thymus; alteration of its expression in these tissues underlies the manifestations of disease at these sites. As with all the severe combined immunodeficiency diseases, the defect in T cells is crucial. These diseases abundantly illustrate the central role of T cells in virtually all adaptive immune responses. In many cases B-cell development is normal, yet the response to nearly all pathogens is profoundly impaired. These diseases of thymic development also illustrate the very complex phenotypes that can be associated with mutations in transcription factors that may control the expression of variable numbers of genes in different tissues and organs and often manifest themselves as disorders of embryological development.

11-13 Defective T-cell signaling, cytokine production, or cytokine action can cause immunodeficiency.

Several gene defects have been described that interfere with signaling through T-cell receptors, and thus with the activation of T cells necessary for an adaptive immune response. Patients who lack CD3γ chains therefore have low levels of surface T-cell receptors and defective T-cell responses. Patients making low levels of mutant CD3ε chains are also deficient in T-cell activation. Patients who make a defective form of the cytosolic protein tyrosine kinase ZAP-70, which transmits signals from the T-cell receptor (see Section 6-10), have been described. CD4 T cells emerge from their thymus in normal numbers, whereas CD8 T cells are absent. However, the CD4 T cells that mature fail to respond to stimuli that normally activate via the T-cell receptor, and the patients are thus very immunodeficient. Another lymphocyte signaling defect that leads to severe immunodeficiency is caused by mutations in the tyrosine phosphatase, CD45. Humans and mice with CD45 deficiency show severely reduced peripheral T-cell numbers and abnormal B-cell maturation.

Another group of patients show a lack of IL-2 production upon receptor ligation, and these patients have a severe immunodeficiency; however, their T-cell development is normal, as it is in mice with mutations in the IL-2 genes made by gene knockout (see Appendix I, Section A-47). These IL-2-negative patients have heterogeneous defects; some of them fail to activate the transcription factor NFAT (see Section 6-12), which induces the transcription of several cytokine genes in addition to that for IL-2. This might explain why their immunodeficiency is more profound than that of mice whose IL-2 gene has been disrupted. IL-2-deficient mice can mount adaptive immune responses through an IL-2-independent pathway that may involve the cytokine IL-15, which shares many activities with IL-2; nevertheless, the mice are susceptible to a variety of infectious agents.

In contrast to the normal development of T cells in patients deficient in IL-2, there is a failure of T-cell and NK-cell development in patients with **X-linked severe combined immunodeficiency** (**X-linked SCID**), which is caused by a defect in the γ chain of the IL-2 receptor. Thus, this disease showed that the common γ chain (γc) must be important in T-cell and NK-cell development for reasons unrelated to IL-2 binding or IL-2 responses. The demonstration that the IL-2 receptor γc chain is also part of other cytokine receptors,

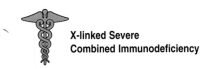

X-linked Severe
Combined Immunodeficiency

including the receptors for IL-7 and IL-15, helps to explain its role in early T-cell and NK-cell development. The γ_c chain seems to function in transducing the signal from this group of receptors, and interacts with a kinase, Jak3 kinase, which is known to be defective in patients with an autosomally inherited severe combined immunodeficiency similar in phenotype to X-linked SCID.

Three additional immunodeficiencies, two in humans and the third engineered in mice, have illuminated part of the role of the different cytokines that share the γ_c chain in T-cell and NK-cell development. Humans with deficiency of the IL-7 receptor α chain have no T cells but normal levels of NK cells, illustrating that IL-7 signaling is essential for the growth of T cells but not for the development of NK cells. In contrast, mice with gene-targeted mutations in IL-15 or the α chain of its receptor have no NK cells and relatively normal T-cell development, although they show reduced T-cell homing to secondary lymphoid tissues and a reduction in the number of CD8-positive T cells. A child reported with SCID lacked NK cells but had normal genes for γ_c and for Jak3 kinase. It transpired that he had a deficiency of the β chain shared by the receptors for IL-2 and IL-15. These mice and the single child define a key role for IL-15 as a growth factor for the development of NK cells, as well as a role for IL-15 in T-cell maturation and trafficking.

As in all serious T-cell deficiencies, X-linked SCID patients do not make effective antibody responses to most antigens, although their B cells seem normal. However, as the gene defect is on the X chromosome, one can determine whether the lack of B-cell function is solely a consequence of the lack of T-cell help by examining X-chromosome inactivation (see Section 11-8) in B cells of unaffected carriers. Most naive IgM-positive B cells from female carriers of X-linked SCID have inactivated the defective X chromosome rather than the normal one, showing that B-cell development is affected by, but is not wholly dependent on, the common γ chain. However, mature memory B cells that have switched to isotypes other than IgM have inactivated the defective X chromosome almost without exception. This might reflect the fact that the IL-2 receptor γ chain is also part of the IL-4 receptor. Thus, B cells that lack this chain will have defective IL-4 receptors and will not proliferate in T-cell-dependent antibody responses. X-linked SCID is so severe that children who inherit it can survive only in a completely pathogen-free environment, unless given antibodies and successfully treated by bone marrow transplantation. A famous case in Houston became known as the 'bubble baby' because of the plastic bubble in which he was enclosed to protect him from infection.

Wiskott–Aldrich Syndrome

Wiskott–Aldrich syndrome (**WAS**) has shed new light on the molecular basis of T-cell signaling and its importance for immune function. The disease affects platelets and was first described as a blood-clotting disorder, but it is also associated with immunodeficiency due to impaired T-cell function, reduced T-cell numbers, and a failure of antibody responses to encapsulated bacteria. WAS is caused by a defective gene on the X chromosome, encoding a protein called WAS protein (WASP). This protein has been shown to bind Cdc42, a small GTP-binding protein that is known to regulate the organization of the actin cytoskeleton and to be important for the effective collaboration of T and B cells. WASP might have a role in regulating changes in the actin cytoskeleton in response to external stimuli. It can bind SH3 domains, which, as we saw in Chapter 6, have an affinity for amino acid sequences rich in proline that are found on some proteins of intracellular signaling pathways. In patients with WAS, and in mice whose WASP gene has been knocked out, T cells fail to respond normally to mitogens or to the cross-linking of surface receptors. Cytotoxic T-cell responses are also impaired, and T-cell help for B-cell responses to polysaccharide antigens is lacking. WASP is expressed in all hematopoietic cell lineages and is likely to be a key regulator of lymphocyte and platelet development and function.

11-14 The normal pathways for host defense against intracellular bacteria are illustrated by genetic deficiencies of IFN-γ and IL-12 and their receptors.

A small number of families have been identified containing several individuals who suffer from persistent and eventually fatal attacks by intracellular pathogens, especially mycobacteria and salmonellae. Typically these patients suffer from the ubiquitous, environmental nontuberculous strains of mycobacteria, such as *Mycobacterium avium*. They may also develop disseminated infection after vaccination with *Mycobacterium bovis* bacillus Calmette–Guérin (BCG), the strain of *M. bovis* that is used as a live vaccine against *M. tuberculosis*. The molecular bases of the susceptibility to these infections are mutations that abolish the function of any of the following proteins: IL-12; the IL-12 receptor β1 chain; or either of the two protein subunits (R1 and R2) of the receptor for interferon (IFN)-γ. A dysfunctional mutant of STAT1, an intracellular protein on the nuclear signaling pathway activated after ligation of the IFN-γ receptor, is also associated in humans with increased susceptibility to mycobacterial infections. Similar susceptibility to intracellular bacterial infection is seen in mice with induced mutations in these same genes, and also in mice lacking tumor necrosis factor (TNF)-α or the TNF p55 receptor gene. All these proteins must therefore have a critical part in the normal mechanisms of host defense against infection by these intracellular bacteria.

Mycobacteria and salmonellae enter dendritic cells and macrophages, where they can reproduce and multiply. At the same time they provoke an immune response that involves several stages and eventually controls the infection with the help of CD4 T cells (Fig. 11.15). First, lipoproteins from the surface of the bacteria ligate receptors on macrophages and dendritic cells as they enter the cells. These receptors include the Toll-like receptors (see Section 2-6), particularly TLR-2, and their ligation stimulates nitric

| Mycobacteria ligate Toll-like receptor 2 (TLR-2) as they infect macrophages | Ligation of TLR-2 induces the macrophage to produce NO intracellularly and to secrete IL-12 | Macrophages present mycobacterial antigens to T cells. In the presence of IL-12, T cells release IFN-γ to stimulate the macrophage | IFN-γ recruits more macrophages, forming a granuloma and activating them to kill intracellular bacteria |

Fig. 11.15 The expression of Toll-like receptor 2 (TLR-2) allows macrophages to respond effectively to mycobacteria. TLR-2 is activated on binding the polysaccharide coat of mycobacteria, stimulating internalization of the bound bacteria and the expression of nitric oxide (NO) and cytokines such as IL-12 by the macrophage. Interaction of macrophages and T cells in the presence of IL-12 leads to the secretion of IFN-γ by T cells; this activates the macrophage, leading to the death of the intracellular mycobacteria.

Interferon-γ
Receptor Deficiency

oxide (NO) production within the cells, which is toxic to the bacteria. Signaling by these Toll-like receptors also stimulates the release of IL-12 which, in turn, stimulates CD4 T cells to release IFN-γ and TNF-α. These cytokines activate and recruit more mononuclear phagocytic cells to the site of infection, resulting in the formation of granulomas. The key role of IFN-γ in activating macrophages to kill intracellular bacteria is illustrated dramatically by the failure to control infection in patients who are genetically deficient in either of the two subunits of this receptor. In the total absence of IFN-γ receptor expression, granuloma formation is much reduced, showing a role for this receptor in the development of granulomas. In contrast, if the underlying mutation is associated with the presence of low levels of functional receptor, granulomas form, but the macrophages within the granulomas are not sufficiently activated to be able to control the division and spread of the mycobacteria. It is important to understand that this cascade of cytokine reactions is occurring in the context of cognate interactions between the macrophages and dendritic cells harboring the intracellular bacteria and antigen-specific CD4 T cells. T-cell receptor ligation and co-stimulation of the phagocyte by, for example, CD40–CD40 ligand interaction send signals that help to activate infected phagocytes sufficiently to kill the intracellular bacteria (see Section 8-26).

11-15 X-linked lymphoproliferative syndrome is associated with fatal infection by Epstein–Barr virus and with the development of lymphomas.

Epstein–Barr virus is a herpes virus that infects the majority of the human race and remains latent in B cells throughout life after primary infection. EBV infection can transform B lymphocytes and is used as a technique for immortalizing clones of B cells in the laboratory. This does not normally happen *in vivo* in humans because EBV infection is actively controlled and maintained in a latent state by cytotoxic T cells with specificity for B cells expressing EBV antigens (see Section 11-2). In the presence of T-cell immunodeficiency this control mechanism can break down and a potentially lethal B-cell lymphoma may develop. One of the situations in which this occurs is the rare immunodeficiency **X-linked lymphoproliferative syndrome**, which results from mutations in a gene named SH2-domain containing gene 1A (*SH2D1A*). This encodes a protein named SAP (an acronym for SLAM-associated protein; SLAM is itself an acronym for signaling lymphocyte activation molecule). Boys with SAP deficiency typically develop overwhelming EBV infection during childhood, and sometimes lymphomas. EBV infection in this condition is usually fatal and is associated with necrosis of the liver. Thus, SAP must have a vital, nonredundant role in the normal control of EBV infection.

X-linked
Lymphoproliferative
Syndrome

The function of SAP is partly understood. The SH2 domain of the protein interacts with the cytoplasmic tails of transmembrane receptors, SLAM and 2B4 (which are structurally homologous to each other), and to the T-cell adhesion molecule CD2 (see Section 8-4). SLAM is expressed on activated T cells, whereas 2B4 is found on T cells, B cells, and NK cells. An activity of SAP is to allow the recruitment of a tyrosine kinase FynT to these receptors. This activates an intracellular signaling cascade that inhibits the production of IFN-γ after T-cell receptor ligation, while not affecting IL-2 production. In the absence of SAP, T cells produce increased amounts of IFN-γ production, and this could lead to a T_H1 skewing of immune responses (see Section 8-13). Boys with X-linked lymphoproliferative syndrome produce markedly more IFN-γ than normal in response to primary infection by EBV. There are two hypotheses to explain the pathogenesis of the fatal EBV infection seen in children with defects in SAP. The first is that the failure of T cells to kill B cells expressing antigens from multiplying EBV allows uncontrolled infection. The second is that the abnormal cytokine response of T cells presented with EBV peptides by infected B cells causes severe inflammatory injury by mechanisms that we discuss in Section 11-16. Some cases of lymphoma in young boys have now been found associated with mutations in the *SH2D1A* gene in the absence of any evidence of EBV infection. This raises the possibility that *SH2D1A* might be a tumor suppressor gene in its own right, in addition to controlling a virus that can contribute to tumor formation.

11-16 Genetic abnormalities in the secretory cytotoxic pathway of lymphocytes cause uncontrolled lymphoproliferation and inflammatory responses to viral infections.

A small group of inherited diseases affect skin pigmentation—causing albinism—as well as the immune system. They have provided insights into the role of cytotoxic lymphocytes in the homeostatic control of immune responses. Many cell types derived from the bone marrow, including lymphocytes, granulocytes, and mast cells, have in common the property of regulated secretion. In response to specific stimuli they exocytose specialized secretory lysosomes that contain specialized collections of proteins. A small number of cell types not derived from the bone marrow also show regulated secretion of secretory lysosomes: melanocytes—the pigment cells of the skin—are prominent among these. The contents of the secretory lysosomes differ according to the cell type. In melanocytes, melanin is the major component, whereas in cytotoxic T lymphocytes, secretory lysosomes contain the cytolytic proteins perforin, granulysin, and granzymes (see Section 8-22). Although the contents of the granules differ between cell types, the fundamental mechanisms for their secretion do not, and this explains how inherited disorders affecting regulated secretion can cause the combination of albinism and immunodeficiency.

We learned in Section 11-15 that X-linked lymphoproliferative syndrome is associated with uncontrolled inflammation in response to EBV infection. In that respect it is very similar to a group of diseases that cause a syndrome known as the **hemophagocytic syndrome**, in which there is a dysregulated expansion of CD8-positive lymphocytes which is associated with macrophage activation. The activated macrophages phagocytose blood cells, including erythrocytes and leukocytes. Some of these hemophagocytic syndromes are inherited, and they can be classified into two types, according to the nature of the gene defect. In the first type the effects of the mutation are confined to lymphocytes or other cells of the immune system because the mutated protein is located within the granules of lymphoid effector cells. In the second, the genetic abnormality is located in the secretory pathway and, in these cases, the skin may be involved as well as the immune system. The inability of melanocytes to secrete melanin-containing lysosomes causes albinism—an obvious phenotypic marker of the disease.

An unpleasant disease named **familial hemophagocytic lymphohistiocytosis** (**FHL**) is caused by an inherited deficiency of perforin. This is an example of a lymphocyte-specific disorder, in which polyclonal CD8-positive T cells accumulate in lymphoid and other organs, associated with hemophagocytic activated macrophages. The progressive inflammation is lethal unless checked by immunosuppressive therapy. When mice were developed that lacked perforin, no spontaneous phenotype was observed. However, if the mice were infected with lymphocytic choriomeningitis virus (LCV) or other viruses, a disease resembling human FHL developed, driven by an uncontrolled virus-specific T-cell response. This rare syndrome demonstrates beautifully that CD8-positive lymphocytes must have a role in limiting T-cell immune responses, for example in response to viral infection, by perforin-dependent cytotoxic mechanisms. When this mechanism fails, uncontrolled activated T cells kill their host.

Examples of inherited diseases that affect the pathway for secretion of secretory lysosomes are Chediak–Higashi syndrome, caused by mutations in a protein, CHS1, that regulates lysosomal trafficking, and **Griscelli syndrome**, caused by mutations in a small GTPase, Rab27a, that controls the movement of vesicles within cells. In Chediak–Higashi syndrome, abnormal giant lysosomes accumulate in melanocytes, neutrophils, lymphocytes, eosinophils, and platelets. The hair is typically a metallic silver color, vision is reduced because of abnormalities in retinal pigment cells, and increased bleeding occurs because of platelet dysfunction. With regard to the immune system, children with the syndrome suffer from recurrent severe infections because of failure of T-cell, neutrophil, and NK-cell function. After a few years, hemophagocytic lymphohistiocytosis develops, with fatal consequences if untreated. Antibiotics are needed to treat and prevent infections, and immunosuppression to deal with the uncontrolled inflammation; only bone marrow transplantation offers any real hope to patients with Chediak–Higashi disease.

Graft-Versus-Host Disease

11-17 Bone marrow transplantation or gene therapy can be useful to correct genetic defects.

It is frequently possible to correct the defects in lymphocyte development that lead to the SCID phenotype by replacing the defective component, generally by bone marrow transplantation. The major difficulties in these therapies result from MHC polymorphism. To be useful, the graft must share some MHC alleles with the host. As we learned in Section 7-20, the MHC alleles expressed by the thymic epithelium determine which T cells can be positively selected. When bone marrow cells are used to restore immune function to individuals with a normal thymic stroma, both the T cells and the antigen-presenting cells are derived from the graft. Therefore, unless the graft shares at least some MHC alleles with the recipient, the T cells that are selected on host thymic epithelium cannot be activated by graft-derived antigen-presenting cells (Fig. 11.16). There is also a danger that mature, post-thymic T cells in donor bone marrow might recognize the host as foreign and attack it, causing **graft-versus-host disease** (**GVHD**) (Fig. 11.17, top panel). This can be overcome by depleting the donor bone marrow of mature T cells. Bone marrow recipients are usually treated with irradiation that kills their own lymphocytes, thus making space for the grafted bone marrow cells and minimizing the threat of **host-versus-graft disease** (**HVGD**) (Fig. 11.17, third panel). In patients with the SCID phenotype, however, there is little problem with the host response to the transplanted bone marrow because the patient is immunodeficient.

Fig. 11.16 Bone marrow donor and recipient must share at least some MHC molecules to restore immune function. In an allogeneic bone marrow transplant, the donor marrow cells share some MHC molecules with the recipient. The shared MHC type is designated b and illustrated in blue, the MHC type of the donor marrow that is not shared is designated a and shown in yellow. Donor lymphocytes are positively selected on MHC^b on thymic epithelial cells and negatively selected by the recipient stromal epithelial cells and at the cortico-medullary junction by encounter with dendritic cells derived from both the donor bone marrow and residual recipient dendritic cells. The negatively selected cells are shown as apoptotic cells. The antigen-presenting cells in the periphery can activate T cells that recognize MHC^b molecules; the activated T cells can then recognize infected MHC^b-bearing cells.

Fig. 11.17 Bone marrow grafting can be used to correct immunodeficiencies caused by defects in lymphocyte maturation, but two problems can arise. First, if there are mature T cells in the bone marrow, they can attack cells of the host by recognizing their MHC antigens, causing graft-versus-host disease (top panel). This can be prevented by T-cell depletion of the donor bone marrow (center panel). Second, if the recipient has competent T cells, these can attack the bone marrow stem cells (bottom panel). This causes failure of the graft by the usual mechanism of transplant rejection (see Chapter 13).

Now that specific gene defects are being identified, a different approach to correcting these inherited immune deficiencies can be attempted. The strategy involves extracting a sample of the patient's own bone marrow cells, inserting a normal copy of the defective gene, and returning them to the patient by transfusion. This approach, called **somatic gene therapy**, should correct the gene defect. Moreover, in immunodeficient patients, it might be possible to reinfuse the bone marrow into the patient without the usual irradiation used to suppress the recipient's bone marrow function. There is no risk of graft-versus-host disease in this case, although the host might respond to the replaced gene product and reject the engineered cells. Although this kind of approach is theoretically attractive, the efficient transfer of genes into bone marrow stem cells is technically difficult.

The first trials of gene therapy for correcting immunodeficiency, such as the treatment of a child with ADA deficiency at the US National Institutes of Health in 1990, used the patient's lymphocytes as the vehicle for gene introduction. However, because most lymphocytes divide regularly, thus diluting out the new gene, the treatment had to be repeated regularly. In another study, bone marrow stem cells obtained from cord blood from three patients with ADA deficiency were transduced with the ADA gene and reinfused. At the age of 4 years, these children expressed up to 10% of normal ADA levels only in T cells and not in other bone marrow derived cells, and they remained immunodeficient in the absence of treatment with ADA enzyme replacement. More recently, however, there has been a striking success in correcting the phenotype of nine X-linked SCID patients by using a Moloney retrovirus-derived construct containing the γ_c chain to infect bone marrow stem cells, with restoration of sufficient immune function to allow the children to lead normal lives. Sadly, this success has been followed by a major setback: two of the nine children whose immunodeficiency was corrected by this gene therapy developed a T-cell tumor. This was caused by integration of the retroviral vector used for the gene therapy close to the promoter for a proto-oncogene called *LMO2*, a gene that regulates hematopoiesis.

11-18 Secondary immunodeficiencies are major predisposing causes of infection and death.

The primary immunodeficiencies have taught us much about the biology of specific molecules of the immune system. However, these conditions are extremely uncommon. In contrast, secondary immunodeficiency is extremely common and important in everyday medical practice. Malnutrition devastates many populations around the world; a major feature of malnutrition is secondary immunodeficiency, which particularly affects cell-mediated immunity, and death in famines is frequently caused by infection. Measles, which is associated with immunosuppression (see Section 11-4), is an important cause of death in malnourished children. In the developed world, measles is an unpleasant illness but major complications are uncommon. In contrast, measles in the malnourished has a high mortality. Tuberculosis is another important infection in the malnourished. In mice, protein starvation causes immunodeficiency by affecting antigen-presenting cell function, but in humans it is not clear how malnourishment specifically affects immune responses: links between the endocrine and immune systems may provide part of the answer. Adipocytes (fat cells) produce the hormone leptin, and leptin levels are related directly to the amount of fat present in the body; leptin levels fall in starvation. Both mice and humans with genetically determined leptin deficiency have reduced T-cell responses and, in addition, in mice the thymus atrophies. Both in starved mice and in mice with inherited leptin deficiency these abnormalities can be reversed by the administration of leptin.

Hematopoietic tumors such as leukemia and lymphoma are each associated with secondary immunodeficiency states. Depending on the specific type, leukemia may be associated with an excess of neutrophils (neutrophilia) or a deficiency of them (neutropenia). In either case, neutrophil dysfunction increases susceptibility to bacterial and fungal infections, as described in Section 11-11. Destruction or invasion of secondary lymphoid tissue caused by lymphoma or metastases from other cancers can promote opportunistic infections. Surgical removal of the spleen, or destruction of spleen function by certain diseases, is associated with a lifelong predisposition to overwhelming infection by *Streptococcus pneumoniae*, graphically illustrating the role of mononuclear phagocytic cells within the spleen in the clearance of this organism from blood. Patients who have lost spleen function should be vaccinated against pneumococcal infection and take prophylactic antibiotics throughout their life.

Congenital
Asplenia

Sadly, a major complication of the immunosuppressive drugs that we consider in Chapters 13 and 14 is infection. The cytotoxic drugs used to treat cancer kill all dividing cells, and cells of the bone marrow and lymphoid systems are the main unwanted targets of these agents. Infection is thus one of the major side effects of cytotoxic drug therapy. Another undesirable side-effect of medical intervention is the increased risk of infection around implanted medical devices such as catheters, artificial heart valves, and artificial joints. These act as privileged sites for the development of infections that resist easy elimination by antibiotics. These implanted materials lack the innate defensive mechanisms of normal body tissues and act as a 'protected' matrix for the growth of bacteria and fungi. Catheters used for peritoneal dialysis or for infusion of drugs or fluids into the circulation can also act as a conduit for bacteria to bypass the normal defensive barrier of the skin.

Summary.

Genetic defects can occur in almost any molecule involved in the immune response. These defects give rise to characteristic deficiency diseases, which, although rare, provide much information about the development and functioning of the immune system in normal humans. Inherited immunodeficiencies illustrate the vital role of the adaptive immune response and T cells in particular, without which both cell-mediated and humoral immunity fail. They have provided information about the separate roles of B lymphocytes in humoral immunity and of T lymphocytes in cell-mediated immunity, the importance of phagocytes and complement in humoral and innate immunity, and the specific functions of several cell-surface or signaling molecules in the adaptive immune response. There are also some inherited immune disorders whose causes we still do not understand. The study of these diseases will undoubtedly teach us more about the normal immune response and its control. Acquired defects in the immune system, the secondary immunodeficiencies, are much commoner than the primary inherited immunodeficiencies, and starvation is a major cause of immunodeficiency and death worldwide. In the next section we consider the pandemic of acquired immune deficiency syndrome caused by infection with the HIV virus.

Acquired immune deficiency syndrome.

The first cases of **acquired immune deficiency syndrome** (**AIDS**) were reported in 1981 but it is now clear that cases of the disease had been occurring without being recognized for at least 4 years before its identification. The disease is characterized by a susceptibility to infection with opportunistic pathogens or by the occurrence of an aggressive form of Kaposi's sarcoma or B-cell lymphoma, accompanied by a profound decrease in the number of CD4 T cells. As the disease seemed to be spread by contact with body fluids, it was soon suspected to be caused by a new virus, and by 1983 the agent now known to be responsible for AIDS, called the **human immunodeficiency virus** (**HIV**), was isolated and identified. It is now clear there are at least two types of HIV—HIV-1 and HIV-2—which are closely related to each other. HIV-2 is endemic in West Africa and is now spreading in India. Most AIDS worldwide, however, is caused by the more virulent HIV-1. Both viruses seem to have spread to humans from other primate species and the best evidence from sequence relationships suggests that HIV-1 has passed to humans on at least three independent occasions from the chimpanzee, *Pan troglodytes*, and HIV-2 from the sooty mangabey, *Cercocebus atys*.

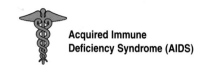

Acquired Immune
Deficiency Syndrome (AIDS)

HIV-1 shows marked genetic variability and is classified on the basis of viral sequences into three major groups named M (main), O (outlier), and N (non-M, non-O). These are only distantly related to each other and, because of this, are thought to have passed into humans by independent transmissions from chimpanzees. The M group of viruses, as implied by its name, is the major cause of AIDS worldwide and is itself genetically diversified into a series of subtypes, sometimes known as clades, that are designated by letters from A to K. In different parts of the world, different subtypes predominate. Phylogenetic trees have been drawn that trace the ancestry of HIV-1 of the M type to a common parent. It is most likely that the evolution of the subtypes of the M virus has occurred within human populations after the original transmission of the virus from a chimpanzee to a human. An alternative explanation is that different subtypes of the M virus crossed into humans on several occasions. It has been estimated that the common ancestor of the M group of HIV-1 may date to as long ago as 1915–1941 and, if this is correct, HIV-1 has been infecting humans for far longer than has been thought and must have been undetected clinically among populations in West Africa.

HIV infection does not immediately cause AIDS, and the issues of how it does, and whether all HIV-infected patients will progress to overt disease, remain controversial. Nevertheless, accumulating evidence clearly implicates the growth of the virus in CD4 T cells, and the immune response to it, as the central keys to the puzzle of AIDS. HIV is now a worldwide pandemic and, although great strides are being made in understanding the pathogenesis and epidemiology of the disease, the number of infected people around the world continues to grow at an alarming rate, presaging the death of many people from AIDS for many years to come. Estimates from the World Health Organization are that 20 million people have died from AIDS since the beginning of the epidemic, and that there are currently around 40 million people alive with HIV infection (Fig. 11.18), of whom most are living in sub-Saharan Africa, where approximately 7% of young adults are infected. In some countries within this region, such as Zimbabwe and Botswana, over 25% of adults are infected. There are growing epidemics of HIV infection and AIDS in China and India, where surveys in several states have shown a 1% to 2% prevalence of HIV infection in pregnant women. The incidence of HIV infection is rising faster in Eastern Europe and Central Asia than in the rest of the world. About one-third of those infected with HIV are aged between 15 and 24, and the majority are unaware that they carry the virus.

Fig. 11.18 HIV infection is spreading on all continents. The number of HIV-infected individuals is large (data are numbers of adults and children living with HIV/AIDS at the end of 2001, as estimated by the World Health Organization) and is increasing rapidly, especially in developing countries. It is estimated that 5 million individuals were newly infected with HIV during 2001.

11-19 Most individuals infected with HIV progress over time to AIDS.

Many viruses cause an acute but limited infection inducing lasting protective immunity. Others, such as herpes viruses, set up a latent infection that is not eliminated but is controlled adequately by an adaptive immune response. However, infection with HIV seems rarely, if ever, to lead to an immune response that can prevent ongoing replication of the virus. Although the initial acute infection does seem to be controlled by the immune system, HIV continues to replicate and infect new cells.

The initial infection with HIV generally occurs after the transfer of body fluids from an infected person to an uninfected one. The virus is carried in infected CD4 T cells, dendritic cells, and macrophages, and as a free virus in blood, semen, vaginal fluid, or mother's milk. It is most commonly spread by sexual intercourse, contaminated needles used for intravenous drug delivery, and the therapeutic use of infected blood or blood products, although this last route of transmission has largely been eliminated in the developed world where blood products are screened routinely for the presence of HIV. An important route of virus transmission is from an infected mother to her baby at birth or through breast milk. In Africa, the perinatal transmission rate is approximately 25%, but this can be substantially reduced by treating infected pregnant women with the drugs zidovudine (AZT) or nevirapine. Mothers who are newly infected and breastfeed their infants transmit HIV 40% of the time, showing that HIV can also be transmitted in breast milk, but transmission is less common after the mother produces antibodies against HIV.

Primary infection with HIV causes an influenza-like illness in up to 80% of cases, with an abundance of virus in the peripheral blood and a marked decrease in the numbers of circulating CD4 T cells. The diagnosis at this stage is usually missed unless there is a high index of suspicion. This acute viremia is associated in virtually all patients with the activation of CD8 T cells, which kill HIV-infected cells, and subsequently with antibody production, or

seroconversion. The cytotoxic T-cell response is thought to be important in controlling virus levels, which peak and then decline, as the CD4 T-cell counts rebound to around 800 cells μl^{-1} (the normal value is 1200 cells μl^{-1}). At present, the best indicator of future disease is the level of virus that persists in the blood plasma once the symptoms of acute viremia have passed.

Most people who are infected with HIV will eventually develop AIDS, after a period of apparent quiescence of the disease known as clinical latency or the asymptomatic period (Fig. 11.19). This period is not silent, however, for there is persistent replication of the virus, and a gradual decline in the function and numbers of CD4 T cells until eventually such patients have few CD4 T cells left. At this point, which can occur anywhere between 2 and 15 years or more after the primary infection, the period of clinical latency ends and opportunistic infections begin to appear.

The typical course of an infection with HIV is illustrated in Fig. 11.20. However, it has become increasingly clear that the course of the disease can vary widely. Thus, although most people infected with HIV go on to develop AIDS and ultimately to die of opportunistic infection or cancer, this is not true of all individuals. Genetic variation in either virus or host can alter the rate of progression of disease. Some naturally attenuated viruses show slower disease progression. Genetic variation in HLA type of the host also modifies disease outcome: HLA-B57 and HLA-B27 are associated with better prognosis and HLA-B35 with more rapid disease progression. Homozygosity of HLA class I expression is associated with more rapid progression, presumably because the T-cell response to infection is less diverse.

A small percentage of people seroconvert, making antibodies against many HIV proteins, but do not seem to have progressive disease, in that their CD4 T-cell counts and other measures of immune competence are maintained. These long-term nonprogressors have unusually low levels of circulating virus and are being studied intensively to determine how they are able to control their HIV infection. A second group consists of seronegative people who have been highly exposed to HIV yet remain disease-free and virus-negative. Some of these people have specific cytotoxic lymphocytes and T_H1 lymphocytes directed against infected cells, which confirms that they have been exposed to HIV or possibly to noninfectious HIV antigens. It is not clear whether this immune response accounts for clearing the infection, but it is a focus of considerable interest for the development and design of vaccines, which we will discuss later. There is a small group of people who are resistant

Fig. 11.19 Most HIV-infected individuals progress to AIDS over a period of years. The incidence of AIDS increases progressively with time after infection. Homosexuals and hemophiliacs are two of the groups at highest risk in the West—homosexuals from sexually transmitted virus, and hemophiliacs from infected human blood used to replace clotting factor VIII. In Africa, spread is mainly by heterosexual intercourse. Hemophiliacs are now protected by the screening of blood products and the use of recombinant factor VIII. Neither homosexuals nor hemophiliacs who have not been infected with HIV show any evidence of AIDS. Most hemophiliacs in Western Europe and North America were exposed to HIV infection by inadvertent administration of contaminated blood products at the start of the HIV epidemic, with the peak of infection occurring in 1982–1983. From this infected population, there are robust cohort data on their progression to the development of AIDS, which are shown here. The age of the individual seems to have a significant role in the rate of progression of the development of HIV. More than 80% of those aged more than 40 at the time of infection progress to AIDS over 13 years, in comparison with approximately 50% of those aged less than 40 over a comparable time. There are a few individuals who, although infected with HIV, seem not to progress to develop AIDS. One protective mechanism is an inherited defect in the major HIV co-receptor, CCR5.

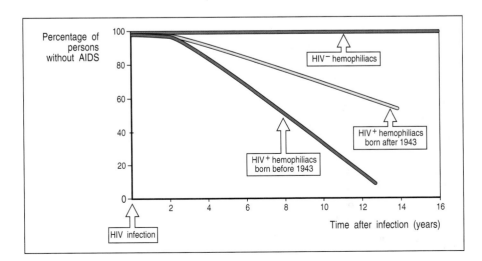

Fig. 11.20 The typical course of untreated infection with HIV. The first few weeks are typified by an acute influenza-like viral illness, sometimes called seroconversion disease, with high titers of virus in the blood. An adaptive immune response follows, which controls the acute illness and largely restores levels of CD4 T cells (CD4+ PBL) but does not eradicate the virus. Opportunistic infections and other symptoms become more frequent as the CD4 T-cell count falls, starting at about 500 cells μl^{-1}. The disease then enters the symptomatic phase. When CD4 T-cell counts fall below 200 cells μl^{-1} the patient is said to have AIDS. Note that CD4 T-cell counts are measured for clinical purposes in cells per microliter (cells μl^{-1}), rather than cells per milliliter (cells ml^{-1}), the unit used elsewhere in this book.

to HIV infection because they carry mutations in a cell-surface chemokine receptor that is used as a co-receptor for viral entry, as we will see below.

We shall return to the interactions of HIV with the immune system and the prospects for manipulating them later in this chapter, but before doing so we must describe the viral life cycle and the genes and proteins on which it depends. Some of these proteins are the targets of the most successful drugs in use at present for the treatment of AIDS.

11-20 HIV is a retrovirus that infects CD4 T cells, dendritic cells, and macrophages.

HIV is an enveloped retrovirus whose structure is shown in Fig. 11.21. Each virus particle, or virion, contains two copies of an RNA genome, which are reverse-transcribed into DNA in the infected cell and then integrate into the host cell chromosome. The RNA transcripts produced from the integrated viral DNA serve both as mRNA to direct the synthesis of the viral proteins and later as the RNA genomes of new viral particles, which escape from the cell by budding from the plasma membrane, each in a membrane envelope. HIV belongs to a group of retroviruses called the **lentiviruses**, from the Latin *lentus*, meaning slow, because of the gradual course of the diseases that they cause. These viruses persist and continue to replicate for many years before causing overt signs of disease.

The ability of HIV to enter particular types of cell, known as the cellular tropism of the virus, is determined by the expression of specific receptors for the virus on the surface of those cells. HIV enters cells by means of a complex of two noncovalently associated viral glycoproteins, gp120 and gp41, in the viral envelope. The gp120 portion of the glycoprotein complex binds with high affinity to the cell-surface molecule CD4. This glycoprotein thereby draws the virus to CD4 T cells and to dendritic cells and macrophages, which also express some CD4. Before fusion and entry of the virus, gp120 must also bind to a co-receptor in the membrane of the host cell. Several different molecules can serve as a co-receptor for HIV entry, but in each case they have been identified as chemokine receptors. The chemokine receptors (see Chapters 2 and 10) are a closely related family of G-protein-coupled receptors with seven transmembrane-spanning domains. Two chemokine receptors—CCR5, predominantly expressed on dendritic cells, macrophages, and CD4 T cells, and CXCR4, expressed on activated T cells—are the major co-receptors for HIV. After binding of gp120 to the receptor and co-receptor, the gp41 then causes fusion of the viral envelope and the plasma membrane of the cell, allowing the viral genome and associated viral proteins to enter the cytoplasm. This fusion process has provided a target for drug therapy. Peptide analogs of the carboxy-terminal peptide of gp41 inhibit fusion of the viral envelope with the plasma membrane of cells and administration of one such peptide, named T-20, to patients with HIV infection caused an approximately 20-fold decline in plasma HIV RNA levels.

There are different variants of HIV, and the cell types that they infect are determined to a large degree by which chemokine receptor they bind as co-receptor. The variants of HIV that are associated with primary infections use CCR5, which binds the CC chemokines CCL3, CCL4, and CCL5, as a co-receptor, and require only a low level of CD4 on the cells they infect. These variants of HIV infect dendritic cells, macrophages, and T cells *in vivo*. They used to be described as 'macrophage-tropic' because they infect macrophage but not T-cell lines *in vitro*, and the cell tropism of different HIV variants was originally defined by their ability to grow in different cell lines. These variants are now usually designated as 'R5' viruses, reflecting their chemokine receptor usage.

In contrast, 'lymphocyte-tropic' variants of HIV infect only CD4 T cells *in vivo* and use CXCR4, which binds the chemokine CXCL12, as a co-receptor. The lymphocyte-tropic variants of HIV can grow *in vitro* in T-cell lines, and require high levels of CD4 on the cells that they infect. These are now known as 'X4' viruses, after their use of CXCR4.

It seems that R5 isolates of HIV are preferentially transmitted by sexual contact, because they are the dominant viral phenotype found in newly infected individuals. Virus is disseminated from an initial reservoir of infected dendritic cells and macrophages, and there is evidence for an important role for mucosal lymphoid tissue in this process. Mucosal epithelia, which are constantly exposed to foreign antigens, provide a milieu of immune system activity in which HIV replication occurs readily. Infection occurs across mucosal surfaces covered by two types of epithelial cell lining. The mucosa of the vagina, penis, cervix, and anus is covered by several layers of epithelial

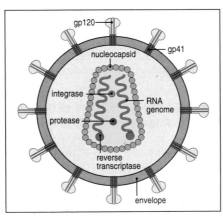

Fig. 11.21 The virion of human immunodeficiency virus (HIV). The virus illustrated is HIV-1, the leading cause of AIDS. The reverse transcriptase, integrase, and viral protease enzymes are packaged in the virion and are shown schematically in the viral capsid. In reality, many molecules of these enzymes are contained in each virion. Some structural proteins of the virus have been omitted for simplicity. Photograph courtesy of H. Gelderblom.

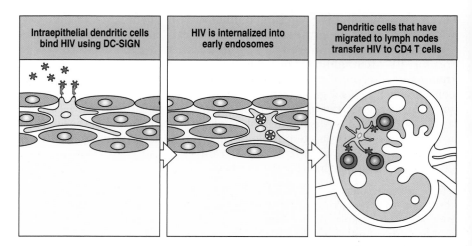

Fig. 11.22 Dendritic cells initiate infection by transporting HIV from mucosal surfaces to lymphoid tissue. On the left is shown the adherence of HIV to the surface of an intraepithelial dendritic cell by the binding of viral gp120 to DC-SIGN. HIV gains access to dendritic cells at sites of mucosal injury or possibly to dendritic cells that have protruded between epithelial cells to sample the external world. The center panel shows a dendritic cell migrating toward lymphoid tissue that has internalized HIV into early endosomes that are mildly acidic. The panel on the right shows dendritic cells transferring HIV that has been translocated back to the cell surface to CD4 T cells within a lymph node.

cells, a stratified squamous epithelium. Within such squamous epithelium, intraepithelial dendritic cells initiate infection by binding HIV and transporting it to lymphoid tissue, where it is transferred to CD4 T cells. HIV attaches to dendritic cells by the binding of viral gp120 to a dendritic cell-surface molecule named DC-SIGN. DC-SIGN mediates the internalization of HIV into a mildly acidic endosomal compartment, which protects the virus during the passage of dendritic cells to lymphoid tissue (Fig. 11.22).

The second type of mucosa in the intestinal tract, including the rectum and the endocervix, is covered by a single layer of epithelial cells. Epithelial cells derived from this type of mucosa have been shown to express CCR5 and yet another HIV-binding molecule, glycosphingolipid galactosyl ceramide, and to selectively translocate R5 HIV variants, and not X4, through the epithelial monolayer, thus allowing HIV to bind to and infect submucosal CD4 T cells and dendritic cells. Infection of CD4 T cells via CCR5 occurs early in the course of infection and continues, with activated CD4 T cells accounting for the major production of HIV throughout infection. Late in infection, in approximately 50% of cases, the viral phenotype switches to the X4 T-lymphocyte-tropic type that uses CXCR4 co-receptors, and this is followed by a rapid decline in CD4 T-cell count and progression to AIDS.

11-21 Genetic deficiency of the macrophage chemokine co-receptor for HIV confers resistance to HIV infection *in vivo*.

Further evidence for the importance of chemokine receptors in HIV infection has come from studies in a small group of individuals with a high risk of exposure to HIV-1 but who remain seronegative. Cultures of lymphocytes and macrophages from these people were relatively resistant to macrophage-tropic HIV infection and were found to secrete high levels of the chemokines CCL3,

CCL4, and CCL5 in response to inoculation with HIV. In other experiments, the addition of these same chemokines to lymphocytes sensitive to HIV blocked their infection because of competition between these CC chemokines and the virus for the cell-surface receptor CCR5.

The resistance of these rare individuals to HIV infection has now been explained by the discovery that they are homozygous for an allelic, nonfunctional variant of CCR5 caused by a 32-base-pair deletion from the coding region that leads to a frameshift and truncation of the translated protein. The gene frequency of this mutant allele in Caucasoid populations is quite high at 0.09 (meaning that about 10% of the Caucasoid population are heterozygous carriers of the allele and about 1% are homozygous). The mutant allele has not been found in Japanese or in black Africans from Western or Central Africa. Heterozygous deficiency of CCR5 might provide some protection against sexual transmission of HIV infection and a modest reduction in the rate of progression of the disease. In addition to the structural polymorphism of the gene, variation of the promoter region of the CCR5 gene has been found in both Caucasian and African Americans. Different promoter variants were associated with different rates of progression of disease.

These results provide a dramatic confirmation of experimental work suggesting that CCR5 is the major macrophage and T-lymphocyte co-receptor used by HIV to establish primary infection *in vivo*, and offers the possibility that primary infection might be blocked by therapeutic antagonists of the CCR5 receptor. Indeed, there is preliminary evidence that low molecular weight inhibitors of this receptor can block infection of macrophages by HIV *in vitro*. Such low molecular weight inhibitors might be the precursors of useful drugs that could be taken by mouth. Such drugs are very unlikely to provide complete protection against infection if used prophylactically, because a very small number of individuals who are homozygous for the nonfunctional variant of CCR5 are infected with HIV. These individuals seem to have suffered from primary infection by CXCR4-using strains of the virus.

11-22 HIV RNA is transcribed by viral reverse transcriptase into DNA that integrates into the host cell genome.

One of the proteins that enters the cell with the viral genome is the viral reverse transcriptase, which transcribes the viral RNA into a complementary DNA (cDNA) copy. The viral cDNA is then integrated into the host cell genome by the viral integrase, which also enters the cell with the viral RNA. The integrated cDNA copy is known as the **provirus**. The infectious cycle up to the integration of the provirus is shown in Fig. 11.23. In activated CD4 T cells, virus replication is initiated by transcription of the provirus, as we discuss in the next section. However, HIV can, like other retroviruses, establish a latent infection in which the provirus remains quiescent. This seems to occur in memory CD4 T cells and in dormant macrophages, and these cells are thought to be an important reservoir of infection.

The entire HIV genome consists of nine genes flanked by long terminal repeat sequences (LTR), which are required for the integration of the provirus into the host cell DNA and contain binding sites for gene regulatory proteins that control the expression of the viral genes. Like other retroviruses, HIV has three major genes—*gag, pol,* and *env*. The *gag* gene encodes the structural proteins of the viral core, *pol* encodes the enzymes involved in viral replication and integration, and *env* encodes the viral envelope glycoproteins. The *gag* and *pol* mRNAs are translated to give polyproteins—long polypeptide chains that are then cleaved by the viral protease (also encoded by *pol*) into individual functional proteins. The product of the *env* gene, gp160, has to be cleaved by a host

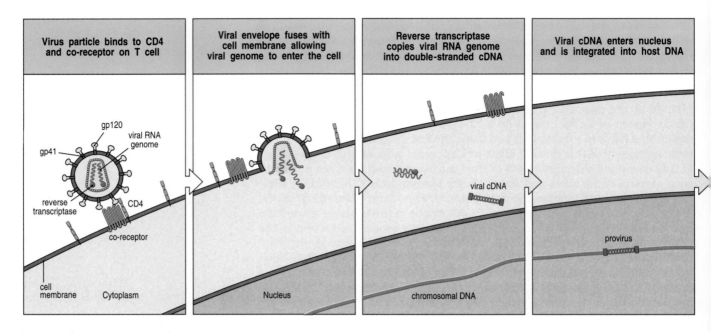

Fig. 11.23 The infection of CD4 T cells by HIV. The virus binds to CD4 using gp120, which is altered by CD4 binding so that it now also binds a specific seven-span chemokine receptor that acts as a co-receptor for viral entry. This binding releases gp41, which then causes fusion of the viral envelope with the cell membrane, and release of the viral core into the cytoplasm.

Once in the cytoplasm, the viral core releases the RNA genome, which is then reverse-transcribed into double-stranded cDNA. The double-stranded cDNA migrates to the nucleus in association with the viral integrase and the Vpr protein, where it is integrated into the cell genome, becoming a provirus.

cell protease into gp120 and gp41, which are then assembled as trimers into the **viral envelope**. As shown in Fig. 11.24, HIV has six other, smaller, genes encoding proteins that affect viral replication and infectivity in various ways. We discuss the function of two of these—Tat and Rev—in the following section.

Fig. 11.24 The genes and proteins of HIV-1. Like all retroviruses, HIV-1 has an RNA genome flanked by long terminal repeats (LTR) involved in viral integration and in regulation of the viral genome. The genome can be read in three frames and several of the viral genes overlap in different reading frames. This allows the virus to encode many proteins in a small genome. The three main protein products—Gag, Pol, and Env—are synthesized by all infectious retroviruses. The known functions of the different genes and their products are listed. The products of *gag*, *pol*, and *env* are known to be present in the mature viral particle, together with the viral RNA. The mRNAs for Tat, Rev, and Nef proteins are produced by splicing of viral transcripts, so their genes are split in the viral genome. In the case of Nef, only one exon, shown in yellow, is translated. The other gene products affect the infectivity of the virus in various ways that are not fully understood.

Gene		Gene product/function
gag	Group-specific antigen	Core proteins and matrix proteins
pol	Polymerase	Reverse transcriptase, protease, and integrase enzymes
env	Envelope	Transmembrane glycoproteins. gp120 binds CD4 and CCR5; gp41 is required for virus fusion and internalization
tat	Transactivator	Positive regulator of transcription
rev	Regulator of viral expression	Allows export of unspliced and partly spliced transcripts from nucleus
vif	Viral infectivity	Affects particle infectivity
vpr	Viral protein R	Transport of DNA to nucleus. Augments virion production. Cell cycle arrest
vpu	Viral protein U	Promotes intracellular degradation of CD4 and enhances release of virus from cell membrane
nef	Negative-regulation factor	Augments viral replication *in vivo* and *in vitro*. Decreases CD4, MHC class I and II expression

T-cell activation induces low-level transcription of provirus	RNA transcripts are multiply spliced, allowing translation of early genes *tat* and *rev*	Tat amplifies transcription of viral RNA. Rev increases transport of singly spliced or unspliced viral RNA to cytoplasm	The late proteins Gag, Pol, and Env are translated and assembled into virus particles which bud from the cell

11-23 Transcription of the HIV provirus depends on host-cell transcription factors induced upon the activation of infected T cells.

The production of infectious virus particles from an integrated HIV provirus is stimulated by a cellular transcription factor that is present in all activated T cells. Activation of CD4 T cells induces the transcription factor NFκB, which binds to promoters not only in the cellular DNA but also in the viral LTR, thereby initiating the transcription of viral RNA by the cellular RNA polymerase. This transcript is spliced in various ways to produce mRNAs for the viral proteins. The Gag and Gag–Pol proteins are translated from unspliced mRNA; Vif, Vpr, Vpu, and Env are translated from singly spliced viral mRNA; Tat, Rev, and Nef are translated from multiply spliced mRNA. At least two of the viral genes, *tat* and *rev*, encode proteins, **Tat** and **Rev** respectively, that promote viral replication in activated T cells. Tat is a potent transcriptional regulator, which functions as an elongation factor that enables the transcription of viral RNA by the RNA polymerase II complex. Tat contains two binding sites, contained in one domain, named the transactivation domain. The first of these allows Tat to bind to a host cellular protein, cyclin T1. This binding reaction promotes the binding of the Tat protein through the second binding site in its transactivation domain to an RNA sequence in the LTR of the virus known as the transcriptional activation region (TAR). The consequence of this interaction is to greatly enhance the rate of viral genome transcription, by causing the removal of negative elongation factors that block the transcriptional activity of RNA polymerase II. The expression of cyclin T1 is greatly increased in activated compared with quiescent T lymphocytes. This, in conjunction with the increased expression of NFκB in activated T cells, may explain the ability of HIV to lie dormant in resting T cells and replicate in activated T cells (Fig. 11.25).

Eukaryotic cells have mechanisms to prevent the export from the cell nucleus of incompletely spliced mRNA transcripts. This could pose a problem for a retrovirus that is dependent on the export of unspliced, singly spliced, and multiply spliced mRNA species to translate the full complement of viral proteins. The Rev protein is the viral solution to this problem. Export from the nucleus and translation of the three HIV proteins encoded by the fully spliced mRNA transcripts, Tat, Nef, and Rev, occurs early after viral infection by means of the normal host cellular mechanisms of mRNA export. The

Fig. 11.25 Cells infected with HIV must be activated for the virus to replicate. Activation of CD4 T cells induces the expression of the transcription factor NFκB, which binds to the proviral LTR and initiates the transcription of the HIV genome into RNA. The first viral transcripts are processed extensively, producing spliced mRNAs encoding several regulatory proteins, including Tat and Rev. Tat both enhances transcription from the provirus and binds to the RNA transcripts, stabilizing them in a form that can be translated. The protein Rev binds the RNA transcripts and transports them to the cytosol. As levels of Rev increase, less extensively spliced and unspliced viral transcripts are transported out of the nucleus. The singly spliced and unspliced transcripts encode the structural proteins of the virus, and the unspliced transcripts, which are the new viral genomes, are packaged with these to form many new virus particles. Photograph courtesy of H. Gelderblom.

expressed Rev protein then enters the nucleus and binds to a specific viral RNA sequence, the Rev response element (RRE). Rev also binds to a host nucleocytoplasmic transport protein named Crm1, which engages a host pathway for exporting mRNA species through nuclear pores into the cytoplasm.

When the provirus is first activated, Rev levels are low, the transcripts are translocated slowly from the nucleus, and thus multiple splicing events can occur. In this way, more Tat and Rev are produced, and Tat in turn ensures that more viral transcripts are made. Later, when Rev levels have increased, the transcripts are translocated rapidly from the nucleus unspliced or only singly spliced. These unspliced or singly spliced transcripts are translated to produce the structural components of the viral core and envelope, together with the reverse transcriptase, the integrase, and the viral protease, all of which are needed to make new viral particles. The complete, unspliced transcripts that are exported from the nucleus late in the infectious cycle are required for the translation of *gag* and *pol* and are also destined to be packaged with the proteins as the RNA genomes of the new virus particles.

11-24 Drugs that block HIV replication lead to a rapid decrease in titer of infectious virus and an increase in CD4 T cells.

Studies with powerful drugs that completely block the cycle of HIV replication indicate that the virus is replicating rapidly at all phases of infection, including the asymptomatic phase. Two viral proteins in particular have been the target of drugs aimed at arresting viral replication. These are the viral reverse transcriptase, which is required for synthesis of the provirus, and the viral protease, which cleaves the viral polyproteins to produce the virion proteins and viral enzymes. Inhibitors of these enzymes prevent the establishment of further infection in uninfected cells. Cells that are already infected can continue to produce virions because, once the provirus is established, reverse transcriptase is not needed to make new virus particles, while the viral protease acts at a very late maturation step of the virus, and inhibition of the protease does not prevent virus from being released. However, in both cases, the released virions are not infectious and further cycles of infection and replication are prevented.

Because of the great efficacy of the protease inhibitors, it is possible to learn much about the kinetics of HIV replication *in vivo* by measuring the decline in viremia after the initiation of protease inhibitor therapy. For the first 2 weeks after starting treatment there is an exponential decrease in plasma virus levels with a half-life of viral decay of about 2 days (Fig. 11.26). This phase reflects the decay in virus production from cells that were actively infected at the start of drug treatment, and indicates that the half-life of productively infected cells is similarly about 2 days. The results also show that free virus is cleared from the circulation very rapidly, with a half-life of about 6 hours. After 2 weeks, levels of virus in plasma have dropped by more than 95%, representing an almost total loss of productively infected CD4 lymphocytes. After this time, the rate of decline of plasma virus levels is much slower, reflecting the very slow decay of virus production from cells that provide a longer-lived reservoir of infection, such as dendritic cells and tissue macrophages, and from latently infected memory CD4 T cells that have been activated. Very long-term sources of infection might be CD4 memory T cells that continue to carry integrated provirus, and virus stored as immune complexes on follicular dendritic cells. These very long-lasting reservoirs of infection are resistant to drug therapy for HIV.

These studies show that most of the HIV present in the circulation of an infected individual is the product of rounds of replication in newly infected cells, and that virus from these productively infected cells is released into,

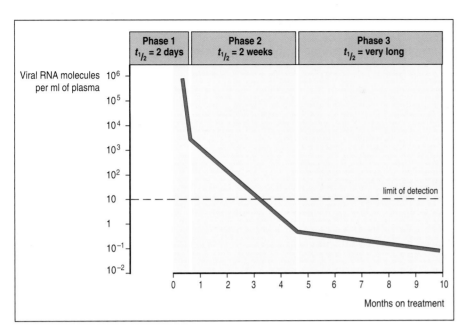

Phase 1 $t_{1/2}$ = 2 days	Phase 2 $t_{1/2}$ = 2 weeks	Phase 3 $t_{1/2}$ = very long

Viral RNA molecules per ml of plasma

10^6, 10^5, 10^4, 10^3, 10^2, 10, 1, 10^{-1}, 10^{-2}

limit of detection

0 1 2 3 4 5 6 7 8 9 10

Months on treatment

Fig. 11.26 Viral decay on drug treatment. The production of new HIV particles can be arrested for prolonged periods by combinations of protease inhibitors and viral reverse-transcriptase inhibitors. After the initiation of such treatment, the virus produced by previously infected cells is no longer infectious, and virus production is curtailed as these cells die and no new cells are infected. The half-life of virus decay occurs in three phases. The first phase has a half-life of about 2 days and lasts for about 2 weeks, during which time viral production declines as the lymphocytes that were productively infected at the onset of treatment die. Released virus is rapidly cleared from the circulation, where it has a half-life ($t_{1/2}$) of 6 hours, and there is a decrease in virus levels in plasma of more than 95% during this first phase. The second phase lasts for about 6 months and has a half-life of about 2 weeks. During this phase, virus is released from infected macrophages and from resting, latently infected CD4 T cells stimulated to divide and develop productive infection. It is thought that there is then a third phase of unknown length that results from the reactivation of integrated provirus in memory T cells and other long-lived reservoirs of infection. This reservoir of latently infected cells might remain present for many years. Measurement of this phase of viral decay is impossible at present as viral levels in plasma are below detectable levels. Data courtesy of G.M. Shaw.

and rapidly cleared from, the circulation at the rate of 10^9 to 10^{10} virions every day. This raises the question of what is happening to these virus particles and how they are removed so rapidly from the circulation. It seems most likely that HIV particles are opsonized by specific antibody and complement and removed by phagocytic cells of the mononuclear phagocyte system. Opsonized HIV particles can also be trapped on the surface of follicular dendritic cells, which are known to capture antigen:antibody complexes and retain them for prolonged periods (see Chapters 9 and 10).

The other issue raised by these studies is the effect of HIV replication on the population dynamics of CD4 T cells. The decline in plasma viremia is accompanied by a steady increase in CD4 T-lymphocyte counts in peripheral blood: what is the source of the new CD4 T cells that appear once treatment is started? Three complementary mechanisms have been established for the recovery in CD4 T-cell numbers. The first of these is a redistribution of CD4 T memory cells from lymphoid tissues into the circulation as viral replication is controlled; this occurs within weeks of starting treatment. The second is the reduction in the abnormal levels of immune activation as the HIV infection is controlled, associated with reduced cytotoxic T lymphocyte killing of infected CD4 T cells. The third is much slower and is caused by the emergence of new naive T cells from the thymus. Although the thymus involutes with aging, evidence that these later-arriving cells are indeed of thymic origin is provided by the observation that they contain T-cell receptor rearrangement excision circles (TRECs) (see Section 4-11), a marker of cells of thymic origin.

11-25 HIV accumulates many mutations in the course of infection in a single individual and drug treatment is soon followed by the outgrowth of drug-resistant variants of the virus.

The rapid replication of HIV, with the generation of 10^9 to 10^{10} virions every day, coupled with a mutation rate of approximately 3×10^{-5} per nucleotide base per cycle of replication, leads to the generation of many variants of HIV in a single infected patient in the course of a day. Replication of a retroviral genome depends on two error-prone steps. Reverse transcriptase lacks the proofreading mechanisms associated with cellular DNA polymerases, and

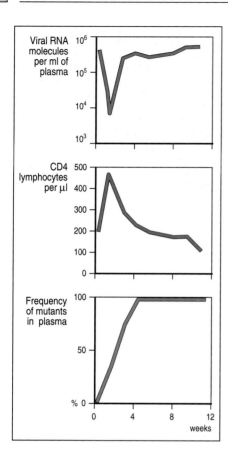

Fig. 11.27 Resistance of HIV to protease inhibitors. After the administration of a single protease inhibitor to a patient with HIV there is a precipitous fall in viral RNA levels in plasma with a half-life of about 2 days (top panel). This is accompanied by an initial rise in the number of CD4 T cells in peripheral blood (center panel). Within days of starting the drug, mutant drug-resistant variants can be detected in plasma (bottom panel) and in peripheral blood lymphocytes. After only 4 weeks of treatment, viral RNA levels and CD4 lymphocyte levels have returned to their original pre-drug levels, and 100% of plasma HIV is present as the drug-resistant mutant.

the RNA genomes of retroviruses are therefore copied into DNA with relatively low fidelity. The transcription of the proviral DNA into RNA copies by the cellular RNA polymerase is similarly a low-fidelity process. A rapidly replicating persistent virus that is going through these two steps repeatedly in the course of an infection can thereby accumulate many mutations, and numerous variants of HIV, sometimes called quasi-species, are found within a single infected individual. This very high variability was first recognized in HIV and has since proved to be common to the other lentiviruses.

As a consequence of its high variability, HIV rapidly develops resistance to antiviral drugs. When antiviral drugs are administered, variants of the virus that carry mutations conferring resistance to their effects emerge and expand until former levels of plasma virus are regained. Resistance to some of the protease inhibitors appears after only a few days (Fig. 11.27). Resistance to some of the nucleoside analogs that are potent inhibitors of reverse transcriptase develops in a similarly short time. By contrast, resistance to the nucleoside zidovudine (AZT), the first drug to be widely used for treating AIDS, takes months to develop. This is not because zidovudine is a more powerful inhibitor but because resistance to it requires three or four mutations in the viral reverse transcriptase, whereas a single mutation can confer resistance to some protease inhibitors and other reverse-transcriptase inhibitors. As a result of the relatively rapid appearance of resistance to all known anti-HIV drugs, successful drug treatment currently depends on combination therapy. It might also be important to begin treatment early in the course of an infection, thereby reducing the chance that a variant virus will have accumulated all the mutations necessary to resist the entire cocktail. Current treatments follow this strategy and use combinations of viral protease inhibitors and nucleoside analogs. The introduction of combination therapy dramatically reduced mortality and morbidity among patients with advanced HIV infection in the United States between the years 1995 and 1997 (Fig. 11.28). However, the downside is that current combination drug treatment is expensive, requires taking many tablets each day, and is accompanied by significant side effects.

11-26 Lymphoid tissue is the major reservoir of HIV infection.

Although viral load and turnover are usually measured by detecting the viral RNA present in viral particles in the blood, a major reservoir of HIV infection is in lymphoid tissue, in which infected CD4 T cells, monocytes, macrophages, and dendritic cells are found. In addition, HIV is trapped in the form of immune complexes on the surface of follicular dendritic cells. These cells are not themselves infected but may act as a store of infective virions.

HIV infection takes different forms within different cells. As we have seen, more than 95% of the virus that can be detected in the plasma is derived from productively infected cells that have a very short half-life of about 2 days. Productively infected CD4 lymphocytes are found in the T-cell areas of lymphoid tissue, and these are thought to succumb to infection in the course of

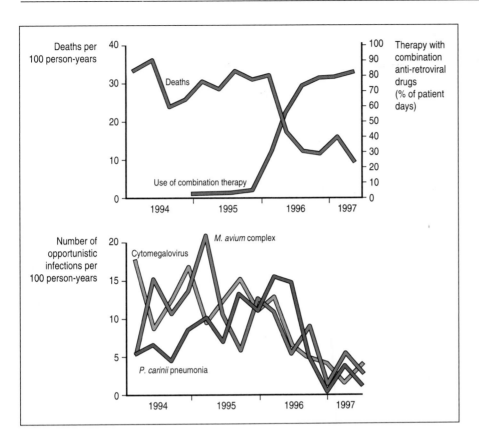

Fig. 11.28 The morbidity and mortality in advanced HIV infection fell in the USA in parallel with the introduction of combination anti-retroviral drug therapy. The upper graph shows the number of deaths, expressed each calendar quarter as the deaths per 100 person-years. The lower graph shows the decline in opportunistic infections caused by cytomegalovirus, *Pneumocystis carinii*, and *Mycobacterium avium*, during the same period of time. Figure based on data from F. Palella.

being activated in an immune response. Latently infected memory CD4 cells that are activated in response to antigen presentation also produce virus that can spread by rounds of replication in other activated CD4 T cells. Unfortunately, latently infected memory CD4 T cells were found to have an extremely long mean half-life of 44 months. This finding means that drug therapy may never be able to eliminate HIV infection and will need to be administered throughout life. In addition to the cells that are infected productively or latently, there is a further large population of cells infected by defective proviruses; such cells are not a source of infectious virus.

Macrophages and dendritic cells seem to be able to harbor replicating virus without necessarily being killed by it, and they are therefore believed to be an important reservoir of infection; they also serve as a means of spreading virus to other tissues such as the brain. Although the function of macrophages as antigen-presenting cells does not seem to be compromised by HIV infection, it is thought that the virus causes abnormal patterns of cytokine secretion that could account for the wasting that commonly occurs in AIDS patients late in their disease.

11-27 An immune response controls but does not eliminate HIV.

Infection with HIV generates an adaptive immune response that contains the virus but only very rarely, if ever, eliminates it. The time course of various elements in the adaptive immune response to HIV is shown, together with the levels of infectious virus in plasma, in Fig. 11.29.

Fig. 11.29 The immune response to HIV. Infectious virus is present at relatively low levels in the peripheral blood of infected individuals during a prolonged asymptomatic phase, during which the virus is replicated persistently in lymphoid tissues. During this period, CD4 T-cell counts gradually decline, although antibodies and CD8 cytotoxic T cells directed against the virus remain at high levels. Two different antibody responses are shown in the figure, one to the envelope protein (Env) of HIV, and one to the core protein p24. Eventually, the levels of antibody and HIV-specific cytotoxic T lymphocytes (CTLs) also decline, and there is a progressive increase in infectious HIV in the peripheral blood.

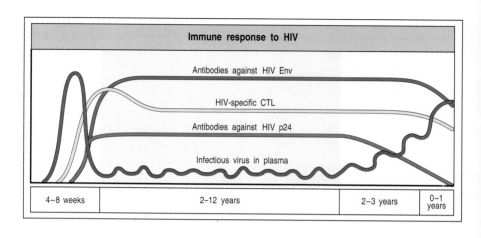

Seroconversion is the clearest evidence for an adaptive immune response to infection with HIV, but the generation of T lymphocytes responding to infected cells is thought by most workers in the field to be central in controlling the infection. Both CD8 cytotoxic T cells and CD4 T_H1 cells specifically responsive to infected cells are associated with the decline in detectable virus after the initial infection. These T-cell responses are unable to clear the infection completely, and it can also cause some pathology. Nevertheless, there is evidence that the virus itself is cytopathic, and T-cell responses that reduce viral spread should therefore, on balance, reduce the pathology of the disease. In this section we consider in turn the roles of CD8 cytotoxic T cells, CD4 T cells, and antibody in the host immunological response to HIV infection that ultimately fails to contain the infection.

The ability of cytotoxic T lymphocytes to destroy HIV-infected cells is demonstrated by studies of peripheral blood cells from infected individuals, in which cytotoxic T cells specific for viral peptides can be shown to kill infected cells *in vitro*. *In vivo*, cytotoxic T cells can be seen to invade sites of HIV replication and they could, in theory, be responsible for killing many productively infected cells before any infectious virus can be released, thereby containing viral load at the quasi-stable levels that are characteristic of the asymptomatic period. Evidence for the clinical importance of the control of HIV-infected cells by CD8 cytotoxic T cells comes from studies relating the numbers and activity of CD8 T cells to viral load. An inverse correlation was found between the number of CD8 T cells carrying a receptor specific for an HLA-A2-restricted HIV peptide and plasma RNA viral load. Similarly, patients with high levels of HIV-specific CD8 T cells showed slower progression of disease than those with low levels. There is also direct evidence from experiments in macaques infected with simian immunodeficiency virus (SIV) that CD8 cytotoxic T cells control retrovirus-infected cells *in vivo*. Treatment of infected animals with depleting anti-CD8 monoclonal antibodies was followed by a large increase in viral load.

In addition to being a major target for HIV infection, CD4 T cells also have an important role in the host response to HIV infected cells, as illustrated by three pieces of evidence. First, an inverse correlation was found between the strength of CD4 T-cell proliferative responses to HIV antigen and viral load. Second, some patients who did not progress to AIDS long after infection by HIV showed strong CD4 T-cell proliferative responses. Third, early treatment with anti-retroviral drugs of acutely infected individuals was associated with a recovery in CD4 proliferative responses to HIV antigens. If this anti-retroviral therapy was stopped, in some of these people the CD4 responses persisted and were associated with reduced levels of viremia. However, the infection persisted in all patients and it is likely that immunological control of the infection will ultimately fail. If CD4 T-cell responses are essential for the control of HIV infection, then the fact that HIV is tropic for these cells and kills them may be the explanation for the long-term inability of the host immune response to control the infection.

Antibodies against gp120 and gp41 envelope viral antigens are produced in response to infection but, as with T cells, are unable to clear the infection. The antibodies react well with purified antigens *in vitro* and with viral debris. In contrast, they bind poorly to intact enveloped virions or to infected cells. This suggests that the native conformation of these antigens, which are heavily glycosylated, is not accessible to naturally produced antibodies. The evidence is strong that antibodies cannot significantly modify established disease. However, as we will learn in Section 11-29, the passive administration of antibodies against HIV can protect experimental animals from mucosal infection by HIV, and this offers hope that an effective vaccine might eventually be developed that could prevent new infections.

Mutations that occur as HIV replicates can allow variants of the virus to escape recognition by antibody or cytotoxic T cells and can contribute to the failure of the immune system to contain the infection in the long term. Direct escape of virus-infected cells from killing by cytotoxic T lymphocytes has been shown by the occurrence of mutations of immunodominant viral peptides presented by MHC class I molecules. In other cases, variant peptides produced by the virus have been found to act as antagonists for T cells responsive to the wild-type epitope (see Section 6-14), thus allowing both mutant and wild-type viruses to survive. Mutant peptides acting as antagonists have also been reported in hepatitis B virus infections, and similar mutant peptides might contribute to the persistence of some viral infections, especially when, as often happens, the immune response of an individual is dominated by T cells specific for a particular epitope.

11-28 HIV infection leads to low levels of CD4 T cells, increased susceptibility to opportunistic infection, and eventually to death.

There are three dominant mechanisms for the loss of CD4 T cells in HIV infection. First, there is evidence for direct viral killing of infected cells; second, there is increased susceptibility to the induction of apoptosis in infected cells; and third, there is killing of infected CD4 T cells by CD8 cytotoxic lymphocytes that recognize viral peptides.

When CD4 T-cell numbers decline below a critical level, cell-mediated immunity is lost, and infections with a variety of opportunistic microbes appear (Fig. 11.30). Typically, resistance is lost early to oral *Candida* species and to *M. tuberculosis*, which is manifest as an increased prevalence of thrush (oral candidiasis) and tuberculosis, respectively. Later, patients suffer from shingles, caused by the activation of latent varicella zoster, from EBV-induced B-cell lymphomas, and from Kaposi's sarcoma, a tumor of endothelial cells that probably represents a response both to cytokines produced in the infection and to a novel herpes virus called HHV-8 that was identified in these lesions. Pneumonia caused by the fungus *P. carinii* is common and was often fatal before effective antifungal therapy was introduced. Co-infection by hepatitis C virus is common and associated with more rapid progression of hepatitis. In the final stages of AIDS, infection with cytomegalovirus or *M. avium* complex is more prominent. It is important to note that not all patients with AIDS get all these infections or tumors, and there are other tumors and infections that are less prominent but still significant. Rather, this is a list of the commonest opportunistic infections and tumors, most of which are normally controlled by robust CD4 T cell-mediated immunity that wanes as the CD4 T-cell counts drop toward zero (see Fig. 11.20).

Infections	
Parasites	*Toxoplasma* spp. *Cryptosporidium* spp. *Leishmania* spp. *Microsporidium* spp.
Intracellular bacteria	*Mycobacterium tuberculosis* *Mycobacterium avium intracellulare* *Salmonella* spp.
Fungi	*Pneumocystis carinii* *Cryptococcus neoformans* *Candida* spp. *Histoplasma capsulatum* *Coccidioides immitis*
Viruses	Herpes simplex Cytomegalovirus Varicella zoster

Malignancies
Kaposi's sarcoma - HHV8 Non-Hodgkin's lymphoma, including EBV-positive Burkitt's lymphoma Primary lymphoma of the brain

Fig. 11.30 A variety of opportunistic pathogens and cancers can kill AIDS patients. Infections are the major cause of death in AIDS, with respiratory infection with *Pneumocystis carinii* and mycobacteria being the most prominent. Most of these pathogens require effective macrophage activation by CD4 T cells or effective cytotoxic T cells for host defense. Opportunistic pathogens are present in the normal environment but cause severe disease primarily in immunocompromised hosts, such as AIDS patients and cancer patients. AIDS patients are also susceptible to several rare cancers, such as Kaposi's sarcoma and various lymphomas, suggesting that immune surveillance of their causative herpes viruses by T cells can normally prevent such tumors (see Chapter 14).

11-29 Vaccination against HIV is an attractive solution but poses many difficulties.

A safe and effective vaccine for the prevention of HIV infection and AIDS is an attractive goal, but its attainment is fraught with difficulties that have not been faced in developing vaccines against other diseases. The main problem is the nature of the infection itself, featuring a virus that proliferates extremely rapidly and causes sustained infection in the face of strong cytotoxic T-cell and antibody responses. As we discussed in Section 11-25, HIV evolves in individual patients by the selective proliferative advantage of mutant virions encoding peptide sequence changes that escape recognition by antibodies and by cytotoxic T lymphocytes. This evolution means that the development of therapeutic vaccination strategies to block the development of AIDS in HIV-infected patients will be extremely difficult. Furthermore, the ability of the virus to persist in latent form as a transcriptionally silent provirus, which is invisible to the immune system, might prevent the immune system from clearing the infection once it has been established. In contrast to therapeutic vaccination, there is more hope for prophylactic vaccination to prevent new infection.

Key among the difficulties is our uncertainty over what form protective immunity to HIV might take. It is not known whether antibodies, responses by CD4 T cells or by cytotoxic T lymphocytes, or all three, are necessary to achieve protective immunity, and which epitopes might provide the targets for protective immunity. If strong cytotoxic responses are necessary to provide protection against HIV, these might be difficult to develop and sustain through vaccination. Other effective viral vaccines rely on the use of live attenuated viruses and there are concerns over the safety of pursuing this approach for HIV. Another possible approach is the use of DNA vaccination, a technique that we discuss in Section 14-27. Both these approaches have been tested in animal models and are now in human trials.

However, against this pessimistic background, there are grounds for hope that successful vaccines can be developed. Of particular interest are rare groups of people who have been exposed often enough to HIV to make it virtually certain that they should have become infected but who have not developed the disease. In some cases this is due to an inherited deficiency in the chemokine receptor used as co-receptor for HIV entry, as we explained in Section 11-21. However, this mutant chemokine receptor does not occur in Africa, where one such group has been identified. A small group of Gambian and Kenyan sex workers who are estimated to have been exposed to many HIV-infected male partners each month for up to 5 years were found to lack antibody responses but to have cytotoxic T lymphocyte responses to a variety of peptide epitopes from HIV. These women seem to have been naturally immunized against HIV. However, follow-up of a number of them showed that about 10% subsequently acquired HIV infection. Paradoxically, HIV infection was found more frequently in women who had reduced their sex work and thereby their regular exposure to the HIV virus. A possible explanation for this was that the absence of repeated HIV antigenic exposure led to loss of the cytotoxic T-cell response, thus rendering them susceptible to infection.

Although there is no perfect animal model for the development of HIV vaccines, one model system is based on simian immunodeficiency virus (SIV), which is closely related to HIV and infects macaques. SIV causes a similar disease to AIDS in Asian macaques such as the cynomolgus monkey, but does not cause disease in African cercopithecus monkeys such as the African green monkey, with which SIV has probably coexisted for up to a million years. Live attenuated SIV vaccines lacking the *nef* gene, and also hybrid

HIV–SIV viruses, have been developed to test the principles of vaccination in primates, and both have proved successful in protecting primates against subsequent infection by fully virulent viruses. For example, the infusion of neutralizing antibodies against HIV into macaques was able to prevent infection after challenge by a pathogenic virus given by the intravenous, or the more physiological mucosal, route.

There are substantial difficulties to be overcome in the development of live attenuated HIV vaccines for use in at-risk populations, not least the worry of recombination between vaccine strains and wild-type viruses leading to reversion to a virulent phenotype. An alternative approach of DNA vaccination followed by the administration of a recombinant modified vaccinia boost has been piloted in primate experiments, and was successful in preventing infection from an intrarectal challenge given 7 months after the booster vaccination. However, for every success in the route to HIV vaccination there is a setback. A cohort of rhesus monkeys was vaccinated with a DNA vaccine given with an IL-2 fusion protein and then challenged with a pathogenic hybrid simian–human immunodeficiency virus. One of the monkeys, 6 months after the challenge, developed an AIDS-like illness that was associated with the emergence of a mutant virus carrying a point mutation in an immunodominant Gag epitope recognized by cytotoxic T cells. This is a beautiful but depressing example of the ability of HIV to escape immune control under the selective pressure of a cytotoxic T lymphocyte response.

Subunit vaccines, which induce immunity to only some proteins in the virus, have also been made. One such vaccine has been made from the envelope protein gp120 and has been tested on chimpanzees. This vaccine proved to be specific to the precise strain of virus used to make it and was therefore useless in protection against natural infection. Subunit vaccines are also less efficient at inducing prolonged cytotoxic T-cell responses. In spite of these results with gp120 in chimpanzees, a recombinant gp120 protein vaccine was used in human volunteers. A small number of volunteers subsequently contracted HIV-1 infection, the course of which was not modified by the previous vaccination.

In addition to all of the biological obstacles to developing effective HIV vaccines, there are difficult ethical issues. It would be unethical to conduct a vaccine trial without trying at the same time to minimize the exposure of a vaccinated population to the virus itself. However, the effectiveness of a vaccine can only be assessed in a population in which the exposure rate to the virus is high enough to assess whether vaccination is protective against infection. This means that initial vaccine trials might have to be conducted in countries where the incidence of infection is very high and public-health measures have not yet succeeded in reducing the spread of HIV.

11-30 Prevention and education are one way in which the spread of HIV and AIDS can be controlled.

The one way in which we know we can protect against infection with HIV is by avoiding contact with body fluids, such as semen, blood, blood products, or milk from people who are infected. Indeed, it has been demonstrated repeatedly that this precaution, simple enough in the developed world, is sufficient to prevent infection, because healthcare workers can take care of AIDS patients for long periods without seroconversion or signs of infection.

For this strategy to work, however, one must be able to test people at risk of infection with HIV periodically, so that they can take the steps necessary to avoid passing the virus to others. This, in turn, requires strict confidentiality and mutual trust. A barrier to the control of HIV is the reluctance of individuals to find out whether or not they are infected, especially as one of the consequences of a positive HIV test is stigmatization by society. As a result, infected individuals can unwittingly infect many others. Balanced against this is the success of therapy with combinations of the new protease inhibitors and reverse-transcriptase inhibitors, which provides an incentive for potentially infected people to identify the presence of infection and gain the benefits of treatment. Responsibility is at the heart of AIDS prevention, and a law guaranteeing the rights of people infected with HIV might go a long way to encouraging responsible behavior. The rights of HIV-infected people are protected in a few countries. The problem in the less-developed nations, where elementary health precautions are extremely difficult to establish, is more profound.

Summary.

Infection with the human immunodeficiency virus (HIV) is the cause of acquired immune deficiency syndrome (AIDS). This worldwide epidemic is now spreading at an alarming rate, especially through heterosexual contact in less-developed countries. HIV is an enveloped retrovirus that replicates in cells of the immune system. Viral entry requires the presence of CD4 and a particular chemokine receptor, and the viral cycle is dependent on transcription factors found in activated T cells. Infection with HIV causes a loss of CD4 T cells and an acute viremia that rapidly subsides as cytotoxic T-cell responses develop, but HIV infection is not eliminated by this immune response. HIV establishes a state of persistent infection in which the virus is continually replicating in newly infected cells. The current treatment consists of combinations of viral protease inhibitors together with nucleoside analogs that inhibit the reverse transcriptase, causing a rapid decrease in virus levels and a slower increase in CD4 T-cell counts. The main effect of HIV infection is the destruction of CD4 T cells, which occurs through the direct cytopathic effects of HIV infection and through killing by CD8 cytotoxic T cells. As the CD4 T-cell counts wane, the body becomes progressively more susceptible to opportunistic infection with intracellular microbes. Eventually, most HIV-infected individuals develop AIDS and die; however, a small minority (3–7%) remain healthy for many years with no apparent ill effects of infection. We hope to be able to learn from these people how infection with HIV can be controlled. The existence of these people, and of others who have been naturally immunized against infection, gives hope that it will be possible to develop effective vaccines against HIV.

Summary to Chapter 11.

Whereas most infections elicit protective immunity, most successful pathogens have developed some means of evading a fully effective immune response, and some result in serious, persistent disease. In addition, some individuals have inherited deficiencies in different components of the immune system, making them highly susceptible to certain classes of infectious agent. Persistent infection and immunodeficiency illustrate the importance of innate and adaptive immunity in an effective host defense against infection, and present huge challenges for future immunological research. HIV combines the characteristics of a persistent infectious agent with the ability to create immunodeficiency in its human host, a combination that is usually slowly lethal to the patient. The key to fighting new pathogens like HIV is to develop our understanding of the basic properties of the immune system and its role in combating infection more fully.

Chapter 11 questions.

11.1   How do viruses evade the immune system?

11.2   What are the causes of immunodeficiencies affecting T lymphocytes?

11.3   What does inherited and acquired immunodeficiency teach us about the normal mechanism of host protection against tuberculosis?

11.4   How does infection by HIV cause AIDS?

11.5   Why can't HIV infection be cured by drug therapy?

General references.

Chapel, H., Geha, R., and Rosen, F.: **Primary immunodeficiency diseases: an update.** Clin. Exp. Immunol. 2003, **132**:9–15.

Cohen, O.J., Kinter, A., and Fauci, A.S.: **Host factors in the pathogenesis of HIV disease.** Immunol. Rev. 1997, **159**:31–48.

De Cock, K.M.: **Epidemiology and the emergence of human immunodeficiency virus and acquired immune deficiency syndrome.** Philos. Trans. R. Soc. Lond B 2001, **356**:795–798.

De Cock, K.M., Mbori-Ngacha, D., and Marum, E.: **Shadow on the continent: public health and HIV/AIDS in Africa in the 21st century.** Lancet 2002, **360**:67–72.

Fischer, A., Cavazzana-Calvo, M., De-Saint-Basile, G., DeVillartay, J.P., Di-Santo, J.P., Hivroz, C., Rieux-Laucat, F., and Le-Deist, F.: **Naturally occurring primary deficiencies of the immune system.** Annu. Rev. Immunol. 1997, **15**:93–124.

Hill, A.V.: **The immunogenetics of human infectious diseases.** Annu. Rev. Immunol. 1998, **16**:593–617.

Korber, B., Muldoon, M., Theiler, J., Gao, F., Gupta, R., Lapedes, A., Hahn, B.H., Wolinsky, S., and Bhattacharya, T.: **Timing the ancestor of the HIV-1 pandemic strains.** Science 2000, **288**:1789–1796.

Kotwal, G.J.: **Microorganisms and their interaction with the immune system.** J. Leukoc. Biol. 1997, **62**:415–429.

Lederberg, J.: **Infectious history.** Science 2000, **288**:287–293.

McNicholl, J.M., Downer, M.V., Udhayakumar, V., Alper, C.A., and Swerdlow, D.L.: **Host–pathogen interactions in emerging and re-emerging infectious diseases: a genomic perspective of tuberculosis, malaria, human immunodeficiency virus infection, hepatitis B, and cholera.** Annu. Rev. Public Health 2000, **21**:15–46.

Royce, R.A., Sena, A., Cates, W., Jr., and Cohen, M.S.: **Sexual transmission of HIV.** N. Engl. J. Med. 1997, **336**:1072–1078.

Tortorella, D., Gewurz, B.E., Furman, M.H., Schust, D.J., and Ploegh, H.L.: **Viral subversion of the immune system.** Annu. Rev. Immunol. 2000, **18**:861–926.

Xu, X.N., Screaton, G.R., and McMichael, A.J.: **Virus infections: escape, resistance, and counterattack.** Immunity 2001, **15**:867–870.

Zinkernagel, R.M.: **Immunology taught by viruses.** Science 1996, **271**:173–178.

Section references.

11-1   Antigenic variation allows pathogens to escape from immunity.

Clegg, S., Hancox, L.S., and Yeh, K.S.: **Salmonella typhimurium fimbrial phase variation and FimA expression.** J. Bacteriol. 1996, **178**:542–545.

Cossart, P.: **Host/pathogen interactions. Subversion of the mammalian cell cytoskeleton by invasive bacteria.** J. Clin. Invest. 1997, **99**:2307–2311.

Donelson, J.E., Hill, K.L., and El-Sayed, N.M.: **Multiple mechanisms of immune evasion by African trypanosomes.** Mol. Biochem. Parasitol. 1998, **91**:51–66.

Gibbs, M.J., Armstrong, J.S., and Gibbs, A.J.: **Recombination in the hemagglutinin gene of the 1918 'Spanish flu'.** Science 2001, **293**:1842–1845.

Hatta, M., Gao, P., Halfmann, P., and Kawaoka, Y.: **Molecular basis for high virulence of Hong Kong H5N1 influenza A viruses.** Science 2001, **293**:1840–1842.

Laver, G., and Garman, E.: **Virology. The origin and control of pandemic influenza.** Science 2001, **293**:1776–1777.

Rudenko, G., Cross, M., and Borst, P.: **Changing the end: antigenic variation orchestrated at the telomeres of African trypanosomes.** Trends Microbiol. 1998, **6**:113–116.

Seifert, H.S., Wright, C.J., Jerse, A.E., Cohen, M.S., and Cannon, J.G.: **Multiple gonococcal pilin antigenic variants are produced during experimental human infections.** J. Clin. Invest. 1994, **93**:2744–2749.

Webster, R.G.: **Virology. A molecular whodunit.** Science 2001, **293**:1773–1775.

11-2   Some viruses persist in vivo by ceasing to replicate until immunity wanes.

Cohen, J.I.: **Epstein–Barr virus infection.** N. Engl. J. Med. 2000, **343**:481–492.

Ehrlich, R.: **Selective mechanisms utilized by persistent and oncogenic viruses to interfere with antigen processing and presentation.** Immunol. Res. 1995, **14**:77–97.

Garcia Blanco, M.A., and Cullen, B.R.: **Molecular basis of latency in pathogenic human viruses.** Science 1991, **254**:815–820.

Hahn, G., Jores, R., and Mocarski, E.S.: **Cytomegalovirus remains latent in a** common precursor of dendritic and myeloid cells. *Proc. Natl. Acad. Sci. USA* 1998, **95**:3937–3942.

Ho, D.Y.: **Herpes simplex virus latency: molecular aspects.** *Prog. Med. Virol.* 1992, **39**:76–115.

Longnecker, R., and Miller, C.L.: **Regulation of Epstein–Barr virus latency by latent membrane protein 2.** *Trends Microbiol.* 1996, **4**:38–42.

Macsween, K.F., and Crawford, D.H.: **Epstein–Barr virus—recent advances.** *Lancet Infect. Dis.* 2003, **3**:131–140.

Mitchell, B.M., Bloom, D.C., Cohrs, R.J., Gilden, D.H., and Kennedy, P.G.: **Herpes simplex virus-1 and varicella-zoster virus latency in ganglia.** *J. Neurovirol.* 2003, **9**:194–204.

Nash, A.A.: **T cells and the regulation of herpes simplex virus latency and reactivation.** *J. Exp. Med.* 2000, **191**:1455–1458.

Wensing, B., and Farrell, P.J.: **Regulation of cell growth and death by Epstein–Barr virus.** *Microbes Infect.* 2000, **2**:77–84.

11-3   Some pathogens resist destruction by host defense mechanisms or exploit them for their own purposes.

Alcami, A., and Koszinowski, U.H.: **Viral mechanisms of immune evasion.** *Trends Microbiol.* 2000, **8**:410–418.

Arvin, A.M.: **Varicella-zoster virus: molecular virology and virus–host interactions.** *Curr. Opin. Microbiol.* 2001, **4**:442–449.

Brander, C., and Walker, B.D.: **Modulation of host immune responses by clinically relevant human DNA and RNA viruses.** *Curr. Opin. Microbiol.* 2000, **3**:379–386.

Cooper, S.S., Glenn, J., and Greenberg, H.B.: **Lessons in defense: hepatitis C, a case study.** *Curr. Opin. Microbiol.* 2000, **3**:363–365.

Gewurz, B.E., Gaudet, R., Tortorella, D., Wang, E.W., and Ploegh, H.L.: **Virus subversion of immunity: a structural perspective.** *Curr. Opin. Immunol.* 2001, **13**:442–450.

Lauer, G.M., and Walker, B.D.: **Hepatitis C virus infection.** *N. Engl. J. Med.* 2001, **345**:41–52.

McFadden, G., and Murphy, P.M.: **Host-related immunomodulators encoded by poxviruses and herpesviruses.** *Curr. Opin. Microbiol.* 2000, **3**:371–378.

Radolf, J.D.: **Role of outer membrane architecture in immune evasion by *Treponema pallidum* and *Borrelia burgdorferi*.** *Trends Microbiol.* 1994, **2**:307–311.

Sinai, A.P., and Joiner, K.A.: **Safe haven: the cell biology of nonfusogenic pathogen vacuoles.** *Annu. Rev. Microbiol.* 1997, **51**:415–462.

11-4   Immunosuppression or inappropriate immune responses can contribute to persistent disease.

Bhardwaj, N.: **Interactions of viruses with dendritic cells: a double-edged sword.** *J. Exp. Med.* 1997, **186**:795–799.

Bloom, B.R., Modlin, R.L., and Salgame, P.: **Stigma variations: observations on suppressor T cells and leprosy.** *Annu. Rev. Immunol.* 1992, **10**:453–488.

Fleischer, B.: **Superantigens.** *APMIS* 1994, **102**:3–12.

Salgame, P., Abrams, J.S., Clayberger, C., Goldstein, H., Convit, J., Modlin, R.L., and Bloom, B.R.: **Differing lymphokine profiles of functional subsets of human CD4 and CD8 T cell clones.** *Science* 1991, **254**:279–282.

11-5   Immune responses can contribute directly to pathogenesis.

Cheever, A.W., and Yap, G.S.: **Immunologic basis of disease and disease regulation in schistosomiasis.** *Chem. Immunol.* 1997, **66**:159–176.

Doherty, P.C., Topham, D.J., Tripp, R.A., Cardin, R.D., Brooks, J.W., and Stevenson, P.G.: **Effector CD4[+] and CD8[+] T-cell mechanisms in the control of respiratory virus infections.** *Immunol. Rev.* 1997, **159**:105–117.

Openshaw, P.J.: **Immunopathological mechanisms in respiratory syncytial virus disease.** *Springer Semin. Immunopathol.* 1995, **17**:187–201.

Varga, S.M., Wang, X., Welsh, R.M., and Braciale, T.J.: **Immunopathology in RSV infection is mediated by a discrete oligoclonal subset of antigen-specific CD4[+] T cells.** *Immunity* 2001, **15**:637–646.

11-6   A history of repeated infections suggests a diagnosis of immunodeficiency.

Rosen, F.S., Cooper, M.D., and Wedgwood, R.J.: **The primary immunodeficiencies.** *N. Engl. J. Med.* 1995, **333**:431–440.

11-7   Inherited immunodeficiency diseases are caused by recessive gene defects.

Fischer, A.: **Inherited disorders of lymphocyte development and function.** *Curr. Opin. Immunol.* 1996, **8**:445–447.

Kokron, C.M., Bonilla, F.A., Oettgen, H.C., Ramesh, N., Geha, R.S., and Pandolfi, F.: **Searching for genes involved in the pathogenesis of primary immunodeficiency diseases: lessons from mouse knockouts.** *J. Clin. Immunol.* 1997, **17**:109–126.

Smart, B.A., and Ochs, H.D.: **The molecular basis and treatment of primary immunodeficiency disorders.** *Curr. Opin. Pediatr.* 1997, **9**:570–576.

Smith, C.I., and Notarangelo, L.D.: **Molecular basis for X-linked immunodeficiencies.** *Adv. Genet.* 1997, **35**:57–115.

11-8   The main effect of low levels of antibody is an inability to clear extracellular bacteria.

Bruton, O.C.: **Agammaglobulinemia.** *Pediatrics* 1952, **9**:722–728.

Burrows, P.D., and Cooper, M.D.: **IgA deficiency.** *Adv. Immunol.* 1997, **65**:245–276.

Desiderio, S.: **Role of Btk in B cell development and signaling.** *Curr. Opin. Immunol.* 1997, **9**:534–540.

Fuleihan, R., Ramesh, N., and Geha, R.S.: **X-linked agammaglobulinemia and immunoglobulin deficiency with normal or elevated IgM: immunodeficiencies of B cell development and differentiation.** *Adv. Immunol.* 1995, **60**:37–56.

Lee, M.L., Gale, R.P., and Yap, P.L.: **Use of intravenous immunoglobulin to prevent or treat infections in persons with immune deficiency.** *Annu. Rev. Med.* 1997, **48**:93–102.

Notarangelo, L.D.: **Immunodeficiencies caused by genetic defects in protein kinases.** *Curr. Opin. Immunol.* 1996, **8**:448–453.

Ochs, H.D., and Wedgwood, R.J.: **IgG subclass deficiencies.** *Annu. Rev. Med.* 1987, **38**:325–340.

Preud'homme, J.L., and Hanson, L.A.: **IgG subclass deficiency.** *Immunodefic. Rev.* 1990, **2**:129–149.

11-9   T-cell defects can also result in low antibody levels.

Doffinger, R., Smahi, A., Bessia, C., Geissmann, F., Feinberg, J., Durandy, A., Bodemer, C., Kenwrick, S., Dupuis-Girod, S., Blanche, S., Wood, P., Rabia, S.H., Headon, D.J., Overbeek, P.A., Le Deist, F., Holland, S.M., Belani, K., Kumararatne, D.S., Fischer, A., Shapiro, R., Conley, M.E., Reimund, E., Kalhoff, H., Abinun, M., Munnich, A., Israel, A., Courtois, G., and Casanova, J.L.: **X-linked anhidrotic ectodermal dysplasia with immunodeficiency is caused by impaired NF-κB signaling.** *Nat. Genet.* 2001, **27**:277–285.

Durandy, A., and Honjo, T.: **Human genetic defects in class-switch recombination (hyper-IgM syndromes).** *Curr. Opin. Immunol.* 2001, **13**:543–548.

Ferrari, S., Giliani, S., Insalaco, A., Al Ghonaium, A., Soresina, A.R., Loubser, M., Avanzini, M.A., Marconi, M., Badolato, R., Ugazio, A.G., Levy, Y., Catalan, N., Durandy, A., Tbakhi, A., Notarangelo, L.D., and Plebani, A.: **Mutations of CD40 gene cause an autosomal recessive form of immunodeficiency with hyper IgM.** *Proc. Natl. Acad. Sci. USA* 2001, **98**:12614–12619.

11-10   Defects in complement components cause defective humoral immune function.

Botto, M., Dell'Agnola, C., Bygrave, A.E., Thompson, E.M., Cook, H.T., Petry, F., Loos, M., Pandolfi, P.P., and Walport, M.J.: **Homozygous C1q deficiency causes glomerulonephritis associated with multiple apoptotic bodies.** *Nat. Genet.* 1998, **19**:56–59.

Colten, H.R., and Rosen, F.S.: **Complement deficiencies.** *Annu. Rev. Immunol.* 1992, **10**:809–834.

Ochsenbein, A.F., and Zinkernagel, R.M.: **Natural antibodies and complement link innate and acquired immunity.** *Immunol. Today* 2000, **21**:624–630.

Walport, M.J.: **Complement. First of two parts.** *N. Engl. J. Med.* 2001, **344**:1058–1066.

Walport, M.J.: **Complement. Second of two parts.** *N. Engl. J. Med.* 2001, **344**:1140–1144.

11-11 Defects in phagocytic cells permit widespread bacterial infections.

Ambruso, D.R., Knall, C., Abell, A.N., Panepinto, J., Kurkchubasche, A., Thurman, G., Gonzalez-Aller, C., Hiester, A., deBoer, M., Harbeck, R.J., Oyer, R., Johnson, G.L., and Roos, D.: **Human neutrophil immunodeficiency syndrome is associated with an inhibitory Rac2 mutation.** *Proc. Natl. Acad. Sci. USA* 2000, **97**:4654–4659.

Aprikyan, A.A., and Dale, D.C.: **Mutations in the neutrophil elastase gene in cyclic and congenital neutropenia.** *Curr. Opin. Immunol.* 2001, **13**:535–538.

Fischer, A., Lisowska Grospierre, B., Anderson, D.C., and Springer, T.A.: **Leukocyte adhesion deficiency: molecular basis and functional consequences.** *Immunodefic. Rev.* 1988, **1**:39–54.

Goldblatt, D., and Thrasher, A.J.: **Chronic granulomatous disease.** *Clin. Exp. Immunol.* 2000, **122**:1–9.

Luhn, K., Wild, M.K., Eckhardt, M., Gerardy-Schahn, R., and Vestweber, D.: **The gene defective in leukocyte adhesion deficiency II encodes a putative GDP-fucose transporter.** *Nat. Genet.* 2001, **28**:69–72.

Malech, H.L., and Nauseef, W.M.: **Primary inherited defects in neutrophil function: etiology and treatment.** *Semin. Hematol.* 1997, **34**:279–290.

Rotrosen, D., and Gallin, J.I.: **Disorders of phagocyte function.** *Annu. Rev. Immunol.* 1987, **5**:127–150.

Spritz, R.A.: **Genetic defects in Chediak–Higashi syndrome and the beige mouse.** *J. Clin. Immunol.* 1998, **18**:97–105.

11-12 Defects in T-cell function result in severe combined immunodeficiencies.

Bosma, M.J., and Carroll, A.M.: **The SCID mouse mutant: definition, characterization, and potential uses.** *Annu. Rev. Immunol.* 1991, **9**:323–350.

Fugmann, S.D.: **DNA repair: breaking the seal.** *Nature* 2002, **416**:691–694.

Gadola, S.D., Moins-Teisserenc, H.T., Trowsdale, J., Gross, W.L., and Cerundolo, V.: **TAP deficiency syndrome.** *Clin. Exp. Immunol.* 2000, **121**:173–178.

Gennery, A.R., Cant, A.J., and Jeggo, P.A.: **Immunodeficiency associated with DNA repair defects.** *Clin. Exp. Immunol.* 2000, **121**:1–7.

Grusby, M.J., and Glimcher, L.H.: **Immune responses in MHC class II-deficient mice.** *Annu. Rev. Immunol.* 1995, **13**:417–435.

Hirschhorn, R.: **Adenosine deaminase deficiency: molecular basis and recent developments.** *Clin. Immunol. Immunopathol.* 1995, **76**:S219–S227.

Lavin, M.F., and Shiloh, Y.: **The genetic defect in ataxia-telangiectasia.** *Annu. Rev. Immunol.* 1997, **15**:177–202.

Masternak, K., Barras, E., Zufferey, M., Conrad, B., Corthals, G., Aebersold, R., Sanchez, J.C., Hochstrasser, D.F., Mach, B., and Reith, W.: **A gene encoding a novel RFX-associated transactivator is mutated in the majority of MHC class II deficiency patients.** *Nat. Genet.* 1998, **20**:273–277.

Moshous, D., Callebaut, I., de Chasseval, R., Corneo, B., Cavazzana-Calvo, M., Le Deist, F., Tezcan, I., Sanal, O., Bertrand, Y., Philippe, N., Fischer, A., and De Villartay, J.P.: **Artemis, a novel DNA double-strand break repair/V(D)J recombination protein, is mutated in human severe combined immune deficiency.** *Cell* 2001, **105**:177–186.

Pignata, C., Gaetaniello, L., Masci, A.M., Frank, J., Christiano, A., Matrecano, E., and Racioppi, L.: **Human equivalent of the mouse Nude/SCID phenotype: long-term evaluation of immunologic reconstitution after bone marrow transplantation.** *Blood* 2001, **97**:880–885.

Schinke, M., and Izumo, S.: **Deconstructing DiGeorge syndrome.** *Nat.Genet.* 2001, **27**:238–240.

Steimle, V., Reith, W., and Mach, B.: **Major histocompatibility complex class II deficiency: a disease of gene regulation.** *Adv. Immunol.* 1996, **61**:327–340.

11-13 Defective T-cell signaling, cytokine production, or cytokine action can cause immunodeficiency.

Arnaiz Villena, A., Timon, M., Corell, A., Perez Aciego, P., Martin Villa, J.M., and Regueiro, J.R.: **Brief report: primary immunodeficiency caused by mutations in the gene encoding the CD3-gamma subunit of the T-lymphocyte receptor.** *N. Engl. J. Med.* 1992, **327**:529–533.

Castigli, E., Pahwa, R., Good, R.A., Geha, R.S., and Chatila, T.A.: **Molecular basis of a multiple lymphokine deficiency in a patient with severe combined immunodeficiency.** *Proc. Natl. Acad. Sci. USA* 1993, **90**:4728–4732.

DiSanto, J.P., Keever, C.A., Small, T.N., Nicols, G.L., O'Reilly, R.J., and Flomenberg, N.: **Absence of interleukin 2 production in a severe combined immunodeficiency disease syndrome with T cells.** *J. Exp. Med.* 1990, **171**:1697–1704.

DiSanto, J.P., Rieux Laucat, F., Dautry Varsat, A., Fischer, A., and de Saint Basile, G.: **Defective human interleukin 2 receptor gamma chain in an atypical X chromosome-linked severe combined immunodeficiency with peripheral T cells.** *Proc. Natl. Acad. Sci. USA* 1994, **91**:9466–9470.

Gilmour, K.C., Fujii, H., Cranston, T., Davies, E.G., Kinnon, C., and Gaspar, H.B.: **Defective expression of the interleukin-2/interleukin-15 receptor beta subunit leads to a natural killer cell-deficient form of severe combined immunodeficiency.** *Blood* 2001, **98**:877–879.

Kung, C., Pingel, J.T., Heikinheimo, M., Klemola, T., Varkila, K., Yoo, L.I., Vuopala, K., Poyhonen, M., Uhari, M., Rogers, M., Speck, S.H., Chatila, T., and Thomas, M.L.: **Mutations in the tyrosine phosphatase CD45 gene in a child with severe combined immunodeficiency disease.** *Nat. Med.* 2000, **6**:343–345.

Leonard, W.J.: **The molecular basis of X linked severe combined immunodeficiency.** *Annu. Rev. Med.* 1996, **47**:229–239.

Ochs, H.D.: **The Wiskott–Aldrich syndrome.** *Springer Semin. Immunopathol.* 1998, **9**:435–458.

Roifman, C.M., Zhang, J., Chitayat, D., and Sharfe, N.: **A partial deficiency of interleukin-7R alpha is sufficient to abrogate T-cell development and cause severe combined immunodeficiency.** *Blood* 2000, **96**:2803–2807.

Snapper, S.B., and Rosen, F.S.: **The Wiskott–Aldrich syndrome protein (WASP): roles in signaling and cytoskeletal organization.** *Annu. Rev. Immunol.* 1999, **17**:905–929.

11-14 The normal pathways for host defense against intracellular bacteria are illustrated by genetic deficiencies of IFN-γ and IL-12 and their receptors.

Casanova, J.L., and Abel, L.: **Genetic dissection of immunity to mycobacteria: the human model.** *Annu. Rev. Immunol.* 2002, **20**:581–620.

Dupuis, S., Dargemont, C., Fieschi, C., Thomassin, N., Rosenzweig, S., Harris, J., Holland, S.M., Schreiber, R.D., and Casanova, J.L.: **Impairment of mycobacterial but not viral immunity by a germline human STAT1 mutation.** *Science* 2001, **293**:300–303.

Keane, J., Gershon, S., Wise, R.P., Mirabile-Levens, E., Kasznica, J., Schwieterman, W.D., Siegel, J.N., and Braun, M.M.: **Tuberculosis associated with infliximab, a tumor necrosis factor α-neutralizing agent.** *N. Engl. J. Med.* 2001, **345**:1098–1104.

Lammas, D.A., Casanova, J.L., and Kumararatne, D.S.: **Clinical consequences of defects in the IL-12-dependent interferon-γ (IFN-γ) pathway.** *Clin. Exp. Immunol.* 2000, **121**:417–425.

Newport, M.J., Huxley, C.M., Huston, S., Hawrylowicz, C.M., Oostra, B.A., Williamson, R., and Levin, M.: **A mutation in the interferon-γ-receptor gene and susceptibility to mycobacterial infection.** *N. Engl. J. Med.* 1996, **335**:1941–1949.

Shtrichman, R., and Samuel, C.E.: **The role of γ interferon in antimicrobial immunity.** *Curr. Opin. Microbiol.* 2001, **4**:251–259.

11-15   X-linked lymphoproliferative syndrome is associated with fatal infection
        by Epstein–Barr virus and with the development of lymphomas.

Latour, S., Gish, G., Helgason, C.D., Humphries, R.K., Pawson, T., and Veillette, A.: Regulation of SLAM-mediated signal transduction by SAP, the X-linked lymphoproliferative gene product. Nat. Immunol. 2001, 2:681–690.

Morra, M., Howie, D., Grande, M.S., Sayos, J., Wang, N., Wu, C., Engel, P., and Terhorst, C.: X-linked lymphoproliferative disease: a progressive immunodeficiency. Annu. Rev. Immunol. 2001, 19:657–682.

Nichols, K.E., Koretzky, G.A., and June, C.H.: SAP: natural inhibitor or grand SLAM of T cell activation? Nat. Immunol. 2001, 2:665–666.

Satterthwaite, A.B., Rawlings, D.J., and Witte, O.N.: DSHP: a 'power bar' for sustained immune responses? Proc. Natl. Acad. Sci. USA 1998, 95:13355–13357.

11-16   Genetic abnormalities in the secretory cytotoxic pathways of
        lymphocytes cause uncontrolled lymphoproliferation and
        inflammatory responses to viral infections.

de Saint, B.G., and Fischer, A.: The role of cytotoxicity in lymphocyte homeostasis. Curr. Opin. Immunol. 2001, 13:549–554.

Dell'Angelica, E.C., Mullins, C., Caplan, S., and Bonifacino, J.S.: Lysosome-related organelles. FASEB J. 2000, 14:1265–1278.

Huizing, M., Anikster, Y., and Gahl, W.A.: Hermansky–Pudlak syndrome and Chediak–Higashi syndrome: disorders of vesicle formation and trafficking. Thromb. Haemost. 2001, 86:233–245.

Menasche, G., Pastural, E., Feldmann, J., Certain, S., Ersoy, F., Dupuis, S., Wulffraat, N., Bianchi, D., Fischer, A., Le Deist, F., and de Saint, B.G.: Mutations in RAB27A cause Griscelli syndrome associated with haemophagocytic syndrome. Nat. Genet. 2000, 25:173–176.

Stinchcombe, J.C., and Griffiths, G.M.: Normal and abnormal secretion by haemopoietic cells. Immunology 2001, 103:10–16.

11-17   Bone marrow transplantation or gene therapy can be useful to correct
        genetic defects.

Anderson, W.F.: Human gene therapy. Nature 1998, 392:25–30.

Candotti, F., and Blaese, R.M.: Gene therapy of primary immunodeficiencies. Springer Semin. Immunopathol. 1998, 19:493–508.

Fischer, A., Hacein-Bey, S., and Cavazzana-Calvo, M.: Gene therapy of severe combined immunodeficiencies. Nat. Rev. Immunol. 2002, 2:615–621.

Fischer, A., Haddad, E., Jabado, N., Casanova, J.L., Blanche, S., Le Deist, F., and Cavazzana-Calvo, M.: Stem cell transplantation for immunodeficiency. Springer Semin. Immunopathol. 1998, 19:479–492.

Hacein-Bey-Abina, S., Le Deist, F., Carlier, F., Bouneaud, C., Hue, C., De Villartay, J.P., Thrasher, A.J., Wulffraat, N., Sorensen, R., Dupuis-Girod, S., Fischer, A., Davies, E.G., Kuis, W., Leiva, L., and Cavazzana-Calvo, M.: Sustained correction of X-linked severe combined immunodeficiency by ex vivo gene therapy. N. Engl. J. Med. 2002, 346:1185–1193.

Hacein-Bey-Abina, S., Von Kalle, C., Schmidt, M., McCormack, M.P., Wulffraat, N., Lebouch, P., Lim, A., Osborne, C.S., Pawliuk, R., Morillon, E., Sorensen, R., Forster, A., Fraser, P., Cohen, J.I., de Saint, B.G., Alexander, I., Wintergerst, U., Frebourg, T., Aurias, A., Stoppa-Lyonnet, D., Romana, S., Radford-Weiss, I., Gross, F., Valensi, F., Delabesse, E., Macintyre, E., Sigaux, F., Soulier, J., Leiva, L.E., Wissler, M., Prinz, C., Rabbitts, T.H., Le Deist, F., Fischer, A., and Cavazzana-Calvo, M.: LMO2-associated clonal T cell proliferation in two patients after gene therapy for SCID-X1. Science 2003, 302:415–419.

Kohn, D.B., Hershfield, M.S., Carbonaro, D., Shigeoka, A., Brooks, J., Smogorzewska, E.M., Barsky, L.W., Chan, R., Burotto, F., Annett, G., Nolta, J.A., Crooks, G., Kapoor, N., Elder, M., Wara, D., Bowen, T., Madsen, E., Snyder, F.F., Bastian, J., Muul, L., Blaese, R.M., Weinberg, K., and Parkman, R.: T lymphocytes with a normal ADA gene accumulate after transplantation of transduced autologous umbilical cord blood CD34+ cells in ADA-deficient SCID neonates. Nat. Med. 1998, 4:775–780.

Onodera, M., Ariga, T., Kawamura, N., Kobayashi, I., Ohtsu, M., Yamada, M.,

Tame, A., Furuta, H., Okano, M., Matsumoto, S., Kotani, H., McGarrity, G.J., Blaese, R.M., and Sakiyama, Y.: Successful peripheral T-lymphocyte-directed gene transfer for a patient with severe combined immune deficiency caused by adenosine deaminase deficiency. Blood 1998, 91:30–36.

Rosen, F.S.: Successful gene therapy for severe combined immunodeficiency. N. Engl. J. Med. 2002, 346:1241–1243.

11-18   Secondary immunodeficiencies are major predisposing causes of
        infection and death

Chandra, R.K.: Nutrition, immunity and infection: from basic knowledge of dietary manipulation of immune responses to practical application of ameliorating suffering and improving survival. Proc. Natl. Acad. Sci. USA 1996, 93:14304–14307.

Lord, G.M., Matarese, G., Howard, J.K., Baker, R.J., Bloom, S.R., and Lechler, R.I.: Leptin modulates the T-cell immune response and reverses starvation-induced immunosuppression. Nature 1998, 394:897–901.

11-19   Most individuals infected with HIV progress over time to AIDS.

Baltimore, D.: Lessons from people with nonprogressive HIV infection. N. Engl. J. Med. 1995, 332:259–260.

Barre-Sinoussi, F.: HIV as the cause of AIDS. Lancet 1996, 348:31–35.

Kirchhoff, F., Greenough, T.C., Brettler, D.B., Sullivan, J.L., and Desrosiers, R.C.: Brief report: absence of intact nef sequences in a long-term survivor with nonprogressive HIV-1 infection. N. Engl. J. Med. 1995, 332:228–232.

Pantaleo, G., Menzo, S., Vaccarezza, M., Graziosi, C., Cohen, O.J., Demarest, J.F., Montefiori, D., Orenstein, J.M., Fox, C., Schrager, L.K., Margolick, J.B., Buchbinder, S., Giorgi, J.V., and Fauci, A.S.: Studies in subjects with long-term nonprogressive human immunodeficiency virus infection. N. Engl. J. Med. 1995, 332:209–216.

Peckham, C., and Gibb, D.: Mother-to-child transmission of the human immunodeficiency virus. N. Engl. J. Med. 1995, 333:298–302.

Rosenberg, P.S., and Goedert, J.J.: Estimating the cumulative incidence of HIV infection among persons with haemophilia in the United States of America. Stat. Med. 1998, 17:155–168.

Volberding, P.A.: Age as a predictor of progression in HIV infection. Lancet 1996, 347:1569–1570.

Wang, W.K., Essex, M., McLane, M.F., Mayer, K.H., Hsieh, C.C., Brumblay, H.G., Seage, G., and Lee, T.H.R.: Pattern of gp120 sequence divergence linked to a lack of clinical progression in human immunodeficiency virus type 1 infection. Proc. Natl. Acad. Sci. USA 1996, 93:6693–6697.

11-20   HIV is a retrovirus that infects CD4 T cells, dendritic cells, and
        macrophages.

Bomsel, M., and David, V.: Mucosal gatekeepers: selecting HIV viruses for early infection. Nat. Med. 2002, 8:114–116.

Cammack, N.: The potential for HIV fusion inhibition. Curr. Opin. Infect. Dis. 2001, 14:13–16.

Chan, D.C., and Kim, P.S.: HIV entry and its inhibition. Cell 1998, 93:681–684.

Connor, R.I., Sheridan, K.E., Ceradini, D., Choe, S., and Landau, N.R.: Change in coreceptor use correlates with disease progression in HIV-1—infected individuals. J. Exp. Med. 1997, 185:621–628.

Farber, J.M., and Berger, E.A.: HIV's response to a CCR5 inhibitor: I'd rather tighten than switch! Proc. Natl. Acad. Sci. USA 2002, 99:1749–1751.

Grouard, G., and Clark, E.A.: Role of dendritic and follicular dendritic cells in HIV infection and pathogenesis. Curr. Opin. Immunol. 1997, 9:563–567.

Kilby, J.M., Hopkins, S., Venetta, T.M., DiMassimo, B., Cloud, G.A., Lee, J.Y., Alldredge, L., Hunter, E., Lambert, D., Bolognesi, D., Matthews, T., Johnson, M.R., Nowak, M.A., Shaw, G.M., and Saag, M.S.: Potent suppression of HIV-1 replication in humans by T-20, a peptide inhibitor of gp41-mediated virus entry. Nat.Med. 1998, 4:1302–1307.

Kwon, D.S., Gregorio, G., Bitton, N., Hendrickson, W.A., and Littman, D.R.:

DC-SIGN-mediated internalization of HIV is required for trans-enhancement of T cell infection. *Immunity* 2002, **16**:135–144.

Moore, J.P., Trkola, A., and Dragic, T.: **Co-receptors for HIV-1 entry.** *Curr. Opin. Immunol.* 1997, **9**:551–562.

Pohlmann, S., Baribaud, F., and Doms, R.W.: **DC-SIGN and DC-SIGNR: helping hands for HIV.** *Trends Immunol.* 2001, **22**:643–646.

Root, M.J., Kay, M.S., and Kim, P.S.: **Protein design of an HIV-1 entry inhibitor.** *Science* 2001, **291**:884–888.

Sol-Foulon, N., Moris, A., Nobile, C., Boccaccio, C., Engering, A., Abastado, J.P., Heard, J.M., van Kooyk, Y., and Schwartz, O.: **HIV-1 Nef-induced upregulation of DC-SIGN in dendritic cells promotes lymphocyte clustering and viral spread.** *Immunity* 2002, **16**:145–155.

Unutmaz, D., and Littman, D.R.: **Expression pattern of HIV-1 coreceptors on T cells: implications for viral transmission and lymphocyte homing.** *Proc. Natl. Acad. Sci. USA* 1997, **94**:1615–1618.

Wyatt, R., and Sodroski, J.: **The HIV-1 envelope glycoproteins: fusogens, antigens, and immunogens.** *Science* 1998, **280**:1884–1888.

11-21 Genetic deficiency of the macrophage chemokine co-receptor for HIV confers resistance to HIV infection *in vivo*.

Berger, E.A., Murphy, P.M., and Farber, J.M.: **Chemokine receptors as HIV-1 coreceptors: roles in viral entry, tropism, and disease.** *Annu. Rev. Immunol.* 1999, **17**:657–700.

Lehner, T.: **The role of CCR5 chemokine ligands and antibodies to CCR5 coreceptors in preventing HIV infection.** *Trends Immunol.* 2002, **23**:347–351.

Littman, D.R.: **Chemokine receptors: keys to AIDS pathogenesis?** *Cell* 1998, **93**:677–680.

Liu, R., Paxton, W.A., Choe, S., Ceradini, D., Martin, S.R., Horuk, R., Macdonald, M.E., Stuhlmann, H., Koup, R.A., and Landau, N.R.: **Homozygous defect in HIV 1 coreceptor accounts for resistance of some multiply exposed individuals to HIV 1 infection.** *Cell* 1996, **86**:367–377.

Murakami, T., Nakajima, T., Koyanagi, Y., Tachibana, K., Fujii, N., Tamamura, H., Yoshida, N., Waki, M., Matsumoto, A., Yoshie, O., Kishimoto, T., Yamamoto, N., and Nagasawa, T.: **A small molecule CXCR4 inhibitor that blocks T cell line-tropic HIV-1 infection.** *J. Exp. Med.* 1997, **186**:1389–1393.

Samson, M., Libert, F., Doranz, B.J., Rucker, J., Liesnard, C., Farber, C.M., Saragosti, S., Lapoumeroulie, C., Cognaux, J., Forceille, C., Muyldermans, G., Verhofstede, C., Burtonboy, G., Georges, M., Imai, T., Rana, S., Yi, Y.J., Smyth, R.J., Collman, R.G., Doms, R.W., Vassart, G., and Parmentier, M.R.: **Resistance to HIV 1 infection in Caucasian individuals bearing mutant alleles of the CCR 5 chemokine receptor gene.** *Nature* 1996, **382**:722–725.

Yang, A.G., Bai, X., Huang, X.F., Yao, C., and Chen, S.: **Phenotypic knockout of HIV type 1 chemokine coreceptor CCR-5 by intrakines as potential therapeutic approach for HIV-1 infection.** *Proc. Natl. Acad. Sci. USA* 1997, **94**:11567–11572.

11-22 HIV RNA is transcribed by viral reverse transcriptase into DNA that integrates into the host cell genome.

Andrake, M.D., and Skalka, A.M.R.: **Retroviral integrase, putting the pieces together.** *J. Biol. Chem.* 1995, **271**:19633–19636.

Baltimore, D.: **The enigma of HIV infection.** *Cell* 1995, **82**:175–176.

McCune, J.M.: **Viral latency in HIV disease.** *Cell* 1995, **82**:183–188.

11-23 Transcription of the HIV provirus depends on host-cell transcription factors induced upon the activation of infected T cells.

Cullen, B.R.: **HIV-1 auxiliary proteins: making connections in a dying cell.** *Cell* 1998, **93**:685–692.

Cullen, B.R.: **Connections between the processing and nuclear export of mRNA: evidence for an export license?** *Proc. Natl. Acad. Sci. USA* 2000, **97**:4–6.

Emerman, M., and Malim, M.H.: **HIV-1 regulatory/accessory genes: keys to unraveling viral and host cell biology.** *Science* 1998, **280**:1880–1884.

Fujinaga, K., Taube, R., Wimmer, J., Cujec, T.P., and Peterlin, B.M.: **Interactions between human cyclin T, Tat, and the transactivation response element (TAR) are disrupted by a cysteine to tyrosine substitution found in mouse cyclin T.** *Proc. Natl. Acad. Sci. USA* 1999, **96**:1285–1290.

Kinoshita, S., Su, L., Amano, M., Timmerman, L.A., Kaneshima, H., and Nolan, G.P.: **The T cell activation factor NF-ATc positively regulates HIV-1 replication and gene expression in T cells.** *Immunity* 1997, **6**:235–244.

Pollard, V.W., and Malim, M.H.: **The HIV-1 Rev protein.** *Annu. Rev. Microbiol.* 1998, **52**:491–532.

Subbramanian, R.A., and Cohen, E.A.: **Molecular biology of the human immuno-deficiency virus accessory proteins.** *J. Virol.* 1994, **68**:6831–6835.

Trono, D.: **HIV accessory proteins: leading roles for the supporting cast.** *Cell* 1995, **82**:189–192.

11-24 Drugs that block HIV replication lead to a rapid decrease in titer of infectious virus and an increase in CD4 T cells.

Carcelain, G., Debre, P., and Autran, B.: **Reconstitution of CD4+ T lymphocytes in HIV-infected individuals following antiretroviral therapy.** *Curr. Opin. Immunol.* 2001, **13**:483–488.

Ho, D.D.: **Perspectives series: host/pathogen interactions. Dynamics of HIV-1 replication *in vivo*.** *J. Clin. Invest.* 1997, **99**:2565–2567.

Lempicki, R.A., Kovacs, J.A., Baseler, M.W., Adelsberger, J.W., Dewar, R.L., Natarajan, V., Bosche, M.C., Metcalf, J.A., Stevens, R.A., Lambert, L.A., Alvord, W.G., Polis, M.A., Davey, R.T., Dimitrov, D.S., and Lane, H.C.: **Impact of HIV-1 infection and highly active antiretroviral therapy on the kinetics of CD4+ and CD8+ T cell turnover in HIV-infected patients.** *Proc. Natl. Acad. Sci. USA* 2000, **97**:13778–13783.

Lipsky, J.J.: **Antiretroviral drugs for AIDS.** *Lancet* 1996, **348**:800–803.

Smith, K.A.: **To cure chronic HIV infection, a new therapeutic strategy is needed.** *Curr. Opin. Immunol.* 2001, **13**:617–624.

Wei, X., Ghosh, S.K., Taylor, M.E., Johnson, V.A., Emini, E.A., Deutsch, P., Lifson, J.D., Bonhoeffer, S., Nowak, M.A., Hahn, B.H., Saag, M.S., and Shaw, G.M.: **Viral dynamics in human immunodeficiency virus type 1 infection.** *Nature* 1995, **373**:117–122.

11-25 HIV accumulates many mutations in the course of infection in a single individual and drug treatment is soon followed by the outgrowth of drug-resistant variants of the virus.

Bonhoeffer, S., May, R.M., Shaw, G.M., and Nowak, M.A.: **Virus dynamics and drug therapy.** *Proc. Natl. Acad. Sci. USA* 1997, **94**:6971–6976.

Condra, J.H., Schleif, W.A., Blahy, O.M., Gabryelski, L.J., Graham, D.J., Quintero, J.C., Rhodes, A., Robbins, H.L., Roth, E., Shivaprakash, M., Titus, D., Yang, T., Teppler, H., Squires, K.E., Deutsch, P.J., and Emini, E.A.: ***In vivo* emergence of HIV-1 variants resistant to multiple protease inhibitors.** *Nature* 1995, **374**:569–571.

Finzi, D., and Siliciano, R.F.: **Viral dynamics in HIV-1 infection.** *Cell* 1998, **93**:665–671.

Katzenstein, D.: **Combination therapies for HIV infection and genomic drug resistance.** *Lancet* 1997, **350**:970–971.

Moutouh, L., Corbeil, J., and Richman, D.D.: **Recombination leads to the rapid emergence of HIV 1 dually resistant mutants under selective drug pressure.** *Proc. Natl. Acad. Sci. USA* 1996, **93**:6106–6111.

11-26 Lymphoid tissue is the major reservoir of HIV infection.

Burton, G.F., Masuda, A., Heath, S.L., Smith, B.A., Tew, J.G., and Szakal, A.K.: **Follicular dendritic cells (FDC) in retroviral infection: host/pathogen perspectives.** *Immunol. Rev.* 1997, **156**:185–197.

Chun, T.W., Carruth, L., Finzi, D., Shen, X., DiGiuseppe, J.A., Taylor, H., Hermankova, M., Chadwick, K., Margolick, J., Quinn, T.C., Kuo, Y.H., Brookmeyer, R., Zeiger, M.A., Barditch-Crovo, P., and Siliciano, R.F.: **Quantification of latent tissue reservoirs and total body viral load in HIV-1 infection.** *Nature* 1997, **387**:183–188.

Clark, E.A.: **HIV: dendritic cells as embers for the infectious fire.** *Curr. Biol.* 1996, **6**:655–657.

Finzi, D., Blankson, J., Siliciano, J.D., Margolick, J.B., Chadwick, K., Pierson, T., Smith, K., Lisziewicz, J., Lori, F., Flexner, C., Quinn, T.C., Chaisson, R.E., Rosenberg, E., Walker, B., Gange, S., Gallant, J., and Siliciano, R.F.: **Latent infection of CD4+ T cells provides a mechanism for lifelong persistence of HIV-1, even in patients on effective combination therapy.** *Nat. Med.* 1999, **5**:512–517.

Haase, A.T.: **Population biology of HIV-1 infection: viral and CD4+ T cell demographics and dynamics in lymphatic tissues.** *Annu. Rev. Immunol.* 1999, **17**:625–656.

Orenstein, J.M., Fox, C., and Wahl, S.M.: **Macrophages as a source of HIV during opportunistic infections.** *Science* 1997, **276**:1857–1861.

Palella, F.J., Jr., Delaney, K.M., Moorman, A.C., Loveless, M.O., Fuhrer, J., Satten, G.A., Aschman, D.J., and Holmberg, S.D.: **Declining morbidity and mortality among patients with advanced human immunodeficiency virus infection. HIV Outpatient Study Investigators.** *N. Engl. J. Med.* 1998, **338**:853–860.

Pierson, T., McArthur, J., and Siliciano, R.F.: **Reservoirs for HIV-1: mechanisms for viral persistence in the presence of antiviral immune responses and antiretroviral therapy.** *Annu. Rev. Immunol.* 2000, **18**:665–708.

Wong, J.K., Hezareh, M., Gunthard, H.F., Havlir, D.V., Ignacio, C.C., Spina, C.A., and Richman, D.D.: **Recovery of replication-competent HIV despite prolonged suppression of plasma viremia.** *Science* 1997, **278**:1291–1295.

11-27 An immune response controls but does not eliminate HIV.

Barouch, D.H., and Letvin, N.L.: **CD8+ cytotoxic T lymphocyte responses to lentiviruses and herpesviruses.** *Curr. Opin. Immunol.* 2001, **13**:479–482.

Evans, D.T., O'Connor, D.H., Jing, P., Dzuris, J.L., Sidney, J., da Silva, J., Allen, T.M., Horton, H., Venham, J.E., Rudersdorf, R.A., Vogel, T., Pauza, C.D., Bontrop, R.E., DeMars, R., Sette, A., Hughes, A.L., and Watkins, D.I.: **Virus-specific cytotoxic T-lymphocyte responses select for amino-acid variation in simian immunodeficiency virus Env and Nef.** *Nat. Med.* 1999, **5**:1270–1276.

Goulder, P.J., Sewell, A.K., Lalloo, D.G., Price, D.A., Whelan, J.A., Evans, J., Taylor, G.P., Luzzi, G., Giangrande, P., Phillips, R.E., and McMichael, A.J.: **Patterns of immunodominance in HIV-1-specific cytotoxic T lymphocyte responses in two human histocompatibility leukocyte antigens (HLA)-identical siblings with HLA-A*0201 are influenced by epitope mutation.** *J. Exp. Med.* 1997, **185**:1423–1433.

Johnson, W.E., and Desrosiers, R.C.: **Viral persistance: HIV's strategies of immune system evasion.** *Annu. Rev. Med.* 2002, **53**:499–518.

Poignard, P., Sabbe, R., Picchio, G.R., Wang, M., Gulizia, R.J., Katinger, H., Parren, P.W., Mosier, D.E., and Burton, D.R.: **Neutralizing antibodies have limited effects on the control of established HIV-1 infection** *in vivo*. *Immunity* 1999, **10**:431–438.

Price, D.A., Goulder, P.J., Klenerman, P., Sewell, A.K., Easterbrook, P.J., Troop, M., Bangham, C.R., and Phillips, R.E.: **Positive selection of HIV-1 cytotoxic T lymphocyte escape variants during primary infection.** *Proc. Natl. Acad. Sci. USA* 1997, **94**:1890–1895.

Schmitz, J.E., Kuroda, M.J., Santra, S., Sasseville, V.G., Simon, M.A., Lifton, M.A., Racz, P., Tenner-Racz, K., Dalesandro, M., Scallon, B.J., Ghrayeb, J., Forman, M.A., Montefiori, D.C., Rieber, E.P., Letvin, N.L., and Reimann, K.A.: **Control of viremia in simian immunodeficiency virus infection by CD8+ lymphocytes.** *Science* 1999, **283**:857–860.

11-28 HIV infection leads to low levels of CD4 T cells, increased susceptibility to opportunistic infection, and eventually to death.

Badley, A.D., Dockrell, D., Simpson, M., Schut, R., Lynch, D.H., Leibson, P., and Paya, C.V.: **Macrophage-dependent apoptosis of CD4+ T lymphocytes from HIV-infected individuals is mediated by FasL and tumor necrosis factor.** *J. Exp. Med.* 1997, **185**:55–64.

Ho, D.D., Neumann, A.U., Perelson, A.S., Chen, W., Leonard, J.M., and Markowitz, M.: **Rapid turnover of plasma virions and CD4 lymphocytes in HIV-1 infection.** *Nature* 1995, **373**:123–126.

Katlama, C., and Dickinson, G.M.: **Update on opportunistic infections.** *AIDS* 1993, **7 Suppl 1**:S185–S194.

Kedes, D.H., Operskalski, E., Busch, M., Kohn, R., Flood, J., and Ganem, D.R.: **The seroepidemiology of human herpesvirus 8 (Kaposi's sarcoma associated herpesvirus): distribution of infection in KS risk groups and evidence for sexual transmission.** *Nat. Med.* 1996, **2**:918–924.

Kolesnitchenko, V., Wahl, L.M., Tian, H., Sunila, I., Tani, Y., Hartmann, D.P., Cossman, J., Raffeld, M., Orenstein, J., Samelson, L.E., and Cohen, D.I.: **Human immunodeficiency virus 1 envelope-initiated G2-phase programmed cell death.** *Proc. Natl. Acad. Sci. USA* 1995, **92**:11889–11893.

Lauer, G.M., and Walker, B.D.: **Hepatitis C virus infection.** *N. Engl. J. Med.* 2001, **345**:41–52.

Miller, R.: **HIV-associated respiratory diseases.** *Lancet* 1996, **348**:307–312.

Pantaleo, G., and Fauci, A.S.: **Apoptosis in HIV infection.** *Nat. Med.* 1995, **1**:118–120.

Zhong, W.D., Wang, H., Herndier, B., and Ganem, D.R.: **Restricted expression of Kaposi sarcoma associated herpesvirus (human herpesvirus 8) genes in Kaposi sarcoma.** *Proc. Natl. Acad. Sci. USA* 1996, **93**:6641–6646.

11-29 Vaccination against HIV is an attractive solution but poses many difficulties.

Amara, R.R., Villinger, F., Altman, J.D., Lydy, S.L., O'Neil, S.P., Staprans, S.I., Montefiori, D.C., Xu, Y., Herndon, J.G., Wyatt, L.S., Candido, M.A., Kozyr, N.L., Earl, P.L., Smith, J.M., Ma, H.L., Grimm, B.D., Hulsey, M.L., Miller, J., McClure, H.M., McNicholl, J.M., Moss, B., and Robinson, H.L.: **Control of a mucosal challenge and prevention of AIDS by a multiprotein DNA/MVA vaccine.** *Science* 2001, **292**:69–74.

Baba, T.W., Liska, V., Hofmann-Lehmann, R., Vlasak, J., Xu, W., Ayehunie, S., Cavacini, L.A., Posner, M.R., Katinger, H., Stiegler, G., Bernacky, B.J., Rizvi, T.A., Schmidt, R., Hill, L.R., Keeling, M.E., Lu, Y., Wright, J.E., Chou, T.C., and Ruprecht, R.M.: **Human neutralizing monoclonal antibodies of the IgG1 subtype protect against mucosal simian–human immunodeficiency virus infection.** *Nat. Med.* 2000, **6**:200–206.

Barouch, D.H., Kunstman, J., Kuroda, M.J., Schmitz, J.E., Santra, S., Peyerl, F.W., Krivulka, G.R., Beaudry, K., Lifton, M.A., Gorgone, D.A., Montefiori, D.C., Lewis, M.G., Wolinsky, S.M., and Letvin, N.L.: **Eventual AIDS vaccine failure in a rhesus monkey by viral escape from cytotoxic T lymphocytes.** *Nature* 2002, **415**:335–339.

Burton, D.R.: **A vaccine for HIV type 1: the antibody perspective.** *Proc. Natl. Acad. Sci. USA* 1997, **94**:10018–10023.

Kaul, R., Rowland-Jones, S.L., Kimani, J., Dong, T., Yang, H.B., Kiama, P., Rostron, T., Njagi, E., Bwayo, J.J., MacDonald, K.S., McMichael, A.J., and Plummer, F.A.: **Late seroconversion in HIV-resistant Nairobi prostitutes despite pre-existing HIV-specific CD8+ responses.** *J. Clin. Invest.* 2001, **107**:341–349.

Letvin, N.L.: **Strategies for an HIV vaccine.** *J. Clin. Invest.* 2002, **110**:15–20.

Letvin, N.L., Barouch, D.H., and Montefiori, D.C.: **Prospects for vaccine protection against HIV-1 infection and AIDS.** *Annu. Rev. Immunol.* 2002, **20**:73–99.

Letvin, N.L., and Walker, B.D.: **HIV versus the immune system: another apparent victory for the virus.** *J. Clin. Invest.* 2001, **107**:273–275.

MacQueen, K.M., Buchbinder, S., Douglas, J.M., Judson, F.N., McKirnan, D.J., and Bartholow, B.: **The decision to enroll in HIV vaccine efficacy trials: concerns elicited from gay men at increased risk for HIV infection.** *AIDS Res. Hum. Retroviruses* 1994, **10 Suppl 2**:S261–S264.

Mascola, J.R., and Nabel, G.J.: **Vaccines for the prevention of HIV-1 disease.** *Curr. Opin. Immunol.* 2001, **13**:489–495.

Mascola, J.R., Stiegler, G., VanCott, T.C., Katinger, H., Carpenter, C.B., Hanson, C.E., Beary, H., Hayes, D., Frankel, S.S., Birx, D.L., and Lewis, M.G.: **Protection of macaques against vaginal transmission of a pathogenic HIV-1/SIV chimeric virus by passive infusion of neutralizing antibodies.** *Nat. Med.* 2000, **6**:207–210.

Robert-Guroff, M.: **IgG surfaces as an important component in mucosal protection.** *Nat. Med.* 2000, **6**:129–130.

Shiver, J.W., Fu, T.M., Chen, L., Casimiro, D.R., Davies, M.E., Evans, R.K.,

Zhang, Z.Q., Simon, A.J., Trigona, W.L., Dubey, S.A., Huang, L., Harris, V.A., Long, R.S., Liang, X., Handt, L., Schleif, W.A., Zhu, L., Freed, D.C., Persaud, N.V., Guan, L., Punt, K.S., Tang, A., Chen, M., Wilson, K.A., Collins, K.B., Heidecker, G.J., Fernandez, V.R., Perry, H.C., Joyce, J.G., Grimm, K.M., Cook, J.C., Keller, P.M., Kresock, D.S., Mach, H., Troutman, R.D., Isopi, L.A., Williams, D.M., Xu, Z., Bohannon, K.E., Volkin, D.B., Montefiori, D.C., Miura, A., Krivulka, G.R., Lifton, M.A., Kuroda, M.J., Schmitz, J.E., Letvin, N.L., Caulfield, M.J., Bett, A.J., Youil, R., Kaslow, D.C., and Emini, E.A.: **Replication-incompetent adenoviral vaccine vector elicits effective anti-immunodeficiency-virus immunity.** *Nature* 2002, **415**:331–335.

11-30 Prevention and education are one way in which the spread of HIV and AIDS can be controlled.

Coates, T.J., Aggleton, P., Gutzwiller, F., Des-Jarlais, D., Kihara, M., Kippax, S., Schechter, M., and van-den-Hoek, J.A.: **HIV prevention in developed countries.** *Lancet* 1996, **348**:1143–1148.

Decosas, J., Kane, F., Anarfi, J.K., Sodji, K.D., and Wagner, H.U.: **Migration and AIDS.** *Lancet* 1995, **346**:826–828.

Dowsett, G.W.: **Sustaining safe sex: sexual practices, HIV and social context.** *AIDS* 1993, **7 Suppl. 1**:S257–S262.

Kimball, A.M., Berkley, S., Ngugi, E., and Gayle, H.: **International aspects of the AIDS/HIV epidemic.** *Annu. Rev. Public. Health* 1995, **16**:253–282.

Kirby, M.: **Human rights and the HIV paradox.** *Lancet* 1996, **348**:1217–1218.

Nelson, K.E., Celentano, D.D., Eiumtrakol, S., Hoover, D.R., Beyrer, C., Suprasert, S., Kuntolbutra, S., and Khamboonruang, C.: **Changes in sexual behavior and a decline in HIV infection among young men in Thailand.** *N. Engl. J. Med.* 1996, **335**:297–303.

Weniger, B.G., and Brown, T.: **The march of AIDS through Asia.** *N. Engl. J. Med.* 1996, **335**:343–345.

Allergy and Hypersensitivity

Allergic reactions occur when an individual who has produced IgE antibody in response to an innocuous antigen, or **allergen**, subsequently encounters the same allergen. The allergen triggers the activation of IgE-binding cells, including mast cells and basophils, in the exposed tissue, leading to a series of responses that are characteristic of **allergy**. As we learned in Chapter 9, IgE is involved in protective immunity, especially in response to parasitic worms, which are prevalent in less economically developed countries. However, in the industrialized countries IgE responses to innocuous antigens predominate, and allergy is an important cause of disease (Fig. 12.1). Almost half the populations of North America and Europe have allergies to one or more common environmental antigens and, although rarely life-threatening, these cause much distress and lost time from school and work. Because of the medical importance of allergy in industrialized societies, much more is known about the pathophysiology of IgE-mediated responses than about the normal physiological role of IgE.

IgE-mediated allergic reactions			
Syndrome	**Common allergens**	**Route of entry**	**Response**
Systemic anaphylaxis	Drugs Serum Venoms Peanuts	Intravenous (either directly or following oral absorption into the blood)	Edema Increased vascular permeability Tracheal occlusion Circulatory collapse Death
Acute urticaria (wheal-and-flare)	Animal hair Insect bites Allergy testing	Through skin	Local increase in blood flow and vascular permeability
Allergic rhinitis (hay fever)	Pollens (ragweed, timothy, birch) Dust-mite feces	Inhalation	Edema of nasal mucosa Irritation of nasal mucosa
Asthma	Danders (cat) Pollens Dust-mite feces	Inhalation	Bronchial constriction Increased mucus production Airway inflammation
Food allergy	Tree nuts Peanuts Shellfish Milk Eggs Fish	Oral	Vomiting Diarrhea Pruritis (itching) Urticaria (hives) Anaphylaxis (rarely)

Fig. 12.1 IgE-mediated reactions to extrinsic antigens. All IgE-mediated responses involve mast-cell degranulation, but the symptoms experienced by the patient can be very different depending on whether the allergen is injected, inhaled, or eaten, and depending also on the dose of the allergen.

	Type I	Type II		Type III	Type IV		
Immune reactant	IgE	IgG		IgG	T_H1 cells	T_H2 cells	CTL
Antigen	Soluble antigen	Cell- or matrix-associated antigen	Cell-surface receptor	Soluble antigen	Soluble antigen	Soluble antigen	Cell-associated antigen
Effector mechanism	Mast-cell activation	Complement, FcR⁺ cells (phagocytes, NK cells)	Antibody alters signaling	Complement, Phagocytes	Macrophage activation	IgE production, Eosinophil activation, Mastocytosis	Cytotoxicity
Example of hypersensitivity reaction	Allergic rhinitis, asthma, systemic anaphylaxis	Some drug allergies (eg, penicillin)	Chronic urticaria (antibody against FCεR1α)	Serum sickness, Arthus reaction	Contact dermatitis, tuberculin reaction	Chronic asthma, chronic allergic rhinitis	Contact dermatitis

Fig. 12.2 There are four types of hypersensitivity reaction mediated by immunological mechanisms that cause tissue damage. Types I–III are antibody-mediated and are distinguished by the different types of antigens recognized and the different classes of antibody involved. Type I responses are mediated by IgE, which induces mast-cell activation, whereas types II and III are mediated by IgG, which can engage complement-mediated and phagocytic effector mechanisms to varying degrees, depending on the subclass of IgG and the nature of the antigen involved. Type II responses are directed against cell-surface or matrix antigens, whereas type III responses are directed against soluble antigens, and the tissue damage involved is caused by responses triggered by immune complexes. A special category of type II responses involves IgG antibodies against cell-surface receptors that disrupt the normal functions of the receptor, either by causing uncontrollable activation or by blocking receptor function. Type IV hypersensitivity reactions are T-cell mediated and can be subdivided into three groups. In the first group, tissue damage is caused by the activation of macrophages by T_H1 cells, which results in an inflammatory response. In the second, damage is caused by the activation by T_H2 cells of inflammatory responses in which eosinophils predominate; in the third, damage is caused directly by cytotoxic T cells (CTL).

The term allergy was originally defined by Clemens Von Pirquet as "an altered capacity of the body to react to a foreign substance," which was an extremely broad definition that included all immunological reactions. Allergy is now defined in a much more restricted manner as "disease following a response by the immune system to an otherwise innocuous antigen." Allergy is one of a class of immune system responses that are termed **hypersensitivity reactions**. These are harmful immune responses that produce tissue injury and can cause serious disease. Hypersensitivity reactions were classified into four types by Coombs and Gell (Fig. 12.2). Allergy is often equated with type I hypersensitivity (immediate-type hypersensitivity reactions mediated by IgE), and will be used in this sense here.

In this chapter we consider first the mechanisms that favor the production of IgE. We then describe the pathophysiological consequences of the interaction between antigen and IgE that is bound by the high-affinity Fcε receptor (FcεRI) on mast cells. Finally, we consider the causes and consequences of other types of immunological hypersensitivity reaction.

Sensitization and the production of IgE.

IgE is produced by plasma cells located in lymph nodes draining the site of antigen entry and also locally, at the sites of allergic reactions, by plasma cells derived from germinal centers developing within the inflamed tissue. IgE differs from other antibody isotypes in being predominantly localized in tissues, where it is tightly bound to mast-cell surfaces through the high-affinity IgE receptor known as **FcεRI**. Binding of antigen to IgE cross-links these receptors and this causes the release of chemical mediators from the mast cells, which can lead to the development of a **type I hypersensitivity reaction**. Basophils also express FcεRI; they can therefore display surface-bound IgE and also take part in the production of type I hypersensitivity reactions. The factors that lead to an antibody response dominated by IgE are still being worked out. Here we describe our current understanding of these processes before turning to the question of how IgE mediates allergic reactions.

12-1   Allergens are often delivered transmucosally at low dose, a route that favors IgE production.

Certain antigens and routes of antigen presentation to the immune system favor the production of IgE. CD4 T_H2 cells can switch the antibody isotype from IgM to IgE, or they can cause switching to IgG2 and IgG4 (human) or IgG1 and IgG3 (mouse) (see Section 9-4). Antigens that selectively evoke T_H2 cells that drive an IgE response are known as allergens.

Much human allergy is caused by a limited number of inhaled small-protein allergens that reproducibly elicit IgE production in susceptible individuals. We inhale many different proteins that do not induce IgE production; this raises the question of what is unusual about the proteins that are common allergens. Although we do not yet have a complete answer, some general principles have emerged (Fig. 12.3). Most allergens are relatively small, highly soluble proteins that are carried on dry particles such as pollen grains or mite feces. On contact with the mucosa of the airways, for example, the soluble allergen elutes from the particle and diffuses into the mucosa. Allergens are typically presented to the immune system at very low doses. It has been estimated that the maximum exposure of a person to the common pollen allergens in ragweed (*Artemisia artemisiifolia*) does not exceed 1 μg per year! Yet many people develop irritating and even life-threatening T_H2-driven IgE antibody responses to these minute doses of allergen. It should be emphasized, however, that only some of the people who are exposed to these substances make IgE antibodies against them.

It seems likely that presenting an antigen transmucosally and at very low doses is a particularly efficient way of inducing T_H2-driven IgE responses. IgE antibody production requires T_H2 cells that produce interleukin-4 (IL-4) and IL-13, and it can be inhibited by T_H1 cells that produce interferon-γ (IFN-γ) (see Fig. 9.7). The presentation of low doses of antigen can favor the activation of T_H2 cells over T_H1 cells (see Section 10-7), and many common allergens are delivered to the respiratory mucosa by the inhalation of a low dose. In the respiratory mucosa these allergens encounter dendritic cells that take up and process protein antigens very efficiently and become activated in the process. These activated cells migrate to regional lymph nodes and differentiate into professional antigen-presenting cells with co-stimulatory activity that favors the differentiation of T_H2 cells. We consider the role of dendritic cells in the stimulation of T_H2 responses in Section 12-3.

Features of inhaled allergens that may promote the priming of T_H2 cells that drive IgE responses	
Protein	Only proteins induce T-cell responses
Enzymatically active	Allergens are often proteases
Low dose	Favors activation of IL-4-producing CD4 T cells
Low molecular weight	Allergen can diffuse out of particle into mucus
Highly soluble	Allergen can be readily eluted from particle
Stable	Allergen can survive in desiccated particle
Contains peptides that bind host MHC class II	Required for T-cell priming

Fig. 12.3 Properties of inhaled allergens. The typical characteristics of inhaled allergens are described in this table.

Fig. 12.4 Scanning electron micrograph of *D. pteronyssimus* with some of its fecal pellets. Photograph courtesy of E.R. Tovey.

12-2   Enzymes are frequent triggers of allergy.

Several lines of evidence suggest that IgE is important in host defense against parasitic worms (see Section 9-23). Many of these invade their hosts by secreting proteolytic enzymes that break down connective tissue and allow the parasite access to host tissues, and it has been proposed that these enzymes are particularly active at promoting T_H2 responses. This idea receives some support from the many examples of allergens that are enzymes. The major allergen in the feces of the house dust mite (*Dermatophagoides pteronyssimus*) (Fig. 12.4), which is responsible for allergy in about 20% of the North American population, is a cysteine protease known as Der p 1. This enzyme has been found to cleave occludin, a protein component of intercellular tight junctions. This reveals one possible reason for the allergenicity of certain enzymes. By destroying the integrity of the tight junctions between epithelial cells, Der p 1 may gain abnormal access to subepithelial antigen-presenting cells, resident mast cells, and eosinophils (Fig. 12.5).

The cysteine protease papain, derived from the papaya fruit, is used as a meat tenderizer and causes allergy in workers preparing the enzyme; such allergies are called **occupational allergies**. Another occupational allergy is the asthma caused by inhalation of the bacterial enzyme subtilisin, the 'biological' component of some laundry detergents. Injection of enzymatically active papain (but not of inactivated papain) into mice stimulates an IgE response. A closely related enzyme, chymopapain, is used medically to destroy intervertebral discs in patients with sciatica; the major (although rare) complication of this procedure is anaphylaxis, an acute systemic response to allergens (see Fig. 12.1).

Not all allergens are enzymes, however; for example, two allergens identified from filarial worms are enzyme inhibitors. Many protein allergens derived from plants have been identified and sequenced, but their functions are currently obscure. Thus, there seems to be no systematic association between enzymatic activity and allergenicity.

Fig. 12.5 The enzymatic activity of some allergens enables the penetration of epithelial barriers. The epithelial barrier of the airways is formed by tight junctions between the epithelial cells. Fecal pellets from the house dust mite, *Dermatophagoides pteronyssimus*, contain a proteolytic enzyme, Der p 1, that acts as an allergen. It cleaves occludin, a protein that helps to maintain the tight junctions, and thus destroys the barrier function of the epithelium. Fecal antigens can then pass through and be taken up by dendritic cells in subepithelial tissue. Der p 1 is taken up by dendritic cells, which are activated and move to lymph nodes (not shown), where they act as antigen-presenting cells, inducing the production of T_H2 cells specific for Der p 1 and the production of Der p 1-specific IgE. Der p 1 can then bind directly to specific IgE on the resident mast cells, triggering mast-cell activation.

Knowledge of the identity of allergenic proteins can be important to public health and can have economic significance, as illustrated by the following cautionary tale. Some years ago, the gene for a protein from brazil nuts that encodes a protein rich in methionine and cysteine was transferred by genetic engineering into soy beans intended for animal feed. This was done to improve the nutritional value of soy beans, which are intrinsically poor in these sulfur-containing amino acids. This experiment led to the discovery that the protein, 2S albumin, was the major brazil nut allergen. Injection of extracts of the genetically modified soy beans into the epidermis triggered an allergic skin response in people with an allergy to brazil nuts. As there could be no guarantee that the modified soy beans could be kept out of the human food chain if they were produced on a large scale, development of this genetically modified food was abandoned.

12-3 Class switching to IgE in B lymphocytes is favored by specific signals.

There are two main components of the immune response leading to IgE production. The first consists of the signals that favor the differentiation of naive T_H0 cells to a T_H2 phenotype. The second comprises the action of cytokines and co-stimulatory signals from T_H2 cells that stimulate B cells to switch to producing IgE antibodies.

The fate of a naive CD4 T cell responding to a peptide presented by a dendritic cell is determined by the cytokines it is exposed to before and during this response, and by the intrinsic properties of the antigen, the antigen dose, and the route of presentation. Exposure to IL-4, IL-5, IL-9, IL-10, and IL-13 favors the development of T_H2 cells, whereas IL-12 and IFN-γ favor T_H1 cell development. IgE antibodies are important in host defense against infection with multicellular parasites. This defense system is anatomically distributed mainly at the sites of entry of such parasites—under the skin, under the epithelial surfaces of the airways (the mucosal-associated lymphoid tissues), and in the submucosa of the gut (the gut-associated lymphoid tissues). Cells of the innate and adaptive immune systems at these sites are specialized to secrete predominantly cytokines that drive T_H2 responses. The dendritic cells at these sites take up antigen and migrate to regional lymph nodes, where their interaction with naive CD4 T cells drives the T cells to become effector T_H2 cells, which themselves secrete T_H2 cytokines that maintain the cytokine environment in which T_H2 cell differentiation is favored.

It is not fully understood how dendritic cells induce this differentiation. It is clear that the environment in which antigen presentation occurs is crucial in influencing the direction of T_H cell development, with chemokines and cytokines having a central and essential role. For example, chemokines CCL2 (MCP-1), CCL7 (MCP-3), and CCL13 (MCP-4) act on monocytes, via their receptor CCR2, to suppress the production of IL-12 by activated monocytes. They thereby promote T_H2 responses. In general, however, it seems that the default interaction between dendritic cells and naive T cells, that is, in the absence of inflammatory stimuli such as might be induced in the presence of infection, directs the polarization of T-cell differentiation toward T_H2 cells. By contrast, if antigen is encountered by dendritic cells in the context of proinflammatory signals, then the dendritic cells are stimulated to produce IL-12, which polarizes the T-cell response to produce T_H1 cells.

T_H2 cells produce a characteristic coordinated array of cytokines and chemokines that maintain and amplify the polarization of the response and stimulate class switching of B cells to IgE production. The cytokines include IL-4, IL-5, IL-9, IL-10, and IL-13. Cytokines IL-4 and IL-13 activate the Janus-family tyrosine kinases Jak1 and Jak3 (see Section 6-19), which ultimately leads to phosphorylation of the transcriptional regulator Stat6 present in

T and B lymphocytes. Mice lacking functional IL-4, IL-13, or Stat6 have impaired T_H2 responses and impaired IgE switching (Fig. 12.6), demonstrating the key importance of these cytokines and their signaling pathways.

IL-4 or IL-13 provides the first signal that switches B cells to IgE production. The second signal is a co-stimulatory interaction between CD40 ligand on the T-cell surface and CD40 on the B-cell surface. This interaction is essential for all antibody class switching (see Section 9-4); patients with the X-linked hyper IgM syndrome have a deficiency of CD40 ligand and produce no IgG, IgA, or IgE.

The IgE response, once initiated, can be amplified by mast cells and basophils, which also drive IgE production (Fig. 12.7). These cells express FcεRI, and when they are activated by antigen cross-linking of their FcεRI-bound IgE they express cell-surface CD40 ligand and secrete IL-4. Like T_H2 cells, therefore, they can drive class switching and IgE production by B cells. The interaction between these specialized granulocytes and B cells can occur at the site of the allergic reaction, because B cells are observed to form germinal centers at inflammatory foci. Blocking this amplification process is a goal of therapy, because allergic reactions can otherwise become self sustaining.

Fig. 12.6 Signaling through the Stat6 pathway is necessary for the development of T_H2 responses. The gene regulatory protein Stat6 is activated in response to IL-4 and IL-13. The key role of this signaling molecule in the development of T_H2 responses is shown by the consequences of Stat6 deficiency. Mice were made deficient in Stat6 by gene targeting. The right-hand panels show the effects of this deficiency; the left-hand panels show the responses of normal mice. The top panels show the levels of different cytokines from T cells grown in the presence of IL-4. This should drive the production of T_H2 cells, but the T cells from mice lacking Stat6 produced high levels of IFN-γ and failed to produce the T_H2 cytokines IL-4, IL-5, and IL-10. The center panels show the frequency of antibody-producing cells of different isotypes produced from lymph node cells stimulated *in vitro* with anti-IgD. Stat6-deficient mice had no IgE-producing cells and had increased numbers of cells producing IgG2a and IgG2b antibodies. This shows that Stat6 is essential for IgE formation and has a negative effect on switching to IgG2a, IgG2b, and IgG3 (not shown). The bottom panels show the effect of Stat6 deficiency on expulsion from the intestine of the parasitic nematode *Nippostrongylus brasiliensis*. Mice lacking Stat6 were unable to develop a normal T_H2 response and expel the worms.

Fig. 12.7 Antigen binding to IgE on mast cells leads to amplification of IgE production. IgE secreted by plasma cells binds to the high-affinity IgE receptor on mast cells (illustrated here) and basophils. When the surface-bound IgE is cross-linked by antigen, these cells express CD40L and secrete IL-4, which in turn binds to IL-4 receptors (IL-4R) on the activated B cell, stimulating isotype switching by B cells and the production of more IgE. These interactions can occur in vivo at the site of allergen-triggered inflammation, for example in bronchial-associated lymphoid tissue.

12-4 Both genetic and environmental factors contribute to the development of IgE-mediated allergy.

As many as 40% of people in Western populations show an exaggerated tendency to mount IgE responses to a wide variety of common environmental allergens. This state is called atopy, has a strong familial basis, and is influenced by several genetic loci. Atopic individuals have higher total levels of IgE in the circulation and higher levels of eosinophils than their normal counterparts. They are more susceptible to allergic diseases such as hay fever and asthma. Studies of atopic families have identified regions on chromosomes 11q and 5q that seem to be important in determining atopy; candidate genes that could affect IgE responses are present in these regions.

The candidate gene on chromosome 11 encodes the β subunit of the high-affinity IgE receptor. On chromosome 5 the situation is more complicated, because genetic studies indicate that the region associated with disease, 5q23–25, contains a plethora of possible candidate genes for increased susceptibility. First, there is a cluster of tightly linked genes for cytokines that promote T_H2 responses by enhancing IgE isotype switching, eosinophil survival, and mast-cell proliferation. This cluster includes the genes for IL-3, IL-4, IL-5, IL-9, IL-13, and granulocyte–macrophage colony-stimulating factor (GM-CSF). Genetic variation in the promoter region of the IL-4 gene has been associated with raised IgE levels in atopic individuals; the variant promoter directs increased expression of a reporter gene in experimental systems. Atopy has also been associated with a gain-of-function mutation of the α subunit of the IL-4 receptor, which causes increased signaling after ligation of the receptor.

A second set of genes on chromosome 5 that are possibly involved in susceptibility to allergy is the TIM family (for T cell, immunoglobulin domain and mucin domain), which encode T-cell surface proteins. Inherited variation in the TIM genes has been correlated with the degree of airway hyper-reactivity and with the production of IL-4 and IL-13 by T cells in mouse strains with varying susceptibility to allergic inflammation of the airways. The third candidate susceptibility gene on chromosome 5 is the gene encoding p40, one of the two subunits of IL-12. This cytokine promotes T_H1 responses, and genetic variation in IL-12 p40 expression that could cause reduced IL-12 production was found to be associated with more severe asthma. Fourth, the β-adrenergic receptor is encoded in this region, and variation in this receptor might be associated with variation in smooth muscle responsiveness to endogenous and pharmacological ligands.

Allergic Asthma

This complexity illustrates a common challenge in identifying the genetic basis of complex disease traits. Relatively small regions of the genome, identified as containing genes for altered disease susceptibility, may contain many good candidates, judged by what is known of their physiological activities. Identifying the correct gene, or genes, may require studies of several very large populations of patients and controls. For chromosome 5q23–25 it is too early to know how important each of these different polymorphisms is in the complex genetics of atopy.

A second type of inherited variation in IgE responses is linked to the MHC class II region and affects responses to specific allergens. Many studies have shown that IgE production in response to particular allergens is associated with certain HLA class II alleles, implying that particular MHC:peptide combinations might favor a strong T_H2 response. For example, IgE responses to several ragweed pollen allergens are associated with haplotypes containing the MHC class II allele *DRB1*1501*. Many people are therefore generally predisposed to make T_H2 responses and are specifically predisposed to respond to some allergens more than others. However, allergies to common drugs such as penicillin show no association with MHC class II or the presence or absence of atopy.

There is evidence that a state of atopy, and the associated susceptibility to asthma, hay fever (rhinitis), and eczema, can be determined by different genes in different populations. Genetic associations found in one group of patients have frequently not been confirmed in patients of a different ethnic origin. There are also likely to be genes that affect only particular aspects of allergic disease. In asthma, for example, there is evidence that different genes affect at least three aspects of the disease—IgE production, the inflammatory response, and clinical responses to particular treatments. Polymorphism of the gene encoding ADAM33, a metalloproteinase expressed by bronchial smooth muscle cells and lung fibroblasts, has been associated with asthma and bronchial hyperreactivity. This is likely to be an example of genetic variation in the pulmonary inflammatory response and the pathological anatomical changes that occur in the airways, leading to increased susceptibility to asthma. Some of the best-characterized genetic polymorphisms of candidate genes associated with asthma are shown in Fig. 12.8, together with possible ways in which the genetic variation might affect the type of disease that develops and its response to drugs.

The prevalence of atopic allergy, and of asthma in particular, is increasing in economically advanced regions of the world, an observation that is best explained by environmental factors. The four main candidate environmental factors are changes in exposure to infectious diseases in early childhood, environmental pollution, allergen levels, and dietary changes. Of these, alterations in exposure to microbial pathogens is the most plausible explanation at present for the increase in atopic allergy. This is known as the 'hygiene hypothesis'. The proposition is that less hygienic environments, specifically environments that predispose to infections early in childhood, help to protect against atopy and asthma (Fig. 12.9). This implies that T_H2 responses predominate over T_H1 responses by default in early childhood, and that the immune system is reprogrammed toward more T_H1-dominated responses by the cytokine response to early infections.

There is much evidence in support of this hypothesis, but also some observations that are difficult to reconcile with it. In favor, there is evidence for a bias toward T_H2 responses in neonates, in whom dendritic cells produce less IL-12 and T cells produce less IFN-γ than in older children and adults. There is also evidence that exposure to childhood infections, with the important exception of some respiratory infections that we consider below, helps to protect against the development of atopic allergic disease. Thus, younger

Gene	Nature of polymorphism	Possible mechanism of association
IL-4	Promoter variant	Variation in expression of IL-4
IL-4 receptor α chain	Structural variant	Increased signaling in response to IL-4
High-affinity IgE receptor β chain	Structural variant	Variation in consequences of IgE ligation by antigen
MHC class II genes	Structural variants	Enhanced presentation of particular allergen-derived peptides
T-cell receptor α locus	Microsatellite markers	Enhanced T-cell recognition of certain allergen-derived peptides
ADAM 33	Structural variants	Variation in airway remodeling
β₂-Adrenergic receptor	Structural variants	Increased bronchial hyperreactivity*
5-Lipoxygenase	Promoter variant	Variation in leukotriene production†

Fig. 12.8 Candidate susceptibility genes for asthma. *May also affect response to bronchodilator therapy with β₂-adrenergic agonists. †Patients with alleles associated with reduced enzyme production failed to show a beneficial response to a drug inhibitor of 5-lipoxygenase. This is an example of a pharmacogenetic effect, in which genetic variation affects the response to medication.

children from families with three or more older siblings, and children aged less than 6 months who are exposed to other children in daycare facilities, each linked to a greater exposure to infections, are somewhat protected against atopy and asthma. Furthermore, early colonization of the gut by commensal bacteria such as lactobacilli and bifidobacteria, or infection by gut pathogens such as *Toxoplasma gondii* (which stimulates a T$_H$1 response) or *Helicobacter pylori*, are associated with a reduced prevalence of allergic disease.

A history of infection with measles or hepatitis A virus, or positive tuberculin skin tests (suggesting previous exposure and an immune response to *Mycobacterium tuberculosis*), also seem to protect against atopy. The human counterpart of the murine *TIM1* gene, which might be important in determining airway hypersensitivity and the production of IL-4 and IL-13 by T cells in mice, is the cellular receptor for hepatitis A virus (hHAVcr-1). The infection of T cells by hepatitis A virus could directly influence their differentiation and cytokine production, limiting the development of T$_H$2 responses.

In contrast to these negative associations between childhood infection and the development of atopy and asthma, there is evidence that children who have had attacks of bronchiolitis associated with respiratory syncytial virus (RSV) infection are more prone to the later development of asthma. This effect of RSV may depend on the age at first infection; infection of neonatal

Fig. 12.9 Genes, the environment, and atopic allergic diseases. Both inherited and environmental factors are important determinants of the likelihood of developing atopic allergic disease. The genes that influence the development of atopic allergic disease are shown in Fig. 12.8. The postulate of the 'hygiene hypothesis' is that exposure to some infectious agents in childhood drives the immune system toward a general state of T$_H$1 responsiveness and nonatopy. In contrast, children with genetic susceptibility to atopic allergic disease who live in an environment with low exposure to infectious disease tend to mount T$_H$2 responses, which naturally predominate in the neonatal period of life. It is these children who are thought to be most susceptible to the development of atopic allergic disease.

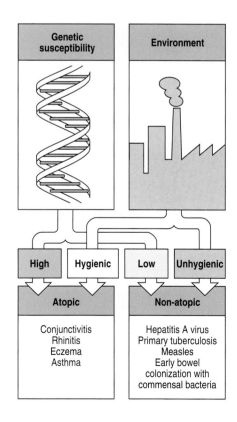

mice with RSV was followed by a decreased IFN-γ response compared with mice challenged at 4 or 8 weeks of age. When these mice were rechallenged at 12 weeks of age with RSV infection, those mice that had been primarily infected as neonates suffered from more severe lung inflammation than mice with primary infection at 4 or 8 weeks of age (Fig. 12.10). Similarly, children hospitalized with RSV infection have a skewed ratio of cytokine production away from IFN-γ toward IL-4, the cytokine that induces T$_H$2 responses. All these findings suggest that an infection that evokes a T$_H$1 immune response early in life might reduce the likelihood of T$_H$2 responses later in life, and vice versa.

It might also be expected that exposure to environmental pollution would worsen the incidence of atopy and asthma. The best evidence shows the opposite, however. Allergic asthma was less prevalent in children from the city of Halle in the former East Germany, which has severe air pollution, than in an ethnically matched population from Munich, exposed to much cleaner air. This does not mean that polluted air is not bad for the lungs. The children from Halle had a higher overall prevalence of respiratory disease than their Munich counterparts, but this was predominantly not allergic in origin.

The biggest 'fly in the ointment' for the hygiene theory, however, is the strong inverse correlation between infection by helminths (such as hookworm and schistosomes) and the development of allergy. Because helminth infections are strong drivers of T$_H$2 responses, an inverse correlation with atopy is very difficult to reconcile with the idea that the polarization of T-cell responses toward T$_H$1 is a general mechanism for the protective effect of infection against the development of atopy. A study in Venezuela showed that children treated for a prolonged period with antihelminthic agents had a higher prevalence of atopy compared with untreated and heavily parasitized children.

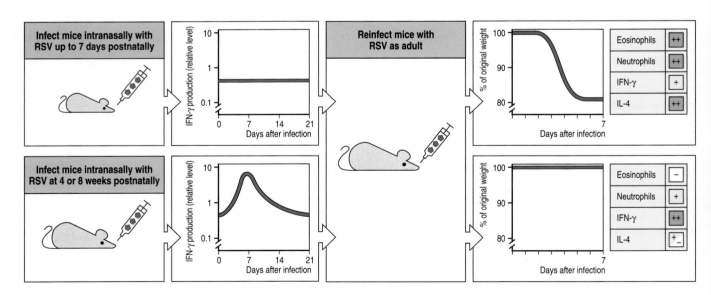

Fig. 12.10 Response to infection and rechallenge of mice with respiratory syncytial virus (RSV) according to the age of primary infection. Mice respond to infection with RSV in different ways according to the age of primary infection. The left-hand panels show the IFN-γ response after either neonatal infection (upper panels) or infection at 4 or 8 weeks of age (lower panels). Mice infected neonatally fail to produce IFN-γ. The right-hand panels show the consequences of reinfection of the two cohorts of mice when adult. The mice that had had the primary infection as neonates show weight loss and a severe inflammatory response to reinfection, with infiltration of the lungs by eosinophils and neutrophils, accompanied by production of the T$_H$2 cytokine IL-4. In contrast, mice that had had the primary infection at 4 or 8 weeks of age show no weight loss, mild neutrophil infiltration, and production of the T$_H$1 cytokine IFN-γ.

These observations have led to a modification of the hygiene hypothesis. This proposes that all types of infection might protect against the development of atopy by driving the production of regulatory cytokines such as IL-10 and TGF-β, which downregulate both T_H1 and T_H2 responses. In hygienic environments, children suffer fewer infections, resulting in a reduced production of these cytokines. As we will learn in Chapter 13, there has also been an increase in autoimmune diseases such as diabetes and systemic lupus erythematosus in the economically advanced parts of the world. This increase could also be explained by the loss of the counter-regulation of immunological responses as a result of a reduced burden of early childhood infection.

Although it is clear that allergy is related to allergen exposure, there is no evidence that the rising prevalence of allergy is due to any systematic change in allergen exposure. Nor is there any evidence that changes in diet can explain the increase in allergy in economically advanced populations.

Summary.

Allergic reactions are the result of the production of specific IgE antibody against common, innocuous antigens. Allergens are small antigens that commonly provoke an IgE antibody response. Such antigens normally enter the body at very low doses by diffusion across mucosal surfaces and therefore trigger a T_H2 response. The differentiation of naive allergen-specific T cells into T_H2 cells is also favored by the presence of an early burst of IL-4. Allergen-specific T_H2 cells produce IL-4 and IL-13, which drive allergen-specific B cells to produce IgE. The specific IgE produced in response to the allergen binds to the high-affinity receptor for IgE on mast cells, basophils, and activated eosinophils. IgE production can be amplified by these cells because, upon activation, they produce IL-4 and CD40 ligand. The tendency to IgE overproduction is influenced by genetic and environmental factors. Once IgE is produced in response to an allergen, reexposure to the allergen triggers an allergic response. We describe the mechanism and pathology of allergic responses in the next part of the chapter.

Effector mechanisms in allergic reactions.

Allergic reactions are triggered when allergens cross-link preformed IgE bound to the high-affinity receptor FcεRI on mast cells. Mast cells line the body surfaces and serve to alert the immune system to local infection. Once activated, they induce inflammatory reactions by secreting chemical mediators stored in preformed granules and by synthesizing prostaglandins, leukotrienes, and cytokines after activation occurs. In allergy, they provoke very unpleasant reactions to innocuous antigens that are not associated with invading pathogens that need to be expelled. The consequences of IgE-mediated mast-cell activation depend on the dose of antigen and its route of entry; symptoms range from the irritating sniffles of hay fever when pollen is inhaled to the life-threatening circulatory collapse that occurs in systemic anaphylaxis (Fig. 12.11). The immediate allergic reaction caused by mast-cell degranulation is followed by a more sustained inflammation, known as the late-phase response. This late response involves the recruitment of other effector cells, notably T_H2 lymphocytes, eosinophils, and basophils, which contribute significantly to the immunopathology of an allergic response.

Fig. 12.11 Mast-cell activation has different effects on different tissues.

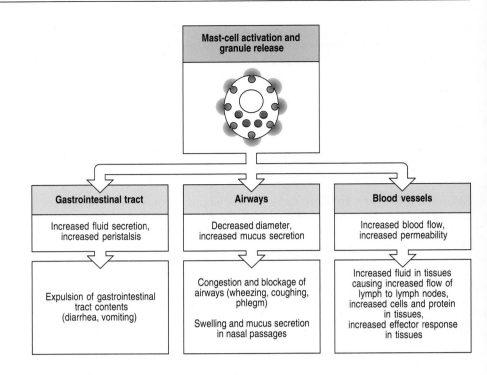

12-5 Most IgE is cell-bound and engages effector mechanisms of the immune system by different pathways from other antibody isotypes.

Most antibodies are found in body fluids and engage effector cells, through receptors specific for the Fc constant regions, only after the antibody variable region has bound specific antigen. IgE is an exception, however, as it is captured by the high-affinity Fcε receptor in the absence of bound antigen. This means that IgE is mostly found fixed in the tissues on mast cells that bear this receptor, as well as on circulating basophils and activated eosinophils. The ligation of cell-bound IgE antibody by specific antigen triggers the activation of these cells at the site of antigen entry into the tissues. The release of inflammatory lipid mediators, cytokines, and chemokines at sites of IgE-triggered reactions recruits eosinophils and basophils to augment the type I response. It also recruits other effector cells, including T lymphocytes that can mediate a local type IV response.

There are two types of IgE-binding Fc receptor. The first, FcεRI, is a high-affinity receptor of the immunoglobulin superfamily that binds IgE on mast cells, basophils, and activated eosinophils (see Section 9-22). When the cell-bound IgE is cross-linked by specific antigen, FcεRI transduces an activating signal. High levels of IgE, such as those that exist in people with allergic diseases or parasite infections, can result in a marked increase in FcεRI on the surface of mast cells, enhanced sensitivity of such cells to activation by low concentrations of specific antigen, and markedly increased IgE-dependent release of chemical mediators and cytokines.

The second IgE receptor, FcεRII, usually known as **CD23**, is a C-type lectin and is structurally unrelated to FcεRI; it binds IgE with low affinity. CD23 is present on many different cell types, including B cells, activated T cells, monocytes, eosinophils, platelets, follicular dendritic cells, and some thymic epithelial cells. This receptor was thought to be crucial for the regulation of IgE levels, but mouse strains in which the CD23 gene has been inactivated still develop relatively normal polyclonal IgE responses. CD23 is, however, involved in enhancing the IgE antibody response against specific antigen in the presence of the same antigen complexed with IgE, because this enhancement fails to occur in mice that lack the CD23 gene. This shows that CD23 on antigen-presenting cells has a role in the capture of antigen by specific IgE.

12-6 Mast cells reside in tissues and orchestrate allergic reactions.

Mast cells were described by Ehrlich in the mesentery of rabbits and named *Mastzellen* ('fattened cells'). Like basophils, mast cells contain granules rich in acidic proteoglycans that take up basic dyes. However, in spite of this resemblance, and the similar range of mediators stored in these basophilic granules, mast cells are derived from a myeloid lineage other than the one that gives rise to basophils and eosinophils. Mast cells are highly specialized and are prominent residents of mucosal and epithelial tissues in the vicinity of small blood vessels and postcapillary venules, where they are well placed to guard against invading pathogens (see Section 9-22). Mast cells are also found in subendothelial connective tissue. They normally home to tissues as agranular or poorly granular cells; their final differentiation, accompanied by granule formation and maturation, occurs after they have arrived in the tissues. The major growth factor for mast cells is stem-cell factor (SCF), which acts on the cell-surface receptor c-Kit (see Section 7-2). Mice with defective c-Kit lack differentiated mast cells and, although they produce IgE, cannot make IgE-mediated inflammatory responses. This shows that such responses depend almost exclusively on mast cells.

Mast cells express FcεRI constitutively on their surface and are activated when antigens cross-link IgE bound to these receptors (see Fig. 9.35). Degranulation begins within seconds, releasing a variety of preformed inflammatory mediators (Fig. 12.12). Among these are **histamine**—a short-lived vasoactive amine

Class of product	Examples	Biological effects
Enzyme	Tryptase, chymase, cathepsin G, carboxypeptidase	Remodel connective tissue matrix
Toxic mediator	Histamine, heparin	Toxic to parasites Increase vascular permeability Cause smooth muscle contraction
Cytokine	IL-4, IL-13	Stimulate and amplify T_H2 cell response
	IL-3, IL-5, GM-CSF	Promote eosinophil production and activation
	TNF-α (some stored preformed in granules)	Promotes inflammation, stimulates cytokine production by many cell types, activates endothelium
Chemokine	CCL3 (MIP-1α)	Attracts monocytes, macrophages, and neutrophils
Lipid mediator	Leukotrienes C4, D4, E4	Cause smooth muscle contraction Increase vascular permeability Stimulate mucus secretion
	Platelet-activating factor	Attracts leukocytes Amplifies production of lipid mediators Activates neutrophils, eosinophils, and platelets

Fig. 12.12 Molecules released by mast cells on activation. Mast cells produce a wide variety of biologically active proteins and other chemical mediators. The enzymes and toxic mediators listed in the first two rows are released from the preformed granules. The cytokines, chemokines, and lipid mediators are synthesized after activation.

that causes an immediate increase in local blood flow and vessel permeability—and enzymes such as mast-cell chymase, tryptase, and serine esterases. These enzymes can in turn activate matrix metalloproteinases, which break down tissue matrix proteins, causing tissue destruction. Large amounts of tumor necrosis factor (TNF)-α are also released by mast cells after activation. Some comes from stores in mast-cell granules; some is newly synthesized by the activated mast cells. TNF-α activates endothelial cells, causing an increased expression of adhesion molecules, which promotes the influx of inflammatory leukocytes and lymphocytes into tissues (see Section 2-22).

On activation, mast cells synthesize and release chemokines, lipid mediators such as prostaglandins, leukotrienes and platelet-activating factor (PAF), and additional cytokines such as IL-4 and IL-13 which perpetuate the T_H2 response. These mediators contribute to both the acute and the chronic inflammatory responses. The lipid mediators, in particular, act rapidly to cause smooth muscle contraction, increased vascular permeability, and the secretion of mucus, and also induce the influx and activation of leukocytes, which contribute to the late phase of the allergic response. The lipid mediators derive from membrane phospholipids, which are cleaved to release the precursor molecule arachidonic acid. This molecule can be modified by two pathways to give rise to prostaglandins, thromboxanes, and leukotrienes. Prostaglandin D_2 is the major prostaglandin produced by mast cells and is a ligand for a chemoattractant receptor named chemoattractant receptor for T_H2 cells (CRTH2), which is expressed by T_H2 cells, eosinophils, and basophils. This is a further example of a mediator and its receptor making a link between the cells responsible for allergic inflammation. The leukotrienes, especially C4, D4, and E4, are also important in sustaining inflammatory responses in tissues. Many anti-inflammatory drugs are inhibitors of arachidonic acid metabolism. Aspirin, for example, is an inhibitor of the enzyme cyclooxygenase and blocks the production of prostaglandins.

IgE-mediated activation of mast cells thus orchestrates an important inflammatory cascade that is amplified by the recruitment of eosinophils, basophils, and T_H2 lymphocytes. The physiological importance of this reaction is as a defense against certain types of infection (see Section 9-23). In allergy, however, the acute and chronic inflammatory reactions triggered by mast-cell activation have important pathophysiological consequences, as seen in the diseases associated with allergic responses to environmental antigens.

12-7 Eosinophils are normally under tight control to prevent inappropriate toxic responses.

Eosinophils are granulocytic leukocytes that originate in bone marrow. They are so called because their granules, which contain arginine-rich basic proteins, are colored bright orange by the acidic stain eosin (Fig. 12.13). Only very small numbers of these cells are normally present in the circulation; most eosinophils are found in tissues, especially in the connective tissue immediately underneath respiratory, gut, and urogenital epithelium, implying a likely role for these cells in defense against invading organisms. Eosinophils

Fig. 12.13 Eosinophils can be detected easily in tissue sections by their bright refractile orange coloration. In this light micrograph a large number of eosinophils are seen in inflamed tissue from a patient with a systemic vasculitis accompanied by asthma, named Churg–Strauss syndrome. The tissue section is stained with hematoxylin and eosin; it is the eosin that imparts the characteristic orange color to the eosinophils. Photograph courtesy of J. Boyle.

have two kinds of effector function. First, on activation they release highly toxic granule proteins and free radicals, which can kill microorganisms and parasites but also cause significant tissue damage in allergic reactions. Second, activation induces the synthesis of chemical mediators such as prostaglandins, leukotrienes, and cytokines. These amplify the inflammatory response by activating epithelial cells and recruiting and activating more eosinophils and leukocytes (Fig. 12.14).

The activation and degranulation of eosinophils is strictly regulated, as their inappropriate activation would be harmful to the host. The first level of control acts on the production of eosinophils by the bone marrow. Few eosinophils are produced in the absence of infection or other immune stimulation. But when T_H2 cells are activated, cytokines such as IL-5 are released that increase the production of eosinophils in the bone marrow and their release into the circulation. However, transgenic animals overexpressing IL-5 have increased numbers of eosinophils (**eosinophilia**) in the circulation but not in their tissues, indicating that the migration of eosinophils from the circulation into tissues is regulated separately, by a second set of controls. The key molecules in this case are CC chemokines (see Section 2-21). Most of these cause chemotaxis of several types of leukocyte, but three are particularly important for eosinophil chemotaxis and have been named **eotaxin 1** (CCL11), **eotaxin 2** (CCL24), and **eotaxin 3** (CCL26).

The eotaxin receptor on eosinophils, CCR3, is a member of the chemokine family of receptors (see Section 6-18). It is quite promiscuous and binds other CC chemokines, including CCL7, CCL13, and CCL5, which also induce eosinophil chemotaxis. The eotaxins and these other CC chemokines also activate eosinophils. Identical or similar chemokines stimulate mast cells and basophils. For example, eotaxins attract basophils and cause their

Class of product	Examples	Biological effects
Enzyme	Eosinophil peroxidase	Toxic to targets by catalyzing halogenation Triggers histamine release from mast cells
	Eosinophil collagenase	Remodels connective tissue matrix
Toxic protein	Major basic protein	Toxic to parasites and mammalian cells Triggers histamine release from mast cells
	Eosinophil cationic protein	Toxic to parasites Neurotoxin
	Eosinophil-derived neurotoxin	Neurotoxin
Cytokine	IL-3, IL-5, GM-CSF	Amplify eosinophil production by bone marrow Cause eosinophil activation
Chemokine	CXCL8 (IL-8)	Promotes influx of leukocytes
Lipid mediator	Leukotrienes C4, D4, E4	Cause smooth muscle contraction Increase vascular permeability Increase mucus secretion
	Platelet-activating factor	Attracts leukocytes Amplifies production of lipid mediators Activates neutrophils, eosinophils, and platelets

Fig. 12.14 Eosinophils secrete a range of highly toxic granule proteins and other inflammatory mediators.

Fig. 12.15 Hypereosinophilia can cause injury to the endocardium. The top panel shows a section of the endocardium from a patient with hypereosinophilic syndrome. There is an organized fibrous exudate and the underlying endocardium is thickened by fibrous tissue. Although there are large numbers of circulating eosinophils, these cells are not seen in the injured endocardium, which is thought to be damaged by granules released from circulating eosinophils. The panel on the bottom shows two partly degranulated eosinophils (center) surrounded by erythrocytes in a peripheral blood film. Photographs courtesy of D. Swirsky and T. Krausz.

degranulation, and CCL2, which binds to CCR2, similarly activates mast cells in both the presence and the absence of antigen. CCL2 can also promote the differentiation of naive T_H0 cells to T_H2 cells; T_H2 cells also carry the receptor CCR3 and migrate toward eotaxins. It is striking that these interactions between different chemokines and their receptors show a high degree of overlap and redundancy; we do not understand the significance of this complexity. However, these findings show that families of chemokines, as well as cytokines, can coordinate certain kinds of immune response.

A third set of controls regulates the state of eosinophil activation. In their nonactivated state, eosinophils do not express high-affinity IgE receptors and have a high threshold for release of their granule contents. After activation by cytokines and chemokines this threshold drops, FcεRI is expressed, and the number of Fcγ receptors and complement receptors on the cell surface also increases. The eosinophil is now primed to carry out its effector activity—for example degranulation in response to antigen that cross-links specific IgE bound to FcεRI on the eosinophil surface.

The potential of eosinophils to cause tissue injury is illustrated by rare syndromes due to abnormally large numbers of eosinophils in the blood (**hypereosinophilia**). These syndromes are sometimes seen in association with T-cell lymphomas, in which unregulated IL-5 secretion drives a marked increase in the numbers of circulating eosinophils. The clinical manifestations of hypereosinophilia are damage to the endocardium (Fig. 12.15) and to nerves, leading to heart failure and neuropathy, both thought to be caused by the toxic effects of eosinophil granule proteins.

12-8   Eosinophils and basophils cause inflammation and tissue damage in allergic reactions.

In a local allergic reaction, mast-cell degranulation and T_H2 activation cause eosinophils to accumulate in large numbers and to become activated. Their continued presence is characteristic of chronic allergic inflammation and they are thought to be major contributors to tissue damage.

Basophils are also present at the site of an inflammatory reaction. Basophils share a common stem-cell precursor with eosinophils; growth factors for basophils are very similar to those for eosinophils and include IL-3, IL-5, and GM-CSF. There is evidence for reciprocal control of the maturation of the stem-cell population into basophils or eosinophils. For example, transforming growth factor (TGF)-β in the presence of IL-3 suppresses eosinophil differentiation and enhances that of basophils. Basophils are normally present in very low numbers in the circulation and seem to have a similar role to that of eosinophils in defense against pathogens. Like eosinophils, they are recruited to the sites of allergic reactions. Basophils express FcεRI on the cell surface and, on activation by cytokines or antigen, they release histamine from the basophilic granules after which they are named; they also produce IL-4 and IL-13.

Eosinophils, mast cells, and basophils can interact with each other. Eosinophil degranulation releases **major basic protein**, which in turn causes degranulation of mast cells and basophils. This effect is augmented by any of the cytokines that affect eosinophil and basophil growth, differentiation, and activation, such as IL-3, IL-5, and GM-CSF.

12-9 Allergic reactions can be divided into immediate and late-phase responses.

The inflammatory response after IgE-mediated mast-cell activation occurs as an immediate reaction, starting within seconds, and a late reaction, which takes up to 8–12 hours to develop. These reactions can be distinguished clinically (Fig. 12.16). The **immediate reaction** is due to the activity of histamine, prostaglandins, and other preformed or rapidly synthesized mediators that cause a rapid increase in vascular permeability and the contraction of smooth muscle. The **late-phase reaction** is caused by the induced synthesis and release of mediators including prostaglandins, leukotrienes, chemokines, and cytokines from the activated mast cells (see Fig. 12.12). These recruit other leukocytes, including eosinophils and T_H2 lymphocytes, to the site of inflammation. Late-phase reactions are associated with a second phase of smooth muscle contraction mediated by T cells, with sustained edema, and with tissue remodeling, such as smooth muscle hypertrophy and hyperplasia.

Fig. 12.16 Allergic reactions can be divided into an immediate response and a late-phase response. A wheal-and-flare allergic reaction develops within a minute or two of superficial injection of antigen into the epidermis and lasts for up to 30 minutes. The reaction to an intracutaneous injection of house dust mite antigen is shown in the upper left panel and is labeled 'HDM;' the area labeled 'saline' shows the absence of any response to a control injection of saline solution. A more widespread edematous response, as shown in the upper right panel, develops approximately 8 hours later and can persist for some hours. Similarly, the response to an inhaled antigen can be divided into early and late responses (bottom panel). An asthmatic response in the lungs with narrowing of the airways caused by the constriction of bronchial smooth muscle can be measured as a fall in the peak expiratory flow rate (PEFR). The immediate response peaks within minutes after antigen inhalation and then subsides. Approximately 8 hours after antigen challenge, there is a late-phase response that also results in a fall in the PEFR. The immediate response is caused by the direct effects on blood vessels and smooth muscle of rapidly metabolized mediators such as histamine and lipid mediators released by mast cells. The late-phase response is caused by the effects of an influx of inflammatory leukocytes attracted by chemokines and other mediators released by mast cells during and after the immediate response. Photographs courtesy of A.B. Kay.

The late-phase reaction and its long-term sequel, chronic allergic inflammation, contribute to much serious long-term illness, as, for example, chronic asthma. This is because the late reaction induces the recruitment of inflammatory leukocytes, especially eosinophils and T_H2 lymphocytes, to the site of the allergen-triggered mast-cell response. This late response can easily convert into a chronic inflammatory response if antigen persists and stimulates allergen-specific T_H2 cells, which in turn promote eosinophilia and further IgE production. This chronic inflammatory response in the lung causes the development of one of the cardinal features of allergic asthma: airway hyperreactivity to immunologically nonspecific bronchoconstrictor stimuli such as histamine and methacholine.

12-10 The clinical effects of allergic reactions vary according to the site of mast-cell activation.

When reexposure to allergen triggers an allergic reaction, the effects are focused on the site at which mast-cell degranulation occurs. In the immediate response, the preformed mediators released are short-lived, and their potent effects on blood vessels and smooth muscles are therefore confined to the vicinity of the activated mast cell. The more sustained effects of the late-phase response are also focused on the site of initial allergen-triggered activation, and the particular anatomy of this site may determine how readily the inflammation can be resolved. Thus, the clinical syndrome produced by an allergic reaction depends critically on three variables: the amount of allergen-specific IgE present; the route by which the allergen is introduced; and the dose of allergen (Fig. 12.17).

**Acute Systemic
Anaphylaxis**

If an allergen is introduced directly into the bloodstream or is rapidly absorbed from the gut, the connective tissue mast cells associated with all blood vessels can become activated. This activation causes a very dangerous syndrome called **systemic anaphylaxis**. Disseminated mast-cell activation has a variety of potentially fatal effects: the widespread increase in vascular permeability leads to a catastrophic loss of blood pressure; airways constrict, causing difficulty in breathing; and swelling of the epiglottis can cause suffocation. This potentially fatal syndrome is called **anaphylactic shock**. It can occur if drugs are administered to people who have IgE specific for that drug, or after an insect bite in individuals allergic to insect venom. Some foods, for example peanuts or brazil nuts, can cause systemic anaphylaxis in susceptible individuals. This syndrome can be rapidly fatal but can usually be controlled by the immediate injection of epinephrine, which relaxes the smooth muscle and inhibits the cardiovascular effects of anaphylaxis.

The most frequent allergic reactions to drugs occur with penicillin and its relatives. In people with IgE antibodies against penicillin, administration of the drug by injection can cause anaphylaxis and even death. Great care should be taken to avoid giving a drug to patients with a past history of allergy to that drug or one that is closely related structurally. Penicillin acts as a hapten (see Section 9-2); it is a small molecule with a highly reactive β-lactam ring that is crucial for its antibacterial activity. This ring reacts with amino groups on host proteins to form covalent conjugates. When penicillin is ingested or injected, it forms conjugates with self proteins, and the penicillin-modified self peptides can provoke a T_H2 response in some individuals. These T_H2 cells then activate penicillin-binding B cells to produce IgE antibody against the penicillin hapten. Thus, penicillin acts both as the B-cell antigen and, by modifying self peptides, as the T-cell antigen. When penicillin is injected intravenously into an allergic individual, the penicillin-modified proteins can cross-link IgE molecules on tissue mast cells and circulating basophils and thus cause anaphylaxis.

Connective tissue mast cells		Mucosal mast cells	
Route of allergen entry			
Intravenous: high dose	Subcutaneous: low dose	Inhalation: low dose	Ingestion

Fig. 12.17 The dose and route of allergen administration determine the type of IgE-mediated allergic reaction that results. There are two main anatomical distributions of mast cells: those associated with vascularized connective tissues, called connective tissue mast cells, and those found in submucosal layers of the gut and respiratory tract, called mucosal mast cells. In an allergic individual all of these are loaded with IgE directed against specific allergens. The overall response to an allergen then depends on which mast cells are activated. Allergen in the bloodstream activates connective tissue mast cells throughout the body, resulting in the systemic release of histamine and other mediators. Subcutaneous administration of allergen activates only local connective tissue mast cells, leading to a local inflammatory reaction. Inhaled allergen, penetrating across epithelia, activates mainly mucosal mast cells, causing smooth muscle contraction in the lower airways; this leads to bronchoconstriction and difficulty in expelling inhaled air. Mucosal mast-cell activation also increases the local secretion of mucus by epithelial cells and causes irritation. Similarly, ingested allergen penetrates across gut epithelia, causing vomiting due to intestinal smooth muscle contraction and diarrhea due to outflow of fluid across the gut epithelium. Food allergens can also be disseminated in the bloodstream, causing urticaria (hives) when the food allergen reaches the skin.

12-11 Allergen inhalation is associated with the development of rhinitis and asthma.

Inhalation is the most common route of allergen entry. Many people have mild allergies to inhaled antigens, manifesting as sneezing and a runny nose. This is called **allergic rhinitis** and results from the activation of mucosal mast cells beneath the nasal epithelium by allergens such as pollens that release their protein contents, which can then diffuse across the mucous membranes of the nasal passages. Allergic rhinitis is characterized by intense itching and sneezing, local edema leading to blocked nasal passages, a nasal discharge, which is typically rich in eosinophils, and irritation of the nose as a result of histamine release. A similar reaction to airborne allergens deposited on the conjunctiva of the eye is called **allergic conjunctivitis**. Allergic rhinitis and conjunctivitis are commonly caused by environmental allergens that are only present during certain seasons of the year. For example, hay fever is caused by a variety of allergens, including certain grass and tree pollens. Summer and autumnal symptoms may be caused by weed pollen, such as that of ragweed or the spores of fungi such as *Alternaria*. Perennial allergens such as cat dander and house dust mites can be a cause of year-round misery.

Allergic Asthma

A more serious syndrome is **allergic asthma**, which is triggered by allergen-induced activation of submucosal mast cells in the lower airways (Fig. 12.18). This leads within seconds to bronchial constriction and an increased secretion of fluid and mucus, making breathing more difficult by trapping inhaled air in the lungs. Patients with allergic asthma usually need treatment, and asthmatic attacks can be life-threatening. The same allergens that cause allergic rhinitis and conjunctivitis commonly cause asthma attacks. For example, respiratory arrest caused by severe attacks of asthma in the summer or autumn has been associated with the inhalation of the spores of *Alternaria*. An important feature of asthma is chronic inflammation of the airways, which is characterized by the continued presence of increased numbers of T_H2 lymphocytes, eosinophils, neutrophils, and other leukocytes (Fig. 12.19). These cells conspire to cause remodeling of the airways, which leads to permanent narrowing of the airways, accompanied by increased mucus secretion. The direct action of T_H2 cytokines such as IL-9 and IL-13 on airway epithelial cells may have a major role in one of the major features of the disease, the induction of goblet-cell metaplasia and the secretion of mucus.

Acute responses		Chronic response

Fig. 12.18 The acute response in allergic asthma leads to T_H2-mediated chronic inflammation of the airways. In sensitized individuals, cross-linking of specific IgE on the surface of mast cells by an inhaled allergen triggers them to secrete inflammatory mediators, causing increased vascular permeability, contraction of bronchial smooth muscle, and increased secretion of mucus. There is an influx of inflammatory cells, including eosinophils and T_H2 cells, from the blood. Activated mast cells and T_H2 cells secrete cytokines that augment eosinophil activation and degranulation, which causes further tissue injury and the entry of more inflammatory cells. The result is chronic inflammation, which can cause irreversible damage to the airways.

Fig. 12.19 Morphological evidence of chronic inflammation in the airways of an asthmatic patient. Panel a shows a section through a bronchus of a patient who died of asthma; there is almost total occlusion of the airway by a mucous plug. In panel b, a close-up view of the bronchial wall shows injury to the epithelium lining the bronchus, accompanied by a dense inflammatory infiltrate that includes eosinophils, neutrophils, and lymphocytes. Photographs courtesy of T. Krausz.

Lung epithelial cells can also produce the chemokine receptor CCR3 and at least two of the ligands for this receptor—CCL5 (RANTES) and eotaxin 1. These chemokines can enhance the T_H2 response by attracting more T_H2 cells and eosinophils to the damaged lungs. The direct effects of T_H2 cytokines and chemokines on airway smooth muscle cells and lung fibroblasts cause airway remodeling due to thickening of the airway walls by hyperplasia and hypertrophy of the smooth muscle layer and mucous glands, with the eventual development of fibrosis. These effects may be independent of the involvement of eosinophils in asthmatic inflammation, and could explain the apparent failure of therapies directed purely at the eosinophil that we consider in Section 12-14.

A disease resembling human asthma develops in mice that lack a transcription factor named T-bet required for T_H1 differentiation and in which T-cell responses are therefore thought to be skewed to T_H2. These mice have increased levels of the T_H2 cytokines IL-4, IL-5, and IL-13 and develop airway inflammation involving lymphocytes and eosinophils. They also develop nonspecific airway hyperreactivity to nonimmunological stimuli, similar to what is seen in human asthma (Fig. 12.20). These changes occurred in the

Fig. 12.20 Mice lacking the transcription factor T-bet develop asthma and T-cell responses polarized toward T_H2. T-bet binds to the promoter of the IL-2 gene and is present in T_H1 but not T_H2 cells. Mice with a gene-targeted deletion of T-bet (T-bet$^{-/-}$) developed a spontaneous asthma-like phenotype in the lungs. Left-hand panels: lung and airways in normal mice. Right-hand panels: T-bet-deficient mice showed lung inflammation, with lymphocytes and eosinophils around the airway and blood vessels (top) and airway remodeling with increased collagen around the airway (bottom). Photographs courtesy of L. Glimcher.

absence of any exogenous inflammatory stimulus and show that, in extreme circumstances, a genetic imbalance toward T_H2 responses can cause allergic disease.

Although allergic asthma is initially driven by a response to a specific allergen, the subsequent chronic inflammation seems to be perpetuated even in the apparent absence of further exposure to allergen. The airways become characteristically hyperreactive, and factors other than reexposure to antigen can trigger asthma attacks. For example, the airways of asthmatics characteristically show hyperresponsiveness to environmental chemical irritants such as cigarette smoke and sulfur dioxide. Viral or, to a smaller extent, bacterial respiratory tract infections can exacerbate the disease by inducing a T_H2-dominated local response.

12-12 Skin allergy is manifest as urticaria or chronic eczema.

The same dichotomy between immediate and delayed responses is seen in cutaneous allergic responses. The skin forms an effective barrier to the entry of most allergens but it can be breached by the local injection of small amounts of allergen, for example by a stinging insect. The entry of allergen into the epidermis or dermis causes a localized allergic reaction. Local mast-cell activation in the skin leads immediately to a local increase in vascular permeability, which causes extravasation of fluid and swelling. Mast-cell activation also stimulates the release of chemicals from local nerve endings by a nerve axon reflex, causing the vasodilation of surrounding cutaneous blood vessels, which causes redness of the surrounding skin. The resulting skin lesion is called a **wheal-and-flare reaction**. About 8 hours later, a more widespread and sustained edematous response appears in some individuals as a consequence of the late-phase response (see Fig. 12.16). A disseminated form of the wheal-and-flare reaction, known as **urticaria** or hives, sometimes appears when ingested allergens enter the bloodstream and reach the skin. Histamine released by mast cells activated by allergen in the skin causes large, itchy, red swellings of the skin.

Allergists take advantage of the immediate response to test for allergy by injecting minute amounts of potential allergens into the epidermal layer of the skin. Although the reaction after the administration of antigen by intraepidermal injection is usually very localized, there is a small risk of inducing systemic anaphylaxis. Another standard test for allergy is to measure levels of IgE antibody specific for a particular allergen in a sandwich ELISA (see Appendix I, Section A-6).

Although acute urticaria is commonly caused by allergens, the causes of chronic urticaria, in which the urticarial rash can recur over long periods, are less well understood. In up to a third of cases, it seems likely that chronic urticaria is an autoimmune disease caused by autoantibodies against the α chain of FcεRI. This is an example of a type II hypersensitivity reaction in which an autoantibody against a cellular receptor triggers cellular activation, in this case causing mast-cell degranulation with resulting urticaria.

Atopic Dermatitis

A more prolonged inflammatory response is sometimes seen in the skin, most often in atopic children. They develop a persistent skin rash called **eczema** or **atopic dermatitis**, due to a chronic inflammatory response similar to that seen in the bronchial walls of patients with asthma. The etiology of eczema is not well understood. Although T_H2 cells and IgE seem to be involved, it usually clears in adolescence, unlike rhinitis and asthma, which can persist throughout life.

12-13 Allergy to foods causes symptoms limited to the gut and systemic reactions.

Genuine food allergy affects about 1% of American and European populations, although food intolerances and dislikes are ubiquitous and often misnamed 'allergy' by the sufferer. About a quarter of true food allergy in the US and Europe is accounted for by allergy to peanuts. Food allergy causes approximately 30,000 anaphylactic reactions each year in the United States, including 200 deaths. This is a significant public health problem, especially in school, where children may be unwittingly exposed to peanuts, which are present in many different foods.

One of the characteristic features of food allergens is a high degree of resistance to digestion by pepsin in the stomach. This allows them to reach the mucosal surface of the small intestine as intact allergens. When an allergen is eaten, two types of allergic response are seen. Activation of mucosal mast cells associated with the gastrointestinal tract leads to transepithelial fluid loss and smooth muscle contraction, causing diarrhea and vomiting. For reasons that are not fully understood, connective tissue mast cells in the dermis and subcutaneous tissues can also be activated after ingestion of allergen, presumably by allergen that has been absorbed into the bloodstream, and this results in urticaria. Urticaria is a common reaction when penicillin is given orally to a patient who already has penicillin-specific IgE antibodies. Ingestion of food allergens can also lead to the development of generalized anaphylaxis, accompanied by cardiovascular collapse and acute asthmatic symptoms. Certain foods, most importantly peanuts, tree nuts, and shellfish, are particularly associated with this type of life-threatening response.

12-14 Allergy can be treated by inhibiting either IgE production or the effector pathways activated by cross-linking of cell-surface IgE.

The approaches to the treatment and prevention of allergy are set out in Fig. 12.21. Two treatments are commonly used in clinical practice—one is desensitization and the other is blockade of the effector pathways. There are also several approaches still in the experimental stage. In **desensitization** the aim is to shift the antibody response away from one dominated by IgE toward one dominated by IgG; the latter can bind to the allergen and thus prevent it from activating IgE-mediated effector pathways. Immune complexes of allergen and IgG might also bind to $Fc\gamma RIIB$ receptors on mast cells. Signaling via $Fc\gamma RIIB$ could downregulate mast-cell activation caused by the binding of allergen to IgE attached to $Fc\varepsilon RI$.

Patients are desensitized by injection with escalating doses of allergen, starting with tiny amounts. This injection schedule gradually diverts the IgE-dominated response, driven by T_H2 cells, to one driven by T_H1 cells, with the consequent downregulation of IgE production. Recent evidence shows that desensitization is also associated with a reduction in the numbers of late-phase inflammatory cells at the site of the allergic reaction. A potential complication of the desensitization approach is the risk of inducing IgE-mediated allergic responses.

An alternative, and still experimental, approach to desensitization is vaccination with peptides derived from common allergens. This procedure induces T-cell anergy (see Section 8-11), which is associated with multiple changes in the T-cell phenotype, including the downregulation of cytokine production and reduced expression of the CD3:T-cell receptor complex. IgE-mediated responses are not induced by the peptides because IgE, in contrast

Fig. 12.21 Approaches to the treatment of allergy. Possible methods of inhibiting allergic reactions are shown. Two approaches are in regular clinical use. The first is the injection of specific antigen in desensitization regimes, which are believed to divert the immune response to the allergen from a T$_H$2 to a T$_H$1 type, so that IgG is produced in place of IgE. The second clinically useful approach is the use of specific inhibitors to block the synthesis or effects of inflammatory mediators produced by mast cells.

Target step	Mechanism of treatment	Specific approach
T$_H$2 activation	Reverse T$_H$2/T$_H$1 balance	Injection of specific antigen or peptides. Administration of cytokines, eg, IFN-γ, IL-10, IL-12, TGF-β. Use of adjuvants such as CpG oligodeoxynucleotides to stimulate T$_H$1 response
Activation of B cell to produce IgE	Block co-stimulation. Inhibit T$_H$2 cytokines	Inhibit CD40L. Inhibit IL-4 or IL-13
Mast-cell activation	Inhibit effects of IgE binding to mast cell	Blockade of IgE receptor
Mediator action	Inhibit effects of mediators on specific receptors. Inhibit synthesis of specific mediators	Antihistamine drugs. Lipoxygenase inhibitors
Eosinophil-dependent inflammation	Block cytokine and chemokine receptors that mediate eosinophil recruitment and activation	Inhibit IL-5. Block CCR3

to T cells, can recognize only the intact antigen. A difficulty with this approach is that an individual's responses to peptides are restricted by their MHC class II alleles (see Section 5-12); patients with different MHC class II molecules therefore respond to different allergen-derived peptides. As the human population is outbred and expresses a wide variety of MHC class II alleles, the number of peptides required to treat all allergic individuals might be very large.

Another vaccination strategy that shows promise in experimental models of allergy is the use of oligodeoxynucleotides rich in unmethylated cytosine guanine dinucleotides (CpG) as adjuvants for desensitization regimes. These oligonucleotides mimic bacterial DNA sequences known as CpG motifs and strongly promote T$_H$1 responses. The mechanism of action of adjuvants is discussed in Sections 8-6 and 14-21, and Appendix I, Section A-4.

The signaling pathways that enhance the IgE response in allergic disease are also potential targets for therapy. Inhibitors of IL-4, IL-5, and IL-13 would be predicted to reduce IgE responses, but redundancy between some of the activities of these cytokines might make this approach difficult to implement in practice. A second approach to manipulating the response is to give cytokines that promote T$_H$1-type responses. IFN-γ, IFN-α, and IL-12 have each been shown to reduce IL-4-stimulated IgE synthesis *in vitro*, and IFN-γ and IFN-α have been shown to reduce IgE synthesis *in vivo*. Administration of IL-12 to patients with mild allergic asthma caused a decrease in the number of eosinophils in blood and sputum but had no effect on immediate or late-phase responses to inhaled allergen. The treatment with IL-12 was accompanied by quite severe flu-like symptoms in most patients, which is likely to limit its possible therapeutic value.

Another target for therapeutic intervention might be the high-affinity IgE receptor. An effective competitor for IgE at this receptor could prevent the binding of IgE to the surfaces of mast cells, basophils, and eosinophils.

Clinical trials have taken place of a humanized mouse anti-IgE monoclonal antibody named omalizumab, which binds to the portion of IgE that ligates the high-affinity IgE receptor. Because IgE is present in plasma at low levels it was possible to give a large molar excess of omalizumab that caused a greater than 95% decrease in IgE levels. This was accompanied by down-regulation of the numbers of high-affinity IgE receptors on basophils and mast cells. This antibody blocked both the immediate and late-phase responses to experimentally inhaled allergen. Patients receiving omalizumab in clinical trials had fewer exacerbations of their asthma than patients on the placebo, and were able to reduce their use of corticosteroids. It is too early to know whether this approach will become important in the treatment of asthma and rhinitis. However, the efficacy of this agent provides a clear-cut demonstration of the importance of IgE in the atopic allergic diseases.

A further approach to treatment would be to block the recruitment of eosinophils to sites of allergic inflammation. The eotaxin receptor CCR3 is a potential target. The production of eosinophils in bone marrow and their exit into the circulation might also be reduced by a blockade of IL-5 action. Preliminary studies using anti-IL-5 treatment have not been encouraging, however: anti-IL-5 did reduce the numbers of blood and sputum eosinophils but did not alter immediate and late-phase responses to inhaled allergen or airway hyperreactivity to histamine.

The current mainstays of therapy are drugs that treat the symptoms of allergic disease and limit the inflammatory response. Anaphylactic reactions are treated with epinephrine, which stimulates the reformation of endothelial tight junctions, promotes the relaxation of constricted bronchial smooth muscle, and also stimulates the heart. Inhaled bronchodilators that act on β-adrenergic receptors to relax constricted muscle are used to relieve acute asthma attacks. Antihistamines that block the histamine H_1 receptor reduce the urticaria that follows histamine release from mast cells and eosinophils. Relevant H_1 receptors include those on blood vessels that cause increased permeability of the vessel wall, and those on unmyelinated nerve fibers that are thought to mediate the itching sensation. In chronic allergic disease it is extremely important to treat and prevent the chronic inflammatory tissue injury. Topical or systemic corticosteroids (see Section 14-1) are used to suppress the chronic inflammatory changes seen in asthma, rhinitis, and eczema. What is really needed, however, is a means of converting the T-cell response to the allergenic peptide antigen from predominantly T_H2 to predominantly T_H1. This topic is also discussed in Chapter 14.

Summary.

The allergic response to innocuous antigens reflects the pathophysiological aspects of a defensive immune response whose physiological role is to protect against helminth parasites. It is triggered by the binding of antigen to IgE antibodies bound to the high-affinity IgE receptor FcεRI on mast cells. Mast cells are strategically distributed beneath the mucosal surfaces of the body and in connective tissue. Antigen cross-linking the IgE on their surface causes them to release large amounts of inflammatory mediators. The resulting inflammation can be divided into early events, characterized by short-lived mediators such as histamine, and later events that involve leukotrienes, cytokines, and chemokines, which recruit and activate eosinophils and basophils. The late phase of this response can evolve into chronic inflammation, characterized by the presence of effector T cells and eosinophils, which is most clearly seen in chronic allergic asthma.

Hypersensitivity diseases.

Immunological responses involving IgG antibodies or specific T cells can also cause adverse hypersensitivity reactions. Although these effector arms of the immune response normally participate in protective immunity to infection, they occasionally react with noninfectious antigens to produce acute or chronic hypersensitivity reactions. We describe common examples of such reactions in this part of the chapter. In addition we consider a newly characterized category of hypersensitivity disease, in which mutations and genetic variations in the molecules regulating inflammatory responses cause the inappropriate triggering of inflammation, leading to severe disease.

12-15 Innocuous antigens can cause type II hypersensitivity reactions in susceptible individuals by binding to the surfaces of circulating blood cells.

Antibody-mediated destruction of red blood cells (hemolytic anemia) or platelets (thrombocytopenia) is an uncommon side-effect associated with the intake of certain drugs such as the antibiotic penicillin, the anti-cardiac arrhythmia drug quinidine, or the antihypertensive agent methyldopa. These are examples of **type II hypersensitivity reactions** in which the drug binds to the cell surface and serves as a target for anti-drug IgG antibodies that cause destruction of the cell (see Fig. 12.2). The anti-drug antibodies are made in only a minority of people and it is not clear why these individuals make them. The cell-bound antibody triggers clearance of the cell from the circulation, predominantly by tissue macrophages in the spleen, which bear Fcγ receptors.

12-16 Systemic disease caused by immune-complex formation can follow the administration of large quantities of poorly catabolized antigens.

Drug-Induced
Serum Sickness

Type III hypersensitivity reactions can arise with soluble antigens. The pathology is caused by the deposition of antigen:antibody aggregates or **immune complexes** in particular tissues and sites. Immune complexes are generated in all antibody responses but their pathogenic potential is determined, in part, by their size and the amount, affinity, and isotype of the responding antibody. Larger aggregates fix complement and are readily cleared from the circulation by the mononuclear phagocyte system. However, the small complexes that form at antigen excess tend to deposit in blood vessel walls. There they can ligate Fc receptors on leukocytes, leading to leukocyte activation and tissue injury.

A local type III hypersensitivity reaction can be triggered in the skin of sensitized individuals who possess IgG antibodies against the sensitizing antigen. When antigen is injected into the skin, circulating IgG antibody that has diffused into the tissues forms immune complexes locally. The immune complexes bind Fc receptors on mast cells and other leukocytes, which creates a local inflammatory response with increased vascular permeability. The enhanced vascular permeability allows fluid and cells, especially polymorphonuclear leukocytes, to enter the site from the local vessels. This reaction is called an **Arthus reaction** (Fig. 12.22). The immune complexes also activate complement, releasing C5a, which contributes to the inflammatory reaction by ligating C5a receptors on leukocytes (see Sections 2-17 and 6-18). This causes their activation and chemotactic attraction to the site of inflammation. The Arthus reaction is absent in mice lacking the α or γ chain of the

| Locally injected antigen in immune individual with IgG antibody | Local immune-complex formation | Activation of FcγRIII on mast cells induces their degranulation | Local inflammation, increased fluid and protein release, phagocytosis, and blood vessel occlusion |

1–2 hours

Fig. 12.22 The deposition of immune complexes in tissues causes a local inflammatory response known as an Arthus reaction (type III hypersensitivity reaction). In individuals who have already made IgG antibody against an antigen, the same antigen injected into the skin forms immune complexes with IgG antibody that has diffused out of the capillaries. Because the dose of antigen is low, the immune complexes are only formed close to the site of injection, where they activate mast cells bearing Fcγ receptors (FcγRIII). As a result of mast-cell activation, inflammatory cells invade the site, and blood vessel permeability and blood flow are increased. Platelets also accumulate inside the vessel at the site, ultimately leading to vessel occlusion.

FcγRIII receptor (CD16) on mast cells, but remains largely unperturbed in complement-deficient mice, showing the primary importance of FcγRIII in triggering inflammatory responses via immune complexes.

A systemic type III hypersensitivity reaction, known as **serum sickness**, can result from the injection of large quantities of a poorly catabolized foreign antigen. This illness was so named because it frequently followed the administration of therapeutic horse antiserum. In the pre-antibiotic era, antiserum made by immunizing horses was often used to treat pneumococcal pneumonia; the specific anti-pneumococcal antibodies in the horse serum would help the patient to clear the infection. In much the same way, **antivenin** (serum from horses immunized with snake venoms) is still used today as a source of neutralizing antibodies to treat people suffering from the bites of poisonous snakes.

Serum sickness occurs 7–10 days after the injection of the horse serum, an interval that corresponds to the time required to mount a primary immune response that switches from IgM to IgG antibody against the foreign antigens in horse serum. The clinical features of serum sickness are chills, fever, rash, arthritis, and sometimes glomerulonephritis (inflammation of the glomeruli of the kidneys). Urticaria is a prominent feature of the rash, implying a role for histamine derived from mast-cell degranulation. In this case, the mast-cell degranulation is triggered by the ligation of cell-surface FcγRIII by IgG-containing immune complexes.

The course of serum sickness is illustrated in Fig. 12.23. The onset of disease coincides with the development of antibodies against the abundant soluble proteins in the foreign serum; these antibodies form immune complexes with their antigens throughout the body. These immune complexes fix complement and can bind to and activate leukocytes bearing Fc and complement receptors; these in turn cause widespread tissue injury. The formation

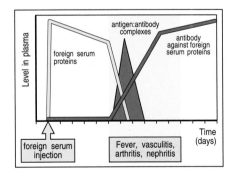

Fig. 12.23 Serum sickness is a classic example of a transient immune complex-mediated syndrome. An injection of a foreign protein or proteins leads to an antibody response. These antibodies form immune complexes with the circulating foreign proteins. The complexes are deposited in small vessels and activate complement and phagocytes, inducing fever and the symptoms of vasculitis, nephritis, and arthritis. All these effects are transient and resolve when the foreign protein is cleared.

of immune complexes causes clearance of the foreign antigen, so serum sickness is usually a self-limiting disease. Serum sickness after a second dose of antigen follows the kinetics of a secondary antibody response, and the onset of disease occurs typically within a day or two. Serum sickness is nowadays seen after the use of anti-lymphocyte globulin, employed as an immunosuppressive agent in transplant recipients, and also, rarely, after the administration of streptokinase, a bacterial enzyme that is used as a thrombolytic agent to treat patients with a myocardial infarction or heart attack.

A similar type of immunopathological response is seen in two other situations in which antigen persists. The first is when an adaptive antibody response fails to clear an infectious agent, for example in subacute bacterial endocarditis or chronic viral hepatitis. In this situation, the multiplying bacteria or viruses are continuously generating new antigen in the presence of a persistent antibody response that fails to eliminate the organism. Immune-complex disease ensues, with injury to small blood vessels in many tissues and organs, including the skin, kidneys, and nerves. Immune complexes also form in autoimmune diseases such as systemic lupus erythematosus in which, because the antigen persists, the deposition of immune complexes continues, and serious disease can result (see Section 13-29).

Some inhaled allergens provoke IgG rather than IgE antibody responses, perhaps because they are present at relatively high levels in inhaled air. When a person is reexposed to high doses of such inhaled antigens, immune complexes form in the alveolar wall of the lung. This leads to the accumulation of fluid, protein, and cells in the alveolar wall, slowing blood–gas interchange and compromising lung function. This type of reaction occurs in certain occupations such as farming, in which there is repeated exposure to hay dust or mold spores. The disease that results is therefore called **farmer's lung**. If exposure to antigen is sustained, the alveolar membranes can become permanently damaged.

12-17 Delayed-type hypersensitivity reactions are mediated by T_H1 cells and CD8 cytotoxic T cells.

Unlike the immediate hypersensitivity reactions described so far, which are mediated by antibodies, **delayed-type hypersensitivity** or **type IV hypersensitivity reactions** are mediated by antigen-specific effector T cells. These function in essentially the same way as during a response to an infectious pathogen, as described in Chapter 8. The causes and consequences of some syndromes in which type IV hypersensitivity responses predominate are listed in Fig. 12.24. These responses can be transferred between experimental animals by purified T cells or cloned T-cell lines.

The prototypic delayed-type hypersensitivity reaction is an artifact of modern medicine—the tuberculin test (see Appendix I, Section A-38). This is used to determine whether an individual has previously been infected with *Mycobacterium tuberculosis*. Small amounts of tuberculin—a complex mixture of peptides and carbohydrates derived from *M. tuberculosis*—are injected intradermally. In people who have previously been exposed to the bacterium, either by infection with the pathogen or by immunization with the BCG vaccine (an attenuated form of *M. tuberculosis*), a local T-cell-mediated inflammatory reaction evolves over 24–72 hours. The response is mediated by T_H1 cells, which enter the site of antigen injection, recognize complexes of peptide:MHC class II molecules on antigen-presenting cells, and release inflammatory cytokines such as IFN-γ and TNF-β. These stimulate the expression of adhesion molecules on endothelium and increase local blood vessel permeability, allowing plasma and accessory cells to enter the site; this causes a visible swelling (Fig. 12.25). Each of these phases takes several hours and so the

Type IV hypersensitivity reactions are mediated by antigen-specific effector T cells		
Syndrome	**Antigen**	**Consequence**
Delayed-type hypersensitivity	Proteins: Insect venom Mycobacterial proteins (tuberculin, lepromin)	Local skin swelling: Erythema Induration Cellular infiltrate Dermatitis
Contact hypersensitivity	Haptens: Pentadecacatechol (poison ivy) DNFB Small metal ions: Nickel Chromate	Local epidermal reaction: Erythema Cellular infiltrate Vesicles Intraepidermal abscesses
Gluten-sensitive enteropathy (celiac disease)	Gliadin	Villous atrophy in small bowel Malabsorption

Fig. 12.24 Type IV hypersensitivity responses. These reactions are mediated by T cells and all take some time to develop. They can be grouped into three syndromes, according to the route by which antigen passes into the body. In delayed-type hypersensitivity the antigen is injected into the skin; in contact hypersensitivity it is absorbed into the skin; and in gluten-sensitive enteropathy it is absorbed by the gut.

fully developed response appears only 24–48 hours after challenge. The cytokines produced by the activated T_H1 cells and their actions are shown in Fig. 12.26.

Very similar reactions are observed in several cutaneous hypersensitivity responses. These can be elicited by either CD4 or CD8 T cells, depending on the pathway by which the antigen is processed. Typical antigens that cause cutaneous hypersensitivity responses are highly reactive small molecules that can easily penetrate intact skin, especially if they cause itching that leads to scratching. These chemicals then react with self proteins, creating protein:hapten complexes that can be processed to hapten:peptide complexes, which can bind to MHC molecules that are recognized by T cells as foreign antigens. There are two phases to a cutaneous hypersensitivity response—sensitization and elicitation. During the sensitization phase, cutaneous Langerhans' cells take up and process antigen, and migrate to regional lymph nodes, where they activate T cells (see Fig. 8.15) with the consequent production of memory T cells, which end up in the dermis. In the elicitation phase, further exposure to the sensitizing chemical leads to antigen presentation to memory T cells in the dermis, with the release of T-cell cytokines such

| Antigen is injected into subcutaneous tissue and processed by local antigen-presenting cells | A T_H1 effector cell recognizes antigen and releases cytokines which act on vascular endothelium | Recruitment of phagocytes and plasma to site of antigen injection causes visible lesion |

24–72 hours

Fig. 12.25 The stages of a delayed-type hypersensitivity reaction. The first phase involves uptake, processing, and presentation of the antigen by local antigen-presenting cells. In the second phase, T_H1 cells that were primed by a previous exposure to the antigen migrate into the site of injection and become activated. Because these specific cells are rare, and because there is little inflammation to attract cells into the site, it can take several hours for a T cell of the correct specificity to arrive. These cells release mediators that activate local endothelial cells, recruiting an inflammatory cell infiltrate dominated by macrophages and causing the accumulation of fluid and protein. At this point the lesion becomes apparent.

Fig. 12.26 The delayed-type (type IV) hypersensitivity response is directed by chemokines and cytokines released by T_H1 cells stimulated by antigen. Antigen in the local tissues is processed by antigen-presenting cells and presented on MHC class II molecules. Antigen-specific T_H1 cells that recognize the antigen locally at the site of injection release chemokines and cytokines that recruit macrophages to the site of antigen deposition. Antigen presentation by the newly recruited macrophages then amplifies the response. T cells can also affect local blood vessels through the release of TNF-α and TNF-β, and stimulate the production of macrophages through the release of IL-3 and GM-CSF. Finally, T_H1 cells activate macrophages through the release of IFN-γ and TNF-α, and kill macrophages and other sensitive cells through the cell-surface expression of the Fas ligand.

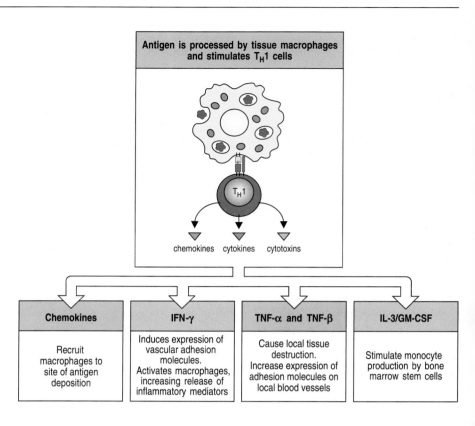

as IFN-γ and IL-17. This stimulates the keratinocytes of the epidermis to release cytokines such as IL-1, IL-6, TNF-α, and GM-CSF, and CXC chemokines including CXCL8 (IL-8) and the interferon-inducible proteins CXCL11 (IP-9), CXCL10 (IP-10), and CXCL9 (Mig; monokine induced by IFN-γ). These cytokines and chemokines enhance the inflammatory response by inducing the migration of monocytes into the lesion and their maturation into macrophages, and by attracting more T cells (Fig. 12.27).

Fig. 12.27 Elicitation of a delayed-type hypersensitivity response to a contact-sensitizing agent. The contact-sensitizing agent is a small highly reactive molecule that can easily penetrate intact skin. It binds covalently as a hapten to a variety of endogenous proteins, which are taken up and processed by Langerhans' cells, the major antigen-presenting cells of skin. These present haptenated peptides to effector T_H1 cells (which must have been previously primed in lymph nodes and then have traveled back to the skin). These secrete cytokines such as IFN-γ that stimulate keratinocytes to secrete further cytokines and chemokines. These in turn attract monocytes and induce their maturation into activated tissue macrophages, which contribute to the inflammatory lesions depicted in Fig. 12.28.

The rash produced by contact with poison ivy (Fig. 12.28) is caused by a T-cell response to a chemical in the poison ivy leaf called pentadecacatechol. This compound is lipid-soluble and can therefore cross the cell membrane and modify intracellular proteins. These modified proteins generate modified peptides within the cytosol, which are translocated into the endoplasmic reticulum and are delivered to the cell surface by MHC class I molecules. These are recognized by CD8 T cells, which can cause damage either by killing the eliciting cell or by secreting cytokines such as IFN-γ. The well-studied chemical picryl chloride produces a CD4 T-cell hypersensitivity reaction. It modifies extracellular self proteins, which are then processed by the exogenous pathway (see Section 5-5) into modified self peptides that bind to self-MHC class II molecules and are recognized by T_H1 cells. When sensitized T_H1 cells recognize these complexes they can produce extensive inflammation by activating macrophages (see Fig. 12.27). As the chemicals in these examples are delivered by contact with the skin, the rash that follows is called a **contact hypersensitivity reaction**.

Some insect proteins also elicit a delayed-type hypersensitivity response. However, the early phases of the host reaction to an insect bite are often IgE-mediated or the result of the direct effects of insect venoms. Important delayed-type hypersensitivity responses to divalent cations such as nickel have also been observed. These divalent cations can alter the conformation or the peptide binding of MHC class II molecules, and thus provoke a T-cell response. Finally, although this section has focused on the role of T cells in inducing delayed-type hypersensitivity reactions, there is evidence that antibody and complement might also have a role. Mice deficient in B cells, antibody, or complement show impaired contact hypersensitivity reactions. These requirements for B cells, antibody, and complement may reflect their role in the early steps of the elicitation of these reactions.

Fig. 12.28 Blistering skin lesions on hand of patient with poison ivy contact dermatitis. Photograph courtesy of R. Geha.

Contact Sensitivity
to Poison Ivy

12-18 Mutation or genetic variation in the molecular regulators of inflammation can cause hypersensitive inflammatory responses resulting in 'autoinflammatory disease'.

We have seen throughout this book that host defense against infection depends on the engagement by the immune system of effector mechanisms that limit the spread of infection and kill the infectious agent. In this chapter we have seen how inappropriate responses to noninfectious immunological stimuli may cause diseases as diverse as asthma and hypersensitivity to nickel. There is a very fine balance between host underresponsiveness to infectious stimuli, allowing the uncontrolled spread of infection, and overresponsiveness, potentially killing not only the infection but also the host. It is our genetic diversity that is one of our most attractive and interesting features, and this extends to variation in our ability to mount inflammatory responses. This variability can be seen in stark form in a small number of diseases in which mutations in proteins that control the life, death, and activities of inflammatory cells are associated with severe inflammatory diseases.

The name familial Mediterranean fever (FMF) describes the key features of one such severe inflammatory illness, inherited as an autosomal recessive disorder. The pathogenesis of FMF was a total mystery until it was discovered to be caused by mutations in the gene encoding the protein pyrin, named to reflect its association with fever. This gene was also discovered by a second group of scientists at much the same time and named marenostrin, after the Latin name *mare nostrum* for the Mediterranean sea. The name pyrin has stuck and has been extended to describe a domain in this protein that is the prototype of 'pyrin domains' found in some proteins involved in the execution of the pathways of apoptosis.

A second disease with similar clinical manifestations is familial Hibernian fever. Although inherited as an autosomal dominant disease, this was romantically thought to have been a variant of FMF brought to Ireland by sailors of the Spanish Armada, until genetic analysis showed it to be caused by mutations in a completely different gene, the TNFR-I receptor for TNF-α. Both illnesses are characterized by episodic attacks of severe inflammation, associated with fever, an acute-phase response, severe malaise and, in FMF, attacks of pleural or peritoneal inflammation known as pleurisy or peritonitis, respectively.

How mutations in pyrin cause FMF is not known, but the pyrin domain is found in proteins that participate in pathways leading to the activation of caspase enzymes and apoptotic cell death. A related protein, named cryopyrin, is mutated in another episodic inflammatory disease that rejoices in the name Muckle–Wells syndrome and in its close relative familial cold autoinflammatory syndrome (FCAS). These dominantly inherited syndromes present with episodes of fever—which is induced by exposure to cold in the case of FCAS—as well as urticarial rash, joint pains, and conjunctivitis. Both pyrin and cryopyrin are predominantly expressed in leukocytes. The mechanism of these diseases is not fully understood, but an attractive hypothesis is that they are caused by a failure to terminate inflammation, which is normally regulated by the death and removal of leukocytes.

In familial Hibernian fever, which has been renamed TNF-receptor associated periodic syndrome (TRAPS), missense mutations in the gene for the receptor TNFR-I are associated with reduced levels of soluble TNF-α receptor in plasma, which can be measured as a diagnostic assay. In normal circumstances, soluble TNFR-I is generated by cleavage of the extracellular portion of the receptor from the cell membrane. Most of the mutations in TRAPS prevent this cleavage, leading to an imbalance between plasma TNFR-I (which inhibits the effects of TNF-α) and membrane-bound receptor (which transduces the effects of TNF-α). The cause of the episodic nature of this and the other illnesses discussed here is not known, but it seems likely that minor inflammatory injuries that would be unnoticed in normal circumstances trigger unregulated inflammation in these people. The name that has been proposed to encompass these syndromes is **autoinflammatory disease** (Fig. 12.29).

Fig. 12.29 The autoinflammatory diseases.

Disease (common abbreviation)	Clinical features	Inheritance	Mutated gene	Protein (alternative name)
Familial Mediterranean fever (FMF)	Periodic fever, serositis (inflammation of the pleural and/or peritoneal cavity), arthritis, acute-phase response	Autosomal recessive	MEFV	Pyrin (marenostrin)
TNF-receptor associated periodic syndrome (TRAPS) (also known as familial Hibernian fever)	Periodic fever, myalgia, rash, acute-phase response	Autosomal dominant	TNFRSF1A	TNF-α 55 kDa receptor (TNFR-I)
Muckle–Wells syndrome	Periodic fever, urticarial rash, joint pains, conjunctivitis, progressive deafness	Autosomal dominant	CIAS1	Cryopyrin
Familial cold autoinflammatory syndrome (FCAS) (familial cold urticaria)	Cold-induced periodic fever, urticarial rash, joint pains, conjunctivitis			
Hyper-IgD syndrome (HIDS)	Periodic fever, elevated IgD levels, lymphadenopathy	Autosomal recessive	MVK	Mevalonate kinase
Blau syndrome	Granulomatous inflammation of skin, eye, and joints	Autosomal dominant	NOD2 (CARD15)	NOD2 (CARD15)
Crohn's disease	Granulomatous inflammatory bowel disease, sometimes eye, skin, and joint granulomata	Complex trait		

Not all autoinflammatory diseases are caused by mutations in genes involved in the regulation of cell death. Hyper-IgD syndrome, which is associated with attacks of fever starting in infancy, high levels of IgD in serum, and lymphadenopathy, is caused by mutations that result in a partial deficiency of mevalonate kinase, an enzyme in the pathway for the synthesis of isoprenoids and cholesterol. It is not known how deficiency of this enzyme causes autoinflammatory disease. However, the activity of the mutant enzyme is dependent on temperature, decreasing in patients with fever. This raises the possibility that minor episodes of fever might cause a decrease in the activity of an already partly deficient enzyme, leading to a fall in the products of the enzyme activity. These include an important posttranslational attachment of a lipophilic prenyl group (prenylation) to many proteins. Some small G proteins such as Rho and Ras are modified by prenylation, thereby enabling them to bind to lipid membranes. It may be that a decrease in the function of certain of these proteins causes the hypersensitive inflammatory responses of hyper-IgD syndrome.

These diseases are fortunately rare, although they are important illustrations of the importance of the precise regulation of inflammatory responses. A much commoner disease of unknown etiology is **Crohn's disease**, one of the two main types of inflammatory bowel disease, the other being ulcerative colitis. Sufferers from Crohn's disease have episodes of severe inflammation that commonly affect the terminal ileum—hence the alternative name of regional ileitis for this disease—but any part of the bowel can be involved. Crohn's disease is characterized by the presence of chronic inflammation affecting the mucosa and submucosa of the bowel that includes the prominent development of granulomatous lesions (Fig. 12.30), similar to those seen in the type IV hypersensitivity responses that we discussed in Section 12-17. Genetic analysis of patients with Crohn's disease and their families has identified a disease susceptibility gene named *NOD2* (also known as *CARD15*) that is expressed predominantly in macrophages. Mutations and uncommon polymorphic variants of the NOD2 protein are strongly associated with the presence of Crohn's disease. Mutations in the same gene have also been discovered as the cause of a dominantly inherited granulomatous disease named Blau syndrome, in which granulomata develop typically in the skin, eye, and joints.

The function of NOD2 is unknown, but it contains some structural motifs that give a clue to its function, in particular the presence of caspase recruitment domain (CARD) motifs that are found in proteins involved in the execution of apoptosis. NOD2 also has a leucine-rich repeat (LRR) domain like those found in other proteins, including the ectodomain of Toll-like receptors. This observation gave rise to the hypothesis that NOD2 might be an intracellular receptor for bacterial LPS and that Crohn's disease could arise as an abnormal response to the gut flora in patients with an abnormal *NOD2* gene. However, macrophages can sense LPS by using Toll-like receptors and the LRRs in NOD2 are arranged in a fashion more similar to that found in ribonuclease inhibitor than in LPS-binding Toll receptors. This has led to the alternative hypothesis that NOD2 is part of a signaling pathway leading to apoptosis and that Crohn's disease is caused by inflammatory macrophages that fail to die normally by apoptotic cell death. This mechanism would be analogous to the autoinflammatory diseases that we have discussed earlier in this section and to the lupus-like illness associated with mutations in the *FAS* or *FAS* ligand genes that we discuss in Section 13-17 and Fig. 13.19.

Analysis of these diseases has opened a new field of study in the medical sciences; it is likely that many other diseases will turn out to be caused or modified by polymorphic genetic variants or mutants in the genes that regulate innate immune responses and the control of inflammation. A minor infection

Fig. 12.30 Granulomatous inflammation in Crohn's disease. A section of bowel wall from a patient with Crohn's disease. The arrow marks a giant cell granuloma. There is a dense infiltrate of lymphocytes throughout the bowel submucosa. Photograph courtesy of H.T. Cook.

or physiological stress with no adverse consequences in most of the population might turn out to have devastating effects in a minority of genetically predisposed people. A second important message from these illnesses is that a more robust classification of disease will be possible when we understand the underlying molecular basis.

Summary.

Hypersensitivity diseases reflect normal immune mechanisms directed against innocuous antigens or inflammatory stimuli. They can be mediated by IgG antibodies bound to modified cell surfaces, or by complexes of antibodies bound to poorly catabolized antigens, as occurs in serum sickness. Hypersensitivity reactions mediated by T cells can be activated by modified self proteins or by injected proteins such as those in the mycobacterial extract tuberculin. These T cell-mediated responses require the induced synthesis of effector molecules and develop more slowly, which is why they are termed delayed-type hypersensitivity. Genetic variation in the molecules that regulate the activity of leukocytes can cause hypersensitive inflammatory responses.

Summary to Chapter 12.

In some people, immune responses to otherwise innocuous antigens produce allergic or hypersensitivity reactions upon reexposure to the same antigen. Most allergies involve the production of IgE antibody against common environmental allergens. Some people are intrinsically prone to making IgE antibodies against many allergens, and such people are said to be atopic. IgE production is driven by antigen-specific T_H2 cells; the response is polarized toward T_H2 by an array of chemokines and cytokines that engage specific signaling pathways. The IgE produced binds to the high-affinity IgE receptor $Fc\epsilon RI$ on mast cells and basophils. The physiological role of this system is to provide front-line defense against parasitic worms, but in economically developed societies in which parasitic infections are uncommon it is almost always involved in allergic reactions. Specific effector T cells, mast cells, and eosinophils, in combination with T_H2 cytokines and chemokines, orchestrate chronic allergic inflammation, which is the major cause of the chronic morbidity of asthma. Antibodies of other isotypes and antigen-specific effector T cells contribute to hypersensitivity to other antigens, as does genetic variation in the molecules that regulate inflammatory responses.

Chapter 12 questions.

12.1   *What is an allergen?*

12.2   *Is allergy due to genetic or environmental factors?*

12.3   *How are T cells programmed toward a T_H2 response?*

12.4   *What is meant by a hypersensitivity response?*

12.5   *What is the difference between autoinflammatory disease and autoimmunity?*

General references.

Bernstein, D.I.: **Allergic reactions to workplace allergens.** *JAMA* 1997, **278**:1907–1913.

Costa, J.J., Weller, P.F., and Galli, S.J.: **The cells of the allergic response: mast cells, basophils, and eosinophils.** *JAMA* 1997, **278**:1815–1822.

Kay, A.B.: *Allergy and Allergic Diseases.* Oxford, Blackwell Science, 1997.

Kay, A.B.: **Allergy and allergic diseases. First of two parts.** *N. Engl. J. Med.* 2001, **344**:30–37.

Kay, A.B.: **Allergy and allergic diseases. Second of two parts.** *N. Engl. J. Med.* 2001, **344**:109–113.

Larche, M., Robinson, D.S., and Kay, A.B.: **The role of T lymphocytes in the pathogenesis of asthma.** *J. Allergy Clin. Immunol.* 2003, **111**:450–463.

Maddox, L., and Schwartz, D.A.: **The pathophysiology of asthma.** *Annu. Rev. Med.* 2002, **53**:477–498.

Oettgen, H.C., and Geha, R.S.: **IgE in asthma and atopy: cellular and molecular connections.** *J. Clin. Invest.* 1999, **104**:829–835.

Papageorgiou, P.S.: **Clinical aspects of food allergy.** *Biochem. Soc. Trans.* 2002, **30**:901–906.

Ring, J., Kramer, U., Schafer, T., and Behrendt, H.: **Why are allergies increasing?** *Curr. Opin. Immunol.* 2001, **13**:701–708.

Romagnani, S.: **The role of lymphocytes in allergic disease.** *J. Allergy Clin. Immunol.* 2000, **105**:399–408.

Rosen, F.S.: **Urticaria, angioedema, and anaphylaxis.** *Pediatr. Rev.* 1992, **13**:387–390.

Section references.

12-1 Allergens are often delivered transmucosally at low dose, a route that favors IgE production.

Holt, P.G.: **The role of airway dendritic cell populations in regulation of T-cell responses to inhaled antigens: atopic asthma as a paradigm.** *J. Aerosol Med.* 2002, **15**:161–168.

Lambrecht, B.N., De Veerman, M., Coyle, A.J., Gutierrez-Ramos, J.C., Thielemans, K., and Pauwels, R.A.: **Myeloid dendritic cells induce Th2 responses to inhaled antigen, leading to eosinophilic airway inflammation.** *J. Clin. Invest.* 2000, **106**:551–559.

O'Hehir, R.E., Garman, R.D., Greenstein, J.L., and Lamb, J.R.: **The specificity and regulation of T-cell responsiveness to allergens.** *Annu. Rev. Immunol.* 1991, **9**:67–95.

Sertl, K., Takemura, T., Tschachler, E., Ferrans, V.J., Kaliner, M.A., and Shevach, E.M.: **Dendritic cells with antigen-presenting capability reside in airway epithelium, lung parenchyma, and visceral pleura.** *J. Exp. Med.* 1986, **163**:436–451.

12-2 Enzymes are frequent triggers of allergy.

Garraud, O., Nkenfou, C., Bradley, J.E., Perler, F.B., and Nutman, T.B.: **Identification of recombinant filarial proteins capable of inducing polyclonal and antigen-specific IgE and IgG4 antibodies.** *J. Immunol.* 1995, **155**:1316–1325.

Grammer, L.C., and Patterson, R.: **Proteins: chymopapain and insulin.** *J. Allergy Clin. Immunol.* 1984, **74**:635–640.

Kauffman, H.F., Tomee, J.F., van de Riet, M.A., Timmerman, A.J., and Borger, P.: **Protease-dependent activation of epithelial cells by fungal allergens leads to morphologic changes and cytokine production.** *J. Allergy Clin. Immunol.* 2000, **105**:1185–1193.

Nordlee, J.A., Taylor, S.L., Townsend, J.A., Thomas, L.A., and Bush, R.K.: **Identification of a Brazil-nut allergen in transgenic soybeans.** *N. Engl. J. Med.* 1996, **334**:688–692.

Shakib, F., Schulz, O., and Sewell, H.: **A mite subversive: cleavage of CD23 and CD25 by Der p 1 enhances allergenicity.** *Immunol. Today* 1998, **19**:313–316.

Thomas, W.R., Smith, W., and Hales, B.J.: **House dust mite allergen characterisation: implications for T-cell responses and immunotherapy.** *Int. Arch. Allergy Immunol.* 1998, **115**:9–14.

Wan, H., Winton, H.L., Soeller, C., Tovey, E.R., Gruenert, D.C., Thompson, P.J., Stewart, G.A., Taylor, G.W., Garrod, D.R., Cannell, M.B., and Robinson, C.: **Der p 1 facilitates transepithelial allergen delivery by disruption of tight junctions.** *J. Clin. Invest.* 1999, **104**:123–133.

12-3 Class switching to IgE in B lymphocytes is favored by specific signals.

Bacharier, L.B., and Geha, R.S.: **Molecular mechanisms of IgE regulation.** *J. Allergy Clin. Immunol.* 2000, **105**:S547–S558.

Burd, P.R., Thompson, W.C., Max, E.E., and Mills, F.C.: **Activated mast cells produce interleukin 13.** *J. Exp. Med.* 1995, **181**:1373–1380.

Corry, D.B., and Kheradmand, F.: **Induction and regulation of the IgE response.** *Nature* 1999, **402**:B18–B23.

Gauchat, J.F., Henchoz, S., Mazzei, G., Aubry, J.P., Brunner, T., Blasey, H., Life, P., Talabot, D., Flores Romo, L., Thompson, J., et al.: **Induction of human IgE synthesis in B cells by mast cells and basophils.** *Nature* 1993, **365**:340–343.

Hoey, T., and Grusby, M.J.: **STATs as mediators of cytokine-induced responses.** *Adv. Immunol.* 1999, **71**:145–162.

Romagnani, S.: **Cytokines and chemoattractants in allergic inflammation.** *Mol. Immunol.* 2002, **38**:881–885.

Romagnani, S., Parronchi, P., D'Elios, M.M., Romagnani, P., Annunziato, F., Piccinni, M.P., Manetti, R., Sampognaro, S., Mavilia, C., De-Carli, M., Maggi, E., and Del-Prete, G.F.: **An update on human Th1 and Th2 cells.** *Int. Arch. Allergy Immunol.* 1997, **113**:153–156.

Sallusto, F., Lenig, D., Mackay, C.R., and Lanzavecchia, A.: **Flexible programs of chemokine receptor expression on human polarized T helper 1 and 2 lymphocytes.** *J. Exp. Med.* 1998, **187**:875–883.

Shimoda, K., van Deursen, J., Sangster, M.Y., Sarawar, S.R., Carson, R.T., Tripp, R.A., Chu, C., Quelle, F.W., Nosaka, T., Vignali, D.A., Doherty, P.C., Grosveld, G., Paul, W.E., and Ihle, J.N.: **Lack of IL-4-induced Th2 response and IgE class switching in mice with disrupted Stat6 gene.** *Nature* 1996, **380**:630–633.

Urban, J.F., Jr, Noben-Trauth, N., Donaldson, D.D., Madden, K.B., Morris, S.C., Collins, M., and Finkelman, F.D.: **IL-13, IL-4Rα, and Stat6 are required for the expulsion of the gastrointestinal nematode parasite *Nippostrongylus brasiliensis*.** *Immunity* 1998, **8**:255–264.

Zhu, J., Guo, L., Watson, C.J., Hu-Li, J., and Paul, W.E.: **Stat6 is necessary and sufficient for IL-4's role in Th2 differentiation and cell expansion.** *J. Immunol.* 2001, **166**:7276–7281.

12-4 Both genetic and environmental factors contribute to the development of IgE-mediated allergy.

Ahmadi, K.R., and Goldstein, D.B.: **Multifactorial diseases: asthma genetics point the way.** *Curr. Biol.* 2002, **12**:R702–R704.

Culley, F.J., Pollott, J., and Openshaw, P.J.: **Age at first viral infection determines the pattern of T cell-mediated disease during reinfection in adulthood.** *J. Exp. Med.* 2002, **196**:1381–1386.

Hershey, G.K., Friedrich, M.F., Esswein, L.A., Thomas, M.L., and Chatila, T.A.: **The association of atopy with a gain-of-function mutation in the alpha subunit of the interleukin-4 receptor.** *N. Engl. J. Med.* 1997, **337**:1720–1725.

Lynch, N.R., Hagel, I., Perez, M., Di Prisco, M.C., Lopez, R., and Alvarez, N.: **Effect of antihelminthic treatment on the allergic reactivity of children in a tropical slum.** *J. Allergy Clin. Immunol.* 1993, **92**:404–411.

Matricardi, P.M., Rosmini, F., Ferrigno, L., Nisini, R., Rapicetta, M., Chionne, P., Stroffolini, T., Pasquini, P., and D'Amelio, R.: **Cross sectional retrospective study of prevalence of atopy among Italian military students with antibodies against hepatitis A virus.** *BMJ* 1997, **314**:999–1003.

McIntire, J.J., Umetsu, S.E., Akbari, O., Potter, M., Kuchroo, V.K., Barsh, G.S., Freeman, G.J., Umetsu, D.T., DeKruyff, R.H.: **Identification of Tapr (an airway** hyperreactivity regulatory locus) and the linked Tim gene family. *Nat. Immunol.* 2001, **2**:1109–1116.

Mitsuyasu, H., Yanagihara, Y., Mao, X.Q., Gao, P.S., Arinobu, Y., Ihara, K., Takabayashi, A., Hara, T., Enomoto, T., Sasaki, S., Kawai, M., Hamasaki, N., Shirakawa, T., Hopkin, J.M., and Izuhara, K.: **Cutting edge: dominant effect of Ile50Val variant of the human IL-4 receptor alpha-chain in IgE synthesis.** *J. Immunol.* 1999, **162**:1227–1231.

Morahan, G., Huang, D., Wu, M., Holt, B.J., White, G.P., Kendall, G.E., Sly, P.D., and Holt, P.G.: **Association of IL12B promoter polymorphism with severity of atopic and non-atopic asthma in children.** *Lancet* 2002, **360**:455–459.

Palmer, L.J., Silverman, E.S., Weiss, S.T., and Drazen, J.M.: **Pharmacogenetics of asthma.** *Am. J. Respir. Crit. Care Med.* 2002, **165**:861–866.

Shaheen, S.O., Aaby, P., Hall, A.J., Barker, D.J., Heyes, C.B., Shiell, A.W., and Goudiaby, A.: **Measles and atopy in Guinea-Bissau.** *Lancet* 1996, **347**:1792–1796.

Shapiro, S.D., and Owen, C.A.: **ADAM-33 surfaces as an asthma gene.** *N. Engl. J. Med.* 2002, **347**:936–938.

Shirakawa, T., Enomoto, T., Shimazu, S., and Hopkin, J.M.: **The inverse association between tuberculin responses and atopic disorder.** *Science* 1997, **275**:77–79.

Umetsu, D.T., McIntire, J.J., Akbari, O., Macaubas, C., and DeKruyff, R.H.: **Asthma: an epidemic of dysregulated immunity.** *Nat. Immunol.* 2002, **3**:715–720.

Van Eerdewegh, P., Little, R.D., Dupuis, J., Del Mastro, R.G., Falls, K., Simon, J., Torrey, D., Pandit, S., McKenny, J., Braunschweiger, K., Walsh, A., Liu, Z., Hayward, B., Folz, C., Manning, S.P., Bawa, A., Saracino, L., Thackston, M., Benchekroun, Y., Capparell, N., Wang, M., Adair, R., Feng, Y., Dubois, J., FitzGerald, M.G., Huang, H., Gibson, R., Allen, K.M., Pedan, A., Danzig, M.R., Umland, S.P., Egan, R.W., Cuss, F.M., Rorke, S., Clough, J.B., Holloway, J.W., Holgate, S.T., and Keith, T.P.: **Association of the ADAM33 gene with asthma and bronchial hyperresponsiveness.** *Nature* 2002, **418**:426–430.

von Mutius, E., Martinez, F.D., Fritzsch, C., Nicolai, T., Roell, G., and Thiemann, H.H.: **Prevalence of asthma and atopy in two areas of West and East Germany.** *Am. J. Respir. Crit Care Med.* 1994, **149**:358–364.

Wills-Karp, M.: **Asthma genetics: not for the TIMid?** *Nat. Immunol.* 2001, **2**:1095–1096.

Wills-Karp, M., Santeliz, J., and Karp, C.L.: **The germless theory of allergic disease: revisiting the hygiene hypothesis.** *Nat. Rev. Immunol.* 2001, **1**:69–75.

12-5 Most IgE is cell-bound and engages effector mechanisms of the immune system by different pathways from other antibody isotypes.

Heyman, B.: **Regulation of antibody responses via antibodies, complement, and Fc receptors.** *Annu. Rev. Immunol.* 2000, **18**:709–737.

Kinet, J.P.: **The high-affinity IgE receptor (FcεRI): from physiology to pathology.** *Annu. Rev. Immunol.* 1999, **17**:931–972.

Metzger, H.: **The receptor with high affinity for IgE.** *Immunol. Rev.* 1992, **125**:37–48.

Payet, M., and Conrad, D.H.: **IgE regulation in CD23 knockout and transgenic mice.** *Allergy* 1999, **54**:1125–1129.

Turner, H., and Kinet, J.P.: **Signalling through the high-affinity IgE receptor FcεRI.** *Nature* 1999, **402**:B24–B30.

12-6 Mast cells reside in tissues and orchestrate allergic reactions.

Austen, K.F.: **The Paul Kallos Memorial Lecture. From slow-reacting substance of anaphylaxis to leukotriene C4 synthase.** *Int. Arch. Allergy Immunol.* 1995, **107**:19–24.

Bingham, C.O., III, and Austen, K.F.: **Mast-cell responses in the development of asthma.** *J. Allergy Clin. Immunol.* 2000, **105**:S527–S534.

Charlesworth, E.N.: **The role of basophils and mast cells in acute and late reactions in the skin.** *Allergy* 1997, **52**:31–43.

Galli, S.J.: **Mast cells and basophils.** *Curr. Opin. Hematol.* 2000, **7**:32–39.

Mekori, Y.A., and Metcalfe, D.D.: **Mast cell–T cell interactions.** *J. Allergy Clin. Immunol.* 1999, **104**:517–523.

Metcalfe, D.D., Baram, D., and Mekori, Y.A.: **Mast cells.** *Physiol. Rev.* 1997, **77**:1033–1079.

Rodewald, H.R., Dessing, M., Dvorak, A.M., and Galli, S.J.: **Identification of a committed precursor for the mast cell lineage.** *Science* 1996, **271**:818–822.

Williams, C.M., and Galli, S.J.: **The diverse potential effector and immunoregulatory roles of mast cells in allergic disease.** *J. Allergy Clin. Immunol.* 2000, **105**:847–859.

12-7 Eosinophils are normally under tight control to prevent inappropriate toxic responses.

Assa'ad, A.H., Spicer, R.L., Nelson, D.P., Zimmermann, N., and Rothenberg, M.E.: **Hypereosinophilic syndromes.** *Chem. Immunol.* 2000, **76**:208–229.

Collins, P.D., Marleau, S., Griffiths Johnson, D.A., Jose, P.J., and Williams, T.J.: **Cooperation between interleukin-5 and the chemokine eotaxin to induce eosinophil accumulation *in vivo*.** *J. Exp. Med.* 1995, **182**:1169–1174.

Dombrowicz, D., and Capron, M.: **Eosinophils, allergy and parasites.** *Curr. Opin. Immunol.* 2001, **13**:716–720.

Kita, H., and Gleich, G.J.: **Eosinophils and IgE receptors: a continuing controversy.** *Blood* 1997, **89**:3497–3501.

Lukacs, N.W.: **Role of chemokines in the pathogenesis of asthma.** *Nat. Rev. Immunol.* 2001, **1**:108–116.

Matthews, A.N., Friend, D.S., Zimmermann, N., Sarafi, M.N., Luster, A.D., Pearlman, E., Wert, S.E., and Rothenberg, M.E.: **Eotaxin is required for the baseline level of tissue eosinophils.** *Proc. Natl. Acad. Sci. USA* 1998, **95**:6273–6278.

Palframan, R.T., Collins, P.D., Williams, T.J., and Rankin, S.M.: **Eotaxin induces a rapid release of eosinophils and their progenitors from the bone marrow.** *Blood* 1998, **91**:2240–2248.

Parker, C.W.: **Lipid mediators produced through the lipoxygenase pathway.** *Annu. Rev. Immunol.* 1987, **5**:65–84.

Rothenberg, M.E.: **Eosinophilia.** *N. Engl. J. Med.* 1998, **338**:1592–1600.

Robinson, D.S., Kay, A.B., and Wardlaw, A.J.: **Eosinophils.** *Clin. Allergy Immunol.* 2002, **16**:43–75.

12-8 Eosinophils and basophils cause inflammation and tissue damage in allergic reactions.

Dvorak, A.M.: **Cell biology of the basophil.** *Int. Rev. Cytol.* 1998, **180**:87–236.

Plager, D.A., Stuart, S., and Gleich, G.J.: **Human eosinophil granule major basic protein and its novel homolog.** *Allergy* 1998, **53**:33–40.

Schroeder, J.T., and MacGlashan, D.W., Jr: **New concepts: the basophil.** *J. Allergy Clin. Immunol.* 1997, **99**:429–433.

Thomas, L.L.: **Basophil and eosinophil interactions in health and disease.** *Chem. Immunol.* 1995, **61**:186–207.

12-9 Allergic reactions can be divided into immediate and late-phase responses.

Bentley, A.M., Kay, A.B., and Durham, S.R.: **Human late asthmatic reactions.** *Clin. Exp. Allergy* 1997, **27 Suppl 1**:71–86.

Cieslewicz, G., Tomkinson, A., Adler, A., Duez, C., Schwarze, J., Takeda, K., Larson, K.A., Lee, J.J., Irvin, C.G., and Gelfand, E.W.: **The late, but not early, asthmatic response is dependent on IL-5 and correlates with eosinophil infiltration.** *J. Clin. Invest.* 1999, **104**:301–308.

Liu, M.C., Hubbard, W.C., Proud, D., Stealey, B.A., Galli, S.J., Kagey Sobotka, A., Bleecker, E.R., and Lichtenstein, L.M.: **Immediate and late inflammatory responses to ragweed antigen challenge of the peripheral airways in allergic asthmatics. Cellular, mediator, and permeability changes.** *Am. Rev. Respir. Dis.* 1991, **144**:51–58.

Macfarlane, A.J., Kon, O.M., Smith, S.J., Zeibecoglou, K., Khan, L.N., Barata, L.T., McEuen, A.R., Buckley, M.G., Walls, A.F., Meng, Q., Humbert, M., Barnes, N.C., Robinson, D.S., Ying, S., and Kay, A.B.: **Basophils, eosinophils, and mast cells in atopic and nonatopic asthma and in late-phase allergic reactions in the lung and skin.** *J. Allergy Clin. Immunol.* 2000, **105**:99–107.

Pearlman, D.S.: **Pathophysiology of the inflammatory response.** *J. Allergy Clin. Immunol.* 1999, **104**:S132–S137.

Varney, V.A., Hamid, Q.A., Gaga, M., Ying, S., Jacobson, M., Frew, A.J., Kay, A.B., and Durham, S.R.: **Influence of grass pollen immunotherapy on cellular infiltration and cytokine mRNA expression during allergen-induced late-phase cutaneous responses.** *J. Clin. Invest.* 1993, **92**:644–651.

12-10 The clinical effects of allergic reactions vary according to the site of mast-cell activation.

Bochner, B.S., and Lichtenstein, L.M.: **Anaphylaxis.** *N. Engl. J. Med.* 1991, **324**:1785–1790.

deShazo, R.D., and Kemp, S.F.: **Allergic reactions to drugs and biologic agents.** *JAMA* 1997, **278**:1895–1906.

Dombrowicz, D., Flamand, V., Brigman, K.K., Koller, B.H., and Kinet, J.P.: **Abolition of anaphylaxis by targeted disruption of the high affinity immunoglobulin E receptor alpha chain gene.** *Cell* 1993, **75**:969–976.

Fernandez, M., Warbrick, E.V., Blanca, M., and Coleman, J.W.: **Activation and hapten inhibition of mast cells sensitized with monoclonal IgE anti-penicillin antibodies: evidence for two-site recognition of the penicillin derived determinant.** *Eur. J. Immunol.* 1995, **25**:2486–2491.

Kemp, S.F., Lockey, R.F., Wolf, B.L., and Lieberman, P.: **Anaphylaxis. A review of 266 cases.** *Arch. Intern. Med.* 1995, **155**:1749–1754.

Martin, T.R., Galli, S.J., Katona, I.M., and Drazen, J.M.: **Role of mast cells in anaphylaxis. Evidence for the importance of mast cells in the cardiopulmonary alterations and death induced by anti-IgE in mice.** *J. Clin. Invest.* 1989, **83**:1375–1383.

Oettgen, H.C., Martin, T.R., Wynshaw Boris, A., Deng, C., Drazen, J.M., and Leder, P.: **Active anaphylaxis in IgE-deficient mice.** *Nature* 1994, **370**:367–370.

Padovan, E.: **T-cell response in penicillin allergy.** *Clin. Exp. Allergy* 1998, **28 Suppl 4**:33–36.

Reisman, R.E.: **Insect stings.** *N. Engl. J. Med.* 1994, **331**:523–527.

Weltzien, H.U., and Padovan, E.: **Molecular features of penicillin allergy.** *J. Invest. Dermatol.* 1998, **110**:203–206.

12-11 Allergen inhalation is associated with the development of rhinitis and asthma.

Bousquet, J., Jeffery, P.K., Busse, W.W., Johnson, M., and Vignola, A.M.: **Asthma. From bronchoconstriction to airways inflammation and remodeling.** *Am. J. Respir. Crit. Care Med.* 2000, **161**:1720–1745.

Busse, W.W., Gern, J.E., and Dick, E.C.: **The role of respiratory viruses in asthma.** *Ciba Found. Symp.* 1997, **206**:208–213.

Busse, W.W., and Lemanske, R.F., Jr: **Asthma.** *N. Engl. J. Med.* 2001, **344**:350–362.

Finotto, S., Neurath, M.F., Glickman, J.N., Qin, S., Lehr, H.A., Green, F.H., Ackerman, K., Haley, K., Galle, P.R., Szabo, S.J., Drazen, J.M., De Sanctis, G.T., and Glimcher, L.H.: **Development of spontaneous airway changes consistent with human asthma in mice lacking T-bet.** *Science* 2002, **295**:336–338.

Grunig, G., Warnock, M., Wakil, A.E., Venkayya, R., Brombacher, F., Rennick, D.M., Sheppard, D., Mohrs, M., Donaldson, D.D., Locksley, R.M., and Corry, D.B.: **Requirement for IL-13 independently of IL-4 in experimental asthma.** *Science* 1998, **282**:2261–2263.

Haselden, B.M., Kay, A.B., and Larche, M.: **Immunoglobulin E-independent major histocompatibility complex-restricted T cell peptide epitope-induced late asthmatic reactions.** *J. Exp. Med.* 1999, **189**:1885–1894.

Jeffery, P.K.: **Remodeling in asthma and chronic obstructive lung disease.** *Am. J. Respir. Crit. Care Med.* 2001, **164**:S28–S38.

Kuperman, D.A., Huang, X., Koth, L.L., Chang, G.H., Dolganov, G.M., Zhu, Z., Elias, J.A., Sheppard, D., and Erle, D.J.: **Direct effects of interleukin-13 on epithelial cells cause airway hyperreactivity and mucus overproduction in asthma.** *Nat. Med.* 2002, **8**:885–889.

Lee, N.A., Gelfand, E.W., and Lee, J.J.: **Pulmonary T cells and eosinophils: coconspirators or independent triggers of allergic respiratory pathology?** *J. Allergy Clin. Immunol.* 2001, **107**:945–957.

Louahed, J., Toda, M., Jen, J., Hamid, Q., Renauld, J.C., Levitt, R.C., and Nicolaides, N.C.: **Interleukin-9 upregulates mucus expression in the airways.** *Am. J. Respir. Cell Mol. Biol.* 2000, **22**:649–656.

Naclerio, R., and Solomon, W.: **Rhinitis and inhalant allergens.** *JAMA* 1997, **278**:1842–1848.

O'Hollaren, M.T., Yunginger, J.W., Offord, K.P., Somers, M.J., O'Connell, E.J., Ballard, D.J., and Sachs, M.I.: **Exposure to an aeroallergen as a possible precipitating factor in respiratory arrest in young patients with asthma.** *N. Engl. J. Med.* 1991, **324**:359–363.

Platts-Mills, T.A.: **The role of allergens in allergic airway disease.** *J. Allergy Clin. Immunol.* 1998, **101**:S364–S366.

Szabo, S.J., Sullivan, B.M., Stemmann, C., Satoskar, A.R., Sleckman, B.P., and Glimcher, L.H.: **Distinct effects of T-bet in TH1 lineage commitment and IFN-gamma production in CD4 and CD8 T cells.** *Science* 2002, **295**:338–342.

Wills-Karp, M., Luyimbazi, J., Xu, X., Schofield, B., Neben, T.Y., Karp, C.L., and Donaldson, D.D.: **Interleukin-13: central mediator of allergic asthma.** *Science* 1998, **282**:2258–2261.

Zureik, M., Neukirch, C., Leynaert, B., Liard, R., Bousquet, J., and Neukirch, F.: **Sensitisation to airborne moulds and severity of asthma: cross sectional study from European Community respiratory health survey.** *BMJ* 2002, **325**:411–414.

12-12 Skin allergy is manifest as urticaria or chronic eczema.

Fiebiger, E., Hammerschmid, F., Stingl, G., and Maurer, D.: **Anti-FcεRIα auto-antibodies in autoimmune-mediated disorders. Identification of a structure–function relationship.** *J. Clin. Invest.* 1998, **101**:243–251.

Fiebiger, E., Stingl, G., and Maurer, D.: **Anti-IgE and anti-FcεRI auto-antibodies in clinical allergy.** *Curr. Opin. Immunol.* 1996, **8**:784–789.

Leung, D.Y.: **Immune mechanisms in atopic dermatitis and relevance to treatment.** *Allergy Proc.* 1991, **12**:339–346.

Ring, J., Bieber, T., Vieluf, D., Kunz, B., and Przybilla, B.: **Atopic eczema, Langerhans cells and allergy.** *Int. Arch. Allergy Appl. Immunol.* 1991, **94**:194–201.

Sabroe, R.A., and Greaves, M.W.: **The pathogenesis of chronic idiopathic urticaria.** *Arch. Dermatol.* 1997, **133**:1003–1008.

12-13 Allergy to foods causes symptoms limited to the gut and systemic reactions.

Astwood, J.D., Leach, J.N., and Fuchs, R.L.: **Stability of food allergens to digestion *in vitro*.** *Nat. Biotechnol.* 1996, **14**:1269–1273.

Bindslev-Jensen, C.: **Food allergy.** *BMJ* 1998, **316**:1299–1302.

Ewan, P.W.: **Clinical study of peanut and nut allergy in 62 consecutive patients: new features and associations.** *BMJ* 1996, **312**:1074–1078.

Rumsaeng, V., and Metcalfe, D.D.: **Food allergy.** *Semin. Gastrointest. Dis.* 1996, **7**:134–143.

Sampson, H.A.: **Food allergy.** *JAMA* 1997, **278**:1888–1894.

12-14 Allergy can be treated by inhibiting either IgE production or the effector pathways activated by cross-linking of cell-surface IgE.

Adkinson, N.F., Jr, Eggleston, P.A., Eney, D., Goldstein, E.O., Schuberth, K.C., Bacon, J.R., Hamilton, R.G., Weiss, M.E., Arshad, H., Meinert, C.L., Tonascia, J., and Wheeler, B.: **A controlled trial of immunotherapy for asthma in allergic children.** *N. Engl. J. Med.* 1997, **336**:324–331.

Ali, F.R., Kay, A.B., and Larche, M.: **The potential of peptide immunotherapy in allergy and asthma.** *Curr. Allergy Asthma Rep.* 2002, **2**:151–158.

Barnes, P.J.: **Therapeutic strategies for allergic diseases.** *Nature* 1999, **402**:B31–B38.

Bertrand, C., and Geppetti, P.: **Tachykinin and kinin receptor antagonists: therapeutic perspectives in allergic airway disease.** *Trends Pharmacol. Sci.* 1996, **17**:255–259.

Bryan, S.A., O'Connor, B.J., Matti, S., Leckie, M.J., Kanabar, V., Khan, J., Warrington, S.J., Renzetti, L., Rames, A., Bock, J.A., Boyce, M.J., Hansel, T.T., Holgate, S.T., and Barnes, P.J.: **Effects of recombinant human interleukin-12 on** eosinophils, airway hyper-responsiveness, and the late asthmatic response. *Lancet* 2000, **356**:2149–2153.

Busse, W.W.: **Anti-immunoglobulin E (omalizumab) therapy in allergic asthma.** *Am. J. Respir. Crit. Care Med.* 2001, **164**:S12–S17.

Creticos, P.S., Reed, C.E., Norman, P.S., Khoury, J., Adkinson, N.F., Jr, Buncher, C.R., Busse, W.W., Bush, R.K., Gadde, J., Li, J.T., et al.: **Ragweed immunotherapy in adult asthma.** *N. Engl. J. Med.* 1996, **334**:501–506.

Drazen, J.: **Clinical pharmacology of leukotriene receptor antagonists and 5-lipoxygenase inhibitors.** *Am. J. Respir. Crit. Care. Med.* 1998, **157**:S233–S237; discussion S247–S248.

Durham, S.R., Walker, S.M., Varga, E.M., Jacobson, M.R., O'Brien, F., Noble, W., Till, S.J., Hamid, Q.A., and Nouri-Aria, K.T.: **Long-term clinical efficacy of grass-pollen immunotherapy.** *N. Engl. J. Med.* 1999, **341**:468–475.

Kline, J.N.: **Effects of CpG DNA on Th1/Th2 balance in asthma.** *Curr. Top. Microbiol. Immunol.* 2000, **247**:211–225.

Leckie, M.J., ten Brinke, A., Khan, J., Diamant, Z., O'Connor, B.J., Walls, C.M., Mathur, A.K., Cowley, H.C., Chung, K.F., Djukanovic, R., Hansel, T.T., Holgate, S.T., Sterk, P.J., and Barnes, P.J.: **Effects of an interleukin-5 blocking monoclonal antibody on eosinophils, airway hyper-responsiveness, and the late asthmatic response.** *Lancet* 2000, **356**:2144–2148.

Oldfield, W.L., Larche, M., and Kay, A.B.: **Effect of T-cell peptides derived from Fel d 1 on allergic reactions and cytokine production in patients sensitive to cats: a randomised controlled trial.** *Lancet* 2002, **360**:47–53.

Sabroe, I., Peck, M.J., Van Keulen, B.J., Jorritsma, A., Simmons, G., Clapham, P.R., Williams, T.J., and Pease, J.E.: **A small molecule antagonist of chemokine receptors CCR1 and CCR3. Potent inhibition of eosinophil function and CCR3-mediated HIV-1 entry.** *J. Biol. Chem.* 2000, **275**:25985–25992.

12-15 Innocuous antigens can cause type II hypersensitivity reactions in susceptible individuals by binding to the surfaces of circulating blood cells.

Greinacher, A., Potzsch, B., Amiral, J., Dummel, V., Eichner, A., and Mueller Eckhardt, C.: **Heparin-associated thrombocytopenia: isolation of the antibody and characterization of a multimolecular PF4-heparin complex as the major antigen.** *Thromb. Haemost.* 1994, **71**:247–251.

Murphy, W.G., and Kelton, J.G.: **Immune haemolytic anaemia and thrombocytopenia: drugs and autoantibodies.** *Biochem. Soc. Trans.* 1991, **19**:183–186.

Petz, L.D.: **Drug-induced autoimmune hemolytic anemia.** *Transfus. Med. Rev.* 1993, **7**:242–254.

Salama, A., Santoso, S., and Mueller Eckhardt, C.: **Antigenic determinants responsible for the reactions of drug-dependent antibodies with blood cells.** *Br. J. Haematol.* 1991, **78**:535–539.

12-16 Systemic disease caused by immune-complex formation can follow the administration of large quantities of poorly catabolized antigens.

Bielory, L., Gascon, P., Lawley, T.J., Young, N.S., and Frank, M.M.: **Human serum sickness: a prospective analysis of 35 patients treated with equine anti-thymocyte globulin for bone marrow failure.** *Medicine (Baltimore)* 1988, **67**:40–57.

Cochrane, C.G., and Koffler, D.: **Immune complex disease in experimental animals and man.** *Adv. Immunol.* 1973, **16**:185–264.

Davies, K.A., Mathieson, P., Winearls, C.G., Rees, A.J., and Walport, M.J.: **Serum sickness and acute renal failure after streptokinase therapy for myocardial infarction.** *Clin. Exp. Immunol.* 1990, **80**:83–88.

Lawley, T.J., Bielory, L., Gascon, P., Yancey, K.B., Young, N.S., and Frank, M.M.: **A prospective clinical and immunologic analysis of patients with serum sickness.** *N. Engl. J. Med.* 1984, **311**:1407–1413.

Ravetch, J.V., and Clynes, R.: **Divergent roles for Fc receptors and complement *in vivo*.** *Annu. Rev. Immunol.* 1998, **16**:421–432.

Schifferli, J.A., Ng, Y.C., and Peters, D.K.: **The role of complement and its receptor in the elimination of immune complexes.** *N. Engl. J. Med.* 1986, **315**:488–495.

Theofilopoulos, A.N., and Dixon, F.J.: **Immune complexes in human diseases: a review.** *Am. J. Pathol.* 1980, **100**:529–594.

12-17 Delayed-type hypersensitivity reactions are mediated by T$_H$1 cells and CD8 cytotoxic T cells.

Bernhagen, J., Bacher, M., Calandra, T., Metz, C.N., Doty, S.B., Donnelly, T., and Bucala, R.: **An essential role for macrophage migration inhibitory factor in the tuberculin delayed-type hypersensitivity reaction.** *J. Exp. Med.* 1996, **183**:277–282.

Grabbe, S., and Schwarz, T.: **Immunoregulatory mechanisms involved in elicitation of allergic contact hypersensitivity.** *Immunol. Today* 1998, **19**:37–44.

Kalish, R.S., Wood, J.A., and LaPorte, A.: **Processing of urushiol (poison ivy) hapten by both endogenous and exogenous pathways for presentation to T cells *in vitro*.** *J. Clin. Invest.* 1994, **93**:2039–2047.

Larsen, C.G., Thomsen, M.K., Gesser, B., Thomsen, P.D., Deleuran, B.W., Nowak, J., Skodt, V., Thomsen, H.K., Deleuran, M., Thestrup Pedersen, K., et al.: **The delayed-type hypersensitivity reaction is dependent on IL-8. Inhibition of a tuberculin skin reaction by an anti-IL-8 monoclonal antibody.** *J. Immunol.* 1995, **155**:2151–2157.

Muller, G., Saloga, J., Germann, T., Schuler, G., Knop, J., and Enk, A.H.: **IL-12 as mediator and adjuvant for the induction of contact sensitivity *in vivo*.** *J. Immunol.* 1995, **155**:4661–4668.

Tsuji, R.F., Geba, G.P., Wang, Y., Kawamoto, K., Matis, L.A., and Askenase, P.W.: **Required early complement activation in contact sensitivity with generation of local C5-dependent chemotactic activity, and late T cell interferon gamma: a possible initiating role of B cells.** *J. Exp. Med.* 1997, **186**:1015–1026.

Vollmer, J., Weltzien, H.U., and Moulon, C.: **TCR reactivity in human nickel allergy indicates contacts with complementarity-determining region 3 but excludes superantigen-like recognition.** *J. Immunol.* 1999, **163**:2723–2731.

12-18 Mutation or genetic variation in the molecular regulators of inflammation can cause hypersensitive inflammatory responses resulting in 'autoinflammatory disease'.

Beutler, B.: **Autoimmunity and apoptosis: the Crohn's connection.** *Immunity* 2001, **15**:5–14.

Bonen, D.K., Ogura, Y., Nicolae, D.L., Inohara, N., Saab, L., Tanabe, T., Chen, F.F., Foster, S.J., Duerr, R.H., Brant, S.R., Cho, J.H., and Nunez, G.: **Crohn's disease-associated NOD2 variants share a signaling defect in response to lipopolysaccharide and peptidoglycan.** *Gastroenterology* 2003, **124**:140–146.

Delpech, M., and Grateau, G.: **Genetically determined recurrent fevers.** *Curr. Opin. Immunol.* 2001, **13**:539–542.

Drenth, J.P. and van der Meer, J.W.: **Hereditary periodic fever.** *N. Engl. J. Med.* 2001, **345**:1748–1757.

Hampe, J., Cuthbert, A., Croucher, P.J., Mirza, M.M., Mascheretti, S., Fisher, S., Frenzel, H., King, K., Hasselmeyer, A., Macpherson, A.J., Bridger, S., van Deventer, S., Forbes, A., Nikolaus, S., Lennard-Jones, J.E., Foelsch, U.R., Krawczak, M., Lewis, C., Schreiber, S., and Mathew, C.G.: **Association between insertion mutation in NOD2 gene and Crohn's disease in German and British populations.** *Lancet* 2001, **357**:1925–1928.

Hoffman, H.M., Mueller, J.L., Broide, D.H., Wanderer, A.A., and Kolodner, R.D.: **Mutation of a new gene encoding a putative pyrin-like protein causes familial cold autoinflammatory syndrome and Muckle–Wells syndrome.** *Nat. Genet.* 2001, **29**:301–305.

Houten, S.M., Frenkel, J., Rijkers, G.T., Wanders, R.J., Kuis, W., and Waterham, H.R.: **Temperature dependence of mutant mevalonate kinase activity as a pathogenic factor in hyper-IgD and periodic fever syndrome.** *Hum. Mol. Genet.* 2002, **11**:3115–3124.

Hugot, J.P., Chamaillard, M., Zouali, H., Lesage, S., Cezard, J.P., Belaiche, J., Almer, S., Tysk, C., O'Morain, C.A., Gassull, M., Binder, V., Finkel, Y., Cortot, A., Modigliani, R., Laurent-Puig, P., Gower-Rousseau, C., Macry, J., Colombel, J.F., Sahbatou, M., and Thomas, G.: **Association of NOD2 leucine-rich repeat variants** with susceptibility to Crohn's disease. *Nature* 2001, **411**:599–603.

Inohara, N., Ogura, Y., and Nunez, G.: **Nods: a family of cytosolic proteins that regulate the host response to pathogens.** *Curr. Opin. Microbiol.* 2002, **5**:76–80.

Kastner, D.L., O'Shea, J.J.: **A fever gene comes in from the cold.** *Nat. Genet.* 2001, **29**:241–242.

McDermott, M.F., and Frenkel, J.: **Hereditary periodic fever syndromes.** *Neth. J. Med.* 2001, **59**:118–125.

McDermott, M.F., Aksentijevich, I., Galon, J., McDermott, E.M., Ogunkolade, B.W., Centola, M., Mansfield, E., Gadina, M., Karenko, L., Pettersson, T., McCarthy, J., Frucht, D.M., Aringer, M., Torosyan, Y., Teppo, A.M., Wilson, M., Karaarslan, H.M., Wan, Y., Todd, I., Wood, G., Schlimgen, R., Kumarajeewa, T.R., Cooper, S.M., Vella, J.P., and Kastner, D.L.: **Germline mutations in the extracellular domains of the 55 kDa TNF receptor, TNFR1, define a family of dominantly inherited autoinflammatory syndromes.** *Cell* 1999, **97**:133–144.

Wang, X., Kuivaniemi, H., Bonavita, G., Mutkus, L., Mau, U., Blau, E., Inohara, N., Nunez, G., Tromp, G., and Williams, C.J.: **CARD15 mutations in familial granulomatosis syndromes: a study of the original Blau syndrome kindred and other families with large-vessel arteritis and cranial neuropathy.** *Arthritis Rheum.* 2002, **46**:3041–3045.

Autoimmunity and Transplantation

13

We have learned in preceding chapters that the adaptive immune response is a critical component of host defense against infection and therefore essential for normal health. Unfortunately, adaptive immune responses are also sometimes elicited by antigens not associated with infectious agents, and this can cause serious disease. These responses are essentially identical to adaptive immune responses to infectious agents; only the antigens differ. In Chapter 12 we saw how responses to certain environmental antigens cause allergic diseases and other hypersensitivity reactions. In this chapter we examine responses to two particularly important categories of antigen: responses to self tissue antigens, called **autoimmunity**, which can lead to **autoimmune diseases** characterized by tissue damage; and responses to transplanted organs that lead to **graft rejection**. In this chapter we also examine the genetic basis of these undesirable adaptive immune responses and the immunological mechanisms involved.

The nature of immune responses to self.

Normally, self-tolerance mechanisms prevent autoimmune disease. Self-tolerance is effected mainly during lymphocyte development, by mechanisms that were described in Chapter 7. The generation of self-tolerance requires that the immune system be able to distinguish self-reactive from nonself-reactive lymphocytes as they develop, but there are no direct means of doing this. As we shall see, the immune system takes advantage of surrogate markers of self and nonself to identify potentially self-reactive lymphocytes. For example, an immature lymphocyte that experiences strong cross-linking of its antigen receptor during development is likely to be self-reactive, and will be subject to mechanisms that produce self-tolerance, such as deletion, receptor editing, and anergy (see Section 7-17). Despite these selective processes, some self-reactive lymphocytes do mature, and they can subsequently be activated to cause autoimmune disease. In part, this is because determination of self-reactivity is indirect and therefore imperfect. In addition, every lymphocyte that has a degree of self-reactivity could also provide an immune response to nonself; if even weakly self-reactive lymphocytes were eliminated, the immune system would be impaired.

Autoimmune responses resemble normal immune responses to pathogens in that they are specifically activated by antigens, in this case self antigens or **autoantigens**. The type of autoimmune disease incited when self-reactive lymphocytes are activated depends in large part on their particular targets. Autoimmune diseases can be broadly divided into organ-specific and systemic. In the former, as in type I insulin-dependent diabetes mellitus

(IDDM), which is caused by immune attack on insulin-producing pancreatic β cells, autoantigens from one or a few organs only are targeted and disease is therefore limited to those organs. In the latter case, the autoantigens are ubiquitous; an example is systemic lupus erythematosus (SLE), in which chromatin is a major target. Hence, systemic autoimmune diseases affect multiple organs and have a tendency to become chronic, because the auto-antigens can never be cleared from the body. Some autoimmune diseases seem to be dominated by one or another immune effector function, either antibodies (**autoantibodies**) or activated T cells, but now that immunologists have studied many autoimmune diseases in detail, it seems that multiple effector functions are usually activated and together contribute to the overall picture of disease.

13-1 A critical function of the immune system is to discriminate self from nonself.

As we have already learned, the immune system has very powerful effector mechanisms that can eliminate a wide variety of pathogens. Early in the study of immunity it was realized that these could, if turned against the host, cause severe tissue damage; **Ehrlich** termed this *horror autotoxicus*. When reactions to self tissues do occur and are then improperly regulated, they can cause a variety of chronic syndromes called autoimmune diseases. These syndromes are quite varied in their severity, the tissues affected, and which effector mechanisms are most important in causing damage.

Yet severe autoimmune diseases are not very common. This is because the immune system has evolved multiple mechanisms to prevent damage to self tissues. Perhaps the most fundamental principle that underlies these mechanisms is discrimination of self from nonself. This poses a major problem because often the differences between self and nonself are subtle. Even pathogens are composed of proteins and other biomolecules that are mostly shared with humans. B cells recognize the three-dimensional shape of an epitope, and these can be indistinguishable in pathogens and humans. Similarly, the short peptides derived from pathogens by antigen processing can be identical to self peptides. We have already learned in Chapter 7 how B and T cells with high affinity for self antigens are eliminated or controlled by the normal immune system. But how does a lymphocyte know what 'self' really is at the molecular level? There are no particular molecular signatures of self, although, as we shall see, there are recognition systems for both self and nonself at the cellular level. The immune system therefore uses a combination of surrogate markers for self, measuring properties of molecules that are more likely to be associated with self than nonself.

The earliest postulate about how the immune system distinguishes self from nonself was that when an immature lymphocyte recognizes antigen, this leads to a negative signal that causes lymphocyte death or inactivation. Thus, self was thought to comprise the molecules recognized by a lymphocyte shortly after it has begun to express its antigen receptor. Indeed, as we have seen in Sections 7-17 and 7-24, this does seem to be an important mechanism in the thymus and bone marrow. Newly formed lymphocytes are especially sensitive to inactivation by strong signals through their antigen receptors, whereas the same signals would activate a mature lymphocyte.

Another antigenic quality that correlates with self is high and constant concentration. Many self proteins are expressed by every cell in the body, often on cell surfaces. These can provide strong signals to lymphocytes; immature lymphocytes are especially sensitive to strong signals. But even mature lymphocytes can be made tolerant to an antigen, or **tolerized**, by strong and constant signals through their antigen receptors. In contrast, foreign pathogens are introduced to the immune system suddenly and the concentrations of their antigens increase rapidly and exponentially as the pathogens replicate in the early stages of an infection. Lymphocytes are tuned to respond by activation to such sudden increases in antigen-receptor signals.

We described in Chapter 2 how the innate immune system provides critical signals that allow the activation of immune responses. This turns out to have an important role in discrimination between self and nonself, particularly in tissues outside the thymus and bone marrow. Encounter of a lymphocyte with antigen in the absence of activation of the innate immune system, particularly when no co-stimulatory molecules are present on the antigen-presenting cell, tends to lead to a negative, inactivating, signal, rather than no signal at all.

Thus, several clues are used by the immune system to distinguish self ligands from nonself ligands: encounter with the ligand when the lymphocyte is still immature, a high and constant concentration of ligand, and binding the ligand in the absence of co-stimulatory signals that are usually dependent on activation of the innate immune system. However, all of these mechanisms are error-prone, because none of them in fact truly distinguishes a self molecule from a nonself one. The immune system therefore has several additional mechanisms to control autoimmune responses should they start.

13-2 Specific adaptive immune responses to self antigens can cause autoimmune disease.

In principle, immune-mediated destruction of self tissues could occur either via specific recognition of self antigens, followed by a typical effector immune response, and/or as a byproduct of unchecked nonspecific inflammation or overly vigorous responses to chronic infections. Although the latter two mechanisms may occasionally come into play, for example in chronic bacterial endocarditis, we believe that most common autoimmune diseases result from the specific activation of self-reactive lymphocytes by self antigens. Because of the spontaneous nature of most autoimmune diseases, however, this is difficult to prove and the inciting autoantigens are difficult to identify.

In certain genetically susceptible strains of experimental animals, autoimmune disease can be induced artificially by the injection of 'self' tissues from a genetically identical animal mixed with strong adjuvants containing bacteria (see Appendix I, Section A-4). This shows directly that autoimmunity can be provoked by inducing a specific, adaptive immune response to self antigens. However, such experimental systems, although useful, are quite artificial, because in humans and genetically autoimmune-prone animals autoimmunity usually arises spontaneously; that is, we do not know what events initiate the immune response to self that leads to the autoimmune disease. Nonetheless, by studying the patterns of autoantibodies and also the particular tissues affected, it has been possible to identify self antigens that are targets of autoimmune disease, although even in these cases it is difficult to say that the immune response was initiated in response to these same antigens. In animal models, and to a lesser degree in humans, it has sometimes been possible to identify self proteins that incite self-reactive T cells.

There is evidence, as we learn in the last part of this chapter, that some autoimmune disorders, such as rheumatic fever, may be triggered by infectious agents. However, there is also evidence, particularly from animal models of autoimmunity, that many autoimmune disorders occur through internal dysregulation of the immune system without the participation of infectious agents.

13-3 Autoimmune diseases can be classified into clusters that are typically either organ-specific or systemic.

The classification of disease is an uncertain science, especially in the absence of a precise understanding of causative mechanisms. This is well illustrated by the difficulty in classifying the autoimmune diseases. It is useful to distinguish two major patterns of autoimmune disease, the diseases in which the expression of autoimmunity is restricted to specific organs of the body, known as 'organ-specific' autoimmune diseases, and those in which many tissues of the body are affected, the 'systemic' autoimmune diseases. Examples of organ-specific autoimmune diseases are Hashimoto's thyroiditis and Graves' disease, each predominantly affecting the thyroid gland, and diabetes—IDDM—which affects the pancreatic islets. Examples of systemic autoimmune disease are SLE and primary Sjögren's syndrome, in which tissues as diverse as the skin, kidneys, and brain may all be affected (Fig. 13.1).

The autoantigens recognized in these two categories of disease are themselves respectively organ-specific and systemic. Thus, Graves' disease is characterized by the production of antibodies against the thyroid-stimulating hormone (TSH) receptor in the thyroid gland, Hashimoto's thyroiditis by antibodies against thyroid peroxidase, and IDDM by anti-insulin antibodies. By contrast, SLE is characterized by the presence of antibodies against antigens that are ubiquitous and abundant in every cell of the body, such as anti-chromatin antibodies and antibodies against proteins of the pre-mRNA splicing machinery—the spliceosome complex—within the cell.

It is likely that the organ-specific and systemic autoimmune diseases have somewhat different etiologies, which provides a biological basis for their division into two broad categories. Evidence for the validity of this classification also comes from observations that different autoimmune diseases cluster within individuals and within families. The organ-specific autoimmune diseases frequently occur together in many combinations; for example, autoimmune thyroid disease and the autoimmune depigmenting disease vitiligo are often found in the same person. Similarly, SLE and Sjögren's syndrome can coexist within a single individual or among different members of a family.

These clusters of autoimmune diseases provide the most useful classification into different subtypes, each of which may turn out to have a distinct mechanism. A working classification of autoimmune diseases based on clustering is given in Fig. 13.1. However, a strict separation of diseases into organ-specific and systemic categories breaks down to some extent. Not all autoimmune diseases can be usefully classified in this manner. Autoimmune hemolytic anemia, for example, sometimes occurs as a solitary entity and could be classified as an organ-specific disease. In other circumstances it can occur in conjunction with SLE as part of a systemic autoimmune disease.

A Kidney Graft for Complications of Autoimmune Insulin-Dependent Diabetes Mellitus

Systemic Lupus Erythematosus

Organ-specific autoimmune diseases
Type I diabetes mellitus
Goodpasture's syndrome
Multiple sclerosis
Graves' disease Hashimoto's thyroiditis Autoimmune pernicious anemia Autoimmune Addison's disease Vitiligo Myasthenia gravis

Systemic autoimmune diseases
Rheumatoid arthritis
Scleroderma
Systemic lupus erythematosus Primary Sjögren's syndrome Polymyositis

Fig. 13.1 Some common autoimmune diseases classified according to their 'organ-specific' or 'systemic' nature. Diseases that tend to occur in clusters are grouped in single boxes. Clustering is defined as more than one disease affecting a single patient or different members of a family. Not all autoimmune diseases can be classified according to this scheme. For example, autoimmune hemolytic anemia can occur in isolation or in association with systemic lupus erythematosus.

Fig. 13.2 Identification of autoantibodies that can transfer disease in patients with myasthenia gravis. Autoantibodies from the serum of patients with myasthenia gravis immunoprecipitate the acetylcholine receptor from lysates of skeletal muscle cells (right-hand panels). Because they can bind to the murine as well as the human acetylcholine receptor, they can transfer disease when injected into mice (bottom panel). This experiment demonstrates that the antibodies are pathogenic. However, to be able to produce antibodies, the same patients should also have CD4 T cells that respond to a peptide derived from the acetylcholine receptor. To detect them, T cells from myasthenia gravis patients are isolated and grown in the presence of the acetylcholine receptor plus antigen-presenting cells of the correct MHC type (left-hand panels). T cells specific for epitopes of the acetylcholine receptor are stimulated to proliferate and can thus be detected.

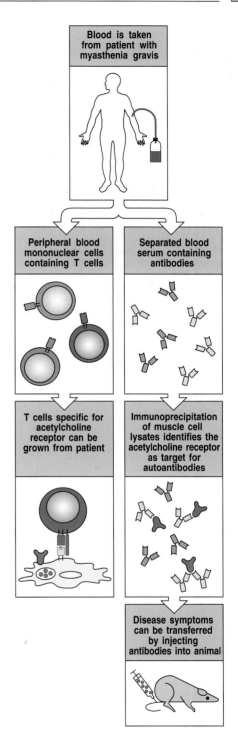

13-4 Multiple limbs of the immune system are typically recruited in autoimmune disease.

Immunologists have long been concerned with the issue of which parts of the immune system are important in causing disease in various autoimmune syndromes. In some, such as SLE, autoantibodies are thought to have a dominant role. In other diseases, such as IDDM, T cells are thought to have the major destructive role. These distinctions can be quite useful in understanding how a disease is caused and how it is maintained, with the ultimate goal of finding effective therapies.

When disease can be transferred from a diseased individual to a healthy one by transferring autoantibodies and/or self-reactive T cells, this proves that the disease is autoimmune in nature. Such experiments also identify which part of the immune system is pathogenic. In **myasthenia gravis**, for example, antibodies against the acetylcholine receptor block its function, resulting in a syndrome of muscle weakness. Serum from affected patients can transfer similar disease symptoms to animal recipients, thus proving the pathogenic role of these autoantibodies (Fig. 13.2). Similarly, in the animal model disease experimental autoimmune encephalomyelitis (EAE), which is a mouse model of multiple sclerosis, T cells isolated from affected animals can transfer disease to normal animals (Fig. 13.3).

Pregnancy is a natural situation in which autoantibodies can be shown to cause disease. IgG antibodies, but not T cells, can cross the placenta (see Section 9-13). For some autoimmune diseases (Fig. 13.4), transmission of autoantibodies across the placenta leads to disease in the fetus or the neonate (Fig. 13.5). This provides proof in humans that such autoantibodies are responsible for at least some of the symptoms of autoimmunity. The symptoms of disease in the newborn typically disappear rapidly as the maternal antibody is catabolized, but in some cases the antibodies cause chronic organ injury before they are removed, such as damage to the heart in babies of mothers with SLE or Sjögren's syndrome. Antibody clearance can be speeded up by exchange of the infant's blood or plasma (plasmapheresis), although this is of no clinical use after permanent injury has occurred, as in congenital heart block.

Although these are clear examples that a particular effector function, once established, can cause a disease syndrome, it is a vast oversimplification to consider most autoimmune diseases to be mediated solely by one or another part of the immune system. It is more useful instead to consider that autoimmune responses, like immune responses to pathogens, engage the

Myasthenia Gravis

| Mouse after induction of EAE (left), compared with normal healthy mouse | Mice injected with myelin basic protein and complete Freund's adjuvant develop EAE and are paralyzed | The disease is mediated by myelin basic protein-specific T_H1 cells | Disease can be transmitted by transfer of T cells from affected animal |

Fig. 13.3 T cells specific for myelin basic protein mediate inflammation of the brain in experimental autoimmune encephalomyelitis (EAE). This disease is produced in experimental animals by injecting them with isolated spinal cord homogenized in complete Freund's adjuvant. EAE is due to an inflammatory reaction in the brain that causes a progressive paralysis affecting first the tail and hind limbs (as shown in the mouse on the left of the photograph, compared with a healthy mouse on the right) before progressing to forelimb paralysis and eventual death. One of the autoantigens identified in the spinal cord homogenate is myelin basic protein (MBP). Immunization with MBP alone in complete Freund's adjuvant can also cause these disease symptoms. Inflammation of the brain and paralysis are mediated by T_H1 cells specific for MBP. Cloned MBP-specific T_H1 cells can transfer symptoms of EAE to naive recipients provided that the recipients carry the correct MHC allele. In this system it has therefore proved possible to identify the peptide:MHC complex recognized by the T_H1 clones that transfer disease. Other purified components of the myelin sheath can also induce the symptoms of EAE, so there is more than one autoantigen in this disease.

Autoimmune diseases transferred across the placenta to the fetus and newborn infant		
Disease	**Autoantibody**	**Symptom**
Myasthenia gravis	Anti-acetylcholine receptor	Muscle weakness
Graves' disease	Anti-thyroid-stimulating hormone (TSH) receptor	Hyperthyroidism
Thrombocytopenic purpura	Anti-platelet antibodies	Bruising and hemorrhage
Neonatal lupus rash and/or congenital heart block	Anti-Ro antibodies Anti-La antibodies	Photosensitive rash and/or bradycardia
Pemphigus vulgaris	Anti-desmoglein-3	Blistering rash

Pemphigus Vulgaris

Fig. 13.4 Some autoimmune diseases that can be transferred across the placenta by pathogenic IgG autoantibodies. These diseases are caused mostly by autoantibodies against cell-surface or tissue-matrix molecules. This suggests that an important factor determining whether an autoantibody that crosses the placenta causes disease in the fetus or newborn baby is the accessibility of the antigen to the autoantibody. Autoimmune congenital heart block is caused by fibrosis of the developing cardiac conducting tissue, which expresses abundant Ro antigen. Ro protein is a constituent of an intracellular small cytoplasmic ribonucleoprotein. It is not yet known whether it is expressed at the cell surface of cardiac conducting tissue to act as a target for autoimmune tissue injury, but in some way autoantibody binding leads to tissue damage and results in slowing of the heart rate (bradycardia).

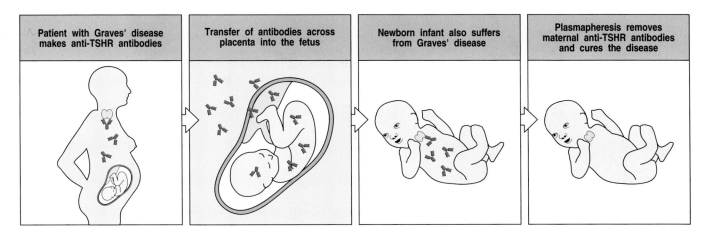

| Patient with Graves' disease makes anti-TSHR antibodies | Transfer of antibodies across placenta into the fetus | Newborn infant also suffers from Graves' disease | Plasmapheresis removes maternal anti-TSHR antibodies and cures the disease |

Fig. 13.5 Antibody-mediated autoimmune diseases can appear in the infants of affected mothers as a consequence of transplacental antibody transfer. In pregnant women, IgG antibodies cross the placenta and accumulate in the fetus before birth (see Fig. 9.22). Babies born to mothers with IgG-mediated autoimmune disease therefore frequently show symptoms similar to those of the mother in the first few weeks of life. Fortunately, there is little lasting damage as the symptoms disappear along with the maternal antibody. In Graves' disease, the symptoms are caused by antibodies against the thyroid-stimulating hormone receptor (TSHR). Children of mothers making thyroid-stimulating antibody are born with hyperthyroidism, but this can be corrected by replacing the plasma with normal plasma (plasmapheresis), thus removing the maternal antibody.

integrated immune system and therefore typically require T cells, B cells, and dendritic cells for initiation and recognition. Also, more than one immune effector function can be involved in causing pathogenesis. For example, murine lupus cannot be initiated without the help of T cells, and T cells can also be directly pathogenic, forming part of the cellular infiltrates in skin and the interstitial areas of the kidney. Similarly, in the NOD (non-obese diabetic) mouse model of IDDM, a disease that is usually thought to be T-cell-mediated, B cells are required for disease initiation. In this case, the B cells are probably functioning as essential antigen-presenting cells for T cells, although the exact details are not clear. A selection of autoimmune diseases showing which parts of the immune response contribute to pathogenesis is given in Fig. 13.6.

Autoimmune diseases involve all aspects of the immune response			
Disease	T cells	B cells	Antibody
Systemic lupus erythematosus	Pathogenic Help for antibody	Present antigen to T cells	Pathogenic
Diabetes	Pathogenic	Present antigen to T cells	–
Myasthenia gravis	Help for antibody	Antibody secretion	Pathogenic
Multiple sclerosis	Pathogenic	Present antigen to T cells	Present, but role unclear

Fig. 13.6 Autoimmune diseases involve all limbs of the immune response. Although some autoimmune diseases have traditionally been thought to be mediated by B cells or T cells, it is useful to consider that, typically, all aspects of the immune system have a role. For four important autoimmune diseases, the figure lists the roles of T cells, B cells, and antibody. In some diseases, such as systemic lupus erythematosus, T cells can have multiple roles such as helping B cells to make autoantibody and directly promoting tissue damage, while B cells can have two roles as well—presenting autoantigens to stimulate T cells and secreting pathogenic autoantibodies.

| Circulating B cell binds self antigens released from injured cells | B cell is activated by a T cell specific for self peptide | B cells differentiate into plasma cells, secreting large amounts of self-antigen specific antibody | At sites of injury, self-antigen specific antibody initiates an inflammatory response, causing more cell injury | More B cells bind self antigens, amplifying the cycle of tissue damage |

Fig. 13.7 Autoantibody-mediated inflammation can lead to release of autoantigens from damaged tissues, which in turn promotes further activation of autoreactive B cells. Autoantigens, particularly intracellular ones that are targets in SLE, stimulate B cells only when released from dying cells (first panel). The result is the activation of autoreactive T and B cells and the eventual secretion of autoantibodies (second and third panels). These autoantibodies can mediate tissue damage through a variety of effector functions (see Chapter 9) and this results in the further death of cells (fourth panel). A positive feedback loop is established because these additional autoantigens recruit and activate additional autoreactive B cells. These in turn can start the cycle over again, as shown in the first panel.

13-5 Initial loss of tolerance and autoimmunity may evolve to a chronic disease state because of positive feedback from inflammation as well as the inability to clear most self antigens.

When normal immune responses are engaged to destroy a pathogen, the typical outcome is the elimination of the foreign invader, after which the immune response ceases, leaving only an expanded cohort of memory lymphocytes (see Chapter 10). However, in autoimmunity the self antigen cannot easily be eliminated, because it is in vast excess or is ubiquitous, as with the SLE autoantigen, chromatin. Thus, a very important mechanism for limiting the extent of an immune response cannot apply to autoimmune diseases. Instead, autoimmune diseases tend to evolve into a chronic state (Fig. 13.7). There is no example of a cure for such diseases once they are well established—short of a bone marrow transplant (see Section 13-38) that completely replaces the active immune system from new cohorts of precursor cells. Even this may not be successful in curing the disease.

In autoimmune disease, the constant presence of autoantigen leads to chronic inflammation. This in turn leads to the release of more autoantigens as a result of tissue damage, and this breaks an important barrier to autoimmunity known as 'sequestration,' by which many self antigens are normally kept apart from the immune system. It also leads to the attraction of nonspecific effector cells such as macrophages and neutrophils that respond to release of cytokines and chemokines (see Fig. 13.7). The result is a continuing and evolving self-destructive process. Self antigens that were not the initial targets of autoreactive lymphocytes at the onset of autoimmunity may become targets at later stages. These secondary targets come into play because of antigen release and because of the presence of more B cells and dendritic cells at the sites of inflammation that can specifically take up and present these antigens to autoreactive T and B cells. This process has been dubbed **epitope spreading** to describe how autoimmunity to a single epitope can lead to more widespread autoimmunity (Fig. 13.8). It has been shown clearly in

EAE, in which injection of a single peptide that matches the sequence of a self protein can ultimately lead to responses to other epitopes from that same protein and even to other proteins expressed in the same tissue.

Another potential mechanism that perpetuates chronic autoimmunity seems paradoxical. In this case, the immune system develops an effective response against the self antigen to the point where the amount available to interact with lymphocytes is reduced substantially. A good example of this is SLE, in which patients make large quantities of autoantibodies against antigens such as chromatin and DNA, which are normally present in small quantities in the serum although present in large quantities in the rest of the body. These auto-antibodies can presumably bind to and clear the circulating autoantigen, thus

**Systemic Lupus
Erythematosus**

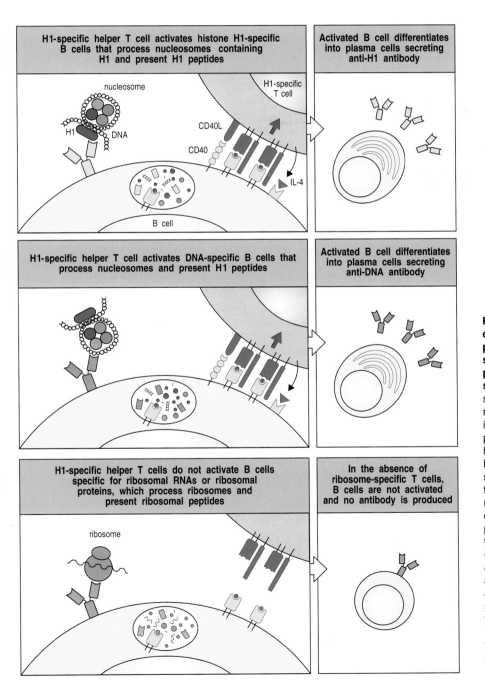

Fig. 13.8 Autoreactive helper T cells of one specificity can drive the production of autoantibodies with several different specificities, in a phenomenon known as epitope spreading. In an SLE patient, a B cell specific for the H1 histone protein in nucleosomes, for example, will bind and internalize the whole nucleosome, and present peptides derived from H1 histone as well as other peptides. This B cell can receive help from a T cell specific for one of the peptides derived from H1 (top panels). A B cell that recognizes the DNA in the nucleosome can also internalize the nucleosome, process it, and present the H1 peptide to that T cell and be activated by it (center panels). Thus, a single autoreactive helper T cell can stimulate a diverse antibody response, but the antibodies will be restricted to those specific for the constituents of a single type of particle. B cells able to bind ribosomes, for example, do not present the H1 peptide and so will not be activated to produce anti-ribosomal antibodies in this patient (bottom panels).

reducing the quantity available to tolerize newly developing T and B cells. The repertoire of developing lymphocytes will therefore not be purged of potentially autoreactive cells, as would have happened in the absence of these autoantibodies. When the self-reactive cells reach maturity in the periphery, they may encounter their cognate self antigen in an immunogenic form, for example in inflamed tissues, where they will be activated and contribute to further autoimmunity.

Summary.

Discrimination between self and nonself is imperfect, partly because of its indirect nature and partly by virtue of the selective pressure of evolution to strike the proper balance between preventing autoimmune disease and preserving immune competence. Thus, self-reactive lymphocytes always exist in the natural immune repertoire but are not often activated. In autoimmune disease, for a variety of reasons these cells become activated by specific autoantigens. If this activation persists, it leads to the generation of effector functions identical to those elicited in response to pathogens: these effector functions cause autoimmune disease. Organ-specific autoimmune diseases include diabetes, multiple sclerosis, myasthenia gravis, and Graves' disease. In each case the effector functions target autoantigens that are restricted to particular organs: insulin-producing β cells of the pancreas (diabetes), the myelin sheath of the central nervous system (multiple sclerosis), and the thyroid-stimulating hormone receptor (Graves' disease). In contrast, systemic diseases such as systemic lupus erythematosus (SLE) cause inflammation in multiple tissues because their autoantigens, such as chromatin or ribonucleoproteins, are found in every cell of the body. These diseases, in particular, tend to be chronically active because their autoantigens cannot be cleared. Some organ-specific diseases, such as multiple sclerosis, are also chronic because their targets, although specific, are distributed throughout the body. Another way of classifying autoimmune diseases is according to the effector functions that are most important in pathogenesis. This distinction can be useful; for example, multiple sclerosis is thought to be mediated by T cells. However, it is becoming more clear that many diseases that were once thought to be mediated solely by one limb or the other actually involve multiple limbs; an example is SLE, which was previously thought to be mediated solely by antibodies and immune complexes but is now known to have a component of T cell-mediated pathogenesis. Again, in this way autoimmune diseases resemble pathogen-directed immune responses that typically elicit multiple effector activities.

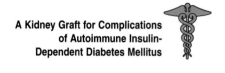

A Kidney Graft for Complications of Autoimmune Insulin-Dependent Diabetes Mellitus

Multiple Sclerosis

Multiple tolerance mechanisms normally prevent autoimmunity.

As discussed above, perfect discrimination between self and nonself is neither possible nor desirable. In particular, the selective pressures that led to the evolution of robust and rapid reactivity to pathogens result in a residual risk of some autoimmunity. The mechanisms that normally prevent autoimmunity are like a succession of layers of control. Each layer is partly effective in preventing anti-self responses, and all of them together act synergistically to provide efficient protection against autoimmunity without inhibiting the ability of the immune system to mount effective responses to pathogens. In this section we discuss these mechanisms and how they work independently and together to prevent autoimmune disease in normal individuals.

13-6   Some degree of autoimmunity is the evolutionary price of being able to make effective responses against pathogens.

One way of preventing autoimmune disease is to eliminate the immune system entirely, as in mice in which the *Rag* genes are knocked out. Of course, this 'solution' would leave no defense against pathogens and, as we have seen in Chapter 11, severe immunodeficiency is uniformly fatal. Nevertheless, this extreme example shows that autoimmunity is an inevitable consequence of vigorous immunity and that the outcome of evolution is a delicate balance between under- and over-responsiveness of the immune system to achieve the greatest possible fitness. Many autoimmune diseases in humans do not manifest themselves until after puberty; rheumatoid arthritis, for example, mainly begins between the ages of 30 and 60 years. The evolutionary 'cost' of late-onset autoimmunity is not as great as that of the relative immunodeficiency that would be needed to prevent autoimmunity more effectively.

Nonetheless, given the potential destructive power of the immune system, mechanisms to control autoimmunity are essential. The immune system has evolved several checkpoints to control autoreactivity. Each of these is only partly effective and each affects the immune response at a different stage. For example, newly formed lymphocytes are eliminated in the thymus and bone marrow if they are strongly autoreactive (see Sections 7-17, and 7-23 to 7-25). At the next stage, self-reactive lymphocytes that do not sense self strongly in the central lymphoid organs, because their cognate self antigens are not expressed there, for example, may be inactivated in the periphery (see Section 7-29). Each individual checkpoint strikes a balance between preventing autoimmunity but not impairing immunity too greatly, and in combination they provide an effective overall defense against autoimmunity. It is relatively easy to find isolated breakdowns of one or even more layers of protection, even in healthy individuals. However, autoimmune disease develops only if enough safeguards are overcome to lead to a sustained reaction to self, including the generation of effectors of tissue destruction. Thus, activation of autoreactive lymphocytes does not necessarily equal autoimmune disease. In fact, this is likely to be an everyday occurrence in a normal healthy person, but the activation is transient and nondestructive because it is controlled by one or more of the many mechanisms of self-tolerance.

13-7   Central deletion or inactivation of newly formed lymphocytes is the first checkpoint of self-tolerance.

The V(D)J recombination that occurs during lymphocyte development in the central lymphoid organs (see Chapter 4) is random, and it thus inevitably results in the generation of lymphocytes with high affinity to ubiquitously expressed self antigens. The solution to this problem also begins in the central lymphoid organs. Developing self-reactive lymphocytes are eliminated there by several mechanisms, including deletion and receptor editing. Similarly, weakly self-reactive lymphocytes are rendered unresponsive, a phenomenon called anergy, which can occur in both central and peripheral lymphoid organs.

These mechanisms, which are covered in detail in Chapter 7, are the first and most important checkpoints in self-tolerance. Without them, the immune system would be strongly self-reactive and lethal autoimmunity would most certainly be present from birth. It is unlikely that the other, later-acting, mechanisms of tolerance would be sufficient to compensate for the failure to remove self-reactive lymphocytes during their primary development. Indeed, there are no known autoimmune diseases attributable to a complete failure of these basic mechanisms, although some diseases are associated with a partial failure of central tolerance, as we shall see.

**Autoimmune
Polyglandular Syndrome**

Fig. 13.9 The 'autoimmune regulator' gene *AIRE* promotes the expression of some tissue-specific antigens in thymic medullary cells, causing the deletion of immature thymocytes that can react to these antigens. Although the thymus expresses many genes, and thus self proteins, common to all cells, it is not obvious how antigens that are specific to specialized tissues, such as retina or ovary (first panel), gain access to the thymus to promote the negative selection of immature autoreactive thymocytes. It was recently discovered that a gene called *AIRE* promotes the expression of many tissue-specific proteins in thymic medullary cells. Peptides from these proteins are presented to developing thymocytes as they undergo negative selection in the thymus (third panel), causing deletion of these cells. In the absence of AIRE, such deletion does not occur and instead the autoreactive thymocytes mature and can be exported to the periphery (fourth panel) where they could cause autoimmune disease. Indeed, people and mice that lack expression of *AIRE* develop a syndrome called APECED, or autoimmune polyendocrinopathy–candidiasis–ectodermal dystrophy.

The ability to tolerize immature lymphocytes as they develop in the central lymphoid organs is relatively easy to understand, because these cells respond differently—that is, negatively—to strong cross-linking of their antigen receptors compared with mature lymphocytes. Because mature cells must be able to respond positively to receptor cross-linking, it is less clear how they distinguish a tolerizing signal from an activating signal. Establishing tolerance in mature lymphocytes that have left the central lymphoid organs is thus more problematic. As we saw in Chapter 10, mature lymphocytes interpret signals through the antigen receptor in the context of whether inflammatory signals that signal the presence of infection, such as certain cytokines, are also present. If there is no inflammatory signal, the lymphocyte responds to signals through its antigen receptor by undergoing deletion by apoptosis or by becoming anergic (see Section 7-29). If inflammatory signals are present, the same signal leads to the proliferation and expression of effector functions.

To the extent that self-tolerance in the central organs is effective, there is less need for peripheral tolerance to the same antigens. But not all self antigens are likely to be expressed in the thymus or bone marrow, which seems to indicate an absolute need for peripheral tolerance. However, it has recently become clear that many (but not all) tissue-specific peripheral antigens, such as insulin, are actually expressed in the thymus by a subset of dendritic-like cells. This expression leads to the presence of many such proteins as tolerogens in the thymus. How these genes are turned on ectopically in the thymus is not yet completely worked out, but an important clue has been found recently. A single transcription factor, AIRE (for *auto*immune *re*gulator), is thought to be responsible for somehow turning on many 'peripheral' genes in the thymus. The *AIRE* gene is defective in patients with a rare inherited form of autoimmunity—**autoimmune polyendocrinopathy–candidiasis–ectodermal dystrophy (APECED)**—that leads to the destruction of multiple endocrine tissues, including insulin-producing islets. Mice that have been engineered to lack this gene have a similar syndrome. Most importantly, these mice no longer express many of the 'peripheral' genes in the thymus. This links the AIRE protein to the expression of these genes as well as suggesting that an inability to express these genes in the thymus leads to autoimmune disease (Fig. 13.9). The fact that AIRE-deficient humans and mice do develop autoimmunity emphasizes the importance of central tolerance, but also that other layers of tolerance control have an important role, because the autoimmunity that accompanies AIRE deficiency takes time to develop and does not always affect all potential organ targets.

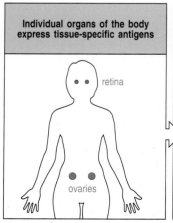

Individual organs of the body express tissue-specific antigens

retina

ovaries

In the thymus, T cells arise capable of recognizing tissue-specific antigens

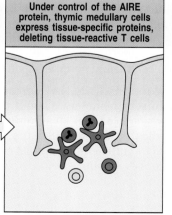

Under control of the AIRE protein, thymic medullary cells express tissue-specific proteins, deleting tissue-reactive T cells

In the absence of AIRE, T cells reactive to tissue-specifc antigens mature and leave the thymus

13-8 Lymphocytes that bind self antigens with relatively low affinity usually ignore them but in some circumstances become activated.

In Section 7-17 we described how some lymphocytes with relatively low affinity for self antigens make no response to them, escape tolerance mechanisms altogether, and simply remain 'ignorant' of self. However, such ignorant but latently self-reactive cells can be recruited into autoimmune responses.

Cells that have low affinity for available self antigens may not react in normal conditions, but their ignorance can be overcome if the stimulus is strong enough. This can occur naturally, for example, in infection. Naive T cells with low affinity for a ubiquitous self antigen can be activated if they encounter an activated dendritic cell expressing high levels of co-stimulatory signals as a result of the presence of infection. Infection can stimulate autoimmunity in a variety of ways, some of which we discuss later; here we describe how infection can activate ignorant cells. Autoantigens for self-reactive B cells, for example, could be ligands for Toll-like receptors (TLRs). These receptors are usually considered simply as specific for pathogen-associated molecular patterns (see Section 2-7), but even these patterns are not exclusive to pathogens and can be found among self molecules. One example is the unmethylated CpG sequences in DNA that are recognized by TLR-9. These are much more common in bacterial than mammalian DNA, but they do exist in mammals and are particularly enriched in activated cells that have undergone substantial DNA demethylation. Fortunately, mammalian CpG DNA is normally at a very low concentration and is ineffective in stimulating TLR-9. However, when there is extensive cell death coupled with inadequate clearance of apoptotic fragments, B cells specific for components of chromatin can internalize these sequences via their B-cell receptor. The CpG sequences then encounter TLR-9 intracellularly, leading to an activation signal that, together with the signal from the B-cell receptor, activates the previously ignorant anti-chromatin B cell (Fig. 13.10). It is believed that this pathway explains why systemic autoimmunity commonly focuses on DNA-related autoantigens. Experiments in mice are also beginning to show that signals through Toll-like receptors could have an important role in systemic autoimmunity.

Another mechanism by which ignorant lymphocytes can be drawn into action is by changing the availability or form of a self antigen. For example, some antigens are normally intracellular and are thus not encountered by lymphocytes, but massive tissue death or inflammation can cause their release. In turn, this can lead to the activation of ignorant T and B cells and resultant

Fig. 13.10 Toll-like receptors, such as TLR-9, that can recognize self antigens provide important co-stimulation for the activation of autoreactive B cells. This example illustrates how TLR-9 promotes the activation of B cells specific for DNA, a common autoantibody in SLE. Although B cells with strong affinity for DNA are eliminated in the bone marrow, some DNA-specific B cells with lower affinity escape and persist in the periphery but are not normally activated. Under some conditions and in genetically susceptible individuals, the concentration of DNA may increase, leading to the ligation of enough B-cell receptors to initiate activation of these B cells (left). B cells signal through their receptor but also take up the DNA (center) and deliver it to an endosomal compartment (right). Here the DNA has access to TLR-9, which recognizes DNA that is enriched in unmethylated CpG DNA sequences. Such CpG-enriched sequences are much more common in microbial than eukaryotic DNA and normally this allows TLR-9 to distinguish pathogens from self. However, the DNA-specific B cell concentrates enough self DNA in the endosomal compartment to activate TLR-9, potentiating the activation of the DNA-specific B cell and ultimately leading to autoantibody production.

B cells with specificity for DNA bind soluble fragments of DNA, sending a signal through the B-cell receptor	The cross-linked B-cell receptor is internalized with the bound DNA molecule	GC-rich fragments from the internalized DNA bind to TLR-9 in an endosomal compartment, sending a co-stimulatory signal

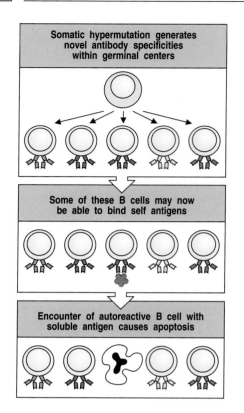

Somatic hypermutation generates novel antibody specificities within germinal centers

Some of these B cells may now be able to bind self antigens

Encounter of autoreactive B cell with soluble antigen causes apoptosis

Rheumatoid Arthritis

Fig. 13.11 Elimination of autoreactive B cells in germinal centers. During somatic hypermutation in germinal centers (top panel), B cells with autoreactive B-cell receptors can arise. Ligation of these receptors by soluble autoantigen (center panel) induces apoptosis of the autoreactive B cell by signaling through the B-cell antigen receptor in the absence of helper T cells (bottom panel).

autoimmunity. This is known to occur in some cases after myocardial infarction, when an autoimmune response is detectable some days after the release of cardiac antigens. Such reactions are typically transient and cease when the autoantigens have been removed; however, when clearance mechanisms are inadequate or genetically deficient, they can continue, causing clinical autoimmune disease.

Some autoantigens are present in great quantity but are usually in a nonimmunogenic form. IgG is a good example, because there are large quantities of it in blood. B cells specific for the IgG constant region are not usually activated because the IgG is monomeric and cannot cross-link the B-cell receptor. However, when immune complexes form after a severe infection or immunization, enough IgG in multivalent form can become available to stimulate these otherwise ignorant B cells to make a response. The autoantibody they produce is known as rheumatoid factor because it is commonly present in rheumatoid arthritis. Again, this response is normally short-lived, as long as the immune complexes are cleared rapidly.

A unique situation occurs in peripheral lymphoid organs when activated B cells undergo somatic hypermutation in germinal centers (see Section 9-7). This could result in some B cells becoming self-reactive or increasing their affinity for a self antigen (Fig. 13.11). Like the ignorant lymphocytes discussed above, such self-reactive B cells would have bypassed all the other tolerance mechanisms, but now would be activated and could be a source of pathogenic autoantibodies. However, there seems to be a mechanism to control germinal-center B cells that have acquired affinity for self. In this case, the self antigen is likely to be present in high concentration in the germinal center whereas a pathogen is not likely to be. So, if a hypermutated self-reactive B cell encounters strong cross-linking of its B-cell receptor at this stage, it undergoes apoptosis rather than further proliferation.

13-9 Antigens in immunologically privileged sites do not induce immune attack but can serve as targets.

Tissue grafts placed in some sites in the body do not elicit immune responses. For instance, the brain and the anterior chamber of the eye are sites in which tissues can be grafted without inducing rejection. Such locations are termed **immunologically privileged sites** (Fig. 13.12). It was originally believed that immunological privilege arose from the failure of antigens to leave privileged sites and induce immune responses. However, subsequent studies have shown that antigens do leave immunologically privileged sites and that they do interact with T cells; but instead of eliciting a destructive immune response, they induce tolerance or a response that is not destructive to the tissue.

Immunologically privileged sites seem to be unusual in three ways. First, the communication between the privileged site and the body is atypical in that extracellular fluid in these sites does not pass through conventional lymphatics, although proteins placed in these sites do leave them and can have immunological effects. Similarly, naive lymphocytes may be excluded by the tissue barriers of privileged sites, such as the blood–brain barrier. Second,

Immunologically privileged sites

Brain

Eye

Testis

Uterus (fetus)

Hamster cheek pouch

Fig. 13.12 Some body sites are immunologically privileged. Tissue grafts placed in these sites often last indefinitely, and antigens placed in these sites do not elicit destructive immune responses.

humoral factors, presumably cytokines, that affect the course of an immune response are produced in privileged sites and leave them together with antigens. The anti-inflammatory cytokine transforming growth factor (TGF)-β seems to be particularly important in this regard: antigens mixed with TGF-β seem to induce mainly T-cell responses that do not damage tissues, such as T_H2 rather than T_H1 responses. Third, the expression of Fas ligand by the tissues of immunologically privileged sites may provide a further level of protection by inducing the apoptosis of Fas-bearing lymphocytes that enter these sites. This mechanism of protection is not fully understood, because it seems that under some circumstances the expression of Fas ligand by tissues may trigger an inflammatory response by neutrophils.

Paradoxically, the antigens sequestered in immunologically privileged sites are often the targets of autoimmune attack; for example, brain autoantigens such as myelin basic protein are targeted in multiple sclerosis. It is therefore clear that this antigen does not induce tolerance attributable to clonal deletion of the self-reactive T cells. Mice become diseased only when they are deliberately immunized with myelin basic protein, in which case they become acutely sick, show severe infiltration of the brain with specific T_H1 cells, and often die.

Thus, at least some antigens expressed in immunologically privileged sites induce neither tolerance nor activation, but if activation is induced elsewhere they can become targets for autoimmune attack. It seems plausible that T cells specific for antigens sequestered in immunologically privileged sites are more likely to remain in a state of immunological ignorance. Further evidence for this comes from the eye disease **sympathetic ophthalmia** (Fig. 13.13). If one eye is ruptured by a blow or other trauma, an autoimmune response to eye proteins can occur, although this happens only rarely. Once the response is induced, it often attacks both eyes. Frequently, immunosuppression—and, rarely, removal of the damaged eye, the source of antigen—is required to preserve vision in the undamaged eye.

It is not surprising that effector T cells can enter immunologically privileged sites: such sites can become infected, and effector cells must be able to enter these sites during infection. As we learned in Chapter 10, effector T cells enter most or all tissues after activation, but accumulations of cells are seen only when antigen is recognized in the site, triggering the production of cytokines that alter tissue barriers.

Trauma to one eye results in the release of sequestered intraocular protein antigens

Released intraocular antigen is carried to lymph nodes and activates T cells

Effector T cells return via bloodstream and encounter antigen in both eyes

Fig. 13.13 Damage to an immunologically privileged site can induce an autoimmune response. In the disease sympathetic ophthalmia, trauma to one eye releases the sequestered eye antigens into the surrounding tissues, making them accessible to T cells. The effector cells that are elicited attack the traumatized eye, and also infiltrate and attack the healthy eye. Thus, although the sequestered antigens do not induce a response by themselves, if a response is induced elsewhere they can serve as targets for attack.

13-10 Autoreactive T cells that express particular cytokines may be nonpathogenic or suppress pathogenic lymphocytes.

In Chapter 8 we learned that during the course of normal immune responses, CD4 T cells can differentiate into two main types of cells, T_H1 and T_H2. These cells secrete different cytokines (interferon (IFN)-γ and tumor necrosis factor (TNF)-α for T_H1, and interleukin (IL)-4, IL-5, IL-10, and IL-13 for T_H2) and have different effects on antigen-presenting cells, on B cells, and on pathogen clearance. A similar paradigm holds true for autoimmunity. In particular, certain T cell-mediated diseases such as IDDM and multiple sclerosis seem to depend on T_H1 cells for disease. Conversely, in SLE, the generation of autoantibodies may require T_H2 cells, although there are T_H1 cells in this disease that are clearly directly pathogenic. In murine models of diabetes, when cytokines were infused to influence T-cell differentiation or when knockout mice that are predisposed to T_H2 differentiation were studied, diabetes was found to be inhibited. The possibility of controlling disease by changing cytokine profiles is termed immune modulation and will be discussed at greater length in Chapter 14. In some cases, potentially pathogenic T cells specific for islet-cell components, which are expressing T_H2 instead of T_H1 cytokines, are actually suppressive of disease caused by T_H1 cells of the same specificity. This and analogous situations may form the basis for the natural regulation of autoimmunity through the dominant effects of certain types of 'regulatory' cells, as we now discuss.

13-11 Autoimmune responses can be controlled at various stages by regulatory T cells.

Autoreactive cells that have broken tolerance can still be regulated so that they do not cause clinical disease. This regulation takes two forms: the first is extrinsic, coming from specific regulatory T cells that exert effects on activated T and B cells as well as on antigen-presenting cells. The second is generally intrinsic and has to do with limits on the size and duration of immune responses of clones of lymphocytes that are inherently programmed into the cells themselves. We shall first discuss the regulatory cells.

The idea of T cells that could regulate immune responses dates back to the 1970s, when many research groups reported the existence of 'T suppressor' cells. These lymphocytes were defined as being able to dominantly inhibit an autoimmune response. Suppressor cells could be induced during the process of tolerance induction, for example by giving a high dose of a soluble antigen in the absence of a pro-inflammatory stimulus. During the 1980s and 1990s the concept of suppressor cells fell out of favor when some of the data could not be reproduced and when immunologists failed to clarify the mechanisms and genetic basis of suppression.

However, very compelling evidence has recently emerged for the existence of suppressor cells—now dubbed **regulatory T cells** (T_{reg}). The reevaluation of suppressor/regulatory cells has been aided by the powerful techniques of modern immunology such as cell sorting, as well as by the greater understanding of immune-system functions that has allowed greater insight into the mechanisms of suppression. A major breakthrough came from experiments in which thymectomized neonatal mice paradoxically developed an autoimmune syndrome. This turned out to be due to the failure of a subset of regulatory T cells, notable for the expression of CD25 (the α chain of the IL-2 receptor), to develop in mice deprived of thymic function early in life. The involvement of regulatory cells was shown by experiments that transferred T cells, and subsequently just CD25 T cells, from adult mice: these cells were effective in preventing the autoimmune disease.

Fig. 13.14 Recessive tolerance occurs when self-reactive T cells are deleted, whereas a dominant form of tolerance mediated by regulatory T cells can inhibit multiple autoreactive T cells that all recognize the same tissue. The best known form of self-tolerance in the thymus results in the deletion of self-reactive T cells by thymic dendritic cells that express self antigens (upper left). However, some autoreactive cells may not be deleted because autoantigen is not available on the deleting cell (upper left, light blue cell). Such T cells can cause damage in the periphery if they encounter their self antigen on an antigen-presenting cell (APC) there (upper right). One mechanism that suppresses this potentially harmful autoreactivity is known as regulatory tolerance (lower panels). This is mediated by specialized regulatory T cells (T_{reg}) that develop in the thymus in response to weak stimulation by self antigen that is not sufficient to cause deletion but is more than required for simple positive selection (lower left). These cells migrate to the periphery where, if they encounter their self antigen (lower right), they secrete inhibitory cytokines such as IL-10 and TGF-β that inhibit all surrounding autoreactive T cells, regardless of their precise autoantigen specificity. This is a dominant form of tolerance in that a single cell can regulate many others.

This experiment illustrates the most important property of tolerance due to regulatory lymphocytes, which distinguishes it from other forms of self-tolerance: regulatory cells act on other cells, and, when mixed or transferred with self-reactive cells, can suppress their activity (Fig. 13.14). This type of tolerance is sometimes known as **regulatory tolerance**, **dominant immune suppression** or **infectious tolerance**. A key feature of dominant regulatory tolerance is that regulatory cells can suppress autoreactive lymphocytes that recognize a variety of different self antigens, as long as the antigens are all on the same tissue or expressed by the same antigen-presenting cell. Many investigators therefore believe that regulatory T cells could have therapeutic potential for the treatment of autoimmune disease if they could be isolated and infused into patients.

13-12   CD4 CD25 T cells are a unique subset of cells that arise in the thymus in response to relatively strong recognition of self antigen.

One of the best characterized and most powerful types of regulatory cell expresses both CD4 and CD25. These cells have been shown in mice to have a role in several autoimmune syndromes, including colitis, diabetes, the experimental model of multiple sclerosis EAE, and even SLE. Experiments in mouse models of these diseases show how CD4 CD25 regulatory T cells suppress disease when transferred *in vivo* and how depletion of these cells exacerbates or causes disease. In addition, these regulatory T cells have been shown to prevent or ameliorate other immunopathologic syndromes, such as graft-versus-host disease and graft rejection, which are described later in this chapter. There is even evidence that normal immune responses can be inhibited by these cells, so they may have a role in controlling the extent, duration, and perhaps even the quality of normal as well as pathologic immune responses.

How do regulatory CD4 CD25 T cells arise? They are present in greater numbers in mice with a transgenic T-cell receptor that recognizes a moderately highly expressed self antigen. This was shown experimentally by using mice expressing a T-cell receptor transgene specific for a peptide from influenza hemagglutinin. When these mice are crossed with another transgenic mouse strain that expresses the hemagglutinin itself at low levels, large numbers of

CD4 CD25 T cells develop that have suppressor function. The affinity of these cells for self must be moderate, because high-affinity self-reactive T cells would be deleted in the thymus. However, the affinity required to produce regulatory cells is clearly much higher than that needed for positive selection. Nonetheless, the selection of CD4 CD25 T cells does depend on recognition of the MHC class II:peptide complex on thymic epithelium, much like the positive selection of conventional CD4 T cells.

By mechanisms that are not yet entirely clear, when CD4 T cells receive this intermediate level of signaling they are induced to express, or to keep on expressing, a gene called *FoxP3*, which encodes a transcription factor that is essential for their differentiation into regulatory CD4 CD25 T cells. How FoxP3 controls differentiation is unknown, but it seems to influence the expression of CD25 itself, as well as of IL-10, an important effector cytokine produced by these regulatory T cells. A rare and severe human autoimmune disease called **IPEX** (immunodysregulation, polyendocrinopathy, and enteropathy, X-linked) has been attributed to a lack of FoxP3, and a similar syndrome is seen in mutant *scurfy* mice, which are deficient in FoxP3. These mice lack CD4 CD25 T cells altogether, but autoimmune disease can be prevented if CD4 CD25 T cells from normal mice are transferred to them at birth. The existence of the human disease and the evidence from the mutant mouse strain establish the crucial role of CD4 CD25 cells in preventing autoimmune disease.

13-13 The mechanisms of regulation are varied and can include cytokine-mediated inhibition, contact-dependent regulation, and cell killing.

In addition to their ability to prevent autoimmune disease *in vivo*, regulatory CD4 CD25 T cells can suppress antigen-specific T-cell proliferation and T-cell proliferation in response to allogeneic stimulator cells *in vitro*. These *in vitro* experiments have shed light on the mechanisms of regulatory T-cell function, although there is still some controversy in this evolving research field. Some of these *in vitro* experiments suggest that regulatory T cells function by directly contacting the target cells that they suppress. However, others suggest that regulatory T cells function by secreting IL-10 and TGF-β, both of which are cytokines that can inhibit T-cell proliferation (see Fig. 13.14). These cytokines in turn may act on the proliferating activated T cells, but there is also evidence they can act on antigen-presenting cells and dendritic cells. In the latter case, IL-10 can affect the differentiation of dendritic cells, inhibiting the secretion of IL-12 and thus impairing the ability of the dendritic cells to promote T-cell activation and T$_H$1 differentiation. *In vivo* also it seems that the secretion of IL-10 and, in some cases, TGF-β are of paramount importance for effective suppression. In any case, it is likely that CD4 CD25 regulatory T cells have multiple mechanisms of mediating suppression, and which ones are important may depend on the biological situation. The potential regulatory mechanisms of these T cells are illustrated by a proposed model for how they cause the resolution of autoimmune colitis in mice (Fig. 13.15).

Among the many controversies concerning regulatory T cells is how they are 'activated' *in vivo* to express their regulatory function. They have conventional α:β T-cell receptors, but whether they are activated by the same ligands that selected them in the thymus or by other self or nonself ligands is simply not clear. Indeed, it is not entirely clear that they need to receive any specific activating signal through their T-cell receptor. *In vitro*, however, regulatory T cells do need to be activated to exert their function; this has been achieved with an antibody against CD3 to stimulate these cells nonspecifically, because the ligands are not known.

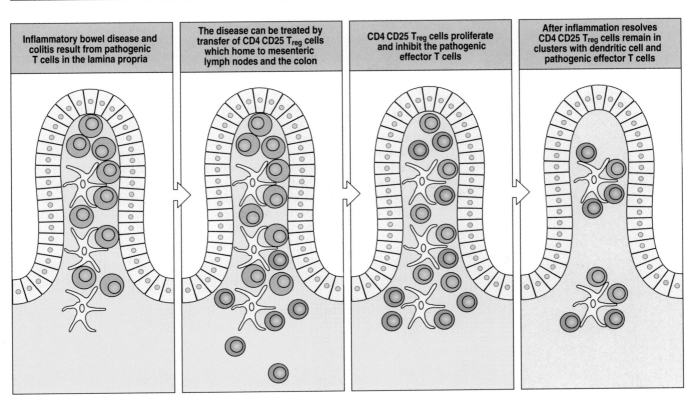

| Inflammatory bowel disease and colitis result from pathogenic T cells in the lamina propria | The disease can be treated by transfer of CD4 CD25 T$_{reg}$ cells which home to mesenteric lymph nodes and the colon | CD4 CD25 T$_{reg}$ cells proliferate and inhibit the pathogenic effector T cells | After inflammation resolves CD4 CD25 T$_{reg}$ cells remain in clusters with dendritic cell and pathogenic effector T cells |

Fig. 13.15 CD4 CD25 regulatory T cells inhibit colitis by migrating to the colon and mesenteric lymph nodes, where they interact with dendritic and effector T cells. Naive T cells that contain some autoreactive clones (see Fig. 13.14) cause colitis when transferred to T-cell-deficient mice (first panel, enlarged pink cells). The naive population lacks CD4 CD25 T$_{reg}$, but if these are also transferred along with the naive T cells (second panel; blue cells are T$_{reg}$), colitis is blocked. The blocking mechanism includes migration of the T$_{reg}$ to mesenteric lymph nodes (not shown) and later to the lamina propria of the colon. The T$_{reg}$ cells proliferate and secrete regulatory cytokines (third panel), including IL-10, which is essential, and interact with both dendritic and autoreactive T cells, reducing activation (indicated by the smaller size of the pink cells) and ultimately reducing inflammation. Once inflammation has been quelled, regulatory T cells remain in the lamina propria (fourth panel). Based on a figure by F. Powrie.

13-14 Other types of regulatory cell also exist.

CD4 CD25 T cells are not the only type of regulatory cell that has been found. In addition to these CD25-positive cells, there are other types of regulatory T cell that are CD25-negative. These include the T$_H$3 and T$_R$1 cells found in the mucosal immune system (see Section 10-21). CD25-negative CD4 T cells with powerful regulatory activity have been found in several instances, including mouse models of diabetes and EAE.

T$_H$3 cells produce IL-4, IL-10, and TGF-β; they are distinguished from T$_H$2 cells by their production of TGF-β. A similar population secretes TGF-β but not IL-4, and is referred to as T$_R$1 (T regulatory 1) cells. These latter cells can be cultured *in vitro* in the presence of high concentrations of IL-10.

The natural origin of both these cell types is not clear. They are found in the mucosal immune system and seem to function to suppress or control immune responses at these sites, which form barriers to the pathogen-laden world. Lack of these cells is linked to autoimmune disease in the gut, and T$_R$1 cells can suppress inflammatory bowel disease in mice. Giving animals large amounts of self antigen orally, which induces so-called oral tolerance (see Section 10-17), can sometimes lead to unresponsiveness to these antigens when given by other routes and can prevent autoimmune disease. Induction of oral tolerance leads to the generation or expansion of T_R1 and/or T_H3 cells, which could have a role in this mechanism.

CD4 T cells are not the only cells to display regulatory activity. Natural killer (NK) cells have been shown to exert a regulatory function, for example in diabetes. NK T cells can also have a regulatory role. CD8 cells can sometimes demonstrate regulatory function, either by cytokine secretion or by direct cytotoxic effects on target cells. Even B cells can regulate experimentally induced autoimmune syndromes, including collagen-induced arthritis and EAE in mice. This regulatory activity is probably mediated in a similar way to that of regulatory CD4 T cells, with the secretion of cytokines that inhibit proliferation and T_H1 differentiation being of major importance. In regulatory B cells, for example, experiments have shown that B cell-derived IL-10 was required for suppression.

13-15 Immune responses have natural brakes that tend to limit damage even when autoimmune cells are activated.

In addition to the extrinsic regulation of autoreactive T and B cells by regulatory cells, lymphocytes have intrinsic limits to proliferation and survival that can help to restrict autoimmune responses as well as normal immune responses. All immune responses end in the death of most of the responding cells, leaving only a small number of resting memory cells (see Chapter 10). This process is sometimes termed **activation-induced cell death**. Activated and effector lymphocytes are notably sensitive to apoptosis throughout their life, as in the case of germinal center B cells or plasmablasts (see Section 9-7). Continuous signals from antigen are likely to have a role in regulating the size and duration of responses, but there is also a natural tendency of responding cells to die. The regulation of the tendency to die involves both the inherent death pathways of all cells as well as sensitivity to extrinsic signals such as Fas ligand, which triggers cell death in activated cells expressing the TNF-receptor family member Fas.

At first glance it is not obvious that this propensity to die helps to control autoimmunity. However, mutations in the pathways that control apoptosis, such as the Bcl-2 pathway or the Fas pathway, lead to spontaneous autoimmunity, as we shall see later in this chapter. Although the mechanism that causes autoimmunity in apoptosis-deficient mice is not completely understood, this autoimmunity does indicate that autoreactive cells are normally generated but then controlled by apoptosis. This is evidently important for both T and B cells.

Summary.

The immune system has a remarkable set of mechanisms that work together to prevent autoimmune disease. These are summarized in Fig. 13.16. This layered approach has the advantage that each layer can compensate for failures of the others. Thus, each layer need not work perfectly nor apply to every possible self-reactive cell. Layers of self-tolerance begin during lymphocyte development, exemplified by deletion of autoreactive T cells in the thymus and B cells in the bone marrow. Because not all self antigens are expressed in the central lymphoid organs, mechanisms of peripheral tolerance, such as peripheral anergy and deletion, exist to complement the central tolerance mechanisms. These are termed 'recessive' mechanisms of tolerance because each autoreactive cell is dealt with individually and its fate does not affect other autoreactive cells (see Fig. 13.14). Weakly self-reactive lymphocytes are

Layers of self-tolerance		
Type of tolerance	**Mechanism**	**Site of action**
Central tolerance	Deletion Editing	Thymus Bone marrow
Antigen segregation	Physical barrier to self-antigen access to lymphoid system	Peripheral organs (eg, thyroid, pancreas)
Peripheral anergy	Cellular inactivation by weak signaling without co-stimulus	Secondary lymphoid tissue
Regulatory cells	Suppression by cytokines, intercellular signals	Secondary lymphoid tissue and sites of inflammation
Cytokine deviation	Differentiation to T_H2 cells, limiting inflammatory cytokine secretion	Secondary lymphoid tissue and sites of inflammation
Clonal exhaustion	Apoptosis post-activation	Secondary lymphoid tissue and sites of inflammation

Fig. 13.16 Self-tolerance is a phenomenon that depends on the concerted action of a variety of mechanisms that operate at different sites and stages of development. Listed are the different ways in which the immune system prevents activation of and damage caused by autoreactive lymphocytes, along with the specific mechanism and where such tolerance predominantly occurs.

not specifically tolerized; extending recessive tolerance mechanisms such as deletion to weakly autoreactive cells would impose too great a limitation on the immune repertoire, resulting in impaired immune responses to pathogens. Instead, other mechanisms to regulate weakly self-reactive cells have evolved that supervene only after these cells are activated. One such mechanism is immune modulation, which refers to the differentiation of T cells to express noninflammatory T_H2 cytokines. In addition, T cells exist that can dominantly regulate autoreactive T and B cells. One major regulatory cell type expresses CD4 and CD25. These regulatory T cells have been shown to regulate a variety of pathogenic autoimmune syndromes and probably work by multiple mechanisms. They are physiologically important, because fairly severe autoimmunity occurs in their absence. It is unclear what activates regulatory T cells, but it is likely that the CD4 CD25 cells are themselves autoreactive, although not pathogenic. Regulatory T cells mediate dominant immune suppression, because in their presence a variety of self-reactive lymphocytes can be inhibited, as long as the regulatory cells are targeting autoantigens located in the same general vicinity of the autoantigens to which the self-reactive lymphocytes respond. In this way the ability of the regulatory cells to recognize autoantigens for the activation of regulatory functions allows them to effectively home to and suppress sites of autoimmune inflammation. A final mechanism that controls autoimmunity is the natural tendency of immune responses to be self-limited. There are inborn programs in activated lymphocytes that make them prone to apoptosis. Activated lymphocytes also acquire sensitivity to external apoptosis-inducing signals, such as those mediated by Fas. In the next section we discuss how both genetic defects and environmental insults can specifically undermine the layers of tolerance to generate autoimmune disease.

The genetic and environmental basis of autoimmunity.

Given the complex and varied mechanisms that exist to prevent autoimmunity, it is not surprising that autoimmune diseases are the result of multiple factors, both genetic and environmental. In this section we discuss some of these. We first discuss the genetic basis of autoimmunity, attempting to understand how genetic defects perturb the various tolerance mechanisms. Genetic defects alone are not always sufficient to cause autoimmune disease. Environmental factors, such as toxins, drugs, and infections, also have a role, and some environmental factors have not yet been identified. As we shall see, genetic and environmental factors together can overcome tolerance mechanisms and result in autoimmune disease.

13-16 Autoimmune diseases have a strong genetic as well as environmental component.

Although the causes of autoimmunity are still being worked out, it is clear that some individuals are genetically predisposed to autoimmunity. Perhaps the clearest demonstration of this is several inbred mouse strains that are prone to various types of autoimmunity. For example, mice of the NOD (non-obese diabetic) strain are very likely to get diabetes. In fact, the female mice become diabetic more quickly than the males (Fig. 13.17). Many autoimmune diseases are more common in females than in males (see Fig. 13.20), although occasionally the opposite is true. Autoimmune diseases in humans also have a genetic component. Some autoimmune diseases, including IDDM, run in families, suggesting that inherited genes have a role. Most convincingly, if one of two identical twins is affected, then the other twin is quite likely to be as well.

However, environmental influences are also clearly involved. For example, although most of a colony of NOD mice are destined to get diabetes, they will do so at different ages (see Fig. 13.17). Moreover, the kinetics of disease onset often differ from one investigator's animal colony to the next. This is true even though all of the mice are genetically identical. Thus, environmental variables must be in part determining which animals are becoming diabetic first; a few even escape the disease entirely. Identical twins tell a similar story. With SLE, although disease occurs in both twins in a quarter to half of twins affected—a rate vastly higher than the normal chance of getting SLE—one can wonder why the concordance rate is so far from 100%. Again, the answer must lie in environmental variables. We know very little about what external factors interact with genetic predisposition to cause autoimmune disease. It has been suggested that exposure to infections or to toxins, or even just random chance, could explain why some but not all genetically identical individuals get the same autoimmune disease.

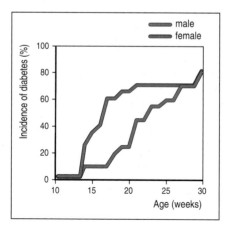

Fig. 13.17 Sex difference in the incidence of autoimmune disease. Many autoimmune diseases are more common in females than males, as illustrated here by the cumulative incidence of diabetes in a population of diabetes-prone NOD mice. Females (red line) get diabetes at a much younger age than do males, indicating their greater predisposition. Data kindly provided by S. Wong.

13-17 Several approaches have given us insight into the genetic basis of autoimmunity.

Predisposition to most of the common autoimmune diseases is due to the combined effects of multiple genes, and there is tremendous interest in identifying these genes. But this has proved difficult. With the use of information from genome sequencing and gene mapping, strategies have now been developed to define the chromosomal locations of genes that contribute to autoimmunity (Fig. 13.18). This is mainly practicable in animals, where large numbers of experimental crosses can be done between a normal strain and one prone to autoimmunity. The degree of autoimmunity in each of the progeny of a backcross can then be correlated with the alleles it has inherited at particular polymorphic loci, such as those of the MHC. This painstaking approach requires many further crosses to isolate each individual gene of interest and to identify its effects. If all goes well, genome sequence information can finally be used to pinpoint a few potential disease-causing genes. To complete such a study, each potential disease gene in the normal and autoimmune-prone strains needs to be sequenced, and this might identify a mutation that is clearly leading to the dysfunction of an important gene. Unfortunately, in some cases, although a genetic locus involved in autoimmunity has been identified, it is not obvious how the differences at this locus between the normal and autoimmune strains cause autoimmunity. Nevertheless, great progress is being made in elucidating the genes responsible for mouse models of SLE and diabetes, and a few candidate genes have been identified.

In some cases, in both humans and experimental animal models, a single gene is responsible for an autoimmune syndrome. This was first realized from the study of naturally occurring mutants. The inheritance of autoimmune syndromes due to such mutations follows a pattern that is consistent with a single gene causing the disease. These genes can be either recessive or dominant, and they are relatively easy to identify. One example of an autoimmune disease caused by a defect in a single gene is the APECED syndrome (see Section 13-7). Another interesting case is the systemic autoimmunity syndrome caused by mutations in the *Fas* gene. Normally, the Fas protein is expressed on activated T and B cells, and when it is ligated it signals a cell to undergo apoptosis. In this way it functions to limit the extent of immune responses. Mutations that eliminate or inactivate the Fas protein lead to an accumulation of lymphocytes, especially T cells, and the production of large quantities of pathogenic autoantibodies. The disease resembles SLE, though

Autoimmune Polyglandular Syndrome

Fig. 13.18 Different types of genetic predispositions in autoimmune disease. Genetics has an important role in determining who will get certain types of autoimmune diseases, as illustrated by these examples. In humans and in animal models, disease is sometimes mediated by a single gene, which has been discovered by relatively straightforward genetic mapping. In other cases, many genes together cause the predisposition; in this case more complex means have been used to try to identify them, with only some success as yet. Another approach to identifying genes that could promote autoimmunity applies only to animal models—experimentally induced mutations in key molecules of the immune system have sometimes led to autoimmune syndromes.

Genetic defect	Examples	Approach
Spontaneous single-gene mutation	Fas (ALPS), AIRE	Backcrossing or family tree studies to map, then positional cloning
Multigenic predisposition	NOD mice (diabetes) Diabetic people NZM2410 mice (lupus)	Genome-wide mapping in families or F2 crosses, then positional cloning
Induced mutation	C1q knockout (lupus) CD22 knockout (lupus) CTLA-4 knockout (multisystem autoimmunity)	Knockouts in mice

Autoimmune
Lymphoproliferative
Syndrome

SLE itself is not caused by mutations in Fas. The role of Fas mutations in autoimmunity was first understood in a spontaneous mutant observed in the mouse strain MRL that was dubbed *lpr*, for lymphoproliferation. Later, researchers studying a rare group of human patients with **autoimmune lymphoproliferative syndrome** (**ALPS**) were able to identify and clone the mutant gene responsible for most of the cases, which also turned out to be that for Fas. The syndrome in humans turned out to be remarkably similar to that in the MRL/*lpr* mouse strain.

Autoimmune diseases caused by single genes are not common. Nonetheless, it is very interesting to know their basis because the mutations that cause such syndromes can provide clues to the genetic pathways that might be disrupted in the more subtle mutations that contribute to multigenic autoimmune diseases.

So far we have discussed naturally occurring mutations that lead to autoimmunity. Since the advent of gene knockout technology in mice, many genes that function in the immune system have been experimentally disrupted. Several of these experimental mutant strains have signs of autoimmune disease, including autoantibodies and, in some cases, T cells infiltrating organs. The study of such strains has greatly expanded our knowledge of the genetic pathways that can potentially contribute to autoimmunity and that therefore might be candidates for naturally occurring mutations.

13-18 Genes that predispose to autoimmunity fall into categories that affect one or more of the layers of tolerance.

Most of the genes identified as predisposing to autoimmunity fall into one of several classes: genes that affect autoantigen availability and clearance, those that affect apoptosis, those that affect signaling thresholds, those involved in cytokine gene expression, and those affecting the expression of costimulatory molecules (Fig. 13.19). The exact details of how mutations in these various categories promote autoimmunity are usually not clear, but it is possible to discuss the general reasons why multiple genes in these pathways are targets.

Genes that control antigen availability and clearance are important either in making self proteins available for inducing tolerance in developing lymphocytes, as with the AIRE gene, or in controlling how self molecules are made available in an immunogenic form to peripheral lymphocytes. In the latter case, some genes might control the expression levels or sites of tissue-specific autoantigens, making them more available than normal. Other genes in this category, such as those for C1q, C3, and C4 of the complement pathway, are important in clearing apoptotic cells and immune complexes. Evidently, if apoptotic cells and immune complexes are not cleared promptly they can be immunogenic for low-affinity self-reactive lymphocytes in the periphery. Genes that control apoptosis, such as *Fas*, are important in regulating the duration and vigor of immune responses. Failure to regulate immune responses properly could cause excessive destruction of self tissues, releasing autoantigens. In addition, because clonal deletion and anergy are not absolute, immune responses can include some self-reactive cells. As long as their numbers are limited by apoptotic mechanisms, they may not be sufficient to cause autoimmune disease, but they could cause a problem if apoptosis is not properly regulated.

Perhaps the largest category of mutations associated with autoimmunity are those associated with signals that control lymphocyte activation. One subset comprises mutations that inactivate negative regulators of lymphocyte activation and lead to the hyperproliferation of lymphocytes and exaggerated immune responses. These include mutations in inhibitory Fc receptors and

Proposed mechanism	Murine models	Disease phenotype	Human gene affected	Disease phenotype
Antigen clearance and presentation	C1q knockout	Lupus-like	C1q	Lupus-like
	C4 knockout		C2 C4	
	Serum amyloid P knockout		Mannan-binding lectin	
	AIRE knockout	Multiorgan autoimmunity resembling APECED	AIRE	APECED
	DNase I knockout	Lupus-like	DNase I	Lupus-like
	Mer knockout			
Signaling	SHP-1 knockout	Lupus-like	TCRζ chain	Lupus-like
	Lyn knockout		TNF-α	
	CD22 knockout			
	CD45 E613R point mutation			
	B cells deficient in all Src-family kinases (triple knockout)			
	Fc-γRIIB knockout (inhibitory signaling molecule)			
Co-stimulatory molecules	CTLA-4 knockout (blocks inhibitory signal)	Lymphocyte infiltration into organs		
	PD-1 knockout (blocks inhibitory signal)	Lupus-like		
	BAFF overexpression (transgenic mouse)			
Apoptosis	Fas knockout (lpr)	Lupus-like with lymphocyte infiltrates	Fas and FasL mutations (ALPS syndrome)	Lupus-like with lymphocyte infiltrates
	FasL knockout (gld)			
	Bcl-2 overexpression (transgenic mouse)	Lupus-like		
	Pten heterozygous deficiency			
Cytokines	IL-2 knockout	Inflammatory bowel disease (gene polymorphism associated with diabetes)		
	IL-10 knockout	Inflammatory bowel disease		

Fig. 13.19 Categories of genetic defects that lead to autoimmune syndromes. With the approaches shown in Fig. 13.18, many genes have been identified in which mutations predispose to autoimmunity in humans and animal models. These are best understood by the type of process affected by the genetic defect. A comprehensive list of such genes is given here, organized by process (see the text for further discussion). In some cases the same gene has been identified in mice and humans. In other cases different genes affecting the same mechanism are implicated in mice and humans. The smaller number of human genes identified so far undoubtedly reflects the difficulty of identifying these in outbred human populations.

receptors containing ITIMs (see Section 6-16), such as CD22 on B cells. Another category of mutations comprises those involved in signal transduction through the antigen receptor itself. Adjusting thresholds in either direction, to make signaling more or less sensitive, can result in autoimmunity, depending on the situation. A decrease in sensitivity in the thymus, for example, can lead to a failure of negative selection and thereby to autoreactivity in the periphery. In contrast, increasing receptor sensitivity in the periphery can lead to greater and prolonged activation, again resulting in an exaggerated immune response with the side-effect of autoimmunity. Inappropriately regulated expression of genes for cytokines and co-stimulatory molecules is yet another example of how failure to control the immune response causes autoimmunity. A particularly interesting example of this involves the protein CTLA-4, a member of the CD28 family that binds to CD80 (B7.1) and CD86 (B7.2) and transduces an inhibitory signal to T cells. When the gene for CTLA-4 is knocked out in mice, a severe and lethal lymphoproliferative autoimmune syndrome results.

13-19 MHC genes have an important role in controlling susceptibility to autoimmune disease.

Among all the genetic loci that could contribute to autoimmunity, susceptibility to autoimmune disease has so far been most consistently associated with MHC genotype. Human autoimmune diseases that show associations with HLA type are shown in Fig. 13.20. For most of these diseases, susceptibility is linked most strongly with MHC class II alleles, but in some cases there are strong associations with particular MHC class I alleles.

Fig. 13.20 Associations of HLA serotype and sex with susceptibility to autoimmune disease. The 'relative risk' for an HLA allele in an autoimmune disease is calculated by comparing the observed number of patients carrying the HLA allele with the number that would be expected, given the prevalence of the HLA allele in the general population. For type I insulin-dependent diabetes mellitus, the association is in fact with the HLA-DQ gene, which is tightly linked to the DR genes but is not detectable by serotyping. Some diseases show a significant bias in the sex ratio; this is taken to imply that sex hormones are involved in pathogenesis. Consistent with this, the difference in the sex ratio in these diseases is greatest between the menarche and the menopause, when levels of such hormones are highest.

Associations of HLA serotype with susceptibility to autoimmune disease			
Disease	HLA allele	Relative risk	Sex ratio (♀:♂)
Ankylosing spondylitis	B27	87.4	0.3
Acute anterior uveitis	B27	10	< 0.5
Goodpasture's syndrome	DR2	15.9	~1
Multiple sclerosis	DR2	4.8	10
Graves' disease	DR3	3.7	4–5
Myasthenia gravis	DR3	2.5	~1
Systemic lupus erythematosus	DR3	5.8	10–20
Type I insulin-dependent diabetes mellitus	DR3/DR4 heterozygote	~25	~1
Rheumatoid arthritis	DR4	4.2	3
Pemphigus vulgaris	DR4	14.4	~1
Hashimoto's thyroiditis	DR5	3.2	4–5

Fig. 13.21 Population studies show association of susceptibility to IDDM with HLA genotype. The HLA genotypes (determined by serotyping) of diabetic patients (bottom panel) are not representative of those found in the population (top panel). Almost all diabetic patients express HLA-DR3 and/or HLA-DR4, and HLA-DR3/DR4 heterozygosity is greatly over-represented in diabetics compared with controls. These alleles are linked tightly to HLA-DQ alleles that confer susceptibility to IDDM. By contrast, HLA-DR2 protects against the development of IDDM and is found only extremely rarely in diabetic patients. The small letter x represents any allele other than DR2, DR3, or DR4.

The association of MHC genotype with disease is assessed initially by comparing the frequency of different alleles in patients with their frequency in the normal population. For IDDM, this approach originally demonstrated an association with the HLA-DR3 and HLA-DR4 alleles identified by serotyping (Fig. 13.21). Such studies also showed that the MHC class II allele HLA-DR2 has a dominant protective effect: individuals carrying HLA-DR2, even in association with one of the susceptibility alleles, rarely develop diabetes. Another way of determining whether MHC genes are important in autoimmune disease is to study the families of affected patients; it has been shown that two siblings affected with the same autoimmune disease are far more likely than expected to share the same MHC haplotypes (Fig. 13.22).

As HLA genotyping has become more exact through the DNA sequencing of HLA alleles, disease associations that were originally discovered through HLA serotyping have been defined more precisely. For example, the association between IDDM and the DR3 and DR4 alleles is now known to be due to their tight genetic linkage to DQβ alleles that actually confer susceptibility to the disease. Indeed, susceptibility is most closely associated with polymorphisms at a particular position in the DQβ amino acid sequence. The most common DQβ amino acid sequence has an aspartic acid residue at position 57 that is able to form a salt bridge across the end of the peptide-binding cleft of the DQ molecule. In contrast, diabetic patients in Caucasoid populations mostly have valine, serine, or alanine at that position, and thus make DQ molecules that lack this salt bridge (Fig. 13.23). The NOD strain of mice, which develops spontaneous diabetes, also has a serine at that position in the homologous mouse MHC class II molecule, known as I-A^{g7}.

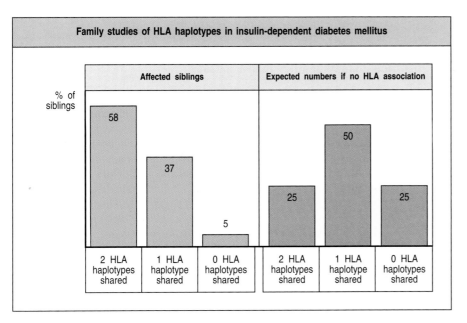

Fig. 13.22 Family studies show strong linkage of susceptibility to IDDM with HLA genotype. In families in which two or more siblings have IDDM, it is possible to compare the HLA genotypes of affected siblings. Affected siblings share two HLA haplotypes much more frequently than would be expected if the HLA genotype did not influence disease susceptibility.

Position 57 of the DQβ chain affects susceptibility to insulin-dependent diabetes mellitus (IDDM)

α chain

Position 57

β chain

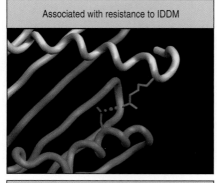

Associated with resistance to IDDM

Associated with susceptibility to IDDM

Fig. 13.23 Amino acid changes in the sequence of an MHC class II protein correlate with susceptibility to and protection from diabetes. The HLA-DQβ₁ chain contains an aspartic acid (Asp) residue at position 57 in most people; in Caucasoid populations, patients with IDDM more often have valine, serine, or alanine at this position instead, as well as other differences. Asp 57, shown in red on the backbone structure of the DQβ chain, forms a salt bridge (shown in green in the center panel) to an arginine residue (shown in pink) in the adjacent α chain (gray). The change to an uncharged residue (for example, alanine, shown in yellow in the bottom panel) disrupts this salt bridge, altering the stability of the DQ molecule. The non-obese diabetic (NOD) strain of mice, which develops spontaneous diabetes, shows a similar substitution of serine for aspartic acid at position 57 of the homologous I-Aβ chain, and NOD mice transgenic for β chains with Asp 57 have a marked reduction in diabetes incidence. Courtesy of C. Thorpe.

The association of MHC genotype with autoimmune disease is not surprising, because autoimmune responses involve T cells, and the ability of T cells to respond to a particular antigen depends on MHC genotype. Thus, the associations can be explained by a simple model in which susceptibility to an autoimmune disease is determined by differences in the ability of different allelic variants of MHC molecules to present autoantigenic peptides to autoreactive T cells. This would be consistent with what we know of T-cell involvement in particular diseases. In diabetes, for example, there are associations with both MHC class I and MHC class II alleles, and this is consistent with the finding that both CD8 and CD4 T cells, which respond to antigens presented by MHC class I and MHC class II molecules, respectively, mediate the autoimmune response.

An alternative hypothesis for the association between MHC genotype and susceptibility to autoimmune diseases emphasizes the role of MHC alleles in shaping the T-cell receptor repertoire (see Chapter 7). This hypothesis proposes that self peptides associated with certain MHC molecules may drive the positive selection of developing thymocytes that are specific for particular autoantigens. Such autoantigenic peptides might be expressed at too low a level or bind too poorly to self MHC molecules to drive negative selection in the thymus, but might be present at a sufficient level or bind strongly enough to drive positive selection. This hypothesis is supported by observations that I-A^{g7}, the disease-associated MHC class II molecule in NOD mice, binds many peptides very poorly and may therefore be less effective in driving intrathymic negative selection of T cells that bind self peptides.

13-20 Molecular pathways promoting autoimmunity are potential targets for the therapy of autoimmune disease.

The identification of genes that are important in promoting autoimmunity has several implications. First, it might help in the diagnosis or prognosis of autoimmune disease and eventually might identify individuals at risk who could benefit from medical intervention before disease starts. Second, it could suggest new therapeutic strategies. Figure 13.24 summarizes several of the strategies that are either being developed in animal models or are already being tried in people. Blockade of co-stimulatory molecule signals has been effective in a number of animal models. One established therapy, the immunosuppressant cyclosporin A (see Section 14-3), exerts its effect by blocking IL-2-mediated T-cell activation. To treat organ-specific autoimmunity, it may be possible to induce regulatory T cells that are specific for critical autoantigens and that could suppress T cells of a variety of autoreactive specificities for the same organ (see Section 13-11). However, manipulation of most of the pathways that are now being elucidated has not yet been developed into therapies. This offers many possibilities in the future for treating autoimmune diseases of all types.

Fig. 13.24 Therapeutic approaches to treating autoimmunity based on genetic and mechanistic insights into disease. New treatment strategies for autoimmunity are emerging that are based on the knowledge that has been gained about the mechanisms of self-tolerance and how they break down in disease, as well as the genetic basis for autoimmunity. Several pathways or mechanisms that can be manipulated to control autoimmune disease are listed on the left and the specific strategies in clinical or preclinical use are given on the right.

Therapeutic approaches to treating autoimmunity	
Genetic/pathogenic pathway	Strategy
Co-stimulatory molecules	B7 blockade (CTLA-4-Ig) CD40L blockade (anti-CD40L) BAFF blockade (soluble receptor or antibody)
T_{reg}	Induction of self-antigen-specific T_{reg} clones for infection
Antigen clearance	Immune complex removal DNase to break up chromatin in SLE
Antigen presentation/ autoantibody secretion	B-cell depletion (with anti-CD20)
Cytokine polarization	Cytokine treatment Oral tolerization to induce cytokine deviation
Inflammatory mediators	Blockade of TNF-α (soluble receptor or antibody)

13-21 Drugs and toxins can cause autoimmune syndromes.

Perhaps some of the clearest evidence of causative agents in human autoimmunity comes from the effects of certain drugs, which elicit autoimmune reactions as side-effects in a small proportion of patients. Procainamide, a drug used to treat arrhythmias, is particularly notable for inducing lupus-like autoantibodies, though these are rarely pathogenic. Several drugs are associated with the development of autoimmune hemolytic anemia (see Section 13-26), in which autoantibodies against surface components of red blood cells attack and destroy these cells. Toxins in the environment can also cause autoimmunity. When heavy metals, such as gold or mercury, are administered to genetically susceptible strains of mice, a predictable autoimmune syndrome, including the production of autoantibodies, ensues. The extent to which heavy metals promote autoimmunity in humans is debatable, but the animal models clearly show that environmental factors such as toxins could have key roles in certain syndromes.

The mechanisms by which drugs and toxins cause autoimmunity are uncertain. However, for certain drugs it is thought that they react chemically with self proteins and form derivatives that the immune system recognizes as foreign. The immune response to these haptenated self proteins can lead to inflammation, complement deposition, destruction of tissue, and finally to immune responses to the original underivatized self proteins.

13-22 Infection can lead to autoimmune disease.

The inflammation that accompanies an infection leads both to tissue destruction and the release of soluble inflammatory mediators such as cytokines and chemokines. During an infection and the consequent immune response, the combination of the release of inflammatory mediators and increased expression of co-stimulatory molecules can have effects on so-called 'bystander' cells—lymphocytes that are not themselves specific for the antigens of the infectious agent. Self-reactive lymphocytes can become activated in these circumstances, particularly if tissue destruction leads to an increase in the availability of self antigen.

Many pathogens also have specific mechanisms that lead to immune-system dysregulation. By preventing the apoptosis of lymphocytes or by secreting their own cytokines, pathogens can alter the normal balance of the immune system. In all these ways, infection can initiate autoimmunity. In most cases it is transient and ends when the infection is cleared. However, it may be sustained in genetically susceptible individuals, for the reasons discussed in Section 13-18. For sustained autoimmunity to occur, it may take a particularly severe infection or combination of infections, or it may result from the cumulative effect of multiple infections. This is a good example of how environment interacts with the genetic background to promote autoimmune disease.

13-23 Cross-reactivity between self molecules and foreign molecules on pathogens can lead to anti-self responses and autoimmune disease.

Infection with particular pathogens is associated with autoimmune sequelae. By chance or design some pathogens express protein or carbohydrate antigens that resemble host molecules, a phenomenon dubbed **molecular mimicry**. In such cases, antibodies produced against a pathogen epitope may cross-react with a self protein. A peptide expressed by the pathogen that was identical or similar to a host peptide could elicit T-cell responses that would recognize host tissues. A model system to demonstrate molecular mimicry has been generated by using transgenic mice that express a viral antigen in the pancreas. Normally, there is no response to this virus-derived 'self' antigen. However, diabetes is induced after infection with the virus that was the source of the transgenic antigen, because the virus activates T cells that are cross-reactive with the 'self' viral antigen (Fig. 13.25).

One might wonder why the self-reactive B or T cells had not been deleted or inactivated by the usual mechanisms of self-tolerance. First, as discussed in Section 13-8, lower-affinity self-reactive B and T cells are not efficiently removed and are present in the naive lymphocyte repertoire. Second, the strong pro-inflammatory stimulus that accompanies an infection could be sufficient to activate even anergic T and B cells in the periphery, thus drawing into the response cells that would usually be silent. Third, pathogens may provide substantially higher local doses of the eliciting antigen in an immunogenic form, whereas normally these would be relatively unavailable to lymphocytes. Some examples of autoimmune syndromes that fit this pattern are **post-streptococcal glomerulonephritis**, **autoimmune hemolytic anemia** after infection with Epstein–Barr virus or mycoplasma, and **rheumatic fever**.

Once self-reactive lymphocytes are activated by such a mechanism, their effector functions can destroy self tissues. Autoimmunity of this type is sometimes transient and remits when the inciting pathogen is eliminated. This is the case in anemia that follows mycoplasma infection, in which case antibodies against the pathogen cross-react with an antigen on red blood cells, leading to their destruction. Recovery from infection leads to the loss of these

Autoimmune Hemolytic Anemia

Rheumatic Fever

Fig. 13.25 Virus infection can break tolerance to a transgenic viral protein expressed in pancreatic β cells. Mice made transgenic for the lymphocytic choriomeningitis virus (LCMV) nucleoprotein under the control of the rat insulin promoter express the nucleoprotein in their pancreatic β cells but do not respond to this protein and therefore do not develop an autoimmune diabetes. However, if the transgenic mice are infected with LCMV, a potent antiviral cytotoxic T-cell response is elicited, and this kills the β cells, leading to diabetes. It is thought that infectious agents can sometimes elicit T-cell responses that cross-react with self peptides (a process known as molecular mimicry) and that this could cause autoimmune disease in a similar way.

Mechanism	Disruption of cell or tissue barrier	Infection of antigen-presenting cell	Binding of pathogen to self protein	Molecular mimicry	Superantigen
Effect	Release of sequestered self antigen; activation of nontolerized cells	Release of inflammatory mediators, notably IFN-α	Pathogen acts as carrier to allow anti-self response	Production of cross-reactive antibodies or T cells	Polyclonal activation of autoreactive T cells
Example	Sympathetic ophthalmia	? SLE	? Interstitial nephritis ? SLE	Rheumatic fever ? Diabetes ? Multiple sclerosis	? Rheumatoid arthritis

autoantibodies. However, sometimes autoimmunity goes on well after the initial cross-reactive pathogen infected the host. This is true in some cases of **rheumatic fever**, a disease in which cross-reaction with streptococcal components after infection leads to antibody-mediated and possibly T cell-mediated damage to a variety of tissues, including heart valves. Although rheumatic fever is often transient, especially with antibiotic treatment, it can sometimes become chronic. Similarly, Lyme disease, an infection with the spirochete *Borrelia burgdorferi*, is followed by later-developing autoimmunity. In this case, the mechanism is not entirely clear, but it is likely to involve cross-reactivity of pathogen and host components, leading to a self-perpetuating autoimmune reaction. Thus, infectious agents can break self-tolerance and cause autoimmunity by a variety of mechanisms (Fig. 13.26).

13-24 Random events may be required for the initiation of autoimmunity.

Although scientists and physicians would like to attribute the onset of 'spontaneous' diseases to some specific cause, this may not always be possible. There may not be one virus or bacterium, or even any understandable pattern of events, that precedes the onset of autoimmune disease. The chance encounter in the peripheral lymphoid tissues of a few autoreactive B and T cells that can interact with each other, at just the moment when an infection is providing pro-inflammatory signals, may be all that is needed. This could be a rare event, and in a genetically resistant individual it could even be brought under control. But in a susceptible individual such events could be more frequent and/or more difficult to control.

Thus, the onset or incidence of autoimmunity can seem to be random. Genetic predisposition in part represents an increased chance of occurrence of this random event. This view, in turn, may explain why many autoimmune diseases appear in early adulthood or later, after enough time has elapsed to allow for a low-frequency random event to occur. It may also explain why after certain kinds of experimental aggressive therapy, such as bone marrow transplantation or B-cell depletion, autoimmune diseases eventually recur after a long interval of remission. In the next part of the chapter we consider what happens after autoimmunity is incited by any of the mechanisms discussed so far. How do the effector functions of autoreactive lymphocytes lead to clinical disease?

Fig. 13.26 There are several ways in which infectious agents could break self-tolerance. Because some antigens are sequestered from the circulation, either behind a tissue barrier or within the cell, an infection that breaks cell and tissue barriers might expose hidden antigens (first panel). A second possibility is that infectious agents might trigger the release of inflammatory mediators from antigen-presenting cells (second panel). In SLE, it is thought that a subset of plasmacytoid dendritic cells release large quantities of interferon-α, a cytokine often induced by viral infection. In some cases, infectious agents might bind to self proteins. Because the infectious agent induces a helper T-cell response, any B cell that recognizes the self protein will also receive help (third panel). Such responses should be self-limiting once the infectious agent is eliminated, because at this point the T-cell help will no longer be provided. Molecular mimicry might result in infectious agents inducing either T- or B-cell responses that can cross-react with self antigens (fourth panel). Polyclonal T-cell activation by a bacterial superantigen could overcome clonal anergy, allowing an autoimmune process to begin (last panel).

Summary.

Multiple genetic factors predispose to autoimmunity. These have a powerful influence, yet even identical twins are not always concordant for autoimmune disease. This is because several environmental factors, in concert with genetic predisposition, are required to elicit autoimmune disease. Our knowledge of the genetic basis for autoimmunity comes from several sources. Natural mutants in mice and humans of single genes such as *Aire* or *Fas* can lead to a genetically determined autoimmune disease, often a severe one. The nature of these mutations, for example in pathways controlling thymic tolerance or apoptosis, have provided insights into how autoimmunity is normally controlled and how it can go wrong during disease. The knockout of single genes in mice has expanded our knowledge in this regard. However, most spontaneous autoimmune diseases in people are the result of more subtle variations or defects in multiple genes, the combination of which predisposes to autoimmunity. Sophisticated genetic mapping approaches are underway in both mice and people to identify these genes, but the process is difficult, and so far only a few genes have been identified. These studies are guided by the likelihood that the defects in multigenic autoimmunity are likely to be in the same pathways as those identified by single-gene defects. These mutations affect certain basic processes, including antigen clearance, co-stimulatory molecule expression, lymphocyte signaling, and apoptosis.

Even individuals with the genes that predispose to a particular autoimmune disease may not get that disease. Environmental factors have at least as strong an influence on the outcome as genetic factors, and are even less well understood. Some toxins and drugs are known to cause autoimmune syndromes, but their role in the common varieties of autoimmune disease is unclear. Similarly, some autoimmune syndromes can follow viral or bacterial infections, and it has long been suspected, but never proven, that such events contribute to the pathogenesis of diseases such as multiple sclerosis, diabetes, and SLE. Pathogens can promote autoimmunity by causing nonspecific inflammation and tissue damage. They can also sometimes elicit responses to self proteins if they express molecules that resemble self, a phenomenon known as molecular mimicry. Much more progress needs to be made to define environmental factors. It may be that there will not be a single, or even an identifiable, environmental factor that contributes to most diseases, and chance may have an important role in determining disease onset.

Mechanisms of pathogenesis in autoimmunity.

Here we describe some of the more common clinical autoimmune syndromes, and the ways in which loss of self-tolerance and expansion of self-reactive lymphocytes lead to tissue damage. These mechanisms of pathogenesis resemble in most ways those that are used to target invading pathogens. Damage by autoantibodies, mediated through the complement and Fc receptor systems, has an important role in some diseases, such as SLE. Similarly, T cells directed at self tissues destroy them much as they would virus-infected cells, and this is one way in which pancreatic β cells are destroyed in diabetes. However, self proteins are not easily eliminated, and typically do not elicit the same types of inflammatory signal as pathogens, so there are important differences. Pathogenesis mechanisms unique to autoimmunity include antibodies against receptors on cell surfaces that affect their function, as in myasthenia gravis, as well as hypersensitivity-type reactions. In this section we describe how some of these mechanisms work to cause common clinical syndromes of autoimmune disease.

13-25 Antibody and T cells can cause tissue damage in autoimmune disease.

Tissue injury in autoimmune disease is caused because the self antigen is an intrinsic component of the body and, consequently, the effector mechanisms of the immune system are directed at the body's own tissues. Also, because the adaptive immune response is incapable of removing the offending autoantigen from the body, the immune response persists, and there is a constant supply of new autoantigen, which amplifies the response. An important exception to this rule is type I diabetes or IDDM, in which the autoimmune response destroys the target organ completely. This leads to a failure to produce insulin—one of the major autoantigens in this disease. Lack of insulin is in turn responsible for the phenotype of IDDM.

The mechanisms of tissue injury in autoimmunity can be classified according to the scheme adopted for hypersensitivity reactions (Fig. 13.27; see also

See various cases in
Case Studies in Immunology

Some common autoimmune diseases classified by immunopathogenic mechanism		
Syndrome	Autoantigen	Consequence
Type II antibody against cell-surface or matrix antigens		
Autoimmune hemolytic anemia	Rh blood group antigens, I antigen	Destruction of red blood cells by complement and FcR⁺ phagocytes, anemia
Autoimmune thrombocytopenic purpura	Platelet integrin GpIIb:IIIa	Abnormal bleeding
Goodpasture's syndrome	Noncollagenous domain of basement membrane collagen type IV	Glomerulonephritis, pulmonary hemorrhage
Pemphigus vulgaris	Epidermal cadherin	Blistering of skin
Acute rheumatic fever	Streptococcal cell-wall antigens. Antibodies cross-react with cardiac muscle	Arthritis, myocarditis, late scarring of heart valves
Type III immune-complex disease		
Mixed essential cryoglobulinemia	Rheumatoid factor IgG complexes (with or without hepatitis C antigens)	Systemic vasculitis
Systemic lupus erythematosus	DNA, histones, ribosomes, snRNP, scRNP	Glomerulonephritis, vasculitis, rash
Rheumatoid arthritis	Rheumatoid factor IgG complexes	Arthritis
Type IV T cell-mediated disease		
Insulin-dependent diabetes mellitus	Pancreatic β-cell antigen	β-cell destruction
Rheumatoid arthritis	Unknown synovial joint antigen	Joint inflammation and destruction
Experimental autoimmune encephalomyelitis (EAE), multiple sclerosis	Myelin basic protein, proteolipid protein, myelin oligodendrocyte glycoprotein	Brain invasion by CD4 T cells, weakness

Fig. 13.27 Autoimmune diseases classified by the mechanism of tissue damage. Autoimmune diseases can be grouped in the same way as hypersensitivity reactions, according to the type of immune response and the mechanism by which it damages tissues. The immunopathological mechanisms are as illustrated for the hypersensitivity reactions in Fig.12.2, with the exception of the type I IgE-mediated responses, which are not a known cause of autoimmune disease. Some additional autoimmune diseases in which the antigen is a cell-surface receptor, and in which the pathology is due to altered signaling, are listed later, in Fig. 13.31. Several immunopathogenic mechanisms operate in parallel to cause many autoimmune diseases. This is illustrated for rheumatoid arthritis, which appears in more than one category of immunopathological mechanism.

Fig. 12.2). As with the hypersensitivity reactions, tissue damage can be mediated by the effector actions of both T cells and B cells. Notably, T cells are almost always required for the production of pathogenic autoantibodies; T cells also directly damage tissues in some diseases. Reciprocally, B cells often have an important role in the maximal activation of T cells that mediate both tissue damage and help autoantibody production. The antigen, or group of antigens, against which the autoimmune response is directed, and the mechanism by which the antigen-bearing tissue is damaged, together determine the pathology and clinical expression of the disease (see Fig. 13.27).

Autoimmune diseases differ from hypersensitivity responses in that type I IgE-mediated responses do not seem to have a major role. By contrast, autoimmunity that damages tissues by mechanisms analogous to type II hypersensitivity reactions is quite common. In this form of autoimmunity, IgG or IgM responses to autoantigens located on cell surfaces or extracellular matrix cause the injury. In other cases of autoimmunity, tissue damage can be due to type III responses, which involve immune complexes containing autoantibodies against soluble autoantigens; these autoimmune diseases are systemic and are characterized by autoimmune vasculitis. In SLE, autoantibodies cause damage by both type II and type III mechanisms. Finally, in a number of organ-specific autoimmune diseases, T-cell responses are directly involved in causing the tissue damage. In most autoimmune diseases, several mechanisms of immunopathogenesis operate. Examples include SLE, IDDM, and rheumatoid arthritis, in which there is evidence that both T-cell and antibody-mediated pathways cause tissue injury. We will examine how autoantibodies cause tissue damage, before ending with a consideration of self-reactive T-cell responses and their role in autoimmune disease.

13-26 Autoantibodies against blood cells promote their destruction.

**Autoimmune
Hemolytic Anemia**

IgG or IgM responses to antigens located on the surface of blood cells lead to the rapid destruction of these cells. An example of this is **autoimmune hemolytic anemia**, in which antibodies against self antigens on red blood cells trigger destruction of the cells, leading to anemia. This can occur in two ways (Fig. 13.28). Red cells with bound IgG or IgM antibody are rapidly cleared from the circulation by interaction with Fc or complement receptors, respectively, on cells of the fixed mononuclear phagocytic system; this occurs particularly in the spleen. Alternatively, the autoantibody-sensitized red cells are lysed by formation of the membrane-attack complex of complement. In **autoimmune thrombocytopenic purpura**, autoantibodies against the GpIIb:IIIa fibrinogen receptor or other platelet-specific surface antigens can cause thrombocytopenia (a depletion of platelets), which can in turn cause hemorrhage.

Lysis of nucleated cells by complement is less common because these cells are better defended by complement regulatory proteins. These proteins protect cells against immune attack by interfering with the activation of complement components and their assembly into a membrane-attack complex (see Section 2-10). Nevertheless, nucleated cells targeted by autoantibodies are still destroyed by cells of the mononuclear phagocytic system. Autoantibodies against neutrophils, for example, cause neutropenia, which increases susceptibility to infection with pyogenic bacteria. In all these cases, accelerated clearance of autoantibody-sensitized cells is the cause of their depletion in the blood. One therapeutic approach to this type of autoimmunity is removal of the spleen, the organ in which the main clearance of red cells, platelets, and leukocytes occurs. Another is the administration of large quantities of nonspecific IgG (termed IVIG, for intravenous immunoglobulin), which inhibits the Fc receptor-mediated uptake of antibody-coated cells.

Red blood cells plus anti-RBC autoantibodies

FcR+ cells in fixed mononuclear phagocytic system

Complement activation and intravascular hemolysis

Phagocytosis and RBC destruction

Lysis and RBC destruction

Fig. 13.28 Antibodies specific for cell-surface antigens can destroy cells. In autoimmune hemolytic anemias, red blood cells (RBC) coated with IgG autoantibodies against a cell-surface antigen are rapidly cleared from the circulation by uptake by Fc receptor-bearing macrophages in the fixed mononuclear phagocytic system (left panel). Red cells coated with IgM autoantibodies fix C3 and are cleared by CR1- and CR3-bearing macrophages in the fixed mononuclear phagocytic system (not shown). Uptake and clearance by these mechanisms occurs mainly in the spleen. The binding of certain rare autoantibodies that fix complement extremely efficiently causes the formation of the membrane-attack complex on the red cells, leading to intravascular hemolysis (right panel).

13-27 The fixation of sublytic doses of complement to cells in tissues stimulates a powerful inflammatory response.

The binding of IgG and IgM antibodies against cells in tissues (in contrast to blood cells) causes inflammatory injury by a variety of mechanisms. As in blood cells, one of these is the fixation of complement. Although nucleated cells are relatively resistant to lysis by complement, the assembly of sublytic amounts of the membrane-attack complex on their surface provides a powerful activating stimulus. Depending on the type of cell, the interaction of sublytic doses of the membrane-attack complex with the cell membrane can cause cytokine release, the generation of a respiratory burst, or the mobilization of membrane phospholipids to generate arachidonic acid—the precursor of prostaglandins and leukotrienes (lipid mediators of inflammation).

Most cells in tissues are fixed in place, and cells of the inflammatory system are attracted to them by chemoattractant molecules. One such molecule is the complement fragment C5a, which is released as a result of complement activation triggered by autoantibody binding. Other chemoattractants, such as leukotriene B4, can be released by the autoantibody-targeted cells. Inflammatory leukocytes are further activated by binding to autoantibody Fc regions and fixed complement C3 fragments on the tissue cells. Tissue injury can then result from the products of the activated leukocytes and by antibody-dependent cellular cytotoxicity mediated by NK cells (see Section 9-21).

A probable example of this type of autoimmunity is **Hashimoto's thyroiditis**, in which autoantibodies against tissue-specific antigens such as thyroid peroxidase and thyroglobulin are found at extremely high levels for prolonged periods. Direct T-cell-mediated cytotoxicity, which we discuss later, is probably also important in this disease.

13-28 Autoimmunity against receptors cause disease by stimulating or blocking receptor function.

A special class of type II hypersensitivity reaction occurs when the autoantibody binds to a cell-surface receptor. Antibody binding to a receptor can either stimulate the receptor or block its stimulation by its natural ligand. In **Graves' disease**, autoantibody against the thyroid-stimulating hormone receptor on thyroid cells stimulates the excessive production of thyroid hormone. The production of thyroid hormone is normally controlled by feedback regulation; high levels of thyroid hormone inhibit the release of thyroid-stimulating hormone (TSH) by the pituitary. In Graves' disease, feedback inhibition fails because the autoantibody continues to stimulate the TSH receptor in the absence of TSH, and the patients become hyperthyroid (Fig. 13.29).

Myasthenia
Gravis

In **myasthenia gravis**, autoantibodies against the α chain of the nicotinic acetylcholine receptor, which is present on skeletal muscle cells at neuromuscular junctions, can block neuromuscular transmission. The antibodies are believed to drive the internalization and intracellular degradation of acetylcholine receptors (Fig. 13.30). Patients with myasthenia gravis develop potentially fatal progressive weakness as a result of their autoimmune disease. Diseases caused by autoantibodies that act as agonists or antagonists for cell-surface receptors are listed in Fig. 13.31.

Fig. 13.29 Feedback regulation of thyroid hormone production is disrupted in Graves' disease. Graves' disease is caused by autoantibodies specific for the receptor for thyroid-stimulating hormone (TSH). Normally, thyroid hormones are produced in response to TSH and limit their own production by inhibiting the production of TSH by the pituitary (left panels). In Graves' disease, the autoantibodies are agonists for the TSH receptor and therefore stimulate the production of thyroid hormones (right panels). The thyroid hormones inhibit TSH production in the normal way but do not affect production of the autoantibody; the excessive thyroid hormone production induced in this way causes hyperthyroidism.

The pituitary gland secretes thyroid-stimulating hormone (TSH), which acts on the thyroid to induce the release of thyroid hormones

Autoimmune B cell makes antibodies against TSH receptor that also stimulate thyroid hormone production

Thyroid hormones act on the pituitary to shut down production of TSH, suppressing further thyroid hormone synthesis (feedback suppression)

Thyroid hormones shut down TSH production but have no effect on autoantibody production, which continues to cause excessive thyroid hormone production

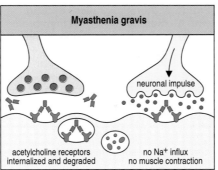

Fig. 13.30 Autoantibodies inhibit receptor function in myasthenia gravis. In normal circumstances, acetylcholine released from stimulated motor neurons at the neuromuscular junction binds to acetylcholine receptors on skeletal muscle cells, triggering muscle contraction (left panel). Myasthenia gravis is caused by autoantibodies against the α subunit of the receptor for acetylcholine. These autoantibodies bind to the receptor without activating it and also cause receptor internalization and degradation (right panel). As the number of receptors on the muscle is decreased, the muscle becomes less responsive to acetylcholine.

13-29 Autoantibodies against extracellular antigens cause inflammatory injury by mechanisms akin to type II and type III hypersensitivity reactions.

Antibody responses to extracellular matrix molecules are infrequent, but can be very damaging when they occur. In **Goodpasture's syndrome**, an example of a type II hypersensitivity reaction (see Fig. 12.2), antibodies are formed against the α_3 chain of basement membrane collagen (type IV collagen). These antibodies bind to the basement membranes of renal glomeruli (Fig. 13.32a) and, in some cases, to the basement membranes of pulmonary alveoli, causing a rapidly fatal disease if untreated. The autoantibodies bound to basement membrane ligate Fcγ receptors, leading to the activation of monocytes, neutrophils, and tissue basophils and mast cells. These release chemokines that attract a further influx of neutrophils into the glomeruli, causing severe tissue injury (Fig. 13.32b). The autoantibodies also cause a local activation of complement, which may amplify the tissue injury.

Immune complexes are produced whenever there is an antibody response to a soluble antigen (see Appendix I, Section A-8). Normally they are cleared efficiently by red blood cells bearing complement receptors and by phagocytes of the mononuclear phagocytic system that have both complement and Fc receptors, and such complexes cause little tissue damage. However, this clearance system can fail in three circumstances. The first follows the injection of large amounts of antigen, leading to the formation of large amounts of immune complexes that overwhelm the normal clearance mechanisms. An example of this is serum sickness (see Section 12-16), which is caused by

Diseases mediated by autoantibodies against cell-surface receptors		
Syndrome	Antigen	Consequence
Graves' disease	Thyroid-stimulating hormone receptor	Hyperthyroidism
Myasthenia gravis	Acetylcholine receptor	Progressive weakness
Insulin-resistant diabetes	Insulin receptor (antagonist)	Hyperglycemia, ketoacidosis
Hypoglycemia	Insulin receptor (agonist)	Hypoglycemia

Fig. 13.31 Autoimmune diseases caused by autoantibodies against cell-surface receptors. These antibodies produce different effects depending on whether they are agonists (which stimulate) or antagonists (which inhibit) the receptor. Note that different autoantibodies against the insulin receptor can either stimulate or inhibit signaling.

Fig. 13.32 Autoantibodies reacting with glomerular basement membrane cause the inflammatory glomerular disease known as Goodpasture's syndrome. The panels show sections of renal glomeruli in serial biopsies taken from patients with Goodpasture's syndrome. Panel a, glomerulus stained for IgG deposition by immuno-fluoresence. Anti-glomerular basement membrane antibody (stained green) is deposited in a linear fashion along the glomerular basement membrane. The autoantibody causes local activation of cells bearing Fc receptors, complement activation, and influx of neutrophils. Panel b, hematoxylin and eosin staining of a section through a renal glomerulus shows that the glomerulus is compressed by the formation of a crescent (C) of proliferating mononuclear cells within the Bowman's capsule (B) and there is an influx of neutrophils (N) into the glomerular tuft. Photographs courtesy of M. Thompson and D. Evans.

Systemic Lupus
Erythematosus

Fig. 13.33 Deposition of immune complexes in the renal glomerulus causes renal failure in systemic lupus erythematosus (SLE). Panel a, a section through a renal glomerulus from a patient with SLE, shows that the deposition of immune complexes has caused thickening of the glomerular basement membrane, seen as the clear 'canals' running through the glomerulus. Panel b, a similar section stained with fluorescent anti-immunoglobulin, reveals immunoglobulin deposits in the basement membrane. In panel c, the immune complexes are seen under the electron microscope as dense protein deposits between the glomerular basement membrane and the renal epithelial cells. Polymorphonuclear neutrophilic leukocytes are also present, attracted by the deposited immune complexes. Photographs courtesy of H.T. Cook and M. Kashgarian.

the injection of large amounts of serum proteins. This is a transient disease, lasting only until the immune complexes have been cleared. The second circumstance is seen in chronic infections such as bacterial endocarditis, in which the immune response to bacteria lodged on a cardiac valve is incapable of clearing the infection. The persistent release of bacterial antigens from the valve infection in the presence of a strong antibacterial antibody response causes widespread immune-complex injury to small blood vessels in organs such as the kidney and the skin.

Thirdly, part of the pathogenesis of SLE can also be attributed to the failure to clear immune complexes. In SLE there is chronic IgG antibody production directed at ubiquitous self antigens present in all nucleated cells, leading to a wide range of autoantibodies against common cellular constituents. The main antigens are three intracellular nucleoprotein particles—the nucleosome, the spliceosome, and a small cytoplasmic ribonucleoprotein complex containing two proteins known as Ro and La (named after the first two letters of the surnames of the two patients in whom autoantibodies against these proteins were discovered). For these autoantigens to participate in immune-complex formation, they must become extracellular. The autoantigens of SLE are exposed on dead and dying cells and released from injured tissues. In SLE, large quantities of antigen are available, so large amounts of small immune complexes are produced continuously and are deposited in the walls of small blood vessels in the renal glomerulus, in glomerular basement membrane (Fig. 13.33), in joints, and in other organs. This leads to the activation of phagocytic cells through their Fc receptors. The consequent tissue damage releases more nucleoprotein complexes, which in turn form more immune complexes. During this process, autoreactive T cells also become activated, although much less is known about their specificity. As we discuss in the next section, they contribute to disease in two ways: by helping B cells to make antibodies, in an analogous manner to a normal T-dependent immune response, and by direct effector functions of T cells as they infiltrate and destroy target tissues such as skin, renal interstitium, and vessels. Eventually, the inflammation induced in these tissues can cause sufficient damage to kill the patient.

Dense protein deposits

13-30 T cells specific for self antigens can cause direct tissue injury and have a role in sustained autoantibody responses.

Activated effector T cells specific for self-peptide:self-MHC complexes can cause local inflammation by activating macrophages or can damage tissue cells directly. Diseases in which these actions of T cells are important include IDDM, rheumatoid arthritis, multiple sclerosis, and most probably SLE. Affected tissues in patients with these diseases are heavily infiltrated by T lymphocytes and activated macrophages. These autoimmune diseases are mediated by T cells specific for the autoantigen presented by self MHC. T cells are, of course, also required to sustain all autoantibody responses.

It is much more difficult to demonstrate the existence of autoreactive T cells than it is to demonstrate the presence of autoantibodies. First, autoreactive human T cells cannot be used to transfer disease to experimental animals because T-cell recognition is MHC-restricted, and animals and humans have different MHC alleles. Second, it is difficult to identify the antigen recognized by a T cell; for example, autoantibodies can be used to stain self tissues to reveal the distribution of the autoantigen, whereas T cells cannot. Nevertheless, there is strong evidence for the involvement of autoreactive T cells in several autoimmune diseases. In IDDM, the insulin-producing β cells of the pancreatic islets are selectively destroyed by specific T cells. When such diabetic patients are transplanted with half a pancreas from an identical twin donor, the β cells in the grafted tissue are rapidly and selectively destroyed by the recipient's T cells. Recurrence of disease can be prevented by the immunosuppressive drug cyclosporin A (see Chapter 14), which inhibits T-cell activation.

Autoantigens recognized by CD4 T cells can be identified by adding cell extracts to cultures of blood mononuclear cells and testing for recognition by CD4 cells derived from an autoimmune patient. If the autoantigen is present in the cell extract, it should be effectively presented, because phagocytes in the blood cultures can take up extracellular protein, degrade it in intracellular vesicles, and present the resulting peptides bound to MHC class II molecules. However, the identification of autoantigenic peptides is particularly difficult in autoimmune diseases in which CD8 T cells have a role, because autoantigens recognized by CD8 T cells are not effectively presented in such cultures. Peptides presented by MHC class I molecules must usually be made by the target cells themselves (see Chapter 5); intact cells of target tissue from the patient must therefore be used to study autoreactive CD8 T cells that cause tissue damage. Conversely, the pathogenesis of the disease can itself give clues to the identity of the antigen in some CD8 T cell-mediated diseases. For example, in IDDM the insulin-producing β cells of the pancreatic islets of Langerhans seem to be specifically targeted and destroyed by CD8 T cells (Fig. 13.34). This suggests that a protein unique to β cells is the source of the peptide recognized by the pathogenic CD8 T cells. Studies in the NOD mouse model of IDDM have shown that peptides from insulin itself are recognized by pathogenic CD8 cells, confirming the role of insulin as one of the principal autoantigens in this diabetes model.

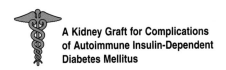

A Kidney Graft for Complications of Autoimmune Insulin-Dependent Diabetes Mellitus

Summary.

For a disease to be defined as autoimmune, the tissue damage must be shown to be caused by an adaptive immune response to self antigens. The most convincing proof that the immune response is causal in autoimmunity is the transfer of disease by transferring the active component of the immune response to an appropriate recipient. Autoimmune diseases can be mediated by autoantibodies and/or by autoreactive T cells, and tissue damage can result from a direct attack on the cells bearing the antigen, from immune-complex

Fig. 13.34 Selective destruction of pancreatic β cells in insulin-dependent diabetes mellitus (IDDM) indicates that the autoantigen is produced in β cells and recognized on their surface. In IDDM there is highly specific destruction of insulin-producing β cells in the pancreatic islets of Langerhans, sparing other islet cell types (α and δ). This is shown schematically in the upper panels. In the lower panels, islets from normal (left) and diabetic (right) mice are stained for insulin (brown), which shows the β cells, and glucagon (black), which shows the α cells. Note the lymphocytes infiltrating the islet in the diabetic mouse (right) and the selective loss of the β cells (brown) whereas the α cells (black) are spared. The characteristic morphology of the islet is also disrupted with the loss of the β cells. Photographs courtesy of I. Visintin.

formation, or from local inflammation. Autoimmune diseases caused by antibodies that bind to cell-surface receptors, causing either excess activity or inhibition of receptor function, fall into a special class. T cells can be involved directly in inflammation or cellular destruction, and they are also required to sustain autoantibody responses. Similarly, B cells may be important antigen-presenting cells for sustaining autoantigen-specific T-cell responses. In spite of our knowledge of the mechanisms of tissue damage and the therapeutic approaches that this information has engendered, the deeper, more important question is how the autoimmune response is induced. Much has been learned about the induction of immune responses to tissue antigens by examining the response to nonself tissues in transplantation experiments. It is therefore appropriate in this final part of the chapter to examine the immune response to grafted tissues, because the lessons learned in the study of graft rejection apply to autoimmunity and vice versa.

Responses to alloantigens and transplant rejection.

The transplantation of tissues to replace diseased organs is now an important medical therapy. In most cases, adaptive immune responses to the grafted tissues are the major impediment to successful transplantation. Rejection is caused by immune responses to alloantigens on the graft, which are proteins that vary from individual to individual within a species and are therefore perceived as foreign by the recipient. When tissues containing nucleated cells are transplanted, T-cell responses to the highly polymorphic MHC molecules almost always trigger a response against the grafted organ. Matching the MHC type of the donor and the recipient increases the success rate of grafts, but perfect matching is possible only when donor and recipient are related and, in these cases, genetic differences at other loci can still trigger rejection, although less severely. In blood transfusion, which was the earliest and is still the most common tissue transplant, MHC matching is not necessary as red blood cells and platelets do not express much MHC I protein and do not express MHC II; thus, they are not targets for the T cells of the recipient. However, blood must be matched for ABO and Rh blood group antigens to avoid the rapid destruction of mismatched red blood cells by antibodies in the recipient (see Appendix I, Section A-11). Because there are only four major ABO types and two Rh types, this is relatively easy. In this section we examine the immune response to tissue grafts and also ask why such responses do not reject the one foreign tissue graft that is tolerated routinely—the mammalian fetus.

13-31 Graft rejection is an immunological response mediated primarily by T cells.

The basic rules of tissue grafting were first elucidated by skin transplantation between inbred strains of mice. Skin can be grafted with 100% success between different sites on the same animal or person (an **autograft**), or between genetically identical animals or people (a **syngeneic graft**). However, when skin is grafted between unrelated or **allogeneic** individuals (an **allograft**), the graft is initially accepted but is then rejected about 10–13 days after grafting (Fig. 13.35). This response is called a **first-set rejection** and is quite consistent. It depends on a T-cell response in the recipient, because skin grafted onto *nude* mice, which lack T cells, is not rejected. The ability to reject skin can be restored to *nude* mice by the adoptive transfer of normal T cells.

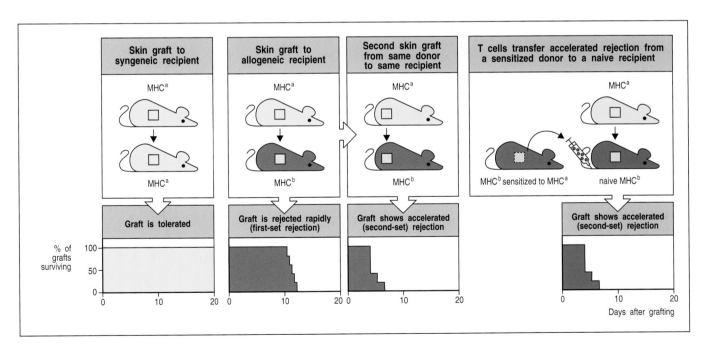

Fig. 13.35 Skin graft rejection is the result of a T cell-mediated anti-graft response. Grafts that are syngeneic are permanently accepted (first panels) but grafts differing at the MHC are rejected about 10–13 days after grafting (first-set rejection, second panels). When a mouse is grafted for a second time with skin from the same donor, it rejects the second graft faster (third panels). This is called a second-set rejection and the accelerated response is MHC-specific; skin from a second donor of the same MHC type is rejected equally fast, whereas skin from an MHC-different donor is rejected in a first-set pattern (not shown). Naive mice that are given T cells from a sensitized donor behave as if they had already been grafted (final panels).

When a recipient that has previously rejected a graft is regrafted with skin from the same donor, the second graft is rejected more rapidly (6–8 days) in a **second-set rejection** (see Fig. 13.35). Skin from a third-party donor grafted onto the same recipient at the same time does not show this faster response but follows a first-set rejection course. The rapid course of second-set rejection can also be transferred to normal or irradiated recipients by T cells from the initial recipient, showing that second-set rejection is caused by a memory-type immune response (see Chapter 10) from clonally expanded and primed T cells specific for the donor skin.

Immune responses are a major barrier to effective tissue transplantation, destroying grafted tissue by an adaptive immune response to its foreign proteins. These responses can be mediated by CD8 T cells, by CD4 T cells, or by both. Antibodies can also contribute to second-set rejection of tissue grafts.

13-32 Matching donor and recipient at the MHC improves the outcome of transplantation.

When donor and recipient differ at the MHC, the immune response, which is known as an **alloreactive** response because it is directed against antigens (**alloantigens**) that differ between members of the same species, is directed at the nonself allogeneic MHC molecule or molecules present on the graft. In most tissues these will be predominantly MHC class I antigens. Once a recipient has rejected a graft of a particular MHC type, any further graft bearing the same nonself MHC molecule will be rapidly rejected in a second-set response. As we learned in Chapter 5, the frequency of T cells specific for any nonself MHC molecule is relatively high, making differences at MHC loci the most potent trigger of the rejection of initial grafts; indeed, the major histocompatibility complex was originally so named because of its central role in graft rejection.

Once it became clear that recognition of nonself MHC molecules is a major determinant of graft rejection, a considerable amount of effort was put into MHC matching between recipient and donor. Although MHC (in humans, known as HLA) matching significantly improves the success rate of clinical organ transplantation, it does not in itself prevent rejection reactions. There are two main reasons for this. First, HLA typing is imprecise, because of the polymorphism and complexity of the human MHC; unrelated individuals who type as HLA-identical with antibodies against MHC proteins rarely have identical MHC genotypes. This should not be a problem with HLA-identical siblings: because siblings inherit their MHC genes as a haplotype, one sibling in four should be truly HLA-identical. Nevertheless, grafts between HLA-identical siblings invariably incite a rejection reaction, albeit more slowly, unless donor and recipient are identical twins. This reaction is the result of differences between minor histocompatibility antigens, which is the second reason for the failure of HLA matching to prevent rejection reactions. These minor histocompatibility antigens, which represent peptides from allelically variable non-MHC proteins, are discussed in the next section.

Thus, unless donor and recipient are identical twins, all graft recipients must be given immunosuppressive drugs to prevent rejection. Indeed, the current success of clinical transplantation of solid organs is more the result of advances in immunosuppressive therapy, discussed in Chapter 14, than of improved tissue matching. The limited supply of cadaveric organs, coupled with the urgency of identifying a recipient once a donor organ becomes available, means that accurate matching of tissue types is achieved only rarely, with the notable exception of matched sibling donation of kidneys.

A Kidney Graft for Complications of Autoimmune Insulin-Dependent Diabetes Mellitus

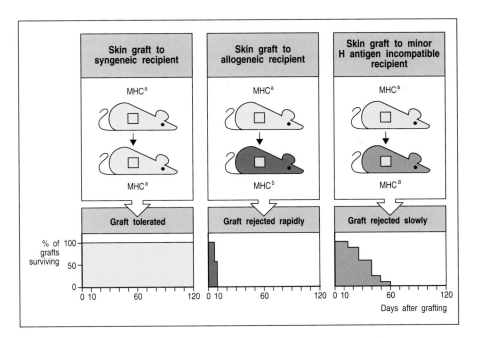

Fig. 13.36 Even complete matching at the MHC does not ensure graft survival. Although syngeneic grafts are not rejected (left panels), MHC-identical grafts from donors that differ at other loci (minor H antigen loci) are rejected (right panels), albeit more slowly than MHC-disparate grafts (center panels).

13-33 In MHC-identical grafts, rejection is caused by peptides from other alloantigens bound to graft MHC molecules.

When donor and recipient are identical at the MHC but differ at other genetic loci, graft rejection is not so rapid (Fig. 13.36). MHC class I molecules bind and present a selection of peptides derived from proteins made in the cell, and if polymorphisms in these proteins mean that different peptides are produced in different members of a species, these can be recognized as **minor histocompatibility antigens** (Fig. 13.37). One set of proteins that induce minor histocompatibility responses is encoded on the male-specific Y chromosome. Responses induced by these proteins are known collectively as H-Y. As these Y-chromosome-specific genes are not expressed in females, female anti-male minor histocompatibility responses occur; however, male

Polymorphic self proteins that differ in amino acid sequence between individuals give rise to minor H antigen differences between donor and recipient

Fig. 13.37 Minor H antigens are peptides derived from polymorphic cellular proteins bound to MHC class I molecules. Self proteins are routinely digested by proteasomes within the cell's cytosol, and peptides derived from them are delivered to the endoplasmic reticulum, where they can bind to MHC class I molecules and be delivered to the cell surface. If a polymorphic protein differs between the graft donor (shown in red on the left) and the recipient (shown in blue on the right), it can give rise to an antigenic peptide (red on the donor cell) that can be recognized by the recipient's T cells as nonself and elicit an immune response. Such antigens are the minor H antigens.

anti-female responses are not seen, because both males and females express X-chromosome genes. One H-Y antigen has been identified in mice and humans as peptides from a protein encoded by the Y-chromosome gene *Smcy*. An X-chromosome homolog of *Smcy*, called *Smcx*, does not contain these peptide sequences, which are therefore expressed uniquely in males. The nature of most minor histocompatibility antigens, encoded by autosomal genes, is unknown, although 10 have now been identified at the genetic level.

The response to minor histocompatibility antigens is in most ways analogous to the response to viral infection. However, an antiviral response eliminates only infected cells, whereas all cells in the graft express these antigens, and thus the entire graft is destroyed in the response against the antigens. Given the virtual certainty of mismatches in minor histocompatibility antigens between any two individuals, and the potency of the reactions they incite, it is no wonder that successful transplantation requires the use of powerful immunosuppressive drugs.

13-34 There are two ways of presenting alloantigens on the transplant to the recipient's T lymphocytes.

Before naive alloreactive T cells can cause rejection, they must be activated by antigen-presenting cells that both bear the allogeneic MHC molecules and have co-stimulatory activity. Organ grafts carry with them antigen-presenting cells of donor origin, known as **passenger leukocytes**, and these are an

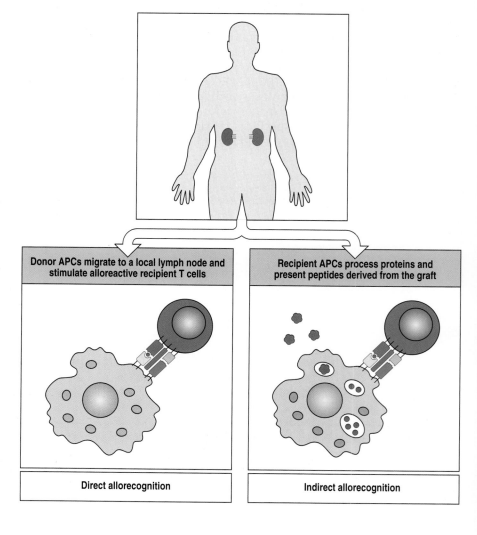

Fig. 13.38 Alloantigens in grafted organs are recognized in two different ways. Direct recognition of a grafted organ (red in upper panel) is mediated by T cells whose receptors have specificity for the allogeneic MHC class I or class II molecule in combination with peptide. These alloreactive T cells are stimulated by donor antigen-presenting cells (APC), which express both the allogeneic MHC molecule and co-stimulatory activity (bottom left panel). Indirect recognition of the graft (bottom right panel) is mediated by T cells whose receptors are specific for allogeneic peptides that are derived from the grafted organ. Proteins from the graft (red) are taken up and processed by the recipient's antigen-presenting cells and are therefore presented by self (recipient) MHC class I or class II molecules.

Donor APCs migrate to a local lymph node and stimulate alloreactive recipient T cells

Recipient APCs process proteins and present peptides derived from the graft

Direct allorecognition

Indirect allorecognition

important stimulus to alloreactivity (Fig. 13.38). This route for sensitization of the recipient to a graft seems to involve donor antigen-presenting cells leaving the graft and migrating via the lymph to regional lymph nodes. Here they can activate those host T cells that bear the corresponding T-cell receptors. The activated alloreactive effector T cells are then carried back to the graft, which they attack directly (Fig. 13.39). This recognition pathway is known as **direct allorecognition**. Indeed, if the grafted tissue is depleted of antigen-presenting cells by treatment with antibodies or by prolonged incubation, rejection occurs only after a much longer time. Also, if the site of grafting lacks lymphatic drainage, no response to the graft results.

A second mechanism of allograft recognition leading to graft rejection is the uptake of allogeneic proteins by the recipient's own antigen-presenting cells and their presentation to T cells by self-MHC molecules (see Fig. 13.38). The recognition of allogeneic proteins presented in this way is known as **indirect allorecognition**, in contrast to the direct recognition by T cells of allogeneic MHC class I and class II molecules expressed on the passenger antigen-presenting cells from the graft itself. Among the graft-derived peptides presented by the recipient's antigen-presenting cells are the minor histocompatibility antigens and also peptides from the foreign MHC molecules themselves, which are a major source of the polymorphic peptides recognized by the recipient's T cells, although in this case only if the graft is MHC-mismatched with the recipient.

The relative contributions of direct and indirect allorecognition in graft rejection are not known. Direct allorecognition is thought to be largely responsible for acute rejection, especially when MHC mismatches mean that the frequency of directly alloreactive recipient T cells is high. Furthermore, a direct cytotoxic T-cell attack on graft cells can be made only by T cells that recognize the graft MHC molecules directly. Nonetheless, T cells with indirect allospecificity can contribute to graft rejection by activating macrophages, which cause tissue injury and fibrosis, and are also likely to be important in the development of an alloantibody response to a graft.

Fig. 13.39 The initiation of graft rejection normally involves the migration of donor antigen-presenting cells from the graft to local lymph nodes. The example of a skin graft is illustrated here, in which Langerhans' cells are the antigen-presenting cells. They display peptides from the graft on their surface. After traveling to a lymph node, these antigen-presenting cells encounter recirculating naive T cells specific for graft antigens, and stimulate these T cells to divide. The resulting activated effector T cells migrate via the thoracic duct to the blood and home to the grafted tissue, which they rapidly destroy. Destruction is highly specific for donor-derived cells, suggesting that it is mediated by direct cytotoxicity and not by nonspecific inflammatory processes.

Fig. 13.40 Preexisting antibody against donor graft antigens can cause hyperacute graft rejection. In some cases, recipients already have antibodies against donor antigens, which are often blood group antigens. When the donor organ is grafted into such recipients, these antibodies bind to vascular endothelium in the graft, initiating the complement and clotting cascades. Blood vessels in the graft become obstructed by clots and leak, causing hemorrhage of blood into the graft. This becomes engorged and turns purple from the presence of deoxygenated blood.

13-35 Antibodies reacting with endothelium cause hyperacute graft rejection.

Antibody responses are also an important potential cause of graft rejection. Preexisting alloantibodies against blood group antigens and polymorphic MHC antigens can cause the rapid rejection of transplanted organs in a complement-dependent reaction that can occur within minutes of transplantation. This type of reaction is known as **hyperacute graft rejection**. Most grafts that are transplanted routinely in clinical medicine are vascularized organ grafts linked directly to the recipient's circulation. In some cases the recipient might already have circulating antibodies against donor graft antigens. Antibodies of the ABO type can bind to all tissues, not just red blood cells. They are preformed and are relevant in all ABO-mismatched individuals. In addition, antibodies against other antigens can be produced in response to a previous transplant or a blood transfusion. All such preexisting antibodies can cause the very rapid rejection of vascularized grafts because they react with antigens on the vascular endothelial cells of the graft and initiate the complement and blood clotting cascades. The vessels of the graft become blocked, causing its immediate death. Such grafts become engorged and purple-colored from hemorrhaged blood, which becomes deoxygenated (Fig. 13.40). This problem can be avoided by ABO-matching as well as **cross-matching** donor and recipient. Cross-matching involves determining whether the recipient has antibodies that react with the white blood cells of the donor. If antibodies of this type are found, they are a serious contraindication to transplantation, as they lead to near-certain hyperacute rejection.

A very similar problem prevents the routine use of animal organs—**xenografts**—in transplantation. If xenogeneic grafts could be used, it would circumvent the major limitation in organ replacement therapy, namely the severe shortage of donor organs. Pigs have been suggested as a potential source of organs for xenografting, because they are of a similar size to humans and are easily farmed. Most humans and other primates have antibodies that react with a ubiquitous cell-surface carbohydrate antigen (α-Gal) of other mammalian species, including pigs. When pig xenografts are placed in humans, these antibodies trigger hyperacute rejection by binding to the endothelial cells of the graft and initiating the complement and clotting cascades. The problem of hyperacute rejection is exacerbated in xenografts because complement-regulatory proteins such as CD59, DAF (CD55), and MCP (CD46) (see Section 2-14) work less efficiently across a species barrier and so pig regulatory proteins, for example, cannot protect the graft from attack by human complement. A recent step toward xenotransplantation has been the development of transgenic pigs expressing human DAF as well as pigs that lack α-Gal. These approaches might one day reduce or eliminate hyperacute rejection in xenotransplantation. However, hyperacute rejection is only the first barrier faced by a xenotransplanted organ. The T lymphocyte-mediated graft rejection mechanisms might be extremely difficult to overcome with the immunosuppressive regimes currently available.

13-36 Chronic organ rejection is caused by inflammatory vascular injury to the graft.

The success of modern immunosuppression means that about 85% of cadaveric kidney grafts are still functioning a year after transplantation. However, there has been no improvement in rates of long-term graft survival: the half-life for functional survival of renal allografts remains about 8 years. The major cause of late organ failure is chronic rejection, characterized by concentric arteriosclerosis of graft blood vessels, accompanied by glomerular and tubular fibrosis and atrophy.

Mechanisms that contribute to chronic rejection can be divided into those due to alloreactivity and those due to other pathways, and into early and late events after transplantation. Alloreactivity can occur days and weeks after transplantation and can cause acute graft rejection. Alloreactive responses can also occur months to years after transplantation, and may be associated with a clinically hard-to-detect gradual loss of graft function. Other important causes of chronic graft rejection include ischemia–reperfusion injury, which occurs at the time of grafting but may have late adverse effects on the grafted organ, and later-developing adverse factors such as chronic cyclosporin toxicity or cytomegalovirus infection.

Infiltration of the graft vessels and tissues by macrophages, followed by scarring, are prominent histological features of late graft rejection. A model of injury has been developed in which alloreactive T cells infiltrating the graft secrete cytokines that stimulate the expression of endothelial adhesion molecules and also secrete chemokines such as CCL5 (RANTES; see Fig. 2.41), which attracts monocytes that mature into macrophages in the graft. A second phase of chronic inflammation then supervenes, dominated by macrophage products including IL-1, TNF-α, and the chemokine CCL2 (MCP-1), which leads to further recruitment of macrophages. These mediators conspire to cause chronic inflammation and scarring, which eventually leads to irreversible organ failure. Animal models of chronic rejection also show that alloreactive IgG antibodies may induce accelerated atherosclerosis in transplanted solid organs.

13-37 A variety of organs are transplanted routinely in clinical medicine.

Although the immune response makes organ transplantation difficult, there are few alternative therapies for organ failure. Three major advances have made it possible to use organ transplantation routinely in the clinic. First, the technical skill to perform organ replacement surgery has been mastered by many people. Second, networks of transplantation centers have been organized to ensure that the few healthy organs that are available are HLA-typed and so are matched with the most suitable recipient. Third, the use of powerful immunosuppressive drugs, especially cyclosporin A and FK-506 (tacrolimus) to inhibit T-cell activation (see Chapter 14), has markedly increased graft survival rates. The different organs that are transplanted in the clinic are listed in Fig. 13.41. Some of these operations are performed routinely with a very high success rate. By far the most frequently transplanted solid organ is the kidney, the organ first successfully transplanted between identical twins in the 1950s. Transplantation of the cornea is even more frequent; this tissue is a special case because it is not vascularized, and corneal grafts between unrelated people are usually successful even without immunosuppression.

However, there are many problems other than graft rejection associated with organ transplantation. First, donor organs are difficult to obtain; this is especially a problem when the organ involved is a vital one, such as the heart or liver. Second, the disease that destroyed the patient's organ might also destroy the graft, as in pancreatic β-cell destruction in diabetes. Third, the immunosuppression required to prevent graft rejection increases the risk of cancer and infection. Finally, the procedure is very costly. All of these problems need to be addressed before clinical transplantation can become commonplace. The problems most amenable to scientific solution are the development of more effective means of immunosuppression, the induction of graft-specific tolerance, and the development of xenografts as a practical solution to organ availability.

Tissue transplanted	5-year graft survival*	No. of grafts in USA (2002)
Kidney	65–75%	15,680
Liver	65–75%	5594
Heart	68%	2231
Pancreas	30%/80%#	1492
Lung	40%	1077
Cornea	~70%	~40,000†
Bone marrow	40%/60%	15,000‡

Fig. 13.41 Tissues commonly transplanted in clinical medicine. All grafts except corneal require long-term immunosuppression. The numbers of organ grafts performed in the United States in 2002 are shown. *Number of grafts includes multiple organ grafts. Data from the United Network for Organ Sharing. #Pancreas survival is 30% when transplanted alone or 80% when transplanted with a kidney. †Data for 2000 courtesy of National Eye Institute. ‡Data for 2000 from the International Bone Marrow Transplant Registry for allogeneic transplants only; survival depends on disease and is 40% for patients with acute and 60% for patients with chronic forms of myelogenous leukemia.

13-38 The converse of graft rejection is graft-versus-host disease.

Graft-Versus-Host Disease

Transplantation of hematopoietic stem cells is a successful therapy for some tumors derived from bone marrow precursors, such as certain leukemias and lymphomas. It can also be used to cure some primary immunodeficiency diseases (see Chapter 11) and inherited hematopoietic stem-cell diseases, such as the severe forms of thalassemia, by replacing genetically defective stem cells with normal donor ones. In leukemia therapy, the recipient's bone marrow, the source of the leukemia, must first be destroyed by aggressive cytotoxic chemotherapy. One of the major complications of allogeneic bone marrow transplantation is **graft-versus-host disease** (**GVHD**), in which mature donor T cells that contaminate the allogeneic bone marrow recognize the tissues of the recipient as foreign, causing a severe inflammatory disease characterized by rashes, diarrhea, and liver disease. GVHD is particularly virulent when there is a mismatch of a major MHC class I or class II antigen. Most transplants are therefore undertaken only when the donor and recipient are HLA-matched siblings or, less frequently, when there is an HLA-matched unrelated donor. However, as in organ transplantation, GVHD also occurs in the context of disparities between minor histocompatibility antigens. For this reason, immunosuppression must be used in every stem-cell transplant.

The presence of alloreactive T cells can easily be demonstrated experimentally by the **mixed lymphocyte reaction** (MLR), in which lymphocytes from a potential donor are mixed with irradiated lymphocytes from the potential recipient. If the donor lymphocytes contain alloreactive T cells, these will respond by cell division (Fig. 13.42). The MLR is sometimes used in the selection of donors for bone marrow transplants, when the lowest possible alloreactive response is essential. However, the limitation of the MLR in selection of bone marrow donors is that the test does not accurately quantify alloreactive T cells. A more accurate test is a version of the limiting-dilution assay (see Appendix I, Section A-25), which precisely counts the frequency of alloreactive T cells.

Fig. 13.42 The mixed lymphocyte reaction (MLR) can be used to detect histoincompatibility. Lymphocytes from the two individuals who are to be tested for compatibility are isolated from peripheral blood. The cells from one person (yellow), which will also contain antigen-presenting cells, are either irradiated or treated with mitomycin C; they will act as stimulator cells but cannot now respond by DNA synthesis and cell division to antigenic stimulation by the other person's cells. The cells from the two individuals are then mixed (top panel). If the unirradiated lymphocytes (the responders, blue) contain alloreactive T cells, these will be stimulated to proliferate and differentiate to effector cells. Between 3 and 7 days after mixing, the culture is assessed for T-cell proliferation (bottom left panel), which is mainly the result of CD4 T cells recognizing differences in MHC class II molecules, and for the generation of activated cytotoxic T cells (bottom right panel), which respond to differences in MHC class I molecules.

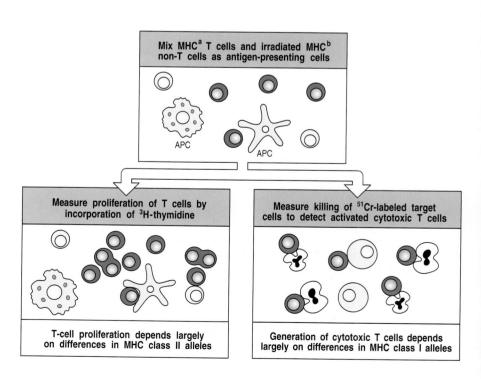

Although GVHD is harmful to the recipient of a bone marrow transplant, there can be some critical beneficial effects. Much of the therapeutic effect of bone marrow transplantation for leukemia can be due to a **graft-versus-leukemia effect**, in which the allogeneic bone marrow recognizes minor histocompatibility antigens or tumor-specific antigens expressed by the leukemic cells, leading the donor cells to kill the leukemic cells. One of the treatment options for suppressing the development of GVHD is the elimination of mature T cells from the donor bone marrow *in vitro* before transplantation, thereby removing alloreactive T cells. Those T cells that subsequently mature from the donor marrow *in vivo* in the recipient are tolerant to the recipient's antigens. Although the elimination of GVHD has benefits for the patient, there is an increase in the risk of leukemic relapse, which provides strong evidence in support of the graft-versus-leukemia effect.

Immunodeficiency is another complication of donor T-cell depletion. Because most of the recipient's T cells are destroyed by the combination of high-dose chemotherapy and irradiation used to treat the recipient before the transplant, donor T cells are the major source for reconstituting mature T cells after the transplant. This is particularly true in adults, who have poor residual thymic function. If too many T cells are depleted from the graft, therefore, transplant recipients experience, and often die from, numerous opportunistic infections. The need to balance the beneficial effects of the graft-versus-leukemia effect and immunocompetence with the adverse effects of GVHD caused by donor T cells has spawned much research. One particularly promising approach is to prevent donor T cells from reacting with recipient antigens that they could meet shortly after the transplant. This is accomplished by depleting the recipient's antigen-presenting cells, chiefly dendritic cells (Fig. 13.43). Evidently, in this situation, the donor T cells are not activated during the initial inflammation that accompanies the transplant, and thereafter they do not promote GVHD. However, it is unclear whether there would be graft-versus-leukemia effect in this context.

| In a hematopoietic stem-cell transplant the recipient receives some mature T cells | Alloreactive T cells are activated by recipient dendritic cells and can cause widespread tissue damage, called graft-versus-host disease (GVHD) | If recipient dendritic cells are absent, donor T cells now only see donor-derived dendritic cells and are not activated to cause GVHD |

Fig. 13.43 Recipient type antigen-presenting cells are required for the efficient initiation of graft-versus-host disease (GVHD). T cells that accompany the hematopoietic stem cells from the donor (left panel) can recognize minor histocompatibility antigens of the recipient and start an immune response against the recipient's tissues. In stem-cell transplantation, minor antigens could be presented by either recipient- or donor-derived antigen-presenting cells, the latter deriving from the stem-cell graft and from precursor cells that differentiate after the transplant. Antigen-presenting cells are shown here as dendritic cells in a lymph node (middle panel). In mice, it has been possible to inactivate the host antigen-presenting cells using gene knockouts. Such recipients are entirely resistant to GVHD mediated by donor CD8 T cells (right panel). Thus, cross-presentation of the recipient's minor histocompatibility antigens on donor dendritic cells is not sufficient to stimulate GVHD; those antigens endogenously synthesized and presented by the recipient's antigen-presenting cells are required to stimulate donor T cells. For this strategy to be useful for preventing GVHD in human patients, ways of depleting the recipient's antigen-presenting cells will be needed. These are the focus of research in a number of laboratories.

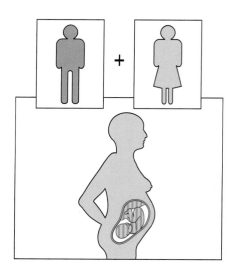

Fig. 13.44 The fetus is an allograft that is not rejected. Although the fetus carries MHC molecules derived from the father, and other foreign antigens, it is not rejected. Even when the mother bears several children to the same father, no sign of immunological rejection is seen.

13-39 The fetus is an allograft that is tolerated repeatedly.

All of the transplants discussed so far are artifacts of modern medical technology. However, one 'foreign' tissue that is repeatedly grafted and repeatedly tolerated is the mammalian fetus. The fetus carries paternal MHC and minor histocompatibility antigens that differ from those of the mother (Fig. 13.44), and yet a mother can successfully bear many children expressing the same nonself MHC proteins derived from the father. The mysterious lack of rejection of the fetus has puzzled generations of immunologists, and no comprehensive explanation has yet emerged. One problem is that acceptance of the fetal allograft is so much the norm that it is difficult to study the mechanism that prevents rejection; if the mechanism for rejecting the fetus is rarely activated, how can one analyze the mechanisms that control it?

Various hypotheses have been advanced to account for the tolerance shown to the fetus. It has been proposed that the fetus is simply not recognized as foreign. There is evidence against this hypothesis, because women who have borne several children usually make antibodies directed against the father's MHC proteins and red blood cell antigens; indeed, this is the best source of antibodies for human MHC typing. However, the placenta, which is a fetus-derived tissue, seems to sequester the fetus away from the mother's T cells. The outer layer of the placenta, the interface between fetal and maternal tissues, is the trophoblast. This does not express classical MHC class I and class II proteins, making it resistant to recognition and attack by maternal T cells. Tissues lacking class I expression are, however, vulnerable to attack by NK cells (see Section 2-28). The trophoblast might be protected from attack by NK cells by the expression of a nonclassical and minimally polymorphic HLA class I molecule—HLA-G. This protein has been shown to bind to the two major inhibitory NK receptors, KIR1 and KIR2, and to inhibit NK killing.

The placenta might also sequester the fetus from the mother's T cells by an active mechanism of nutrient depletion. The enzyme indoleamine 2,3-dioxygenase (IDO) is expressed at a high level by cells at the maternal–fetal interface. This enzyme catabolizes, and thereby depletes, the essential amino acid tryptophan at this site. T cells starved of tryptophan show reduced responsiveness. Inhibition of IDO in pregnant mice, using the inhibitor 1-methyltryptophan, causes rapid rejection of allogeneic but not syngeneic fetuses. This supports the hypothesis that maternal T cells, alloreactive to paternal MHC proteins, might be held in check in the placenta by tryptophan depletion.

It is likely that fetal tolerance is a multifactorial process. The trophoblast does not act as an absolute barrier between mother and fetus, and fetal blood cells can cross the placenta and be detected in the maternal circulation, albeit in very low numbers. There is direct evidence from experiments in mice for specific T-cell tolerance against paternal MHC alloantigens. Pregnant female mice whose T cells bear a transgenic receptor specific for a paternal alloantigen showed reduced expression of this T-cell receptor during pregnancy. These same mice lost the ability to control the growth of an experimental tumor bearing the same paternal MHC alloantigen. After pregnancy, tumor growth was controlled and the level of the T-cell receptor increased. This experiment demonstrates that the maternal immune system must have been exposed to paternal MHC alloantigens and that the immune response to these antigens was temporarily suppressed.

Yet another factor that might contribute to maternal tolerance of the fetus is the secretion of cytokines at the maternal–fetal interface. Both the uterine epithelium and the trophoblast secrete cytokines, including TGF-β, IL-4, and IL-10. This cytokine pattern tends to suppress T_H1 responses (see Chapter 10). The induction or injection of cytokines such as IFN-γ and IL-12, which promote T_H1 responses in experimental animals, promotes fetal resorption, the equivalent of spontaneous abortion in humans. Finally, it is possible that regulatory T cells could have a role in suppressing responses to the fetus.

The fetus is thus tolerated for two main reasons: it occupies a site protected by a nonimmunogenic tissue barrier, and it promotes a local immunosuppressive response in the mother. Several sites in the body, such as the eye, have these characteristics and allow the prolonged acceptance of foreign tissue grafts. They are usually called immunologically privileged sites (see Section 13-9).

Summary.

Clinical transplantation is now an everyday reality, its success built on MHC matching, immunosuppressive drugs, and technical skill. However, even accurate MHC matching does not prevent graft rejection; other genetic differences between host and donor can result in allogeneic proteins whose peptides are presented as minor histocompatibility antigens by MHC molecules on the grafted tissue, and responses to these can lead to rejection. As we lack the ability to specifically suppress the response to the graft without compromising host defense, most transplants require generalized immunosuppression of the recipient. This can be toxic and increases the risk of cancer and infection. The fetus is a natural allograft that must be accepted—it almost always is—or the species will not survive. Tolerance to the fetus might hold the key to inducing specific tolerance to grafted tissues, or it might be a special case not applicable to organ replacement therapy.

Summary to Chapter 13.

Ideally, the effector functions of the immune system would be targeted only to foreign pathogens and never to self tissues. In practice, because foreign and self proteins are chemically similar, strict discrimination between self and nonself is impossible. Yet the immune system maintains tolerance to self tissues. This is accomplished by layers of regulation, all of which use surrogate markers to distinguish self from nonself, thus properly directing the immune response. When these regulatory mechanisms break down, autoimmune disease can result. Minor breaches of single regulatory barriers probably occur every day but are quelled by the effects of other regulatory layers: thus, tolerance operates at the level of the overall immune system. For disease to occur, multiple layers of tolerance have to be overcome and the effect needs to be chronic. These layers begin with central tolerance in the bone marrow and thymus, and include peripheral mechanisms such as anergy, cytokine deviation, and regulatory T cells. Sometimes immune responses do not occur simply because the antigens are not available, as in immune sequestration.

Perhaps because of selective pressure to mount effective immune responses to pathogens, the damping of immune responses to promote self-tolerance is limited and prone to failure. Genetic predisposition has an important role in determining which individuals will get an autoimmune disease. The MHC region, not surprisingly, has a dominant effect in many diseases. There are numerous additional genes, most of which are not clearly identified, that contribute to immune regulation and thus, when defective, can cause or predispose to autoimmune disease. Environmental forces also have a significant role, because even identical twins are not always both affected by the same autoimmune disease. Influences from the environment could include infections, toxins, and chance events.

When self-tolerance is broken and autoimmune disease ensues, the effector mechanisms are quite similar to those used in pathogen responses. Although the details vary from disease to disease, both antibody and T cells can be involved. Transplantation of solid organs and bone marrow have brought on syndromes of rejection that are in many ways similar to autoimmune disease, but the targets are either major or minor histocompatibility antigens. The latter come from polymorphic genes. T cells are the main effectors in graft rejection and graft-versus-host disease.

For each of the undesirable categories of response discussed here (along with allergy, discussed in Chapter 12), the question is how to control the response without adversely affecting protective immunity to infection. The answer might lie in a more complete understanding of the regulation of the immune response, especially the suppressive mechanisms that seem to be important in tolerance. The deliberate control of the immune response is examined further in Chapter 14.

Chapter 13 questions.

13.1 (a) Discuss the multiple layers of self-tolerance. (b) Name at least four of them and describe the mechanism of each in a few sentences.

13.2 What is the difference between 'dominant' and 'recessive' tolerance? Explain, and give an example of each.

13.3 What is the evidence that genetic predisposition has an important role in autoimmune disease? Give two examples, and for each explain why the example implicates genetics.

13.4 (a) Discuss one compelling piece of evidence that environment also has a role in the development of autoimmunity. (b) Name two potential environmental factors, and for one of them describe in more detail how it might work to incite autoimmunity.

13.5 There are several different pathogenesis mechanisms in autoimmunity. Provide an example of four, and briefly describe an example of each. Include both antibody- and T-cell-dependent mechanisms.

13.6 A person with leukemia receives a bone marrow transplant from his HLA-identical brother. Two weeks later he develops a skin rash and nausea, although his leukemia is in remission. (a) What is this syndrome called? (b) What type of lymphocyte causes it? (c) What antigens are being recognized?

Section references.

13-1   A critical function of the immune system is to discriminate self from nonself.

Ehrlich, P., and Morgenroth, J.: **On haemolysins**, in Himmelweit, F. (ed): *The Collected Papers of Paul Ehrlich*. London, Pergamon, 1957: 246–255.

Janeway, C.A., Jr.: **The immune system evolved to discriminate infectious nonself from noninfectious self.** *Immunol. Today* 1992, **13**:11–16.

13-2   Specific adaptive immune responses to self antigens can cause autoimmune disease.

Hardin, J.A., and Craft, J.E.: **Patterns of autoimmunity to nucleoproteins in patients with systemic lupus erythematosus.** *Rheum. Dis. Clinics N. Am.* 1987, **13**:37–46.

Plotz, P.H.: **The autoantibody repertoire: searching for order.** *Nat. Rev. Immunol.* 2003, **3**:73–78.

Shlomchik, M.J., Marshak-Rothstein, A., Wolfowicz, C.B., Rothstein, T.L., and Weigert, M.G.: **The role of clonal selection and somatic mutation in autoimmunity.** *Nature* 1987, **328**:805–811.

Steinman, L.: **Multiple sclerosis: a coordinated immunological attack against myelin in the central nervous system.** *Cell* 1996, **85**:299–302.

13-3   Autoimmune diseases can be classified into clusters that are typically either organ-specific or systemic.

Bach, J.F.: **Organ-specific autoimmunity.** *Immunol. Today* 1995, **16**:353–355.

King, C., and Sarvetnick, N.: **Organ-specific autoimmunity.** *Curr. Opin. Immunol.* 1997, **9**:863–871.

13-4   Multiple limbs of the immune system are typically recruited in autoimmune disease.

Couser, W.G.: **Pathogenesis of glomerulonephritis.** *Kidney Int. Suppl.* 1993, **42**:S19–S26.

Green, E.A., and Flavell, R.A.: **The initiation of autoimmune diabetes.** *Curr. Opin. Immunol.* 1999, **11**:663–669.

Huang, X.R., Tipping, P.G., Apostolopoulos, C., Oettinger, C., D'Souza, M., Milton, G., and Holdsworth, S.R.: **Mechanisms of T cell-induced glomerular injury in anti-glomerular basement membrane (GBM) glomerulonephritis in rats.** *Clin. Exp. Immunol.* 1997, **157**:134–142.

Shlomchik, M.J., and Madaio, M.P.: **The role of antibodies and B cells in the pathogenesis of lupus nephritis.** *Springer Semin. Immunopathol.* 2003, **24**:363–375.

13-5   Initial loss of tolerance and autoimmunity may evolve to a chronic disease state because of positive feedback from inflammation as well as the inability to clear most self antigens.

Shlomchik, M.J., Craft, J., and Mamula, M.J.: **From T to B and back again: positive feedback in systemic autoimmune disease.** *Nat. Rev. Immunol.* 2001, **1**:147–153.

Steinman, L.: **A few autoreactive cells in an autoimmune infiltrate control a vast population of nonspecific cells: a tale of smart bombs and the infantry.** *Proc. Natl. Acad. Sci. USA* 1996, **93**:2253–2256.

13-6   Some degree of autoimmunity is the evolutionary price of being able to make effective responses against pathogens.

Goodnow, C.C.: **Balancing immunity and tolerance: deleting and tuning lymphocyte repertoires.** *Proc. Natl. Acad. Sci. USA* 1996, **93**:2264–2271.

13-7   Central deletion or inactivation of newly formed lymphocytes is the first checkpoint of self-tolerance.

Goodnow, C.C., Adelstein, S., and Basten, A.: **The need for central and peripheral tolerance in the B cell repertoire.** *Science* 1990, **248**:1373–1379.

Kisielow, P., Bluthmann, H., Staerz, U.D., Steinmetz, M., and von Boehmer, H.: **Tolerance in T-cell-receptor transgenic mice involves deletion of nonmature CD4+8+ thymocytes.** *Nature* 1988, **333**:742–746.

Nemazee, D.A., and Burki, K.: **Clonal deletion of B lymphocytes in a transgenic mouse bearing anti-MHC class-I antibody genes.** *Nature* 1989, **337**:562–566.

Nossal, G.J.V., and Pike, B.L.: **Clonal anergy: persistence in tolerant mice of antigen-binding B lymphocytes incapable of responding to antigen or mitogen.** *Proc. Natl. Acad. Sci. USA* 1980, **77**:1602–1606.

Nossal, G.J.V., and Pike, B.L.: **Mechanisms of clonal abortion tolerogenesis: I. Response of immature hapten-specific B lymphocytes.** *J. Exp. Med.* 1978, **148**:1161–1170.

13-8   Lymphocytes that bind self antigens with relatively low affinity usually ignore them but in some circumstances become activated.

Billingham, R.E., Brent, L., and Medawar, P.B.: **Actively acquired tolerance of foreign cells.** *Nature* 1953, **172**:603–606.

Goverman, J., Woods, A., Larson, L., Weiner, L.P., Hood, L., and Zaller, D.M.: **Transgenic mice that express a myelin basic protein-specific T cell receptor develop spontaneous autoimmunity.** *Cell* 1993, **72**:551–560.

Hannum, L.G., Ni, D., Haberman, A.M., Weigert, M.G., and Shlomchik, M.J.: **A disease-related RF autoantibody is not tolerized in a normal mouse: implications for the origins of autoantibodies in autoimmune disease.** *J. Exp. Med.* 1996, **184**:1269–1278.

Katz, J.D., Wang, B., Haskins, K., Benoist, C., and Mathis, D.: **Following a diabetogenic T cell from genesis through pathogenesis.** *Cell* 1993, **74**:1089–1100.

Kurts, C., Sutherland, R.M., Davey, G., Li, M., Lew, A.M., Blanas, E., Carbone, F.R., Miller, J.F., and Heath, W.R.: **CD8 T cell ignorance or tolerance to islet antigens depends on antigen dose.** *Proc. Natl. Acad. Sci. USA* 1999, **96**:12703–12707.

Miller, J.F., and Heath, W.R.: **Self-ignorance in the peripheral T-cell pool.** *Immunol. Rev.* 1993, **133**:131–150.

13-9   Antigens in immunologically privileged sites do not induce immune attack but can serve as targets.

Alison, J., Georgiou, H.M., Strasser, A., and Vaux, D.L.: **Transgenic expression of CD95 ligand on islet β cells induces a granulocytic infiltration but does not confer immune privilege upon islet allografts.** *Proc. Natl. Acad. Sci. USA* 1997, **94**: 3943–3947.

Ferguson, T.A., and Griffith, T.S.: **A vision of cell death: insights into immune privilege.** *Immunol. Rev.* 1997, **156**:167–184.

Green, D.R., and Ware, C.F.: **Fas-ligand: privilege and peril.** *Proc. Natl. Acad. Sci. USA* 1997, **94**:5986–5990.

Streilein, J.W., Ksander, B.R., and Taylor, A.W.: **Immune deviation in relation to ocular immune privilege.** *J. Immunol.* 1997, **158**:3557–3560.

13-10   Autoreactive T cells that express particular cytokines may be nonpathogenic or suppress pathogenic lymphocytes.

von Herrath, M.G., and Harrison, L.C.: **Antigen-induced regulatory T cells in autoimmunity.** *Nat. Rev. Immunol.* 2003, **3**:223–232.

Qin, S., Cobbold, S.P., Pope, H., Elliott, J., Kioussis, D., Davies, J., and Waldmann, H.: **'Infectious' transplantation tolerance.** *Science* 1993, **259**:974–977.

Rocken, M., and Shevach E.M.: **Immune deviation—the third dimension of nondeletional T cell tolerance.** *Immunol. Rev.* 1996, **149**:175–194.

13-11 Autoimmune responses can be controlled at various stages by regulatory T cells.

Asano, M., Toda, M., Sakaguchi, N., and Sakaguchi, S.: **Autoimmune disease as a consequence of developmental abnormality of a T cell subpopulation.** *J. Exp. Med.* 1996, **184**:387–396.

Sakaguchi, S.: **Regulatory T cells: key controllers of immunologic self-tolerance.** *Cell* 2000, **101**:455–458.

13-12 CD4 CD25 T cells are a unique subset of cells that arise in the thymus in response to relatively strong recognition of self antigen.

Fontenot, J.D., Gavin, M.A., and Rudensky, A.Y.: **Foxp3 programs the development and function of CD4+CD25+ regulatory T cells.** *Nat. Immunol.* 2003, **4**:330–336.

Johnson, B.D., Becker, E.E., LaBelle, J.L., and Truitt, R.L.: **Role of immunoregulatory donor T cells in suppression of graft-versus-host disease following donor leukocyte infusion therapy.** *J. Immunol.* 1999, **163**:6479–6487.

Jordan, M.S., Boesteanu, A., Reed, A.J., Petrone, A.L., Holenbeck, A.E., Lerman, M.A., Naji, A., and Caton, A.J.: **Thymic selection of CD4+CD25+ regulatory T cells induced by an agonist self-peptide.** *Nat. Immunol.* 2001, **2**:301–306.

Khattri, R., Cox, T., Yasayko, S.A., and Ramsdell, F.: **An essential role for Scurfin in CD4+CD25+ T regulatory cells.** *Nat. Immunol.* 2003, **4**:337–342.

Maloy, K.J., and Powrie, F.: **Regulatory T cells in the control of immune pathology.** *Nat. Immunol.* 2001, **2**:816–822.

Seo, S.J., Fields, M.L., Buckler, J.L., Reed, A.J., Mandik-Nayak, L., Nish, S.A., Noelle, R.J., Turka, L.A., Finkelman, F.D., Caton, A.J., and Erikson, J.: **The impact of T helper and T regulatory cells on the regulation of anti-double-stranded DNA B cells.** *Immunity* 2002, **16**:535–546.

Shevach, E.M.: **Regulatory T cells in autoimmmunity.** *Annu. Rev. Immunol.* 2000, **18**:423–449.

Wildin, R.S., Ramsdell, F., Peake, J., Faravelli, F., Casanova, J.L., Buist, N., Levy-Lahad, E., Mazzella, M., Goulet, O., Perroni, L., Bricarelli, F.D., Byrne, G., McEuen, M., Proll, S., Appleby, M., and Brunkow, M.E.: **X-linked neonatal diabetes mellitus, enteropathy and endocrinopathy syndrome is the human equivalent of mouse scurfy.** *Nat. Genet.* 2001, **27**:18–20.

13-13 The mechanisms of regulation are varied and can include cytokine-mediated inhibition, contact-dependent regulation, and cell killing.

Hara, M., Kingsley, C.I., Niimi, M., Read, S., Turvey, S.E., Bushell, A.R., Morris, P.J., Powrie, F., and Wood, K.J.: **IL-10 is required for regulatory T cells to mediate tolerance to alloantigens** *in vivo.* *J. Immunol.* 2001, **166**:3789–3796.

Mottet, C., Uhlig, H.H., and Powrie, F.: **Cutting edge: cure of colitis by CD4+CD25+ regulatory T cells.** *J. Immunol.* 2003, **170**:3939–3943.

Shevach, E.M.: **CD4+ CD25+ suppressor T cells: more questions than answers.** *Nat. Rev. Immunol.* 2002, **2**:389–400.

13-14 Other types of regulatory cell also exist.

Faria, A.M., and Weiner, H.L.: **Oral tolerance: mechanisms and therapeutic applications.** *Adv. Immunol.* 1999, **73**:153–264.

Fillatreau, S., Sweenie, C.H., McGeachy, M.J., Gray, D., and Anderton, S.M.: **B cells regulate autoimmunity by provision of IL-10.** *Nat. Immunol.* 2002, **3**:944–950.

Roncarolo, M.G., Bacchetta, R., Bordignon, C., Narula, S., and Levings, M.K.: **Type 1 T regulatory cells.** *Immunol. Rev.* 2001, **182**:68–79.

Roncarolo, M.G., and Levings, M.K.: **The role of different subsets of T regulatory cells in controlling autoimmunity.** *Curr. Opin. Immunol.* 2000, **12**:676–683.

Wang, B., Geng, Y.B., and Wang, C.R.: **CD1-restricted NK T cells protect nonobese diabetic mice from developing diabetes.** *J. Exp. Med.* 2001, **194**:313–320.

Weiner, H.L.: **Oral tolerance: immune mechanisms and the generation of Th3-type TGF-β-secreting regulatory cells.** *Microbes Infect.* 2001, **3**:947–954.

13-15 Immune responses have natural brakes that tend to limit damage even when autoimmune cells are activated.

Ku, C.C., Murakami, M., Sakamoto, A., Kappler, J., and Marrack, P.: **Control of homeostasis of CD8+ memory T cells by opposing cytokines.** *Science* 2000, **288**:675–678.

Plas, D.R., Rathmell, J.C., and Thompson, C.B.: **Homeostatic control of lymphocyte survival: potential origins and implications.** *Nat. Immunol.* 2002, **3**:515–521.

Singer, G.G., and Abbas, A.K.: **The fas antigen is involved in peripheral but not thymic deletion of T lymphocytes in T cell receptor transgenic mice.** *Immunity* 1994, **1**:365–371.

13-16 Autoimmune diseases have a strong genetic as well as environmental component.

Gonzalez, A., Katz, J.D., Mattei, M.G., Kikutani, H., Benoist, C., and Mathis D.: **Genetic control of diabetes progression.** *Immunity* 1997, **7**:873–883.

Morel, L., Rudofsky, U.H., Longmate, J.A., Schiffenbauer, J., and Wakeland, E.K.: **Polygenic control of susceptibility to murine systemic lupus erythematosus.** *Immunity* 1994, **1**:219–229.

13-17 Several approaches have given us insight into the genetic basis of autoimmunity.

Vyse, T.J., and Todd, J.A.: **Genetic analysis of autoimmune disease.** *Cell* 1996, **85**:311–318.

Wakeland, E.K., Wandstrat, A.E., Liu, K., and Morel, L.: **Genetic dissection of systemic lupus erythematosus.** *Curr. Opin. Immunol.* 1999, **11**:701–707.

13-18 Genes that predispose to autoimmunity fall into categories that affect one or more of the layers of tolerance.

Goodnow, C.C.: **Polygenic autoimmune traits: Lyn, CD22, and SHP-1 are limiting elements of a biochemical pathway regulating BCR signaling and selection.** *Immunity* 1998, **8**:497–508.

Singer, G.G., Carrera, A.C., Marshak-Rothstein, A., Martinez, C., and Abbas, A.K.: **Apoptosis, Fas and systemic autoimmunity: the MRL-lpr/lpr model.** *Curr. Opin. Immunol.* 1994, **6**:913–920.

Tivol, E.A., Borriello, F., Schweitzer, A.N., Lynch, W.P., Bluestone, J.A., and Sharpe, A.H.: **Loss of CTLA-4 leads to massive lymphoproliferation and fatal multiorgan tissue destruction, revealing a critical negative regulatory role of CTLA-4.** *Immunity* 1995, **3**:541–547.

Wakeland, E.K., Liu, K., Graham, R.R., and Behrens, T.W.: **Delineating the genetic basis of systemic lupus erythematosus.** *Immunity* 2001, **15**:397–408.

Walport, M.J.: **Lupus, DNase and defective disposal of cellular debris.** *Nat. Genet.* 2000, **25**:135–136.

Whitacre, C.C., Reingold, S.C., and O'Looney, P.A.: **A gender gap in autoimmunity.** *Science* 1999, **283**:1277–1278.

13-19 MHC genes have an important role in controlling susceptibility to autoimmune disease.

Haines, J.L., Ter Minassian, M., Bazyk, A., Gusella, J.F., Kim, D.J., Terwedow, H., Pericak-Vance, M.A., Rimmler, J.B., Haynes, C.S., Roses, A.D., Lee, A., Shaner, B., Menold, M., Seboun, e., Fitoussi, R.P., Gartioux, C., Reyes, C., Ribierre, F., Gyapay, G., Weissenbach, J., Hauser, S.L., Goodkin, D.E., Lincoln, R., Usuku, K., Oksenberg, J.R., et al.: **A complete genomic screen for multiple sclerosis underscores a role for the major histocompatibility complex. The Multiple Sclerosis Genetics Group.** *Nat. Genet.* 1996, **13**:469–471.

McDevitt, H.O.: **Discovering the role of the major histocompatibility complex in the immune response.** *Annu. Rev. Immunol.* 2000, **18**:1–17.

13-20 Molecular pathways promoting autoimmunity are potential targets for the therapy of autoimmune disease.

Blazar, B.R., Taylor, P.A., Panoskaltsis-Mortari, A., Buhlman, J., Xu, J., Flavell, R.A., Korngold, R., Noelle, R., and Vallera, D.A.: **Blockade of CD40 ligand-CD40 interaction impairs CD4+ T cell-mediated alloreactivity by inhibiting mature donor T cell expansion and function after bone marrow transplantation.** *J. Immunol.* 1997, **158**:29–39.

Kalled, S.L., Cutler, A.H., Datta, S.K., and Thomas, D.W.: **Anti-CD40 ligand antibody treatment of SNF$_1$ mice with established nephritis: preservation of kidney function.** *J. Immunol.* 1998, **160**:2158–2165.

Wang, X., Huang, W., Mihara, M., Sinha, J., and Davidson, A.: **Mechanism of action of combined short-term CTLA4Ig and anti-CD40 ligand in murine systemic lupus erythematosus.** *J. Immunol.* 2002, **168**:2046–2053.

Wiederrecht, G., Lam, E., Hung, S., Martin, M., and Sigal, N.: **The mechanism of action of FK-506 and cyclosporin A.** *Ann. N.Y. Acad. Sci.* 1993, **696**:9–19.

13-21   Drugs and toxins can cause autoimmune syndromes.

Bagenstose, L.M., Salgame, P., and Monestier, M.: **Murine mercury-induced autoimmunity: a model of chemically related autoimmunity in humans.** *Immunol. Res.* 1999, **20**:67–78.

Yoshida, S., and Gershwin, M.E.: **Autoimmunity and selected environmental factors of disease induction.** *Semin. Arthritis Rheum.* 1993, **22**:399–419.

13-22   Infection can lead to autoimmune disease.

Aichele, P., Bachmann, M.F., Hengarter, H., and Zinkernagel, R.M.: **Immunopathology or organ-specific autoimmunity as a consequence of virus infection.** *Immunol. Rev.* 1996, **152**:21–45.

von Herrath, M.G., Evans, C.F., Horwitz, M.S., and Oldstone, M.B.: **Using transgenic mouse models to dissect the pathogenesis of virus-induced autoimmune disorders of the islets of Langerhans and the central nervous system.** *Immunol. Rev.* 1996, **152**:111–143.

von Herrath, M.G., Holz, A., Homann, D., and Oldstone, M.B.: **Role of viruses in type I diabetes.** *Semin. Immunol.* 1998, **10**:87–100.

Moens, U., Seternes, O.M., Hey, A.W., Silsand, Y., Traavik, T., Johansen, B., and Rekvig, O.P.: **In vivo expression of a single viral DNA-binding protein generates systemic lupus erythematosus-related autoimmunity to double-stranded DNA and histones.** *Proc. Natl. Acad. Sci. USA* 1995, **92**:12393–12397.

Steinman, L., and Conlon, P.: **Viral damage and the breakdown of self-tolerance.** *Nat. Med.* 1997, **3**:1085–1087.

13-23   Cross-reactivity between self molecules and foreign molecules on pathogens can lead to anti-self responses and autoimmune disease.

Barnaba, V., and Sinigaglia, F.: **Molecular mimicry and T cell-mediated autoimmune disease.** *J. Exp. Med.* 1997, **185**:1529–1531.

Rose, N.R., Herskowitz, A., Neumann, D.A., and Neu, N.: **Autoimmune myocarditis: a paradigm of post-infection autoimmune disease.** *Immunol. Today* 1988, **9**:117–120.

Rose, N.R.: **Infection, mimics, and autoimmune disease.** *J. Clin. Invest.* 2001, **107**:943–944.

Steinman, L., and Oldstone, M.B.: **More mayhem from molecular mimics.** *Nat. Med.* 1997, **3**:1321–1322.

13-24   Random events may be required for the initiation of autoimmunity.

Eisenberg, R.A., Craven, S.Y., Warren, R.W., and Cohen, P.L.: **Stochastic control of anti-Sm autoantibodies in MRL/Mp-lpr/lpr mice.** *J. Clin. Invest.* 1987, **80**:691–697.

Todd, J.A., and Steinman, L.: **The environment strikes back.** *Curr. Opin. Immunol.* 1993, **5**:863–865.

13-25   Antibody and T cells can cause tissue damage in autoimmune disease.

Chan, O.T.M., Madaio, M.P., and Shlomchik, M.J.: **The central and multiple roles of B cells in lupus pathogenesis.** *Immunol. Rev.* 1999, **169**:107–121.

Naparstek, Y., and Plotz, P.H.: **The role of autoantibodies in autoimmune disease.** *Annu. Rev. Immunol.* 1993, **11**:79–104.

Vlahakos, D., Foster, M.H., Ucci, A.A., Barrett, K.J., Datta, S.K., and Madaio, M.P.: **Murine monoclonal anti-DNA antibodies penetrate cells, bind to nuclei, and induce glomerular proliferation and proteinuria in vivo.** *J. Am. Soc. Nephrol.* 1992, **2**:1345–1354.

13-26   Autoantibodies against blood cells promote their destruction.

Beardsley, D.S., and Ertem, M.: **Platelet autoantibodies in immune thrombocytopenic purpura.** *Transfus. Sci.* 1998, **19**:237–244.

Clynes, R., and Ravetch, J.V.: **Cytotoxic antibodies trigger inflammation through Fc receptors.** *Immunity* 1995, **3**:21–26.

Domen, R.E.: **An overview of immune hemolytic anemias.** *Cleveland Clin. J. Med.* 1998, **65**:89–99.

Silberstein, L.E.: **Natural and pathologic human autoimmune responses to carbohydrate antigens on red blood cells.** *Springer Semin. Immunopathol.* 1993, **15**:139–153.

13-27   The fixation of sublytic doses of complement to cells in tissues stimulates a powerful inflammatory response.

Brandt, J., Pippin, J., Schulze, M., Hansch, G.M., Alpers, C.E., Johnson, R.J., Gordon, K., and Couser, W.G.: **Role of the complement membrane attack complex (C5b-9) in mediating experimental mesangioproliferative glomerulonephritis.** *Kidney Int.* 1996, **49**:335–343.

Hansch, G.M.: **The complement attack phase: control of lysis and non-lethal effects of C5b-9.** *Immunopharmacol.* 1992, **24**:107–117.

Shin, M.L., and Carney, D.F.: **Cytotoxic action and other metabolic consequences of terminal complement proteins.** *Prog. Allergy* 1988, **40**:44–81.

13-28   Autoantibodies against receptors cause disease by stimulating or blocking receptor function.

Bahn, R.S., and Heufelder, A.E.: **Pathogenesis of Graves' ophthalmopathy.** *N. Engl. J. Med.* 1993, **329**:1468–1475.

Feldmann, M., Dayan, C., Grubeck Loebenstein, B., Rapoport, B., and Londei, M.: **Mechanism of Graves thyroiditis: implications for concepts and therapy of autoimmunity.** *Int. Rev. Immunol.* 1992, **9**:91–106.

Vincent, A., Lily, O., and Palace, J.: **Pathogenic autoantibodies to neuronal proteins in neurological disorders.** *J. Neuroimmunol.* 1999, **100**:169–180.

13-29   Autoantibodies against extracellular antigens cause inflammatory injury by mechanisms akin to type II and type III hypersensitivity reactions.

Casciola-Rosen, L.A., Anhalt, G., and Rosen, A.: **Autoantigens targeted in systemic lupus erythematosus are clustered in two populations of surface structures on apoptotic keratinocytes.** *J. Exp. Med.* 1994, **179**:1317–1330.

Clynes, R., Dumitru, C., and Ravetch, J.V.: **Uncoupling of immune complex formation and kidney damage in autoimmune glomerulonephritis.** *Science* 1998, **279**:1052–1054.

Kotzin, B.L.: **Systemic lupus erythematosus.** *Cell* 1996, **85**:303–306.

Lawley, T.J., Bielory, L., Gascon, P., Yancey, K.B., Young, N.S., and Frank, M.M.: **A prospective clinical and immunologic analysis of patients with serum sickness.** *N. Engl. J. Med.* 1984, **311**:1407–1413.

Tan, E.M.: **Antinuclear antibodies: diagnostic markers for autoimmune diseases and probes for cell biology.** *Adv. Immunol.* 1989, **44**:93–151.

13-30   T cells specific for self antigens can cause direct tissue injury and have a role in sustained autoantibody responses.

Haskins, K., and Wegmann, D.: **Diabetogenic T-cell clones.** *Diabetes* 1996, **45**:1299–1305.

Peng, S.L., Madaio, M.P., Hughes, D.P., Crispe, I.N., Owen, M.J., Wen, L., Hayday, A.C., and Craft, J.: **Murine lupus in the absence of alpha beta T cells.** *J. Immunol.* 1996, **156**:4041–4049.

Zamvil, S., Nelson, P., Trotter, J., Mitchell, D., Knobler, R., Fritz, R., and Steinman, L.: **T-cell clones specific for myelin basic protein induce chronic relapsing paralysis and demyelination.** *Nature* 1985, **317**:355–358.

Zekzer, D., Wong, F.S., Ayalon, O., Altieri, M., Shintani, S., Solimena, M., and Sherwin, R.S.: **GAD-reactive CD4+ Th1 cells induce diabetes in NOD/SCID mice.** *J. Clin. Invest.* 1998, **101**:68–73.

13-31 Graft rejection is an immunological response mediated primarily by T cells.

Arakelov, A., and Lakkis, F.G.: **The alloimmune response and effector mechanisms of allograft rejection.** *Semin. Nephrol.* 2000, **20**:95–102.

Rosenberg, A.S., and Singer, A.: **Cellular basis of skin allograft rejection: an *in vivo* model of immune-mediated tissue destruction.** *Annu. Rev. Immunol.* 1992, **10**:333–358.

Strom, T.B., Roy-Chaudhury, P., Manfro, R., Zheng, X.X., Nickerson, P.W., Wood, K., and Bushell, A.: **The Th1/Th2 paradigm and the allograft response.** *Curr. Opin. Immunol.* 1996, **8**:688–693.

Zelenika, D., Adams, E., Humm, S., Lin, C.Y., Waldmann, H., and Cobbold, S.P.: **The role of CD4+ T-cell subsets in determining transplantation rejection or tolerance.** *Immunol. Rev.* 2001, **182**:164–179.

13-32 Matching donor and recipient at the MHC improves the outcome of transplantation.

Opelz, G.: **Factors influencing long-term graft loss. The Collaborative Transplant Study.** *Transplant. Proc.* 2000, **32**:647–649.

Opelz, G., and Wujciak, T.: **The influence of HLA compatibility on graft survival after heart transplantation. The Collaborative Transplant Study.** *N. Engl. J. Med.* 1994, **330**:816–819.

13-33 In MHC-identical grafts, rejection is caused by peptides from other alloantigens bound to graft MHC molecules.

den Haan, J.M., Meadows, L.M., Wang, W., Pool, J., Blokland, E., Bishop, T.L., Reinhardus, C., Shabanowitz, J., Offringa, R., Hunt, D.F., Engelhard, V.H., and Goulmy, E.: **The minor histocompatibility antigen HA-1: a diallelic gene with a single amino acid polymorphism.** *Science* 1998, **279**:1054–1057.

Mutis, T., Gillespie, G., Schrama, E., Falkenburg, J.H., Moss, P., and Goulmy, E.: **Tetrameric HLA class I–minor histocompatibility antigen peptide complexes demonstrate minor histocompatibility antigen-specific cytotoxic T lymphocytes in patients with graft-versus-host disease.** *Nat. Med.* 1999, **5**:839–842.

13-34 There are two ways of presenting alloantigens on the transplant to the recipient's T lymphocytes.

Benichou, G., Takizawa, P.A., Olson, C.A., McMillan, M., and Sercarz, E.E.: **Donor major histocompatibility complex (MHC) peptides are presented by recipient MHC molecules during graft rejection.** *J. Exp. Med.* 1992, **175**:305–308.

Carbone, F.R., Kurts, C., Bennett, S.R., Miller, J.F., and Heath, W.R.: **Cross-presentation: a general mechanism for CTL immunity and tolerance.** *Immunol. Today* 1998, **19**:368–373.

13-35 Antibodies reacting with endothelium cause hyperacute graft rejection.

Kissmeyer Nielsen, F., Olsen, S., Petersen, V.P., and Fjeldborg, O.: **Hyperacute rejection of kidney allografts, associated with pre-existing humoral antibodies against donor cells.** *Lancet* 1966, **2**:662–665.

Robson, S.C., Schulte am Esche, J., and Bach, F.H.: **Factors in xenograft rejection.** *Ann. N.Y. Acad. Sci.* 1999, **875**:261–276.

Sharma, A., Okabe, J., Birch, P., McClellan, S.B., Martin, M.J., Platt, J.L., and Logan, J.S.: **Reduction in the level of Gal(α1,3)Gal in transgenic mice and pigs by the expression of an α(1,2)fucosyltransferase.** *Proc. Natl. Acad. Sci. USA* 1996, **93**:7190–7195.

Williams, G.M., Hume, D.M., Hudson, R.P., Jr., Morris, P.J., Kano, K., and Milgrom, F.: **'Hyperacute' renal-homograft rejection in man.** *N. Engl. J. Med.* 1968, **279**:611–618.

13-36 Chronic organ rejection is caused by inflammatory vascular injury to the graft.

Orosz, C.G., and Peletier, R.P.: **Chronic remodeling pathology in grafts.** *Curr. Opin. Immunol.* 1997, **9**:676–680.

Paul, L.C.: **Current knowledge of the pathogenesis of chronic allograft dysfunction.** *Transplant. Proc.* 1999, **31**:1793–1795.

Womer, K.L., Vella, J.P., and Sayegh, M.H.: **Chronic allograft dysfunction: mechanisms and new approaches to therapy.** *Semin. Nephrol.* 2000, **20**:126–147.

13-37 A variety of organs are transplanted routinely in clinical medicine.

Murray, J.E.: **Human organ transplantation: background and consequences.** *Science* 1992, **256**:1411–1416.

13-38 The converse of graft rejection is graft-versus-host disease.

Dazzi, F., and Goldman, J.: **Donor lymphocyte infusions.** *Curr. Opin. Hematol.* 1999, **6**:394–399.

Goulmy, E., Schipper, R., Pool, J., Blokland, E., Flakenburg, J.H., Vossen, J., Grathwohl, A., Vogelsang, G.B., van Houwelingen, H.C., and van Rood, J.J.: **Mismatches of minor histocompatibility antigens between HLA-identical donors and recipients and the development of graft-versus-host disease after bone marrow transplantation.** *N. Engl. J. Med.* 1996, **334**:281–285.

Murphy, W.J., and Blazar, B.R.: **New strategies for preventing graft-versus-host disease.** *Curr. Opin. Immunol.* 1999, **11**:509–515.

Porter, D.L., and Antin, J.H.: **The graft-versus-leukemia effects of allogeneic cell therapy.** *Annu. Rev. Med.* 1999, **50**:369–386.

Ruggeri, L., Capanni, M., Urbani, E., Perruccio, K., Shlomchik, W.D., Tosti, A., Posati, S., Rogaia, D., Frassoni, F., Aversa, F., Martelli, M.F., and Velardi, A.: **Effectiveness of donor natural killer cell alloreactivity in mismatched hematopoietic transplants.** *Science* 2002, **295**:2097–2100.

Shlomchik, W.D., Couzens, M.S., Tang, C.B., McNiff, J., Robert, M.E., Liu, J., Shlomchik, M.J., and Emerson, S.G.: **Prevention of graft versus host disease by inactivation of host antigen-presenting cells.** *Science* 1999, **285**:412–415.

13-39 The fetus is an allograft that is tolerated repeatedly.

Carosella, E.D., Rouas-Freiss, N., Paul, P., and Dausset, J.: **HLA-G: a tolerance molecule from the major histocompatibility complex.** *Immunol. Today* 1999, **20**:60–62.

Mellor, A.L., and Munn, D.H.: **Immunology at the maternal–fetal interface: lessons for T cell tolerance and suppression.** *Annu. Rev. Immunol.* 2000, **18**:367–391.

Munn, D.H., Zhou, M., Attwood, J.T., Bondarev, I., Conway, S.J., Marshall, B., Brown, C., and Mellor, A.L.: **Prevention of allogeneic fetal rejection by tryptophan catabolism.** *Science* 1998, **281**:1191–1193.

Parham, P.: **Immunology: keeping mother at bay.** *Curr. Biol.* 1996, **6**:638–641.

Schust, D.J., Tortorella, D., and Ploegh, H.L.: **HLA-G and HLA-C at the feto-maternal interface: lessons learned from pathogenic viruses.** *Semin. Cancer Biol.* 1999, **9**:37–46.

Manipulation of the Immune Response

Most of this book has been concerned with the mechanisms whereby the immune system successfully protects us from disease. In the preceding three chapters, however, we have seen examples of the failure of immunity to some important infections; conversely, with allergy and autoimmunity we have seen how inappropriate immune responses can themselves cause disease. We have also discussed the problems arising from immune responses to grafted tissues.

In this chapter we consider the ways in which the immune system can be manipulated or controlled, both to suppress unwanted immune responses in autoimmunity, allergy, and graft rejection, and to stimulate protective immune responses to some of the diseases that, at present, largely elude the immune system. It has long been felt that it should be possible to deploy the powerful and specific mechanisms of adaptive immunity to destroy tumors, and we discuss the present state of progress toward that goal. In the final section of the chapter we discuss current vaccination strategies and how a more rational approach to the design and development of vaccines promises to increase their efficacy and widen their usefulness and application.

Extrinsic regulation of unwanted immune responses.

The unwanted immune responses that occur in autoimmune disease, transplant rejection, and allergy present slightly different problems, and the approach to developing effective treatment is correspondingly different for each. We have already discussed the treatment of allergy in Chapter 12; the problems in this case are due to the production of IgE, and the goals are, accordingly, to treat the adverse consequences of an IgE response or to induce the production of IgG instead of IgE against the allergenic antigens. In autoimmune disease and graft rejection the problem is an immune response to tissue antigens, and the goal is to downregulate the response so as to avoid damage to the tissues or disruption of their function. From the point of view of management, the single most important difference between allograft rejection and autoimmunity is that allografts are a deliberate surgical intervention and the immune response to them can be foreseen, whereas autoimmune responses are not detected until they are already established. Effective treatment of an established immune response is much harder to achieve than prevention of a response before it has had a chance to develop, and autoimmune diseases are generally harder to control than a *de novo* immune response to an allograft. The relative difficulty of suppressing established immune responses is seen in animal models of autoimmunity, in which methods able to prevent the induction of autoimmune disease generally fail to halt established disease.

Current treatments for immunological disorders are nearly all empirical in origin, using immunosuppressive drugs identified by screening large numbers of natural and synthetic compounds. The drugs currently used to suppress the immune system can be divided into three categories: first, powerful anti-inflammatory drugs of the corticosteroid family such as prednisone; second, cytotoxic drugs such as azathioprine and cyclophosphamide; and third, fungal and bacterial derivatives such as cyclosporin A, tacrolimus (FK506), and rapamycin (sirolimus), which inhibit signaling events within T lymphocytes. These drugs are all very broad in their actions and inhibit protective functions of the immune system as well as harmful ones. Opportunistic infection is therefore a common complication of immunosuppressive drug therapy. The ideal immunosuppressive agent would be one that targets the specific part of the adaptive immune response that causes tissue injury. Paradoxically, antibodies themselves, by virtue of their exquisite specificity, might offer the best possibility for the therapeutic inhibition of specific immune responses. We also consider experimental approaches to controlling specific immune responses by manipulating the local cytokine environment or by manipulating antigen so as to divert the response from a pathogenic pathway to an innocuous one. We have discussed in Chapters 12 and 13 how the pathological responses that cause allergy, autoimmunity, or graft rejection can be prevented by innocuous, nonpathological T-cell responses.

14-1 Corticosteroids are powerful anti-inflammatory drugs that alter the transcription of many genes.

Corticosteroid drugs are powerful anti-inflammatory agents that are used widely to suppress the harmful effects of immune responses of autoimmune or allergic origin, as well as those induced by graft rejection. **Corticosteroids** are pharmacological derivatives of members of the glucocorticoid family of steroid hormones; one of the most widely used is **prednisone**, which is a synthetic analogue of cortisol (Fig. 14.1). Cortisol acts through intracellular receptors that are expressed in almost every cell of the body. On binding hormone, these receptors regulate the transcription of specific genes, as illustrated in Fig. 14.2.

The expression of as many as 1% of genes in the genome may be regulated by glucocorticoids, which can either induce, or less commonly suppress, the transcription of responsive genes. The pharmacological effects of corticosteroid drugs result from exposure of the glucocorticoid receptors to supraphysiological concentrations of ligand. The abnormally high level of ligation of glucocorticoid receptors causes exaggerated glucocorticoid-mediated responses, which have both beneficial and toxic effects.

Given the large number of genes regulated by corticosteroids and the fact that different genes are regulated in different tissues, it is hardly surprising that the effects of steroid therapy are very complex. The beneficial effects are anti-inflammatory and are summarized in Fig. 14.3; however, there are also many adverse effects, including fluid retention, weight gain, diabetes, bone mineral loss, and thinning of the skin. The use of corticosteroids to control disease requires a careful balance between helping the patient by reducing the inflammatory manifestations of disease and avoiding harm from the toxic

Fig. 14.1 The structure of the anti-inflammatory corticosteroid drug prednisone. Prednisone is a synthetic analogue of the natural adrenocorticosteroid cortisol. Introduction of the 1,2 double bond into the A ring increases anti-inflammatory potency approximately fourfold compared with cortisol, without modifying the sodium-retaining activity of the compound.

| Steroid receptors are found in the cytoplasm complexed with a heat-shock protein Hsp90 | Steroids cross the cell membrane and bind to the steroid receptor complex, releasing Hsp90 | The steroid:receptor complex can now cross the nuclear membrane | In the nucleus the steroid receptor binds to specific gene regulatory sequences and activates transcription |

Fig. 14.2 Mechanism of steroid action. Corticosteroids are lipid-soluble molecules that enter cells by diffusing across the plasma membrane and bind to their receptors in the cytosol. Binding of corticosteroid to the receptor displaces a dimer of a heat-shock protein named Hsp90, exposing the DNA-binding region of the receptor. The steroid:receptor complex then enters the nucleus and binds to specific DNA sequences in the promoter regions of steroid-responsive genes. Corticosteroids exert their numerous effects by modulating the transcription of a wide variety of genes.

side-effects of the drug. For this reason, corticosteroids used in transplant recipients and to treat inflammatory autoimmune and allergic disease are often administered in combination with other drugs in an effort to keep the dose and toxic effects to a minimum. In autoimmunity and allograft rejection, corticosteroids are commonly combined with cytotoxic immunosuppressive drugs.

14-2 Cytotoxic drugs cause immunosuppression by killing dividing cells and have serious side-effects.

The three cytotoxic drugs most commonly used as immunosuppressants are **azathioprine**, **cyclophosphamide** and **mycophenolate**. These drugs interfere with DNA synthesis and have their major pharmacological action on dividing tissues. They were developed originally to treat cancer and, after observations that they were cytotoxic to dividing lymphocytes, were found to be immunosuppressive as well. The use of these compounds is limited by a range of toxic effects on tissues that have in common the property of continuous cell division. These effects include decreased immune function, as well as anemia, leukopenia, thrombocytopenia, damage to intestinal epithelium, hair loss, and fetal death or injury. As a result of their toxicity, these drugs are used at high doses only when the aim is to eliminate all dividing lymphocytes, and in these cases treated patients require subsequent bone marrow transplantation to restore their hematopoietic function. They are used at lower doses and in combination with other drugs such as corticosteroids to treat unwanted immune responses.

Azathioprine is converted *in vivo* to a purine antagonist that interferes with the synthesis of nucleic acids and is toxic to dividing cells. It is metabolized to 6-thioinosinic acid, which competes with inosine monophosphate, thereby blocking the *de novo* synthesis of adenosine monophosphate and guanosine monophosphate and thus inhibiting DNA synthesis. Mycophenolate mofetil, the newest addition to the family of cytotoxic immunosuppressive drugs, works in a similar fashion to azathioprine. It is metabolized to mycophenolic acid, which is an inhibitor of the enzyme inosine monophosphate dehydrogenase. This blocks the *de novo* synthesis of guanosine monophosphate.

Corticosteroid therapy	
Effect on	**Physiological effects**
$\downarrow$ IL-1, TNF-α, GM-CSF $\downarrow$ IL-3, IL-4, IL-5, CXCL8	$\downarrow$ Inflammation $\downarrow$ caused by cytokines
$\downarrow$ NOS	$\downarrow$ NO
$\downarrow$ Phospholipase A$_2$ $\downarrow$ Cyclooxygenase type 2 $\uparrow$ Lipocortin-1	$\downarrow$ Prostaglandins and $\downarrow$ Leukotrienes
$\downarrow$ Adhesion molecules	Reduced emigration of leukocytes from vessels
$\uparrow$ Endonucleases	Induction of apoptosis in lymphocytes and eosinophils

Fig. 14.3 Anti-inflammatory effects of corticosteroid therapy. Corticosteroids regulate the expression of many genes, with a net anti-inflammatory effect. First, they reduce the production of inflammatory mediators, including cytokines, prostaglandins, and nitric oxide. Second, they inhibit inflammatory cell migration to sites of inflammation by inhibiting the expression of adhesion molecules. Third, corticosteroids promote the death by apoptosis of leukocytes and lymphocytes.

Azathioprine and mycophenolate are less toxic than cyclophosphamide, which is metabolized to phosphoramide mustard, which alkylates DNA. Cyclophosphamide is a member of the nitrogen mustard family of compounds, which were originally developed as chemical weapons. With this pedigree goes a range of highly toxic effects including inflammation of and hemorrhage from the bladder, known as hemorrhagic cystitis, and induction of bladder neoplasia.

14-3 Cyclosporin A, tacrolimus (FK506), and rapamycin (sirolimus) are powerful immunosuppressive agents that interfere with T-cell signaling.

There are now relatively nontoxic alternatives to the cytotoxic class of drugs that can be used for immunosuppression in transplant patients. The systematic study of products from bacteria and fungi has led to the development of a large number of important medicines, including the three immunosuppressive drugs **cyclosporin A**, **tacrolimus** (previously known as **FK506**), and **rapamycin** (also known as **sirolimus**), which are now widely used to treat transplant recipients. Cyclosporin A is a cyclic decapeptide derived from a soil fungus from Norway, *Tolypocladium inflatum*. Tacrolimus is a macrolide compound from the filamentous bacterium *Streptomyces tsukabaensis* found in Japan; macrolides are compounds that contain a many-membered lactone ring to which is attached one or more deoxysugars. Rapamycin, another *Streptomyces* macrolide, is likely to become important in the prevention of transplant rejection; rapamycin is derived from *Streptomyces hygroscopicus*, found on Easter Island ('Rapa ui' in Polynesian—hence the name of the drug). All three compounds exert their pharmacological effects by binding to members of a family of intracellular proteins known as the immunophilins, forming complexes that interfere with signaling pathways important for the clonal expansion of lymphocytes.

Cyclosporin A and tacrolimus block T-cell proliferation by inhibiting the phosphatase activity of a Ca^{2+}-activated enzyme called **calcineurin** at nanomolar concentrations. Their mechanism of action, which we discuss further in the next section, revealed a role for calcineurin in transmitting signals from the T-cell receptor to the nucleus. Both drugs reduce the expression of several cytokine genes that are normally induced on T-cell activation (Fig. 14.4). These include interleukin (IL)-2, whose synthesis by T lymphocytes is

Immunological effects of cyclosporin A and tacrolimus	
Cell type	**Effects**
T lymphocyte	Reduced expression of IL-2, IL-3, IL-4, GM-CSF, TNF-α Reduced proliferation following decreased IL-2 production Reduced Ca^{2+}-dependent exocytosis of granule-associated serine esterases Inhibition of antigen-driven apoptosis
B lymphocyte	Inhibition of proliferation secondary to reduced cytokine production by T lymphocytes Inhibition of proliferation following ligation of surface immunoglobulin Induction of apoptosis following B-cell activation
Granulocyte	Reduced Ca^{2+}-dependent exocytosis of granule-associated serine esterases

Fig. 14.4 Cyclosporin A and tacrolimus inhibit lymphocyte and some granulocyte responses.

an important growth signal for T cells. Cyclosporin A and tacrolimus inhibit T-cell proliferation in response to either specific antigens or allogeneic cells and are used extensively in medical practice to prevent the rejection of allogeneic organ grafts. Although the major immunosuppressive effects of both drugs are probably the result of inhibition of T-cell proliferation, they also act on other cells and have a large variety of other immunological effects (see Fig. 14.4), some of which might turn out to be important pharmacologically.

Cyclosporin A and tacrolimus are effective, but they are not problem-free. First, as with the cytotoxic agents, they affect all immune responses indiscriminately. The only way of controlling their immunosuppressive action is by varying the dose; at the time of grafting, high doses are required but, once a graft is established, the dose can be decreased to allow useful protective immune responses while maintaining adequate suppression of the residual response to the grafted tissue. This is a difficult balance that is not always achieved. Furthermore, although T cells are particularly sensitive to the actions of these drugs, their molecular targets are found in other cell types and therefore these drugs have effects on many other tissues. Cyclosporin A and tacrolimus are both toxic to kidneys and other organs. Finally, treatment with these drugs is expensive because they are complex natural products that must be taken for prolonged periods. Thus, there is room for improvement in these compounds, and better and less expensive analogues are being sought. Nevertheless, at present they are the drugs of choice in clinical transplantation, and they are also being tested in a variety of autoimmune diseases, especially those that, like graft rejection, are mediated by T cells.

14-4 Immunosuppressive drugs are valuable probes of intracellular signaling pathways in lymphocytes.

The mechanism of action of cyclosporin A and tacrolimus is now fairly well understood. Each binds to a different group of immunophilins: cyclosporin A to the cyclophilins, and tacrolimus to the FK-binding proteins (FKBP). These immunophilins are peptidyl-prolyl *cis–trans* isomerases but their isomerase activity does not seem to be relevant to the immunosuppressive activity of the drugs that bind them. Rather, the immunophilin:drug complexes bind and inhibit the Ca^{2+}-activated serine/threonine phosphatase calcineurin. Calcineurin is activated in T cells when intracellular calcium ion levels rise after T-cell receptor binding; on activation it dephosphorylates the NFATc family of transcription factors in the cytoplasm, allowing them to migrate to the nucleus, where they form complexes with nuclear partners, including the transcription factor AP-1, and induce the transcription of genes that include those for IL-2, CD40 ligand, and Fas ligand (Fig. 14.5, and see Sections 6-12 and 8-10). This pathway is inhibited by cyclosporin A and tacrolimus, which thus inhibit the clonal expansion of activated T cells. Calcineurin is found in other cells besides T cells but at higher levels; T cells are therefore particularly susceptible to the inhibitory effects of these drugs.

Rapamycin has a different mode of action from either cyclosporin A or tacrolimus. Like tacrolimus it binds to the FKBP family of immunophilins. However, the rapamycin:immunophilin complex has no effect on calcineurin activity but, instead, blocks the signal transduction pathway triggered by ligation of growth factor receptors. Rapamycin blocks the late stages of T-cell activation after T-cell receptor engagement (signal 1 of T-cell activation) and co-stimulatory signals (signal 2 of T-cell activation; see Fig. 8.10). It therefore allows the activation of T lymphocytes by antigen but blocks their proliferation. It causes arrest of the cells in the G_1 phase of the cell cycle; these cells die by apoptosis. The drug similarly inhibits lymphocyte proliferation driven by

Fig. 14.5 Cyclosporin A and tacrolimus inhibit T-cell activation by interfering with the serine/threonine-specific phosphatase calcineurin. Signaling via T-cell receptor-associated tyrosine kinases leads to the activation and increased synthesis of the transcription factor AP-1 and other partner proteins, as well as increasing the concentration of Ca^{2+} in the cytoplasm (left panels). The Ca^{2+} binds to calcineurin and thereby activates it to dephosphorylate the cytoplasmic form of members of the family of nuclear factors of activated T cells (NFATc). Once dephosphorylated, the active NFATc family members migrate to the nucleus to form a complex with AP-1 and other partner proteins; the NFATc:AP-1 complexes can then induce the transcription of genes required for T-cell activation, including the IL-2 gene. When cyclosporin A (CsA) or tacrolimus are present, they form complexes with their immunophilin targets, cyclophilin (CyP) and FK-binding protein (FKBP), respectively (right panels). The complex of cyclophilin with cyclosporin A can bind to calcineurin and block its ability to activate NFATc family members. The complex of tacrolimus with FKBP binds to calcineurin at the same site, also blocking its activity.

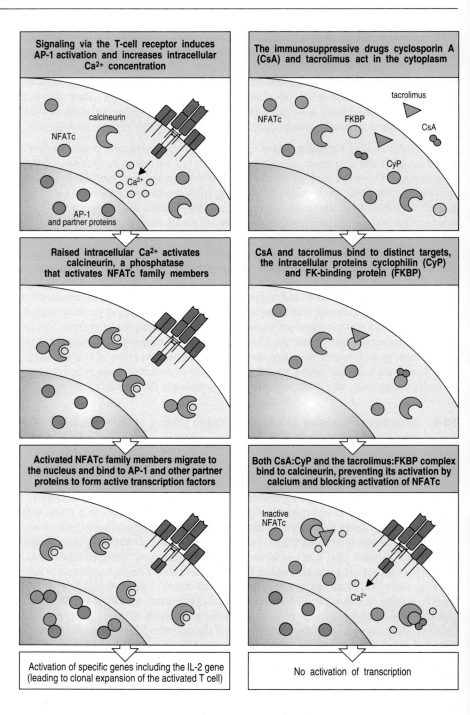

growth factors such as IL-2, IL-4, and IL-6. These effects are in contrast to those of the calcineurin antagonists, cyclosporin A and tacrolimus, which block all T-cell receptor mediated signals (signal 1).

The rapamycin:immunophilin complex acts by binding to and inhibiting the downstream effects of a protein kinase named mTOR (mammalian target of rapamycin; also known as FRAP, RAFT1, or RAPT1), which is a regulator of protein translation and essential to the control of the cell cycle. Because rapamycin has different pharmacological activities from cyclosporin A and tacrolimus, clinical trials indicate that it should be used in combination with cyclosporin A and corticosteroids. The rationale for combination therapy is that it might be possible to use smaller amounts of each drug in combination compared with the amounts required for treatment with a single agent. This might be a method of reducing unwanted side-effects.

14-5 Antibodies against cell-surface molecules have been used to remove specific lymphocyte subsets or to inhibit cell function.

Cytotoxic drugs kill all proliferating cells and therefore indiscriminately affect all types of activated lymphocyte and any other dividing cells. Cyclosporin A, tacrolimus, and rapamycin are more selective, but still inhibit most adaptive immune responses. In contrast, antibodies can interfere with immune responses in a nontoxic and much more specific manner. The potential of antibodies for the removal of unwanted lymphocytes is demonstrated by **anti-lymphocyte globulin**, a preparation of immunoglobulin from horses immunized with human lymphocytes, which has been used for many years to treat acute graft rejection episodes. Anti-lymphocyte globulin does not, however, discriminate between useful lymphocytes and those responsible for unwanted responses. Moreover, horse immunoglobulin is highly antigenic in humans, and the large doses used in therapy are often followed by the development of serum sickness, caused by the formation of immune complexes of horse immunoglobulin and human anti-horse immunoglobulin antibodies (see Chapter 12). Nevertheless, anti-lymphocyte globulins are still in use to treat acute rejection and have stimulated the quest for monoclonal antibodies to achieve more specifically targeted effects.

Immunosuppressive monoclonal antibodies act by one of two general mechanisms. Some monoclonal antibodies trigger the destruction of lymphocytes *in vivo*, and are referred to as **depleting antibodies**, whereas others are **nondepleting** and act by blocking the function of their target protein without killing the cell that bears it. Monoclonal IgG antibodies that cause lymphocyte depletion target these cells to macrophages and NK cells, which bear Fc receptors and kill the lymphocytes by phagocytosis and antibody-dependent cytotoxicity, respectively. Many antibodies are being tested for their ability to inhibit allograft rejection and to modify the expression of autoimmune disease. We will discuss some of these examples after looking at the measures being taken to prepare monoclonal antibodies for therapy in humans.

14-6 Antibodies can be engineered to reduce their immunogenicity in humans.

The major impediment to therapy with monoclonal antibodies in humans is that these antibodies are most readily made by using mouse cells, and humans rapidly develop antibody responses to mouse antibodies. This not only blocks the actions of the mouse antibodies but also leads to allergic reactions, and if treatment is continued it can result in anaphylaxis (see Section 12-10). Once this has happened, future treatment with any mouse monoclonal antibody is ruled out. This problem can, in principle, be avoided by making antibodies that are not recognized as foreign by the human immune system, and three strategies for their construction are being explored. One approach is to clone human V regions into a phage display library and select for binding to human cells, as described in Appendix I (see Section A-13).

In this way, monoclonal antibodies that are entirely human in origin can be obtained. Second, mice lacking endogenous immunoglobulin genes can be made transgenic (see Appendix I, Section A-46) for human immunoglobulin heavy- and light-chain loci by using yeast artificial chromosomes. B cells in these mice, sometimes known as humanized mice, have receptors encoded by human immunoglobulin genes but are not tolerant to most human proteins. In these mice, it is possible to induce human monoclonal antibodies against epitopes on human cells or proteins.

Finally, one can graft the complementarity-determining regions (CDRs) of a mouse monoclonal antibody, which form the antigen-binding loops, onto the framework of a human immunoglobulin molecule, a process known as **humanization**. Because antigen-binding specificity is determined by the structure of the CDRs (see Chapter 3), and because the overall frameworks of mouse and human antibodies are so similar, this approach produces a monoclonal antibody that is antigenically identical to human immunoglobulin but binds the same antigen as the mouse monoclonal antibody from which the CDR sequences were derived. These recombinant antibodies are far less immunogenic in humans than the parent mouse monoclonal antibodies, and thus they can be used to treat humans with far less risk of anaphylaxis.

14-7   Monoclonal antibodies can be used to inhibit allograft rejection.

Antibodies specific for various physiological targets have been used in attempts to prevent the development of allograft rejection by inhibiting the development of harmful inflammatory and cytotoxic responses. One approach is to perfuse the organ, before transplantation, with antibodies that react with antigen-presenting cells, thus targeting them for destruction within the mononuclear phagocytic system. Depletion of antigen-presenting cells in the graft by this method is effective at preventing allograft rejection in animal models, although there is no convincing evidence that it is successful in humans. Antibodies have, however, been used to treat episodes of graft rejection in humans. Anti-CD3 antibodies are moderately effective as an adjunct to immunosuppressive drugs in the treatment of episodes of transplanted kidney rejection.

A further approach to inhibiting allograft rejection is the blockade of the costimulatory signals needed to activate T cells that recognize donor antigens. In animal studies of graft rejection, a fusion protein CTLA4Ig (made from CTLA-4 and the Fc portion of human immunoglobulin) that binds to both B7.1 and B7.2 (see Section 8-5), has allowed the long-term survival of certain grafted tissues. Even more effective in a primate model of renal allograft rejection was the use of a humanized monoclonal antibody against the CD40 ligand (CD154) on T cells (see Section 8-5). CD40 ligand binds to CD40, expressed on dendritic and endothelial cells, stimulating these cells to secrete cytokines such as IL-6, IL-8, and IL-12. The mechanism of the immunosuppressive effect of anti-CD40 ligand antibody is not known, but it is most likely to be a consequence of blocking the activation of dendritic cells by T helper cells recognizing donor antigens. There have been only preliminary studies of the use of anti-CD40 ligand antibodies in humans. One antibody was associated with thromboembolic complications and was withdrawn; a different antibody was administered to patients with systemic lupus erythematosus (SLE) without significant complications but also with little evidence of effectiveness.

Various forms of combination therapy have been tried in experimental models. For example, the combination of CTLA4Ig with anti-CD40 ligand was synergistic in murine models of allograft rejection. Addition of rapamycin to this combination therapy caused massive apoptosis of alloreactive

T lymphocytes and allowed the permanent engraftment of skin allografts. By contrast, a combination of co-stimulatory blockade with cyclosporin A was no more effective than either cyclosporin A or co-stimulatory blockade alone. The difference can be explained as follows. Rapamycin allows T-cell receptor engagement and enhanced signaling for activation-induced cell death in the absence of co-stimulation. In contrast, cyclosporin A blocks signals from the engagement of T-cell receptors of alloreactive cells and prevents activation-induced cell death. These contrasting effects of cyclosporin A and rapamycin raise the possibility that they could be mutually antagonistic if administered together. However, the proof of the pudding lies in the eating and studies of renal transplant therapy in humans suggest that combination therapy that includes rapamycin, cyclosporin A, and corticosteroids (see Section 14-4) is beneficial.

Monoclonal antibodies against other targets have also had some success in preventing graft rejection in animals. Of particular interest are certain non-depleting anti-CD4 antibodies: when given for a short time during primary exposure to grafted tissue, these lead to a state of tolerance in the recipient (Fig. 14.6). This tolerant state is an example of the dominant immune suppression discussed in Section 13-11. It is long lived and can be transferred to

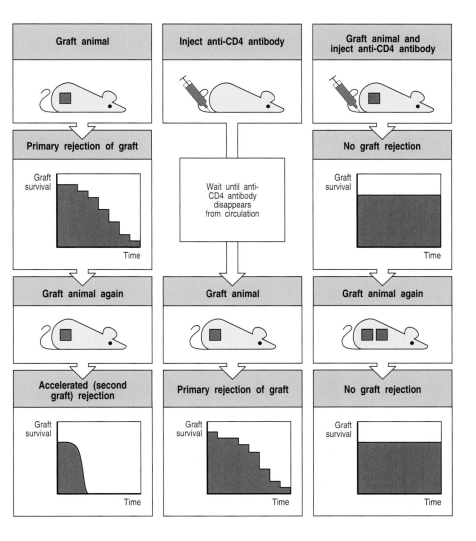

Fig. 14.6 A tissue graft given together with anti-CD4 antibody can induce specific tolerance. Mice grafted with tissue from a genetically different mouse reject that graft. Having been primed to respond to the antigens in the graft, they then reject a subsequent graft of identical tissue more rapidly (left panels). Mice injected with anti-CD4 antibody alone can recover immune competence when the antibody disappears from the circulation, as shown by a normal primary rejection of graft tissue (center panels). However, when tissue is grafted and anti-CD4 antibody is administered at the same time, the primary rejection response is markedly inhibited (right panels). An identical graft made later in the absence of anti-CD4 antibody is not rejected, showing that the animal has become tolerant to the graft antigen. This tolerance can be transferred with T cells to naive recipients (not shown).

naive recipients by CD4 T cells producing cytokines typical of T_H2 cells, although T cells producing other patterns of cytokines might also be involved. The most effective tolerance-inducing cells have the phenotype CD4$^+$ CD25$^+$, the so-called T regulatory cells (see Section 13-12), although subpopulations of CD4$^+$ CD25$^-$ T cells may have similar but much weaker effects. The tolerance is specific. Thus, animals of strain A, tolerant to strain B, reject grafts of strain C. This tolerance is 'infectious'—naive T cells exposed to allografts in the presence of regulatory T cells acquire dominant tolerance. It is not known how treatment with nondepleting anti-CD4 antibodies at the time of exposure to an allograft causes this effect. The presence of anti-CD4 antibody at the time of transplantation might favor the development of a nondamaging T_H2 response, rather than an inflammatory T_H1 response, because of a reduced strength of interaction between the graft cell antigens and responding naive T cells, as discussed in Section 10-7.

In human bone marrow transplantation, depleting antibodies directed at mature T lymphocytes have proved particularly useful. Elimination of mature T lymphocytes from donor bone marrow before infusion into a recipient is very effective at reducing the incidence of graft-versus-host disease (see Section 13-38). In this disease, the T lymphocytes in the donor bone marrow recognize the recipient as foreign and mount a damaging alloreaction against the recipient, causing rashes, diarrhea, and pneumonia, which is often fatal.

14-8 Biological agents can be used to alleviate and suppress autoimmune disease.

Autoimmune disease is detected only once the autoimmune response has caused tissue damage or has disturbed specific physiological functions. There are three main approaches to treatment. First, anti-inflammatory therapy can reduce tissue injury caused by an inflammatory autoimmune response; second, therapy can be aimed at modifying and reducing the autoimmune response; and third, treatment can be directed specifically at compensating for the damage. An example of the third approach is the use of injected insulin to treat diabetes, which is induced by autoimmune attack on pancreatic β cells, causing loss of physiological insulin secretion. In addition to the drugs discussed in Sections 14-1 to 14-3, there is a new class of therapy that has been named **biological therapy**. This somewhat clumsy term applies to treatments comprising natural proteins such as antibodies and cytokines or fragments of proteins or synthetic peptides. The term also encompasses the use of cells such as bone marrow derived cells for treatment.

The first line of anti-inflammatory therapy for autoimmune disease is normally drug therapy. The typical sequence is to start with anti-inflammatory agents such as aspirin, other nonsteroidal anti-inflammatory drugs, and sometimes low-dose corticosteroids. For more severe disease, immunosuppressive and anti-inflammatory therapy are combined, with the use of corticosteroids at higher doses often combined with the use of one of the cytotoxic drugs described in Section 14-2. Biological therapy has become established as part of the anti-inflammatory treatment of certain autoimmune diseases, especially treatments directed toward neutralizing the effects of TNF-α.

Anti-TNF-α antibodies were found to induce striking remissions in rheumatoid arthritis (Fig. 14.7) and to reduce tissue inflammation in Crohn's disease, an inflammatory bowel disease (see Section 12-18). There are two established means of antagonizing TNF-α in clinical practice. The first is the use of humanized monoclonal antibodies, such as infliximab, that bind to TNF-α and block its activity. The second is the use of a recombinant human tumor necrosis factor receptor (TNFR) p75:Fc fusion protein, named etanercept, that binds TNF-α, thereby neutralizing its activity. These biological agents are

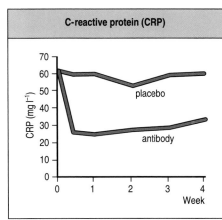

Fig. 14.7 Anti-inflammatory effects of anti-TNF-α therapy in rheumatoid arthritis. The clinical course of 24 patients was followed for 4 weeks after treatment with either a placebo or a monoclonal antibody against TNF-α at a dose of 10 mg kg⁻¹. The antibody therapy was associated with a reduction in both subjective and objective parameters of disease activity (as measured by pain score and swollen-joint count, respectively) and in the systemic inflammatory acute-phase response, measured as a fall in the concentration of the acute-phase C-reactive protein. Data courtesy of R.N. Maini.

extremely potent anti-inflammatories, and the number of diseases in which they have been shown to be effective is increasing as further clinical trials are performed. In addition to rheumatoid arthritis, the rheumatic diseases ankylosing spondylitis, psoriatic arthropathy, and juvenile chronic arthritis each respond well to blockade of TNF-α. In medicine, most treatments that have powerful effects also carry the risk of major side-effects. With TNF-α blockade there is an increased risk to patients of developing clinically manifest tuberculosis. This is an excellent illustration of the physiological action of TNF-α in host defense against tuberculosis, as noted in Section 11-14.

Rheumatoid Arthritis

Anti-TNF therapy was the first specific biological therapeutic to enter the clinical armamentarium. Close behind as a licensed treatment is anti-IL-1 therapy. The IL-1 receptor antagonist IL-1Ra is a natural antagonist of IL-1. It competes with IL-1 for binding to the IL-1 receptor and blocks signaling through the receptor. A recombinant IL-1Ra protein, with a slight modification to the native protein structure, named anakinra, is effective in the treatment of rheumatoid arthritis. Other antagonists to cytokines are being used in clinical trials, for example a humanized antibody against the IL-6 receptor that blocks the effects of IL-6.

Antibodies can also block cell migration to sites of inflammation. A humanized monoclonal antibody called natalizumab that binds to the α_4 integrins VLA-4 (α_4:β_1) and α_4:β_7 (lamina propria-associated molecule 1) has been developed for clinical use. Natalizumab prevents the interaction of these integrins with their respective ligands VCAM-1 and MAdCAM-1 (Fig. 14.8) (see Sections 8-12 and 8-3). This antibody showed therapeutic efficacy in placebo-controlled trials in patients with Crohn's disease or multiple sclerosis. The α_4 integrins direct the adhesion of lymphocytes expressing VLA-4 to VCAM-1 on endothelium in the central nervous system and of those expressing α_4:β_7 to MAdCAM-1 on endothelium in the gut. The early signs that this treatment could be successful illustrate the fact that disease depends on the continuing emigration of lymphocytes, monocytes, and macrophages from the circulation into the tissues of the brain in multiple sclerosis, and into the gut wall in Crohn's disease. Chemokines and their receptors are also excellent drug targets for the prevention of migration of immune effector cells to sites of autoimmune disease. It is likely that the next edition of this book will be able to cite successes in inhibiting these targets.

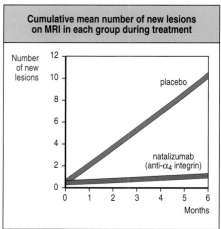

Fig. 14.8 Treatment with anti-α_4 integrin humanized monoclonal antibody reduces relapses of multiple sclerosis. Left panel: interaction between $\alpha_4{:}\beta_1$ integrin (VLA-4) on lymphocytes and macrophages and VCAM-1 expressed on endothelial cells allows the adhesion of these cells to brain endothelium. This facilitates migration of these cells into the plaques of inflammation in multiple sclerosis. Center panel: the monoclonal antibody natalizumab binds to the α_4 chain of the integrin and blocks adhesive interactions between lymphocytes and monocytes and VCAM-1 on endothelial cells, thus preventing the cells entering the tissue and exacerbating the inflammation. Right panel: the number of new lesions detected on MRI of the brain is greatly reduced in patients treated with natalizumab compared with a placebo. Data courtesy of D. Miller.

14-9 Depletion or inhibition of autoreactive lymphocytes can treat autoimmune disease.

Pathogenic lymphocytes can be removed in a crude way by depleting whole populations of lymphocytes, of which only a small subfraction are actually pathogenic. Polyclonal anti-lymphocyte globulin is one means of doing this; we considered the effects and side-effects of this treatment in Section 14-5. Here we look at the use of antibodies that are more selective in their massacre of lymphocytes. Alternatively, if the clonally restricted T-cell receptors or immunoglobulin on lymphocytes that cause disease can be identified, cells bearing them can be targeted with antibodies against idiotypic determinants on the relevant antigen receptor.

Monoclonal antibodies that react with lymphocytes have various effects on the target cells. Some cause cell depletion, either by antibody-dependent cytotoxicity (see Section 9-21) or by means of complement activation and cell lysis (see Section 9-17). Nondepleting antibodies, in contrast, are not associated with any change in cell numbers. It is an apparent paradox that some nondepleting antibodies seem to be more effective treatments than depleting antibodies that bind to the identical target proteins on lymphocytes. The most likely explanation is that nondepleting antibodies exert their effects by modifying the function of the cells that they have bound. Some examples of the effects of this latter type of antibody will be considered in the next section.

Treatment with anti-CD4 antibodies that cause depletion of helper T cells has been tried experimentally in rheumatoid arthritis and multiple sclerosis, with disappointing results. In controlled studies the antibodies showed only small therapeutic effects but caused depletion of T lymphocytes from peripheral blood for more than 6 years after treatment. Subsequent studies showed that the likely explanation for treatment failure was that these antibodies failed to delete primed CD4 T_H1 cells secreting interferon (IFN)-γ, and may have missed their target. This cautionary tale shows that it is possible to deplete large numbers of lymphocytes and yet completely fail to kill the cells that matter.

Another monoclonal antibody, Campath-1H, a humanized anti-CD52 antibody also known as alemtuzumab, binds to most lymphocytes and monocytes. This antibody, similarly to the depleting anti-CD4 antibodies, causes long-standing lymphopenia. Campath-1H did show some beneficial effect in studies of small numbers of patients with multiple sclerosis, but immediately after its infusion most patients suffered a frightening, although fortunately brief, flare-up of their illness. This flare illustrates another potential complication of antibody therapy. While Campath-1H was binding and killing cells by complement- and Fc-dependent mechanisms, cytokines were released, including TNF-α, IFN-γ, and IL-6. One of the effects of this was the transient blockade of nerve conduction in nerve fibers previously affected by demyelination.

It has also been possible to explore the effects of depleting B cells by the use of a chimeric mouse/human monoclonal anti-CD20 antibody, named rituximab, that was originally developed for treating B-cell lymphomas. Infusions of rituximab cause B-cell depletion for several months and are being tested experimentally in autoimmune diseases in which autoantibody-mediated pathogenesis is believed to be important. There is early evidence of efficacy of this antibody in some patients with autoimmune hemolytic anemia, SLE, rheumatoid arthritis, or type II mixed cryoglobulinemia (see Chapter 13).

A more specific approach to inhibition of specific autoreactive lymphocytes is to identify particular MHC class I or class II molecules responsible for presenting peptides from autoantigens and to inhibit their antigen-presenting function selectively with antibodies or blocking peptides. This approach has been successful in some animal models of autoimmunity, for example experimental autoimmune encephalomyelitis (EAE) (Fig. 14.9), in which it seems that a limited number of clones of T cells, responding to a single peptide, might cause disease. However, autoimmune disease in humans and most animal models is driven by a polyclonal response to autoantigens by T and B lymphocytes. For this reason, immunotherapy based on the identification

| Macrophage processes myelin basic protein (MBP) from oligodendrocytes | T$_H$1 cells with receptors for MBP peptides are activated and secrete products that activate macrophages | Activated macrophages damage oligodendrocytes | Antibodies against MHC class II molecules block T-cell activation |

Fig. 14.9 Anti-MHC class II antibody can inhibit the development of experimental autoimmune encephalomyelitis. In mice with experimental autoimmune encephalomyelitis (EAE), macrophages process myelin basic protein (MBP) and present MBP peptides to T$_H$1 lymphocytes in conjunction with co-stimulatory signals. Activated T$_H$1 cells secrete cytokines, which activate macrophages. The activated macrophages can, in turn, injure the oligodendrocytes. Antibodies against MHC class II molecules block this process by blocking the interaction between T$_H$1 cells and antigen-presenting macrophages.

of specific receptors carried by pathogenic lymphocytes is unlikely to succeed. Immunotherapy based on the identification of the particular MHC molecules that drive an autoimmune response is more likely to be effective, but such therapy could also inhibit some protective immune responses.

14-10 Interference with co-stimulatory pathways for the activation of lymphocytes could be a treatment for autoimmune disease.

We learned in Section 14-7 that interference with the co-stimulatory pathways that lead to lymphocyte activation could be a useful therapy to prevent allograft rejection. Similar principles apply to the treatment of autoimmune disease. CD28 and its homologue CD152 (CTLA-4) are expressed by CD4 T cells and some CD8 T cells. The co-stimulatory partners for these molecules are CD80 (B7.1) and CD86 (B7.2), which are expressed by antigen-presenting cells at variable levels according to their state of activation. This pathway is an obvious target for therapy and various biological agents are undergoing trials. For example a soluble recombinant chimeric CTLA4Ig has been developed (see Section 14-7) that binds to B7.1 (CD80) and B7.2 (CD86) on antigen-presenting cells and thereby inhibits co-stimulatory signals provided by these cells to T cells. When CTLA4Ig was given to patients with psoriasis, there was an improvement in the psoriatic rash and histological evidence of loss of activation of keratinocytes, T lymphocytes, and dendritic cells within the damaged skin.

Another co-stimulatory pathway that has been targeted in psoriasis is the interaction between CD2 on T cells and CD58 (LFA-3) on antigen-presenting cells. Patients were treated with a recombinant LFA-3-IgG1 fusion protein, called alefacept, that inhibited the interaction between CD2 and CD58, or with placebo. There was a marked therapeutic response that could be attributed to the active treatment and a reduction in both CD4 and CD8 memory effector lymphocytes detected in peripheral blood.

These approaches to inhibition of co-stimulation have given very encouraging results in the treatment of psoriasis and tell us something important about this disease. They demonstrate the importance of T lymphocytes in the induction of the skin lesions, which fits with the fact that cyclosporin A is an established treatment for this disease.

14-11 Modulation of the cytokines expressed by T lymphocytes can inhibit autoimmune disease.

The ultimate goal of immunotherapy for autoimmune disease is specific intervention to restore tolerance to the relevant autoantigens. The aim is to try to turn a pathological autoimmune response into an innocuous one. This approach is being pursued experimentally because, as discussed in Chapter 13, tolerance to tissue antigens does not always depend on the absence of a T-cell response; instead, it can be actively maintained by T cells secreting cytokines that suppress the development of a harmful, inflammatory T-cell response. Because the pattern of cytokines expressed by T lymphocytes is critical in determining the perpetuation and expression of autoimmune disease, the manipulation of cytokine expression offers a way of controlling the disease. There are various techniques, collectively known as **immune modulation**, that can affect cytokine expression by T lymphocytes. These involve manipulating the cytokine environment in which T-cell activation takes place, or manipulating the way antigen is presented, because these factors have been observed to influence the differentiation and cytokine-secreting function of the activated T cells (see Sections 8-13, 10-5, and 10-6).

As discussed in earlier chapters, CD4 T lymphocytes can be subdivided into two major subsets, the T_H1 cells, which secrete IFN-γ, and the T_H2 cells, which secrete IL-4, IL-5, IL-10, and transforming growth factor (TGF)-β. In many cases, autoimmune disease is associated with the activation of T_H1 cells, which activate macrophages and drive an inflammatory immune response. In animal models of experimentally induced autoimmune disease, such as EAE, the relative activation of the T_H1 and T_H2 subsets of T lymphocytes can be manipulated to give either a T_H1 response and disease, or a T_H2 response that confers protection against disease. The preferential activation of T_H1 or T_H2 cells can be achieved by direct manipulation of the cytokine environment or by administering antigen by particular routes, for example by feeding.

Recent evidence shows that patterns of cytokines secreted by T lymphocytes are very complicated and that the T_H1 and T_H2 subdivision of T lymphocytes is a considerable oversimplification. An additional three subsets of CD4 T cells have been characterized that have been designated regulatory T cells; these cells downregulate immune responses by the secretion of cytokines such as IL-10 and TGF-β and by mechanisms that are not yet understood. As we saw in Sections 13-11 to 13-14, loss of these regulatory CD4 T-cell subsets might be associated with the development of autoimmunity.

The first of these subsets of CD4 T cells is designated T_R1 cells, and these secrete IL-10 and TGF-β. The development of T_R1 cells from uncommitted T cells is favored by IL-10 in the type of autocrine positive-feedback loop that we have learned about in the context of the development of T_H1 and T_H2 cells (see Sections 10-5 and 10-6). Development of T_R1 cells is also favored by IFN-α. Immature dendritic cells presenting antigens in the absence of inflammatory stimuli could be the origin of the IFN-α and IL-10 that initiate the development of this subset of cells.

IL-10 suppresses T-cell responses directly by reducing T cells' production of IL-2, TNF-α, and IL-5, and indirectly by inhibiting antigen presentation by reducing the expression of MHC and co-stimulatory molecules by antigen-presenting cells. TGF-β similarly blocks T-cell cytokine production, cell division, and killing. However, the situation is complex because not all the effects of IL-10 and TGF-β are immunosuppressive. IL-10 can upregulate B-cell survival and maturation into plasma cells and increase the activity of CD8 T cells, and TGF-β can similarly have positive as well as negative effects on antigen-presenting cells, depending on the milieu of other cytokines. However, the dominant effects *in vivo* of both IL-10 and TGF-β are immunosuppressive, because mice lacking either cytokine are prone to autoimmune disease.

The second subset of regulatory CD4 T cells are those bearing the α chain of the IL-2 receptor (CD25), and high levels of the L-selectin receptor CD62L. $CD4^+$ $CD25^+$ $CD62L^{hi}$ T cells represent about 10–15% of the CD4 T cells in the human circulation. These cells seem to be positively selected in the thymus by high-affinity binding to MHC molecules containing self peptides and are activated by the binding of cognate peptide via their T-cell receptor. Once activated, however, they mediate their effects in a contact-dependent but antigen-nonspecific fashion. These cells are profoundly immunosuppressive, inhibiting IL-2 production and the proliferation of both CD4 and CD8 T cells. Although their pattern of cytokine production is similar to that of T_R1 cells, they can mediate their immunosuppressive effects independently of IL-10 and TGF-β. These cells may be the major effectors of the infectious transplant tolerance that can be induced experimentally by transient treatment with nondepleting anti-CD4 monoclonal antibodies (see Section 14-7). Depletion of these cells in mice is associated with the development of the organ-specific autoimmune diseases (see Section 13-12).

The third subset of T cells with immunosuppressive bystander effects secretes TGF-β as the dominant cytokine and has been designated T_H3 (see Section 13-14). Such cells might be predominantly of mucosal origin and be activated by the mucosal presentation of antigen (see Section 10-21). The challenge for the immunotherapy of autoimmune disease is to alter the balance between different subsets of responding T cells such that helpful responses are promoted and damaging responses are suppressed. As a therapy for autoimmunity it has the advantage that one might not need to know the precise nature of the autoantigen stimulating the autoimmune disease. This is because the administration of cytokines or antigen to modulate the immune response causes changes in the pattern of cytokine expression that have bystander effects on lymphocytes with the presumed autoreactive receptors. However, the drawback of this approach is the unpredictability of the results. In murine models of diseases such as diabetes and EAE, most of the results suggest that a T_H2 response can protect against T_H1-mediated disease, but there is evidence that T_H2 lymphocytes can also contribute to the pathology of these diseases.

An additional problem is the difficulty of modulating established immune responses. Experiments in animals have shown that anti-cytokine antibodies (or recombinant cytokines) present at the time of immunization with an autoantigen can sometimes divert a pathogenic immune response. In contrast, the modification of an ongoing immune response is much harder to achieve with this approach.

In spite of these caveats there are a few glimmers of hope that immune modulation may work in the treatment of autoimmune disease in humans. An important example is the preliminary study of the use of a nondepleting antibody to CD3 to treat patients in the early stages of type 1 diabetes mellitus. Patients were studied within 6 weeks of the diagnosis of disease and were randomly allocated to either a single course of treatment with anti-CD3 or no antibody. For a whole year after treatment there was a significant difference in the rate of progression of diabetes, with maintenance of endogenous insulin production in the majority of the patients treated with anti-CD3. Treatment with this antibody was associated with the production of IL-10 and IL-5 in the absence of significant IFN-γ production. A second example is the use of IL-10 in psoriasis: this led to an improvement in skin lesions and suppression of T_H1 but not T_H2 cytokine production by cells from treated patients.

14-12 Controlled administration of antigen can be used to manipulate the nature of an antigen-specific response.

When the target antigen of an unwanted response is identified, it is possible to manipulate the response by using antigen directly rather than using antibodies or relying on the bystander effects discussed in the previous section. This is because the way in which antigen is presented to the immune system affects the nature of the response, and the induction of one type of response to an antigen can inhibit a pathogenic response to the same antigen.

As mentioned in Chapter 12, this principle has been applied with some success to the treatment of allergies caused by an IgE response to very low doses of antigen. Repeated treatment of allergic individuals with higher doses of allergen seems to divert the allergic response to one dominated by T cells that favor the production of IgG and IgA antibodies. These antibodies are thought to desensitize the patient by binding the small amounts of allergen normally encountered and preventing it from binding to IgE.

There has been considerable interest in using peptide antigens to suppress pathogenic responses in T cell-mediated autoimmune disease. The type of CD4 T-cell response induced by a peptide depends on the way in which it is presented to the immune system. For instance, peptides given orally tend to prime T_H2 T cells that make IL-4 or T cells that make predominantly TGF-β, without activating T_H1 cells or inducing a great deal of systemic antibody. These mucosal immune responses have relatively little pathogenic potential. Indeed, experiments in animal models indicate that they can protect against induced autoimmune disease. EAE in mice is induced by the injection of myelin basic protein in complete Freund's adjuvant and resembles multiple sclerosis, whereas collagen arthritis is similarly induced in mice by injection of collagen type II and has features in common with rheumatoid arthritis. Oral administration of myelin basic protein or type II collagen inhibits the development of disease in animals, and has some beneficial effects in reducing the activity of already established disease. Trials of this approach in people with multiple sclerosis or rheumatoid arthritis have found marginal therapeutic effect. Similarly, a large study to examine whether giving low-dose parenteral insulin to those at high risk of developing diabetes could delay the onset of the disease showed absolutely no protective effect of this treatment. Intravenous delivery of peptides can also inhibit inflammatory responses stimulated by the same peptide presented in a different context. When a soluble peptide is given intravenously, it binds preferentially to MHC class II molecules on resting B cells and tends to induce anergy in T_H1 cells. Thus, a careful choice of the dose or structure of antigen, or its route of administration, could allow us to control the type of response that results. Whether such approaches can be effective in manipulating the established immune responses that drive human autoimmune diseases remains to be seen.

Summary.

Existing treatments for unwanted immune responses, such as allergic reactions, autoimmunity, and graft rejection, depend largely on three types of drug. Anti-inflammatory drugs, of which the most potent are the corticosteroids, are used for all three types of response. However, these have a broad spectrum of actions and a correspondingly wide range of toxic side-effects; their dose must be controlled carefully. They are therefore normally used in combination with either cytotoxic or immunosuppressive drugs. The cytotoxic drugs kill all dividing cells and thereby prevent lymphocyte proliferation, but they suppress all immune responses indiscriminately and also kill other types of dividing cells. The immunosuppressive drugs act by intervening in the intracellular signaling pathways of T cells. They are less generally toxic than the cytotoxic drugs, but they also suppress all immune responses indiscriminately. They are also much more expensive than cytotoxic drugs.

Immunosuppressive drugs are now the drugs of choice in the treatment of transplant patients: they can be used to suppress the immune response to the graft before it has become established. Autoimmune responses are already well established at the time of diagnosis and, in consequence, are much more difficult to suppress. They are therefore less responsive to the immunosuppressive drugs and, for that reason, they are usually controlled with a combination of corticosteroids and cytotoxic drugs. In animal experiments, attempts have been made to target immunosuppression more specifically, by blocking the response to autoantigen with the use of antibodies or antigenic peptides, or by diverting the immune response into a nonpathogenic pathway by manipulating the cytokine environment, or by administering antigen through the oral route, where a nonpathogenic immune response is likely to be invoked. Many of these approaches to treatment are now being tried in humans, in some cases with great success. The development and introduction of antagonists to TNF-α has been one of the triumphs of immunotherapy. Many biological agents are under development and some will enter clinical practice. All have the disadvantage that they are expensive to produce and cumbersome to administer. An important goal of the pharmaceutical industry is to produce small-molecule drugs that have targets and effects similar to those of current biological therapies.

Using the immune response to attack tumors.

Cancer is one of the three leading causes of death in industrialized nations. As treatments for infectious diseases and the prevention of cardiovascular disease continue to improve, and the average life expectancy increases, cancer is likely to become the most common fatal disease in these countries. Cancers are caused by the progressive growth of the progeny of a single transformed cell. Curing cancer therefore requires that all the malignant cells be removed or destroyed without killing the patient. An attractive way of achieving this would be to induce an immune response against the tumor that would discriminate between the cells of the tumor and their normal cell counterparts. Immunological approaches to the treatment of cancer have been attempted for over a century, with tantalizing but unsustainable results. Experiments in animals have, however, provided evidence for immune responses to tumors and have shown that T cells are a critical mediator of tumor immunity. More recently, advances in our understanding of antigen presentation and the molecules involved in T-cell activation have provided new immunotherapeutic strategies based on a better molecular understanding of the immune response. These are showing some success in animal models and are now being tested in human patients.

14-13 The development of transplantable tumors in mice led to the discovery that mice could mount a protective immune response against tumors.

The finding that tumors could be induced in mice after treatment with chemical carcinogens or irradiation, coupled with the development of inbred strains of mice, made it possible to undertake the key experiments that led to the discovery of immune responses to tumors. These tumors could be transplanted between mice, and the experimental study of tumor rejection has generally been based on the use of such tumors. If these bear MHC molecules foreign to the mice into which they are transplanted, the tumor cells are readily recognized and destroyed by the immune system, a fact that was exploited to develop the first MHC-congenic strains of mice. Specific immunity to tumors must therefore be studied within inbred strains, so that host and tumor can be matched for their MHC type.

Transplantable tumors in mice exhibit a variable pattern of growth when injected into syngeneic recipients. Most tumors grow progressively and eventually kill the host. However, if mice are injected with irradiated tumor cells that cannot grow, they are frequently protected against subsequent injection with a normally lethal dose of viable cells of the same tumor. There seems to be a spectrum of immunogenicity among transplantable tumors: injections of irradiated tumor cells seem to induce varying degrees of protective immunity against a challenge injection of viable tumor cells at a distant site. These protective effects are not seen in T-cell deficient mice but can be conferred by adoptive transfer of T cells from immune mice, showing the need for T cells to mediate all these effects.

Fig. 14.10 Tumor rejection antigens are specific to individual tumors. Mice immunized with irradiated tumor cells and challenged with viable cells of the same tumor can, in some cases, reject a lethal dose of that tumor (left panels). This is the result of an immune response to tumor rejection antigens. If the immunized mice are challenged with viable cells of a different tumor, there is no protection and the mice die (right panels).

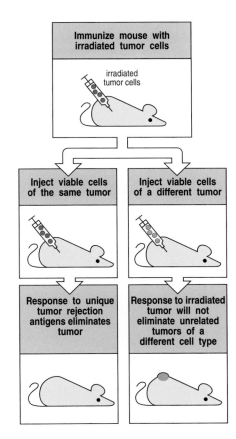

These observations indicate that the tumors express antigenic peptides that can become targets of a tumor-specific T-cell response. The antigens expressed by experimentally induced murine tumors, often termed **tumor-specific transplantation antigens** (**TSTAs**), or **tumor rejection antigens** (**TRAs**), are usually specific for an individual tumor. Thus, immunization with irradiated tumor cells from tumor X protects a syngeneic mouse from challenge with live cells from tumor X but not from challenge with a different syngeneic tumor Y, and vice versa (Fig. 14.10).

14-14 T lymphocytes can recognize specific antigens on human tumors.

Tumor rejection antigens are peptides of tumor-cell proteins that are presented to T cells by MHC molecules. These peptides can become the targets of a tumor-specific T-cell response because they are not displayed on the surface of normal cells, at least not at levels sufficient to be recognized by T cells. Six different categories of tumor rejection antigens can be distinguished, and examples of each are given in Fig. 14.11. The first category consists of antigens that are strictly tumor specific. These antigens are the result of point mutations or gene rearrangements, which often arise as part of the process of oncogenesis. Point mutations may evoke a T-cell response either by allowing *de novo* binding of a peptide to MHC class I molecules or by creating a new epitope for T cells by modification of a peptide that already binds class I molecules (Fig. 14.12). A special class of tumor-specific antigen in the case of B- and T-cell tumors, which are derived from single clones of lymphocytes, is the idiotypic sequences unique to the antigen receptor expressed by the clone.

The second category comprises proteins encoded by genes that are normally expressed only in male germ cells, which do not express MHC molecules and therefore cannot present peptides from these molecules to T lymphocytes. Tumor cells show widespread abnormalities of gene expression, including the activation of these genes and thus the presentation of these proteins to T cells; these proteins are therefore effectively tumor specific in their expression as antigens (Fig. 14.13).

The third category of tumor rejection antigen comprises differentiation antigens encoded by genes that are expressed only in particular types of tissue. The best examples of these are the differentiation antigens expressed in melanocytes and melanoma cells; several of these antigens are proteins involved in the pathways of production of the black pigment melanin. The fourth category consists of antigens that are strongly overexpressed in tumor cells compared with their normal counterparts (see Fig. 14.13). An example is HER-2/neu (also known as c-Erb-2), which is a receptor tyrosine kinase homologous to the epidermal growth factor receptor (EGFR). This receptor is overexpressed in many adenocarcinomas, including breast and ovarian cancers, where it is linked with a poor prognosis. MHC class I-restricted, CD8-positive cytotoxic T lymphocytes have been found infiltrating solid tumors overexpressing HER-2/neu but are not capable of destroying such tumors *in vivo*. The fifth category of tumor rejection antigens comprises molecules that display abnormal posttranslational modifications. An example is underglycosylated mucin, MUC-1, which is expressed by several tumors, including breast and pancreatic cancers.

Fig. 14.11 Proteins selectively expressed in human tumors are candidate tumor rejection antigens. The molecules listed here have all been shown to be recognized by cytotoxic T lymphocytes raised from patients with the tumor type listed.

Potential tumor rejection antigens have a variety of origins			
Class of antigen	**Antigen**	**Nature of antigen**	**Tumor type**
Tumor-specific mutated oncogene or tumor suppressor	Cyclin-dependent kinase 4	Cell-cycle regulator	Melanoma
	β-Catenin	Relay in signal transduction pathway	Melanoma
	Caspase-8	Regulator of apoptosis	Squamous cell carcinoma
Germ cell	MAGE-1 MAGE-3	Normal testicular proteins	Melanoma Breast Glioma
Differentiation	Tyrosinase	Enzyme in pathway of melanin synthesis	Melanoma
	Surface Ig	Specific antibody after gene rearrangements in B-cell clone	Lymphoma
Abnormal gene expression	HER-2/neu	Receptor tyrosine kinase	Breast Ovary
Abnormal post-translational modification	MUC-1	Underglycosylated mucin	Breast Pancreas
Oncoviral protein	HPV type 16, E6 and E7 proteins	Viral transforming gene products	Cervical carcinoma

Proteins encoded by viral oncogenes comprise the sixth category of tumor rejection antigen. These oncoviral proteins may have a critical role in the oncogenic process and, because they are foreign, they can evoke a T-cell response. Examples of such proteins are the human papilloma virus type 16 proteins, E6 and E7, which are expressed in cervical carcinoma.

Although each of these categories of tumor rejection antigen may evoke an antitumor response *in vitro* and *in vivo*, it is exceptional for such a response to be able to eliminate an established tumor spontaneously. It is the goal of tumor immunotherapy to harness and augment such responses to treat cancer more effectively. In this respect, the spontaneous remission occasionally observed in cases of malignant melanoma and renal cell carcinoma, even when disease is quite advanced, offers hope that this goal is achievable.

In melanoma, tumor-specific antigens were discovered by culturing irradiated tumor cells with autologous lymphocytes, a reaction known as the mixed lymphocyte–tumor cell culture. From such cultures, cytotoxic T lymphocytes could be identified that would kill, in an MHC-restricted fashion, tumor cells bearing the relevant tumor-specific antigen. Melanomas have been studied in detail with this approach. Cytotoxic T cells reactive against melanoma peptides have been cloned and used to characterize melanomas by the array of tumor-specific antigens displayed. These studies have yielded three important findings. The first is that melanomas carry at least five different antigens

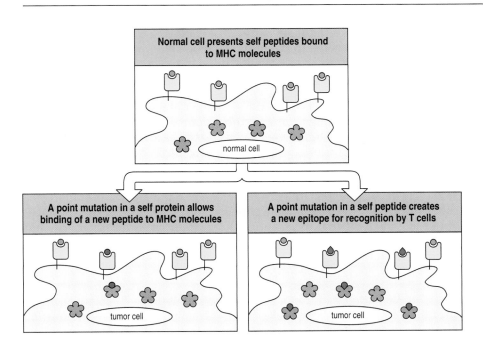

Fig. 14.12 Tumor rejection antigens may arise by point mutations in self proteins, which occur during the process of oncogenesis. In some cases a point mutation in a self protein may allow a new peptide to associate with MHC class I molecules (lower left panel). In other cases, a point mutation occurring within a self peptide that can bind self MHC proteins causes the expression of a new epitope for T-cell binding (lower right panel). In both cases, these mutated peptides will not have induced tolerance by the clonal deletion of developing T cells and can be recognized by mature T cells.

that can be recognized by cytotoxic T lymphocytes. The second is that cytotoxic T lymphocytes reactive against melanoma antigens are not expanded *in vivo*, suggesting that these antigens are not immunogenic *in vivo*. The third is that the expression of these antigens can be selected against *in vitro* and possibly also *in vivo* by the presence of specific cytotoxic T cells. These discoveries offer hope for tumor immunotherapy, an indication that these antigens are not naturally strongly immunogenic, and also a caution about the possibility of selecting, *in vivo*, tumor cells that can escape recognition and killing by cytotoxic T cells.

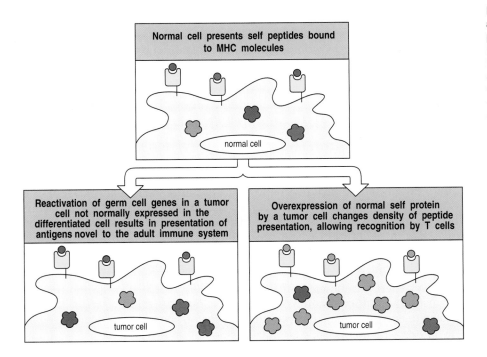

Fig. 14.13 Tumor rejection antigens are peptides of cell proteins presented by self MHC class I molecules. This figure shows two ways in which tumor rejection antigens may arise from unmutated proteins. In some cases, proteins that are normally expressed only in male germ cell tissues are reexpressed by the tumor cells (lower left panel). As these proteins are normally expressed only during germ cell development, and in cells lacking MHC antigens, T cells are not tolerant of these self antigens and can respond to them as though they were foreign proteins. In other tumors, overexpression of a self protein increases the density of presentation of a normal self peptide on tumor cells (lower right panel). Such peptides are then presented at high enough levels to be recognized by T cells. It is often the case that the same germ cell or self proteins are overexpressed in many tumors of a given tissue origin, giving rise to shared tumor rejection antigens.

Consistent with these findings is the observation that melanoma-specific T cells can be propagated from peripheral blood lymphocytes, from tumor-infiltrating lymphocytes, or by draining the lymph nodes of patients in whom the melanoma is growing. Interestingly, none of the peptides recognized by these T cells derives from the mutant proto-oncogenes or tumor suppressor genes that are likely to be responsible for the initial transformation of the cell into a cancer cell, although a few are the products of mutant genes. The rest derive from normal genes but are displayed at levels detectable by T cells for the first time on tumor cells, as illustrated in Fig. 14.13. Antigens of the MAGE family are not expressed in any normal adult tissues, with the exception of the testis, which is an immunologically privileged site. They probably represent early developmental antigens reexpressed in the process of tumorigenesis. Only a minority of melanoma patients have T cells reactive to the MAGE antigens, indicating that these antigens are either not expressed or are not immunogenic in most cases. The most common melanoma antigens are peptides from the enzyme tyrosinase or from three other proteins—gp100, MART1, and gp75. These are differentiation antigens specific to the melanocyte lineage from which melanomas arise. It is likely that overexpression of these antigens in tumor cells leads to an abnormally high density of specific peptide:MHC complexes and this makes them immunogenic. Although in most cases tumor rejection antigens are presented as peptides complexed with MHC class I molecules, tyrosinase has been shown to stimulate CD4 T-cell responses in some melanoma patients by being ingested and presented by cells expressing MHC class II molecules. It is important to note that both CD4 and CD8 T cells are likely to be important in achieving immunological control of tumors. CD4 T cells have a role in the activation of CD8 cytotoxic T cells; CD4 T cells may also kill tumor cells by means of the cytokines, such as TNF-α, that they secrete.

Tumor rejection antigens shared by most examples of a tumor, and against which tolerance can be broken, represent candidate antigens for tumor vaccines. The MAGE antigens are candidates because of their limited tissue distribution and their expression by many melanomas. It might seem dangerous to use tumor vaccines based on antigens that are not truly tumor-specific, because of the risk of inducing autoimmunity. Often, however, the tissues from which tumors arise are dispensable: the prostate is perhaps the best example. With melanoma, however, some melanocyte-specific tumor rejection antigens are also expressed in certain retinal cells, in the inner ear, in the brain, and in the skin. Despite this, melanoma patients receiving immunotherapy with whole tumor cells or tumor-cell extracts, although occasionally developing vitiligo—a destruction of pigmented cells in the skin that correlates well with a good response to the tumor—do not develop abnormalities in the visual, vestibular, and central nervous systems, perhaps because of the low level of expression of MHC class I molecules in these sites.

In addition to the human tumor antigens that have been shown to induce cytotoxic T-cell responses (see Fig. 14.11), many other candidate tumor rejection antigens have been identified by studies of the molecular basis of cancer development. These include the products of mutated cellular oncogenes or tumor suppressors, such as Ras and p53, and also fusion proteins, such as the Bcr–Abl tyrosine kinase that results from the chromosomal translocation (t9;22) found in chronic myeloid leukemia (CML). It is intriguing that, in each case, no specific cytotoxic T-cell response has been identified in cultures of autologous lymphocytes with tumor cells bearing these mutated antigens.

However, there are encouraging data that suggest that T-cell immunotherapy against tumor antigens could be a feasible clinical approach. CML cells were shown to carry a peptide derived from the fusion site between Bcr and Abl in the groove of HLA class I molecules of the common type HLA-A*0301. This peptide was detected with the use of a powerful technique known as 'reverse' immunogenetics. In this technique, peptides eluted from the grooves of polymorphic variants of MHC molecules are recovered and sequenced using highly sensitive mass spectrometry. This allows the peptide sequences spontaneously bound by MHC molecules to be identified. The technique has been used to detect HLA-bound peptides from other tumor antigens, for example peptides derived from the MART1 and gp100 tumor antigens of melanomas. It has also been used to identify candidate peptide sequences for vaccination in infectious disease.

In the case of the Bcr–Abl fusion protein, T cells specific for this peptide antigen could be identified in peripheral blood from patients with CML by using, as specific ligands, tetramers of HLA-A*0301 carrying the fusion peptide (see Appendix I, Section A-28). Cytotoxic T lymphocytes specific for this and other tumor antigens can be developed *in vitro* by using peptide sequences derived either from the mutated sequence or from the fusion sequence of these common oncogenic proteins; these cytotoxic T cells are able to recognize and kill tumor cells.

After treatment and bone marrow transplantation to treat CML, mature lymphocytes from the bone marrow donor infused into the patient can help to eliminate any residual tumor. This technique is known as donor lymphocyte infusion (DLI). At present, it is not clear to what extent the clinical response is due to a graft-versus-host effect, where the donor lymphocytes are responding to alloantigens expressed on the leukemia cells, or whether a specific antileukemic response has important effects. It is encouraging that it has been possible to separate T lymphocytes *in vitro* that mediate either a graft-versus-host effect or a graft-versus-leukemia effect. The ability to prime the donor cells against leukemia-specific peptides offers the prospect of enhancing the antileukemic effect while minimizing the risk of graft-versus-host disease. It is a challenge for immunologists to understand why these mutated proteins do not spontaneously prime cytotoxic T cells in the patients in which the tumors arise. They are excellent targets for therapy, because they are unique to the tumor and have a causal role in oncogenesis.

14-15 Tumors can escape rejection in many ways.

Burnet called the ability of the immune system to detect tumor cells and destroy them '**immune surveillance**.' However, it has been difficult to show that tumors are subject to surveillance by the immune system; after all, cancer is a common disease, and most tumors show little evidence of immunological control. The study of mice with targeted gene deletions that remove specific components of innate and adaptive immunity has provided the best evidence that immune surveillance does influence the development of certain types of tumor, although even in cases of extreme immunodeficiency the typical onset of tumors is in murine old age. For example, mice lacking perforin, part of the killing mechanism of NK cells and CD8 cytotoxic T cells, showed an increase in lymphomas, tumors of the lymphoid system. Strains of mice lacking the RAG and STAT-1 proteins, and thus deficient in both adaptive and certain innate immune mechanisms, developed gut epithelial and breast tumors. Mice lacking T lymphocytes expressing $\gamma{:}\delta$ receptors showed markedly increased susceptibility to skin tumors induced by the topical application of carcinogens, illustrating a physiological role for intra-epithelial lymphocytes in surveying and killing abnormal epithelial cells (see Section 10-15).

The major tumor types that occur with increased frequency in immunodeficient mice or humans are virus-associated tumors; immune surveillance therefore seems to be critical for the control of virus-associated tumors, but

Mechanisms by which tumors escape immune recognition				
Low immunogenicity	**Tumor treated as self antigen**	**Antigenic modulation**	**Tumor-induced immune suppression**	**Tumor-induced privileged site**
No peptide:MHC ligand No adhesion molecules No co-stimulatory molecules	Tumor antigens taken up and presented by APCs in absence of co-stimulation tolerize T cells	Antibody against tumor cell-surface antigens can induce endocytosis and degradation of the antigen. Immune selection of antigen-loss variants	Factors (eg,TGF-β) secreted by tumor cells inhibit T cells directly	Factors secreted by tumor cells create a physical barrier to the immune system

Fig. 14.14 Tumors can escape immune surveillance in a variety of ways. First panel: tumors can have low immunogenicity. Some tumors do not have peptides of novel proteins that can be presented by MHC molecules, and therefore appear normal to the immune system. Others have lost one or more MHC molecules, and most do not express co-stimulatory proteins, which are required to activate naive T cells. Second panel: tumor antigens presented in the absence of co-stimulatory signals will make the responding T cells tolerant to that antigen.

Third panel: tumors can initially express antigens to which the immune system responds but lose them by antibody-induced internalization or antigenic variation. When tumors are attacked by cells responding to a particular antigen, any tumor that does not express that antigen will have a selective advantage. Fourth panel: tumors often secrete molecules, such as TGF-β, that suppress immune responses directly. Fifth panel: tumor cells can secrete molecules such as collagen that form a physical barrier around the tumor, preventing lymphocyte access.

Fig. 14.15 Loss of MHC class I expression in a prostatic carcinoma. Some tumors can evade immune surveillance by loss of expression of MHC class I molecules, preventing their recognition by CD8 T cells. A section of a human prostate cancer that has been stained with a peroxidase-conjugated antibody to HLA class I is shown. The brown stain correlating with HLA class I expression is restricted to infiltrating lymphocytes and tissue stromal cells. The tumor cells that occupy most of the section show no staining. Photograph courtesy of G. Stamp.

the immune system does not normally respond to the novel antigens deriving from the multiple genetic alterations in spontaneous tumors. The goal in the development of anticancer vaccines is to break the tolerance of the immune system for antigens expressed mainly or exclusively by the tumor.

It is not surprising that tumors arising spontaneously are rarely rejected by T cells, because in general they probably lack either distinctive antigenic peptides or the adhesion or co-stimulatory molecules needed to elicit a primary T-cell response (Fig. 14.14). Even tumors that express tumor-specific antigens may be treated as 'self' if they cause no inflammation, being taken up by antigen-presenting cells such as immature dendritic cells and presented to T lymphocytes in the absence of co-stimulatory signals, causing T-cell anergy or deletion.

Moreover, there are other mechanisms whereby tumors can avoid immune attack or evade it when it occurs (see Fig. 14.14). Tumors tend to be genetically unstable and can lose their antigens by mutation; in the event of an immune response this instability might generate mutants that can escape the immune response. Some tumors, such as colon and cervical cancers, lose the expression of a particular MHC class I molecule (Fig. 14.15), perhaps through immunoselection by T cells specific for a peptide presented by that MHC class I molecule. In experimental studies, when a tumor loses expression of all MHC class I molecules it can no longer be recognized by cytotoxic T cells, although it might become susceptible to NK cells (Fig. 14.16). However, tumors that lose only one MHC class I molecule might be able to avoid recognition by specific CD8 cytotoxic T cells while remaining resistant to NK cells, conferring a selective advantage *in vivo*.

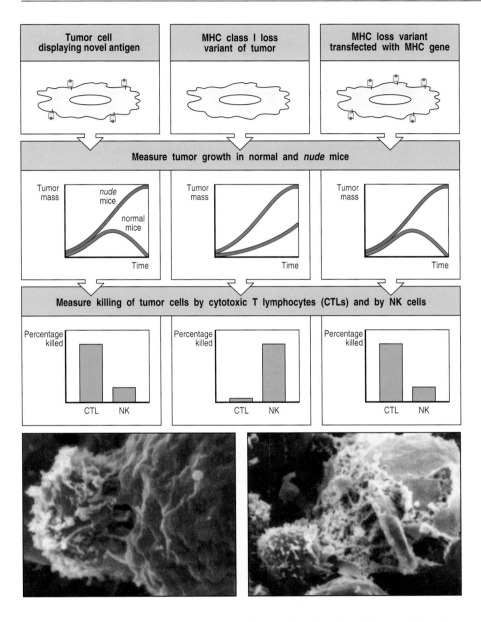

Fig. 14.16 Tumors that lose expression of all MHC class I molecules as a mechanism of escape from immune surveillance are more susceptible to NK cell killing. Regression of transplanted tumors is largely due to the actions of cytotoxic T cells (CTLs), which recognize novel peptides bound to MHC class I antigens on the surface of the cell (left panels). NK cells have inhibitory receptors that bind MHC class I molecules, so variants of the tumor that have low levels of MHC class I, although less sensitive to CD8 cytotoxic T cells, become susceptible to NK cells (center panels). Although *nude* mice lack T cells, they have higher than normal levels of NK cells, and so tumors that are sensitive to NK cells grow less well in *nude* mice than in normal mice. Transfection with MHC class I genes can restore both resistance to NK cells and susceptibility to CD8 cytotoxic T cells (right panels). However, tumors that lose only one MHC class I molecule can escape a specific cytotoxic CD8 T-cell response while remaining NK cell resistant. The bottom panels show scanning electron micrographs of NK cells attacking leukemia cells. Left panel: shortly after binding to the target cell, the NK cell has put out numerous microvillous extensions and established a broad zone of contact with the leukemia cell. The NK cell is the smaller cell on the left in both photographs. Right panel: 60 minutes after mixing, long microvillous processes can be seen extending from the NK cell (bottom left) to the leukemia cell and there is extensive damage to the leukemia cell membrane; the plasma membrane of the leukemia cell has rolled up and fragmented under the NK cell attack. Photographs courtesy of J.C. Hiserodt.

Yet another way in which tumors might evade rejection is by making immunosuppressive cytokines. Many tumors make these, although in most cases little is known of their precise nature. TGF-β was first identified in the culture supernatant of a tumor (hence its name, transforming growth factor-β) and, as we have seen, tends to suppress inflammatory T-cell responses and cell-mediated immunity, which are needed to control tumor growth. Several tumors of different tissue origins, such as melanoma, ovarian carcinoma, and B-cell lymphoma, have been shown to produce the immunosuppressive cytokine IL-10, which can reduce dendritic cell development and activity.

A further type of evasion of the immune system is the creation by some tumors of their own immunologically privileged sites (see Section 13-9). Such tumors grow in nodules surrounded by physical barriers such as collagen and fibrin. These tumors may be invisible to the immune system, which is ignorant to their existence; they may grow in this way until the tumor mass is too great to be controlled, even if the physical barrier is destroyed or inflammation ensues. Thus, there are many different ways in which tumors avoid recognition and destruction by the immune system.

14-16 Monoclonal antibodies against tumor antigens, alone or linked to toxins, can control tumor growth.

The advent of monoclonal antibodies suggested the possibility of targeting and destroying tumors by making antibodies against tumor-specific antigens (Fig. 14.17). This depends on finding a tumor-specific antigen that is a cell-surface molecule. Some of the cell-surface molecules that have been targeted in experimental clinical trials are shown in Fig. 14.18. So far there has been limited success with this approach, although, as an adjunct to other therapies, it holds promise. Some striking initial results have been reported in the treatment of breast cancer with a humanized monoclonal antibody, known as trastuzumab or Herceptin, which targets a growth factor receptor, HER-2/neu, that is overexpressed in about one-quarter of breast cancer patients. As we discussed in Section 14-14, this overexpression accounts for HER-2/neu evoking an antitumor T-cell response, although HER-2/neu is also associated with a poorer prognosis. It is thought that Herceptin acts by blocking interaction between the receptor and its natural ligand and by downregulating the level of expression of the receptor. The effects of this antibody can be potentiated when it is combined with conventional chemotherapy. A second monoclonal antibody that has promise for the treatment of non-Hodgkin's B-cell lymphoma binds to CD20 and is known as rituximab. Ligation and clustering of CD20 transduces a signal that causes lymphocyte apoptosis. Monoclonal antibodies coupled to γ-emitting radioisotopes have also been used to image tumors, for the purpose of diagnosis and monitoring tumor spread (Fig. 14.19).

The first reported successful treatment of a tumor with monoclonal antibodies used anti-idiotypic antibodies to target B-cell lymphomas whose surface immunoglobulin expressed the corresponding idiotype. The initial course of treatment usually leads to a remission, but the tumor always reappears in a mutant form that no longer binds to the antibody used for the initial treatment. This case represents a clear example of genetic instability enabling a tumor to evade treatment.

Fig. 14.17 Monoclonal antibodies that recognize tumor-specific antigens might be used in a variety of ways to help eliminate tumors. Tumor-specific antibodies of the correct isotypes might be able to direct the lysis of the tumor cells by NK cells, activating the NK cells via their Fc receptors (left panels). A more useful strategy might be to couple the antibody to a powerful toxin (center panels). When the antibody binds to the tumor cell and is endocytosed, the toxin is released from the antibody and can kill the tumor cell. If the antibody is coupled to a radioisotope (right panels), binding of the antibody to a tumor cell will deliver a dose of radiation sufficient to kill the tumor cell. In addition, nearby tumor cells could also receive a lethal radiation dose, even though they do not bind the antibody.

Tumor tissue origin	Type of antigen	Antigen	Tumor type
Lymphoma/ leukemia	Differentiation antigen	CD5 Idiotype CAMPATH-1 (CDw52)	T-cell lymphoma B-cell lymphoma T- and B-cell lymphoma
	B-cell signaling receptor	CD20	Non-Hodgkin's B-cell lymphoma
Solid tumors	Cell-surface antigens Glycoprotein Carbohydrate	CEA, mucin-1 Lewis^y CA-125	Epithelial tumors (breast, colon, lung) Epithelial tumors Ovarian carcinoma
	Growth factor receptor	Epidermal growth factor receptor p185^{HER2} IL-2 receptor	Lung, breast, head, and neck tumors Breast, ovarian tumors T- and B-cell tumors
	Stromal extracellular antigen	FAP-α Tenascin Metalloproteinases	Epithelial tumors Glioblastoma multiforme Epithelial tumors

Fig. 14.18 Examples of tumor antigens that have been targeted by monoclonal antibodies in therapeutic trials. CEA, carcinoembryonic antigen.

Other problems with tumor-specific or tumor-selective monoclonal antibodies as therapeutic agents include inefficient killing of cells after binding of the monoclonal antibody and inefficient penetration of the antibody into the tumor mass. The first problem can often be circumvented by linking the antibody to a toxin, producing a reagent called an **immunotoxin**; two favored toxins are ricin A chain and *Pseudomonas* toxin. Both approaches require the antibody to be internalized to allow the cleavage of the toxin from the antibody in the endocytic compartment, allowing the toxin chain to penetrate and kill the cell. An example of a successful immunotoxin is a recombinant Fv anti-CD22 antibody fused to a fragment of *Pseudomonas* toxin. This induced complete remissions in two-thirds of a group of patients with a type of B-cell leukemia known as hairy-cell leukemia, in which the disease was resistant to conventional chemotherapy.

Two other approaches using monoclonal antibody conjugates involve linking the antibody molecule to chemotherapeutic drugs such as adriamycin or to radioisotopes. In the first case, the specificity of the monoclonal antibody for a cell-surface antigen on the tumor concentrates the drug to the site of the tumor. After internalization, the drug is released in the endosomes and exerts its cytostatic or cytotoxic effect. A variation on this approach is to link an antibody to an enzyme that metabolizes a nontoxic pro-drug to the active cytotoxic drug, a technique known as ADEPT, the acronym for antibody-directed enzyme/pro-drug therapy. This technique has the potential advantage that a small amount of enzyme, localized by the antibody to the tumor, can generate much larger amounts of active cytotoxic drug in the immediate vicinity of tumor cells than could be coupled directly to the targeting antibody. Monoclonal antibodies linked to radioisotopes (see Fig. 14.17) concentrate the radioactive source in the tumor site. Each of these approaches has the advantage of also killing neighboring tumor cells, because the released drug or radioactive emissions can affect cells adjacent to those that actually bind the antibody. Ultimately, combinations of toxin-, drug-, or radioisotope-linked monoclonal antibodies, together with vaccination strategies aimed at inducing T cell-mediated immunity, might provide the most effective cancer immunotherapy.

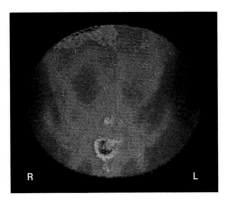

Fig. 14.19 Recurrent colorectal cancer can be detected with a radiolabeled monoclonal antibody against carcinoembryonic antigen. A patient with a possible recurrence of a colorectal cancer was injected intravenously with an indium-111-labeled monoclonal antibody to carcinoembryonic antigen. The recurrent tumor is seen as two red spots located in the pelvic region. The blood vessels are faintly outlined by circulating antibody that has not bound to the tumor. Courtesy of A.M. Peters.

14-17 Enhancing the immunogenicity of tumors holds promise for cancer therapy.

Vaccines based on tumor antigens are, in principle, the ideal approach to T cell-mediated cancer immunotherapy. However, such vaccines are difficult to develop; it is not clear how widely the relevant epitopes will be shared between tumors, and peptides of tumor rejection antigens will be presented only by particular MHC alleles. To be effective, a tumor vaccine may therefore need to include a range of tumor antigens. MAGE-1 antigens, for example, are recognized only by T cells in melanoma patients expressing the HLA-A1 haplotype. However, the range of MAGE-type proteins that has now been characterized encompasses peptide epitopes presented by many HLA class I and II molecules.

Until recently, most cancer vaccines have used the individual patient's tumor removed at surgery as a source of vaccine antigens. These cell-based vaccines are prepared by mixing either irradiated tumor cells or tumor extracts with bacterial adjuvants such as BCG or *Corynebacterium parvum*, which enhance their immunogenicity (see Appendix I, Section A-4). Such vaccines have generated modest therapeutic results in melanomas but have, in general, been disappointing.

Where candidate tumor rejection antigens have been identified, for example in melanoma, experimental vaccination strategies include the use of whole proteins, peptide vaccines based on sequences recognized by cytotoxic T lymphocytes (either administered alone or presented by the patient's own dendritic cells), and recombinant viruses encoding these peptide epitopes. A novel experimental approach to tumor vaccination is the use of heat-shock proteins isolated from tumor cells. The underlying principle of this therapy is that one of the physiological activities of heat-shock proteins is to act as intracellular chaperones of antigenic peptides. There is evidence for receptors on the surface of professional antigen-presenting cells that take up certain heat-shock proteins together with any bound peptides. Uptake of heat-shock proteins via these receptors delivers the accompanying peptide into the antigen-processing pathways leading to peptide presentation by MHC class I molecules. This experimental technique for tumor vaccination has the advantage that it does not depend on any prior knowledge of the nature of the relevant tumor rejection antigens, but the disadvantage that the heat-shock proteins purified from the cell carry very many peptides, so that any tumor rejection antigen might constitute only a tiny fraction of the peptides bound to the heat-shock protein.

A further experimental approach to tumor vaccination in mice is to increase the immunogenicity of tumor cells by introducing genes that encode co-stimulatory molecules or cytokines. This is intended to make the tumor itself more immunogenic. The basic scheme of such experiments is shown in Fig. 14.20. A tumor cell transfected with the gene encoding the co-stimulatory molecule B7 (see Section 8-5) is implanted in a syngeneic animal. These B7-positive cells can activate tumor-specific naive T cells to become effector T cells able to reject the tumor cells. They are also able to stimulate further proliferation of the effector cells that reach the site of implantation. These T cells can then target the tumor cells whether they express B7 or not; this can be shown by reimplanting nontransfected tumor cells, which are also rejected.

The second strategy, that of introducing cytokine genes into tumors so that they secrete the relevant cytokine, is aimed at attracting antigen-presenting cells to the tumor and takes advantage of the paracrine nature of cytokines. In mice, the most effective tumor vaccines so far are tumor cells that secrete granulocyte-macrophage colony-stimulating factor (GM-CSF), which induces the differentiation of hematopoietic precursors into dendritic cells

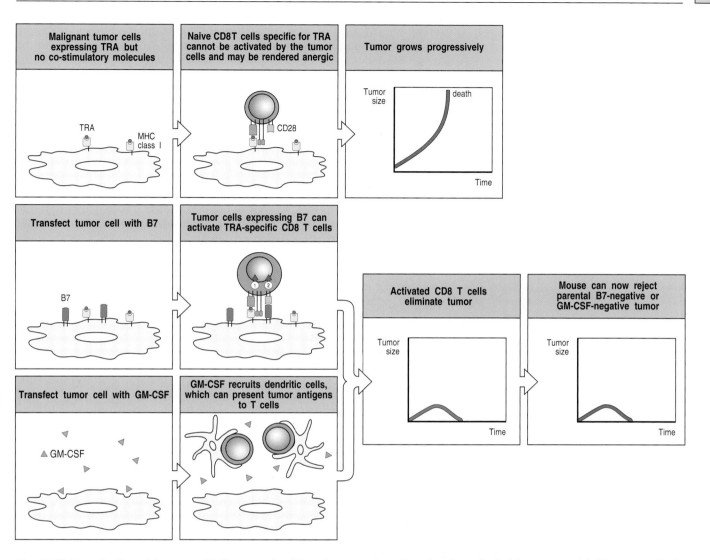

Fig. 14.20 Transfection of tumors with the gene for B7 or for GM-CSF enhances tumor immunogenicity. A tumor that does not express co-stimulatory molecules will not induce an immune response, even though it might express tumor rejection antigens (TRAs), because naive CD8 T cells specific for the TRA cannot be activated by the tumor. The tumor therefore grows progressively in normal mice and eventually kills the host (top panels). If such tumor cells are transfected with a co-stimulatory molecule, such as B7, TRA-specific CD8 T cells now receive both signal 1 and signal 2 from the same cell (see Section 8-5) and can therefore be activated (center panels). The same effect can be obtained by transfecting the tumor with the gene encoding GM-CSF, which attracts and stimulates the differentiation of dendritic cell precursors (bottom panels). Both these strategies have been tested in mice and shown to elicit memory T cells, although results with GM-CSF are more impressive. Because TRA-specific CD8 cells have now been activated, even the original B7-negative or GM-CSF-negative tumor cells can be rejected.

and attracts these to the site. GM-CSF is also thought to function as an adjuvant, activating the dendritic cells. It is believed that these cells process the tumor antigens and migrate to the local lymph nodes, where they induce potent antitumor responses. The B7-transfected cells seem less potent in inducing antitumor responses, perhaps because the bone marrow derived dendritic cells express more of the molecules required to activate naive T cells than do B7-transfected tumor cells. In addition, the tumor cells do not share the dendritic cells' special ability to migrate into the T-cell areas of the lymph nodes, where they are optimally placed to interact with passing naive T cells (see Section 8-6).

The potency of dendritic cells in activating T-cell responses provides the rationale for yet another strategy for vaccinating against tumors. The use of antigen-loaded autologous dendritic cells to stimulate therapeutically useful cytotoxic T-cell responses to tumors has been developed in experimental models, and there have been initial trials in humans with cancer. Other methods under trial include loading dendritic cells *ex vivo* with DNA encoding the tumor antigen (see Section 14-27) or with mRNA derived from tumor cells, and the use of apoptotic or necrotic tumor cells as sources of antigens. The field of dendritic cell vaccination against tumors is very active, and many variables are being explored in early-phase studies in patients. There is a worry that effective immunotherapy against tumors may bring with it an autoimmune response against the normal tissue from which the tumor derived. However, this has not been a significant problem so far, although it is too early to judge the therapeutic value in clinical practice of this potentially powerful approach to cancer immunotherapy.

Summary.

Tumors represent outgrowths of a single abnormal cell, and animal studies have shown that some tumors elicit specific immune responses that suppress their growth. These seem to be directed at MHC-bound peptides derived from antigens that might be mutated, inappropriately expressed, or overexpressed in the tumor cells. T-cell deficient individuals, however, do not develop more tumors than normal individuals. This is probably chiefly because most tumors do not make distinctive antigenic proteins or do not express the co-stimulatory molecules necessary to initiate an adaptive immune response, promoting tolerance rather than protective immunity. Tumors also have other ways of avoiding or suppressing immune responses, such as ceasing to express MHC class I molecules, making immunosuppressive cytokines, or creating barriers akin to those expressed at immunologically privileged sites in the body. Monoclonal antibodies have been developed for tumor immunotherapy by conjugation to toxins, cytotoxic drugs, or radioisotopes, which are thereby delivered at high dose specifically to the tumor cells. More recently, attempts have been made to develop vaccines based on tumor cells taken from patients and made immunogenic by the addition of adjuvants, or by pulsing autologous dendritic cells with modified tumor cells or tumor antigens. This approach has been extended in animal experiments to the transfection of tumor cells with genes encoding co-stimulatory molecules or cytokines that attract and activate dendritic cells.

Manipulating the immune response to fight infection.

Infection is the leading cause of death in humans. The two most important contributions to public health in the past 100 years have been sanitation and vaccination, which together have dramatically reduced deaths from infectious disease. Modern immunology grew from the success of Jenner's and Pasteur's vaccines against smallpox and chicken cholera, respectively, and its greatest triumph has been the global eradication of smallpox, announced by the World Health Organization in 1980. Unfortunately, we may not have seen the last of this lethal disease, if laboratory stocks of the organism have been illegally held and fall into the hands of terrorists. As part of a state of cautious preparedness, smallpox vaccine doses are once more being stockpiled around the world. A global campaign to eradicate polio is now under way.

Adaptive immunity to a specific infectious agent can be achieved in several ways. One early strategy was to deliberately cause a mild infection with the unmodified pathogen. This was the principle of variolation, in which the inoculation of a small amount of dried material from a smallpox pustule would cause a mild infection followed by long-lasting protection against reinfection. However, infection after variolation was not always mild: fatal smallpox ensued in about 3% of cases, which would not meet modern criteria of safety. Jenner's achievement was the realization that infection with a bovine analogue of smallpox, vaccinia (from *vacca*, Latin for cow), which caused cowpox, would provide protective immunity against smallpox in humans without the risk of significant disease. He named the process **vaccination**, and Pasteur, in his honour, extended the term to the stimulation of protection to other infectious agents. Humans are not a natural host of vaccinia, which establishes only a brief and limited subcutaneous infection. But it contains antigens that stimulate an immune response that is cross-reactive with smallpox antigens and thereby confers protection from the human disease.

This established the general principles of safe and effective vaccination, and vaccine development in the early part of the 20th century followed two empirical pathways. The first was the search for **attenuated** organisms with reduced pathogenicity, which would stimulate protective immunity; the second was the development of vaccines based on killed organisms and, subsequently, on purified components of organisms that would be as effective as live whole organisms. Killed vaccines were desirable because any live vaccine, including vaccinia, can cause lethal systemic infection in the immunosuppressed.

Immunization is now considered so safe and so important that most states in the United States require all children to be immunized against measles, mumps, and polio viruses with live-attenuated vaccines as well as against tetanus (caused by *Clostridium tetani*), diphtheria (caused by *Corynebacterium diphtheriae*), and whooping cough (caused by *Bordetella pertussis*), with inactivated toxins or toxoids prepared from these bacteria (see Fig. 1.33). More recently, a vaccine has become available against *Haemophilus influenzae* type b, one of the causative agents of meningitis. Current vaccination schedules for children in the United States are shown in Fig. 14.21. Impressive as these accomplishments are, there are still many diseases for

Fig. 14.21 Recommended childhood vaccination schedules (in red) in the United States. Each red bar denotes a time range during which a vaccine dose should be given. Bars spanning multiple months indicate a range of times during which the vaccine may be given. *Tetanus and diphtheria toxoids only.

Current immunization schedule for children (USA)									
Vaccine given	1 month	2 months	4 months	6 months	12 months	15 months	18 months	4–6 years	11–12 years	14–16 years
Diphtheria–tetanus–pertussis (DTP/DTaP)		■	■	■		■	■	■	■ *	
Inactivated polio vaccine		■	■	■	■	■	■	■		
Measles/mumps/rubella (MMR)					■	■		■		
Pneumococcal conjugate		■	■	■	■	■				
Haemophilus B conjugate (HiBC)		■	■	■	■	■				
Hepatitis B	■	■		■	■	■	■			
Varicella					■	■	■			

Fig. 14.22 Diseases for which effective vaccines are still needed.
*The number of people infected is estimated at ~200 million, of which 20 million have severe disease. †Current measles vaccines are effective but heat-sensitive, which makes their use difficult in tropical countries. Estimated mortality data for 2001 from *World Health Report 2002* (World Health Organization).

Some diseases for which effective vaccines are not yet available		
Disease	**Estimated annual mortality**	**Estimated annual incidence**
Malaria*	1,124,000	300–500 million
Schistosomiasis	15,000	no numbers available
Worm infestation	12,000	no numbers available
Tuberculosis	1,644,000	~8 million
Diarrheal disease	2,001,000	~4,100 million
Respiratory disease	3,947,000	~362 million
HIV/AIDS	2,866,000	~2 million
Measles†	745,000	~44 million

which we lack effective vaccines, as shown in Fig. 14.22. Even when a vaccine such as measles or polio can be used effectively in developed countries, technical and economic problems can prevent its widespread use in developing countries, where mortality from these diseases is still high. The development of vaccines therefore remains an important goal of immunology, and the latter half of the 20th century saw a shift to a more rational approach based on a detailed molecular understanding of microbial pathogenicity, analysis of the protective host response to pathogenic organisms, and the understanding of the regulation of the immune system to generate effective T- and B-lymphocyte responses.

14-18 There are several requirements for an effective vaccine.

The particular requirements for successful vaccination vary depending on the nature of the infecting organism. For extracellular organisms, antibody provides the most important adaptive mechanism of host defense, whereas for the control of intracellular organisms an effective CD8 T-lymphocyte response is also essential. The ideal vaccination provides host defense at the point of entry of the infectious agent; stimulation of mucosal immunity is therefore an important goal of vaccination against those many organisms that enter through mucosal surfaces.

Effective protective immunity against some microorganisms requires the presence of preexisting antibody at the time of exposure to the infection. For example, the clinical manifestations of tetanus and diphtheria are due entirely to the effects of extremely powerful exotoxins (see Fig. 9.23). Indeed, the tetanus exotoxin is so powerful that the tiny amount that can cause disease may be insufficient to lead to a protective immune response. This means that survivors of tetanus require vaccination to be protected against the risk of developing a subsequent attack. Preexisting antibody against the bacterial exotoxin is necessary to provide a defense against tetanus and diphtheria. Preexisting antibodies are also required to protect against some intracellular pathogens, such as the poliomyelitis virus, which infect critical host cells within a short period after entering the body and are not easily controlled by T lymphocytes once intracellular infection has been established.

Immune responses to infectious agents usually involve antibodies directed at multiple epitopes, and only some of these antibodies confer protection. The particular T-cell epitopes recognized can also affect the nature of the response. For example, as we saw in Chapter 11, the predominant epitope recognized by T cells after vaccination with respiratory syncytial virus induces a vigorous inflammatory response but fails to elicit neutralizing antibodies and thus causes pathology without protection. Thus, an effective vaccine must lead to the generation of antibodies and T cells directed at the correct epitopes of the infectious agent. For some of the modern vaccine techniques, in which only one or a few epitopes are used, this consideration is particularly important.

Several very important additional constraints need to be satisfied by a successful vaccine (Fig. 14.23). First, it must be safe. Vaccines must be given to huge numbers of people, relatively few of whom are likely to die of, or sometimes even catch, the disease that the vaccine is designed to prevent. This means that even a low level of toxicity is unacceptable. Second, the vaccine must be able to produce protective immunity in a very high proportion of the people to whom it is given. Third, because it is impracticable to give large or dispersed rural populations regular 'booster' vaccinations, a successful vaccine must generate long-lived immunological memory. This means that the vaccine must prime both B and T lymphocytes. Fourth, vaccines must be very cheap if they are to be administered to large populations. Vaccines are one of the most cost-effective measures in health care, but this benefit is eroded as the cost per dose rises.

An effective vaccination program provides herd immunity—by lowering the number of susceptible members of a population, the natural reservoir of infected individuals in that population falls, reducing the probability of transmission of infection. Thus, even nonvaccinated members of a population can be protected from infection if the majority are vaccinated.

Features of effective vaccines	
Safe	Vaccine must not itself cause illness or death
Protective	Vaccine must protect against illness resulting from exposure to live pathogen
Gives sustained protection	Protection against illness must last for several years
Induces neutralizing antibody	Some pathogens (such as poliovirus) infect cells that cannot be replaced (eg, neurons). Neutralizing antibody is essential to prevent infection of such cells
Induces protective T cells	Some pathogens, particularly intracellular, are more effectively dealt with by cell-mediated responses
Practical considerations	Low cost per dose Biological stability Ease of administration Few side-effects

Fig. 14.23 There are several criteria for an effective vaccine.

14-19 The history of vaccination against *Bordetella pertussis* illustrates the importance of developing an effective vaccine that is perceived to be safe.

The history of vaccination against the bacterium that causes whooping cough, *Bordetella pertussis*, provides a good example of the challenges of developing and disseminating an effective vaccine. At the turn of the 20th century, whooping cough killed approximately 0.5% of American children under the age of 5 years. In the early 1930s, a trial of a killed, whole bacterial cell vaccine on the Faroe Islands provided evidence of a protective effect. In the United States, systematic use of a whole-cell vaccine in combination with diphtheria and tetanus toxoids (the DTP vaccine) from the 1940s resulted in a decline in the annual infection rate from 200 to less than 2 cases per 100,000 of the population. First vaccination with DTP was typically given at the age of 3 months.

Whole-cell pertussis vaccine causes side-effects, typically redness, pain, and swelling at the site of the injection; less commonly, vaccination is followed by high temperature and persistent crying. Very rarely, fits and a short-lived sleepiness or a floppy unresponsive state ensue. During the 1970s, widespread concern developed after several anecdotal observations that encephalitis leading to irreversible brain damage might very rarely follow pertussis vaccination. In Japan, in 1972, approximately 85% of children were given the pertussis vaccine, and fewer than 300 cases of whooping cough and no deaths were reported. As a result of two deaths after vaccination in Japan in 1975, DTP was temporarily suspended and then reintroduced with the first vaccination at 2 years of age rather than 3 months. In 1979 there were approximately 13,000 cases of whooping cough and 41 deaths. The possibility that pertussis vaccine very rarely causes severe brain damage has been studied extensively and expert consensus is that pertussis vaccine is not a primary cause of brain injury. There is no doubt that there is greater morbidity from whooping cough than from the vaccine.

The public and medical perception that whole-cell pertussis vaccination might be unsafe provided a powerful incentive to develop safer pertussis vaccines. Study of the natural immune response to *B. pertussis* showed that infection induced antibodies against four components of the bacterium—pertussis toxin, filamentous hemagglutinin, pertactin, and fimbrial antigens. Immunization of mice with these antigens in purified form protected them against challenge with pertussis. This has led to the development of acellular pertussis vaccines, all of which contain purified pertussis toxoid, that is, toxin inactivated by chemical treatment, for example with hydrogen peroxide or formaldehyde, or more recently by genetic engineering of the toxin. Some also contain one or more of the filamentous hemagglutinin, pertactin, and fimbrial antigens. Current evidence shows that these are probably as effective as whole-cell pertussis vaccine and are free of the common minor side-effects of the whole-cell vaccine.

The main messages of the history of pertussis vaccination are, first, that vaccines must be extremely safe and free of side-effects; second, that the public and the medical profession must perceive the vaccine to be safe; and third, that careful study of the nature of the protective immune response can lead to acellular vaccines that are safer than whole-cell vaccines but still as effective.

Public concerns about vaccination remain high. Unwarranted fears of a link between the combined live-attenuated vaccine against measles, mumps, and rubella (MMR) and autism have seen the uptake of MMR vaccine in England fall from a peak of 92% of children in 1995–1996 to 84% in 2001–2002. Small clustered outbreaks of measles during 2002 in London show that there is a danger of a recrudescence of epidemics of measles in the UK.

14-20 Conjugate vaccines have been developed as a result of understanding how T and B cells collaborate in an immune response.

Although acellular vaccines are inevitably safer than vaccines based on whole organisms, a fully effective vaccine cannot normally be made from a single isolated constituent of a microorganism, and it is now clear that this is because of the need to activate more than one cell type to initiate an immune response. One consequence of this insight has been the development of conjugate vaccines. We have already described briefly one of the most important of these in Section 9-2.

Many bacteria, including *Neisseria meningitidis* (meningococcus), *Streptococcus pneumoniae* (pneumococcus), and *Haemophilus* species, have an outer capsule composed of polysaccharides that are species- and type-specific for particular strains of the bacterium. The most effective defense against these microorganisms is opsonization of the polysaccharide coat with antibody. The aim of vaccination is therefore to elicit antibodies against the polysaccharide capsules of the bacteria.

Capsular polysaccharides can be harvested from bacterial growth medium and, because they are T-cell independent antigens, they can be used on their own as vaccines. However, young children under the age of 2 years cannot make good T-cell independent antibody responses and cannot be vaccinated effectively with polysaccharide vaccines. An efficient way of overcoming this problem (see Fig. 9.5) is to conjugate bacterial polysaccharides chemically to protein carriers, which provide peptides that can be recognized by antigen-specific T cells, thus converting a T-cell independent response into a T-cell dependent anti-polysaccharide antibody response. By using this approach, various conjugate vaccines have been developed against *Haemophilus influenzae* type b, an important cause of serious childhood chest infections and meningitis, and against *Neisseria meningitidis* serogroup C, and these are now widely applied.

14-21 The use of adjuvants is another important approach to enhancing the immunogenicity of vaccines.

Purified antigens are not usually strongly immunogenic on their own, and most acellular vaccines require the addition of **adjuvants**, which are defined as substances that enhance the immunogenicity of antigens (see Appendix I, Section A-4). For example, tetanus toxoid is not immunogenic in the absence of adjuvants, and tetanus toxoid vaccines often contain aluminum salts, which bind polyvalently to the toxoid by ionic interactions and selectively stimulate antibody responses. Pertussis toxin, produced by *B. pertussis*, has adjuvant properties in its own right and, when given mixed as a toxoid with tetanus and diphtheria toxoids, not only vaccinates against whooping cough but also acts as an adjuvant for the other two toxoids. This mixture makes up the DTP triple vaccine given to infants in the first year of life.

Many important adjuvants are sterile constituents of bacteria, particularly of their cell walls. For example, Freund's complete adjuvant, widely used in experimental animals to augment antibody responses, is an oil and water emulsion containing killed mycobacteria. A complex glycolipid, muramyl dipeptide, which can be extracted from mycobacterial cell walls or synthesized, contains much of the adjuvant activity of whole killed mycobacteria. Other bacterial adjuvants include killed *B. pertussis*, bacterial polysaccharides, bacterial heat-shock proteins, and bacterial DNA. Many of these adjuvants cause quite marked inflammation and are not suitable for use in vaccines for humans.

It is thought that most, if not all, adjuvants act on antigen-presenting cells, especially on dendritic cells, and reflect the importance of these cells in initiating immune responses. As we saw in Section 8-6, dendritic cells are widely distributed throughout the body, acting as sentinels to detect potential pathogens at their portals of entry. These tissue dendritic cells take up antigens from their environment by phagocytosis and macropinocytosis, and they are tuned to respond to the presence of infection by migrating into lymphoid tissue and presenting these antigens to T cells. They seem to detect the presence of pathogens in two main ways. The first of these is direct, and follows the ligation and activation of receptors for invading microorganisms. These include receptors of the complement system, Toll-like receptors (TLRs), and other pattern recognition receptors of the innate immune system (see Chapter 2).

The discovery that the effects of many adjuvants are mediated by the activation of TLRs on dendritic cells opens the door to the rational development of novel adjuvants for vaccine therapy. Lipopolysaccharide (LPS) is a component of the cell wall of Gram-negative bacteria. It has adjuvant effects but these are limited by its toxicity. Small amounts of injected LPS can induce a state of shock and systemic inflammation that mimics Gram-negative sepsis. A key question is: can the adjuvant effects of LPS be separated from the toxic effects? A derivative of LPS, monophosphoryl lipid A, partly achieves this, retaining adjuvant effects but being associated with much lower toxicity than parental LPS. Both LPS and monophosphoryl lipid A are ligands for TLR-4, which seems to be the most important receptor mediating the adjuvant effect of LPS and its derivatives. Other adjuvants use other TLRs. Unmethylated CpG DNA binds to TLR-9, lipoprotein components of many Gram-positive bacteria bind to TLR-2, and muramyl dipeptide binds to Nod2, which is implicated in the intracellular recognition of bacteria (see Section 12-18).

These discoveries have transformed our understanding of the mechanisms of action of adjuvants. When dendritic cells are activated through the ligation of TLRs, they respond by secreting cytokines and expressing co-stimulatory molecules, which in turn stimulate the activation and differentiation of antigen-specific T cells. However, even with this greater understanding of the mechanisms of adjuvants, it is likely that the therapeutic window between efficacy and toxicity of adjuvants will remain narrow. This is because both the pharmacological and toxicological effects of adjuvants are mediated in identical fashions. The physiological function of TLRs is to stimulate an inflammatory and immune response to infection. Pharmacological ligation of these receptors by adjuvants in the context of vaccination therefore steers a fine course between stimulating beneficial immunity or damaging inflammation.

The second mechanism of stimulation of dendritic cells by invading organisms is indirect and involves their activation by cytokine signals derived from the inflammatory response triggered by infection (see Chapter 2). Cytokines such as GM-CSF are particularly effective in activating dendritic cells to express co-stimulatory signals and, in the context of viral infection, dendritic cells also express IFN-α and IL-12.

Adjuvants trick the immune system into responding as though there were an active infection, and just as different classes of infectious agent stimulate different types of immune response (see Chapter 10), different adjuvants may promote different types of response, for example, an inflammatory T_H1 response or an antibody-dominated response. Some adjuvants, for example pertussis toxin, cholera toxin, and *E. coli* heat-labile enterotoxin, stimulate mucosal immune responses, which are particularly important in defense against organisms entering through the digestive or respiratory tracts. These adjuvants are discussed further in Section 14-26.

Following our increased understanding of the mechanisms of action of adjuvants, rational approaches to improving the activity of vaccines in clinical settings are being implemented. One approach is to coadminister cytokines. For example, IL-12 is a cytokine produced by macrophages, dendritic cells, and B cells that stimulates T lymphocytes and NK cells to release IFN-γ and promotes a T_H1 response. It has been used as an adjuvant to promote protective immunity against the protozoan parasite *Leishmania major*. Certain strains of mice are susceptible to severe cutaneous and systemic infection by *L. major*; these mice mount an immune response that is predominantly T_H2 in type and is ineffective in eliminating the organism (see Section 10-6). The coadministration of IL-12 with a vaccine containing leishmania antigens generated a T_H1 response and protected the mice against challenge with *L. major*. The use of IL-12 to promote a T_H1 response has also proved valuable in reducing the pathogenic consequences of experimental parasitic infection by *Schistosoma mansoni* and is considered in Sections 14-29 and 14-30. These are important examples of how an understanding of the regulation of immune responses can enable rational intervention to enhance the effectiveness of vaccines.

14-22 Live-attenuated viral vaccines are usually more potent than 'killed' vaccines and can be made safer by using recombinant DNA technology.

Most antiviral vaccines currently in use consist of inactivated or live attenuated viruses. Inactivated, or 'killed,' viral vaccines consist of viruses treated so that they are unable to replicate. Live-attenuated viral vaccines are generally far more potent, perhaps because they elicit a greater number of relevant effector mechanisms, including cytotoxic CD8 T cells: inactivated viruses cannot produce proteins in the cytosol, so peptides from the viral antigens cannot be presented by MHC class I molecules and thus cytotoxic CD8 T cells are not generated by these vaccines. Attenuated viral vaccines are now in use for polio, measles, mumps, rubella, and varicella.

Traditionally, attenuation is achieved by growing the virus in cultured cells. Viruses are usually selected for preferential growth in nonhuman cells and, in the course of selection, become less able to grow in human cells (Fig. 14.24). Because these attenuated strains replicate poorly in human hosts, they induce immunity but not disease when given to people. Although attenuated virus strains contain multiple mutations in genes encoding several of their proteins, it might be possible for a pathogenic virus strain to reemerge by a further series of mutations. For example, the type 3 Sabin polio vaccine strain differs at only 10 of 7429 nucleotides from a wild-type progenitor strain. On extremely rare occasions, reversion of the vaccine to a neurovirulent strain can occur, causing paralytic disease in the unfortunate recipient.

Attenuated viral vaccines can also pose particular risks to immunodeficient recipients, in whom they often behave as virulent opportunistic infections. Immunodeficient infants who are vaccinated with live attenuated polio before their inherited immunoglobulin deficiencies have been diagnosed are at risk because they cannot clear the virus from their gut, and there is therefore an increased chance that mutation of the virus associated with its continuing uncontrolled replication in the gut will lead to fatal paralytic disease. For the same reason, patients with immunoglobulin deficiencies show an abnormal susceptibility to chronic infection by opportunistic enteroviruses and can develop chronic, and ultimately lethal, echovirus encephalitis if mutation of the virus leads to neurovirulence.

Fig. 14.24 Viruses are traditionally attenuated by selecting for growth in nonhuman cells. To produce an attenuated virus, the virus must first be isolated by growing it in cultured human cells. The adaptation to growth in cultured human cells can cause some attenuation in itself; the rubella vaccine, for example, was made in this way. In general, however, the virus is then adapted to growth in cells of a different species, until it grows only poorly in human cells. The adaptation is a result of mutation, usually a combination of several point mutations. It is usually hard to tell which of the mutations in the genome of an attenuated viral stock are critical to attenuation. An attenuated virus will grow poorly in the human host and will therefore produce immunity but not disease.

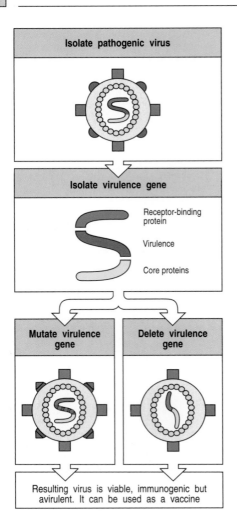

Isolate pathogenic virus

Isolate virulence gene

Receptor-binding protein

Virulence

Core proteins

Mutate virulence gene

Delete virulence gene

Resulting virus is viable, immunogenic but avirulent. It can be used as a vaccine

Fig. 14.25 Attenuation can be achieved more rapidly and reliably with recombinant DNA techniques. If a gene in the virus that is required for virulence but not for growth or immunogenicity can be identified, this gene can be either multiply mutated (left lower panel) or deleted from the genome (right lower panel) by using recombinant DNA techniques. This procedure creates an avirulent (nonpathogenic) virus that can be used as a vaccine. The mutations in the virulence gene are usually large, so that it is very difficult for the virus to revert to the wild type.

An empirical approach to attenuation is still in use but might be superseded by two new approaches that use recombinant DNA technology. One is the isolation and *in vitro* mutagenesis of specific viral genes. The mutated genes are used to replace the wild-type gene in a reconstituted virus genome, and this deliberately attenuated virus can then be used as a vaccine (Fig. 14.25). The advantage of this approach is that mutations can be engineered so that reversion to wild type is virtually impossible.

Such an approach might be useful in developing live influenza vaccines. As described in Chapter 11, the influenza virus can reinfect the same host several times, because it undergoes antigenic shift and thus escapes the original immune response. The current approach to vaccination against influenza is to use a killed virus vaccine that is reformulated annually on the basis of the prevalent strains of virus. The vaccine is moderately effective, reducing mortality in elderly people and illness in healthy adults. The ideal influenza vaccine would be an attenuated live organism that matched the prevalent virus strain. This could be created by first introducing a series of attenuating mutations into the gene encoding a viral polymerase protein, PB2. The mutated gene segment from the attenuated virus could then be substituted for the wild-type gene in a virus carrying the relevant hemagglutinin and neuraminidase antigenic variants of the current epidemic or pandemic strain. This last procedure could be repeated as necessary to keep pace with the antigenic shift of the virus.

14-23 Live-attenuated bacterial vaccines can be developed by selecting nonpathogenic or disabled mutants.

Similar approaches are being used for bacterial vaccine development. *Salmonella typhi*, the causative agent of typhoid, has been manipulated to develop a live vaccine. A strain of wild-type bacteria was mutated with nitrosoguanidine; a new strain was selected to be defective in the enzyme UDP-galactose epimerase, thus blocking the pathway for the synthesis of LPS, an important determinant of bacterial pathogenesis. Recent approaches to the rational design of attenuated *Salmonella* vaccines have involved the specific targeting of genes encoding enzymes in the pathways that synthesize amino acids containing aromatic rings, such as tyrosine and phenylalanine. Mutating these genes generates auxotrophs— organisms that need an external supply of an essential nutrient that wild-type bacteria can make themselves. These bacteria grow poorly in the gut but should survive long enough as a vaccine to induce an effective immune response.

It is not only vaccination of humans against *Salmonella* that is important. Modern methods of mass production of chickens for food has led to extensive infection of poultry with *Salmonella* strains that are pathogenic to humans and an increasingly important cause of food poisoning. Thus, in parts of the world where typhoid is prevalent, vaccinating humans has a high priority. In other parts, where food poisoning caused by *Salmonella typhimurium* and *S. enteritidis* infection is common, vaccination of chickens would contribute to public health.

14-24 Attenuated microorganisms can serve as vectors for vaccination against many pathogens.

An effective live-attenuated typhoid vaccine would not only be valuable in its own right but could also serve as a vector for presenting antigens from other organisms. Attenuated strains of *Salmonella* have been used as carriers of heterologous genes encoding tetanus toxoid and antigens from organisms as diverse as *Listeria monocytogenes, Bacillus anthracis, Leishmania major,*

Yersinia pestis, and *Schistosoma mansoni.* Each of these has been used as an oral vaccine to protect mice against experimental challenge with the respective pathogen.

Viral vectors can similarly be engineered to carry heterologous peptides or proteins from other microorganisms. Although vaccinia is no longer needed to protect against smallpox, it remains a candidate for an avirulent carrier of heterologous antigens. Genes encoding protective antigens from several different organisms could be placed in a single vaccine strain. This approach makes it possible to immunize individuals against several different pathogens at once, but such a vaccine could not be used twice because the vaccinia vector itself generates long-lasting immunity that would neutralize its effectiveness on a second administration. The development of successful heterologous vaccines requires the identification of protective antigens; it therefore depends on the analytical power of recombinant DNA methods, as well as their use to manipulate gene structure.

Plant viruses, which are nonpathogenic to humans, have been used as a source of novel vaccine vectors. These viruses can be engineered to incorporate heterologous peptide antigens into chimeric coat proteins. The success of this approach relies on the successful identification of protective peptide antigens as well as the immunogenicity of the vaccine. With the use of this strategy, mice have been protected against lethal challenge with rabies virus by prior feeding with spinach leaves infected by recombinant alfalfa mosaic virus incorporating a rabies virus peptide.

14-25 Synthetic peptides of protective antigens can elicit protective immunity.

One route to vaccine development is the identification of the T-cell peptide epitopes that stimulate protective immunity. This can be approached in two ways. One possibility is to synthesize systematically overlapping peptides from immunogenic proteins and to test each in turn for its ability to stimulate protective immunity. An alternative, but no less arduous approach— 'reverse' immunogenetics—has been used in developing a vaccine against malaria (Fig. 14.26). We met this approach earlier in Section 14-14 of this chapter in the context of the characterization of tumor antigens.

The immunogenicity of T-cell peptide epitopes depends on their specific associations with particular polymorphic variants of MHC molecules. The starting point for the studies on malaria was an association between the human MHC class I molecule HLA-B53 and resistance to cerebral malaria— a relatively infrequent complication of infection but one that is usually fatal. The hypothesis is that these MHC molecules are protective because they present peptides that are particularly good at evoking cytotoxic T lymphocytes. A direct route to identifying the relevant peptides is to elute them from

Fig. 14.26 'Reverse' immunogenetics can be used to identify protective T-cell epitopes against infectious diseases. Population studies show that the MHC class I variant HLA-B53 is associated with resistance to cerebral malaria. Self nonapeptides were eluted from HLA-B53 and found to have a strong preference for proline at the second position. Candidate nonapeptide sequences containing proline at position 2 were then identified in several malarial protein sequences and synthesized. These synthetic nonapeptides were then tested to see whether they fitted well into the peptide groove of HLA-B53 by assaying whether HLA-B53 would assemble to form a stable cell-surface heterodimer in the presence of peptide. Peptide sequences identified by this approach were then tested to see whether they would induce the proliferation of T cells from patients infected by malaria. Such sequences are good candidates for incorporation into vaccines.

MHC molecules of cells infected with the pathogen. In HLA-B53, a high proportion of the peptides eluted had proline in the second of nine positions; this information was used to identify candidate protective peptides from four proteins of *Plasmodium falciparum* expressed in the early phase of hepatocyte infection, an important phase of infection to target in an effective immune response. One of the candidate peptides, from liver stage antigen-1, is recognized by cytotoxic T cells when bound to HLA-B53.

This approach is being extended to other MHC class I and class II molecules associated with protective immune responses against infection. Recently, a protective peptide epitope was eluted from MHC class II molecules in *Leishmania*-infected macrophages and used as a guide to isolate the gene from *Leishmania*. The gene was then used to make a protein-based vaccine that primed mice from susceptible strains for responses to *Leishmania*.

These results show considerable promise, but they also illustrate one of the major drawbacks to the approach. A malaria peptide that is restricted by HLA-B53 might not be immunogenic in an individual lacking HLA-B53: indeed, this presumably accounts for the higher susceptibility of these individuals to natural infections. Because of the very high polymorphism of MHC molecules in humans it will be necessary to identify panels of protective T-cell epitopes and construct vaccines containing arrays of these to develop vaccines that will protect the majority of a susceptible population.

There are other problems with peptide vaccines. Peptides are not strongly immunogenic and it is particularly difficult to generate MHC class I-specific responses by *in vivo* immunization with peptides. One approach to this problem is to integrate peptides by genetic engineering into carrier proteins within a viral vector, such as hepatitis B core antigen, which are then processed *in vivo* through natural antigen-processing pathways. A second possible technique is the use of **ISCOMs** (immune stimulatory complexes). These are lipid carriers that act as adjuvants but have minimal toxicity. They seem to load peptides and proteins into the cell cytoplasm, allowing MHC class I-restricted T-cell responses to peptides to develop (Fig. 14.27). These carriers are being developed for use in human immunization. Another approach to delivering protective peptides, which is discussed in the previous section, is the genetic engineering of infectious microorganisms to create vaccines that stimulate immunity without causing disease.

Fig. 14.27 ISCOMs can be used to deliver peptides to the MHC class I processing pathway. ISCOMs (immune stimulatory complexes) are lipid micelles that will fuse with cell membranes. Peptides trapped in ISCOMs can be delivered to the cytosol of an antigen-presenting cell (APC), allowing the peptide to be transported into the endoplasmic reticulum, where it can be bound by newly synthesized MHC class I molecules and hence transported to the cell surface as peptide:MHC class I complexes. This is a possible means for delivering vaccine peptides to activate CD8 cytotoxic T cells. ISCOMs can also be used to deliver proteins to the cytosol of other types of cell, where they can be processed and presented as though they were a protein produced by the cell.

14-26 The route of vaccination is an important determinant of success.

Most vaccines are given by injection. This route has two disadvantages: the first is practical, the second immunological. Injections are painful and expensive, requiring needles, syringes, and a trained injector. They are unpopular with the recipient, reducing vaccine uptake, and mass vaccination by this approach is laborious. The immunological drawback is that injection may not be the most effective way of stimulating an appropriate immune response because it does not mimic the usual route of entry of the majority of pathogens against which vaccination is directed.

Many important pathogens infect mucosal surfaces or enter the body through mucosal surfaces. Examples include respiratory microorganisms such as *B. pertussis*, rhinoviruses, and influenza viruses, and enteric microorganisms such as *Vibrio cholerae*, *Salmonella typhi*, enteropathogenic *E. coli*, and *Shigella*. The enteric microorganisms are particularly important pathogens in underdeveloped countries. It is therefore important to understand how these organisms stimulate mucosal immunity and to develop vaccines that behave similarly. To this end, there are efforts to develop vaccines that can be administered to the mucosa orally or by nasal inhalation.

The power of this approach is illustrated by the effectiveness of live-attenuated polio vaccines. The Sabin polio vaccine consists of three attenuated polio virus strains and is highly immunogenic. Moreover, just as polio itself can be transmitted by fecal contamination of public swimming pools and other failures of hygiene, the vaccine can be transmitted from one individual to another by the orofecal route. Infection with *Salmonella* likewise stimulates a powerful mucosal and systemic immune response and, as we saw in Section 14-24, has been attenuated for use as a vaccine and carrier of heterologous antigens for presentation to the mucosal immune system.

The rules of mucosal immunity are poorly understood. On the one hand, presentation of soluble protein antigens by the oral route often results in tolerance, which is important given the enormous load of foodborne and airborne antigens presented to the gut and respiratory tract. As discussed in Section 14-12, the ability to induce tolerance by oral or nasal administration of antigens is being explored as a therapeutic mechanism for reducing unwanted immune responses. On the other hand, the mucosal immune system can respond to and eliminate mucosal infections such as pertussis, cholera, and polio. The proteins from these microorganisms that stimulate immune responses are therefore of special interest. One group of powerfully immunogenic proteins at mucosal surfaces is a group of bacterial toxins that have the property of binding to eukaryotic cells and are protease-resistant. A recent finding of potential practical importance is that certain of these molecules, such as the *E. coli* heat-labile toxin and pertussis toxin, have adjuvant properties that are retained even when the parent molecule has been engineered to eliminate its toxic properties. These molecules can be used as adjuvants for oral or nasal vaccines. In mice, nasal insufflation of either of these mutant toxins together with tetanus toxoid resulted in the development of protection against lethal challenge with tetanus toxin.

14-27 Protective immunity can be induced by injecting DNA encoding microbial antigens and human cytokines into muscle.

The latest development in vaccination has come as a surprise even to the scientists who first developed the method. The story begins with attempts to use nonreplicating bacterial plasmids encoding proteins for gene therapy: proteins expressed *in vivo* from these plasmids were found to stimulate an immune response. When DNA encoding a viral immunogen is injected

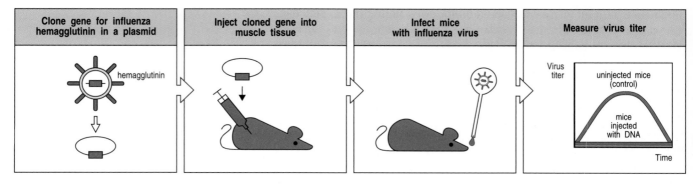

Clone gene for influenza hemagglutinin in a plasmid	Inject cloned gene into muscle tissue	Infect mice with influenza virus	Measure virus titer

Fig. 14.28 DNA vaccination by injection of DNA encoding a protective antigen and cytokines directly into muscle. Influenza hemagglutinin contains both B- and T-cell epitopes. When a DNA plasmid containing the gene for hemagglutinin is injected directly into muscle, an influenza-specific immune response consisting of both antibody and cytotoxic CD8 T cells results. The response can be enhanced by including a plasmid encoding GM-CSF in the injection. The plasmid DNAs are presumably expressed by some of the cells in the muscle tissue into which they are injected, provoking an immune response that involves both antibody and cytotoxic T cells. The details of this process are not yet understood.

intramuscularly, it leads to the development of antibody responses and cytotoxic T cells that allow the mice to reject a later challenge with whole virus (Fig. 14.28). This response does not seem to damage the muscle tissue, is safe and effective, and, because it uses only a single microbial gene or DNA encoding sets of antigenic peptides, does not carry the risk of active infection. This procedure has been termed **DNA vaccination**. DNA coated onto minute metal projectiles can be administered by 'biolistic' (biological ballistic) gun, so that several metal particles penetrate the skin and enter the muscle beneath. This technique has been shown to be effective in animals and might be suitable for mass immunization. Mixing in plasmids that encode cytokines such as GM-CSF makes immunization with genes encoding protective antigens much more effective, as was seen earlier for tumor immunity. As we saw earlier, unmethylated CpG DNA is a ligand for TLR-9 (see Section 2-7), and the targets for DNA vaccines are probably dendritic cells that take up and express the DNA, undergoing activation through TLR-9 in the process. DNA vaccines are being used in trials for the prevention of malaria and HIV.

14-28 The effectiveness of a vaccine can be enhanced by targeting it to sites of antigen presentation.

An important way of enhancing the effectiveness of a vaccine is to target it efficiently to antigen-presenting cells. This is an important mechanism of action of vaccine adjuvants. There are three complementary approaches. The first is to prevent proteolysis of the antigen on its way to antigen-presenting cells. Preserving antigen structure is an important reason why so many vaccines are given by injection rather than by the oral route, which exposes the vaccine to digestion in the gut. The second and third approaches are to target the vaccine selectively, once in the body, to antigen-presenting cells and to devise methods of engineering the selective uptake of the vaccine into antigen-processing pathways within the cell.

Techniques to enhance the uptake of antigens by antigen-presenting cells include coating the antigen with mannose to enhance uptake by mannose receptors on antigen-presenting cells, and presenting the antigen as an immune complex to take advantage of antibody and complement binding by Fc and complement receptors. The effects of DNA vaccination have been enhanced experimentally by injecting DNA encoding antigen coupled to CTLA-4, which enables the selective binding of the expressed protein to antigen-presenting cells carrying B7, the receptor for CTLA-4 (see Section 8-5).

A more complicated set of strategies involves targeting vaccine antigens selectively into antigen-presenting pathways within the cell. For example, human papillomavirus E7 antigen has been coupled to the signal peptide that targets a lysosomal-associated membrane protein to lysosomes and endosomes. This directs the E7 antigen directly to the intracellular compartments in which antigens are cleaved to peptides before binding to MHC class

II molecules (see Section 5-5). A vaccinia virus incorporating this chimeric antigen induced a greater response in mice to E7 antigen than did vaccinia incorporating wild-type E7 antigen alone. A second approach is the use of ISCOMs, which seem to encourage the entry of peptides into the cytoplasm, thus enhancing the loading of peptides onto MHC class I molecules (see Section 14-25).

An improved understanding of the mechanisms of mucosal immunity (see Chapter 10) has led to the development of techniques to target antigens to M cells overlying the Peyer's patches (see Fig. 1.10). These specialized epithelial cells lack the mucin barrier and digestive properties of other mucosal epithelial cells. Instead, they can bind and endocytose macromolecules and microorganisms, which are transcytosed intact and delivered to the underlying lymphoid tissue. In view of these properties, it is not surprising that some pathogens target M cells to gain entry to the body. The counterattack by immunologists is to gain a detailed molecular understanding of this mechanism of bacterial pathogenesis and subvert it as a delivery system for vaccines. For example, the outer membrane fimbrial proteins of *Salmonella typhimurium* have a key role in the binding of these bacteria to M cells. It might be possible to use these fimbrial proteins or, ultimately, just their binding motifs, as targeting agents for vaccines. A related strategy to encourage the uptake of mucosal vaccines by M cells is to encapsulate antigens in particulate carriers that are taken up selectively by M cells.

14-29 An important question is whether vaccination can be used therapeutically to control existing chronic infections.

There are many chronic diseases in which infection persists because of a failure of the immune system to eliminate disease. These can be divided into two groups: those infections in which there is an obvious immune response that fails to eliminate the organism, and those in which the infection seems to be invisible to the immune system and evokes a barely detectable immune response.

In the first category, the immune response is often partly responsible for the pathogenic effects. Infection by the helminth *Schistosoma mansoni* is associated with a powerful T_H2-type response, characterized by high IgE levels, circulating and tissue eosinophilia, and a harmful fibrotic response to schistosome ova, leading to hepatic fibrosis. Other common parasites, such as *Plasmodium* and *Leishmania* species, cause damage because they are not eliminated effectively by the immune response in many patients. Mycobacteria causing tuberculosis and leprosy cause persistent intracellular infection; a T_H1 response helps to contain these infections but also causes granuloma formation and tissue necrosis (see Fig. 8.42). Among viruses, hepatitis B and hepatitis C infections are commonly followed by persistent viral carriage and hepatic injury, resulting in death from hepatitis or from hepatoma. HIV infection, as we have seen in Chapter 11, persists despite an ongoing immune response.

There is a second category of chronic infection, predominantly viral, in which the immune response fails to clear infection because of the relative invisibility of the infectious agent to the immune system. A good example is herpes simplex type 2, which is transmitted venereally, becomes latent in nerve tissue, and causes genital herpes, which is frequently recurrent. This invisibility seems to be caused by a viral protein, ICP-47, that binds to the TAP complex (see Section 5-2) and inhibits peptide transport into the endoplasmic reticulum in infected cells. Thus, viral peptides are not presented to the immune system by MHC class I molecules. Another example in this category of chronic infection is genital warts, caused by certain papilloma viruses to which very little immune response is evoked.

Fig. 14.29 Treatment with anti-IL-4 antibody at the time of infection with *Leishmania major* allows normally susceptible mice to clear the infection. The top panel shows a hematoxylin–eosin-stained section through the footpad of a mouse of the BALB/c strain infected with *Leishmania major* (small red dots). Large numbers of parasites are present in tissue macrophages. The bottom panel shows a similar preparation from a mouse infected in the same experiment but simultaneously treated with a single injection of anti-IL-4 monoclonal antibody. Very few parasites are present. Photographs courtesy of R.M. Locksley.

There are two main immunological approaches to the treatment of chronic infection. One is to try to boost or change the pattern of the host immune response by using cytokine therapy. The second is to attempt therapeutic vaccination to see whether the host immune response can be supercharged by immunization with antigens from the infectious agent in combination with adjuvant. There has been substantial pharmaceutical investment in therapeutic vaccination but it is too early to know whether the approach will be successful.

Some promise for the cytokine therapy approach comes from the experimental treatment of leprosy: one can clear certain leprosy lesions by the injection of cytokines directly into the lesion, which may cause reversal of the type of leprosy seen. Another example in which cytokine therapy has been shown to be effective in treating an established infection depends on combining a cytokine with an antiparasitic drug. In a proportion of mice infected with *Leishmania* and subsequently treated with a combination of drug therapy and IL-12, the immune response deviated from a T_H2 to a T_H1 pattern and the infection was cleared. In most of the animal studies, however, it seems that the anti-cytokine antibody or the cytokine needs to be present at the first encounter with the antigen to modulate the response effectively. For example, in experimental leishmaniasis in mice, susceptible BALB/c mice injected with anti-IL-4 antibody at the time of infection clear their infection (Fig. 14.29). However, if administration of anti-IL-4 antibody is delayed by just 1 week, there is progressive growth of the parasite and a dominant T_H2 response.

14-30 Modulation of the immune system might be used to inhibit immunopathological responses to infectious agents.

We have mentioned several times the possibility of modulating immunity by cytokine manipulation of the immune response. This approach is being explored as a means of inhibiting harmful immune responses to a number of important infections. As we have seen in the preceding section, the liver fibrosis in schistosomiasis results from the powerful T_H2-type response. The coadministration of *S. mansoni* ova together with IL-12 does not protect mice against subsequent infection with *S. mansoni* cercariae but has a striking effect in reducing hepatic granuloma formation and fibrosis in response to ova. IgE levels are reduced, with reduced tissue eosinophilia, and the cytokine response indicates the activation of T_H1 rather than T_H2 cells. Although these results indicate that it might be possible to use a combination of antigen and cytokines to vaccinate against the pathology of diseases for which a fully protective vaccine is unavailable, they do not solve the difficulty of applying this approach in patients whose infection is already established.

Summary.

The greatest triumphs of modern immunology have come from vaccination, which has eradicated or virtually eliminated several human diseases. It is the single most successful manipulation of the immune system so far, because it takes advantage of the immune system's natural specificity and inducibility. Nevertheless, there are many important infectious diseases for which there is still no effective vaccine. The most effective vaccines are based on attenuated live microorganisms, but these carry some risk and are potentially lethal to immunosuppressed or immunodeficient individuals. Better techniques for developing live-attenuated vaccines, or vaccines that incorporate both immunogenic components and protective antigens of pathogens, are therefore being sought. Most current viral vaccines are based on live-attenuated virus, but many bacterial vaccines are based on components of the microorganism, including components of the toxins that it produces. Protective responses to carbohydrate antigens can be enhanced by conjugation to a protein. Vaccines based on peptide epitopes are still at an experimental stage and have the problem that the peptide is likely to be specific for particular variants of the MHC molecules to which they must bind, as well as being only very weakly immunogenic. A vaccine's immunogenicity often depends on adjuvants that can help, directly or indirectly, to activate antigen-presenting cells that are necessary for the initiation of immune responses. Adjuvants activate these cells by engaging the innate immune system and providing ligands for Toll-like and other receptors on antigen-presenting cells. The development of oral vaccines is particularly important for stimulating immunity to the many pathogens that enter through the mucosa. Cytokines have been used experimentally as adjuvants to boost the immunogenicity of vaccines or to bias the immune response along a specific path.

Summary to Chapter 14.

One of the great future challenges of immunology is the control of the immune response, so that unwanted immune responses can be suppressed and desirable responses elicited. Current methods of suppressing unwanted responses rely, to a great extent, on drugs that suppress adaptive immunity indiscriminately and are thus inherently flawed. We have seen in this book that the immune system can suppress its own responses in an antigen-specific manner and, by studying these endogenous regulatory events, it might be possible to devise strategies to manipulate specific responses while sparing general immune competence. This is starting to allow the development of new treatments that selectively suppress the responses that lead to allergy, autoimmunity, or the rejection of grafted organs. Similarly, as we understand more about tumors and infectious agents, better strategies to mobilize the immune system against cancer and infection are becoming possible. To achieve all this, we need to learn more about the induction of immunity and the biology of the immune system, and to apply what we have learned to human disease.

Chapter 14 questions.

14.1   How is a transplant recognized by the immune system?

14.2   What are the roles of antibodies in the treatment of disease?

14.3   What are regulatory T lymphocytes?

14.4   Discuss the question of whether immunotherapy is a realistic approach to the treatment of tumors.

14.5   What is an adjuvant and how does it work?

General references.

Ada, G.: **Vaccines and vaccination.** *N. Engl. J. Med.* 2001, **345**:1042–1053.

Curtiss, R., III: **Bacterial infectious disease control by vaccine development.** *J. Clin. Invest.* 2002, **110**:1061–1066.

Goodnow, C.C.: **Pathways for self-tolerance and the treatment of autoimmune diseases.** *Lancet* 2001, **357**:2115–2121.

Nepom, G.T.: **Therapy of autoimmune diseases: clinical trials and new biologics.** *Curr. Opin. Immunol.* 2002, **14**:812–815.

Steinman, L.: **Immunotherapy of multiple sclerosis: the end of the beginning.** *Curr. Opin. Immunol.* 2001, **13**:597–600.

Ulmer, J.B., and Liu, M.A.: **Ethical issues for vaccines and immunization.** *Nat. Rev. Immunol.* 2002, **2**:291–296.

Yu, X., Carpenter, P., and Anasetti, C.: **Advances in transplantation tolerance.** *Lancet* 2001, **357**:1959–1963.

Section references.

14-1 Corticosteroids are powerful anti-inflammatory drugs that alter the transcription of many genes.

Barnes, P.J.: **Anti-inflammatory actions of glucocorticoids: molecular mechanisms.** *Clin. Sci. (Colch.)* 1998, **94**:557–572.

Boumpas, D.T., Chrousos, G.P., Wilder, R.L., Cupps, T.R., and Balow, J.E.: **Glucocorticoid therapy for immune-mediated diseases: basic and clinical correlates.** *Ann. Intern. Med.* 1993, **119**:1198–1208.

Cronstein, B.N., Kimmel, S.C., Levin, R.I., Martiniuk, F., and Weissmann, G.: **Corticosteroids are transcriptional regulators of acute inflammation.** *Trans. Assoc. Am. Physicians* 1992, **105**:25–35.

Cupps, T.R., and Fauci, A.S.: **Corticosteroid-mediated immunoregulation in man.** *Immunol. Rev.* 1982, **65**:133–155.

14-2 Cytotoxic drugs cause immunosuppression by killing dividing cells and have serious side-effects.

Aarbakke, J., Janka-Schaub, G., and Elion, G.B.: **Thiopurine biology and pharmacology.** *Trends Pharmacol. Sci.* 1997, **18**:3–7.

Smak Gregoor, P.J., van Gelder, T., and Weimar, W.: **Mycophenolate mofetil, Cellcept, a new immunosuppressive drug with great potential in internal medicine.** *Neth. J. Med.* 2000, **57**:233–246.

Zhu, L.P., Cupps, T.R., Whalen, G., and Fauci, A.S.: **Selective effects of cyclophosphamide therapy on activation, proliferation, and differentiation of human B cells.** *J. Clin. Invest.* 1987, **79**:1082–1090.

14-3 Cyclosporin A, tacrolimus (FK506), and rapamycin (sirolimus) are powerful immunosuppressive agents that interfere with T-cell signaling.

Brazelton, T.R., and Morris, R.E.: **Molecular mechanisms of action of new xenobiotic immunosuppressive drugs: tacrolimus (FK506), sirolimus (rapamycin), mycophenolate mofetil and leflunomide.** *Curr. Opin. Immunol.* 1996, **8**:710–720.

Crabtree, G.R.: **Generic signals and specific outcomes: signaling through Ca²⁺, calcineurin, and NF-AT.** *Cell* 1999, **96**:611–614.

14-4 Immunosuppressive drugs are valuable probes of intracellular signaling pathways in lymphocytes.

Bierer, B.E., Mattila, P.S., Standaert, R.F., Herzenberg, L.A., Burakoff, S.J., Crabtree, G., and Schreiber, S.L.: **Two distinct signal transmission pathways in T lymphocytes are inhibited by complexes formed between an immunophilin and either FK506 or rapamycin.** *Proc. Natl. Acad. Sci. USA* 1990, **87**:9231–9235.

Brown, E.J., and Schreiber, S.L.: **A signaling pathway to translational control.** *Cell* 1996, **86**:517–520.

Crespo, J.L., and Hall, M.N.: **Elucidating TOR signaling and rapamycin action: lessons from *Saccharomyces cerevisiae*.** *Microbiol. Mol. Biol. Rev.* 2002, **66**:579–591.

Cutler, N.S., Heitman, J., and Cardenas, M.E.: **TOR kinase homologs function in a signal transduction pathway that is conserved from yeast to mammals.** *Mol. Cell Endocrinol.* 1999, **155**:135–142.

Gingras, A.C., Raught, B., and Sonenberg, N.: **Regulation of translation initiation by FRAP/mTOR.** *Genes Dev.* 2001, **15**:807–826.

14-5 Antibodies against cell-surface molecules have been used to remove specific lymphocyte subsets or to inhibit cell function.

Cobbold, S.P., Qin, S., Leong, L.Y., Martin, G., and Waldmann, H.: **Reprogramming the immune system for peripheral tolerance with CD4 and CD8 monoclonal antibodies.** *Immunol. Rev.* 1992, **129**:165–201.

Honey, K., Cobbold, S.P., and Waldmann, H.: **Dominant regulation: a common mechanism of monoclonal antibody induced tolerance?** *Immunol. Res.* 1999, **20**:1–14.

14-6 Antibodies can be engineered to reduce their immunogenicity in humans.

Hayden, M.S., Gilliland, L.K., and Ledbetter, J.A.: **Antibody engineering.** *Curr. Opin. Immunol.* 1997, **9**:201–212.

Little, M., Kipriyanov, S.M., Le Gall, F., and Moldenhauer, G.: **Of mice and men: hybridoma and recombinant antibodies.** *Immunol. Today* 2000, **21**:364–370.

Winter, G., Griffiths, A.D., Hawkins, R.E., and Hoogenboom, H.R.: **Making antibodies by phage display technology.** *Annu. Rev. Immunol.* 1994, **12**:433–455.

14-7 Monoclonal antibodies can be used to inhibit allograft rejection.

Charlton, B., Auchincloss, H., Jr., and Fathman, C.G.: **Mechanisms of transplantation tolerance.** *Annu. Rev. Immunol.* 1994, **12**:707–734.

Graca, L., Cobbold, S.P., and Waldmann, H.: **Identification of regulatory T cells in tolerated allografts.** *J. Exp. Med.* 2002, **195**:1641–1646.

Graca, L., Thompson, S., Lin, C.Y., Adams, E., Cobbold, S.P., and Waldmann, H.: **Both CD4⁺CD25⁺ and CD4⁺CD25⁻ regulatory cells mediate dominant transplantation tolerance.** *J. Immunol.* 2002, **168**:5558–5565.

Kirk, A.D., Burkly, L.C., Batty, D.S., Baumgartner, R.E., Berning, J.D., Buchanan, K., Fechner, J.H., Jr., Germond, R.L., Kampen, R.L., Patterson, N.B., Swanson, S.J., Tadaki, D.K., TenHoor, C.N., White, L., Knechtle, S.J., and Harlan, D.M.: **Treatment with humanized monoclonal antibody against CD154 prevents acute renal allograft rejection in nonhuman primates.** *Nat. Med.* 1999, **5**:686–693.

Li, X.C., Strom, T.B., Turka, L.A., and Wells, A.D.: **T-cell death and transplantation tolerance.** *Immunity* 2001, **14**:407–416.

Li, Y., Li, X.C., Zheng, X.X., Wells, A.D., Turka, L.A., and Strom, T.B.: **Blocking both signal 1 and signal 2 of T-cell activation prevents apoptosis of alloreactive T cells and induction of peripheral allograft tolerance.** *Nat. Med.* 1999, **5**:1298–1302.

Lin, C.Y., Graca, L., Cobbold, S.P., and Waldmann, H.: **Dominant transplantation tolerance impairs CD8⁺ T cell function but not expansion.** *Nat. Immunol.* 2002, **3**:1208–1213.

Waldmann, H.: **Therapeutic approaches for transplantation.** *Curr. Opin. Immunol.* 2001, **13**:606–610.

Waldmann, H.: **Reprogramming the immune system.** *Immunol. Rev.* 2002, **185**:227–235.

14-8 Biological agents can be used to alleviate and suppress autoimmune disease.

Feldmann, M., Elliott, M.J., Woody, J.N., and Maini, R.N.: **Anti-tumor necrosis factor-α therapy of rheumatoid arthritis.** *Adv. Immunol.* 1997, **64**:283–350.

Ghosh, S., Goldin, E., Gordon, F.H., Malchow, H.A., Rask-Madsen, J., Rutgeerts, P., Vyhnalek, P., Zadorova, Z., Palmer, T., and Donoghue, S.: **Natalizumab for active Crohn's disease.** *N. Engl. J. Med.* 2003, **348**:24–32.

Hallegua, D.S., and Weisman, M.H.: **Potential therapeutic uses of interleukin 1 receptor antagonists in human diseases.** *Ann. Rheum. Dis.* 2002, **61**:960–967.

Mackay, C.R.: **New avenues for anti-inflammatory therapy.** *Nat. Med.* 2002, **8**:117–118.

Miller, D.H., Khan, O.A., Sheremata, W.A., Blumhardt, L.D., Rice, G.P., Libonati, M.A., Willmer-Hulme, A.J., Dalton, C.M., Miszkiel, K.A., and O'Connor, P.W.: **A controlled trial of natalizumab for relapsing multiple sclerosis.** *N. Engl. J. Med.* 2003, **348**:15–23.

Sandborn, W.J., and Targan, S.R.: **Biologic therapy of inflammatory bowel disease.** *Gastroenterology* 2002, **122**:1592–1608.

Taylor, P.C., Williams, R.O., Maini, R.N.: **Immunotherapy for rheumatoid arthritis.** *Curr. Opin. Immunol.* 2001, **13**:611–616.

14-9 Depletion or inhibition of autoreactive lymphocytes can treat autoimmune disease.

Choy, E.H., Kingsley, G.H., and Panayi, G.S.: **Monoclonal antibody therapy in rheumatoid arthritis.** *Br. J. Rheumatol.* 1998, **37**:484–490.

Edwards, J.C., Leandro, M.J., and Cambridge, G.: **B-lymphocyte depletion therapy in rheumatoid arthritis and other autoimmune disorders.** *Biochem. Soc. Trans.* 2002, **30**:824–828.

Moreau, T., Coles, A., Wing, M., Thorpe, J., Miller, D., Moseley, I., Isaacs, J., Hale, G., Clayton, D., Scolding, N., Waldmann, H., and Compston, A.: **CAMPATH-IH in multiple sclerosis.** *Mult. Scler.* 1996, **1**:357–365.

Rep, M.H., van Oosten, B.W., Roos, M.T., Ader, H.J., Polman, C.H., and van Lier, R.A.: **Treatment with depleting CD4 monoclonal antibody results in a preferential loss of circulating naive T cells but does not affect IFN-γ secreting TH1 cells in humans.** *J. Clin. Invest.* 1997, **99**:2225–2231.

Riethmuller, G., Rieber, E.P., Kiefersauer, S., Prinz, J., van der Lubbe, P., Meiser, B., Breedveld, F., Eisenburg, J., Kruger, K., Deusch, K. et al.: **From antilymphocyte serum to therapeutic monoclonal antibodies: first experiences with a chimeric CD4 antibody in the treatment of autoimmune disease.** *Immunol. Rev.* 1992, **129**:81–104.

Willis, F., Marsh, J.C., Bevan, D.H., Killick, S.B., Lucas, G., Griffiths, R., Ouwehand, W., Hale, G., Waldmann, H., and Gordon-Smith, E.C.: **The effect of treatment with Campath-1H in patients with autoimmune cytopenias.** *Br. J. Haematol.* 2001, **114**:891–898.

Zaja, F., De Vita, S., Mazzaro, C., Sacco, S., Damiani, D., De Marchi, G., Michelutti, A., Baccarani, M., Fanin, R., and Ferraccioli, G.: **Efficacy and safety of rituximab in type II mixed cryoglobulinemia.** *Blood* 2003, **101**: 3827–3834.

14-10 Interference with co-stimulatory pathways for the activation of lymphocytes could be a treatment for autoimmune disease.

Abrams, J.R., Kelley, S.L., Hayes, E., Kikuchi, T., Brown, M.J., Kang, S., Lebwohl, M.G., Guzzo, C.A., Jegasothy, B.V., Linsley, P.S., and Krueger, J.G.: **Blockade of T lymphocyte costimulation with cytotoxic T lymphocyte-associated antigen 4-immunoglobulin (CTLA4Ig) reverses the cellular pathology of psoriatic plaques, including the activation of keratinocytes, dendritic cells, and endothelial cells.** *J. Exp. Med.* 2000, **192**:681–694.

Aruffo, A., and Hollenbaugh, D.: **Therapeutic intervention with inhibitors of co-stimulatory pathways in autoimmune disease.** *Curr. Opin. Immunol.* 2001, **13**:683–686.

Ellis, C.N., and Krueger, G.G.: **Treatment of chronic plaque psoriasis by selective targeting of memory effector T lymphocytes.** *N. Engl. J. Med.* 2001, **345**:248–255.

Kraan, M.C., van Kuijk, A.W., Dinant, H.J., Goedkoop, A.Y., Smeets, T.J., de Rie, M.A., Dijkmans, B.A., Vaishnaw, A.K., Bos, J.D., and Tak, P.P.: **Alefacept treatment in psoriatic arthritis: reduction of the effector T cell population in peripheral blood and synovial tissue is associated with improvement of clinical signs of arthritis.** *Arthritis Rheum.* 2002, **46**:2776–2784.

14-11 Modulation of the cytokines expressed by T lymphocytes can inhibit autoimmune disease.

Chatenoud, L., Salomon, B., and Bluestone, J.A.: **Suppressor T cells—they're back and critical for regulation of autoimmunity!** *Immunol. Rev.* 2001, **182**:149–163.

Coffman, R.L., Mocci, S., and O'Garra, A.: **The stability and reversibility of Th1 and Th2 populations.** *Curr. Top. Microbiol. Immunol.* 1999, **238**:1–12.

Curotto de Lafaille, M.A., and Lafaille, J.J.: **CD4⁺ regulatory T cells in autoimmunity and allergy.** *Curr. Opin. Immunol.* 2002, **14**:771–778.

Fukaura, H., Kent, S.C., Pietrusewicz, M.J., Khoury, S.J., Weiner, H.L., and Hafler, D.A.: **Induction of circulating myelin basic protein and proteolipid protein-specific transforming growth factor-β1-secreting Th3 T cells by oral administration of myelin in multiple sclerosis patients.** *J. Clin. Invest.* 1996, **98**:70–77.

Hafler, D.A., Kent, S.C., Pietrusewicz, M.J., Khoury, S.J., Weiner, H.L., and Fukaura, H.: **Oral administration of myelin induces antigen-specific TGF-β 1 secreting T cells in patients with multiple sclerosis.** *Ann. N.Y. Acad. Sci.* 1997, **835**:120–131.

Herold, K.C., Burton, J.B., Francois, F., Poumian-Ruiz, E., Glandt, M., and Bluestone, J.A.: **Activation of human T cells by FcR nonbinding anti-CD3 mAb, hOKT3γ1(Ala-Ala).** *J. Clin. Invest.* 2003, **111**:409–418.

Herold, K.C., Hagopian, W., Auger, J.A., Poumian-Ruiz, E., Taylor, L., Donaldson, D., Gitelman, S.E., Harlan, D.M., Xu, D., Zivin, R.A., and Bluestone, J.A.: **Anti-CD3 monoclonal antibody in new-onset type 1 diabetes mellitus.** *N. Engl. J. Med.* 2002, **346**:1692–1698.

Masteller, E.L., and Bluestone, J.A.: **Immunotherapy of insulin-dependent diabetes mellitus.** *Curr. Opin. Immunol.* 2002, **14**:652–659.

O'Garra, A.: **Cytokines induce the development of functionally heterogeneous T helper cell subsets.** *Immunity* 1998, **8**:275–283.

Roncarolo, M.G., Bacchetta, R., Bordignon, C., Narula, S., and Levings, M.K.: **Type 1 T regulatory cells.** *Immunol. Rev.* 2001, **182**:68–79.

14-12 Controlled administration of antigen can be used to manipulate the nature of an antigen-specific response.

Diabetes Prevention Trial: Type 1 Diabetes Study Group: **Effects of insulin in relatives of patients with type 1 diabetes mellitus.** *N. Engl. J. Med.* 2002, **346**:1685–1691.

Fairchild, P.J.: **Altered peptide ligands: prospects for immune intervention in autoimmune disease.** *Eur. J. Immunogenet.* 1997, **24**:155–167.

Liblau, R., Tisch, R., Bercovici, N., and McDevitt, H.O.: **Systemic antigen in the treatment of T-cell-mediated autoimmune diseases.** *Immunol. Today* 1997, **18**:599–604.

Magee, C.C., and Sayegh, M.H.: **Peptide-mediated immunosuppression.** *Curr. Opin. Immunol.* 1997, **9**:669–675.

Weiner, H.L.: **Oral tolerance for the treatment of autoimmune diseases.** *Annu. Rev. Med.* 1997, **48**:341–351.

14-13 The development of transplantable tumors in mice led to the discovery that mice could mount a protective immune response against tumors.

Jaffee, E.M., and Pardoll, D.M.: **Murine tumor antigens: is it worth the search?** *Curr. Opin. Immunol.* 1996, **8**:622–627.

14-14 T lymphocytes can recognize specific antigens on human tumors.

Boon, T., Coulie, P.G., and Van den Eynde, B.: **Tumor antigens recognized by T cells.** *Immunol. Today* 1997, **18**:267–268.

Chaux, P., Vantomme, V., Stroobant, V., Thielemans, K., Corthals, J., Luiten, R., Eggermont, A.M., Boon, T., and van der Bruggen, P.: **Identification of MAGE-3 epitopes presented by HLA-DR molecules to CD4⁺ T lymphocytes.** *J. Exp. Med.* 1999, **189**:767–778.

Clark, R.E., Dodi, I.A., Hill, S.C., Lill, J.R., Aubert, G., Macintyre, A.R., Rojas, J., Bourdon, A., Bonner, P.L., Wang, L., Christmas, S.E., Travers, P.J., Creaser, C.S.,

Rees, R.C., and Madrigal, J.A.: **Direct evidence that leukemic cells present HLA-associated immunogenic peptides derived from the BCR-ABL b3a2 fusion protein.** *Blood* 2001, **98**:2887–2893.

de Smet, C., Lurquin, C., Lethe, B., Martelange, V., and Boon, T.: **DNA methylation is the primary silencing mechanism for a set of germ line- and tumor-specific genes with a CpG-rich promoter.** *Mol. Cell. Biol.* 1999, **19**:7327–7335.

Disis, M.L., and Cheever, M.A.: **HER-2/neu oncogenic protein: issues in vaccine development.** *Crit. Rev. Immunol.* 1998, **18**:37–45.

Disis, M.L., and Cheever, M.A.: **Oncogenic proteins as tumor antigens.** *Curr. Opin. Immunol.* 1996, **8**:637–642.

Michalek, J., Collins, R.H., Durrani, H.P., Vaclavkova, P., Ruff, L.E., Douek, D.C., and Vitetta, E.S.: **Definitive separation of graft-versus-leukemia- and graft-versus-host-specific CD4+ T cells by virtue of their receptor beta loci sequences.** *Proc. Natl. Acad. Sci. USA* 2003, **100**:1180–1184.

Robbins, P.F., and Kawakami, Y.: **Human tumor antigens recognized by T cells.** *Curr. Opin. Immunol.* 1996, **8**:628–636.

14-15 Tumors can escape rejection in many ways.

Bodmer, W.F., Browning, M.J., Krausa, P., Rowan, A., Bicknell, D.C., and Bodmer, J.G.: **Tumor escape from immune response by variation in HLA expression and other mechanisms.** *Ann N.Y. Acad. Sci.* 1993, **690**:42–49.

Girardi, M., Oppenheim, D.E., Steele, C.R., Lewis, J.M., Glusac, E., Filler, R., Hobby, P., Sutton, B., Tigelaar, R.E., and Hayday, A.C.: **Regulation of cutaneous malignancy by γδ T cells.** *Science* 2001, **294**:605–609.

Ikeda, H., Lethe, B., Lehmann, F., van Baren, N., Baurain, J.F., de Smet, C., Chambost, H., Vitale, M., Moretta, A., Boon, T., and Coulie, P.G.: **Characterization of an antigen that is recognized on a melanoma showing partial HLA loss by CTL expressing an NK inhibitory receptor.** *Immunity* 1997, **6**:199–208.

Koopman, L.A., Corver, W.E., van der Slik, A.R., Giphart, M.J., and Fleuren, G.J.: **Multiple genetic alterations cause frequent and heterogeneous human histocompatibility leukocyte antigen class I loss in cervical cancer.** *J. Exp. Med.* 2000, **191**:961–976.

Ochsenbein, A.F., Klenerman, P., Karrer, U., Ludewig, B., Pericin, M., Hengartner, H., and Zinkernagel, R.M.: **Immune surveillance against a solid tumor fails because of immunological ignorance.** *Proc. Natl. Acad. Sci. USA* 1999, **96**:2233–2238.

Ochsenbein, A.F., Sierro, S., Odermatt, B., Pericin, M., Karrer, U., Hermans, J., Hemmi, S., Hengartner, H., and Zinkernagel, R.M.: **Roles of tumour localization, second signals and cross priming in cytotoxic T-cell induction.** *Nature* 2001, **411**:1058–1064.

Pardoll, D.: **T cells and tumours.** *Nature* 2001, **411**:1010–1012.

Tada, T., Ohzeki, S., Utsumi, K., Takiuchi, H., Muramatsu, M., Li, X.F., Shimizu, J., Fujiwara, H., and Hamaoka, T.: **Transforming growth factor-β-induced inhibition of T cell function. Susceptibility difference in T cells of various phenotypes and functions and its relevance to immunosuppression in the tumor-bearing state.** *J. Immunol.* 1991, **146**:1077–1082.

Torre Amione, G., Beauchamp, R.D., Koeppen, H., Park, B.H., Schreiber, H., Moses, H.L., and Rowley, D.A.: **A highly immunogenic tumor transfected with a murine transforming growth factor type β1 cDNA escapes immune surveillance.** *Proc. Natl. Acad. Sci. USA* 1990, **87**:1486–1490.

14-16 Monoclonal antibodies against tumor antigens, alone or linked to toxins, can control tumor growth.

Bagshawe, K.D., Sharma, S.K., Burke, P.J., Melton, R.G., and Knox, R.J.: **Developments with targeted enzymes in cancer therapy.** *Curr. Opin. Immunol.* 1999, **11**:579–583.

Cragg, M.S., French, R.R., and Glennie, M.J.: **Signaling antibodies in cancer therapy.** *Curr. Opin. Immunol.* 1999, **11**:541–547.

Fan, Z., and Mendelsohn, J.: **Therapeutic application of anti-growth factor receptor antibodies.** *Curr. Opin. Oncol.* 1998, **10**:67–73.

Houghton, A.N., and Scheinberg, D.A.: **Monoclonal antibody therapies—a 'constant' threat to cancer.** *Nat. Med.* 2000, **6**:373–374.

Kreitman, R.J., Wilson, W.H., Bergeron, K., Raggio, M., Stetler-Stevenson, M., FitzGerald, D.J., and Pastan, I.: **Efficacy of the anti-CD22 recombinant immunotoxin BL22 in chemotherapy-resistant hairy-cell leukemia.** *N. Engl. J. Med.* 2001, **345**:241–247.

White, C.A., Weaver, R.L., and Grillo-Lopez, A.J.: **Antibody-targeted immunotherapy for treatment of malignancy.** *Annu. Rev. Med.* 2001, **52**:125–145.

14-17 Enhancing the immunogenicity of tumors holds promise for cancer therapy.

Bendandi, M., Gocke, C.D., Kobrin, C.B., Benko, F.A., Sternas, L.A., Pennington, R., Watson, T.M., Reynolds, C.W., Gause, B.L., Duffey, P.L., Jaffe, E.S., Creekmore, S.P., Longo, D.L., and Kwak, L.W.: **Complete molecular remissions induced by patient-specific vaccination plus granulocyte-monocyte colony-stimulating factor against lymphoma.** *Nat. Med.* 1999, **5**:1171–1177.

Hellstrom, K.E., Gladstone, P., and Hellstrom, I.: **Cancer vaccines: challenges and potential solutions.** *Mol. Med. Today* 1997, **3**:286–290.

Kugler, A., Stuhler, G., Walden, P., Zoller, G., Zobywalski, A., Brossart, P., Trefzer, U., Ullrich, S., Muller, C.A., Becker, V., Gross, A.J., Hemmerlein, B., Kanz, L., Muller, G.A., and Ringert, R.H.: **Regression of human metastatic renal cell carcinoma after vaccination with tumor cell-dendritic cell hybrids.** *Nat. Med.* 2000, **6**:332–336.

Li, Y., Hellstrom, K.E., Newby, S.A., and Chen, L.: **Costimulation by CD48 and B7–1 induces immunity against poorly immunogenic tumors.** *J. Exp. Med.* 1996, **183**:639–644.

Melief, C.J., Offringa, R., Toes, R.E., and Kast, W.M.: **Peptide-based cancer vaccines.** *Curr. Opin. Immunol.* 1996, **8**:651–657.

Nestle, F.O., Banchereau, J., and Hart, D.: **Dendritic cells: on the move from bench to bedside.** *Nat. Med.* 2001, **7**:761–765.

Pardoll, D.M.: **Cancer vaccines.** *Nat. Med.* 1998, **4**:525–531.

Pardoll, D.M.: **Paracrine cytokine adjuvants in cancer immunotherapy.** *Annu. Rev. Immunol.* 1995, **13**:399–415.

Przepiorka, D., and Srivastava, P.K.: **Heat shock protein–peptide complexes as immunotherapy for human cancer.** *Mol. Med. Today* 1998, **4**:478–484.

Ragnhammar, P.: **Anti-tumoral effect of GM-CSF with or without cytokines and monoclonal antibodies in solid tumors.** *Med. Oncol.* 1996, **13**:167–176.

Steinman, R.M., and Pope, M.: **Exploiting dendritic cells to improve vaccine efficacy.** *J. Clin. Invest.* 2002, **109**:1519–1526.

14-18 There are several requirements for an effective vaccine.

Ada, G.L.: **The immunological principles of vaccination.** *Lancet* 1990, **335**:523–526.

Anderson, R.M., Donnelly, C.A., and Gupta, S.: **Vaccine design, evaluation, and community-based use for antigenically variable infectious agents.** *Lancet* 1997, **350**:1466–1470.

Levine, M.M., and Levine, O.S.: **Influence of disease burden, public perception, and other factors on new vaccine development, implementation, and continued use.** *Lancet* 1997, **350**:1386–1392.

Nichol, K.L., Lind, A., Margolis, K.L., Murdoch, M., McFadden, R., Hauge, M., Magnan, S., and Drake, M.: **The effectiveness of vaccination against influenza in healthy, working adults.** *N. Engl. J. Med.* 1995, **333**:889–893.

Palese, P., and Garcia-Sastre, A.: **Influenza vaccines: present and future.** *J. Clin. Invest.* 2002, **110**:9–13.

Rabinovich, N.R., McInnes, P., Klein, D.L., and Hall, B.F.: **Vaccine technologies: view to the future.** *Science* 1994, **265**:1401–1404.

14-19 The history of vaccination against *Bordetella pertussis* illustrates the importance of developing an effective vaccine that is perceived to be safe.

Decker, M.D., and Edwards, K.M.: **Acellular pertussis vaccines.** *Pediatr. Clin. North Am.* 2000, **47**:309–335.

Madsen, K.M., Hviid, A., Vestergaard, M., Schendel, D., Wohlfahrt, J., Thorsen, P., Olsen, J., and Melbye, M.: **A population-based study of measles, mumps, and rubella vaccination and autism.** *N. Engl. J. Med.* 2002, **347**:1477–1482.

Mortimer, E.A.: Pertussis vaccines, in Plotkin, S.A., and Mortimer, E.A.: *Vaccines*, 2nd edn. Philadelphia, W.B. Saunders Co., 1994.

Poland, G.A.: **Acellular pertussis vaccines: new vaccines for an old disease.** *Lancet* 1996, **347**:209–210.

14-20 Conjugate vaccines have been developed as a result of understanding how T and B cells collaborate in an immune response.

van den Dobbelsteen, G.P., and van Rees, E.P.: **Mucosal immune responses to pneumococcal polysaccharides: implications for vaccination.** *Trends Microbiol.* 1995, **3**:155–159.

Kroll, J.S., and Booy, R.: *Haemophilus influenzae*: **capsule vaccine and capsulation genetics.** *Mol. Med. Today* 1996, **2**:160–165.

Peltola, H., Kilpi, T., and Anttila, M.: **Rapid disappearance of** *Haemophilus influenzae* **type b meningitis after routine childhood immunisation with conjugate vaccines.** *Lancet* 1992, **340**:592–594.

Rosenstein, N.E., and Perkins, B.A.: **Update on** *Haemophilus influenzae* **serotype b and meningococcal vaccines.** *Pediatr. Clin. N. Am.* 2000, **47**:337–352.

14-21 The use of adjuvants is another important approach to enhancing the immunogenicity of vaccines.

Alving, C.R., Koulchin, V., Glenn, G.M., and Rao, M.: **Liposomes as carriers of peptide antigens: induction of antibodies and cytotoxic T lymphocytes to conjugated and unconjugated peptides.** *Immunol. Rev.* 1995, **145**:5–31.

Gupta, R.K., and Siber, G.R.: **Adjuvants for human vaccines—current status, problems and future prospects.** *Vaccine* 1995, **13**:1263–1276.

Hartmann, G., Weiner, G.J., and Krieg, A.M.: **CpG DNA: a potent signal for growth, activation, and maturation of human dendritic cells.** *Proc. Natl. Acad. Sci. USA* 1999, **96**:9305–9310.

Kersten, G.F., and Crommelin, D.J.: **Liposomes and ISCOMs.** *Vaccine* 2003, **21**:915–920.

Persing, D.H., Coler, R.N., Lacy, M.J., Johnson, D.A., Baldridge, J.R., Hershberg, R.M., and Reed, S.G.: **Taking toll: lipid A mimetics as adjuvants and immunomodulators.** *Trends Microbiol.* 2002, **10**:S32–S37.

Scott, P., and Trinchieri, G.: **IL-12 as an adjuvant for cell-mediated immunity.** *Semin. Immunol.* 1997, **9**:285–291.

Takeda, K., Kaisho, T., and Akira, S.: **Toll-like receptors.** *Annu. Rev. Immunol.* 2003, **21**:335–376.

Vogel, F.R.: **Immunologic adjuvants for modern vaccine formulations.** *Ann. N.Y. Acad. Sci.* 1995, **754**:153–160.

14-22 Live-attenuated viral vaccines are usually more potent than 'killed' vaccines and can be made safer by using recombinant DNA technology.

Brochier, B., Kieny, M.P., Costy, F., Coppens, P., Bauduin, B., Lecocq, J.P., Languet, B., Chappuis, G., Desmettre, P., Afiademanyo, K., et al.: **Large-scale eradication of rabies using recombinant vaccinia–rabies vaccine.** *Nature* 1991, **354**:520–522.

Murphy, B.R., and Collins, P.L.: **Live-attenuated virus vaccines for respiratory syncytial and parainfluenza viruses: applications of reverse genetics.** *J. Clin. Invest.* 2002, **110**:21–27.

Parkin, N.T., Chiu, P., and Coelingh, K.: **Genetically engineered live attenuated influenza A virus vaccine candidates.** *J. Virol.* 1997, **71**:2772–2778.

14-23 Live-attenuated bacterial vaccines can be developed by selecting nonpathogenic or disabled mutants.

Guleria, I., Teitelbaum, R., McAdam, R.A., Kalpana, G., Jacobs, W.R., Jr., and Bloom, B.R.: **Auxotrophic vaccines for tuberculosis.** *Nat. Med.* 1996, **2**:334–337.

Hassan, J.O., and Curtiss, R., III.: **Effect of vaccination of hens with an aviru-**
lent strain of *Salmonella typhimurium* **on immunity of progeny challenged with wild-type** *Salmonella* **strains.** *Infect. Immun.* 1996, **64**:938–944.

Levine, M.M., Galen, J., Barry, E., Noriega, F., Tacket, C., Sztein, M., Chatfield, S., Dougan, G., Losonsky, G., and Kotloff, K.: **Attenuated** *Salmonella typhi* **and** *Shigella* **as live oral vaccines and as live vectors.** *Behring Inst. Mitt.* 1997, **98**:120–123.

14-24 Attenuated microorganisms can serve as vectors for vaccination against many pathogens.

Chatfield, S.N., Roberts, M., Dougan, G., Hormaeche, C., and Khan, C.M.: **The development of oral vaccines against parasitic diseases utilizing live attenuated** *Salmonella*. *Parasitology* 1995, **110 Suppl**:S17–S24.

Cirillo, J.D., Stover, C.K., Bloom, B.R., Jacobs, W.R., Jr., and Barletta, R.G.: **Bacterial vaccine vectors and bacillus Calmette–Guerin.** *Clin. Infect. Dis.* 1995, **20**:1001–1009.

Moss, B.: **Genetically engineered poxviruses for recombinant gene expression, vaccination, and safety.** *Proc. Natl. Acad. Sci. USA* 1996, **93**:11341–11348.

Paoletti, E.: **Applications of pox virus vectors to vaccination: an update.** *Proc. Natl. Acad. Sci. USA* 1996, **93**:11349–11353.

14-25 Synthetic peptides of protective antigens can elicit protective immunity.

Berzofsky, J.A.: **Mechanisms of T cell recognition with application to vaccine design.** *Mol. Immunol.* 1991, **28**:217–223.

Berzofsky, J.A.: **Epitope selection and design of synthetic vaccines. Molecular approaches to enhancing immunogenicity and cross-reactivity of engineered vaccines.** *Ann. N.Y. Acad. Sci.* 1993, **690**:256–264.

Davenport, M.P., and Hill, A.V.: **Reverse immunogenetics: from HLA-disease associations to vaccine candidates.** *Mol. Med. Today* 1996, **2**:38–45.

Hoffman, S.L., Rogers, W.O., Carucci, D.J., and Venter, J.C.: **From genomics to vaccines: malaria as a model system.** *Nat. Med.* 1998, **4**:1351–1353.

Modelska, A., Dietzschold, B., Sleysh, N., Fu, Z.F., Steplewski, K., Hooper, D.C., Koprowski, H., and Yusibov, V.: **Immunization against rabies with plant-derived antigen.** *Proc. Natl. Acad. Sci. USA* 1998, **95**:2481–2485.

14-26 The route of vaccination is an important determinant of success.

Burnette, W.N.: **Bacterial ADP-ribosylating toxins: form, function, and recombinant vaccine development.** *Behring Inst. Mitt.* 1997, **98**:434–441.

Douce, G., Fontana, M., Pizza, M., Rappuoli, R., and Dougan, G.: **Intranasal immunogenicity and adjuvanticity of site-directed mutant derivatives of cholera toxin.** *Infect. Immun.* 1997, **65**:2821–2828.

Dougan, G.: **The molecular basis for the virulence of bacterial pathogens: implications for oral vaccine development.** *Microbiology* 1994, **140**:215–224.

Dougan, G., Ghaem-Maghami, M., Pickard, D., Frankel, G., Douce, G., Clare, S., Dunstan, S., and Simmons, C.: **The immune responses to bacterial antigens encountered** *in vivo* **at mucosal surfaces.** *Phil. Trans. R. Soc. Lond. B* 2000, **355**:705–712.

Eriksson, K., and Holmgren, J.: **Recent advances in mucosal vaccines and adjuvants.** *Curr. Opin. Immunol.* 2002, **14**:666–672.

Ivanoff, B., Levine, M.M., and Lambert, P.H.: **Vaccination against typhoid fever: present status.** *Bull. World Health Org.* 1994, **72**:957–971.

Levine, M.M.: **Modern vaccines. Enteric infections.** *Lancet* 1990, **335**:958–961.

14-27 Protective immunity can be induced by injecting DNA encoding microbial antigens and human cytokines into muscle.

Donnelly, J.J., Ulmer, J.B., Shiver, J.W., and Liu, M.A.: **DNA vaccines.** *Annu. Rev. Immunol.* 1997, **15**:617–648.

Gurunathan, S., Klinman, D.M., and Seder, R.A.: **DNA vaccines: immunology, application, and optimization.** *Annu. Rev. Immunol.* 2000, **18**:927–974.

14-28 The effectiveness of a vaccine can be enhanced by targeting it to sites of antigen presentation.

Deliyannis, G., Boyle, J.S., Brady, J.L., Brown, L.E., and Lew, A.M.: **A fusion DNA vaccine that targets antigen-presenting cells increases protection from viral challenge.** *Proc. Natl. Acad. Sci. USA* 2000, **97**:6676–6680.

Hahn, H., Lane-Bell, P.M., Glasier, L.M., Nomellini, J.F., Bingle, W.H., Paranchych, W., and Smit, J.: **Pilin-based anti-Pseudomonas vaccines: latest developments and perspectives.** *Behring Inst. Mitt.* 1997, **98**:315–325.

Neutra, M.R.: **Current concepts in mucosal immunity. V. Role of M cells in transepithelial transport of antigens and pathogens to the mucosal immune system.** *Am. J. Physiol.* 1998, **274**:G785–G791.

Shen, Z., Reznikoff, G., Dranoff, G., and Rock, K.L.: **Cloned dendritic cells can present exogenous antigens on both MHC class I and class II molecules.** *J. Immunol.* 1997, **158**:2723–2730.

Tan, M.C., Mommaas, A.M., Drijfhout, J.W., Jordens, R., Onderwater, J.J., Verwoerd, D., Mulder, A.A., van der Heiden, A.N., Scheidegger, D., Oomen, L.C., et al.: **Mannose receptor-mediated uptake of antigens strongly enhances HLA class II-restricted antigen presentation by cultured dendritic cells.** *Eur. J. Immunol.* 1997, **27**:2426–2435.

Thomson, S.A., Burrows, S.R., Misko, I.S., Moss, D.J., Coupar, B.E., and Khanna, R.: **Targeting a polyepitope protein incorporating multiple class II-restricted viral epitopes to the secretory/endocytic pathway facilitates immune recognition by CD4+ cytotoxic T lymphocytes: a novel approach to vaccine design.** *J. Virol.* 1998, **72**:2246–2252.

14-29 An important question is whether vaccination can be used therapeutically to control existing chronic infections.

Burke, R.L.: **Contemporary approaches to vaccination against herpes simplex virus.** *Curr. Top. Microbiol. Immunol.* 1992, **179**:137–158.

Grange, J.M., and Stanford, J.L.: **Therapeutic vaccines.** *J. Med. Microbiol.* 1996, **45**:81–83.

Hill, A., Jugovic, P., York, I., Russ, G., Bennink, J., Yewdell, J., Ploegh, H., and Johnson, D.: **Herpes simplex virus turns off the TAP to evade host immunity.** *Nature* 1995, **375**:411–415.

Modlin, R.L.: **Th1–Th2 paradigm: insights from leprosy.** *J. Invest. Dermatol.* 1994, **102**:828–832.

Plebanski, M., Proudfoot, O., Pouniotis, D., Coppel, R.L., Apostolopoulos, V., and Flannery, G.: **Immunogenetics and the design of *Plasmodium falciparum* vaccines for use in malaria-endemic populations.** *J. Clin. Invest.* 2002, **110**:295–301.

Reiner, S.L., and Locksley, R.M.: **The regulation of immunity to *Leishmania major*.** *Annu. Rev. Immunol.* 1995, **13**:151–177.

Stanford, J.L.: **The history and future of vaccination and immunotherapy for leprosy.** *Trop. Geogr. Med.* 1994, **46**:93–107.

14-30 Modulation of the immune system might be used to inhibit immunopathological responses to infectious agents.

Biron, C.A., and Gazzinelli, R.T.: **Effects of IL-12 on immune responses to microbial infections: a key mediator in regulating disease outcome.** *Curr. Opin. Immunol.* 1995, **7**:485–496.

Grau, G.E., and Modlin, R.L.: **Immune mechanisms in bacterial and parasitic diseases: protective immunity versus pathology.** *Curr. Opin. Immunol.* 1991, **3**:480–485.

Kaplan, G.: **Recent advances in cytokine therapy in leprosy.** *J. Infect. Dis.* 1993, **167 Suppl 1**:S18–S22.

Locksley, R.M.: **Interleukin 12 in host defense against microbial pathogens.** *Proc. Natl. Acad. Sci. USA* 1993, **90**:5879–5880.

Murray, H.W.: **Interferon-γ and host antimicrobial defense: current and future clinical applications.** *Am. J. Med.* 1994, **97**:459–467.

Sher, A., Gazzinelli, R.T., Oswald, I.P., Clerici, M., Kullberg, M., Pearce, E.J., Berzofsky, J.A., Mosmann, T.R., James, S.L., and Morse, H.C.: **Role of T-cell derived cytokines in the downregulation of immune responses in parasitic and retroviral infection.** *Immunol. Rev.* 1992, **127**:183–204.

Sher, A., Jankovic, D., Cheever, A., and Wynn, T.: **An IL-12-based vaccine approach for preventing immunopathology in schistosomiasis.** *Ann. N.Y. Acad. Sci.* 1996, **795**:202–207.

PART VI

THE ORIGINS OF IMMUNE RESPONSES

Evolution of the Immune System

We began this book with an overview of immunology and its fascination for scientists throughout the 20th century. In this chapter we will reexamine the basic machinery of immunology in terms of how it has evolved over eons. We will start, as we started this book, with the innate immune system, some aspects of which are as old as the first multicellular organisms. We will then look at the fascinating question of the evolution of the adaptive immune system in vertebrates, of which much has been learned over the past few years, especially from the study of the mechanism of gene rearrangement.

In its present state, the immune system of mammals is a coherent system of interacting cells and molecules, but this state has been pieced together like a jigsaw, with individual pieces being coopted from different physiological functions and shaped by evolutionary pressures to fit relatively seamlessly together. The problem with evolutionary studies is that the direct ancestors of the animals alive today are no longer available to study, and thus it is never possible to say exactly what molecules or what immunological functions were present in these organisms. However, this does not mean that we can know nothing of the evolutionary past, and in this chapter we will make use of the fact that the distribution of the individual components of the immune system in different species can shed light on its overall evolutionary history.

An evolutionary 'tree' showing the organisms discussed in this chapter, and the order in which the different lineages diverged, is shown in Fig. 15.1. Thus, the divergence of plants from their common ancestor with animals occurred earlier than the divergence of the insect lineage from that leading to the deuterostomes (echinoderms and chordates). When studying the evolution of a particular system such as the immune system, the underlying assumption that we make in this is that if a gene is found in the same (or similar) form in two different species, then that gene must also be present in the common ancestor of those species. The more widely diverged the species, the more distant is the common ancestor. Thus, we are able to trace the evolution of host-defense mechanisms from our more ancient ancestors, such as those we have in common with insects, through our common ancestor with echinoderms and eventually to our common ancestor with the urochordate ascidians (the

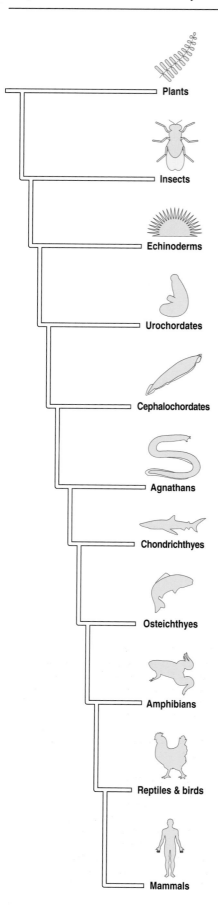

Plants

Insects

Echinoderms

Urochordates

Cephalochordates

Agnathans

Chondrichthyes

Osteichthyes

Amphibians

Reptiles & birds

Mammals

Fig. 15.1 The evolutionary history of the organisms mentioned in this chapter. The branching of the schematic evolutionary 'tree' represents the order of divergence of the different lineages, so that the lineage of plants diverged from its last common ancestor with animals before the separation of the insect lineage, and so on. Note that the tree does not show the relative times involved.

tunicates or sea squirts), a sister group of the lineage that leads to the vertebrates. Within the vertebrates, we can trace the development of immune functions from the jawless fishes (lampreys and hagfishes), through the cartilaginous fish (sharks, skates, and rays) to the bony fish, then to the amphibians, to reptiles and birds, and finally to mammals. In some cases we do not yet know whether a particular immune-system gene is present in all the 'intermediate' groups. However, if it is present in, for example, mammals and invertebrates, then we would assume that it is also present (or was at one time) in all vertebrate lineages. It is not quite as straightforward to draw the opposite conclusion—that a gene absent from one species must therefore not be present in the common ancestor—because it is possible for genes and functions to be lost in individual lineages.

It seems likely that the concept of an immune system—the defense of the individual against infectious agents—is ubiquitous, because all organisms are attacked by pathogens, and natural selection will always provide a pressure to develop protection against those pathogens. Thus, even bacteria have some protection against the parasites (plasmids) and pathogens (bacteriophages) that may infect them: these are the restriction enzymes that cleave incoming DNA and the modification systems that modify the bacterium's own DNA so that the enzymes cannot cleave it. It is unlikely, however, that such systems have any direct counterparts in the immune systems of higher organisms. But bacteria also produce antimicrobial peptides that are active against competing bacteria, and this type of host defense does have a counterpart in multicellular organisms. Nevertheless, when evaluating similarities between organisms, one always has to keep in mind the possibility that they may represent convergent evolution—the independent evolution of similar solutions to the same problem. The antimicrobial peptides of higher organisms might therefore represent independent evolution of the same function, rather than direct evolution from a common ancestral peptide in bacteria.

To avoid such problems we will concern ourselves here only with the evolution of an immune system in multicellular organisms that have a defined body that can be invaded and colonized by pathogens. We shall also not consider the specialized forms of host defense that have arisen in individual species or groups of species, but will confine ourselves to trying to trace the roots of the mammalian immune system.

The most ancient immune defenses lie within the innate immune system. The history of the immune system is one of a stepwise diversification by the addition of new recognition systems and effector pathways, punctuated by the sudden explosion of new functions that was marked by the acquisition of somatic gene rearrangement and the capacity to produce clones of cells bearing receptors for different antigens. The advent of somatic rearrangement marked the origin of the adaptive immune system, and although the precise nature of the molecular recognition system into which this capacity was introduced is unknown, we can speculate about what it might have been. In time, advances in sequencing the genomes of the evolutionarily 'intermediate' organisms and a better understanding of their biology will reveal the various evolutionary strands that intersected to create the immune system of present-day mammals.

Evolution of the innate immune system.

An innate immune system is well developed in the fruitfly *Drosophila melanogaster*, a favorite model organism for many aspects of biological research, and in many other invertebrates. What *Drosophila* shares with vertebrates are invariant cell-surface receptors—the so-called pattern-recognition receptors—that recognize common molecular patterns of pathogens, and intracellular signaling pathways leading from these receptors to the activation of the transcription factor NFκB (see Chapters 2 and 6). Many multicellular animal species have a cassette of genes that encode the proteins of this pathway. This suggests that the activation of NFκB is the original and central signaling pathway of activation in innate immunity, leading in turn to the activation of a set of genes that depend on NFκB for their transcription. This is an almost universal pathway that leads to the activation of many different host-defense systems.

15-1 Antimicrobial peptides are likely to be the most ancient immune defenses.

One form of host defense, found in both plants and animals and therefore predating the separation of the plant and animal lineages, is the production of antimicrobial peptides. There are many different antimicrobial peptides, with a great variety of physical and chemical characteristics and a variety of effects on different microbial pathogens. One broadly distributed class of antimicrobial peptides are the small peptides known as defensins (see Section 2-2). Although the precise structures of defensins are different in mammals and in insects and plants (Fig. 15.2) it is clear that they are all structurally related and derive from the same ancestral system of host defense. The defensins themselves are thought to act by disrupting the cell membranes of bacteria and fungi, and the membrane envelope of some viruses, although some may be able to cross microbial cell membranes and enter the cell.

Most multicellular organisms make many different defensins—the plant *Arabidopsis thaliana* produces 13, *Drosophila* at least 15, and in humans a single gut cell can make as many as 21 different defensins. The various defensins have distinct activities, some being active against Gram-positive bacteria and some against Gram-negative bacteria, whereas others are specific for fungal pathogens. All these organisms make other types of antimicrobial peptide in addition to defensins.

Fig. 15.2 The antimicrobial defensins of plants, insects, and mammals are structurally related. The structures of the plant defensin AFP-1 from the radish *Raphanus sativus* (left panel), the insect antimicrobial peptide drosomycin (center panel) from *Drosophila*, and the human β_2-defensin (right panel) are shown. The colors indicate the nature of the peptide structure, with the α helices shown in purple and the β strands in yellow. Unstructured regions are shown in cyan; turns are shown in white. All three defensins have a similar structure, with a short segment of α helix resting against two or three strands of antiparallel β sheet, which has been conserved since the divergence of the plant and animal kingdoms.

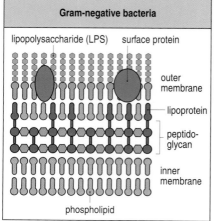

Fig. 15.3 The organization of the cell walls of Gram-positive and Gram-negative bacteria. Gram-positive bacteria, as shown in the upper panel, have a cell wall composed of an outer layer of a repeating matrix of peptidoglycan molecules in which repeating *N*-acetylglucosamine (light blue hexagons) and *N*-acetylmuramic acid (purple hexagons) are cross-linked by peptide bridges into a dense three-dimensional network. Bacterial surface proteins and other molecules, such as teichoic acid, are embedded within this peptidoglycan layer, and lipoteichoic acids link the peptidoglycan layer to the bacterial cell membrane itself. The cell wall of Gram-negative bacteria is composed of two lipid membranes, between which a thin matrix of peptidoglycan is sandwiched. The outer membrane contains lipopolysaccharide (LPS), and in this layer the outer-membrane proteins are also embedded.

The production of antimicrobial peptides in the plant and animal kingdoms suggests that this means of defense must have evolved before the plant and animal lineages diverged. The common precursor of plants and animals is likely to have been a single-celled organism. Many of the other lineages that diverged around that time are single-celled eukaryotic organisms known generally as protists (some of which, such as the parasitic protozoa, cause human disease today; see Fig. 10.3).Whether antimicrobial peptides exist in extant protists is not known, nor is it clear whether such peptides would necessarily have a protective function in these organisms. Many free-living protists regard bacteria as a source of food rather than a threat to their well-being.

However, when we consider the behavior of phagocytic cells in multicellular organisms, such as macrophages in vertebrates, it is not unreasonable to speculate that at least some aspects of innate immunity evolved from the phagocytic feeding mechanisms of single-celled eukaryotes. All vertebrates, and many invertebrates, have phagocytic cells that patrol their blood vessels and tissues, as described in Chapter 2, and that have much in common with protists such as amoebae. It is possible that phagocytic cells in animals could have derived from a population of cells that retained an ancestral, unicellular morphology and behavior.

15-2 Toll-like receptors may represent the most primitive pathogen-recognition system.

If antimicrobial peptides are thought to be the earliest form of defense against infection, then receptors that recognize pathogens and induce the production of antimicrobial peptides have a good claim to be among the first receptors dedicated to host defense. Such receptors have been discovered, and seem also to be conserved over a long evolutionary period. The Toll receptor, first discovered in the fruitfly *Drosophila*, induces the expression of several host defenses, including antimicrobial peptides, primarily those acting against Gram-positive bacteria and fungal pathogens.

The Toll receptor gene was first identified as a gene that acted during *Drosophila* embryonic development to specify correct dorso-ventral patterning. Only later was the function of the Toll receptor in host defense in the adult insect recognized with the observation that mutations in Toll or in the signaling molecules downstream of Toll affected the production of the antimicrobial peptide drosomycin, and the consequent susceptibility of *Drosophila* to fungal infections. Later, homologs of Toll were found in other species, ranging from plants to mammals, in which they are associated with resistance to viral, bacterial, and fungal infection. In plants, as in insects, they are involved in the production of antimicrobial peptides, indicating their ancient association with this means of host defense. They have acquired additional functions in vertebrates (see Chapter 2), but because of their apparently ancient origin they are good candidates for at least one type of primordial pathogen receptor.

We now know that the mouse has more than 10 Toll-like receptors, each seemingly involved in a variety of host defense functions (see Chapter 2). The first one isolated, now known as Toll-like receptor-4 (TLR-4), is required for mice to make an early response to bacterial lipopolysaccharide (LPS), a component of the cell surface of Gram-negative bacteria (Fig. 15.3). Mice lacking TLR-4 are consequently exceptionally susceptible to infection with Gram-negative bacteria. Like mice, humans have at least 10 functional Toll-like receptors. They recognize components of pathogens such as bacterial, yeast, and fungal cell walls, bacterial flagella, viral RNA, and bacterial DNA (see Fig. 2.12).

The signaling pathway through the Toll receptor also seems to be conserved between widely different species, and there is a good correspondence between its components in *Drosophila* and mammals, as shown in Fig. 15.4. The end result of the pathway in *Drosophila* is the activation of transcription factors of the Rel family (homologs of the mammalian NFκB transcription factors), which then translocate to the nucleus to induce new gene transcription. In *Drosophila* the transcription factors of the Rel family involved in the induction of antimicrobial peptides seem to be the dorsal-related immunity factor (DIF) and, to a smaller extent, the Dorsal transcription factor. A third member of the Rel family, Relish, also induces the transcription of antimicrobial peptides but in response to a different signaling pathway, which we will describe later.

One significant difference between the recognition of pathogens by Toll receptors in *Drosophila* and mammals is that most of the mammalian receptors seem to be capable of directly recognizing pathogen products. *Drosophila* Toll does not, instead binding a cleaved version of a self protein, spätzle. The exact sequence of events that leads to the cleavage of spätzle during *Drosophila* immune responses is not known, as the best-described activation pathway operates during embryogenesis but has no role in the host-defense functions of Toll. The immune-response pathway seems to involve specific pattern-recognition molecules that interact with serine proteases to initiate the cleavage of spätzle. One such molecule has been identified, a peptidoglycan-binding protein encoded by a gene known as *semmelweis* (in honor of **Ignaz Semmelweis**, a pioneer of the prevention of infection in hospitals). The protein is a member of a protein family that binds peptidoglycans, components of bacterial cell walls. *Drosophila* has some 13 genes encoding members of this family of peptidoglycan-recognition proteins (PGRPs). The protein encoded by *semmelweis*, PGRP-SA, is involved in the recognition of Gram-positive bacteria, but not of fungi. A second family of *Drosophila* proteins, the Gram-negative binding proteins (GNBPs), which recognize β-1–3-linked glucans, also has a function in the recognition of Gram-positive bacteria similar to that of PGRP-SA, interacting with serine proteases to activate the Toll pathway. The serine protease of the Gram-positive bacterial recognition pathway has not yet been identified, but a serine protease involved in the recognition of fungal infections in *Drosophila* has. This protease, called Persephone, has similarities to the proteases of the clotting pathway of both insect hemolymph and mammalian blood. There is, presumably, an as-yet unidentified fungal-specific pattern-recognition molecule analogous to PGRP-SA that will activate Persephone.

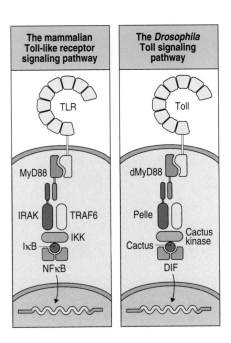

Fig. 15.4 A comparison of the *Drosophila* and mammalian Toll signaling pathways. The components of the mammalian Toll-like receptor signaling pathway that culminates in the activation of NFκB have direct parallels in the components of the signaling pathway from the Toll receptor of *Drosophila*. The intracellular domain of the Toll-like receptors interacts with a homologous domain in the adaptor protein MyD88. A similar interaction occurs between the intracellular domain of Toll and dMyD88. The next step in both signaling pathways occurs via the interaction of death domains, between MyD88 and IRAK in the mammalian cells and between dMyD88 and Pelle in *Drosophila*. Both IRAK and Pelle are serine kinases. At this point the mammalian signaling pathway passes through an adaptor, TRAF6, which is activated by IRAK and in turn activates IKK. IKK phosphorylates the inhibitor of NFκB, IκB, targeting it for degradation and releasing the active dimeric transcription factor, NFκB. In *Drosophila*, homologs of MyD88, TRAF6, and of a kinase homologous to IKK that phosphorylates the *Drosophila* IκB homolog Cactus are found. Moreover, the terminal parts of the pathway are also homologous between *Drosophila* and mammals; phosphorylation of Cactus initiates its degradation and the release of the DIF dimer, which is a transcription factor and a homolog of NFκB.

Of the mammalian Toll-like receptors, the one whose mode of recognition most closely resembles that of *Drosophila* Toll may be TLR-4, which rather than binding the bacterial ligand LPS directly, instead binds it indirectly through a soluble LPS-binding protein, which in turn binds TLR-4. A more relevant functional parallel, however, might be with the complement system, in which the proteolytic activation of a series of proteases generates ligands for cell-surface receptors; in the case of complement, these receptors are involved in stimulating phagocytosis (see Chapter 2).

15-3   A second recognition system in *Drosophila* homologous to the mammalian tumor necrosis factor receptor pathway provides protection from Gram-negative bacteria.

In mammals, the Toll-like receptors recognize a variety of pathogens including Gram-positive and Gram-negative bacteria as well as fungi. In *Drosophila*, the Toll receptor does not seem to be involved in the recognition of Gram-negative bacteria (see Fig. 15.3). Instead, a second pathway, the more recently discovered Imd (immunodeficiency) pathway, is used. Two receptors that recognize Gram-negative bacteria have recently been identified in *Drosophila*, and both are members of the PGRP family. One is PGRP-LC, which is associated with the cell membrane; the other, PGRP-LE, is secreted. Some of the steps in the signaling pathway from these receptors have been determined through the analysis of mutants of *Drosophila* that are susceptible to infections with Gram-negative, but not Gram-positive, bacteria. The Imd pathway is shown in Fig. 15.5 and is strikingly similar to at least part of the mammalian tumor necrosis factor (TNF) receptor pathway. The Imd protein itself is homologous to the TNF receptor binding protein RIP, whereas another component, DREDD, is a caspase homologous to the mammalian caspase-8. The end result of the Imd pathway is the activation of the transcription factor Relish, another member of the Rel family. Relish activates the expression of several immune-response genes, some of which encode the antimicrobial peptides diptericin, attacin, and cecropin; these are distinct from the peptides induced by Toll signaling. Thus, the Toll and Imd pathways activate equivalent effector mechanisms to eliminate infections. It is likely that these two distinct signaling pathways have arisen by the duplication of a more ancient common pathway of host defense, but it is impossible to say whether that pathway resembled the Toll or the Imd pathway. In mammals, however, it seems that the host-defense functions of the Imd pathway have been taken over by mammalian Toll pathway equivalents.

The *Drosophila* Imd pathway detects Gram-negative bacteria through a pathway analogous to mammalian TNF receptor pathway

Fig. 15.5 *Drosophila* detects Gram-negative bacteria through the Imd signaling receptor pathway, which is analogous to the mammalian TNF receptor pathway. The TNF receptor transduces signals that lead either to new gene expression or to cell death. In the mammalian TNFR-I pathway, ligand binding to the receptor leads to the recruitment of the adaptors TRADD (TNF receptor-associated death-domain protein), which in turn recruits FADD (Fas-associated death-domain protein), RIP (receptor-interacting protein), and TRAF2 (TNF receptor-associated factor 2). Each of these initiates different signaling pathways. FADD activates caspase-8, initiating a protease cascade that leads to apoptosis, whereas RIP binds and, through a separate kinase, MEKK3, activates the Iκ kinase IKK, leading ultimately to the activation of NFκB and the induction of new gene expression. TRAF2 also activates a kinase cascade, leading to the activation of the Jun transcription factor and the induction of new gene expression. The Imd pathway seems to be a *Drosophila* homolog of the TNFR pathway and leads to the same outcomes. Imd itself is a homolog of RIP, whereas DmFADD is a homolog of FADD, and DREDD is a homolog of caspase-8. In this pathway, dTAK1 may be the homolog of MEKK3, activating the Iκ kinase and resulting in the activation of Relish and the induction of several immune-related genes, including those for defensins.

15-4 An ancestral complement system opsonizes pathogens for uptake by phagocytic cells.

Another ancient means of host defense is represented by the complement system (see Chapter 2). The most primitive function of complement is likely to have been opsonization, a means of increasing the efficiency of uptake of pathogens by the scavenger phagocytes that survey animal body spaces for the presence of infection. Even before complement components were discovered in invertebrates, it had been suggested that a primitive complement system would contain a minimum of three components. The central component would be C3, which would be activated spontaneously, as it is in the alternative pathway of complement activation in mammals today (see Section 2-14). Activated C3 would bind the equivalent of factor B, forming a C3 convertase that would amplify the original signal by cleaving and activating many more molecules of C3 (see Section 2-15). The third component of this system would be a C3 receptor expressed by phagocytes and capable of activating phagocytosis of the C3-coated pathogens.

This prediction has been borne out with the discovery of complement components in invertebrates, as shown in Fig. 15.6. A homolog of C3 has been found in echinoderms: it is produced by amoeboid coelomocytes, phagocytic cells in the echinoderm coelomic fluid, and its expression is increased when bacteria are present. A homolog of factor B has also been identified in echinoderms. In mammals, factor B is activated by another protease—factor D—and, although no equivalent of factor D has yet been identified in echinoderms, the site at which factor D cleaves is conserved in echinoderm factor B. Thus, the echinoderms seem to possess the components of the amplification loop of the alternative pathway of complement activation, in which spontaneously activated C3 binds factor B, which is then cleaved by factor D to create an active C3 convertase, which cleaves more C3. As far as the function of the cleaved C3 is concerned, although no echinoderm C3 receptor has yet been identified, it is known that cells coated with C3 are taken up more efficiently than uncoated cells by echinoderm phagocytes, and so it seems that a functional, opsonizing complement system equivalent to the predicted ancestral system does exist in these invertebrates.

The spontaneous activation of C3 and its amplification by factor B poses the same problem for the echinoderms as it does in mammals (see Section 2-19): how might such a system be regulated to prevent autoimmunity? How this is achieved in echinoderms is not known, although there is indirect evidence for the presence of a 'factor I' that can inactivate C3, and it is possible that the relevant genes and their complement regulatory products are present but have not yet been identified. The factor I cleavage site is conserved in echinoderm C3, and fragments of C3 consistent with cleavage at that site can be found in the coelomic fluid. However, in echinoderms the C3 and factor B proteins are produced by the phagocytic cells themselves (see Fig. 15.6), and it is possible that they are secreted directly onto the surface of microbes, much as mammalian T cells secrete their effector molecules directly into the interface between the T cell and its target. In such a case there would be less need for regulatory proteins that prevent complement from attacking the organism's own cells.

With the emergence of the chordates, the main components of the complement system seem to be well established. In the urochordate *Ciona*, for which the complete genome sequence has been determined, homologs of C3 and factor B have been identified, as well as several genes homologous to integrins, which could encode complement receptors. In another urochordate, *Halocynthia*, an integrin family CR3-like receptor is known to have a function in C3-mediated phagocytosis.

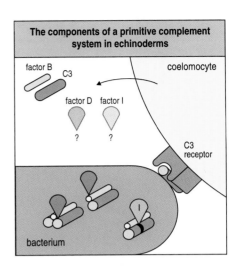

The components of a primitive complement system in echinoderms

Fig. 15.6 The components of a simple complement system are present in echinoderms. The complement system of echinoderms resembles the alternative pathway of complement activation in mammals. Echinoderms possess equivalents of the complement components C3 and factor B, which are produced by coelomocytes, and are also thought to possess equivalents of factor D and the complement regulatory protein factor I. In this system, spontaneously activated C3 would bind to pathogen surfaces, where it would in turn bind factor B. Cleavage of factor B by a proteinase in the coelomic fluid, an as-yet unidentified equivalent of factor D, would create the C3 convertase C3bBb, which can cleave and activate many more molecules of C3. As echinoderm coelomocytes are phagocytes that will readily take up cells coated with C3, it is thought that they must express a C3 receptor. Finally, the C3 convertase is inactivated by another unidentified humoral proteinase, thought to be the equivalent of factor I.

The characteristic marker of many mammalian complement regulatory proteins is a small domain called a short consensus repeat (SCR) or complement control protein (CCP) repeat (see Section 2-19). Several genes encoding proteins bearing such SCR domains have been identified in the *Ciona* genome, and it is expected that some of these will have complement regulatory functions.

It is not known how ancient this opsonizing complement system is. C3 homologs have been found in invertebrates more distantly related to vertebrates than are echinoderms or urochordates, notably horseshoe crabs and *Drosophila*, but their function has not been defined. C3, which is cleaved and activated by serine proteases, is clearly evolutionarily related to, and seems to have been duplicated from, the serine protease inhibitor α_2-macroglobulin. In *Drosophila* there seem to be at least four C3 homologs containing the thioester linkage characteristic of this family of proteins (see Section 2-13); this linkage allows the activated protein to bind to pathogen surfaces. These molecules are known as thioester-containing proteins (TEPs).

The TEPs are thought to have some immune function in *Drosophila*, because the expression of at least three of them increases when *Drosophila* is infected with bacteria. *Drosophila* has phagocytic cells but there is as yet no evidence to suggest that there is any opsonizing activity in the hemolymph, the *Drosophila* equivalent of blood. Moreover, the TEPs are synthesized by the *Drosophila* fat body, the equivalent of the mammalian liver, rather than by phagocytic cells themselves, as is the case for the echinoderm C3 homolog. Thus, although the *Drosophila* TEPs are clearly evolutionarily related to C3 they might have some quite different role. A different picture is revealed in a second insect, the *Anopheles* mosquito, in which a TEP protein, aTEP-1, has been identified. aTEP-1 is produced by hemocytes (phagocytic cells in the hemolymph) and is induced in response to infection. There is also direct evidence of binding of aTEP-1 to bacterial surfaces, and of the involvement of TEP molecules in the phagocytosis of Gram-negative bacteria. The origin of the complement system might therefore predate the ancient separation of the Bilateria (multicellular animals other than the sponges and the coelenterates) into the protostomes, which include the insects, and the deuterostomes, which include the echinoderms and chordates (and thus the vertebrates).

15-5   The lectin pathway of complement activation evolved in invertebrates.

After its initial appearance, the complement system seems to have evolved by the acquisition of new activation pathways, allowing microbial surfaces to be specifically targeted. The first of these new complement-activating systems to appear was the ficolin pathway, which is present both in vertebrates and in some 'higher' invertebrates, such as the urochordates. Ficolins are related to the collectins (see Section 2-12), the family to which the vertebrate mannose-binding lectin (MBL) belongs. Like the collectins, the ficolins have a collagen-like domain and a carbohydrate-binding domain and form a similar 'bunch of tulips' multimeric structure. However, the carbohydrate-binding domain of ficolins is not related to C-type lectins, as in MBL, but is similar to fibrinogen. The ficolin carbohydrate-binding domain is able to bind *N*-acetylglucosamine, as does MBL, although the latter is also able to bind mannose-containing carbohydrates, which the ficolins do not recognize. Evolutionarily, the ficolins seem to predate the collectins, which are first seen in the chordates and have been identified in *Ciona*. Both MBL and homologs of the classical pathway complement component C1q, another collectin, have been identified in the *Ciona* genome. This suggests that in the evolution of the antibody-mediated classical pathway of complement activation (see

Section 2-11) the ancestral immunoglobulin molecule, which does not appear until much later in evolution, took advantage of an already diversified family of collectins rather than driving the diversification of C1q from an MBL-like ancestor.

The activation of complement by ficolins and collectins is mediated through serine proteases called MASPs—MBL-associated serine proteases—which are able to cleave and activate C2, C4, and C3. In vertebrates, two different MASPs—MASP1 and MASP2—are associated with the ficolins and collectins, and this seems also to be true of the invertebrate ficolins. Two distinct invertebrate homologs of mammalian MASPs have been identified in the same ascidian species from which the ficolins were identified. The specificity of the invertebrate MASPs has not been determined, but it seems likely that they are able to cleave and activate C3. This invertebrate ficolin complement system, illustrated in Fig. 15.7, is functionally identical to the ficolin and MBL-mediated pathways found in mammals. Thus, the minimal complement system of the echinoderms has been supplemented in the urochordates by the recruitment of a specific activation system that can target the deposition of C3 onto microbial surfaces. The complement activation system evolved further by diversification of a C1q-like collectin and its associated MASPs to become the initiating components (C1q, C1r, and C1s) of the classical complement pathway. This could occur only after the evolution of the specific antigen-recognition molecules of the adaptive immune system, and it is to those that we now turn.

Summary.

The innate immune system exists to provide early defense against pathogen attack and to alert the adaptive immune system to the fact that a pathogen invasion has begun. This dual function seems to operate through a very ancient signaling pathway, the Toll pathway, that long predates the adaptive immune system, and is present in invertebrates as well as in vertebrates. The first defense molecules in evolutionary terms were probably antimicrobial peptides, which are produced by both plants and animals. Another component of innate immunity in animals, the phagocytic cells that scavenge incoming pathogens, could have had their origins in unicellular amoeba-like eukaryotes. The complement system also predates the vertebrates, being found in echinoderms and urochordates.

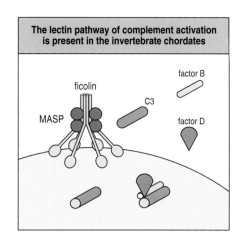

The lectin pathway of complement activation is present in the invertebrate chordates

Fig. 15.7 A lectin pathway of complement activation is present in invertebrate chordates. A lectin-mediated pathway of complement activation has been defined in a urochordate ascidian. Ficolin, which uses a fibrinogen-like domain rather than a C-type lectin domain to bind carbohydrate ligands on a pathogen surface, is associated with serine proteases homologous to the MBL-associated serine proteases, MASP1 and MASP2. Binding of ficolin to a cell surface allows the MASPs to cleave and activate C3. Activated C3b binds to the pathogen and initiates an amplification loop, in which the bound C3b binds factor B, allowing it to be cleaved by factor D to create a C3 convertase, C3bBb, which cleaves C3 to produce more C3b.

Evolution of the adaptive immune response.

The evolution of adaptive immunity is a fascinating problem in immunology. For a long time the origin of adaptive immunity was obscure, partly because it seemed to emerge suddenly as a complete biological system at roughly the same time as the vertebrates. The picture is now becoming clearer, particularly as molecular methods are applied to a wider range of species. As we will see in this part of the chapter, the evolution of adaptive immunity seems to have been made possible by the invasion of a putative immunoglobulin-like gene by a transposable genetic element. This conferred on the ancestral immunoglobulin gene the ability to undergo somatic gene rearrangement, and thus to generate diversity. When a mobile DNA element excises itself from a piece of DNA, alterations in the original sequence are introduced in the 'host' DNA when the cut ends are rejoined; this is the origin of the diversity of antigen receptors in the adaptive immune system.

There are, however, many unanswered questions, and probably many others that have not yet been thought of. The first key question is: what was the nature of the gene that was invaded? It must have resembled a member of the immunoglobulin gene superfamily, and may have already been functioning as some type of antigen receptor, which would have enabled it to operate appropriately in its changed form. This should help to narrow the search considerably.

A second question is: what was the function of the cell type in which this immunoglobulin ancestor was expressed, and which could make good use of this new ability to generate a diversity of antigen-recognition molecules? It may have already been something like a lymphocyte, but it could equally have been a phagocytic cell like a macrophage or a polymorphonuclear leukocyte that then lost the capacity to phagocytose as it evolved new functions made possible by the expression of a variable antigen receptor. The answer is that we really do not know. It might even have resembled a primitive NK cell, in which an invariant immunoglobulin superfamily receptor was already involved in the recognition of a primordial MHC-like molecule. Or perhaps it was some quite different cell type that no longer exists in vertebrates.

15-6   Adaptive immunity appeared abruptly in the cartilaginous fish.

It has been known for at least 50 years that all jawed fish can mount an adaptive immune response. In contrast, hagfish and lampreys, which are jawless vertebrates, lack all signs of an adaptive immune system: they do not have organized lymphoid tissue, they lack primary immune responses, and, most importantly, they do not exhibit immunological memory. By contrast, even the cartilaginous fish, the earliest group of jawed fishes to survive to the present day, have organized lymphoid tissue, T-cell receptors and immunoglobulins, and the ability to mount adaptive immune responses.

In jawed fish and all 'higher' vertebrates, adaptive immunity is possible because of a specific event that occurred in some ancestor of the jawed fish in which a transposon carrying the ancestral *RAG* recombinases inserted itself into a stretch of DNA, presumably into a gene that was similar to an immunoglobulin gene or a T-cell receptor gene V region. Both prokaryotic and eukaryotic genomes contain mobile DNA elements known generally as transposable elements, which can move themselves, or copies of themselves, to different positions on the chromosomes. Transposons contain two essential elements—a sequence encoding an enzyme, called a transposase, which is a DNA recombinase that is able to cut double-stranded DNA to insert and excise the element, and terminal repeat sequences that are recognized by the transposase and are required for the element to be able to undergo excision and insertion (Fig. 15.8).

A key feature of transposition is that both the insertion and excision processes cause changes to the 'host' target DNA. Insertion of a transposon leads to the formation of short additional sequences at each end of the integrated element; the excision process leaves these sequences in the DNA and also makes a gap in the host DNA that is repaired by the cell's error-prone DNA repair mechanisms. In the original transposon, the transposase is thought to have been the ancestral *RAG* recombinase. After the original integration event, it seems that the transposon sequences encoding the recombinase became separated from the recognition sequences for the enzyme. This could have occurred most simply by the deletion of the transposase genes from the transposon integrated into the primordial immune-receptor gene, while another copy of the transposon elsewhere in the genome retained the transposase genes but lost the associated terminal repeats. The terminal repeats left in the immune-receptor gene became the recombination signal

| Transposons encode enzymes—transposases—that allow them to move and integrate sequences recognized by the transposase | The transposase cleaves host DNA and inserts the transposon. | During the evolution of the immunoglobulin and TCR loci, rearrangement of the integrated transposon has separated the integration sites from the transposase genes |

Fig. 15.8 The integration of a transposable element into a receptor gene ultimately gave rise to the immunoglobulin and T-cell receptor genes and their capacity for somatic recombination. Transposons are specialized DNA sequences that can move around the genome by excising themselves from one site and inserting into another. A transposable element must contain two functional elements, the first being sequences encoding a transposase, the enzyme that mediates the excision and integration of the transposon in the genome. The second is specific recognition sequences for the transposase, which are present at each end of the transposon and are required for the transposon to excise from or integrate into DNA (left panel). After excising from DNA (not shown) the transposon reinserts elsewhere: the transposase cleaves genomic DNA at a random site, and then joins the free ends of the transposon to the cut ends of the genomic DNA (center panel). A transposon excises by the reverse of this process, the transposase bringing the terminal sequences together and then cutting the transposon out of the genomic DNA. In the evolution of the immunoglobulin and T-cell receptor (TCR) genes, an initial integration event into the middle of a cell-surface receptor has been followed by DNA rearrangements that separated the transposase genes, which we now know as the *RAG-1* and *RAG-2* genes, from the transposon terminal sequences, which we now term the recombination signal sequences, or RSSs (right panel). However, the enzymes retain their ancestral function and the *RAG* gene products have been shown to be able to catalyze the insertion of RSS-containing fragments of DNA into another piece of DNA.

sequences (RSSs) flanking gene segments in immunoglobulin and T-cell receptor genes, whereas the sequences encoding the transposases became the *RAG-1* and *RAG-2* genes, which now encode the recombinase essential for the rearrangement of the antigen-receptor genes (see Section 4-5). A transposon had been proposed for many years as the origin of the *RAG* genes, because, unusually for mammals, these genes lack introns; however, this is a feature of transposons. That the action of the RAG proteins on the RSSs was similar to the mechanism of excision of transposons was well known, but it has only quite recently been demonstrated that the present-day RAG proteins can catalyze the insertion into DNA of a DNA fragment containing the RSSs, a process identical to that of transposition.

The origin of somatic gene rearrangement in the excision of a transposable element makes sense of an apparent paradox in the rearrangement of immune-system genes. This is that the RSSs are joined precisely in the excised DNA, which has no further function and whose fate is irrelevant to the cell, whereas the cut ends in the genomic DNA, which form part of the immunoglobulin or T-cell receptor gene, are joined by an error-prone process, which could be viewed as a disadvantage. However, when looked at from the transposon's point of view this makes sense because the transposon preserves its integrity by this excision mechanism, and the fate of the DNA it leaves behind is of no significance to it. As it turned out, the error-prone joining in the primitive immunoglobulin gene generated useful diversity in molecules used for antigen recognition and was clearly strongly selected for. Subsequent duplication, reduplication, and recombination of the immune-receptor gene and its inserted RSSs eventually led to the multisegmented immunoglobulin and T-cell receptor loci of present-day vertebrates.

15-7 The target of the transposon is likely to have been a gene encoding a cell-surface receptor containing an immunoglobulin-like V domain.

Proteins containing immunoglobulin-like domains are ubiquitous throughout the plant, animal, and bacterial kingdoms, making this one of the most abundant protein superfamilies. Moreover, in species whose genomes have been fully sequenced, the immunoglobulin superfamily is found to be one of the largest families of protein domains in the genome. The functions of the members of this superfamily are very disparate, and they are a striking example of natural selection taking a useful structure—the basic immunoglobulin-domain fold—and adapting it to a wide variety of different purposes.

The immunoglobulin superfamily domains can be divided into four families—V (resembling an immunoglobulin variable domain), C1 and C2 (resembling constant-region domains), and the more diverse I domains—on the basis of differences in structure and sequence. V, C1, and C2 domains are found in many immune-system molecules. For example, immunoglobulins and T-cell receptors have V and C1 domains, CD4 and CD8 molecules have V and, in the case of CD4, C2 domains, and MHC class I and class II molecules have C1 domains. The adhesion molecules VCAM and ICAM contain C2 and I domains. The I domains seem to be the most disparate. As well as being found in adhesion molecules of the immune system, they are also present in proteins outside the immune system, such as the muscle proteins titin and twitchin.

When we come to consider the evolution of the adaptive immune system, we find that, until very recently, only I-family immunoglobulin superfamily molecules had been found in invertebrates. Yet the ancestral domain into which the transposon inserted to create the capacity for rearrangement was certainly a V domain. This domain was most probably linked to a C1 domain to form a transmembrane receptor, as this is the basic organization of both T-cell receptors and immunoglobulins. It is possible that the original receptor could have been a V domain coupled to a C2 domain, a combination found, for example, in the KIR receptors of NK cells and in other members of the extended leukocyte receptor family (see Section 2-28), with a subsequent evolution of the C2 domain into a C1 domain within the lineage that led to the immunoglobulins and T-cell receptors, although this is less likely.

Genes with both of these types of organization have now been found in invertebrates. In the urochordate *Ciona*, four genes containing V domains paired with C domains have been identified. Two of these contain V domains in association with C2 domains, while the other two contain V domains linked to C1-like and C2 domains. It is these latter two genes that are the most likely candidates for the ancestor of the vertebrate antigen receptors.

Two additional invertebrate protein families containing V domains have been identified, in the cephalochordate *Branchiostoma* (the amphioxus). A family of secreted molecules containing immunoglobulin V domains has been found in this species, although in this case the V domain is associated with chitin-binding domains rather than with immunoglobulin C domains. It remains to be determined whether these molecules have any immune function. The second family is represented by a protein containing a V domain linked to a multispan transmembrane domain. Again, there is no evidence for any immune function associated with this protein.

15-8 Different species generate immunoglobulin diversity in different ways.

Most of the animals that we are familiar with generate a large part of their antigen receptor diversity in the same way as humans, by putting together gene segments in different combinations, as described in Chapters 3 and 4. However, we noted a few exceptions in passing (see Section 4-10), and it is useful to return to these now. Some animals use gene rearrangement to always join together the same V and J gene segment initially, and then go on to diversify this recombined V region in various ways. In chickens and rabbits, the recombined V region is diversified by gene conversion (see Section 4-10) in the bursa of Fabricius (in chickens) or another intestinal lymphoid organ (in rabbits). The various strategies used by different groups are outlined in Fig. 15.9. Other animals may generate their diverse repertoire mainly by somatic hypermutation of a fairly invariant recombined V region. The generation of some immunoglobulin diversity within the sheep ileal Peyer's patch may depend on this mechanism, although gene conversion also has a role in this species.

The immunoglobulin loci in bony fish and higher vertebrates are organized such that separate blocks containing repeated V regions lie upstream of blocks of D regions (in the V_H locus) and blocks of J regions. In contrast, the cartilaginous fish have multiple copies of discrete V_L–J_L–C_L and V_H–D_H–J_H–C_H cassettes, and activate rearrangement within individual cassettes. Although these mechanisms differ from the canonical process described in Chapter 4, where diversity is generated through combinatorial gene rearrangement, in most cases there is still a requirement for a somatic rearrangement event.

In cartilaginous fish such as rays and carcharine sharks, however, some of the immunoglobulin genes are not generated by rearrangement. Instead these organisms have multiple 'rearranged' V_L regions (and sometimes rearranged V_H regions) in the germline genome and apparently generate diversity by activating the transcription of different copies. These are examples of non-combinatorial immunoglobulin systems, although in the strict sense there is still combinatorial diversity, which is generated by the subsequent pairing of heavy and light chains. This organization of the light-chain loci is unlikely to

Fig. 15.9 The organization of immunoglobulin genes is different in different species, but all can generate a diverse repertoire of receptors. The organization of the immunoglobulin heavy-chain genes in mammals, in which there are separated clusters of repeated V, D, and J gene segments, is not the only solution to the problem of generating a diverse repertoire of receptors. Other animals have found alternative solutions. In 'primitive' groups, such as the sharks, the locus consists of multiple repeats of a basic unit composed of a V gene segment, one or two D gene segments, a J gene segment, and a C gene segment. A more extreme version of this organization is found in the λ-like light-chain locus of some elasmobranch species such as sharks and rays, in which the repeated unit consists of already rearranged VJ–C genes, from which a random choice is made for expression. Finally, in chickens, there is a single rearranging set of gene segments at the heavy-chain locus, but multiple copies of V-segment pseudogenes. Diversity in this system is created by gene conversion, in which sequences from the V_H pseudogenes are copied onto the single rearranged V_H gene.

represent an intermediate evolutionary stage, because for this to be the case the heavy-chain and light-chain genes must have independently acquired the capacity for rearrangement by a process of convergent rather than divergent evolution. It is very much more likely that, after the divergence of the cartilaginous fish, some of the immunoglobulin loci in the common ancestor of this group became rearranged in the germline through activation of the *RAG* genes in germ cells, with the consequent inheritance of rearranged loci by the offspring. In these species, the rearranged germline loci may confer some advantages, perhaps in early development before a complex repertoire becomes established, or in ensuring rapid responses to common pathogens by using a preformed set of immunoglobulin chains.

The predominant form of immunoglobulin in cartilaginous fish is IgM, and this is also true of the bony fish. However, the cartilaginous fishes have at least two additional types of immunoglobulin heavy chain not found in more recent species. One, IgW, has six constant-region domains, whereas the second, IgNAR (for new antigen receptor) seems to be related to IgW but has lost the first constant domain and does not pair with light chains, instead forming a homodimer in which each V domain forms a separate antigen-binding site. The IgW molecule is thought to be present only as a cell-surface receptor on B cells, and this function may have been taken over by IgD, which is first found in the bony fish. This variability does suggest that in the early cartilaginous fish the immunoglobulins had only recently evolved and were throwing up variants to be tested by natural selection.

15-9 Both α:β and γ:δ T-cell receptors are present in cartilaginous fish.

Many studies have now identified the key receptors of the adaptive immune system—the T-cell receptors and immunoglobulins—in a wide variety of vertebrate species. Neither of these proteins has been found in any species evolutionarily earlier than the cartilaginous fishes. What is surprising, however, is that by the time we first observe them in the cartilaginous fish, the adaptive components of the cellular immune system have essentially the same form that we see in mammals. The identification of TCRβ-chain and δ-chain homologs from sharks, and of distinct TCRα, β, γ, and δ chains from a skate, show that even at the earliest time that these adaptive immune system receptors can be identified they have already diversified into at least two recognition systems. Moreover, each shows diversity resulting from combinatorial somatic rearrangement. Although we still do not fully understand the role of γ:δ T cells in the mammalian adaptive immune system, the very early divergence of the two sets of T-cell receptors and their conservation through subsequent evolution suggests that there was an early clear separation of the functions of these receptors.

15-10 MHC class I and class II molecules are also first found in the cartilaginous fishes.

One corollary of the appearance of the T-cell receptors is that at the same time one should see the emergence of their specific ligands, the MHC molecules. Indeed, these are present in cartilaginous fishes and in all 'higher' species but, like the T-cell receptors, no MHC molecule has been found in any jawless fish or in an invertebrate. Both MHC class I and class II α-chain and β-chain genes are present in sharks and their products seem to function in an identical way to the mammalian MHC molecules. The key residues of the peptide-binding cleft that interact with the ends of the peptide, in MHC class I molecules, or with the central region of the peptide, in MHC class II molecules, are conserved in shark MHC molecules.

Moreover, the MHC genes are also polymorphic in sharks, with multiple alleles of class I and class II loci having been identified. In some species more than 20 MHC class I alleles have been identified so far. For the shark MHC class II molecules, both the class II α and the class II β chains are polymorphic. Thus, not only has the function of the MHC molecules in selecting peptides for presentation evolved between the agnathans and the cartilaginous fishes, but the continuous selection imposed by pathogens has resulted in the polymorphism that is a characteristic feature of the MHC.

The MHC class I genes can be classified into the classical MHC class I genes (sometimes called class IA) and the nonclassical MHC class IB genes (see Section 5-10). This is also true in cartilaginous fishes, because the class I genes of sharks include some that resemble mammalian class IB molecules. However, it is thought that the shark class IB genes are not the ancestors of the class IB genes found in more recent species. Instead, some class IB genes, notably CD1 and some that have functions distinct from antigen presentation, such as zinc-α_2-glycoprotein and the MHC-like Fc receptor (see Section 9-13), seem to have evolved early, before the divergence of the cartilaginous fishes from the vertebrate line, and are likely to have homologs in all vertebrates. For the other class I genes, it seems that within each of the five major vertebrate lineages studied (cartilaginous fishes, lobe-finned fishes, ray-finned fishes, amphibians, and mammals) the class I genes have independently separated into classical and nonclassical loci.

Thus, the characteristic features of the MHC molecules are all present when these molecules are first encountered, and there are no evolutionarily intermediate forms that may guide our understanding of their evolution. Thus, although we can trace the evolution of the components of the innate immune system, the mystery of the origin of the adaptive immune system still largely persists.

15-11 Are adaptive immune systems dependent on the emergence of the jaw?

In this part of the chapter we have discussed both the event that made adaptive immunity possible—the insertion of a transposon into an unknown receptor gene—and the sudden emergence of the adaptive immune system, apparently already well developed, at the time of the appearance of the jawed fishes. What one must realize, however, is that these events were not necessarily simultaneous. The insertion of a transposon may have created the capacity to generate diversity in a receptor, but to understand the evolution of the adaptive immune system we have to understand the processes of natural selection that shaped the adaptive immune system into the form in which we can first detect it. The insertion of a transposon tells us how it exists, not why it exists.

One possible scenario is that the original insertion event occurred in a receptor that recognized an ancestor of the MHC molecules. As discussed previously, both T-cell and NK-cell receptors would meet this criterion, and the function of this hypothetical ancestral receptor may have been more like that of the NK-cell receptors—an invariant receptor recognizing an essentially invariant ligand, and perhaps activating a cellular response to stress or to viral infection. If so, the stage would be set for the introduction of variability, but what would be the selective force?

One intriguing speculation is that the development of adaptive immunity was a side-effect of acquiring jaws, and hence the ability to eat a wider variety of foodstuffs, including animals with hard shells or chitinous exoskeletons. This would expose the animal to damage to the gut tissue and a higher risk of infection. However, some invertebrates, notably the beaked cephalopods such as octopuses and squid, also eat shelled or bony prey and so this feature by itself does not seem to be a sufficient selective force for the development of adaptive immunity. Moreover, the evolution of immunological memory as well as antigen-receptor diversity suggests that repeated exposure to pathogens, rather than simply exposure to a greater variety of pathogens, was an important selecting pressure. The acquisition of a jaw was only one of several changes taking place during the transition from agnathans to jawed vertebrates, both in the organization of the vertebrate body and in the development and lifestyle of the organisms. Vertebrates tend to have slower development and longer life-spans than invertebrates, and to reproduce more than once. Animals with these characteristics are more at risk from repeated infection and have a greater reproductive benefit from a prolonged life-span, and these may have been the selective pressures that drove the development of the adaptive immune system.

Summary.

The 'immunological Big Bang' represented by the evolution of an adaptive immune response has been recognized for some years, and its relation to the acquisition of somatic gene rearrangement in some primordial antigen receptor has been the subject of much speculation. It is thought that gene rearrangement in the antigen-receptor loci arose as the result of a chance insertion of a transposon into a member of the immunoglobulin superfamily of genes. This event must have taken place in a germline cell in some ancestor of the vertebrates. By a lucky chance, the transposon terminal sequences were placed in an appropriate location within this gene to enable intramolecular somatic recombination, thus paving the way for the full-blown somatic gene rearrangement seen in the immunoglobulin and T-cell receptor genes today. At the same time, the transposase genes (the *RAG* genes), presumably from the same transposon, were preserved, but became separated from the transposon terminal sequences and are now carried on a different chromosome. However, even with the advent of somatic recombination, adaptive immunity would not have arisen had not the transposon inserted into a suitable receptor gene. That ancestral receptor gene is as yet unknown, and so the search for the evolutionary origins of the adaptive immune system continues.

Summary to Chapter 15.

The evolution of the immune system, summarized in Fig. 15.10, has mostly been a gradual process of increasing diversification from a small number of very ancient recognition and effector pathways, this gradual process being broken into by the cataclysmic acquisition of adaptive immunity. After that, the gradual pace of steady development and diversification returned. From the time of the common ancestors of animals and plants, antimicrobial peptides have been a basic defense mechanism, supplemented in later organisms by the retention of mobile, phagocytic cells capable of eating invading microbes. Systems of innate immunity evolved that targeted pathogens to phagocytes more efficiently; the first of these was a simple version of the alternative pathway of complement activation, which was followed by the evolution of a lectin-mediated pathway. At this point, adaptive immunity emerged from an as-yet unknown ancestral immune system, with the rapid evolution of a full complement of T-cell and immunoglobulin receptors, together with the MHC class I and class II antigen-presenting molecules. The subsequent development of the immune system has served to refine the adaptive immune system, but its essential nature has remained unchanged.

	Drosophila (insect)	Sea urchin (echinoderm)	Sea squirts (ascidian)	Lamprey (agnathan)	Shark (chon drichthyes)	Carp (teleost)	Frog (amphibian)	Snake (reptile)	Chicken (bird)	Human (mammal)
Acquired immunity	No	No	No	No	Yes	Yes	Yes	Yes	Yes	Yes
Immunoglobulin rearrangement	No	No	No	No	Yes	Yes	Yes	Yes	Yes	Yes
Combinatorial T-cell receptor rearrangement	No	No	No	No	Yes	Yes	Yes	Yes	Yes	Yes
Polymorphic MHC molecules	No	No	No	No	Yes	Yes	Yes	Yes	Yes	Yes
Classical complement pathway	No	No	No	No	Yes	Yes	Yes	Yes	Yes	Yes
C3 and factor B	No	Yes	Yes	Yes	Yes	Yes	Yes	Yes	Yes	Yes
Mannose-binding lectin	No	?	Yes	Inferred	Inferred	Yes	Inferred	Inferred	Yes	Yes
Ficolins	No	?	Yes	Inferred	Inferred	Inferred	Inferred	Inferred	Inferred	Yes
MASPs	No	?	Yes	Yes	Yes	Yes	Yes	Yes	Yes	Yes
Toll-like receptors	Yes	Yes	Yes	Yes	Yes	Yes	Yes	Yes	Yes	Yes
Antibacterial peptides	Yes	Inferred	Inferred	Inferred	Inferred	Inferred	Yes	Yes	Yes	Yes

Fig. 15.10 Summary of the evolutionary emergence of innate and adaptive immune characteristics.

Section references.

15-1 Antimicrobial peptides are likely to be the most ancient immune defenses.

Ganz, T.: Defensins and host defense. *Science* 1999, **286**:420–421.

Ganz, T.: **Defensins: antimicrobial peptides of innate immunity.** *Nat. Rev. Immunol.* 2003, **3**:710–720.

Gura, T.: Innate immunity. Ancient system gets new respect. *Science* 2001, **291**:2068–2071.

Hoffmann, J. A.: **Innate immunity of insects.** *Curr. Opin. Immunol.* 1995, **7**:4–10.

Thomma, B.P., Cammue, B.P., and Thevissen, K.: **Plant defensins.** *Planta* 2002, **216**:193–202.

15-2 Toll-like receptors may represent the most primitive pathogen-recognition system.

Hetru, C., Troxler, L., and Hoffmann, J.A.: ***Drosophila melanogaster* antimicrobial defense.** *J. Infect. Dis.* 2003, **187 Suppl 2**:S327–S334.

Hoffmann, J.A., Kafatos, F.C., Janeway, C.A., and Ezekowitz, R.A.: **Phylogenetic perspectives in innate immunity.** *Science* 1999, **284**:1313–1318.

Imler, J.L., and Hoffmann, J.A.: **Toll and Toll-like proteins: an ancient family of receptors signaling infection.** *Rev. Immunogenet.* 2000, **2**:294–304.

Imler, J.L., and Hoffmann, J.A.: **Toll receptors in innate immunity.** *Trends Cell Biol.* 2001, **11**:304–311.

Imler, J.L., and Hoffmann, J.A.: **Toll signaling: the TIReless quest for specificity.** *Nat. Immunol.* 2003, **4**:105–106.

15-3 A second recognition system in *Drosophila* homologous to the mammalian tumor necrosis factor receptor pathway provides protection from Gram-negative bacteria.

Ferrandon, D., Jung, A.C., Criqui, M., Lemaitre, B., Uttenweiler-Joseph, S., Michaut, L., Reichhart, J., and Hoffmann, J.A.: **A drosomycin-GFP reporter transgene reveals a local immune response in *Drosophila* that is not dependent on the Toll pathway.** *EMBO J.* 1998, **17:**1217–1227.

Georgel, P., Naitza, S., Kappler, C., Ferrandon, D., Zachary, D., Swimmer, C., Kopczynski, C., Duyk, G., Reichhart, J.M., and Hoffmann, J.A.: ***Drosophila* immune deficiency (IMD) is a death domain protein that activates antibacterial defense and can promote apoptosis.** *Dev. Cell* 2001, **1:**503–514.

Hoffmann, J.A., and Reichhart, J.M.: ***Drosophila* innate immunity: an evolutionary perspective.** *Nat. Immunol.* 2002, **3:**121–126.

Rutschmann, S., Jung, A.C., Zhou, R., Silverman, N., Hoffmann, J.A., and Ferrandon, D.: **Role of *Drosophila* IKKγ in a toll-independent antibacterial immune response.** *Nat. Immunol.* 2000, **1:**342–347.

15-4 An ancestral complement system opsonizes pathogens for uptake by phagocytic cells.

Gross, P.S., Al-Sharif, W.Z., Clow, L.A., and Smith, L.C.: **Echinoderm immunity and the evolution of the complement system.** *Dev. Comp. Immunol.* 1999, **23:**429–442.

Smith, L.C.: **The complement system in sea urchins.** *Adv. Exp. Med. Biol.* 2001, **484:**363–372.

Smith, L.C., Clow, L.A., and Terwilliger, D.P.: **The ancestral complement system in sea urchins.** *Immunol. Rev.* 2001, **180:**16–34.

Smith, L.C., Shih, C.S., and Dachenhausen, S.G.: **Coelomocytes express SpBf, a homologue of factor B, the second component in the sea urchin complement system.** *J. Immunol.* 1998, **161:**6784–6793.

15-5 The lectin pathway of complement activation evolved in invertebrates.

Fujita, T.: **Evolution of the lectin-complement pathway and its role in innate immunity.** *Nat. Rev. Immunol.* 2002, **2:**346–353.

Holmskov, U., Thiel, S., and Jensenius, J.C.: **Collections and ficolins: humoral lectins of the innate immune defense.** *Annu. Rev. Immunol.* 2003, **21:**547–578.

Matsushita, M., and Fujita, T.: **Ficolins and the lectin complement pathway.** *Immunol. Rev.* 2001, **180:**78–85.

Matsushita, M., and Fujita, T.: **The role of ficolins in innate immunity.** *Immunobiology* 2002, **205:**490–497.

Nonaka, M., Azumi, K., Ji, X., Namikawa-Yamada, C., Sasaki, M., Saiga, H., Dodds, A.W., Sekine, H., Homma, M.K., Matsushita, M., Endo, Y., and Fujita, T.: **Opsonic complement component C3 in the solitary ascidian, *Halocynthia roretzi.*** *J. Immunol.* 1999, **162:**387–391.

Raftos, D., Green, P., Mahajan, D., Newton, R., Pearce, S., Peters, R., Robbins, J., and Nair, S.: **Collagenous lectins in tunicates and the proteolytic activation of complement.** *Adv. Exp. Med. Biol.* 2001, **484:**229–236.

Smith, L.C., Azumi, K., and Nonaka, M.: **Complement systems in invertebrates. The ancient alternative and lectin pathways.** *Immunopharmacology* 1999, **42:**107–120.

15-6 Adaptive immunity appeared abruptly in the cartilaginous fish.

Agrawal, A.: **Amersham Pharmacia Biotech & Science Prize. Transposition and evolution of antigen-specific immunity.** *Science* 2000, **290:**1715–1716.

Agrawal, A., Eastman, Q.M., and Schatz, D.G.: **Transposition mediated by RAG1 and RAG2 and its implications for the evolution of the immune system.** *Nature* 1998, **394:**744–751.

Hansen, J.D., and McBlane, J.F.: **Recombination-activating genes, transposition, and the lymphoid-specific combinatorial immune system:** a common evolutionary connection. *Curr. Top. Microbiol. Immunol.* 2000, **248:**111–135.

van Gent, D.C., Mizuuchi, K., and Gellert, M.: **Similarities between initiation of V(D)J recombination and retroviral integration.** *Science* 1996, **271:**1592–1594.

Schatz, D.G.: **Transposition mediated by RAG1 and RAG2 and the evolution of the adaptive immune system.** *Immunol. Res.* 1999, **19:**169–182.

15-7 The target of the transposon is likely to have been a gene encoding a cell-surface receptor containing an immunoglobulin-like V domain.

Cannon, J.P., Haire, R.N., and Litman, G.W.: **Identification of diversified genes that contain immunoglobulin-like variable regions in a protochordate.** *Nat. Immunol.* 2002, **3:**1200–1207.

Rast, J.P., and Litman, G.W.: **Towards understanding the evolutionary origins and early diversification of rearranging antigen receptors.** *Immunol. Rev.* 1998, **166:**79–86.

15-8 Different species generate immunoglobulin diversity in different ways.

Anderson, M.K., Shamblott, M.J., Litman, R.T., and Litman, G.W.: **Generation of immunoglobulin light chain gene diversity in *Raja erinacea* is not associated with somatic rearrangement, an exception to a central paradigm of B cell immunity.** *J. Exp. Med.* 1995, **182:**109–119.

Anderson, M.K., Strong, S.J., Litman, R.T., Luer, C.A., Amemiya, C.T., Rast, J.P., and Litman, G.W.: **A long form of the skate IgX gene exhibits a striking resemblance to the new shark IgW and IgNARC genes.** *Immunogenetics* 1999, **49:**56–67.

Rast, J.P., Amemiya, C.T., Litman, R.T., Strong, S.J., and Litman, G.W.: **Distinct patterns of IgH structure and organization in a divergent lineage of chrondrichthyan fishes.** *Immunogenetics* 1998, **47:**234–245.

Yoder, J.A., and Litman, G.W.: **Immune-type diversity in the absence of somatic rearrangement.** *Curr. Top. Microbiol. Immunol.* 2000, **248:**271–282.

15-9 Both α:β and γ:δ T-cell receptors are present in cartilaginous fish.

Rast, J.P., and Litman, G.W.: **T-cell receptor gene homologs are present in the most primitive jawed vertebrates.** *Proc. Natl. Acad. Sci. USA* 1994, **91:**9248–9252.

Rast, J.P., Anderson, M.K., Strong, S.J., Luer, C., Litman, R.T., and Litman, G.W. **α, β, γ, and δ T-cell antigen receptor genes arose early in vertebrate phylogeny.** *Immunity* 1997, **6:**1–11.

15-10 MHC class I and class II molecules are also first found in the cartilaginous fishes.

Hashimoto, K., Okamura, K., Yamaguchi, H., Ototake, M., Nakanishi, T., and Kurosawa, Y.: **Conservation and diversification of MHC class I and its related molecules in vertebrates.** *Immunol. Rev.* 1999, **167:**81–100.

Kurosawa, Y., and Hashimoto, K.: **How did the primordial T cell receptor and MHC molecules function initially?** *Immunol. Cell Biol.* 1997, **75:**193–196.

Ohta, Y., Okamura, K., McKinney, E.C., Bartl, S., Hashimoto, K., and Flajnik, M.F.: **Primitive synteny of vertebrate major histocompatibility complex class I and class II genes.** *Proc. Natl. Acad. Sci. USA* 2000, **97:**4712–4717.

Okamura, K., Ototake, M., Nakanishi, T., Kurosawa, Y., and Hashimoto, K.: **The most primitive vertebrates with jaws possess highly polymorphic MHC class I genes comparable to those of humans.** *Immunity* 1997, **7:**777–790.

15-11 Are adaptive immune systems dependent on the emergence of the jaw?

Matsunaga, T., and Rahman, A.: **What brought the adaptive immune system to vertebrates? The jaw hypothesis and the seahorse.** *Immunol. Rev.* 1998, **166:**177–186.

Immunologists' Toolbox

APPENDIX I

Immunization.

Natural adaptive immune responses are normally directed at antigens borne by pathogenic microorganisms. The immune system can, however, also be induced to respond to simple nonliving antigens, and experimental immunologists have focused on the responses to these simple antigens in developing our understanding of the immune response. The deliberate induction of an immune response is known as **immunization**. Experimental immunizations are routinely carried out by injecting the test antigen into the animal or human subject. The route, dose, and form in which antigen is administered can profoundly affect whether a response occurs and the type of response that is produced, and are considered in Sections A-1–A-4. The induction of protective immune responses against common microbial pathogens in humans is often called **vaccination**, although this term is correctly only applied to the induction of immune responses against smallpox by immunizing with the cross-reactive cowpox virus, vaccinia (see Chapter 14).

To determine whether an immune response has occurred and to follow its course, the immunized individual is monitored for the appearance of immune reactants directed at the specific antigen. Immune responses to most antigens elicit the production of both specific antibodies and specific effector T cells. Monitoring the antibody response usually involves the analysis of relatively crude preparations of **antiserum** (plural: **antisera**). The **serum** is the fluid phase of clotted blood, which, if taken from an immunized individual, is called antiserum because it contains specific antibodies against the immunizing antigen as well as other soluble serum proteins. To study immune responses mediated by T cells, blood lymphocytes or cells from lymphoid organs such as the spleen are tested; T-cell responses are more commonly studied in experimental animals than in humans.

Any substance that can elicit an immune response is said to be **immunogenic** and is called an **immunogen**. There is a clear operational distinction between an immunogen and an antigen. An **antigen** is defined as any sustance that can bind to a specific antibody. All antigens therefore have the potential to elicit specific antibodies, but some need to be attached to an immunogen in order to do so. This means that although all immunogens are antigens, not all antigens are immunogenic. The antigens used most frequently in experimental immunology are proteins, and antibodies to proteins are of enormous utility in experimental biology and medicine. Purified proteins are, however, not always highly immunogenic and to provoke an immune response have to be administered with an adjuvant (see Section A-4). Carbohydrates, nucleic acids, and other types of molecule are all potential antigens, but will often only induce an immune response if attached to a protein carrier. Thus, the immunogenicity of protein antigens determines the outcome of virtually every immune response.

Fig. A.1 The dose of antigen used in an initial immunization affects the primary and secondary antibody response. The typical antigen dose–response curve shown here illustrates the influence of dose on both a primary antibody response (amounts of antibody produced expressed in arbitrary units) and the effect of the dose used for priming on a secondary antibody response elicited by a dose of antigen of 10^3 arbitrary mass units. Very low doses of antigen do not cause an immune response at all. Slightly higher doses appear to inhibit specific antibody production, an effect known as low-zone tolerance. Above these doses there is a steady increase in the response with antigen dose to reach a broad optimum. Very high doses of antigen also inhibit immune responsiveness to a subsequent challenge, a phenomenon known as high-zone tolerance.

Antisera generated by immunization with even the simplest antigen will contain many different antibody molecules that bind to the immunogen in slightly different ways. Some of the antibodies in an antiserum are cross-reactive. A **cross-reaction** is defined as the binding of an antibody to an antigen other than the immunogen; most antibodies cross-react with closely related antigens but, on occasion, some bind antigens having no clear relationship to the immunogen. These cross-reacting antibodies can create problems when the antiserum is used to detect a specific antigen. They can be removed from an antiserum by **absorption** with the cross-reactive antigen, leaving behind the antibodies that bind only to the immunogen. Absorption can be performed by affinity chromatography using immobilized antigen, a technique that is also used for purification of antibodies or antigens (see Section A-5). Most problems of cross-reactivity can be avoided, however, by making monoclonal antibodies (see Section A-12).

Although almost any structure can be recognized by antibody as an antigen, usually only proteins elicit fully developed adaptive immune responses. This is because proteins have the ability to engage T cells, which contribute to inducing most antibody responses and are required for immunological memory. Proteins engage T cells because the T cells recognize antigens as peptide fragments of proteins bound to major histocompatibility complex (MHC) molecules (see Section 3-11). An adaptive immune response that includes immunological memory can be induced by nonpeptide antigens only when they are attached to a protein carrier that can engage the necessary T cells (see Section 9-2 and Fig. 9.4).

Immunological memory is produced as a result of the initial or **primary immunization**, which evokes the **primary immune response**. This is also known as **priming**, as the animal or person is now 'primed' like a pump to mount a more potent response to subsequent challenges with the same antigen. The response to each immunization is increasingly intense, so that **secondary**, **tertiary**, and subsequent responses are of increasing magnitude (Fig. A.1). Repetitive challenge with antigen to achieve a heightened state of immunity is known as **hyperimmunization**.

Certain properties of a protein that favor the priming of an adaptive immune response have been defined by studying antibody responses to simple natural proteins like hen egg-white lysozyme and to synthetic polypeptide antigens (Fig. A.2). The larger and more complex a protein, and the more distant its relationship to self proteins, the more likely it is to elicit a response. This is because such responses depend on the proteins being degraded into peptides that can bind to MHC molecules, and on the subsequent recognition of these peptide:MHC complexes by T cells. The larger and more distinct the protein antigen, the more likely it is to contain such peptides. Particulate or aggregated antigens are more immunogenic because they are taken up more efficiently by the specialized antigen-presenting cells responsible for initiating a response. Indeed small soluble proteins are unable to induce a response unless they are made to aggregate in some way. Many vaccines, for example, use aggregated protein antigens to potentiate the immune response.

A-1   Haptens.

Small organic molecules of simple structure, such as phenyl arsonates and nitrophenyls, do not provoke antibodies when injected by themselves. However, antibodies can be raised against them if the molecule is attached covalently, by simple chemical reactions, to a protein carrier. Such small molecules were termed **haptens** (from the Greek *haptein*, to fasten) by the immunologist Karl Landsteiner, who first studied them in the early 1900s. He found that animals immunized with a hapten–carrier conjugate produced

Factors that influence the immunogenicity of proteins		
Parameter	**Increased immunogenicity**	**Decreased immunogenicity**
Size	Large	Small (MW<2500)
Dose	Intermediate	High or low
Route	Subcutaneous > intraperitoneal > intravenous or intragastric	
Composition	Complex	Simple
Form	Particulate	Soluble
	Denatured	Native
Similarity to self protein	Multiple differences	Few differences
Adjuvants	Slow release	Rapid release
	Bacteria	No bacteria
Interaction with host MHC	Effective	Ineffective

Fig. A.2 Intrinsic properties and extrinsic factors that affect the immunogenicity of proteins.

three distinct sets of antibodies (Fig. A.3). One set comprised hapten-specific antibodies that reacted with the same hapten on any carrier, as well as with free hapten. The second set of antibodies was specific for the carrier protein, as shown by their ability to bind both the hapten-modified and unmodified carrier protein. Finally, some antibodies reacted only with the specific conjugate of hapten and carrier used for immunization. Landsteiner studied mainly the antibody response to the hapten, as these small molecules could be synthesized in many closely related forms. He observed that antibodies raised against a particular hapten bind that hapten but, in general, fail to bind even very closely related chemical structures. The binding of haptens by anti-hapten antibodies has played an important part in defining the precision of antigen binding by antibody molecules. Anti-hapten antibodies are also important medically as they mediate allergic reactions to penicillin and other compounds that elicit antibody responses when they attach to self proteins (see Section 12-10).

Fig. A.3 Antibodies can be elicited by small chemical groups called haptens only when the hapten is linked to an immunogenic protein carrier. Three types of antibodies are produced. One set (blue) binds the carrier protein alone and is called carrier-specific. One set (red) binds to the hapten on any carrier or to free hapten in solution and is called hapten-specific. One set (purple) only binds the specific conjugate of hapten and carrier used for immunization, apparently binding to sites at which the hapten joins the carrier, and is called conjugate-specific. The amount of antibody of each type in this serum is shown schematically in the graphs at the bottom; note that the original antigen binds more antibody than the sum of anti-hapten and anti-carrier antibodies owing to the additional binding of conjugate-specific antibody.

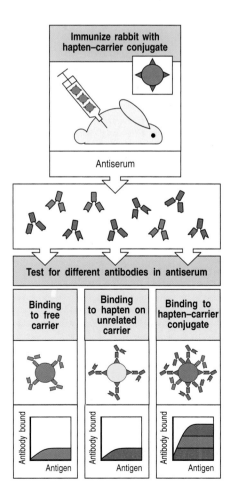

Immunize rabbit with hapten–carrier conjugate

Antiserum

Test for different antibodies in antiserum

Binding to free carrier

Binding to hapten on unrelated carrier

Binding to hapten–carrier conjugate

Antibody bound — Antigen

A-2   Routes of immunization.

The route by which antigen is administered affects both the magnitude and the type of response obtained. The most common routes by which antigen is introduced experimentally or as a vaccine into the body are injection into tissue by **subcutaneous (s.c.)** injection between the epidermis and dermal layers, or by **intradermal (i.d.)** injection, or **intramuscular (i.m.)** injection; by **intravenous (i.v.)** injection or transfusion directly into the bloodstream; into the gastrointestinal tract by **oral** administration; into the respiratory tract by **intranasal (i.n.)** administration or inhalation.

Antigens injected subcutaneously generally elicit the strongest responses, most probably because the antigen is taken up by Langerhans' cells and efficiently presented in local lymph nodes, and so this is the method most commonly used when the object of the experiment is to elicit specific antibodies or T cells against a given antigen. Antigens injected or transfused directly into the bloodstream tend to induce immune unresponsiveness or tolerance unless they bind to host cells or are in the form of aggregates that are readily taken up by antigen-presenting cells.

Antigen administration via the gastrointestinal tract is used mostly in the study of allergy. It has distinctive effects, frequently eliciting a local antibody response in the intestinal lamina propria, while producing a systemic state of tolerance that manifests as a diminished response to the same antigen if subsequently administered in immunogenic form elsewhere in the body. This 'split tolerance' may be important in avoiding allergy to antigens in food, as the local response prevents food antigens from entering the body, while the inhibition of systemic immunity helps to prevent the formation of IgE antibodies, which are the cause of such allergies (see Chapter 12).

Introduction of antigen into the respiratory tract is also used mainly in the study of allergy. Protein antigens that enter the body through the respiratory epithelium tend to elicit allergic responses, for reasons that are not clear.

A-3   Effects of antigen dose.

The magnitude of the immune response depends on the dose of immunogen administered. Below a certain threshold dose, most proteins do not elicit any immune response. Above the threshold dose, there is a gradual increase in the response as the dose of antigen is increased, until a broad plateau level is reached, followed by a decline at very high antigen doses (see Fig. A.1). As most infectious agents enter the body in small numbers, immune responses are generally elicited only by pathogens that multiply to a level sufficient to exceed the antigen dose threshold. The broad response optimum allows the system to respond to infectious agents across a wide range of doses. At very high antigen doses the immune response is inhibited, which may be important in maintaining tolerance to abundant self proteins such as plasma proteins. In general, secondary and subsequent immune responses occur at lower antigen doses and achieve higher plateau values, which is a sign of immunological memory. However, under some conditions, very low or very high doses of antigen may induce specific unresponsive states, known respectively as acquired **low-zone** or **high-zone tolerance**.

A-4   Adjuvants.

Most proteins are poorly immunogenic or nonimmunogenic when administered by themselves. Strong adaptive immune responses to protein antigens almost always require that the antigen be injected in a mixture known as an

adjuvant. An adjuvant is any substance that enhances the immunogenicity of substances mixed with it. Adjuvants differ from protein carriers in that they do not form stable linkages with the immunogen. Furthermore, adjuvants are needed primarily for initial immunizations, whereas carriers are required to elicit not only primary but also subsequent responses to haptens. Commonly used adjuvants are listed in Fig. A.4.

Adjuvants can enhance immunogenicity in two different ways. First, adjuvants convert soluble protein antigens into particulate material, which is more readily ingested by antigen-presenting cells such as macrophages. For example, the antigen can be adsorbed on particles of the adjuvant (such as alum), made particulate by emulsification in mineral oils, or incorporated into the colloidal particles of ISCOMs. This enhances immunogenicity somewhat, but such adjuvants are relatively weak unless they also contain bacteria or bacterial products. Such microbial constituents are the second means by which adjuvants enhance immunogenicity, and although their exact contribution to enhancing immunogenicity is unknown, they are clearly the more important component of an adjuvant. Microbial products may signal macrophages or dendritic cells to become more effective antigen-presenting cells (see Chapter 2). One of their effects is to induce the production of inflammatory cytokines and potent local inflammatory responses; this effect is probably intrinsic to their activity in enhancing responses, but precludes their use in humans.

Nevertheless, some human vaccines contain microbial antigens that can also act as effective adjuvants. For example, purified constituents of the bacterium *Bordetella pertussis*, which is the causal agent of whooping cough, are used as both antigen and adjuvant in the triplex DPT (diphtheria, pertussis, tetanus) vaccine against these diseases.

Adjuvants that enhance immune responses		
Adjuvant name	**Composition**	**Mechanism of action**
Incomplete Freund's adjuvant	Oil-in-water emulsion	Delayed release of antigen; enhanced uptake by macrophages
Complete Freund's adjuvant	Oil-in-water emulsion with dead mycobacteria	Delayed release of antigen; enhanced uptake by macrophages; induction of co-stimulators in macrophages
Freund's adjuvant with MDP	Oil-in-water emulsion with muramyldipeptide (MDP), a constituent of mycobacteria	Similar to complete Freund's adjuvant
Alum (aluminum hydroxide)	Aluminum hydroxide gel	Delayed release of antigen; enhanced macrophage uptake
Alum plus *Bordetella pertussis*	Aluminum hydroxide gel with killed *B. pertussis*	Delayed release of antigen; enhanced uptake by macrophages; induction of co-stimulators
Immune stimulatory complexes (ISCOMs)	Matrix of Quil A containing viral proteins	Delivers antigen to cytosol; allows induction of cytotoxic T cells

Fig. A.4 Common adjuvants and their use. Adjuvants are mixed with the antigen and usually render it particulate, which helps to retain the antigen in the body and promotes uptake by macrophages. Most adjuvants include bacteria or bacterial components that stimulate macrophages, aiding in the induction of the immune response. ISCOMs (immune stimulatory complexes) are small micelles of the detergent Quil A; when viral proteins are placed in these micelles, they apparently fuse with the antigen-presenting cell, allowing the antigen to enter the cytosol. Thus, the antigen-presenting cell can stimulate a response to the viral protein, much as a virus infecting these cells would stimulate an anti-viral response.

The detection, measurement, and characterization of antibodies and their use as research and diagnostic tools.

B cells contribute to adaptive immunity by secreting antibodies, and the response of B cells to an injected immunogen is usually measured by analyzing the specific antibody produced in a **humoral immune response**. This is most conveniently achieved by assaying the antibody that accumulates in the fluid phase of the blood or **plasma**; such antibodies are known as circulating antibodies. Circulating antibody is usually measured by collecting blood, allowing it to clot, and then isolating the serum from the clotted blood. The amount and characteristics of the antibody in the resulting antiserum are then determined using the assays we will describe in Sections A-5–A-11.

The most important characteristics of an antibody response are the specificity, amount, isotype or class, and affinity of the antibodies produced. The **specificity** determines the ability of the antibody to distinguish the immunogen from other antigens. The amount of antibody can be determined in many different ways and is a function of the number of responding B cells, their rate of antibody synthesis, and the persistence of the antibody after production. The persistence of an antibody in the plasma and extracellular fluid bathing the tissues is determined mainly by its **isotype** (see Sections 4-15 and 9-12); each isotype has a different half-life *in vivo*. The isotypic composition of an antibody response also determines the biological functions these antibodies can perform and the sites in which antibody will be found. Finally, the strength of binding of the antibody to its antigen in terms of a single antigen-binding site binding to a monovalent antigen is termed its **affinity** (the total binding strength of a molecule with more than one binding site is called its **avidity**). Binding strength is important, since the higher the affinity of the antibody for its antigen, the less antibody is required to eliminate the antigen, as antibodies with higher affinity will bind at lower antigen concentrations. All these parameters of the humoral immune response help to determine the capacity of that response to protect the host from infection.

Antibody molecules are highly specific for their corresponding antigen, being able to detect one molecule of a protein antigen out of more than 10^8 similar molecules. This makes antibodies both easy to isolate and study, and invaluable as probes of biological processes. Whereas standard chemistry would have great difficulty in distinguishing between two such closely related proteins as human and pig insulin, or two such closely related structures as *ortho*- and *para*-nitrophenyl, antibodies can be made that discriminate between these two structures absolutely. The value of antibodies as molecular probes has stimulated the development of many sensitive and highly specific techniques to measure their presence, to determine their specificity and affinity for a range of antigens, and to ascertain their functional capabilities. Many standard techniques used throughout biology exploit the specificity and stability of antigen binding by antibodies. Comprehensive guides to the conduct of these antibody assays are available in many books on immunological methodology; we will illustrate here only the most important techniques, especially those used in studying the immune response itself.

Some assays for antibody measure the direct binding of the antibody to its antigen. Such assays are based on **primary interactions**. Others determine the amount of antibody present by the changes it induces in the physical state

| Antibody to antigen A bound to beads | Add a mixture of molecules | Wash away unbound molecules | Elute specifically bound molecules |

Mixture depleted of antigen A

Purified antigen A

Fig. A.5 Affinity chromatography uses antigen–antibody binding to purify antigens or antibodies. To purify a specific antigen from a complex mixture of molecules, a monoclonal antibody is attached to an insoluble matrix, such as chromatography beads, and the mixture of molecules is passed over the matrix. The specific antibody binds the antigen of interest; other molecules are washed away. Specific antigen is then eluted by altering the pH, which can usually disrupt antibody–antigen bonds. Antibodies can be purified in the same way on beads coupled to antigen (not shown).

of the antigen, such as the precipitation of soluble antigen or the clumping of antigenic particles; these are called secondary interactions. Both types of assay can be used to measure the amount and specificity of the antibodies produced after immunization, and both can be applied to a wide range of other biological questions.

As assays for antibody were originally conducted with antisera from immune individuals, they are commonly referred to as **serological assays**, and the use of antibodies is often called **serology**. The amount of antibody is usually determined by antigen-binding assays after titration of the antiserum by serial dilution, and the point at which binding falls to 50% of the maximum is usually referred to as the **titer** of an antiserum.

A-5 Affinity chromatography.

Specific antibody can be isolated from an antiserum by **affinity chromatography**, which exploits the specific binding of antibody to antigen held on a solid matrix (Fig. A.5). Antigen is bound covalently to small, chemically reactive beads, which are loaded into a column, and the antiserum is allowed to pass over the beads. The specific antibodies bind, while all the other proteins in the serum, including antibodies to other substances, can be washed away. The specific antibodies are then eluted, typically by lowering the pH to 2.5 or raising it to greater than 11. Antibodies bind stably under physiological conditions of salt concentration, temperature, and pH, but the binding is reversible as the bonds are noncovalent. Affinity chromatography can also be used to purify antigens from complex mixtures by using beads coated with specific antibody. The technique is known as affinity chromatography because it separates molecules on the basis of their affinity for one another.

A-6 Radioimmunoassay (RIA), enzyme-linked immunosorbent assay (ELISA), and competitive inhibition assay.

Radioimmunoassay (RIA) and **enzyme-linked immunosorbent assay (ELISA)** are direct binding assays for antibody (or antigen) and both work on the same principle, but the means of detecting specific binding is different. Radioimmunoassays are commonly used to measure the levels of hormones in blood and tissue fluids, while ELISA assays are frequently used in viral diagnostics, for example in detecting cases of HIV infection. For both these

Fig. A.6 The principle of the enzyme-linked immunosorbent assay (ELISA).
To detect antigen A, purified antibody specific for antigen A is linked chemically to an enzyme. The samples to be tested are coated onto the surface of plastic wells to which they bind nonspecifically; residual sticky sites on the plastic are blocked by adding irrelevant proteins (not shown). The labeled antibody is then added to the wells under conditions where nonspecific binding is prevented, so that only binding to antigen A causes the labeled antibody to be retained on the surface. Unbound labeled antibody is removed from all wells by washing, and bound antibody is detected by an enzyme-dependent color-change reaction. This assay allows arrays of wells known as microtiter plates to be read in fiberoptic multichannel spectrometers, greatly speeding the assay. Modifications of this basic assay allow antibody or antigen in unknown samples to be measured as shown in Figs A.7 and A.29 (see also Section A-10).

methods one needs a pure preparation of a known antigen or antibody, or both, in order to standardize the assay. We will describe the assay with a sample of pure antibody, which is the more usual case, but the principle is similar if pure antigen is used instead. In RIA for an antigen, pure antibody against that antigen is radioactively labeled, usually with ^{125}I; for the ELISA, an enzyme is linked chemically to the antibody. The unlabeled component, which in this case would be antigen, is attached to a solid support, such as the wells of a plastic multiwell plate, which will adsorb a certain amount of any protein.

The labeled antibody is allowed to bind to the unlabeled antigen, under conditions where nonspecific adsorption is blocked, and any unbound antibody and other proteins are washed away. Antibody binding in RIA is measured directly in terms of the amount of radioactivity retained by the coated wells, whereas in ELISA, binding is detected by a reaction that converts a colorless substrate into a colored reaction product (Fig. A.6). The color change can be read directly in the reaction tray, making data collection very easy, and ELISA also avoids the hazards of radioactivity. This makes ELISA the preferred method for most direct-binding assays. Labeled anti-immunoglobulin antibodies (see Section A-10) can also be used in RIA or ELISA to detect binding of unlabeled antibody to unlabeled antigen-coated plates. In this case, the labeled anti-immunoglobulin antibody is used in what is termed a 'second layer.' The use of such a second layer also amplifies the signal, as at least two molecules of the labeled anti-immunoglobulin antibody are able to bind to each unlabeled antibody. RIA and ELISA can also be carried out with unlabeled antibody stuck to the plates and labeled antigen added.

A modification of ELISA known as a **capture** or **sandwich ELISA** (or more generally as an **antigen-capture assay**) can be used to detect secreted products such as cytokines. Rather than the antigen being directly attached to a plastic plate, antigen-specific antibodies are bound to the plate. These are able to bind antigen with high affinity, and thus concentrate it on the surface of the plate, even with antigens that are present in very low concentrations in the initial mixture. A separate labeled antibody that recognizes a different epitope to the immobilized first antibody is then used to detect the bound antigen.

These assays illustrate two crucial aspects of all serological assays. First, at least one of the reagents must be available in a pure, detectable form in order to obtain quantitative information. Second, there must be a means of separating the bound fraction of the labeled reagent from the unbound, free fraction so that the percentage of specific binding can be determined. Normally, this separation is achieved by having the unlabeled partner trapped on a solid support. Labeled molecules that do not bind can then be washed away, leaving just the labeled partner that has bound. In Fig. A.6, the unlabeled antigen is attached to the well and the labeled antibody is trapped by binding to it. The separation of bound from free is an essential step in every assay that uses antibodies.

RIA and ELISA do not allow one to measure directly the amount of antigen or antibody in a sample of unknown composition, as both depend on the binding of a pure labeled antigen or antibody. There are various ways around this problem, one of which is to use a **competitive inhibition assay**, as shown in Fig. A.7. In this type of assay, the presence and amount of a particular antigen in an unknown sample is determined by its ability to compete with a labeled reference antigen for binding to an antibody attached to a plastic well. A standard curve is first constructed by adding varying amounts of a known, unlabeled standard preparation; the assay can then measure the amount of antigen in unknown samples by comparison with the standard. The competitive binding assay can also be used for measuring antibody in a sample of unknown composition by attaching the appropriate antigen to the plate and measuring the ability of the test sample to inhibit the binding of a labeled specific antibody.

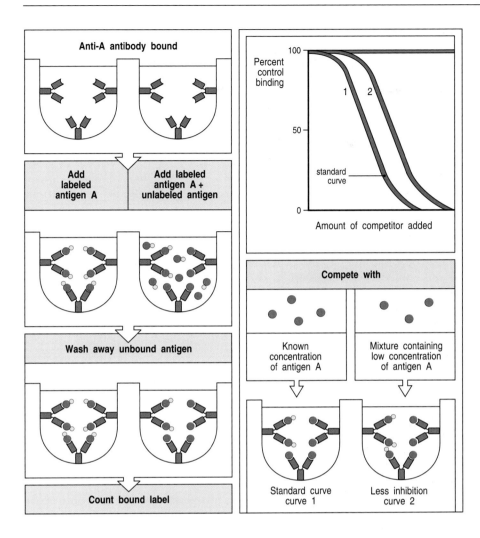

Fig. A.7 Competitive inhibition assay for antigen in unknown samples. A fixed amount of unlabeled antibody is attached to a set of wells, and a standard reference preparation of a labeled antigen is bound to it. Unlabeled standard or test samples are then added in various amounts and the displacement of labeled antigen is measured, generating characteristic inhibition curves. A standard curve is obtained by using known amounts of unlabeled antigen identical to that used as the labeled species, and comparison with this curve allows the amount of antigen in unknown samples to be calculated. The green line on the graph represents a sample lacking any substance that reacts with anti-A antibodies.

A-7 Hemagglutination and blood typing.

The direct measurement of antibody binding to antigen is used in most quantitative serological assays. However, some important assays are based on the ability of antibody binding to alter the physical state of the antigen it binds to. These secondary interactions can be detected in a variety of ways. For instance, when the antigen is displayed on the surface of a large particle such as a bacterium, antibodies can cause the bacteria to clump or **agglutinate**. The same principle applies to the reactions used in blood typing, only here the target antigens are on the surface of red blood cells and the clumping reaction caused by antibodies against them is called **hemagglutination** (from the Greek *haima*, blood).

Hemagglutination is used to determine the ABO blood group of blood donors and transfusion recipients. Clumping or agglutination is induced by antibodies or agglutinins called anti-A or anti-B that bind to the A or B blood-group substances, respectively (Fig. A.8). These blood-group antigens are arrayed in many copies on the surface of the red blood cell, allowing the cells to agglutinate when cross-linked by antibodies. Because hemagglutination involves the cross-linking of blood cells by the simultaneous binding of antibody molecules to identical antigens on different cells, this reaction demonstrates that each antibody molecule has at least two identical antigen-binding sites.

Fig. A.8 Hemagglutination is used to type blood groups and match compatible donors and recipients for blood transfusion. Common gut bacteria bear antigens that are similar or identical to blood-group antigens, and these stimulate the formation of antibodies to these antigens in individuals who do not bear the corresponding antigen on their own red blood cells (left column); thus, type O individuals, who lack A and B, have both anti-A and anti-B antibodies, while type AB individuals have neither. The pattern of agglutination of the red blood cells of a transfusion donor or recipient with anti-A and anti-B antibodies reveals the individual's ABO blood group. Before transfusion, the serum of the recipient is also tested for antibodies that agglutinate the red blood cells of the donor, and vice versa, a procedure called a cross-match, which may detect potentially harmful antibodies to other blood groups that are not part of the ABO system.

Serum from individuals of type	Red blood cells from individuals of type			
	O	**A**	**B**	**AB**
	Express the carbohydrate structures			
	R–GlcNAc–Gal $\overset{\mid}{Fuc}$	R–GlcNAc–Gal–GalNAc $\overset{\mid}{Fuc}$	R–GlcNAc–Gal–Gal $\overset{\mid}{Fuc}$	R–GlcNAc–Gal–GalNAc $\overset{\mid}{Fuc}$ + R–GlcNAc–Gal–Gal $\overset{\mid}{Fuc}$
O Anti-A and anti-B antibodies	no agglutination	agglutination	agglutination	agglutination
A Anti-B antibodies	no agglutination	no agglutination	agglutination	agglutination
B Anti-A antibodies	no agglutination	agglutination	no agglutination	agglutination
AB No antibodies to A or B	no agglutination	no agglutination	no agglutination	no agglutination

A-8 Precipitin reaction.

When sufficient quantities of antibody are mixed with soluble macromolecular antigens, a visible precipitate consisting of large aggregates of antigen cross-linked by antibody molecules can form. The amount of precipitate depends on the amounts of antigen and antibody, and on the ratio between them (Fig. A.9). This **precipitin reaction** provided the first quantitative assay for antibody, but is now seldom used in immunology. However, it is important to understand the interaction of antigen with antibody that leads to this reaction, as the production of **antigen:antibody complexes**, also known as **immune complexes**, *in vivo* occurs in almost all immune responses and occasionally can cause significant pathology (see Chapters 12 and 13).

In the precipitin reaction, various amounts of soluble antigen are added to a fixed amount of serum containing antibody. As the amount of antigen added increases, the amount of precipitate generated also increases up to a maximum and then declines (see Fig. A.9). When small amounts of antigen are added,

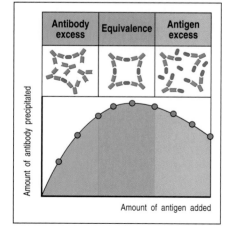

Fig. A.9 Antibody can precipitate soluble antigen. Analysis of the precipitate can generate a precipitin curve. Different amounts of antigen are added to a fixed amount of antibody, and precipitates form by antibody cross-linking of antigen molecules. The precipitate is recovered and the amount of precipitated antibody measured; the supernatant is tested for residual antigen or antibody. This defines zones of antibody excess, equivalence, and antigen excess. At equivalence, the largest antigen:antibody complexes form. In the zone of antigen excess, some of the immune complexes are too small to precipitate. These soluble immune complexes can cause pathological damage to small blood vessels when they form *in vivo* (see Chapter 13).

Fig. A.10 Different antibodies bind to distinct epitopes on an antigen molecule. The surface of an antigen possesses many potential antigenic determinants or epitopes, distinct sites to which an antibody can bind. The number of antibody molecules that can bind to a molecule of antigen at one time defines the antigen's valence. Steric considerations can limit the number of different antibodies that bind to the surface of an antigen at any one time (center and bottom panels) so that the number of epitopes on an antigen is always greater than or equal to its valence.

Small antigen, 2 epitopes: antigen valence = 2

Intermediate antigen, 6 epitopes: antigen valence = 4

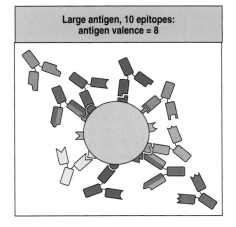

Large antigen, 10 epitopes: antigen valence = 8

antigen:antibody complexes are formed under conditions of antibody excess so that each molecule of antigen is bound by antibody and cross-linked to other molecules of antigen. When large amounts of antigen are added, only small antigen:antibody complexes can form and these are often soluble in this zone of antigen excess. Between these two zones, all of the antigen and antibody is found in the precipitate, generating a zone of equivalence. At equivalence, very large lattices of antigen and antibody are formed by cross-linking. While all antigen:antibody complexes can potentially produce disease, the small, soluble immune complexes formed in the zone of antigen excess may persist and cause pathology *in vivo*.

The precipitin reaction is affected by the number of binding sites that each antibody has for antigen, and by the maximum number of antibodies that can be bound by an antigen molecule or particle at any one time. These quantities are defined as the **valence** of the antibody and the valence of the antigen: the valence of both the antibodies and the antigen must be two or greater before any precipitation can occur. The valence of an antibody depends on its structural class (see Section 4-19).

Antigen will be precipitated only if it has several antibody-binding sites. This condition is usually satisfied in macromolecular antigens, which have a complex surface with binding sites for several different antibodies. The site on an antigen to which each distinct antibody molecule binds is called an **antigenic determinant** or an **epitope**. Steric considerations limit the number of distinct antibody molecules that can bind to a single antigen molecule at any one time however, because antibody molecules binding to epitopes that partially overlap will compete for binding. For this reason, the valence of an antigen is almost always less than the number of epitopes on the antigen (Fig. A.10).

A-9   Equilibrium dialysis: measurement of antibody affinity and avidity.

The affinity of an antibody is the strength of binding of a monovalent ligand to a single antigen-binding site on the antibody. The affinity of an antibody that binds small antigens, such as haptens, that can diffuse freely across a dialysis membrane can be determined directly by the technique of **equilibrium dialysis**. A known amount of antibody, whose molecules are too large to cross a dialysis membrane, is placed in a dialysis bag and offered various amounts of antigen. Molecules of antigen that bind to the antibody are no longer free to diffuse across the dialysis membrane, so only the unbound molecules of antigen equilibrate across it. By measuring the concentration of antigen inside the bag and in the surrounding fluid, one can determine the amount of the antigen that is bound as well as the amount that is free when equilibrium has been achieved. Given that the amount of antibody present is known, the affinity of the antibody and the number of specific binding sites for the antigen per molecule of antibody can be determined from this information. The data are usually analyzed using **Scatchard analysis** (Fig. A.11); such analyses were used to demonstrate that a molecule of IgG antibody has two identical antigen-binding sites.

Fig. A.11 The affinity and valence of an antibody can be determined by equilibrium dialysis. A known amount of antibody is placed in the bottom half of a dialysis chamber and exposed to different amounts of a diffusible monovalent antigen, such as a hapten. At equilibrium, the concentration of free antigen will be the same on each side of the membrane, so that at each concentration of antigen added, the fraction of the antigen bound is determined from the difference in concentration of total antigen in the top and bottom chambers. This information can be transformed into a Scatchard plot as shown here. In Scatchard analysis, the ratio r/c (where r = moles of antigen bound per mole of antibody and c = molar concentration of free antigen) is plotted against r. The number of binding sites per antibody molecule can be determined from the value of r at infinite free-antigen concentration, where r/free = 0, in other words at the x-axis intercept. The analysis of a monoclonal IgG antibody molecule, in which there are two identical antigen-binding sites per molecule, is shown in the left panel. The slope of the line is determined by the affinity of the antibody molecule for its antigen; if all the antibody molecules in a preparation are identical, as for this monoclonal antibody, then a straight line is obtained whose slope is equal to $-K_a$, where K_a is the association (or affinity) constant and the dissociation constant $K_d = 1/K_a$. However, antiserum raised even against a simple antigenic determinant such as a hapten contains a heterogeneous population of antibody molecules (see Section A-1). Each antibody molecule would, if isolated, make up part of the total and give a straight line whose x-axis intercept is less than two, as this antibody molecule contains only a fraction of the total binding sites in the population (middle panel). As a mixture, they give curved lines with an x-axis intercept of two for which an average affinity ($\overline{K}_a$) can be determined from the slope of this line at a concentration of antigen where 50% of the sites are bound, or at x = 1 (right panel). The association constant determines the equilibrium state of the reaction Ag + Ab = Ag:Ab, where antigen = Ag and antibody = Ab, and $K_a =$ [Ag:Ab]/[Ag][Ab]. This constant reflects the 'on' and 'off' rates for antigen binding to the antibody; with small antigens such as haptens, binding is usually as rapid as diffusion allows, whereas differences in 'off' rates determine the affinity constant. However, with larger antigens the 'on' rate may also vary as the interaction becomes more complex.

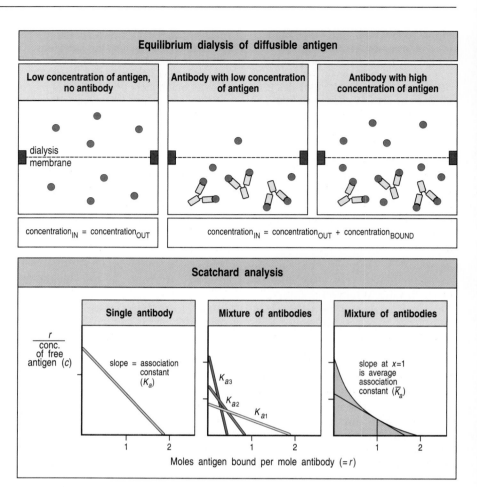

Whereas affinity measures the strength of binding of an antigenic determinant to a single antigen-binding site, an antibody reacting with an antigen that has multiple identical epitopes or with the surface of a pathogen will often bind the same molecule or particle with both of its antigen-binding sites. This increases the apparent strength of binding, since both binding sites must release at the same time in order for the two molecules to dissociate. This is often referred to as **cooperativity** in binding, but it should not be confused with the cooperative binding found in a protein such as hemoglobin, in which binding of ligand at one site enhances the affinity of a second binding site for its ligand. The overall strength of binding of an antibody molecule to an antigen or particle is called its avidity (Fig. A.12). For IgG antibodies, bivalent binding can significantly increase avidity; in IgM antibodies, which have ten identical antigen-binding sites, the affinity of each site for a monovalent antigen is usually quite low, but the avidity of binding of the whole antibody to a surface such as a bacterium that displays multiple identical epitopes can be very high.

A-10 Anti-immunoglobulin antibodies.

A general approach to the detection of bound antibody that avoids the need to label each preparation of antibody molecules is to detect bound, unlabeled antibody with a labeled antibody specific for immunoglobulins themselves. Immunoglobulins, like other proteins, are immunogenic when used to immunize individuals of another species. The majority of **anti-immunoglobulin antibodies** raised in this way recognize conserved features shared by all

Fig. A.12 The avidity of an antibody is its strength of binding to intact antigen. When an IgG antibody binds a ligand with multiple identical epitopes, both binding sites can bind the same molecule or particle. The overall strength of binding, called avidity, is greater than the affinity, the strength of binding of a single site, since both binding sites must dissociate at the same time for the antibody to release the antigen. This property is very important in the binding of antibody to bacteria, which usually have multiple identical epitopes on their surfaces.

immunoglobulin molecules of the immunizing species. Others can be specific for immunoglobulin chains, heavy or light chains, for example, or for individual isotypes. Antibodies raised by immunization of goats with mouse IgG are commonly used in experimental immunology. Such goat anti-mouse IgG antibodies can be purified using affinity chromatography, then labeled and used as a general probe for bound IgG antibodies. Anti-immunoglobulin antisera have found many uses in clinical medicine and biological research since their introduction. Fluorescently labeled anti-immunoglobulin antibodies are now widely used both in immunology and other areas of biology as secondary reagents for detecting specific antibodies bound, for example, to cell structures (see Sections A-14 and A-16). Labeled anti-immunoglobulin antibodies can also be used in radioimmunoassay or ELISA (see Section A-6) to detect binding of unlabeled antibody to antigen-coated plates.

Antibodies specific for individual immunoglobulin isotypes can be produced by immunizing an animal of a different species with a pure preparation of one isotype and then removing those antibodies that cross-react with immunoglobulins of other isotypes by using affinity chromatography (see Section A-5). **Anti-isotype antibodies** can be used to measure how much antibody of a particular isotype in an antiserum reacts with a given antigen. This reaction is particularly important for detecting small amounts of specific antibodies of the IgE isotype, which are responsible for most allergies. The presence in an individual's serum of IgE binding to an antigen correlates with allergic reactions to that antigen.

An alternative approach to detecting bound antibodies exploits bacterial proteins that bind to immunoglobulins with high affinity and specificity. One of these, **Protein A** from the bacterium *Staphylococcus aureus*, has been exploited widely in immunology for the affinity purification of immunoglobulin and for the detection of bound antibody. The use of standard second reagents such as labeled anti-immunoglobulin antibodies or Protein A to detect antibody bound specifically to its antigen allows great savings in reagent labeling costs, and also provides a standard detection system so that results in different assays can be compared directly.

A-11   Coombs tests and the detection of Rhesus incompatibility.

These tests use anti-immunoglobulin antibodies (see Section A-10) to detect the antibodies that cause **hemolytic disease of the newborn**, or **erythroblastosis fetalis**. Anti-immunoglobulin antibodies were first developed by Robin Coombs and the test for this disease is still called the Coombs test. Hemolytic disease of the newborn occurs when a mother makes IgG antibodies specific for the **Rhesus** or **Rh blood group antigen** expressed on the red blood cells of her fetus. Rh-negative mothers make these antibodies when they are exposed to Rh-positive fetal red blood cells bearing the paternally inherited Rh antigen. Maternal IgG antibodies are normally transported across the placenta to the fetus, where they protect the newborn infant against infection. However, IgG anti-Rh antibodies coat the fetal red blood cells, which are then destroyed by phagocytic cells in the liver, causing a hemolytic anemia in the fetus and newborn infant.

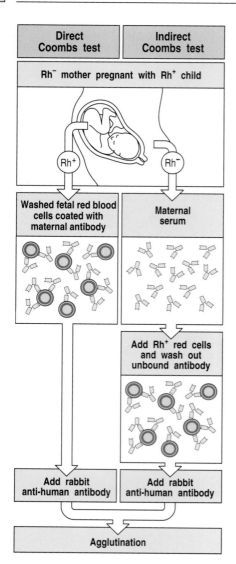

Direct Coombs test	Indirect Coombs test

Rh⁻ mother pregnant with Rh⁺ child

Washed fetal red blood cells coated with maternal antibody

Maternal serum

Add Rh⁺ red cells and wash out unbound antibody

Add rabbit anti-human antibody

Add rabbit anti-human antibody

Agglutination

Fig. A.13 The Coombs direct and indirect anti-globulin tests for antibody to red blood cell antigens. A Rh⁻ mother of a Rh⁺ fetus can become immunized to fetal red blood cells that enter the maternal circulation at the time of delivery. In a subsequent pregnancy with a Rh⁺ fetus, IgG anti-Rh antibodies can cross the placenta and damage the fetal red blood cells. In contrast to anti-Rh antibodies, maternal anti-ABO antibodies are of the IgM isotype and cannot cross the placenta, and so do not cause harm. Anti-Rh antibodies do not agglutinate red blood cells but their presence on the fetal red blood cell surface can be shown by washing away unbound immunoglobulin and then adding antibody to human immuno-globulin, which agglutinates the antibody-coated cells. Anti-Rh antibodies can be detected in the mother's serum in an indirect Coombs test; the serum is incubated with Rh⁺ red blood cells, and once the antibody binds, the red blood cells are treated as in the direct Coombs test.

Since the Rh antigens are widely spaced on the red blood cell surface, the IgG anti-Rh antibodies cannot fix complement and cause lysis of red blood cells *in vitro*. Furthermore, for reasons that are not fully understood, antibodies to Rh blood group antigens do not agglutinate red blood cells as do antibodies to the ABO blood group antigens. Thus, detecting these antibodies was difficult until anti-human immunoglobulin antibodies were developed. With these, maternal IgG antibodies bound to the fetal red blood cells can be detected after washing the cells to remove unbound immunoglobulin that is present in the fetal serum. Adding anti-human immunoglobulin antibodies to the washed fetal red blood cells agglutinates any cells to which maternal antibodies are bound. This is the **direct Coombs test** (Fig. A.13), so called because it directly detects antibody bound to the surface of the fetal red blood cells. An **indirect Coombs test** is used to detect nonagglutinating anti-Rh antibody in maternal serum; the serum is first incubated with Rh-positive red blood cells, which bind the anti-Rh antibody, after which the antibody-coated cells are washed to remove unbound immunoglobulin and are then agglutinated with anti-immunoglobulin antibody (see Fig. A.13). The indirect Coombs test allows Rh incompatibilities that might lead to hemolytic disease of the newborn to be detected, and this knowledge allows the disease to be prevented (see Section 10-25). The Coombs test is also commonly used to detect antibodies to drugs that bind to red blood cells and cause hemolytic anemia.

A-12 Monoclonal antibodies.

The antibodies generated in a natural immune response or after immunization in the laboratory are a mixture of molecules of different specificities and affinities. Some of this heterogeneity results from the production of antibodies that bind to different epitopes on the immunizing antigen, but even antibodies directed at a single antigenic determinant such as a hapten can be markedly heterogeneous, as shown by **isoelectric focusing**. In this technique, proteins are separated on the basis of their isoelectric point, the pH at which their net charge is zero. By electrophoresing proteins in a pH gradient for long enough, each molecule migrates along the pH gradient until it reaches the pH at which it is neutral and is thus concentrated (focused) at that point. When antiserum containing anti-hapten antibodies is treated in this way and then transferred to a solid support such as nitrocellulose paper, the anti-hapten antibodies can be detected by their ability to bind labeled hapten. The binding of antibodies of various isoelectric points to the hapten shows that even antibodies that bind the same antigenic determinant can be heterogeneous.

Antisera are valuable for many biological purposes but they have certain inherent disadvantages that relate to the heterogeneity of the antibodies they contain. First, each antiserum is different from all other antisera, even if raised in a genetically identical animal by using the identical preparation of antigen and the same immunization protocol. Second, antisera can be produced in only limited volumes, and thus it is impossible to use the identical serological reagent in a long or complex series of experiments or clinical tests. Finally, even antibodies purified by affinity chromatography (see Section A-5) may include minor populations of antibodies that give unexpected cross-reactions, which confound the analysis of experiments. To avoid these problems, and to harness the full potential of antibodies, it was necessary to develop a way of making an unlimited supply of antibody molecules of homogeneous structure and known specificity. This has been achieved through the production of monoclonal antibodies from cultures of hybrid antibody-forming cells or, more recently, by genetic engineering.

Biochemists in search of a homogeneous preparation of antibody that they could subject to detailed chemical analysis turned early to proteins produced by patients with multiple myeloma, a common tumor of plasma cells. It was known that antibodies are normally produced by plasma cells and since this disease is associated with the presence of large amounts of a homogeneous gamma globulin called a **myeloma protein** in the patient's serum, it seemed likely that myeloma proteins would serve as models for normal antibody molecules. Thus, much of the early knowledge of antibody structure came from studies on myeloma proteins. These studies showed that monoclonal antibodies could be obtained from immortalized plasma cells. However, the antigen specificity of most myeloma proteins was unknown, which limited their usefulness as objects of study or as immunological tools.

This problem was solved by Georges Köhler and Cesar Milstein, who devised a technique for producing a homogeneous population of antibodies of known antigenic specificity. They did this by fusing spleen cells from an immunized mouse to cells of a mouse myeloma to produce hybrid cells that both proliferated indefinitely and secreted antibody specific for the antigen used to immunize the spleen cell donor. The spleen cell provides the ability to make specific antibody, while the myeloma cell provides the ability to grow indefinitely in culture and secrete immunoglobulin continuously. By using a myeloma cell partner that produces no antibody proteins itself, the antibody produced by the hybrid cells comes only from the immune spleen cell partner. After fusion, the hybrid cells are selected using drugs that kill the myeloma parental cell, while the unfused parental spleen cells have a limited life-span and soon die, so that only hybrid myeloma cell lines or **hybridomas** survive. Those hybridomas producing antibody of the desired specificity are then identified and cloned by regrowing the cultures from single cells (Fig. A.14). Since each hybridoma is a **clone** derived from fusion with a single B cell, all the antibody molecules it produces are identical in structure, including their antigen-binding site and isotype. Such antibodies are called **monoclonal antibodies**. This technology has revolutionized the use of antibodies by providing a limitless supply of antibody of a single and known specificity. Monoclonal antibodies are now used in most serological assays, as diagnostic probes, and as therapeutic agents. So far, however, only mouse monoclonals are routinely produced and efforts to use this same approach to make human monoclonal antibodies have met with very limited success.

A-13 Phage display libraries for antibody V-region production.

This is a technique for producing antibody-like molecules. Gene segments encoding the antigen-binding variable or V domains of antibodies are fused to genes encoding the coat protein of a bacteriophage. Bacteriophage containing such gene fusions are used to infect bacteria, and the resulting phage particles have coats that express the antibody-like fusion protein, with

Spleen cells producing antibody from mouse immunized with antigen A	Myeloma cells (immortal) lacking antibody secretion and the enzyme HGPRT

Mix and fuse cells with PEG

Transfer to HAT medium

Immortal hybridomas proliferate; mortal spleen cells and unfused HGPRT⁻ myeloma cells die

Select hybridoma that makes antibody specific for antigen A

Clone selected hybridoma

Fig. A.14 The production of monoclonal antibodies. Mice are immunized with antigen A and given an intravenous booster immunization three days before they are killed, in order to produce a large population of spleen cells secreting specific antibody. Spleen cells die after a few days in culture. In order to produce a continuous source of antibody they are fused with immortal myeloma cells by using polyethylene glycol (PEG) to produce a hybrid cell line called a hybridoma. The myeloma cells are selected beforehand to ensure that they are not secreting antibody themselves and that they are sensitive to the hypoxanthine-aminopterin-thymidine (HAT) medium that is used to select hybrid cells because they lack the enzyme hypoxanthine:guanine phosphoribosyl transferase (HGPRT). The HGPRT gene contributed by the spleen cell allows hybrid cells to survive in the HAT medium, and only hybrid cells can grow continuously in culture because of the malignant potential contributed by the myeloma cells. Therefore, unfused myeloma cells and unfused spleen cells die in the HAT medium, as shown here by cells with dark, irregular nuclei. Individual hybridomas are then screened for antibody production, and cells that make antibody of the desired specificity are cloned by growing them up from a single antibody-producing cell. The cloned hybridoma cells are grown in bulk culture to produce large amounts of antibody. As each hybridoma is descended from a single cell, all the cells of a hybridoma cell line make the same antibody molecule, which is thus called a monoclonal antibody.

the antigen-binding domain displayed on the outside of the bacteriophage. A collection of recombinant phage, each displaying a different antigen-binding domain on its surface, is known as a **phage display library**. In much the same way that antibodies specific for a particular antigen can be isolated from a complex mixture by affinity chromatography (see Section A-5), phage expressing antigen-binding domains specific for a particular antigen can be isolated by selecting the phage in the library for binding to that antigen. The phage particles that bind are recovered and used to infect fresh bacteria. Each phage isolated in this way will produce a monoclonal antigen-binding particle analogous to a monoclonal antibody (Fig. A.15). The genes encoding the antigen-binding site, which are unique to each phage, can then be recovered from the phage DNA and used to construct genes for a complete antibody molecule by joining them to parts of immunoglobulin genes that encode the invariant parts of an antibody. When these reconstructed antibody genes are introduced into a suitable host cell line, such as the nonantibody-producing myeloma cells used for hybridomas, the transfected cells can secrete antibodies with all the desirable characteristics of monoclonal antibodies produced from hybridomas.

In much the same way that a collection of phage can display a wide variety of potential antigen-binding sites, the phage can also be engineered to display a wide variety of antigens; such a library is known as an **antigen display library**. In such cases, the antigens displayed are often short peptides encoded by chemically synthesized DNA sequences that have mixtures of all four nucleotides in some positions, so that all possible amino acids are incorporated. It is not usual for every position in a peptide to be allowed to vary in this way, since the number of different peptide sequences increases dramatically with the number of variable positions; there are over 2×10^{10} possible sequences of eight amino acids.

A-14   Immunofluorescence microscopy.

Since antibodies bind stably and specifically to their corresponding antigen, they are invaluable as probes for identifying a particular molecule in cells, tissues, or biological fluids. Antibody molecules can be used to locate their target molecules accurately in single cells or in tissue sections by a variety of

| Isolate population of genes encoding antibody variable regions | Construct fusion protein of V region with a bacteriophage coat protein | Cloning a random population of variable regions gives rise to a mixture of bacteriophage—a phage-display library | Select phage with desired V regions by specific binding to antigen |

different labeling techniques. When the antibody itself, or the anti-immunoglobulin antibody used to detect it, is labeled with a fluorescent dye the technique is known as **immunofluorescence microscopy**. As in all serological techniques, the antibody binds stably to its antigen, allowing unbound antibody to be removed by thorough washing. As antibodies to proteins recognize the surface features of the native, folded protein, the native structure of the protein being sought usually needs to be preserved, either by using only the most gentle chemical fixation techniques or by using frozen tissue sections that are fixed only after the antibody reaction has been performed. Some antibodies, however, bind proteins even if they are denatured, and such antibodies will bind specifically even to protein in fixed tissue sections.

The fluorescent dye can be covalently attached directly to the specific antibody, but more commonly, the bound antibody is detected by fluorescent anti-immunoglobulin, a technique known as **indirect immunofluorescence**. The dyes chosen for immunofluorescence are excited by light of one wavelength, usually blue or green, and emit light of a different wavelength in the visible spectrum. The most common fluorescent dyes are fluorescein, which emits green light, Texas Red and Peridinin chlorophyll protein (PerCP), which emit red light, and rhodamine and phycoerythrin (PE) which emit orange/red light (Fig. A.16). By using selective filters, only the light coming from the dye or fluorochrome used is detected in the fluorescence microscope (Fig. A.17). Although Albert Coons first devised this technique to identify the plasma cell as the source of antibody, it can be used to detect the distribution of any protein. By attaching different dyes to different antibodies, the distribution of two or more molecules can be determined in the same cell or tissue section (see Fig. A.17).

The recent development of the **confocal fluorescent microscope**, which uses computer-aided techniques to produce an ultrathin optical section of a cell or tissue, gives very high resolution immunofluorescence microscopy without the need for elaborate sample preparation. The resolution of the confocal microscope can be further increased using low-intensity illumination so that two photons are required to excite the fluorochrome. A pulsed laser beam is used, and only when it is focused into the focal plane of the microscope is the intensity sufficient to excite fluorescence. In this way the fluorescence emission itself can be restricted to the optical section.

One important development in the area of microscopy has been the use of **time-lapse video microscopy**, in which sensitive digital video cameras record the movement of fluorescently labeled molecules in cell membranes and their redistribution when cells come into contact with each other. Cell-surface molecules can be fluorescently labeled in two main ways. One is by the binding of fluorochrome-labeled Fab fragments of antibodies specific for

Fig. A.15 The production of antibodies by genetic engineering. Short primers to consensus sequences in heavy- and light-chain variable (V) regions of immunoglobulin genes are used to generate a library of heavy- and light-chain V-region DNAs by the polymerase chain reaction, with spleen DNA as the starting material. These heavy- and light-chain V-region genes are cloned randomly into a filamentous phage such that each phage expresses one heavy-chain and one light-chain V region as a surface fusion protein with antibody-like properties. The resulting phage display library is multiplied in bacteria, and the phage are then bound to a surface coated with antigen. The unbound phage are washed away; the bound phage are recovered, multiplied in bacteria, and again bound to antigen. After a few cycles, only specific high-affinity antigen-binding phage are left. These can be used like antibody molecules, or their V genes can be recovered and engineered into antibody genes to produce genetically engineered antibody molecules (not shown). This technology may replace the hybridoma technology for producing monoclonal antibodies and has the advantage that humans can be used as the source of DNA.

Fig. A.16 Excitation and emission wavelengths for common fluorochromes.

Excitation and emission wavelengths of some commonly used fluorochromes		
Probe	Excitation (nm)	Emission (nm)
R-phycoerythrin (PE)	480; 565	578
Fluorescein	495	519
PerCP	490	675
Texas Red	589	615
Rhodamine	550	573

the protein of interest; the other is by generating a fusion protein, in which the protein of interest has been attached to one of a family of fluorescent proteins obtained from jellyfish. The first of these fluorescent proteins to come into wide use was green fluorescent protein (GFP), isolated from the jellyfish, *Aequorea victoria*. Other variants of this protein with different properties are now available, and the list of available fluorescent labels now includes red, blue, cyan, or yellow fluorescent proteins. Using cells transfected with the genes encoding such fusion proteins, it is possible to show the redistribution of T-cell receptors, co-receptors, adhesion molecules, and other signaling molecules, such as CD45, that takes place when a T cell makes contact with a target cell. It is clear from these observations that the interface between the T cell and its target does not represent a simple apposition of two cell membranes, but is an actively organized and dynamic structure, often now referred to as the 'immunological synapse.'

A-15 Immunoelectron microscopy.

Antibodies can be used to detect the intracellular location of structures or particular proteins at high resolution by electron microscopy, a technique known as **immunoelectron microscopy**. Antibodies against the required antigen are labeled with gold particles and then applied to ultrathin sections, which are then examined in the transmission electron microscope. Antibodies labeled with gold particles of different diameters enable two or more proteins to be studied simultaneously (see Fig. 5.8). The difficulty with this technique is in staining the ultrathin section adequately, as few molecules of antigen are present in each section.

Fig. A.17 Immunofluorescence microscopy. Antibodies labeled with a fluorescent dye such as fluorescein (green triangle) are used to reveal the presence of their corresponding antigens in cells or tissues. The stained cells are examined in a microscope that exposes them to blue or green light to excite the fluorescent dye. The excited dye emits light at a characteristic wavelength, which is captured by viewing the sample through a selective filter. This technique is applied widely in biology to determine the location of molecules in cells and tissues. Different antigens can be detected in tissue sections by labeling antibodies with dyes of distinctive color. Here, antibodies to the protein glutamic acid decarboxylase (GAD) coupled to a green dye are shown to stain the β cells of pancreatic islets of Langerhans. The α cells do not make this enzyme and are labeled with antibodies to the hormone glucagon coupled with an orange fluorescent dye. GAD is an important antigen in diabetes, a disease in which the insulin-secreting β cells of the islets of Langerhans are destroyed by an immune attack on self tissues (see Chapter 13). Photograph courtesy of M. Solimena and P. De Camilli.

A-16 Immunohistochemistry.

An alternative to immunofluorescence (see Section A-14) for detecting a protein in tissue sections is **immunohistochemistry**, in which the specific antibody is chemically coupled to an enzyme that converts a colorless substrate into a colored reaction product *in situ*. The localized deposition of the colored product where antibody has bound can be directly observed under a light microscope. The antibody binds stably to its antigen, allowing unbound antibody to be removed by thorough washing. This method of detecting bound antibody is analogous to ELISA (see Section A-6) and frequently uses the same coupled enzymes, the difference in detection being primarily that in immunohistochemistry the colored products are insoluble and precipitate at the site where they are formed. Horseradish peroxidase and alkaline phosphatase are the two enzymes most commonly used in these applications. Horseradish peroxidase oxidises the substrate diaminobenzidine to produce a brown precipitate, while alkaline phosphatase can produce red or blue dyes depending on the substrates used; a common substrate is 5-bromo-4-chloro-3-indolyl phosphate plus nitroblue tetrazolium (BCIP/NBT), which gives rise to a dark blue or purple stain. As with immunofluorescence, the native structure of the protein being sought usually needs to be preserved, so that it will be recognized by the antibody. Tissues are fixed by the most gentle chemical fixation techniques or frozen tissue sections are used that are fixed only after the antibody reaction has been performed.

A-17 Immunoprecipitation and co-immunoprecipitation.

In order to raise antibodies to membrane proteins and other cellular structures that are difficult to purify, mice are often immunized with whole cells or crude cell extracts. Antibodies to the individual molecules are then obtained by using these immunized mice to produce hybridomas making monoclonal antibodies (see Section A-12) that bind to the cell type used for immunization. To characterize the molecules identified by the antibodies, cells of the same type are labeled with radioisotopes and dissolved in nonionic detergents that disrupt cell membranes but do not interfere with antigen–antibody interactions. This allows the labeled protein to be isolated by binding to the antibody in a reaction known as **immunoprecipitation**. The antibody is usually attached to a solid support, such as the beads that are used in affinity chromatography (see Section A-5), or to Protein A. Cells can be labeled in two main ways for immunoprecipitation analysis. All the proteins in a cell can be labeled metabolically by growing the cell in radioactive amino acids that are incorporated into cellular protein (Fig. A.18). Alternatively, one can label only

Fig. A.18 Cellular proteins reacting with an antibody can be characterized by immunoprecipitation of labeled cell lysates. All actively synthesized cellular proteins can be labeled metabolically by incubating cells with radioactive amino acids (shown here for methionine) or one can label just the cell-surface proteins by using radioactive iodine in a form that cannot cross the cell membrane or by a reaction with the small molecule biotin, detected by its reaction with labeled avidin (not shown). Cells are lysed with detergent and individual labeled cell-associated proteins can be precipitated with a monoclonal antibody attached to beads. After unbound proteins have been washed away, the bound protein is eluted in the detergent sodium dodecyl sulfate (SDS), which dissociates it from the antibody and also coats the protein with a strong negative charge, allowing it to migrate according to its size in polyacrylamide gel electrophoresis (PAGE). The positions of the labeled proteins are determined by auto-radiography using X-ray film. This technique of SDS-PAGE can be used to determine the molecular weight and subunit composition of a protein. Patterns of protein bands observed with metabolic labeling are usually more complex than those revealed by radioiodination, owing to the presence of precursor forms of the protein (right panel). The mature form of a surface protein can be identified as being the same size as that detected by surface iodination or biotinylation (not shown).

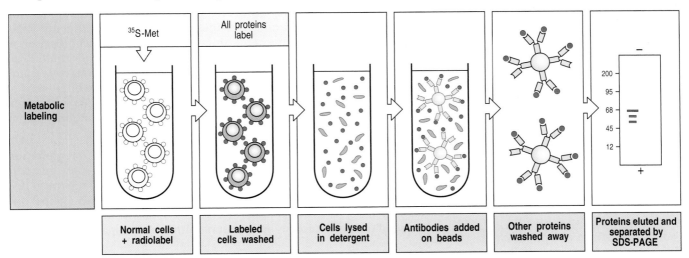

| Metabolic labeling | Normal cells + radiolabel | Labeled cells washed | Cells lysed in detergent | Antibodies added on beads | Other proteins washed away | Proteins eluted and separated by SDS-PAGE |

Fig. A.19 Two-dimensional gel electrophoresis of MHC class II molecules. Proteins in mouse spleen cells have been labeled metabolically (see Fig. A.18), precipitated with a monoclonal antibody against the mouse MHC class II molecule H2-A, and separated by isoelectric focusing in one direction and SDS-PAGE in a second direction at right angles to the first; hence the term two-dimensional gel electrophoresis. This allows one to distinguish molecules of the same molecular weight on the basis of their charge. The separated proteins are detected by autoradiography. The MHC class II molecules are composed of two chains, α and β, and in the different MHC class II molecules these have different isoelectric points (compare upper and lower panels). The MHC genotype of mice is indicated by lower case superscripts (k,p). Actin, a common contaminant, is marked a. Photographs courtesy of J.F. Babich.

the cell-surface proteins by radioiodination under conditions that prevent iodine from crossing the plasma membrane and labeling proteins inside the cell, or by a reaction that labels only membrane proteins with biotin, a small molecule that is detected readily by labeled avidin, a protein found in egg whites that binds biotin with very high affinity.

Once the labeled proteins have been isolated by the antibody, they can be characterized in several ways. The most common is polyacrylamide gel electrophoresis (PAGE) of the proteins after dissociating them from antibody in the strong ionic detergent sodium dodecyl sulfate (SDS), a technique generally abbreviated as **SDS-PAGE**. SDS binds relatively homogeneously to proteins, conferring a charge that allows the electrophoretic field to drive protein migration through the gel. The rate of migration is controlled mainly by protein size (see Fig. A.18). Proteins of differing charges can be separated using isoelectric focusing (see Section A-12). This technique can be combined with SDS-PAGE in a procedure known as **two-dimensional gel electrophoresis**. For this, the immunoprecipitated protein is eluted in urea, a nonionic solubilizing agent, and run on an isoelectric focusing gel in a narrow tube of polyacrylamide. This first-dimensional isoelectric focusing gel is then placed across the top of an SDS-PAGE slab gel, which is then run vertically to separate the proteins by molecular weight (Fig. A.19). Two-dimensional gel electrophoresis is a powerful technique that allows many hundreds of proteins in a complex mixture to be distinguished from one another.

Immunoprecipitation and the related technique of immunoblotting (see Section A-18) are useful for determining the molecular weight and isoelectric point of a protein as well as its abundance, distribution, and whether, for example, it undergoes changes in molecular weight and isoelectric point as a result of processing within the cell.

A-18 Immunoblotting (Western blotting).

Like immunoprecipitation (see Section A-17), **immunoblotting** is used for identifying the presence of a given protein in a cell lysate, but it avoids the problem of having to label large quantities of cells with radioisotopes. Unlabeled cells are placed in detergent to solubilize all cell proteins and the lysate is run on SDS-PAGE to separate the proteins (see Section A-17). The size-separated proteins are then transferred from the gel to a stable support such as a nitrocellulose membrane. Specific proteins are detected by treatment with antibodies able to react with SDS-solubilized proteins (mainly those that react with denatured sequences); the bound antibodies are revealed by anti-immunoglobulin antibodies labeled with radioisotopes or an enzyme. The term **Western blotting** as a synonym for immunoblotting arose because the comparable technique for detecting specific DNA sequences is known as Southern blotting, after Ed Southern who devised it, which in turn provoked the name Northern for blots of size-separated RNA, and Western for blots of size-separated proteins. Western blots have many applications in basic research and clinical diagnosis. They are often used to test sera for the presence of antibodies to specific proteins, for example to detect antibodies to different constituents of the human immunodeficiency virus, HIV (Fig. A.20).

Co-immunoprecipitation is an extension of the immunoprecipitation technique which is used to determine whether a given protein interacts physically with another given protein. Cell extracts containing the presumed interaction complex are first immunoprecipitated with antibody against one of the proteins. The material identified by this means is then tested for the presence of the other protein by immunoblotting with a specific antibody.

Fig. A.20 Western blotting is used to identify antibodies to the human immunodeficiency virus (HIV) in serum from infected individuals. The virus is dissociated into its constituent proteins by treatment with the detergent SDS, and its proteins are separated using SDS-PAGE. The separated proteins are transferred to a nitrocellulose sheet and reacted with the test serum. Anti-HIV antibodies in the serum bind to the various HIV proteins and are detected with enzyme-linked anti-human immunoglobulin, which deposits colored material from a colorless substrate. This general methodology will detect any combination of antibody and antigen and is used widely, although the denaturing effect of SDS means that the technique works most reliably with antibodies that recognize the antigen when it is denatured.

A-19 Use of antibodies in the isolation and identification of genes and their products.

As a first step in isolating the gene that codes for a particular protein, antibodies specific for the protein can be used to isolate the purified protein from cells using affinity chromatography (see Section A-5). Small amounts of amino acid sequence can then be obtained from the protein's amino-terminal end or from peptide fragments generated by proteolysis. The information in these amino acid sequences is used to construct a set of synthetic oligonucleotides corresponding to the possible DNA sequences, which are then used as probes to isolate the gene encoding the protein from either a library of DNA sequences complementary to mRNA (a cDNA library) or a genomic DNA library (a library of chromosomal DNA fragments).

An alternative approach to gene identification uses antibodies to identify the protein product of a gene that has been introduced into a cell that does not normally express it. This technique is most commonly applied to the identification of genes encoding cell-surface proteins. A set of cDNA-containing expression vectors is first made from a cDNA library prepared from the total mRNA from a cell type that does express the protein of interest. The vectors are used to transfect a cell type that does not normally express the protein of interest, and the vector drives expression of the cDNA it contains without integrating into the host cell DNA. Cells expressing the required protein after transfection are then isolated by binding to specific antibodies that detect the presence of the protein on the cell surface. The vector containing the required gene can then be recovered from these cells (Fig. A.21).

The recovered vectors are then introduced into bacterial cells where they replicate rapidly, and these amplified vectors are used in a second round of transfection in mammalian cells. After several cycles of transfection, isolation, and amplification in bacteria, single colonies of bacteria are picked and the vectors prepared from cultures of each colony are used in a final transfection to identify a cloned vector carrying the cDNA of interest, which is then isolated and characterized. This methodology has been used to isolate many genes encoding cell-surface molecules.

The full amino acid sequence of the protein can be deduced from the nucleotide sequence of its cDNA, and this often gives clues to the nature of the protein and its biological properties. The nucleotide sequence of the gene and its regulatory regions can be determined from genomic DNA clones. The gene can be manipulated and introduced into cells by transfection for larger-scale production and functional studies. This approach has been used to characterize many immunologically important proteins, such as the MHC glycoproteins.

The converse approach is taken to identify the unknown protein product of a cloned gene. The gene sequence is used to construct synthetic peptides of 10–20 amino acids that are identical to part of the deduced protein sequence,

| Clone cDNAs obtained from cell mRNAs into expression vectors | Transfect the cDNAs into fibroblast cells where they propagate as episomes | Antibodies identify the cells expressing the desired protein | The cells are purified and disrupted, releasing the vector containing the desired cDNA clone |

Fig. A.21 The gene encoding a cell-surface molecule can be isolated by expressing it in fibroblasts and detecting its protein product with monoclonal antibodies. Total mRNA from a cell line or tissue expressing the protein is isolated, converted into cDNA, and cloned as cDNAs in a vector designed to direct expression of the cDNA in fibroblasts. The entire cDNA library is used to transfect cultured fibroblasts. Fibroblasts that have taken up cDNA encoding a cell-surface protein express the protein on their surface; they can be isolated by binding a monoclonal antibody against that protein. The vector containing the gene is isolated from the cells that express the antigen and used for more rounds of transfection and reisolation until uniform positive expression is obtained, ensuring that the correct gene has been isolated. The cDNA insert can then be sequenced to determine the sequence of the protein it encodes and can also be used as the source of material for large-scale expression of the protein for analysis of its structure and function. The method illustrated is limited to cloning genes for single-chain proteins (that is, those encoded by only one gene) that can be expressed in fibroblasts. It has been used to clone many genes of immunological interest such as that for CD4.

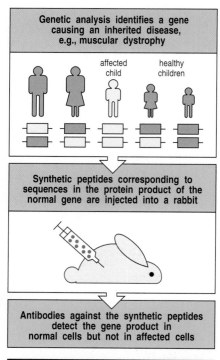

| Genetic analysis identifies a gene causing an inherited disease, e.g., muscular dystrophy |

affected child   healthy children

| Synthetic peptides corresponding to sequences in the protein product of the normal gene are injected into a rabbit |

| Antibodies against the synthetic peptides detect the gene product in normal cells but not in affected cells |

and antibodies are then raised against these peptides by coupling them to carrier proteins; the peptides behave as haptens. These anti-peptide antibodies often bind the native protein and so can be used to identify its distribution in cells and tissues and to try to ascertain its function (Fig. A.22). This approach to identifying the function of a gene is often called 'reverse genetics' as it works from gene to phenotype rather than from phenotype to gene, which is the classical genetic approach. The great advantage of reverse genetics over the classical approach is that it does not require a detectable phenotypic genetic trait in order to identify a gene.

Antibodies can also be used in the determination of the function of gene products. Some antibodies are able to act as agonists, when the binding of the antibody to the molecule mimics the binding of the natural ligand and activates the function of the gene product. For example, antibodies to the CD3 molecule have been used to stimulate T cells, replacing the interaction of the T-cell receptor with MHC:peptide antigens in cases where the specific peptide antigen is not known. Conversely, antibodies can function as antagonists, inhibiting the binding of the natural ligand and thus blocking the function.

Fig. A.22 The use of antibodies to detect the unknown protein product of a known gene is called reverse genetics. When the gene responsible for a genetic disorder such as Duchenne muscular dystrophy is isolated, the amino acid sequence of the unknown protein product of the gene can be deduced from the nucleotide sequence of the gene, and synthetic peptides representing parts of this sequence can be made. Antibodies are raised against these peptides and purified from the antiserum by affinity chromatography on a peptide column (see Fig. A.5). Labeled antibody is used to stain tissue from individuals with the disease and from unaffected individuals to determine differences in the presence, amount, and distribution of the normal gene product. The product of the dystrophin gene is present in normal mouse skeletal muscle cells, as shown in the bottom panel (red fluorescence), but is missing from the cells of mice bearing the mutation *mdx*, the mouse equivalent of Duchenne muscular dystrophy (not shown). Photograph (× 15) courtesy of H.G.W. Lidov and L. Kunkel.

Isolation of lymphocytes.

A-20   Isolation of peripheral blood lymphocytes by Ficoll-Hypaque™ gradient.

The first step in studying lymphocytes is to isolate them so that their behavior can be analyzed *in vitro*. Human lymphocytes can be isolated most readily from peripheral blood by density centrifugation over a step gradient consisting of a mixture of the carbohydrate polymer Ficoll™ and the dense iodine-containing compound metrizamide. This yields a population of mononuclear cells at the interface that has been depleted of red blood cells and most polymorphonuclear leukocytes or granulocytes (Fig. A.23). The resulting population, called **peripheral blood mononuclear cells**, consists mainly of lymphocytes and monocytes. Although this population is readily accessible, it is not necessarily representative of the lymphoid system, as only recirculating lymphocytes can be isolated from blood.

A particular cell population can be isolated from a sample or culture by binding to antibody-coated plastic surfaces, a technique known as **panning**, or by removing unwanted cells by treatment with specific antibody and complement to kill them. Cells can also be passed over columns of antibody-coated, nylon-coated steel wool and different populations differentially eluted. This technique extends affinity chromatography to cells, and is now a very popular way to separate cells. All these techniques can also be used as a pre-purification step prior to sorting out highly purified populations by FACS (see Section A-22).

A-21   Isolation of lymphocytes from tissues other than blood.

In experimental animals, and occasionally in humans, lymphocytes are isolated from lymphoid organs, such as spleen, thymus, bone marrow, lymph nodes, or mucosal-associated lymphoid tissues, most commonly the palatine tonsils in humans (see Fig. 1.7). A specialized population of lymphocytes resides in surface epithelia; these cells are isolated by fractionating the epithelial layer after its detachment from the basement membrane. Finally, in situations where local immune responses are prominent, lymphocytes can be isolated from the site of the response itself. For example, in order to study the autoimmune reaction that is thought to be responsible for rheumatoid arthritis, an inflammatory response in joints, lymphocytes are isolated from the fluid aspirated from the inflamed joint space.

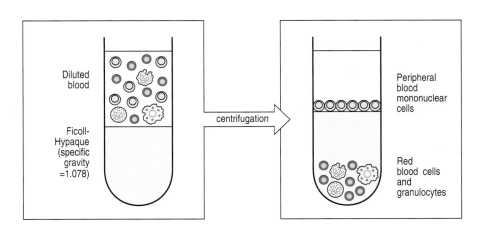

Diluted blood

Ficoll-Hypaque (specific gravity =1.078)

centrifugation

Peripheral blood mononuclear cells

Red blood cells and granulocytes

Fig. A.23 Peripheral blood mononuclear cells can be isolated from whole blood by Ficoll-Hypaque™ centrifugation. Diluted anticoagulated blood (left panel) is layered over Ficoll-Hypaque™ and centrifuged. Red blood cells and polymorphonuclear leukocytes or granulocytes are more dense and centrifuge through the Ficoll-Hypaque™, while mononuclear cells consisting of lymphocytes together with some monocytes band over it and can be recovered at the interface (right panel).

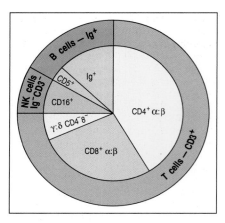

Fig. A.24 The distribution of lymphocyte subpopulations in human peripheral blood. As shown on the outside of the circle, lymphocytes can be divided into T cells bearing T-cell receptors (detected with anti-CD3 antibodies), B cells bearing immuno-globulin receptors (detected with anti-immunoglobulin antibodies), and null cells including natural killer (NK) cells, that label with neither. Further divisions of the T-cell and B-cell populations are shown inside. Using anti-CD4 and anti-CD8 antibodies, α:β T cells can be subdivided into two populations, whereas γ:δ T cells are identified with antibodies against the γ:δ T-cell receptor and mainly lack CD4 and CD8. A minority population of B cells express CD5 on their surface (see Section 7-28).

A-22 Flow cytometry and FACS analysis.

Resting lymphocytes present a deceptively uniform appearance, all being small round cells with a dense nucleus and little cytoplasm (see Fig. 1.5). However, these cells comprise many functional subpopulations, which are usually identified and distinguished from each other on the basis of their differential expression of cell-surface proteins, which can be detected using specific antibodies (Fig. A.24). B and T lymphocytes, for example, are identified unambiguously and separated from each other by antibodies to the constant regions of the B- and T-cell antigen receptors. T cells are further subdivided on the basis of expression of the co-receptor proteins CD4 and CD8.

An immensely powerful tool for defining and enumerating lymphocytes is the flow cytometer, which detects and counts individual cells passing in a stream through a laser beam. A flow cytometer equipped to separate the identified cells is called a **fluorescence-activated cell sorter** (**FACS**). These instruments are used to study the properties of cell subsets identified using monoclonal antibodies to cell-surface proteins. Individual cells within a mixed population are first tagged by treatment with specific monoclonal antibodies labeled with fluorescent dyes, or by specific antibodies followed by labeled anti-immunoglobulin antibodies. The mixture of labeled cells is then forced with a much larger volume of saline through a nozzle, creating a fine stream of liquid containing cells spaced singly at intervals. As each cell passes through a laser beam it scatters the laser light, and any dye molecules bound to the cell will be excited and will fluoresce. Sensitive photomultiplier tubes detect both the scattered light, which gives information on the size and granularity of the cell, and the fluorescence emissions, which give information on the binding of the labeled monoclonal antibodies and hence on the expression of cell-surface proteins by each cell (Fig. A.25).

In the cell sorter, the signals passed back to the computer are used to generate an electric charge, which is passed from the nozzle through the liquid stream at the precise time that the stream breaks up into droplets, each containing no more than a single cell; droplets containing a charge can then be deflected from the main stream of droplets as they pass between plates of opposite charge, so that positively charged droplets are attracted to a negatively charged plate, and vice versa. In this way, specific subpopulations of cells, distinguished by the binding of the labeled antibody, can be purified from a mixed population of cells. Alternatively, to deplete a population of cells, the same fluorochrome can be used to label different antibodies directed at marker proteins expressed by the various undesired cell types. The cell sorter can be used to direct labeled cells to a waste channel, retaining only the unlabeled cells.

When cells are labeled with a single fluorescent antibody, the data from a flow cytometer are usually displayed in the form of a histogram of fluorescence intensity versus cell numbers. If two or more antibodies are used, each coupled to different fluorescent dyes, then the data are more usually displayed in the form of a two-dimensional scatter diagram or as a contour diagram, where the fluorescence of one dye-labeled antibody is plotted against that of a second, with the result that a population of cells labeling with one antibody can be further subdivided by its labeling with the second antibody (see Fig. A.25). By examining large numbers of cells, flow cytometry can give quantitative data on the percentage of cells bearing different molecules, such as surface immunoglobulin, which characterizes B cells, the T-cell receptor-associated molecules known as CD3, and the CD4 and CD8 co-receptor proteins that distinguish the major T-cell subsets. Likewise, FACS analysis has been instrumental in defining stages in the early development of B and T cells. As the power of the FACS technology has grown, progressively more anti-bodies labeled with distinct fluorescent dyes can be used at the same time. Three-, four-, and even five-color analyses can now be handled by very powerful machines. FACS analysis has been applied to a broad range of problems in immunology; indeed, it played a vital role in the early identification of AIDS as a disease in which T cells bearing CD4 are depleted selectively (see Chapter 11).

Fig. A.25 The FACS™ allows individual cells to be identified by their cell-surface antigens and to be sorted. Cells to be analyzed by flow cytometry are first labeled with fluorescent dyes (top panel). Direct labeling uses dye-coupled antibodies specific for cell-surface antigens (as shown here), while indirect labeling uses a dye-coupled immunoglobulin to detect unlabeled cell-bound antibody. The cells are forced through a nozzle in a single-cell stream that passes through a laser beam (second panel). Photomultiplier tubes (PMTs) detect the scattering of light, which is a sign of cell size and granularity, and emissions from the different fluorescent dyes. This information is analyzed by computer (CPU). By examining many cells in this way, the number of cells with a specific set of characteristics can be counted and levels of expression of various molecules on these cells can be measured. The lower part of the figure shows how this data can be represented, using the expression of two surface immunoglobulins, IgM and IgD, on a sample of B cells from a mouse spleen. The two immunoglobulins have been labeled with different colored dyes. When the expression of just one type of molecule is to be analyzed (IgM or IgD), the data is usually displayed as a histogram, as in the left-hand panels. Histograms display the distribution of cells expressing a single measured parameter (for example, size, granularity, fluorescence intensity). When two or more parameters are measured for each cell (IgM and IgD), various types of two-color plots can be used to display the data, as shown in the right-hand panel. All four plots represent the same data. The horizontal axis represents intensity of IgM fluorescence and the vertical axis the intensity of IgD fluorescence. Two-color plots provide more information than histograms; they allow recognition, for example, of cells that are 'bright' for both colors, 'dull' for one and bright for the other, dull for both, negative for both, and so on. For example, the cluster of dots in the extreme lower left portions of the plots represents cells that do not express either immunoglobulin, and are mostly T cells. The standard dot plot (upper left) places a single dot for each cell whose fluorescence is measured. It is good for picking up cells that lie outside the main groups but tends to saturate in areas containing a large number of cells of the same type. A second means of presenting these data is the color dot plot (lower left), which uses color density to indicate high-density areas. A contour plot (upper right) draws 5% 'probability' contours, with 5% of the cells lying between each contour providing the best monochrome visualization of regions of high and low density. The lower right plot is a 5% probability contour map which also shows outlying cells as dots.

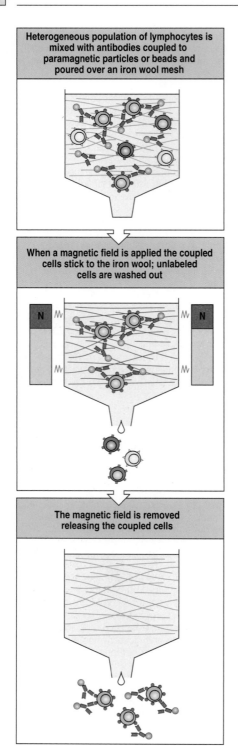

Heterogeneous population of lymphocytes is mixed with antibodies coupled to paramagnetic particles or beads and poured over an iron wool mesh

When a magnetic field is applied the coupled cells stick to the iron wool; unlabeled cells are washed out

The magnetic field is removed releasing the coupled cells

Fig. A.26 Lymphocyte subpopulations can be separated physically by using antibodies coupled to paramagnetic particles or beads. A mouse monoclonal antibody specific for a particular cell-surface molecule is coupled to paramagnetic particles or beads. It is mixed with a heterogeneous population of lymphocytes and poured over an iron wool mesh in a column. A magnetic field is applied so that the antibody-bound cells stick to the iron wool while cells which have not bound antibody are washed out; these cells are said to be negatively selected for lack of the molecule in question. The bound cells are released by removing the magnetic field; they are said to be positively selected for presence of the antigen recognized by the antibody.

A-23   Lymphocyte isolation using antibody-coated magnetic beads.

Although the FACS is superb for isolating small numbers of cells in pure form, when large numbers of lymphocytes must be prepared quickly, mechanical means of separating cells are preferable. A powerful and efficient way of isolating lymphocyte populations is to couple paramagnetic beads to monoclonal antibodies that recognize distinguishing cell-surface molecules. These antibody-coated beads are mixed with the cells to be separated, and run through a column containing material that attracts the paramagnetic beads when the column is placed in a strong magnetic field. Cells binding the magnetically labeled antibodies are retained; cells lacking the appropriate surface molecule can be washed away (Fig. A.26). The bound cells are positively selected for expression of the particular cell-surface molecule, while the unbound cells are negatively selected for its absence.

A-24   Isolation of homogeneous T-cell lines.

The analysis of specificity and effector function in T cells depends heavily on the study of monoclonal populations of T lymphocytes. These can be obtained in four distinct ways. First, as for B-cell hybridomas (see Section A-12), normal T cells proliferating in response to specific antigen can be fused to malignant T-cell lymphoma lines to generate **T-cell hybrids**. The hybrids express the receptor of the normal T cell, but proliferate indefinitely owing to the cancerous state of the lymphoma parent. T-cell hybrids can be cloned to yield a population of cells all having the same T-cell receptor. When stimulated by their specific antigen these cells release cytokines such as the T-cell growth factor interleukin-2 (IL-2), and the production of cytokines is used as an assay to assess the antigen specificity of the T-cell hybrid.

T-cell hybrids are excellent tools for the analysis of T-cell specificity, as they grow readily in suspension culture. However, they cannot be used to analyze the regulation of specific T-cell proliferation in response to antigen because they are continually dividing. T-cell hybrids also cannot be transferred into an animal to test for function *in vivo* because they would give rise to tumors. Functional analysis of T-cell hybrids is also confounded by the fact that the malignant partner cell affects their behavior in functional assays. Therefore, the regulation of T-cell growth and the effector functions of T cells must be studied using **T-cell clones**. These are clonal cell lines of a single T-cell type and antigen specificity, which are derived from cultures of heterogeneous T cells, called **T-cell lines**, whose growth is dependent on periodic restimulation with specific antigen and, frequently, on the addition of T-cell growth factors (Fig. A.27). T-cell clones also require periodic restimulation with antigen and are more tedious to grow than T-cell hybrids but, because their growth depends on specific antigen recognition, they maintain antigen specificity, which is often lost in T-cell hybrids. Cloned T-cell lines can be used for studies of effector function both *in vitro* and *in vivo*. In addition, the proliferation of T cells, a critical aspect of clonal selection, can be characterized only in cloned T-cell lines, where such growth is dependent on antigen recognition. Thus, both types of monoclonal T-cell line have valuable applications in experimental studies.

Studies of human T cells have relied largely on T-cell clones because a suitable fusion partner for making T-cell hybrids has not been identified. However, a human T-cell lymphoma line, called Jurkat, has been characterized extensively because it secretes IL-2 when its antigen receptor is cross-linked with anti-receptor monoclonal antibodies. This simple assay system has yielded much information about signal transduction in T cells. One of the Jurkat cell line's most interesting features, shared with T-cell hybrids, is that it stops growing when its antigen receptor is cross-linked. This has allowed mutants lacking the receptor or having defects in signal transduction pathways to be selected simply by culturing the cells with anti-receptor antibody and selecting those that continue to grow. Thus, T-cell tumors, T-cell hybrids, and cloned T-cell lines all have valuable applications in experimental immunology.

Finally, primary T cells from any source can be isolated as single, antigen-specific cells by limiting dilution rather than by first establishing a mixed population of T cells in culture as a T-cell line and then deriving clonal subpopulations. During the growth of T-cell lines, particular T-cell clones can come to dominate the cultures and give a false picture of the number and specificities in the original sample. Direct cloning of primary T cells avoids this artifact.

Characterization of lymphocyte specificity, frequency, and function.

B cells are relatively easy to characterize as they have only one function—antibody production. T cells are more difficult to characterize as there are several different classes with different functions. It is also technically more difficult to study the membrane-bound T-cell receptors than the antibodies secreted in large amounts by B cells. All the methods in this part of the appendix can be used for T cells. Some are also used to detect and count B cells.

On many occasions it is important to know the frequency of antigen-specific lymphocytes, especially T cells, in order to measure the efficiency with which an individual responds to a particular antigen, for example, or the degree to which specific immunological memory has been established. There are a number of methods for doing this, either by detecting the cells directly by the specificity of their receptor, or by detecting activation of the cells to provide some particular function, such as cytokine secretion or cytotoxicity.

The first technique of this type to be established was the limiting-dilution culture (see Section A-25), in which the frequency of specific T or B cells responding to a particular antigen could be estimated by plating the cells into 96-well plates at increasing dilutions and measuring the number of wells in which there was no response. However, in this type of assay it became laborious to ask detailed questions about the phenotype of the responding cells, and to compare responses from different cell subpopulations.

A simpler assay for measuring the responses of T-cell populations has been developed from a variant of the antigen-capture ELISA method (see Section A-6), called the ELISPOT assay (see Section A-26). It assays T cells on the basis of cytokine production. In the ELISPOT assay, cytokine secreted by individual

T cells from an immunized animal comprise a mixture of cells with different specificities

The T cells are placed into culture with antigen-presenting cells and antigen. Antigen-specific T cells proliferate while T cells that do not recognize the antigen do not proliferate

Antigen-specific T cells can be cloned by limiting-dilution culture in IL-2

Fig. A.27 Production of cloned T-cell lines. T cells from an immune donor, comprising a mixture of cells with different specificities, are activated with antigen and antigen-presenting cells. Single responding cells are cultured by limiting dilution in the T-cell growth factor IL-2, which selectively stimulates the responding cells to proliferate. From these single cells, cloned lines specific for antigen are identified and can be propagated by culture with antigen, antigen-presenting cells, and IL-2.

Fig. A.28 The frequency of specific lymphocytes can be determined using limiting-dilution assay. Varying numbers of lymphoid cells from normal or immunized mice are added to individual culture wells and stimulated with antigen and antigen-presenting cells (APCs) or polyclonal mitogen and added growth factors. After several days, the wells are tested for a specific response to antigen, such as cytotoxic killing of target cells. Each well that initially contained a specific T cell will make a response to its target, and from the Poisson distribution one can determine that when 37% of the wells are negative, each well contained, on average, one specific T cell at the beginning of the culture. In the example shown, for the unimmunized mouse 37% of the wells are negative when 160,000 T cells have been added to each well; thus the frequency of antigen-specific T cells is 1 in 160,000. When the mouse is immunized, 37% of the wells are negative when only 1100 T cells have been added; hence the frequency of specific T cells after immunization is 1 in 1100, an increase in responsive cells of 150-fold.

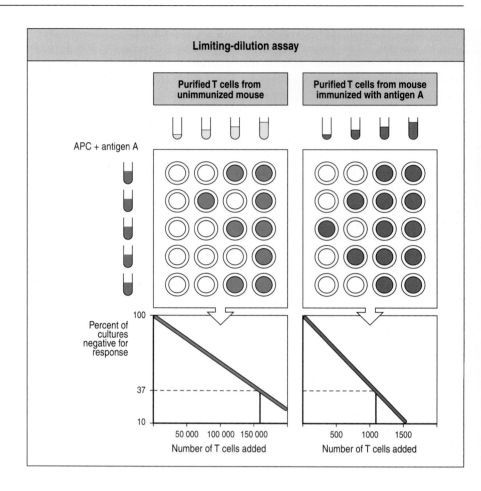

activated T cells is immobilized as discrete spots on a plastic plate, which are counted to give the number of activated T cells. The ELISPOT assay suffers from many of the same problems as the limiting-dilution assay in giving information about the nature of the activated cells, and it can be difficult to determine whether individual cells are capable of secreting mixtures of cytokines. It was therefore important to develop assays that could make these measurements on single cells. Measurements based on flow cytometry (see Section A-22) proved the answer, with the development of methods for detecting fluorescently labeled cytokines within activated T cells. The draw-back of intracellular cytokine staining (see Section A-27) was that the T cells have to be killed and permeabilized by detergents to enable the cytokines to be detected. This led to the more sophisticated technique of capturing secreted labeled cytokines on the surfaces of the living T cells (see Section A-27).

Finally, methods for directly detecting T cells on the basis of the specificity of their receptor, using fluorochrome-tagged tetramers of specific MHC:peptide complexes (see Section A-28), have revolutionized the study of T-cell responses in a similar way to the use of monoclonal antibodies.

A-25   Limiting-dilution culture.

The response of a lymphocyte population is a measure of the overall response, but the frequency of lymphocytes able to respond to a given antigen can be determined only by limiting-dilution culture. This assay makes use of the Poisson distribution, a statistical function that describes how objects are distributed at random. For instance, when a sample of heterogeneous T cells is distributed equally into a series of culture wells, some wells will receive no T cells specific for a given antigen, some will receive one specific T cell, some two, and so on. The T cells in the wells are activated with specific antigen, antigen-presenting cells, and growth factors. After allowing several days for their growth and differentiation, the cells in each well are tested for a response to antigen, such as cytokine release or the ability to kill specific target cells (Fig. A.28). The assay is replicated with different numbers of T cells in the samples. The logarithm of the proportion of wells in which there is no response is plotted against the number of cells initially added to each well. If cells of one type, typically antigen-specific T cells because of their rarity, are the only limiting factor for obtaining a response, then a straight line is obtained. From the Poisson distribution, it is known that there is, on average, one antigen-specific cell per well when the proportion of negative wells is 37%. Thus, the frequency of antigen-specific cells in the population equals the reciprocal of the number of cells added to each well when 37% of the wells are negative. After priming, the frequency of specific cells goes up substantially, reflecting the antigen-driven proliferation of antigen-specific cells. The limiting-dilution assay can also be used to measure the frequency of B cells that can make antibody to a given antigen.

A-26   ELISPOT assays.

A modification of the ELISA antigen-capture assay (see Section A-6), called the **ELISPOT assay**, has provided a powerful tool for measuring the frequency of T-cell responses. Populations of T cells are stimulated with the antigen of interest, and are then allowed to settle onto a plastic plate coated with antibodies to the cytokine that is to be assayed (Fig. A.29). If an activated T cell is secreting that cytokine, it is captured by the antibody on the plastic plate. After a period the cells are removed, and a second antibody to the cytokine is added to the plate to reveal a circle of bound cytokine surrounding the position of each activated T cell; counting each spot, and knowing the number of T cells originally added to the plate allows a simple calculation of the frequency of T cells secreting that particular cytokine, giving the ELISPOT assay its name. ELISPOT can also be used to detect specific antibody secretion by B cells, in this case by using antigen-coated surfaces to trap specific antibody and labeled anti-immunoglobulin to detect the bound antibody.

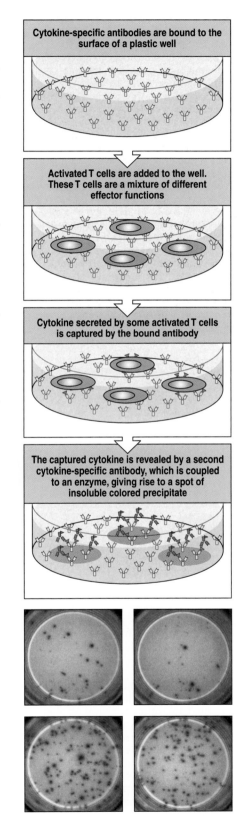

Fig. A.29 The frequency of cytokine-secreting T cells can be determined by the ELISPOT assay. The ELISPOT assay is a variant of the ELISA assay in which antibodies bound to a plastic surface are used to capture cytokines secreted by individual T cells. Usually, cytokine specific antibodies are bound to the surface of a plastic tissue-culture well and the unbound antibodies are removed (top panel). Activated T cells are then added to the well and settle onto the antibody-coated surface (second panel). If a T cell is secreting the appropriate cytokine, this will then be captured by the antibody molecules on the plate surrounding the T cell (third panel). After a period of time the T cells are removed, and the presence of the specific cytokine is detected using an enzyme-labeled second antibody specific for the same cytokine. Where this binds, a colored reaction product can be formed (fourth panel). Each T cell that originally secreted cytokine gives rise to a single spot of color, hence the name of the assay. The results of such an ELISPOT assay for T cells secreting IFN-γ in response to different stimuli are shown in the last panel. In this example, T cells from a stem cell transplant recipient were treated with a control peptide (top two panels) or a peptide from cytomegalovirus (bottom two panels). You can see a greater number of spots in the bottom two panels, indicating clearly that the patient's T cells are able to respond to the viral peptide and produce IFNγ. Photographs courtesy of Ms S. Nowack.

Fig. A.30 Cytokine-secreting cells can be identified by intracellular cytokine staining. The cytokines secreted by activated T cells can be determined by using fluorochrome-labeled antibodies to detect cytokine molecules that have been allowed to accumulate inside the cell. The accumulation of cytokine molecules, to allow them to reach a high enough concentration for efficient detection, is achieved by treating the activated T cells with inhibitors of protein export. In such treated cells, proteins destined to be secreted are instead retained within the endoplasmic reticulum (first panel). These treated cells are then fixed, to cross-link the proteins inside the cell and in the cell membranes, so that they are not lost when the cell is permeabilized by dissolving the cell membrane in a mild detergent (center panel). Fluorochrome-labeled antibodies can now enter the permeabilized cell and bind to the cytokines inside the cell (last panel). Cells labeled in this way can also be labeled with antibodies that bind to cell-surface proteins to determine which subsets of T cells are secreting particular cytokines.

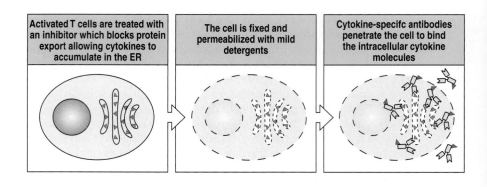

| Activated T cells are treated with an inhibitor which blocks protein export allowing cytokines to accumulate in the ER | The cell is fixed and permeabilized with mild detergents | Cytokine-specifc antibodies penetrate the cell to bind the intracellular cytokine molecules |

A-27   Identification of functional subsets of T cells by staining for cytokines.

One problem with the detection of cytokine production on a single-cell level is that the cytokines are secreted by the T cells into the surrounding medium, and any association with the originating cell is lost. Two methods have been devised that allow the cytokine profile produced by individual cells to be determined. The first, that of **intracellular cytokine staining** (Fig. A.30), relies on the use of metabolic poisons that inhibit protein export from the cell. The cytokine thus accumulates within the endoplasmic reticulum and vesicular network of the cell. If the cells are subsequently fixed and rendered permeable by the use of mild detergents, antibodies can gain access to these intracellular compartments and detect the cytokine. The T cells can be stained for other markers simultaneously, and thus the frequency, for example, of IL-10-producing CD25+ CD4 T cells can be easily obtained.

A second method, which has the advantage that the cells being analyzed are not killed in the process, is called **cytokine capture**. This technique uses hybrid antibodies, in which the two separate heavy- and light-chain pairs from different antibodies are combined to give a mixed antibody molecule in which the two antigen-binding sites recognize different ligands (Fig. A.31).

| A hybrid antibody is made from antibodies specific for a cytokine and a common cell-surface protein such as MHC class I | The hybrid antibodies bind to a population of activated T cells | If the T cells secrete the cytokine it is captured by the hybrid antibody bound to the cell surface | Cytokine secreting T cells are detected using a labeled second antibody specific for the cytokine of interest |

Fig. A.31 Hybrid antibodies containing cell-specific and cytokine-specific binding sites can be used to assay cytokine secretion by living cells and to purify cells secreting particular cytokines. Hybrid antibodies can be made by mixing together heavy- and light-chain pairs from antibodies of different specificities, for example, an antibody to an MHC class I molecule and an antibody specific for a cytokine such as IL-4 (first panel). The hybrid antibodies are then added to a population of activated T cells, and bind to each cell via the MHC class I binding arm (second panel). If some of the cells in the population are secreting the appropriate cytokine, IL-4, this is captured by the cytokine specific arm of the hybrid antibody (third panel). The presence of the cytokine can then be revealed, for example using a fluorochrome-labeled second antibody specific for the same cytokine, but binding to a different site to the one used for the hybrid antibody (last panel). Such labeled cells may be analyzed by flow cytometry, or can be isolated using a fluorescence activated cell sorter. Alternatively, the second cytokine specific antibody may be coupled to magnetic beads, and the cytokine producing cells isolated magnetically.

In the bispecific antibodies used to detect cytokine production, one of the antigen-binding sites is specific for a T-cell surface marker, while the other is specific for the cytokine in question. The bispecific antibody binds to the T cells through the binding site for the cell-surface marker, leaving the cytokine-binding site free. If that T cell is secreting the particular cytokine, it is captured by the bound antibody before it diffuses away from the surface of the cell. It can then be detected by adding a fluorochrome-labeled second antibody specific for the cytokine to the cells.

A-28 Identification of T-cell receptor specificity using MHC:peptide tetramers.

For many years, the ability to identify antigen-specific T cells directly through their receptor specificity eluded immunologists. Foreign antigen could not be used directly to identify T cells, since, unlike B cells, they do not recognize antigen alone but rather the complexes of peptide fragments of antigen bound to self MHC molecules. Moreover, the affinity of interaction between the T-cell receptor and the MHC:peptide complex was in practice so low that attempts to label T cells with their specific MHC:peptide complexes routinely failed. The breakthrough in labeling antigen-specific T cells came with the idea of making multimers of the MHC:peptide complex, so as to increase the avidity of the interaction.

Peptides can be biotinylated using the bacterial enzyme BirA, which recognizes a specific amino acid sequence. Recombinant MHC molecules containing this target sequence are used to make MHC:peptide complexes which are then biotinylated. Avidin, or the bacterial counterpart streptavidin, contains four sites that bind biotin with extremely high affinity. Mixing the biotinylated MHC:peptide complex with avidin or streptavidin results in the formation of an **MHC:peptide tetramer**—four specific MHC:peptide complexes bound to a single molecule of streptavidin (Fig. A.32). Routinely, the streptavidin moiety is labeled with a fluorochrome to allow detection of those T cells capable of binding the MHC:peptide tetramer.

Fig. A.32 MHC:peptide complexes coupled to streptavidin to form tetramers are able to stain antigen-specific T cells. MHC:peptide tetramers are formed from recombinant refolded MHC:peptide complexes containing a single defined peptide epitope. The MHC molecules can be chemically derivatized to contain biotin, but more usually, the recombinant MHC heavy chain is linked to a bacterial biotinylation sequence, a target for the *E. coli* enzyme BirA, which is used to add a single biotin group to the MHC molecule. Streptavidin is a tetramer, each subunit having a single binding site for biotin, hence the streptavidin/MHC:peptide complex creates a tetramer of MHC:peptide complexes (top panel). While the affinity between the T-cell receptor and its MHC:peptide ligand is too low for a single complex to bind stably to a T cell, the tetramer, by being able to make a more avid interaction with multiple MHC:peptide complexes binding simultaneously, is able to bind to T cells whose receptors are specific for the particular MHC:peptide complex (center panel). Routinely, the streptavidin molecules are coupled to a fluorochrome, so that the binding to T cells can be monitored by flow cytometry. In the example shown in the bottom panel, T cells have been stained simultaneously with antibodies specific for CD3 and CD8, and with a tetramer of HLA-A2 molecules containing a cytomegalovirus peptide. Only the CD3+ cells are shown, with the staining of CD8 displayed on the vertical axis and the tetramer staining displayed along the horizontal axis. The CD8− cells (mostly CD4+) on the bottom left of the figure show no specific tetramer staining, while the bulk of the CD8+ cells, on the top left, likewise show no tetramer staining. However, a discrete population of tetramer positive CD8+ cells, at the top right of the panel, comprising some 5% of the total CD8+ cells, can clearly be demonstrated. Data courtesy of Ms G. Aubert

MHC:peptide tetramers have been used to identify populations of antigen-specific T cells in, for example, patients with acute Epstein–Barr virus infections (infectious mononucleosis), showing that up to 80% of the peripheral T cells in infected individuals can be specific for a single MHC:peptide complex. They have also been used to follow responses over longer timescales in individuals with HIV or, in the example we show, cytomegalovirus infections. These reagents have also been important in identifying the cells responding, for example, to nonclassical class I molecules such as HLA-E or HLA-G, in both cases showing that these nonclassical molecules are recognized by subsets of NK receptors.

A-29   Assessing the diversity of the T-cell repertoire by 'spectratyping.'

The extent of the diversity of the T-cell repertoire, either generally or during specific immune responses, is often of interest. In particular, as T cells do not undergo somatic hypermutation and affinity maturation in the same way that B cells do, the relationship between the repertoire of T cells making a primary response to antigen and the repertoire of T cells involved in secondary and subsequent responses to antigen has been difficult to determine. This information has usually been obtained through the laborious process of cloning the T cells involved in specific responses (see Section A-24), and the cloning and sequencing of their T-cell receptors.

It is possible, however, to estimate the diversity of T-cell responses by making use of the junctional diversity generated when T-cell receptors are created by somatic recombination, a technique known as **spectratyping**. Variability in the length of the CDR3 segments is created during the recombination process, both by variation in the exact positions at which the junctions between gene segments occur, and by variation in the number of N-nucleotides added. Both these processes result in the length of the V_β CDR3 varying by up to nine amino acids. The problem in detecting this variability is that there are 24 families of V_β gene segments in humans and it is not possible to design a single oligonucleotide primer that will anneal to all of these families. Specific oligonucleotide primers can, however, be designed for each family, and these can be used in the polymerase chain reaction (PCR), together with a primer specific for the C_β region, to amplify, for each individual family, a segment of the mRNA for the T-cell receptor β chain that spans the CDR3 region. A population of TCR V_β genes will therefore show a distribution, or 'spectrum,' of CD3 lengths, and will give rise to PCR products of different lengths that can be resolved, usually by polyacrylamide gel electrophoresis (Fig. A.33). The deletion and addition of nucleotides during the generation of T-cell receptors by rearrangement is random, and so in a normal individual the CDR3 lengths follow a Gaussian distribution. Deviations from this Gaussian distribution, such as an excess of one particular CDR3 length, indicate the presence of clonal expansions of T cells, such as occurs during a T-cell response.

A-30   Biosensor assays for measuring the rates of association and disassociation of antigen receptors for their ligands.

Two of the important questions that are always asked of any receptor–ligand interaction is: what is the strength of binding, or affinity, of the interaction, and what are the rates of association and disassociation? Traditionally, measurements of affinity have been made by equilibrium binding measurements (see Section A-9), and measurements of rates of binding have been difficult to obtain. Equilibrium binding assays also cannot be performed on T-cell receptors, which have large macromolecular ligands and which cannot be isolated and purified in large quantity.

| T cells express a diverse repertoire of receptors | Receptors exressing the same V segment have CDR3 regions of different lengths | The different lengths of the CDR3 regions can be displayed by denaturing gel electrophoresis | From a diverse population of T cells the pattern of CDR3 lengths is approximately Gaussian |

Fig. A.33 The diversity of the T-cell receptor repertoire can be displayed by spectratyping, a PCR-based technique that separates different receptors on the basis of their CDR3 length. The process of generation of T-cell receptors is stochastic, giving rise to a population of mature T cells whose receptors are clonally distributed (first panel). In each of the cells expressing a particular V_β gene segment, all of the differences between the unique receptors are restricted to the CDR3 region, where there will be differences in length as well as sequence as a consequence of the imprecision of the rearrangement process (second panel). Using sets of primers for the PCR reaction that are specific for individual V_β gene segments at one end and for a conserved part of the C region at the other, it is possible to generate a set of DNA fragments that span the CDR3 region. If these are separated by denaturing acrylamide gel electrophoresis then a series of bands are formed or, since these fragments can be labeled with fluorochromes and analyzed by automated gel readers, a series of peaks corresponding to the different length fragments (third panel). The pattern of peaks obtained in this way is known as a spectratype. From a diverse population of cells, the distribution of fragment lengths is Gaussian, as shown in the last panel, where the spectratypes of two different V_β regions from the same individual are shown. In this case, both of the patterns are approximately Gaussian; deviations from a Gaussian distribution may indicate expansion of particular clones of T cells, perhaps in response to antigenic challenge. Data courtesy of Dr. L. McGreavey.

It is now possible to measure binding rates directly, by following the binding of ligands to receptors immobilized on gold-plated glass slides, using a phenomenon known as surface plasmon resonance to detect the binding (Fig. A.34). A full explanation of surface plasmon resonance is beyond the scope of this textbook, as it is based on advanced physical and quantum mechanical principles. Briefly, it relies on the total internal reflection of a beam of light from the surface of a gold-coated glass slide. As the light is reflected, some of its energy excites electrons in the gold coating and these excited electrons are in turn affected by the electric field of any molecules binding to the surface of the glass coating. The more molecules that bind to the surface, the greater the effect on the excited electrons, and this in turn affects the reflected light beam. The reflected light thus becomes a sensitive measure of the number of atoms bound to the gold surface of the slide.

If a purified receptor is immobilized on the surface of the gold-coated glass slide, to make a biosensor 'chip,' and a solution containing the ligand is flowed over that surface, the binding of ligand to the receptor can be followed until it reaches equilibrium (see Fig. A.34). If the ligand is then washed out, dissociation of ligand from the receptor can easily be followed and the dissociation rate calculated. A new solution of the ligand at a different concentration can then be flowed over the chip and the binding once again measured. The affinity of binding can be calculated in a number of ways in this type of assay. Most simply, the ratio of the rates of association and dissociation will give an estimate of the affinity, but more accurate estimates can be obtained from the measurements of the binding at different concentrations of ligand. From measurements of binding at equilibrium, a Scatchard plot (see Fig. A.11) will give a measurement of the affinity of the receptor–ligand interaction.

| The ligand to be tested, in this case MHC:peptide complexes, is immobilized on a special gold-plated surface | Soluble T-cell receptors are allowed to flow over the surface and bind to the MHC:peptide complex | Receptor binding reaches equilibrium | Unbound receptors are washed away; continued washing removes receptors as they dissociate from the MHC:peptide complex |

Fig. A.34 Measurement of receptor–ligand interactions can be made in real time using a biosensor. Biosensors are able to measure the binding of molecules on the surface of gold-plated glass chips through the indirect effects of the binding on the total internal reflection of a beam of polarized light at the surface of the chip. Changes in the angle and intensity of the reflected beam are measured in 'resonance units' (Ru) and plotted against time in what is termed a 'sensorgram.' Depending on the exact nature of the receptor–ligand pair to be analyzed, either the receptor or the ligand can be immobilized on the surface of the chip. In the example shown, MHC:peptide complexes are immobilized on such a surface (first panel).

T-cell receptors in solution are now allowed to flow over the surface, and to bind to the immobilized MHC:peptide complexes (second panel). As the T-cell receptors bind, the sensorgram (inset panel below the main panel) reflects the increasing amount of protein bound. As the binding reaches either saturation or equilibrium (third panel), the sensorgram shows a plateau, as no more protein binds. At this point, unbound receptors can be washed away. With continued washing, bound receptors now start to dissociate and are removed in the flow of the washing solution (last panel). The sensorgram now shows a declining curve, reflecting the rate at which the receptor and ligand dissociation occurs.

A-31   Stimulation of lymphocyte proliferation by treatment with polyclonal mitogens or specific antigen.

To function in adaptive immunity, rare antigen-specific lymphocytes must proliferate extensively before they differentiate into functional effector cells in order to generate sufficient numbers of effector cells of a particular specificity. Thus, the analysis of induced lymphocyte proliferation is a central issue in their study. It is, however, difficult to detect the proliferation of normal lymphocytes in response to specific antigen because only a minute proportion of cells will be stimulated to divide. Great impetus was given to the field of lymphocyte culture by the finding that certain substances induce many or all lymphocytes of a given type to proliferate. These substances are referred to collectively as **polyclonal mitogens** because they induce mitosis in lymphocytes of many different specificities or clonal origins. T and B lymphocytes are stimulated by different polyclonal mitogens (Fig. A.35). Polyclonal mitogens seem to trigger essentially the same growth response mechanisms as antigen. Lymphocytes normally exist as resting cells in the G_0 phase of the cell cycle. When stimulated with polyclonal mitogens, they rapidly enter the G_1 phase and progress through the cell cycle. In most studies, lymphocyte proliferation is most simply measured by the incorporation of ^{3}H-thymidine into DNA. This assay is used clinically for assessing the ability of lymphocytes from patients with suspected immunodeficiencies to proliferate in response to a nonspecific stimulus.

Mitogen	Responding cells
Phytohemagglutinin (PHA) (red kidney bean)	T cells
Concanavalin (ConA) (Jack bean)	T cells
Pokeweed mitogen (PWM) (Pokeweed)	T and B cells
Lipopolysaccharide (LPS) (*Escherichia coli*)	B cells (mouse)

Fig. A.35 Polyclonal mitogens, many of plant origin, stimulate lymphocyte proliferation in tissue culture. Many of these mitogens are used to test the ability of lymphocytes in human peripheral blood to proliferate.

Once lymphocyte culture had been optimized using the proliferative response to polyclonal mitogens as an assay, it became possible to detect antigen-specific T-cell proliferation in culture by measuring ^{3}H-thymidine uptake in response to an antigen to which the T-cell donor had been previously immunized (Fig. A.36). This is the assay most commonly used for assessing T-cell responses after immunization, but it reveals little about the functional capabilities of the responding T cells. These must be ascertained by functional assays, as outlined in Sections A-33 and A-34.

A-32   Measurements of apoptosis by the TUNEL assay.

Apoptotic cells can be detected by a procedure known as TUNEL staining. In this technique, the 3′ ends of the DNA fragments generated in apoptotic cells are labeled with biotin-coupled uridine by using the enzyme terminal deoxynucleotidyl transferase (TdT). The biotin label is then detected with enzyme tagged streptavidin, which binds to biotin. When the colorless substrate of the enzyme is added to a tissue section or cell culture, it is reacted upon to produce a colored precipitate only in cells that have undergone apoptosis (Fig. A.37). This technique has revolutionized the detection of apoptotic cells.

A-33   Assays for cytotoxic T cells.

Activated CD8 T cells generally kill any cells that display the specific peptide:MHC class I complex they recognize. Thus CD8 T-cell function can be determined using the simplest and most rapid T-cell bioassay—the killing of a target cell by a cytotoxic T cell. This is usually detected in a ^{51}Cr-release assay. Live cells will take up, but do not spontaneously release, radioactively labeled sodium chromate, $Na_2{}^{51}CrO_4$. When these labeled cells are killed, the radioactive chromate is released and its presence in the supernatant of mixtures of target cells and cytotoxic T cells can be measured (Fig. A.38). In a similar assay, proliferating target cells such as tumor cells can be labeled with ^{3}H-thymidine, which is incorporated into the replicating DNA. On attack by a cytotoxic T cell, the DNA of the target cells is rapidly fragmented and retained in the filtrate, while large, unfragmented DNA is collected on a filter, and one can measure either the release of these fragments or the retention of ^{3}H-thymidine in chromosomal DNA. These assays provide a rapid, sensitive, and specific measure of the activity of cytotoxic T cells.

A-34   Assays for CD4 T cells.

CD4 T-cell functions usually involve the activation rather than the killing of cells bearing specific antigen. The activating effects of CD4 T cells on B cells or macrophages are mediated in large part by nonspecific mediator proteins called cytokines, which are released by the T cell when it recognizes antigen. Thus, CD4 T-cell function is usually studied by measuring the type and amount of these released proteins. As different effector T cells release different amounts and types of cytokines, one can learn about the effector potential of that T cell by measuring the proteins it produces.

Cytokines can be detected by their activity in biological assays of cell growth, where they serve either as growth factors or growth inhibitors. A more specific assay is a modification of ELISA known as a capture or sandwich ELISA (see Section A-6). In this assay, the cytokine is characterized by its ability to bridge between two monoclonal antibodies reacting with different epitopes on the cytokine molecule. Cytokine-secreting cells can also be detected by ELISPOT (see Section A-26).

Sandwich ELISA and ELISPOT avoid a major problem of cytokine bioassays, the ability of different cytokines to stimulate the same response in a bioassay. Bioassays must always be confirmed by inhibition of the response with neutralizing monoclonal antibodies specific for the cytokine. Another way of

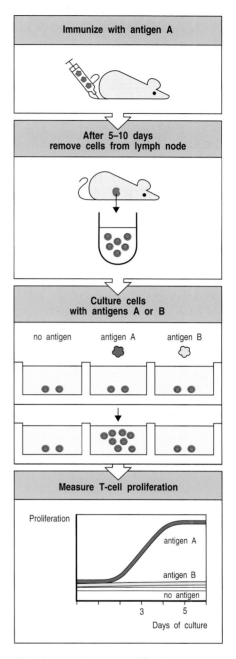

Fig. A.36 Antigen-specific T-cell proliferation is used frequently as an assay for T-cell responses. T cells from mice or humans that have been immunized with an antigen (A) proliferate when they are exposed to antigen A and antigen-presenting cells but not when cultured with unrelated antigens to which they have not been immunized (antigen B). Proliferation can be measured by incorporation of ^{3}H-thymidine into the DNA of actively dividing cells. Antigen-specific proliferation is a hallmark of specific CD4 T-cell immunity.

Fig. A.37 Fragmented DNA can be labeled by terminal deoxynucleotidyl transferase (TdT) to reveal apoptotic cells. When cells undergo programmed cell death, or apoptosis, their DNA becomes fragmented (left panel). The enzyme TdT is able to add nucleotides to the ends of DNA fragments; most commonly in this assay, biotin-labeled nucleotides (usually dUTP) are added (second panel). The biotinylated DNA can be detected by using streptavidin, which binds to biotin, coupled to enzymes that convert a colorless substrate into a colored insoluble product (third panel). Cells stained in this way can be detected by light microscopy, as shown in the photograph of apoptotic cells (stained red) in the thymic cortex. Photograph courtesy of R. Budd and J. Russell.

identifying cells actively producing a given cytokine is to stain them with a fluorescently tagged anti-cytokine monoclonal antibody and identify and count them by FACS (see Section A-22).

A quite different approach to detecting cytokine production is to determine the presence and amount of the relevant cytokine mRNA in stimulated T cells. This can be done for single cells by *in situ* hybridization and for cell populations by **reverse transcriptase–polymerase chain reaction** (**RT–PCR**). Reverse transcriptase is an enzyme used by certain RNA viruses, such as the human immunodeficiency virus (HIV-1) that causes AIDS, to convert an RNA genome into a DNA copy, or cDNA. In RT–PCR, mRNA is isolated from cells and cDNA copies made using reverse transcriptase. The desired cDNA is then selectively amplified by PCR using sequence-specific primers. When the products of the reaction are subjected to electrophoresis on an agarose gel, the amplified DNA can be visualized as a band of a specific size. The amount of amplified cDNA sequence will be proportional to its representation in the mRNA; stimulated T cells actively producing a particular cytokine will produce large amounts of that particular mRNA and thus give correspondingly large amounts of the selected cDNA on RT–PCR. The level of cytokine mRNA in the original tissue is usually determined by comparison with the outcome of RT–PCR on the mRNA produced by a so-called 'housekeeping gene' expressed by all cells.

A-35   DNA microarrays.

Any cell expresses, at any one time, many hundreds or even thousands of genes. Some of the products are expressed at high levels, the actin that forms the cytoskeleton of the cell is one example, while others may only be expressed in a few copies per cell. Different cell types, or cells at different stages of

Fig. A.38 Cytotoxic T-cell activity is often assessed by chromium release from labeled target cells. Target cells are labeled with radioactive chromium as $Na_2^{51}CrO_4$, washed to remove excess radioactivity and exposed to cytotoxic T cells. Cell destruction is measured by the release of radioactive chromium into the medium, detectable within 4 hours of mixing target cells with T cells.

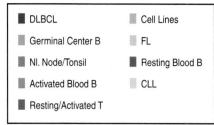

Fig. A.39 DNA microarrays allow a rapid, simultaneous screening of a great many genes for changes in expression between different cells. In the experiment whose results are shown here, nearly 18,000 cDNA clones made from lymphoid cells and lymphoid tumors were arrayed horizontally across the chip. Some of these cDNAs represent the products of known genes, and examples of these are indicated on the right hand edge of the diagram. To these cDNAs mRNA was hybridized from 96 normal cells, cell lines and lymphoid tumor cells, with the mRNA from each individual cell arrayed vertically. The types of cells used are indicated by the colored bars at the top, with the colors explained in the key. The malignant cells used were from diffuse large B-cell lymphoma (DLBCL), follicular lymphoma (FL) or mantle cell lymphoma, and chronic lymphocytic leukemia (CLL). A number of established lymphoid cell lines were included. Normal cells are represented by resting B cells from peripheral blood (Resting Blood B), B cells activated by cross-linking cell-surface IgM with or without additional cytokines and co-stimulation (Activated blood B) germinal center B cells from tonsil (Germinal Center B), and normal, noninflamed tonsil and lymph node (Nl. Node/Tonsil) were used as representatives of different stages in B-cell maturation. Normal T cells, CD4 T cells, either resting or stimulated with PMA and ionomycin (Resting/Activated T) were also used. Each point on the array represents, therefore, the hybridization of the mRNA from one of these cell lines to one of the cDNAs, and is displayed in color to represent the level of expression of the mRNA in question, green being those expressed at lower levels than in a control cell, while red represents those expressed at a higher level. The data shown has been clustered by patterns of expression of the various genes, to give clusters of genes upregulated in proliferating cells, germinal center B cells, lymph node B cells, and in T cells. Courtesy of Dr. L. M. Staudt.

maturation, or even tumor cells compared to their normal counterparts, will express different sets of genes, and trying to identify these differences is an important field of research, in immunology as well as in other areas of biology. One important new technique in analyzing these differences makes use of arrays of hundreds of DNA sequences attached to a glass surface—a so-called **DNA microarray** or 'DNA chip.' The array contains a range of DNA sequences from known genes, arranged in a fixed pattern, and the differential expression of those genes in a particular cell type or tissue is tested by exposing the array to labeled mRNA (or cDNA made from it) from the tissue. Hybridization of labeled mRNAs to their corresponding DNA sequences in the array is detected by standard techniques and the whole technique is readily automated. Many different samples can be examined in parallel, which makes this a powerful analytical technique, as can be seen from the example we illustrate in Fig. A.39. Here the DNA microarray has been constructed with almost 18,000 cDNA clones known to be expressed in either B or T cells and B-cell tumors. This array was then probed with fluorochrome-labeled cDNAs from 96 normal and malignant cells, and the level of expression of approximately 18,000 genes in each of the cell lines was measured simultaneously. In this particular case the patterns of expression of the different genes revealed that the malignant B cells formed discrete subtypes, which were then found to have different clinical prognoses.

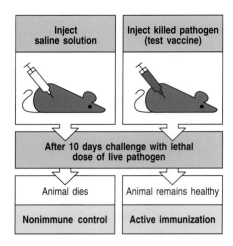

Fig. A.40 *In vivo* assay for the presence of protective immunity after vaccination in animals. Mice are injected with the test vaccine or a control such as saline solution. Different groups are then challenged with lethal or pathogenic doses of the test pathogen or with an unrelated pathogen as a specificity control (not shown). Unimmunized animals die or become severely infected. Successful vaccination is seen as specific protection of immunized mice against infection with the test pathogen. This is called active immunity and the process is called active immunization.

Detection of immunity *in vivo*.

A-36   Assessment of protective immunity.

An adaptive immune response against a pathogen often confers long-lasting immunity against infection with that pathogen; successful vaccination achieves the same end. The very first experiment in immunology, Jenner's successful vaccination against smallpox, is still the model for assessing the presence of such protective immunity. The assessment of protective immunity conferred by vaccination has three essential steps. First, an immune response is elicited by immunization with a candidate vaccine. Second, the immunized individuals, along with unimmunized controls, are challenged with the infectious agent (Fig. A.40). Finally, the prevalence and severity of infection in the immunized individual is compared with the course of the disease in the unimmunized controls. For obvious reasons, such experiments are usually carried out first in animals, if a suitable animal model for the infection exists. However, eventually a trial must be carried out in humans. In this case, the infectious challenge is usually provided naturally by carrying out the trial in a region where the disease is prevalent. The efficacy of the vaccine is determined by assessing the prevalence and severity of new infections in the immunized and control populations. Such studies necessarily give less precise results than a direct experiment but, for most diseases, they are the only way of assessing a vaccine's ability to induce protective immunity in humans.

A-37   Transfer of protective immunity.

The tests described in Section A-36 show that protective immunity has been established, but cannot show whether it involves humoral immunity, cell-mediated immunity, or both. When these studies are carried out in inbred mice, the nature of protective immunity can be determined by transferring serum or lymphoid cells from an immunized donor animal to an unimmunized syngeneic recipient (that is, a genetically identical animal of the same inbred strain) (Fig. A.41). If protection against infection can be conferred by the transfer of serum, the immunity is provided by circulating antibodies and is called **humoral immunity**. Transfer of immunity by antiserum or purified antibodies provides immediate protection against many pathogens and against toxins such as those of tetanus and snake venom. However, although protection is immediate, it is temporary, lasting only so long as the transferred antibodies remain active in the recipient's body. This type of transfer is therefore called **passive immunization**. Only **active immunization** with antigen can provide lasting immunity. Moreover, the recipient may become immunized to the antiserum used to transfer immunity. Horse or sheep sera are the usual sources of anti-snake venoms used in humans, and repeated administration can lead either to serum sickness (see Section 12-16) or, if the recipient becomes allergic to the foreign serum, to anaphylaxis (see Section 12-10).

Protection against many diseases cannot be transferred with serum but can be transferred by lymphoid cells from immunized donors. The transfer of lymphoid cells from an immune donor to a normal syngeneic recipient is called **adoptive transfer** or **adoptive immunization**, and the immunity transferred is called **adoptive immunity**. Immunity that can be transferred only with lymphoid cells is called **cell-mediated immunity**. Such cell transfers must be between genetically identical donors and recipients, such as members of the same inbred strain of mouse, so that the donor lymphocytes are not rejected by the recipient and do not attack the recipient's tissues. Adoptive transfer of immunity is used clinically in humans in experimental approaches to cancer therapy or as an adjunct to bone marrow transplantation; in these cases, the patient's own T cells, or the T cells of the bone marrow donor, are given.

A-38   The tuberculin test.

Local responses to antigen can indicate the presence of active immunity. Active immunity is often studied *in vivo*, especially in humans, by injecting antigens locally in the skin. If a reaction appears, this indicates the presence of antibodies or immune lymphocytes that are specific for that antigen; the **tuberculin test** is an example of this. When people have had tuberculosis they develop cell-mediated immunity that can be detected as a local response when their skin is injected with a small amount of tuberculin, an extract of *Mycobacterium tuberculosis*, the pathogen that causes tuberculosis. The response typically appears a day or two after the injection and consists of a raised, red, and hard (or indurated) area in the skin, which then disappears as the antigen is degraded.

A-39   Testing for allergic responses.

Local **intracutaneous** injections of minute doses of the antigens that cause allergies are used to determine which antigen triggers a patient's allergic reactions. Local responses that happen in the first few minutes after antigen injection in immune recipients are called **immediate hypersensitivity reactions**, and they can be of several forms, one of which is the wheal-and-flare response (see Fig. 12.14). Immediate hypersensitivity reactions are mediated by specific antibodies of the IgE class formed as a result of earlier exposures to the antigen. Responses that take hours to days to develop, such as the tuberculin test, are referred to as **delayed-type hypersensitivity** responses and are caused by preexisting immune T cells. This latter type of response was observed by Jenner when he tested vaccinated individuals with a local injection of vaccinia virus.

These tests work because the local deposit of antigen remains concentrated in the initial site of injection, eliciting responses in local tissues. They do not cause generalized reactions if sufficiently small doses of antigen are used. However, local tests carry a risk of systemic allergic reactions, and they should be used with caution in people with a history of hypersensitivity.

A-40   Assessment of immune responses and immunological competence in humans.

The methods used for testing immune function in humans are necessarily more limited than those used in experimental animals, but many different tests are available. They fall into several groups depending on the reason the patient is being studied.

Assessment of protective immunity in humans generally relies on tests conducted *in vitro*. To assess humoral immunity, specific antibody levels in the patient's serum are assayed by RIA or, more commonly, ELISA (see Section A-6), using the test microorganism or a purified microbial product as antigen. To test for humoral immunity against viruses, antibody production is often measured by the ability of serum to neutralize the infectivity of live virus for tissue culture cells. In addition to providing information about protective

Fig. A.41 Immunity can be transferred by antibodies or by lymphocytes. Successful vaccination leads to a long-lived state of protection against the specific immunizing pathogen. If this immune protection can be transferred to a normal syngeneic recipient with serum from an immune donor, then immunity is mediated by antibodies; such immunity is called humoral immunity and the process is called passive immunization. If immunity can only be transferred by infusing lymphoid cells from the immune donor into a normal syngeneic recipient, then the immunity is called cell-mediated immunity and the transfer process is called adoptive transfer or adoptive immunization. Passive immunity is short-lived, as antibody is eventually catabolized, but adoptively transferred immunity is mediated by immune cells, which can survive and provide longer-lasting immunity.

immunity, the presence of antibody to a particular pathogen indicates that the patient has been exposed to it, making such tests of crucial importance in epidemiology. At present, testing for antibody to HIV is the main screening test for infection with this virus, critical both for the patient and in blood banking, where blood from infected donors must be excluded from the supply. Essentially similar tests are used in investigating allergy, where allergens are used as the antigens in tests for specific IgE antibody by ELISA or RIA (see Section A-6), which may be used to confirm the results of skin tests.

Cell-mediated immunity, that is immunity mediated by T cells, is technically more difficult to measure than humoral immunity. This is principally because T cells do not make a secreted antigen-binding product, so there is no simple binding assay for their antigen-specific responses. T-cell activity can be divided into an induction phase, in which T cells are activated to divide and differentiate, and an effector phase, in which their function is expressed. Both phases require that the T cell interacts with another cell and that it recognizes specific antigen displayed in the form of peptide:MHC complexes on the surface of this interacting cell. In the induction phase, the interaction must be with an antigen-presenting cell able to deliver co-stimulatory signals, whereas, in the effector phase, the nature of the target cell depends on the type of effector T cell that has been activated. Most commonly, the presence of T cells that have responded to a specific antigen is detected by their subsequent *in vitro* proliferation when reexposed to the same antigen (see Section A-31).

T-cell proliferation indicates only that cells able to recognize that antigen have been activated previously; it does not reveal what effector function they mediate. The effector function of a T cell is assayed by its effect on an appropriate target cell. Assays for cytotoxic CD8 T cells (see Section A-33) and for cytokine production by CD4 T cells (see Sections A-26, A-27, and A-34) are used to characterize the immune response. Cell-mediated immunity to infectious agents can also be tested by skin test with extracts of the pathogen, as in the tuberculin test (see Section A-36). These tests provide information about the exposure of the patient to the disease and also about their ability to mount an adaptive immune response to it.

Patients with immune deficiency (see Chapter 11) are usually detected clinically by a history of recurrent infection. To determine the competence of the immune system in such patients, a battery of tests are usually conducted (see Appendix V); these focus with increasing precision as the nature of the defect is narrowed down to a single element. The presence of the various cell types in blood is determined by routine hematology, often followed by FACS analysis of lymphocyte subsets (see Section A-22), and the measurement of serum immunoglobulins. The phagocytic competence of freshly isolated polymorphonuclear leukocytes and monocytes is tested, and the efficiency of the complement system (see Chapters 2 and 9) is determined by testing the dilution of serum required for lysis of 50% of antibody-coated red blood cells (this is denoted the CH_{50}).

In general, if such tests reveal a defect in one of the broad compartments of immune function, more specialized testing is then needed to determine the precise nature of the defect. Tests of lymphocyte function are often valuable, starting with the ability of polyclonal mitogens to induce T-cell proliferation and B-cell secretion of immunoglobulin in tissue culture (see Section A-31). These tests can eventually pinpoint the cellular defect in immunodeficiency.

In patients with autoimmune diseases (see Chapter 13), the same parameters are usually analyzed to determine whether there is a gross abnormality in the immune system. However, most patients with such diseases show few abnormalities in general immune function. To determine whether a patient is producing antibody against their own cellular antigens, the most informative test is to react their serum with tissue sections, which are then examined for bound antibody by indirect immunofluorescence using anti-human immunoglobulin labeled with fluorescent dye (see Section A-14). Most autoimmune diseases are associated with the production of broadly characteristic patterns of autoantibodies directed at self tissues. These patterns aid in the diagnosis of the disease and help to distinguish autoimmunity from tissue inflammation due to infectious causes.

It is also possible to investigate allergies by administration of possible allergens by routes other than intracutaneous administration. Allergen may be given by inhalation to test for asthmatic allergic responses (see Fig. 12.14); this is mainly done for experimental purposes in studies of the mechanisms and treatment of asthma. Similarly, food allergens may be given by mouth. The administration of allergens is potentially very dangerous because of the risk of causing anaphylaxis, and must only be carried out by trained and experienced investigators in an environment in which full resuscitation facilities are available.

A-41 The Arthus reaction.

This is an experimental method using only animal models for studying the formation of immune complexes in tissues and how immune complexes cause inflammation (see Section 12-16). The original reaction described by Maurice Arthus was induced by the repeated injection of horse serum into rabbits. Initial injections of horse serum into the skin induced no reaction, but later injections, following the production of antibodies to the proteins in horse serum, induced an inflammatory reaction at the site of injection after several hours, characterized by the presence of edema, hemorrhage, and neutrophil infiltration, which frequently progressed to tissue necrosis. Most investigators now use passive models of the Arthus reaction in which either antibody is infused systemically and antigen given locally (passive Arthus reaction) or antigen is infused systemically and antibody injected locally (reverse passive Arthus reaction).

Manipulation of the immune system.

A-42 Adoptive transfer of lymphocytes.

Ionizing radiation from X-ray or γ-ray sources kills lymphoid cells at doses that spare the other tissues of the body. This makes it possible to eliminate immune function in a recipient animal before attempting to restore immune function by adoptive transfer, and allows the effect of the adoptively transferred cells to be studied in the absence of other lymphoid cells. James Gowans originally used this technique to prove the role of the lymphocyte in immune responses. He showed that all active immune responses could be transferred to irradiated recipients by small lymphocytes from immunized donors. This technique can be refined by transferring only certain lymphocyte subpopulations, such as B cells, CD4 T cells, and so on. Even cloned T-cell lines have been tested for their ability to transfer immune function, and have been shown to confer adoptive immunity to their specific antigen. Such adoptive transfer studies are a cornerstone in the study of the intact immune system, as they can be carried out rapidly, simply, and in any strain of mouse.

A-43 Hematopoietic stem-cell transfers.

All cells of hematopoietic origin can be eliminated by treatment with high doses of X rays, allowing replacement of the entire hematopoietic system, including lymphocytes, by transfusion of donor bone marrow or purified hematopoietic stem cells from another animal. The resulting animals are called **radiation bone marrow chimeras** from the Greek word *chimera*, a mythical animal that had the head of a lion, the tail of a serpent, and the body of a goat. This technique is used experimentally to examine the development of lymphocytes, as opposed to their effector functions, and has been particularly important in studying T-cell development. Essentially the same technique is used in humans to replace the hematopoietic system when it fails, as in aplastic anemia or after nuclear accidents, or to eradicate the bone marrow and replace it with normal marrow in the treatment of certain cancers. In man, bone marrow is the main source of hematopoietic stem cells, but increasingly they are being obtained from peripheral blood after the donor has been treated with hematopoietic growth factors such as GM-CSF, or from umbilical cord blood, which is rich in such stem cells.

A-44 *In vivo* depletion of T cells.

The importance of T-cell function *in vivo* can be ascertained in mice with no T cells of their own. Under these conditions, the effect of a lack of T cells can be studied, and T-cell subpopulations can be restored selectively to analyze their specialized functions. T lymphocytes originate in the thymus, and neonatal **thymectomy**, the surgical removal of the thymus of a mouse at birth, prevents T-cell development from occurring because the export of most functionally mature T cells only occurs after birth in the mouse. Alternatively, adult mice can be thymectomized and then irradiated and reconstituted with bone marrow; such mice will develop all hematopoietic cell types except mature T cells.

The recessive *nude* mutation in mice is caused by a mutation in the gene for the transcription factor Wnt and in homozygous form causes hairlessness and absence of the thymus. Consequently, these animals fail to develop T cells from bone marrow progenitors. Grafting thymectomized or *nude/nude* mice with thymic epithelial elements depleted of lymphocytes allows the graft recipients to develop normal mature T cells. This procedure allows the role of the nonlymphoid thymic stroma to be examined; it has been crucial in determining the role of thymic stromal cells in T-cell development (see Chapter 7).

A-45 *In vivo* depletion of B cells.

There is no single site of B-cell development in mice, so techniques such as thymectomy cannot be applied to the study of B-cell function and development in rodents. However, **bursectomy**, the surgical removal of the Bursa of Fabricius in birds, can inhibit the development of B cells in these species. In fact, it was the effect of thymectomy versus bursectomy that led to the naming

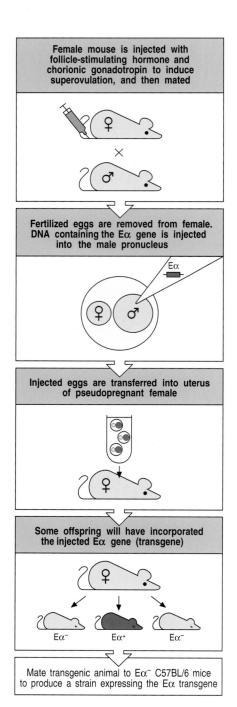

Fig. A.42 The function and expression of genes can be studied *in vivo* by using transgenic mice. DNA encoding a protein of interest, here the mouse MHC class II protein Eα, is purified and microinjected into the male pronuclei of fertilized eggs. The eggs are then implanted into pseudopregnant female mice. The resulting offspring are screened for the presence of the transgene in their cells, and positive mice are used as founders that transmit the transgene to their offspring, establishing a line of transgenic mice that carry one or more extra genes. The function of the Eα gene used here is tested by breeding the transgene into C57BL/6 mice that carry an inactivating mutation in their endogenous Eα gene.

Figure panels:

Female mouse is injected with follicle-stimulating hormone and chorionic gonadotropin to induce superovulation, and then mated

Fertilized eggs are removed from female. DNA containing the Eα gene is injected into the male pronucleus

Injected eggs are transferred into uterus of pseudopregnant female

Some offspring will have incorporated the injected Eα gene (transgene)

Eα⁻   Eα⁺   Eα⁻

Mate transgenic animal to Eα⁻ C57BL/6 mice to produce a strain expressing the Eα transgene of T cells for thymus-derived lymphocytes and B cells for bursal-derived lymphocytes. There are no known spontaneous mutations (analogous to the *nude* mutation) in mice that produce animals with T cells but no B cells. However, such mutations exist in humans, leading to a failure to mount humoral immune responses or make antibody. The diseases produced by such mutations are called agammaglobulinemias because they were originally detected as the absence of gamma globulins. The genetic basis for one form of this disease in humans has now been established (see Chapter 11), and some features of the disease can be reproduced in mice by targeted disruption of the corresponding gene (see Section A-47). Several different mutations in crucial regions of immunoglobulin genes have already been produced by gene targeting and have provided mice lacking B cells.

A-46   Transgenic mice.

The function of genes has traditionally been studied by observing the effects of spontaneous mutations in whole organisms and, more recently, by analyzing the effects of targeted mutations in cultured cells. The advent of gene cloning and *in vitro* mutagenesis now make it possible to produce specific mutations in whole animals. Mice with extra copies or altered copies of a gene in their genome can be generated by **transgenesis**, which is now a well established procedure. To produce **transgenic mice**, a cloned gene is introduced into the mouse genome by microinjection into the male pronucleus of a fertilized egg, which is then implanted into the uterus of a pseudopregnant female mouse. In some of the eggs, the injected DNA becomes integrated randomly into the genome, giving rise to a mouse that has an extra genetic element of known structure, the transgene (Fig. A.42).

The transgene, to be studied in detail, needs to be introduced onto a stable, well-characterized genetic background. However, it is difficult to prepare transgenic embryos successfully in inbred strains of mice, and transgenic mice are routinely prepared in F_2 embryos (that is, the embryo formed after the mating of two F_1 animals). The transgene must then be bred onto a well-characterized genetic background; this requires 10 generations of back-crossing with an inbred strain to assure that the integrated transgene is largely (>99%) free of heterogeneous genes from the founder mouse of the transgenic mouse line (Fig. A.43).

This technique allows one to study the impact of a newly discovered gene on development, to identify the regulatory regions of a gene required for its normal tissue-specific expression, to determine the effects of its over-expression or expression in inappropriate tissues, and to find out the impact of mutations on gene function. Transgenic mice have been particularly useful in studying the role of T-cell and B-cell receptors in lymphocyte development, as described in Chapter 7.

Fig. A.43 The breeding of transgenic co-isogeneic or congenic mouse strains. Transgenic mouse strains are routinely made in F_2 mice. To produce mice on an inbred background, the transgene is introgressively back-crossed onto a standard strain, usually C57BL/6 (B6). The presence of the transgene is tracked by carrying out PCR on genomic DNA extracted from the tail of young mice. After 10 generations of back-crossing, mice are >99% genetically identical, so that any differences observed between the mice are likely to be due to the transgene itself. The same technique can be used to breed a gene knockout into a standard strain of mice, as most gene knockouts are made in the 129 strain of mice (see Fig. A.45). The mice are then intercrossed and homozygous knockout mice detected by an absence of an intact copy of the gene of interest (as determined by PCR).

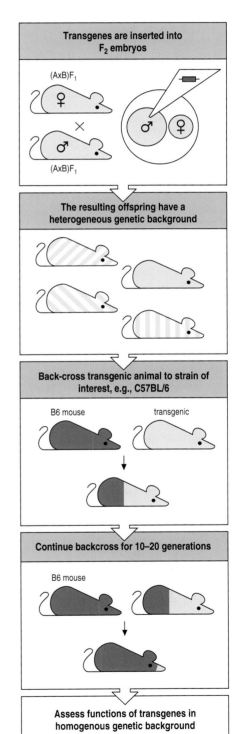

Transgenes are inserted into F_2 embryos

$(AxB)F_1$ ♀

×

$(AxB)F_1$ ♂

The resulting offspring have a heterogeneous genetic background

Back-cross transgenic animal to strain of interest, e.g., C57BL/6

B6 mouse   transgenic

Continue backcross for 10–20 generations

B6 mouse

Assess functions of transgenes in homogenous genetic background

Fig. A.44 The deletion of specific genes can be accomplished by homologous recombination. When pieces of DNA are introduced into cells, they can integrate into cellular DNA in two different ways. If they randomly insert into sites of DNA breaks, the whole piece is usually integrated, often in several copies. However, extrachromosomal DNA can also undergo homologous recombination with the cellular copy of the gene, in which case only the central, homologous region is incorporated into cellular DNA. Inserting a selectable marker gene such as resistance to neomycin (*neo^r*) into the coding region of a gene does not prevent homologous recombination, and it achieves two goals. First, any cell that has integrated the injected DNA is protected from the neomycin-like antibiotic G418. Second, when the gene recombines with homologous cellular DNA, the *neo^r* gene disrupts the coding sequence of the modified cellular gene. Homologous recombinants can be discriminated from random insertions if the gene for herpes simplex virus thymidine kinase (HSV-tk) is placed at one or both ends of the DNA construct, which is often known as a 'targeting construct' because it targets the cellular gene. In random DNA integrations, HSV-tk is retained. HSV-tk renders the cell sensitive to the antiviral agent ganciclovir. However, as HSV-tk is not homologous to the target DNA, it is lost from homologous recombinants. Thus, cells that have undergone homologous recombination are uniquely both G418 and ganciclovir resistant, and survive in a mixture of the two antibiotics. The presence of the disrupted gene has to be confirmed by Southern blotting or by PCR using primers in the *neo^r* gene and in cellular DNA lying outside the region used in the targeting construct. By using two different resistance genes one can disrupt the two cellular copies of a gene, making a deletion mutant (not shown).

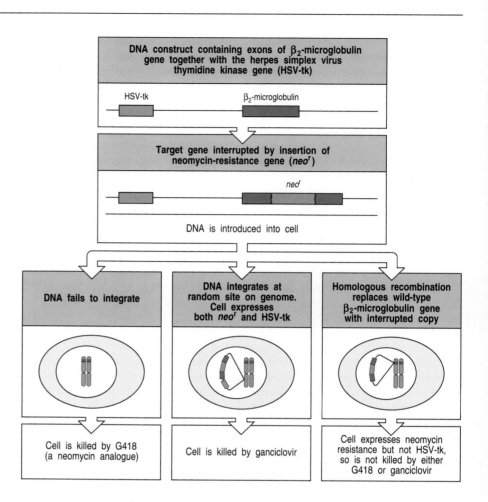

A-47   Gene knockout by targeted disruption.

In many cases, the functions of a particular gene can be fully understood only if a mutant animal that does not express the gene can be obtained. Whereas genes used to be discovered through identification of mutant phenotypes, it is now far more common to discover and isolate the normal gene and then determine its function by replacing it *in vivo* with a defective copy. This procedure is known as **gene knockout**, and it has been made possible by two fairly recent developments: a powerful strategy to select for targeted mutation by homologous recombination, and the development of continuously growing lines of **embryonic stem cells** (**ES cells**). These are embryonic cells which, on implantation into a blastocyst, can give rise to all cell lineages in a chimeric mouse.

The technique of **gene targeting** takes advantage of the phenomenon known as **homologous recombination** (Fig. A.44). Cloned copies of the target gene are altered to make them nonfunctional and are then introduced into the ES cell where they recombine with the homologous gene in the cell's genome, replacing the normal gene with a nonfunctional copy. Homologous recombination is a rare event in mammalian cells, and thus a powerful selection strategy is required to detect those cells in which it has occurred. Most commonly, the introduced gene construct has its sequence disrupted by an inserted antibiotic-resistance gene such as that for neomycin resistance. If this construct undergoes homologous recombination with the endogenous copy of the gene, the endogenous gene is disrupted but the antibiotic-resistance gene remains functional, allowing cells that have incorporated the gene to be selected in culture for resistance to the neomycin-like drug G418. However, antibiotic resistance on its own shows only that the cells have taken up and integrated the neomycin-resistance gene. To be able to select for those cells in which homologous recombination has occurred, the ends of the construct usually carry the thymidine kinase gene from the herpes simplex virus (HSV-tk). Cells that incorporate DNA randomly usually retain the entire DNA construct including HSV-tk, whereas homologous recombination between the construct and cellular DNA, the desired result, involves the exchange of homologous DNA sequences so that the nonhomologous HSV-tk genes at the ends of the construct are eliminated. Cells carrying HSV-tk are killed by the antiviral drug ganciclovir, and so cells with homologous recombinations have the unique feature of being resistant to both neomycin and ganciclovir, allowing them to be selected efficiently when these drugs are added to the cultures (see Fig. A.44).

This technique can be used to produce homozygous mutant cells in which the effects of knocking-out a specific gene can be analyzed. Diploid cells in which both copies of a gene have been mutated by homologous recombination can be selected after transfection with a mixture of constructs in which the gene to be targeted has been disrupted by one or other of two different antibiotic-resistance genes. Having obtained a mutant cell with a functional defect, the defect can be ascribed definitively to the mutated gene if the mutant phenotype can be reverted with a copy of the normal gene transfected into the mutant cell. Restoration of function means that the defect in the mutant gene has been complemented by the normal gene's function. This technique is very powerful as it allows the gene that is being transferred to be mutated in precise ways to determine which parts of the protein are required for function.

To knock out a gene *in vivo*, it is only necessary to disrupt one copy of the cellular gene in an ES cell. ES cells carrying the mutant gene are produced by targeted mutation (see Fig. A.44), and injected into a blastocyst which is reimplanted into the uterus. The cells carrying the disrupted gene become incorporated into the developing embryo and contribute to all tissues of the resulting chimeric offspring, including those of the germline. The mutated gene can therefore be transmitted to some of the offspring of the original chimera, and further breeding of the mutant gene to homozygosity produces mice that completely lack the expression of that particular gene product (Fig. A.45). The effects of the absence of the gene's function can then be studied. In addition, the parts of the gene that are essential for its function can be identified by determining whether function can be restored by introducing different mutated copies of the gene back into the genome by transgenesis.

Fig. A.45 Gene knockout in embryonic stem cells enables mutant mice to be produced. Specific genes can be inactivated by homologous recombination in cultures of embryonic stem cells (ES cells). Homologous recombination is carried out as described in Fig. A.44. In this example, the gene for β2-microglobulin in ES cells is disrupted by homologous recombination with a targeting construct. Only a single copy of the gene needs to be disrupted. ES cells in which homologous recombination has taken place are injected into mouse blastocysts. If the mutant ES cells give rise to germ cells in the resulting chimeric mice (striped in the figure), then the mutant gene can be transferred to their offspring. By breeding the mutant gene to homozygosity, a mutant phenotype is generated. These mutant mice are usually of the 129 strain as gene knockout is generally conducted in ES cells derived from the 129 strain of mice. In this case, the homozygous mutant mice lack MHC class I molecules on their cells, as MHC class I molecules have to pair with β2-microglobulin for surface expression. The β2-microglobulin-deficient mice can then be bred with mice transgenic for subtler mutants of the deleted gene, allowing the effect of such mutants to be tested *in vivo*.

ES cells with a mutation that is lethal in a homozygote are injected into a *RAG⁻* blastocyst

The resultant mouse is chimeric, with lymphocytes derived from the ES cells

The *RAG⁻* cells cannot give rise to lymphocytes. All lymphocytes in the chimera are derived from the injected ES cells

Fig. A.46 The role of recessive lethal genes in lymphocyte function can be studied using *RAG*-deficient chimeric mice. ES cells homozygous for the lethal mutation are injected into a *RAG*-deficient blastocyst (top panel). The *RAG*-deficient cells can give rise to all the tissues of a normal mouse except lymphocytes, and so can compensate for any deficiency in the developmental potential of the mutant ES cells (middle panel). If the mutant ES cells are capable of differentiating into hemato-poietic stem cells, that is, if the gene function that has been deleted is not essential for this developmental pathway, then all the lymphocytes in the chimeric mouse will be derived from the ES cells (bottom panel), as *RAG*-deficient mice cannot make lymphocytes of their own.

The manipulation of the mouse genome by gene knockout and transgenesis is revolutionizing our understanding of the role of individual genes in lympho-cyte development and function.

Because the most commonly used ES cells are derived from a poorly character-ized strain of mice known as strain 129, the analysis of the function of a gene knockout often requires extensive back-crossing to another strain, just as in transgenic mice (see Fig. A.43). One can track the presence of the mutant copy of the gene by the presence of the *neo*ʳ gene. After sufficient back-crossing, the mice are intercrossed to produce mutants on a stable genetic background.

A problem with gene knockouts arises when the function of the gene is essential for the survival of the animal; in such cases the gene is termed a **recessive lethal gene** and homozygous animals cannot be produced. However, by making chimeras with mice that are deficient in B and T cells, it is possible to analyze the function of recessive lethal genes in lymphoid cells. To do this, ES cells with homozygous lethal loss-of-function mutations are injected into blastocysts of mice lacking the ability to rearrange their antigen-receptor genes because of a mutation in their recombinase-activating genes (*RAG* knockout mice). As these chimeric embryos develop, the *RAG*-deficient cells can compensate for any developmental failure resulting from the gene knockout in the ES cells in all except the lymphoid lineage. So long as the mutated ES cells can develop into hematopoietic progenitors in the bone marrow, the embryos will survive and all of the lymphocytes in the resulting chimeric mouse will be derived from the mutant ES cells (Fig. A.46).

A second powerful technique achieves tissue-specific or developmentally regulated gene deletion by employing the DNA sequences and enzymes used by bacteriophage P1 to excise itself from a host cell's genome. Integrated bacteriophage P1 DNA is flanked by recombination signal sequences called *loxP* sites. A recombinase, Cre, recognizes these sites, cuts the DNA and joins the two ends, thus excising the intervening DNA in the form of a circle. This mechanism can be adapted to allow the deletion of specific genes in a transgenic animal only in certain tissues or at certain times in development. First, *loxP* sites flanking a gene, or perhaps just a single exon, are introduced by homologous recombination (Fig. A.47). Usually, the introduction of these sequences into flanking or intronic DNA does not disrupt the normal function of the gene. Mice containing such *loxP* mutant genes are then mated with mice made transgenic for the Cre recombinase, under the control of a tissue-specific or inducible promoter. When the Cre recombinase is active, either in the appropriate tissue or when induced, it excises the DNA between the inserted *loxP* sites, thus inactivating the gene or exon. Thus, for example, using a T-cell specific promoter to drive expression of the Cre recombinase, a gene can be deleted only in T cells, while remaining functional in all other cells of the animal. This is an extremely powerful genetic technique that while still in its infancy, was used to demonstrate the importance of B-cell receptors in B-cell survival. It is certain to yield exciting results in the future.

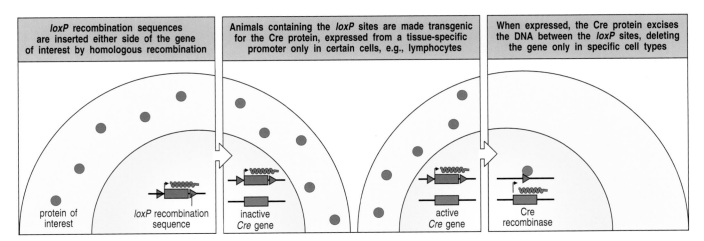

loxP recombination sequences are inserted either side of the gene of interest by homologous recombination	Animals containing the *loxP* sites are made transgenic for the Cre protein, expressed from a tissue-specific promoter only in certain cells, e.g., lymphocytes	When expressed, the Cre protein excises the DNA between the *loxP* sites, deleting the gene only in specific cell types

protein of interest   *loxP* recombination sequence   inactive *Cre* gene   active *Cre* gene   Cre recombinase

Fig. A.47 The P1 bacteriophage recombination system can be used to eliminate genes in particular cell lineages. The P1 bacteriophage protein Cre excises DNA that is bounded by recombination signal sequences called *loxP* sequences. These sequences can be introduced at either end of a gene by homologous recombination (left panel). Animals carrying genes flanked by *loxP* can also be made transgenic for the gene for the Cre protein, which is placed under the control of a tissue-specific promoter so that it is expressed only in certain cells or only at certain times during development (middle panel). In the cells in which the Cre protein is expressed, it recognizes the *loxP* sequences and excises the DNA lying between them (right panel). Thus, individual genes can be deleted only in certain cell types or only at certain times. In this way, genes that are essential for the normal development of a mouse can be analyzed for their function in the developed animal and/or in specific cell types. Genes are shown as boxes, RNA as squiggles, and proteins as colored balls.

APPENDICES II – V

Appendix II. CD antigens.					
CD antigen	**Cellular expression**	**Molecular weight (kDa)**	**Functions**	**Other names**	**Family relationships**
CD1a,b,c,d	Cortical thymocytes, Langerhans' cells, dendritic cells, B cells (CD1c), intestinal epithelium, smooth muscle, blood vessels (CD1d)	43–49	MHC class I-like molecule, associated with β_2-microglobulin. Has specialized role in presentation of lipid antigens		Immunoglobulin
CD2	T cells, thymocytes, NK cells	45–58	Adhesion molecule, binding CD58 (LFA-3). Binds Lck intracellularly and activates T cells	T11, LFA-2	Immunoglobulin
CD3	Thymocytes, T cells	γ: 25–28 δ: 20 ε: 20	Associated with the T-cell antigen receptor (TCR). Required for cell-surface expression of and signal transduction by the TCR	T3	Immunoglobulin
CD4	Thymocyte subsets, T_H1 and T_H2 T cells (about two thirds of peripheral T cells), monocytes, macrophages	55	Co-receptor for MHC class II molecules. Binds Lck on cytoplasmic face of membrane. Receptor for HIV-1 and HIV-2 gp120	T4, L3T4	Immunoglobulin
CD5	Thymocytes, T cells, subset of B cells	67		T1, Ly1	Scavenger receptor
CD6	Thymocytes, T cells, B cells in chronic lymphatic leukemia	100–130	Binds CD166	T12	Scavenger receptor
CD7	Pluripotential hematopoietic cells, thymocytes, T cells	40	Unknown, cytoplasmic domain binds PI 3-kinase on cross-linking. Marker for T cell acute lymphatic leukemia and pluripotential stem cell leukemias		Immunoglobulin
CD8	Thymocytes subsets, cytotoxic T cells (about one third of peripheral T cells)	α: 32–34 β: 32–34	Co-receptor for MHC class I molecules. Binds Lck on cytoplasmic face of membrane	T8, Lyt2,3	Immunoglobulin
CD9	Pre-B cells, monocytes, eosinophils, basophils, platelets, activated T cells, brain and peripheral nerves, vascular smooth muscle	24	Mediates platelet aggregation and activation via FcγRIIa, may play a role in cell migration		Tetraspanning membrane protein, also called transmembrane 4 (TM4)
CD10	B- and T-cell precursors, bone marrow stromal cells	100	Zinc metalloproteinase, marker for pre-B acute lymphatic leukemia (ALL)	Neutral endopeptidase, common acute lymphocytic leukemia antigen (CALLA)	
CD11a	Lymphocytes, granulocytes, monocytes and macrophages	180	αL subunit of integrin LFA-1 (associated with CD18); binds to CD54 (ICAM-1), CD102 (ICAM-2), and CD50 (ICAM-3)	LFA-1	Integrin α

CD antigen	Cellular expression	Molecular weight (kDa)	Functions	Other names	Family relationships
CD11b	Myeloid and NK cells	170	αM subunit of integrin CR3 (associated with CD18): binds CD54, complement component iC3b, and extracellular matrix proteins	Mac-1	Integrin α
CD11c	Myeloid cells	150	αX subunit of integrin CR4 (associated with CD18); binds fibrinogen	CR4, p150, 95	Integrin α
CD11d	Leukocytes	125	αD subunits of integrin; associated with CD18; binds to CD50		Integrin α
CDw12	Monocytes, granulocytes, platelets	90–120	Unknown		
CD13	Myelomonocytic cells	150–170	Zinc metalloproteinase	Aminopeptidase N	
CD14	Myelomonocytic cells	53–55	Receptor for complex of lipopolysaccharide and lipopolysaccharide binding protein (LBP)		
CD15	Neutrophils, eosinophils, monocytes		Terminal trisaccharide expressed on glycolipids and many cell-surface glycoproteins	Lewis^x (Le^x)	
CD15s	Leukocytes, endothelium		Ligand for CD62E, P	Sialyl-Lewis^x (sLe^x)	poly-N-acetyl-lactosamine
CD15u			Sulphated CD15		Carbohydrate structures
CD16	Neutrophils, NK cells, macrophages	50–80	Component of low affinity Fc receptor, FcγRIII, mediates phagocytosis and antibody-dependent cell-mediated cytotoxicity	FcγRIII	Immunoglobulin
CDw17	Neutrophils, monocytes, platelets		Lactosyl ceramide, a cell-surface glycosphingolipid		
CD18	Leukocytes	95	Intergrin β2 subunit, associates with CD11a, b, c, and d		Integrin β
CD19	B cells	95	Forms complex with CD21 (CR2) and CD81 (TAPA-1); co-receptor for B cells—cytoplasmic domain binds cytoplasmic tyrosine kinases and PI 3-kinase		Immunoglobulin
CD20	B cells	33–37	Oligomers of CD20 may form a Ca^{2+} channel; possible role in regulating B-cell activation		Contains 4 transmembrane segments
CD21	Mature B cells, follicular dendritic cells	145	Receptor for complement component C3d, Epstein–Barr virus. With CD19 and CD81, CD21 forms co-receptor for B cells	CR2	Complement control protein (CCP)
CD22	Mature B cells	α: 130 β: 140	Binds sialoconjugates	BL-CAM	Immunoglobulin
CD23	Mature B cells, activated macrophages, eosinophils, follicular dendritic cells, platelets	45	Low-affinity receptor for IgE, regulates IgE synthesis; ligand for CD19:CD21:CD81 co-receptor	FcϵRII	C-type lectin
CD24	B cells, granulocytes	35–45	Unknown	Possible human homologue of mouse heat stable antigen (HSA)	
CD25	Activated T cells, B cells, and monocytes	55	IL-2 receptor α chain	Tac	CCP
CD26	Activated B and T cells, macrophages	110	Exopeptidase, cleaves N terminal X-Pro or X-Ala dipeptides from polypeptides	Dipeptidyl peptidase IV	Type II transmembrane glycoprotein

CD antigen	Cellular expression	Molecular weight (kDa)	Functions	Other names	Family relationships
CD27	Medullary thymocytes, T cells, NK cells, some B cells	55	Binds CD70; can function as a co-stimulator for T and B cells		TNF receptor
CD28	T-cell subsets, activated B cells	44	Activation of naive T cells, receptor for co-stimulatory signal (signal 2) binds CD80 (B7.1) and CD86 (B7.2)	Tp44	Immunoglobulin and CD86 (B7.2)
CD29	Leukocytes	130	Integrin $\beta1$ subunit, associates with CD49a in VLA-1 integrin		Integrin β
CD30	Activated T, B, and NK cells, monocytes	120	Binds CD30L (CD153); cross-linking CD30 enhances proliferation of B and T cells	Ki-1	TNF receptor
CD31	Monocytes, platelets, granulocytes, T-cell subsets, endothelial cells	130–140	Adhesion molecule, mediating both leukocyte–endothelial and endothelial–endothelial interactions	PECAM-1	Immunoglobulin
CD32	Monocytes, granulocytes, B cells, eosinophils	40	Low affinity Fc receptor for aggregated immunoglobulin:immune complexes	FcγRII	Immunoglobulin
CD33	Myeloid progenitor cells, monocytes	67	Binds sialoconjugates		Immunoglobulin
CD34	Hematopoietic precursors, capillary endothelium	105–120	Ligand for CD62L (L-selectin)		Mucin
CD35	Erythrocytes, B cells, monocytes, neutrophils, eosinophils, follicular dendritic cells	250	Complement receptor 1, binds C3b and C4b, mediates phagocytosis	CR1	CCP
CD36	Platelets, monocytes, endothelial cells	88	Platelet adhesion molecule; involved in recognition and phagocytosis of apoptosed cells	Platelet GPIV, GPIIIb	
CD37	Mature B cells, mature T cells, myeloid cells	40–52	Unknown, may be involved in signal transduction; forms complexes with CD53, CD81, CD82, and MHC class II		Transmembrane 4
CD38	Early B and T cells, activated T cells, germinal center B cells, plasma cells	45	NAD glycohydrolase, augments B cell proliferation	T10	
CD39	Activated B cells, activated NK cells, macrophages, dendritic cells	78	Unknown, may mediate adhesion of B cells		
CD40	B cells, macrophages, dendritic cells, basal epithelial cells	48	Binds CD154 (CD40L); receptor for co-stimulatory signal for B cells, promotes growth, differentiation, and isotype switching of B cells, and cytokine production by macrophages and dendritic cells		TNF receptor
CD41	Platelets, megakaryocytes	Dimer: GPIIba: 125 GPIIbb: 22	αIIb integrin, associates with CD61 to form GPIIb, binds fibrinogen, fibronectin, von Willebrand factor, and thrombospondin	GPIIb	Integrin α
CD42a,b,c,d	Platelets, megakaryocytes	a: 23 b: 135, 23 c: 22 d: 85	Binds von Willebrand factor, thrombin; essential for platelet adhesion at sites of injury	a: GPIX b: GPIbα c: GPIbβ d: GPV	Leucine-rich repeat
CD43	Leukocytes, except resting B cells	115–135 (neutrophils) 95–115 (T cells)	Has extended structure, approx. 45 nm long and may be anti-adhesive	Leukosialin, sialophorin	Mucin
CD44	Leukocytes, erythrocytes	80–95	Binds hyaluronic acid, mediates adhesion of leukocytes	Hermes antigen, Pgp-1	Link protein

CD antigen	Cellular expression	Molecular weight (kDa)	Functions	Other names	Family relationships
CD45	All hematopoietic cells	180–240 (multiple isoforms)	Tyrosine phosphatase, augments signaling through antigen receptor of B and T cells, multiple isoforms result from alternative splicing (see below)	Leukocyte common antigen (LCA), T200, B220	Fibronectin type III
CD45RO	T-cell subsets, B-cell subsets, monocytes, macrophages	180	Isoform of CD45 containing none of the A, B, and C exons		Fibronectin type II
CD45RA	B cells, T-cell subsets (naive T cells), monocytes	205–220	Isoforms of CD45 containing the A exon		Fibronectin type II
CD45RB	T-cell subsets, B cells, monocytes, macrophages, granulocytes	190–220	Isoforms of CD45 containing the B exon	T200	Fibronectin type II
CD46	Hematopoietic and non-hematopoietic nucleated cells	56/66 (splice variants)	Membrane co-factor protein, binds to C3b and C4b to permit their degradation by Factor I	MCP	CCP
CD47	All cells	47–52	Adhesion molecule, thrombospondin receptor	IAP, MER6, OA3	Immunoglobulin superfamily
CD48	Leukocytes	40–47	Putative ligand for CD244	Blast-1	Immunoglobulin
CD49a	Activated T cells, monocytes, neuronal cells, smooth muscle	200	α1 integrin, associates with CD29, binds collagen, laminin-1	VLA-1	Integrin α
CD49b	B cells, monocytes, platelets, megakaryocytes, neuronal, epithelial and endothelial cells, osteoclasts	160	α2 integrin, associates with CD29, binds collagen, laminin	VLA-2, platelet GPIa	Integrin α
CD49c	B cells, many adherent cells	125, 30	α3 integrin, associates with CD29, binds laminin-5, fibronectin, collagen, entactin, invasin	VLA-3	Integrin α
CD49d	Broad distribution includes B cells, thymocytes, monocytes, granulocytes, dendritic cells	150	α4 integrin, associates with CD29, binds fibronectin, MAdCAM-1, VCAM-1	VLA-4	Integrin α
CD49e	Broad distribution includes memory T cells, monocytes, platelets	135, 25	α5 integrin, associates with CD29, binds fibronectin, invasin	VLA-5	Integrin α
CD49f	T lymphocytes, monocytes, platelets, megakaryocytes, trophoblasts	125, 25	α6 integrin, associates with CD29, binds laminin, invasin, merosine	VLA-6	Integrin α
CD50	Thymocytes, T cells, B cells, monocytes, granulocytes	130	Binds integrin CD11a/CD18	ICAM-3	Immunoglobulin
CD51	Platelets, megakaryocytes	125, 24	αV integrin, associates with CD61, binds vitronectin, von Willebrand factor, fibrinogen, and thrombospondin; may be receptor for apoptotic cells	Vitronectin receptor	Integrin α
CD52	Thymocytes, T cells, B cells (not plasma cells), monocytes, granulocytes, spermatozoa	25	Unknown, target for antibodies used therapeutically to deplete T cells from bone marrow	CAMPATH-1, HE5	
CD53	Leukocytes	35–42	Unknown	MRC OX44	Transmembrane 4
CD54	Hematopoietic and non-hematopoietic cells	75–115	Intercellular adhesion molecule (ICAM)-1 binds CD11a/CD18 integrin (LFA-1) and CD11b/CD18 integrin (Mac-1), receptor for rhinovirus	ICAM-1	Immunoglobulin
CD55	Hematopoietic and non-hematopoietic cells	60–70	Decay accelerating factor (DAF), binds C3b, disassembles C3/C5 convertase	DAF	CCP
CD56	NK cells	135–220	Isoform of neural cell-adhesion molecule (NCAM), adhesion molecule	NKH-1	Immunoglobulin
CD57	NK cells, subsets of T cells, B cells, and monocytes		Oligosaccharide, found on many cell-surface glycoproteins	HNK-1, Leu-7	

CD antigen	Cellular expression	Molecular weight (kDa)	Functions	Other names	Family relationships
CD58	Hematopoietic and non-hematopoietic cells	55–70	Leukocyte function-associated antigen-3 (LFA-3), binds CD2, adhesion molecule	LFA-3	Immunoglobulin
CD59	Hematopoietic and non-hematopoietic cells	19	Binds complement components C8 and C9, blocks assembly of membrane-attack complex	Protectin, Mac inhibitor	Ly-6
CD60a			Disialyl ganglioside D3 (GD3)		Carbohydrate structures
CD60b			9-O-acetyl-GD3		Carbohydrate structures
CD60c			7-O-acetyl-GD3		Carbohydrate structures
CD61	Platelets, megakaryocytes, macrophages	110	Intergrin β3 subunit, associates with CD41 (GPIIb/IIIa) or CD51 (vitronectin receptor)		Integrin β
CD62E	Endothelium	140	Endothelium leukocyte adhesion molecule (ELAM), binds sialyl-Lewis^x, mediates rolling interaction of neutrophils on endothelium	ELAM-1, E-selectin	C-type lectin, EGF, and CCP
CD62L	B cells, T cells, monocytes, NK cells	150	Leukocyte adhesion molecule (LAM), binds CD34, GlyCAM, mediates rolling interactions with endothelium	LAM-1, L-selectin, LECAM-1	C-type lectin, EGF, and CCP
CD62P	Platelets, megakaryocytes, endothelium	140	Adhesion molecule, binds CD162 (PSGL-1), mediates interaction of platelets with endothelial cells, monocytes and rolling leukocytes on endothelium	P-selectin, PADGEM	C-type lectin, EGF, and CCP
CD63	Activated platelets, monocytes, macrophages	53	Unknown, is lysosomal membrane protein translocated to cell surface after activation	Platelet activation antigen	Transmembrane 4
CD64	Monocytes, macrophages	72	High-affinity receptor for IgG, binds IgG3>IgG1>IgG4>>>IgG2, mediates phagocytosis, antigen capture, ADCC	FcγRI	Immunoglobulin
CD65	Myeloid cells		Oligosaccharide component of a ceramide dodecasaccharide		
CD66a	Neutrophils	160–180	Unknown, member of carcino-embryonic antigen (CEA) family (see below)	Biliary glyco-protein-1 (BGP-1)	Immunoglobulin
CD66b	Granulocytes	95–100	Unknown, member of carcino-embryonic antigen (CEA) family	Previously CD67	Immunoglobulin
CD66c	Neutrophils, colon carcinoma	90	Unknown, member of carcino-embryonic antigen (CEA) family	Nonspecific cross-reacting antigen (NCA)	Immunoglobulin
CD66d	Neutrophils	30	Unknown, member of carcino-embryonic antigen (CEA) family		Immunoglobulin
CD66e	Adult colon epithelium, colon carcinoma	180–200	Unknown, member of carcino-embryonic antigen (CEA) family	Carcino-embryonic antigen (CEA)	Immunoglobulin
CD66f	Unknown		Unknown, member of carcino-embryonic antigen (CEA) family	Pregnancy specific glycoprotein	Immunoglobulin
CD68	Monocytes, macrophages, neutrophils, basophils, large lymphocytes	110	Unknown	Macrosialin	Mucin

CD antigen	Cellular expression	Molecular weight (kDa)	Functions	Other names	Family relationships
CD69	Activated T and B cells, activated macrophages and NK cells	28, 32 homodimer	Unknown, early activation antigen	Activation inducer molecule (AIM)	C-type lectin
CD70	Activated T and B cells, and macrophages	75, 95, 170	Ligand for CD27, may function in co-stimulation of B and T cells	Ki-24	TNF
CD71	All proliferating cells, hence activated leukocytes	95 homodimer	Transferrin receptor	T9	
CD72	B cells (not plasma cells)	42 homodimer	Unknown	Lyb-2	C-type lectin
CD73	B-cell subsets, T-cell subsets	69	Ecto-5′-nucleotidase, dephosphorylates nucleotides to allow nucleoside uptake		
CD74	B cells, macrophages, monocytes, MHC class II positive cells	33, 35, 41, 43 (alternative initiation and splicing)	MHC class II-associated invariant chain	Ii, Iγ	
CD75	Mature B cells, T-cells subsets		Lactosamines, ligand for CD22, mediates B-cell–B-cell adhesion		
CD75s			α-2,6-sialylated lactosamines		Carbohydrate structures
CD77	Germinal center B cells		Neutral glycosphingolipid (Galα1→4Galβ1→4Galcβ1→ceramide), binds Shiga toxin, cross-linking induces apoptosis	Globotriaocyl-ceramide (Gb3) Pk blood group	
CD79α,β	B cells	α: 40–45 β: 37	Components of B-cell antigen receptor analogous to CD3, required for cell-surface expression and signal transduction	Igα, Igβ	Immunoglobulin
CD80	B-cell subset	60	Co-stimulator, ligand for CD28 and CTLA-4	B7 (now B7.1), BB1	Immunoglobulin
CD81	Lymphocytes	26	Associates with CD19, CD21 to form B cell co-receptor	Target of anti-proliferative antibody (TAPA-1)	Transmembrane 4
CD82	Leukocytes	50–53	Unknown	R2	Transmembrane 4
CD83	Dendritic cells, B cells, Langerhans' cells	43	Unknown	HB15	Immunoglobulin
CDw84	Monocytes, platelets, circulating B cells	73	Unknown	GR6	Immunoglobulin
CD85	Dendritic cells		ILT/LIR family	GR4	Immunoglobulin superfamily
CD86	Monocytes, activated B cells, dendritic cells	80	Ligand for CD28 and CTLA4	B7.2	Immunoglobulin
CD87	Granulocytes, monocytes, macrophages, T cells, NK cells, wide variety of nonhematopoietic cell types	35–59	Receptor for urokinase plasminogen activator	uPAR	Ly-6
CD88	Polymorphonuclear leukocytes, macrophages, mast cells	43	Receptor for complement component C5a	C5aR	G protein-coupled receptor
CD89	Monocytes, macrophages, granulocytes, neutrophils, B-cell subsets, T-cell subsets	50–70	IgA receptor	FcαR	Immunoglobulin
CD90	CD34+ prothymocytes (human), thymocytes, T cells (mouse)	18	Unknown	Thy-1	Immunoglobulin
CD91	Monocytes, many non-hematopoietic cells	515, 85	α2-macroglobulin receptor		EGF, LDL receptor

CD antigen	Cellular expression	Molecular weight (kDa)	Functions	Other names	Family relationships
CD92	Neutrophils, monocytes, platelets, endothelium	70	Unknown	GR9	
CD93	Neutrophils, monocytes, endothelium	120	Unknown	GR11	
CD94	T-cell subsets, NK cells	43	Unknown	KP43	C-type lectin
CD95	Wide variety of cell lines, *in vivo* distribution uncertain	45	Binds TNF-like Fas ligand, induces apoptosis	Apo-1, Fas	TNF receptor
CD96	Activated T cells, NK cells	160	Unknown	T-cell activation increased late expression (TACTILE)	Immunoglobulin
CD97	Activated B and T cells, monocytes, granulocytes	75–85	Binds CD55	GR1	EGF, G protein-coupled receptor
CD98	T cells, B cells, natural killer cells, granulocytes, all human cell lines	80, 45 heterodimer	May be amino acid transporter	4F2, FRP-1	
CD99	Peripheral blood lymphocytes, thymocytes	32	Unknown	MIC2, E2	
CD100	Hematopoietic cells	150 homodimer	Unknown	GR3	Semaphorin
CD101	Monocytes, granulocytes, dendritic cells, activated T cells	120 homodimer	Unknown	BPC#4	Immunoglobulin
CD102	Resting lymphocytes, monocytes, vascular endothelium cells (strongest)	55–65	Binds CD11a/CD18 (LFA-1) but not CD11b/CD18 (Mac-1)	ICAM-2	Immunoglobulin
CD103	Intraepithelial lymphocytes, 2–6% peripheral blood lymphocytes	150, 25	αE integrin	HML-1, α6, αE integrin	Integrin α
CD104	CD4⁻ CD8⁻ thymocytes, neuronal, epithelial, and some endothelial cells, Schwann cells, trophoblasts	220	Integrin β4 associates with CD49f, binds laminins	β4 integrin	Integrin β
CD105	Endothelial cells, activated monocytes and macrophages, bone marrow cell subsets	90 homodimer	Binds TGF-β	Endoglin	
CD106	Endothelial cells	100–110	Adhesion molecule, ligand for VLA-4 ($\alpha_4\beta_1$ integrin)	VCAM-1	Immunoglobulin
CD107a	Activated platelets, activated T cells, activated neutrophils, activated endothelium	110	Unknown, is lysosomal membrane protein translocated to the cell surface after activation	Lysosomal associated membrane protein-1 (LAMP-1)	
CD107b	Activated platelets, activated T cells, activated neutrophils, activated endothelium	120	Unknown, is lysosomal membrane protein translocated to the cell surface after activation	LAMP-2	
CD108	Erythrocytes, circulating lymphocytes, lymphoblasts	80	Unknown	GR2, John Milton-Hagen blood group antigen	
CD109	Activated T cells, activated platelets, vascular endothelium	170	Unknown	Platelet activation factor, GR56	
CD110	Platelets		MPL, TPO R		
CD111	Myeloid cells		PPR1/Nectin1		
CD112	Myeloid cells		PRR2		
CD114	Granulocytes, monocytes	150	Granulocytes colony-stimulating factor (G-CSF) receptor		Immunoglobulin, fibronectin type III

CD antigen	Cellular expression	Molecular weight (kDa)	Functions	Other names	Family relationships
CD115	Monocytes, macrophages	150	Macrophage colony-stimulating factor (M-CSF) receptor	M-CSFR, c-fms	Immunoglobulin, tyrosine kinase
CD116	Monocytes, neutrophils, eosinophils, endothelium	70–85	Granulocyte-macrophage colony-stimulating factor (GM-CSF) receptor α chain	GM-CSFRα	Cytokine receptor, fibronectin type III
CD117	Hematopoietic progenitors	145	Stem-cell factor (SCF) receptor	c-Kit	Immunoglobulin, tyrosine kinase
CD118	Broad cellular expression		Interferon-α, β receptor	IFN-α, βR	
CD119	Macrophages, monocytes, B cells, endothelium	90–100	Interferon-γ receptor	IFN-γR	Fibronectin type III
CD120a	Hematopoietic and nonhematopoietic cells, highest on epithelial cells	50–60	TNF receptor, binds both TNF-α and TNF-β	TNFR-I	TNF receptor
CD120b	Hematopoietic and nonhematopoietic cells, highest on myeloid cells	75–85	TNF receptor, binds both TNF-α and TNF-β	TNFR-II	TNF receptor
CD121a	Thymocytes, T cells	80	Type I interleukin-1 receptor, binds IL-1α and IL-1β	IL-1R type I	Immunoglobulin
CDw121b	B cells, macrophages, monocytes	60–70	Type II interleukin-1 receptor, binds IL-1α and IL-1β	IL-1R type II	Immunoglobulin
CD122	NK cells, resting T-cell subsets, some B-cell lines	75	IL-2 receptor β chain	IL-2Rβ	Cytokine receptor, fibronectin type III
CD123	Bone marrow stem cells, granulocytes, monocytes, megakaryocytes	70	IL-3 receptor α chain	IL-3Rα	Cytokine receptor, fibronectin type III
CD124	Mature B and T cells, hematopoietic precursor cells	130–150	IL-4 receptor	IL-4R	Cytokine receptor, fibronectin type III
CD125	Eosinophils, basophils, activated B cells	55–60	IL-5 receptor	IL-5R	Cytokine receptor, fibronectin type III
CD126	Activated B cells and plasma cells (strong), most leukocytes (weak)	80	IL-6 receptor α subunit	IL-6Rα	Immunoglobulin, cytokine receptor, fibronectin type III
CD127	Bone marrow lymphoid precursors, pro-B cells, mature T cells, monocytes	68–79, possibly forms homodimers	IL-7 receptor	IL-7R	Fibronectin type III
CDw128	Neutrophils, basophils, T-cell subsets	58–67	IL-8 receptor	IL-8R	G protein-coupled receptor
CD129	Not yet assigned				
CD130	Most cell types, strong on activated B cells and plasma cells	130	Common subunit of IL-6, IL-11, oncostatin-M (OSM) and leukemia inhibitory factor (LIF) receptors	IL-6Rβ, IL-11Rβ, OSMRβ, LIFRβ, IFRβ	Immunoglobulin, cytokine receptor, fibronectin type III
CDw131	Myeloid progenitors, granulocytes	140	Common β subunit of IL-3, IL-5, and GM-CSF receptors	IL-3Rβ, IL-5Rβ, GM-CSFRβ	Cytokine receptor, fibronectin type III
CD132	B cells, T cells, NK cells, mast cells, neutrophils	64	IL-2 receptor γ chain, common subunit of IL-2, IL-4, IL-7, IL-9, and IL-15 receptors		Cytokine receptor
CD133	Stem/progenitor cells		AC133		
CD134	Activated T cells	50	May act as adhesion molecule costimulator	OX40	TNF receptor
CD135	Multipotential precursors, myelomonocytic and B-cell progenitors	130, 155	Growth factor receptor	FLK2, STK-1	Immunoglobulin, tyrosine kinase
CDw136	Monocytes, epithelial cells, central and peripheral nervous system	180	Chemotaxis, phagocytosis, cell growth, and differentiation	MSP-R, RON	Tyrosine kinase

CD antigen	Cellular expression	Molecular weight (kDa)	Functions	Other names	Family relationships
CDw137	T and B lymphocytes, monocytes, some epithelial cells		Co-stimulator of T-cell proliferation	ILA (induced by lymphocyte activation), 4-1BB	TNF receptor
CD138	B cells		Heparan sulphate proteoglycan binds collagen type I	Syndecan-1	
CD139	B cells	209, 228	Unknown		
CD140a,b	Stromal cells, some endothelial cells	a: 180 b: 180	Platelet derived growth factor (PDGF) receptor α and β chains		
CD141	Vascular endothelial cells	105	Anticoagulant, binds thrombin, the complex then activates protein C	Thrombomodulin fetomodulin	C-type lectin, EGF
CD142	Epidermal keratinocytes, various epithelial cells, astrocytes, Schwann cells. Absent from cells in direct contact with plasma unless induced by inflammatory mediators	45–47	Major initiating factor of clotting. Binds Factor VIIa; this complex activates Factors VII, IX, and X	Tissue factor, thromboplastin	Fibronectin type III
CD143	Endothelial cells, except large blood vessels and kidney, epithelial cells of brush borders of kidney and small intestine, neuronal cells, activated macrophages and some T cells. Soluble form in plasma	170–180	Zn^{2+} metallopeptidase dipeptidyl peptidase, cleaves angiotensin I and bradykinin from precursor forms	Angiotensin converting en-zyme (ACE)	
CD144	Endothelial cells	130	Organizes adherens junction in en-dothelial cells	Cadherin-5, VE-cadherin	Cadherin
CD145	Endothelial cells, some stromal cells	25, 90, 110	Unknown		
CD146	Endothelium	130	Potential adhesion molecule, localized at cell–cell junctions	MCAM, MUC18, S-ENDO	Immunoglobulin
CD147	Leukocytes, red blood cells, platelets, endothelial cells	55–65	Potential adhesion molecule	M6, neurothelin, EMMPRIN, basigin, OX-47	Immunoglobulin
CD148	Granulocytes, monocytes, dendritic cells, T cells, fibroblasts, nerve cells	240–260	Contact inhibition of cell growth	HPTPη	Fibronectin type III, protein tyro-sine phosphatase
CD150	Thymocytes, activated lymphocytes	75–95	Unknown	SLAM	Immunoglobulin
CD151	Platelets, megakaryocytes, epithelial cells, endothelial cells	32	Associates with β1 integrins	PETA-3, SFA-1	Transmembrane 4
CD152	Activated T cells	33	Receptor for B7.1 (CD80), B7.2 (CD86); negative regulator of T-cell activation	CTLA-4	Immunoglobulin
CD153	Activated T cells, activated macrophages, neutrophils, B cells	38–40	Ligand for CD30, may co-stimulate T cells	CD30L	TNF
CD154	Activated CD4 T cells	30 trimer	Ligand for CD40, inducer of B cell proliferation and activation	CD40L, TRAP, T-BAM, gp39	TNF receptor
CD155	Monocytes, macrophages, thymocytes, CNS neurons	80–90	Normal function unknown; receptor for poliovirus	Poliovirus receptor	Immunoglobulin
CD156a	Neutrophils, monocytes	69	Unknown, may be involved in integrin leukocyte extravasation	MS2, ADAM 8 (A disintegrin and metallo-protease)	
CD156b			TACE/ADAM17. Adhesion structures		
CD157	Granulocytes, monocytes, bone marrow stromal cells, vascular endothelial cells, follicular dendritic cells	42–45 (50 on monocytes)	ADP-ribosyl cyclase, cyclic ADP-ribose hydrolase	BST-1	
CD158	NK cells		KIR family		

CD antigen	Cellular expression	Molecular weight (kDa)	Functions	Other names	Family relationships
CD158a	NK-cell subsets	50 or 58	Inhibits NK cell cytotoxicity on binding MHC class I molecules	p50.1, p58.1	Immunoglobulin
CD158b	NK-cell subsets	50 or 58	Inhibits NK cell cytotoxicity on binding HLA-Cw3 and related alleles	p50.2, p58.2	Immunoglobulin
CD159a	NK cells		Binds CD94 to form NK receptor; inhibits NK cell cytotoxicity on binding MHC class I moolecules	NKG2A	
CD160	T cells			BY55	
CD161	NK cells, T cells	44	Regulates NK cytotoxicity	NKRP1	C-type lectin
CD162	Neutrophils, lymphocytes, monocytes	120 homodimer	Ligand for CD62P	PSGL-1	Mucin
CD162R	NK cells			PEN5	
CD163	Monocytes, macrophages	130	Unknown	M130	
CD164	Epithelial cells, monocytes, bone marrow stromal cells	80	Unknown	MUC-24 (multi-glycosylated protein 24)	Mucin
CD165	Thymocytes, thymic epithelial cells, CNS neurons, pancreatic islets, Bowman's capsule	37	Adhesion between thymocytes and thymic epithelium	Gp37, AD2	
CD166	Activated T cells, thymic epithelium, fibroblasts, neurons	100–105	Ligand for CD6, involved integrin neurite extension	ALCAM, BEN, DM-GRASP, SC-1	Immunoglobulin
CD167a	Normal and transformed epithelial cells	63, 64 dimer	Binds collagen	DDR1, trkE, cak, eddr1	Receptor tyrosine kinase, discoidin-related
CD168	Breast cancer cells	Five isoforms: 58, 60, 64, 70, 84	Adhesion molecule. Receptor for hyaluronic acid-mediated motility—mediated cell migration	RHAMM	
CD169	Subsets of macrophages	185	Adhesion molecule. Binds sialylated carbohydrates. May mediate macrophage binding to granulocytes and lymphocytes	Sialoadhesin	Immunoglobulin superfamily, sialoadhesin family
CD170	Neutrophils	67 homodimer	Adhesion molecule. **S**ialic acid-binding **I**g-like **lec**tin (Siglec). Cytoplasmic tail contains ITIM motifs	Siglec-5, OBBP2, CD33L2	Immunoglobulin superfamily, sialoadhesin family
CD171	Neurons, Schwann cells, lymphoid and myelomonocytic cells, B cells, CD4 T cells (not CD8 T cells)	200–220, exact MW varies with cell type	Adhesion molecule, binds CD9, CD24, CD56, also homophilic binding	L1, NCAM-L1	Immunoglobulin superfamily
CD172a		115–120	Adhesion molecule; the transmembrane protein is a substrate of activated receptor tyrosine kinases (RTKs) and binds to SH2 domains	SIRP, SHPS1, MYD-1, SIRP-α-1, protein tyrosine phosphatase, non-receptor type substrate 1 (PTPNS1)	Immunoglobulin superfamily
CD173	All cells		Blood group H type 2. Carbohydrate moiety		
CD174	All cells		Lewis y Blood group. Carbohydrate moiety		
CD175	All cells		Tn Blood group. Carbohydrate moiety		
CD175s	All cells		Sialyl-Tn Blood group. Carbohydrate moiety		
CD176	All cells		TF Blood group. Carbohydrate moiety		

CD antigen	Cellular expression	Molecular weight (kDa)	Functions	Other names	Family relationships
CD177	Myeloid cells	56–64	NB1 is a GPI-linked neutrophil-specific antigen, found on only a subpopulation of neutrophils present in NB1-positive adults (97% of healthy donors) NB1 is first expressed at the myelocyte stage of myeloid differentiation	NB1	
CD178	Activated T cells	38–42	Fas ligand; binds to Fas to induce apoptosis	FasL	TNF superfamily
CD179a	Early B cells	16–18	Immunoglobulin iota chain associates noncovalently with CD179b to form a surrogate light chain which is a component of the pre-B-cell receptor that plays a critical role in early B-cell differentiation	VpreB, IGVPB, IGι	Immunoglobulin superfamily
CD179b	B cells	22	Immunoglobulin λ-like polypeptide 1 associates noncovalently with CD179a to form a surrogate light chain that is selectively expressed at the early stages of B-cell development. Mutations in the CD179b gene have been shown to result in impairment of B-cell development and agammaglobulinemia in humans	IGLL1, λ5 (IGL5), IGVPB, 14.	Immunoglobulin superfamily
CD180	B cells	95–105	Type 1 membrane protein consisting of extracellular leucine-rich repeats (LRR). Is associated with a molecule called MD-1 and forms the cell-surface receptor complex, RP105/MD-1, which by working in concert with TLR4, controls B-cell recognition and signaling of lipopolysaccharide (LPS)	LY64, RP105	Toll-like receptors (TLR)
CD183	Particularly on malignant B cells from chronic lymphoproliferative disorders	46–52	CXC chemokine receptor involved in chemotaxis of malignant B lymphocytes. Binds INP10 and MIG[3]	CXCR3, G protein-coupled receptor 9 (GPR 9)	Chemokine receptors, G protein-coupled receptor superfamily
CD184	Preferentially expressed on the more immature CD34+ haematopoietic stem cells	46–52	Binding to SDF-1 (LESTR/fusin); acts as a cofactor for fusion and entry of T-cell line; trophic strains of HIV-1	CXCR4, NPY3R, LESTR, fusin, HM89	Chemokine receptors, G protein-coupled receptor superfamily
CD195	Promyelocytic cells	40	Receptor for a CC type chemokine. Binds to MIP-1α, MIP-1β and RANTES. May play a role in the control of granulocytic lineage proliferation or differentiation. Acts as co-receptor with CD4 for primary macrophage-tropic isolates of HIV-1	CMKBR5, CCR5, CKR-5, CC-CKR-5, CKR5	Chemokine receptors, G protein-coupled receptor superfamily
CDw197	Activated B and T lymphocytes, strongly upregulated in B cells infected with EBV and T cells infected with HHV6 or 7	46–52	Receptor for the MIP-3β chemokine; probable mediator of EBV effects on B lymphocytes or of normal lymphocyte functions	CCR7. EBI1 (Epstein–Barr virus induced gene 1), CMKBR7, BLR2	Chemokine receptors, G protein-coupled receptor superfamily
CD200	Normal brain and B-cell lines	41 (rat thymocytes) 47 (rat brain)	Antigen identified by MoAb MRC OX-2. Nonlineage molecules. Function unknown	MOX-2, MOX-1	Immunoglobulin superfamily
CD201	Endothelial cells	49	Endothelial cell-surface receptor (EPCR) that is capable of high-affinity binding of protein C and activated protein C. It is downregulated by exposure of endothelium to tumor necrosis factor	EPCR	CD1major histocompatibility complex family
CD202b	Endothelial cells	140	Receptor tyrosine kinase, binds angiopoietin-1; important in angiogenesis, particularly for vascular network formation in endothelial cells. Defects in TEK are associated with inherited venous malformations; the TEK signaling pathway appears to be critical for endothelial cell–smooth muscle cell communication in venous morphogenesis	VMCM, TEK (tyrosine kinase, endothelial), TIE2 (tyrosine kinase with Ig and EGF homology domains), VMCM1 NPP3, B10,	Immunoglobulin superfamily, tyrosine kinase

CD antigen	Cellular expression	Molecular weight (kDa)	Functions	Other names	Family relationships
CD203c	Myeloid cells (uterus, basophils, and mast cells)	101	Belongs to a series of ectoenzymes that are involved in hydrolysis of extracellular nucleotides. They catalyze the cleavage of phosphodiester and phosphosulfate bonds of a variety of molecules, including deoxynucleotides, NAD, and nucleotide sugars	PDNP3, PD-Iβ, gp130RB13-6	Type II transmembrane proteins, Ecto-nucleotide pyrophosphatase/phosphodiesterase (E-NPP) family
CD204	Myeloid cells	220	Mediate the binding, internalization, and processing of a wide range of negatively charged macromolecules. Implicated in the pathologic deposition of cholesterol in arterial walls during atherogenesis	Macrophage scavenger R (MSR1)	Scavenger receptor family, collagen-like
CD205	Dendritic cells	205	Lymphocyte antigen 75; putative antigen-uptake receptor on dendritic cells	LY75, DEC-205, GP200-MR6	Type I transmembrane protein
CD206	Macrophages, endothelial cells	175–190	Type I membrane glycoprotein; only known example of a C-type lectin that contains multiple C-type CRDs (carbohydrate-recognition domains); it binds high-mannose structures on the surface of potentially pathogenic viruses, bacteria, and fungi	Macrophage mannose receptor (MMR), MRC1	C-type lectin superfamily
CD207	Langerhans' cells	40	Type II transmembrane protein; Langerhans' cell specific C-type lectin; potent inducer of membrane superimposition and zippering leading to BG (Birbeck granules) formation	Langerin	C-type lectin superfamily
CD208	Interdigitating dendritic cells in lymphoid organs	70–90	Homologous to CD68, DC-LAMP is a lysosomal protein involved in remodeling of specialized antigen-processing compartments and in MHC class II-restricted antigen presentation. Upregulated in mature DCs induced by CD40L, TNF-α and LPS.	D lysosome-associated membrane protein, DC-LAMP	Major histocompatibility complex family
CD209	Dendritic cells	44	C-type lectin; binds ICAM3 and HIV-1 envelope glycoprotein gp120 enables T-cell receptor engagement by stabilization of the DC/T-cell contact zone, promotes efficient infection in *trans* cells that express CD4 and chemokine receptors; type II transmembrane protein	DC-SIGN (dendritic cell-specific ICAM3-grabbing non-integrin)	C-type lectin superfamily
CDw210	B cells, T helper cells, and cells of the monocyte/macrophage lineage	90–110	Interleukin 10 receptor α and β	IL-10Rα, IL-10RA, HIL-10R, IL-10Rβ, IL-10RB, CRF2-4, CRFB4	Class II cytokine receptor family
CD212	Activated CD4, CD8, and NK cells	130	IL-12 receptor β chain; a type I transmembrane protein involved in IL-12 signal transduction.	IL-12R IL-12RB	Haemopoietin cytokine receptor superfamily
CD213a1	B cells, monocytes, fibroblasts, endothelial cells	60–70	Receptor which binds Il-13 with a low affinity; together with IL-4Rα can form a functional receptor for IL-13, also serves as an alternate accessory protein to the common cytokine receptor gamma chain for IL-4 signaling	IL-13Rα 1, NR4, IL-13Ra	Haemopoietic cytokine receptor superfamily
CD213a2	B cells, monocytes, fibroblasts, endothelial cells		IL-13 receptor which binds as a monomer with high affinity to interleukin-13 (IL-13), but not to IL-4; human cells expressing IL-13RA2 show specific IL-13 binding with high affinity	IL-13Rα 2, IL-13BP	Haemopoietic cytokine receptor superfamily
CDw217	Activated memory T cells	120	Interleukin 17 receptor homodimer	IL-17R, CTLA-8 Insulin receptor	Chemokine/ cytokine receptors

CD antigen	Cellular expression	Molecular weight (kDa)	Functions	Other names	Family relationships
CD220	Nonlineage molecules	α: 130 β: 95	Insulin receptor; integral transmembrane glycoprotein comprised of two α and two β subunits; this receptor binds insulin and has a tyrosine-protein kinase activity—autophosphorylation activates the kinase activity		Insulin receptor family of tyrosine-protein kinases, EGFR family
CD221	Nonlineage molecules	α: 135 β: 90	Insulin-like growth factor I receptor binds insulin-like growth factor with a high affinity. It has tyrosine kinase activity and plays a critical role in transformation events. Cleavage of the precursor generates α and β subunits.	IGF1R, JTK13	Insulin receptor family of tyrosine-protein kinases, EGFR family
CD222	Nonlineage molecules	250	Ubiquitously expressed multifunctional type I transmembrane protein. Its main functions include internalization of IGF-II, internalization or sorting of lysosomal enzymes and other M6P-containing proteins	IGF2R, CIMPR, CI-MPR, IGF2R, M6P-R (Mannose-6-phosphate receptor)	Mammalian lectins
CD223	Activated T and NK cells	70	Involved in lymphocyte activation; binds to HLA class-II antigens; role in down-regulating antigen specific response; close relationship of LAG3 to CD4	Lymphocyte-activation gene 3 LAG-3	Immunoglobulin superfamily
CD224	Nonlineage molecules	62 (un-processed precursor)	Predominantly a membrane-bound enzyme; plays a key role in the γ-glutamyl cycle, a pathway for the synthesis and degradation of glutathione. This enzyme consists of two polypeptide chains, which are synthesized in precursor form from a single polypeptide	γ-glutamyl transferase, GGT1, D22S672 D22S732	γ-glutamyl transferase protein family
CD225	Leukocytes and endothelial cells	16–17	Interferon-induced transmembrane protein 1 is implicated in the control of cell growth. It is a component of a multimeric complex involved in the transduction of antiproliferative and homotypic adhesion signals	Leu 13, IFITM1, IFI17	IFN-induced transmembrane proteins
CD226	NK cells, platelets, monocytes, and a subset of T cells	65	Adhesion glycoprotein; mediates cellular adhesion to other cells bearing an unidentified ligand and cross-linking CD226 with antibodies causes cellular activation	DNAM-1 (PTA1), DNAX, TLiSA1	Immunoglobulin superfamily
CD227	Human epithelial tumors, such as breast cancer	122 (nonglyco-sylated)	Epithelial mucin containing a variable number of repeats with a length of twenty amino acids, resulting in many different alleles. Direct or indirect interaction with actin cytoskeleton.	PUM (peanut-reactive urinary mucin), MUC.1, mucin 1	Mucin
CD228	Predominantly in human melanomas	97	Tumor-associated antigen (melanoma) identified by monoclonal antibodies 133.2 and 96.5, involved in cellular iron uptake.	Melanotransferrin, P97	Transferrin superfamily
CD229	Lymphocytes	90–120	May participate in adhesion reactions between T lymphocytes and accessory cells by homophilic interaction	Ly9	Immunoglobulin superfamily (CD2 subfamily)
CD230	Expressed both in normal and infected cells	27–30	The function of PRP is not known. It is encoded in the host genome found in high quantity in the brain of humans and animals infected with neurodegenerative diseases known as transmissible spongiform encephalopathies or prion diseases (Creutzfeld–Jakob disease, Gerstmann–Strausler–Scheinker syndrome, fatal familial insomnia)	CJD, PRIP, prion protein (p27-30) TALLA-1,	Prion family

CD antigen	Cellular expression	Molecular weight (kDa)	Functions	Other names	Family relationships
CD231	T-cell acute lymphoblastic leukemia, neuroblastoma cells and normal brain neuron	150	The function of CD231 is currently unknown. It is cell-surface glycoprotein which is a specific marker for T-cell acute lymphoblastic leukemia. Also found on neuroblastomas	TM4SF2, A15, MXS1, CCG-B7	Transmembrane 4 superfamily (TM4SF also known as tetraspanins)
CD232	Nonlineage molecules	200	Receptor for an immunologically active semaphorin (virus-encoded semaphorin protein receptor)	VESPR, PLXN, PLXN-C1	Plexin family
CD233	Erythroid cells	93	Band 3 is the major integral glycoprotein of the erythrocyte membrane. It has two functional domains. Its integral domain mediates a 1:1 exchange of inorganic anions across the membrane, whereas its cytoplasmic domain provides binding sites for cytoskeletal proteins, glycolytic enzymes, and hemoglobin. Multifunctional transport protein	SLC4A1, Diego blood group, D1, AE1, EPB3	Anion exchanger family
CD234	Erythroid cells and nonerythroid cells	35	Fy-glycoprotein; Duffy blood group antigen; nonspecific receptor for many chemokines such as IL-8, GRO, RANTES, MCP-1 and TARC. It is also the receptor for the human malaria parasites *Plasmodium vivax* and *Plasmodium knowlesi* plays a role in inflammation and in malaria infection	GPD, CCBP1, DARC (duffy antigen/receptor for chemokines)	Family 1 of G protein-coupled receptors, chemokine receptors superfamily
CD235a	Erythroid cells	31	Major carbohydrate rich sialoglycoprotein of human erythrocyte membrane which bears the antigenic determinants for the MN and Ss blood groups. The N-terminal glycosylated segment, which lies outside the erythrocyte membrane, has MN blood group receptors and also binds influenza virus	Glycophorin A, GPA, MNS	Glycophorin A family
CD235b	Erythroid cells	GYPD is smaller than GYPC (24 kD vs 32 kD)	This protein is a minor sialoglycoprotein in human erythrocyte membranes. Along with GYPA, GYPB is responsible for the MNS blood group system. The Ss blood group antigens are located on glycophorin B	Glycophorin B, MNS, GPB	Glycophorin A family
CD236	Erythroid cells	24	Glycophorin C (GPC) and glycophorin D (GPD) are closely related sialoglycoproteins in the human red blood cell (RBC) membrane. GPD is a ubiquitous shortened isoform of GPC, produced by alternative splicing of the same gene. The Webb and Duch antigens, also known as glycophorin D, result from single point mutations of the glycophorin C gene	Glycophorin D, GPD, GYPD	Type III membrane proteins
CD236R	Erythroid cells	32	Glycophorin C (GPC) is associated with the Gerbich (Ge) blood group deficiency. It is a minor red cell-membrane component, representing about 4% of the membrane sialoglycoproteins, but shows very little homology with the major red cell-membrane glycophorins A and B. It plays an important role in regulating the mechanical stability of red cells and is a putative receptor for the merozoites of *Plasmodium falciparum*	Glycophorin C, GYPC, GPC	Type III membrane proteins
CD238	Erythroid cells	93	KELL blood group antigen; homology to a family of zinc metalloglycoproteins with neutral endopeptidase activity, type II transmembrane glycoprotein	KELL	Belongs to peptidase family m13 (zinc metalloprotease); also known as the neprilysin subfamily

CD antigen	Cellular expression	Molecular weight (kDa)	Functions	Other names	Family relationships
CD239	Erythroid cells	78	A type I membrane protein. The human F8/G253 antigen, B-CAM, is a cell surface glycoprotein that is expressed with restricted distribution pattern in normal fetal and adult tissues, and is upregulated following malignant transformation in some cell types. Its overall structure is similar to that of the human tumor marker MUC 18 and the chicken neural adhesion molecule SC1	B-CAM (B-cell adhesion molecule), LU, Lutheran blood group	Immunoglobulin superfamily
CD240CE	Erythroid cells	45.5	Rhesus blood group, CcEe antigens. May be part of an oligomeric complex which is likely to have a transport or channel function in the erythrocyte membrane. It is highly hydrophobic and deeply buried within the phospholipid bilayer	RHCE, RH30A, RHPI, Rh4	Rh family
CD240D	Erythroid cells	45.5 (product—30)	Rhesus blood group, D antigen. May be part of an oligomeric complex which is likely to have a transport or channel function in the erythrocyte membrane. Absent in the Caucasian RHD-negative phenotype	RhD, Rh4, RhPI, RhII, Rh30D	Rh family
CD241	Erythroid cells	50	Rhesus blood group-associated glycoprotein RH50, component of the RH antigen multisubunit complex; required for transport and assembly of the Rh membrane complex to the red blood cell surface. highly homologous to RH, 30kD components. Defects in RhAg are a cause of a form of chronic hemolytic anemia associated with stomatocytosis, and spherocytosis, reduced osmotic fragility, and increased cation permeability	RhAg, RH50A	Rh family
CD242	Erythroid cells	42	Intercellular adhesion molecule 4, Landsteiner-Wiener blood group. LW molecules may contribute to the vaso-occlusive events associated with episodes of acute pain in sickle cell disease	ICAM-4, LW	Immunoglobulin superfamily, intercellular adhesion molecules (ICAMs)
CD243	Stem/progenitor cells	170	Multidrug resistance protein 1 (P-glycoprotein). P-gp has been shown to utilise ATP to pump hydrophobic drugs out of cells, thus increasing their intracellular concentration and hence their toxicity. The MDR 1 gene is amplified in multidrug resistant cell lines	MDR-1, p-170	ABC superfamily of ATP-binding transport proteins
CD244	NK cells	66	2B4 is a cell-surface glycoprotein related to CD2 and implicated in the regulation of natural killer and T-lymphocyte function. It appears that the primary function of 2B4 is to modulate other receptor–ligand interactions to enhance leukocyte activation	2B4, NK cell activation inducing ligand (NAIL)	Immunoglobulin superfamily
CD245	T cells	220–240	Cyclin E/Cdk2 interacting protein p220. NPAT is involved in a key S phase event and links cyclical cyclin E/Cdk2 kinase activity to replication-dependent histone gene transcription. NPAT gene may be essential for cell maintenance and may be a member of	NPAT ALK	

CD antigen	Cellular expression	Molecular weight (kDa)	Functions	Other names	Family relationships
CD246	Expressed in the small intestine, testis, and brain but not in normal lymphoid cells	177 kDa; after glycosylation, produces a 200 kDa mature glycoprotein	the housekeeping genes Anaplastic (CD30+ large cell) lymphoma kinase; plays an important role in brain development, involved in anaplastic nodal non Hodgkin lymphoma or Hodgkin's disease with translocation t(2;5)(p23;q35) or inv2(23;q35). Oncogenesis via the kinase function is activated by oligomerization of NPM1-ALK mediated by the NPM1 part		Insulin receptor family of tyrosine-protein kinases
CD247	T cells, NK cells	16	T-cell receptor ζ; has a probable role in assembly and expression of the TCR complex as well as signal transduction upon antigen triggering. TCRζ together with TCRα:β and γ:δ heterodimers and CD3-γ, -δ, and -ϵ, forms the TCR-CD3 complex. The ζ chain plays an important role in coupling antigen recognition to several intracellular signal-transduction pathways. Low expression of the antigen results in impaired immune response	ζ chain, CD3Z	Immunoglobulin superfamily

Compiled by Laura Herbert, Royal Free Hospital, London. Data based on CD designations made at the 7th Workshop on Human Leucocyte Differentiation Antigens, provided by Protein Reviews on the Web (www.ncbi.nlm.nih.gov/prow/).

			Appendix III. Cytokines and their receptors.			
Family	Cytokine (alternative names)	Size (no. of amino acids) and form	Receptors (c denotes common subunit)	Producer cells	Actions	Effect of cytokine or receptor knock-out (where known)
Hematopoietins (four-helix bundles)	Epo (erythropoietin)	165, monomer*	EpoR	Kidney cells hepatocytes	Stimulates erythroid progenitors	Epo or EpoR: embryonic lethal
	IL-2 (T-cell growth factor)	133, monomer	CD25 (α), CD122 (β), CD132 (γc)	T cells	T-cell proliferation	IL-2: deregulated T-cell proliferation, colitis IL-2Rα: incomplete T-cell development IL-2Rβ: increased T-cell autoimmunity IL-2γc: severe combined immunodeficiency
	IL-3 (multicolony CSF)	133, monomer	CD123, βc	T cells, thymic epithelial cells	Synergistic action in early hematopoiesis	IL-3: impaired eosinophil development. Bone marrow unresponsive to IL-5, GM-CSF
	IL-4 (BCGF-1, BSF-1)	129, monomer	CD124, CD132 (γc)	T cells, mast cells	B-cell activation, IgE switch, induces differentiation into T$_H$2 cells	IL-4: decreased IgE synthesis
	IL-5 (BCGF-2)	115, homodimer	CD125, βc	T cells, mast cells	Eosinophil growth, differentiation	IL-5: decreased IgE, IgG1 synthesis (in mice); decreased levels of IL-9, IL-10, and eosinophils
	IL-6 (IFN-β_2, BSF-2, BCDF)	184, monomer	CD126, CD130	T cells, macrophages, endothelial cells	T- and B-cell growth and differentiation, acute phase protein production, fever	IL-6: decreased acute phase reaction, reduced IgA production
	IL-7	152, monomer*	CD127, CD132 (γc)	Non-T cells	Growth of pre-B cells and pre-T cells	IL-7: early thymic and lymphocyte expansion severely impaired
	IL-9	125, monomer	IL-9R, CD132 (γc)	T cells	Mast-cell enhancing activity stimulates T$_H$2	
	IL-11	178, monomer	IL-11R, CD130	Stromal fibroblasts	Synergistic action with IL-3 and IL-4 in hematopoiesis	
	IL-13 (P600)	132, monomer	IL-13R, CD132 (γc) (may also include CD24)	T cells	B-cell growth and differentiation, inhibits macrophage inflammatory cytokine production and T$_H$1 cells, induces allergy/asthma	IL-13: defective regulation of isotype-specific responses
	G-CSF	?, monomer*	G-CSFR	Fibroblasts and monocytes	Stimulates neutrophil development and differentiation	Defective myelopoiesis, neutropenia
	IL-15 (T-cell growth factor)	114, monomer	IL-15R, CD122 (IL-Rβ) CD132 (γc)	Many non-T cells	IL-2-like, stimulates growth of intestinal epithelium, T cells, and NK cells, enhances CD8 memory T cell survival	
	IL-21	133	IL-21R +IL-2Rγc	T$_H$2 cells	Induces proliferation of B, T and NK cells	
	GM-CSF (granulocyte-macrophage colony-stimulating factor)	127, monomer*	CD116, βc	Macrophages, T cells	Stimulates growth and differentiation of myelomonocytic lineage cells, particularly dendritic cells	GM-CSF, GM-CSFR: pulmonary alveolar proteinosis
	OSM (OM, oncostatin M)	196, monomer	OSMR or LIFR, CD130	T cells, macrophages	Stimulates Kaposi's sarcoma cells, inhibits melanoma growth	
	LIF (leukemia inhibitory factor)	179, monomer	LIFR, CD130	Bone marrow stroma, fibroblasts	Maintains embryonic stem cells, like IL-6, IL-11, OSM	LIFR: die at or soon after birth; decreased hematopoietic stem cells

*May function as dimers

Family	Cytokine (alternative names)	Size (no. of amino acids) and form	Receptors (c denotes common subunit)	Producer cells	Actions	Effect of cytokine or receptor knock-out (where known)
Interferons	IFN-γ	143, homodimer	CD119, IFNGR2	T cells, natural killer cells	Macrophage activation, increased expression of MHC molecules and antigen processing components, Ig class switching, supresses T$_H$2	IFN-γ, IFN-γR: decreased resistance to bacterial infection, especially mycobacteria and certain viruses, impaired T$_H$1 responses
	IFN-α	166, monomer	CD118, IFNAR2	Leukocytes, dendritic cells	Antiviral, increased MHC class I expression	IFN-α: impaired antiviral defences
	IFN-β	166, monomer	CD118, IFNAR2	Fibroblasts	Antiviral, increased MHC class I expression	
TNF family	TNF-α (cachectin)	157, trimers	p55, p75 CD120a, CD120b	Macrophages, NK cells, T cells	Local inflammation, endothelial activation	TNF-αR: resistance to septic shock, susceptibility to *Listeria* STNFαR: periodic febrile attacks
	TNF-β (lymphotoxin, LT, LT-α)	171, trimers	p55, p75 CD120a, CD120b	T cells, B cells	Killing, endothelial activation	TNF-β: absent lymph nodes, decreased antibody, increased IgM
	LT-β	Transmembrane, trimerizes with TNF-β, (LT-α)	LTβR or HVEM	T cells, B cells	Lymph node development	Defective development of peripheral lymph nodes, Peyer's patches, and spleen
	CD40 ligand (CD40L)	Trimers	CD40	T cells, mast cells	B-cell activation, class switching	CD40L: poor antibody response, no class switching, diminished T-cell priming (hyper IgM syndrome)
	Fas ligand (FasL)	Trimers	CD95 (Fas)	T cells, stroma?	Apoptosis, Ca^{2+}-independent cytotoxicity	Fas, FasL: mutant forms lead to lymphoproliferation, and autoimmunity
	CD27 ligand (CD27L)	Trimers (?)	CD27	T cells	Stimulates T-cell proliferation	
	CD30 ligand (CD30L)	Trimers (?)	CD30	T cells	Stimulates T- and B-cell proliferation	CD30: increased thymic size, alloreactivity
	4-1BBL	Trimers (?)	4-1BB	T cells	Co-stimulates T and B cells	
	Trail	281, aa trimers	DR4, DR5 DCR1, DCR2 and OPG	T cells, monocytes	Apoptosis of activated T cells and tumor cells	
	OPG-L (RANK-L)	316 aa trimers	RANK/OPG	Osteoblasts, T cells	Stimulates osteoclasts and bone resorption	OPG-L: osteopetrotic runted, toothless OPG: osteoporosis
	APRIL	86	TAC1 and BCMA		B-cell proliferation	
	LIGHT	240		Activated T cells	Dendritic cell activation	
	TWEAK	102	TWEAKR (Fn14)		Angiogenesis	
	BlyS		TAC1 and BCMA		B-cell proliferation	BlyS: B-cell dysfunction
IL-10	IL-10 (cytokine synthesis inhibitory factor)	160, homodimer	IL-10Rα +IL–20Rβc	T cells, macrophages, EBV-transformed B cells	Potent suppressant of macrophage functions	IL-10: reduced growth, anemia, chronic enterocolitis
	IL-19	153, monomer	IL-20Rα +IL–20Rβc	Monocytes	Induces IL-6 and TNF-α expression by monocytes	
	IL-20	152	IL-20Rα +IL20Rβc; IL-22Rαc +IL-20Rβc	Monocytes	Stimulates keratinocyte proliferation and TNF-α production	
	IL-22 (IL-TIF)	146	IL-22Rαc+ IL-10Rβc	T cells (type 1), NK cells	Induces liver acute-phase proteins, pro-inflammatory agents	

Family	Cytokine (alternative names)	Size (no. of amino acids) and form	Receptors (c denotes common subunit)	Producer cells	Actions	Effect of cytokine or receptor knock-out (where known)
	IL-24 (MDA7)	157	IL-22Rαc +IL-20Rβc; IL-20Rα+ IL-20Rβc	Monocytes, T cells	Inhibits tumor growth	
	IL26(AK155)	150	IL-20Rα +IL-10Rβc	T cells (type 1), NK cells		
	IL-28A,B (IFN-λ2,3)	175	IL-28Rαc +IL-10Rβc		Antiviral	
	IL-29 (IFN-λ1)	181	IL-28Rαc +IL-10Rβc		Antiviral	
IL-12	IL-12 (NK-cell stimulatory factor)	197 (p35) and 306 (p40c), heterodimer	IL-12Rβ1c +IL-12Rβ2	Macrophages, dendritic cells	Activates NK cells, induces CD4 T-cell differentiation into T_H1-like cells	IL-12: impaired in IFN-γ production and in T_H1 responses
	IL-23	170 (p19) and 306 (p40c), heterodimer	IL-12Rβ1c +IL-23R	Dendritic cells	Induces proliferation of memory T cells, increased IFN-γ production	
	IL-27	142 (p28) and 209 (EBI3), heterodimer	WSX-1 +CD130c	Monocytes, macrophages, dendritic cells	Induces IL-12R on T cells via T-bet induction	EBI3: reduced NK T cells. WSX-1: over-reaction to *Toxoplasma gondii* infection and death from inflammation
Unassigned	TGF-β	112, homo- and heterotrimers	TGF-βR	Chondrocytes, monocytes, T cells	Inhibits cell growth, anti-inflammatory, induces switch to IgA production	TGFβ: lethal inflammation
	IL-1α	159, monomer	CD121a (IL-1RI) and CD121b (IL-1RII)	Macrophages, epithelial cells	Fever, T-cell activation, macrophage activation	IL-1RI: decreased IL-6 production
	IL-1β	153, monomer	CD121a (IL-1RI) and CD121b (IL-1RII)	Macrophages, epithelial cells	Fever, T-cell activation, macrophage activation	IL-1β: impaired acute phase response
	IL-1 RA	?, monomer	CD121a	Monocytes, macrophages, neutrophils, hepatocytes	Binds to but doesn't trigger IL-1 receptor, acts as a natural antagonist of IL-1 function	IL-1RA: reduced body mass, increased sensitivity to endotoxins (septic shock)
	MIF	115, monomer		T cells, pituitary cells	Inhibits macrophage migration, stimulates macrophage activation, induces steroid resistance	MIF: resistance to septic shock
	IL-16	130, homotetramer	CD4	T cells, mast cells, eosinophils	Chemoattractant for CD4 T cells, monocytes, and eosinophils, antiapoptotic for IL-2-stimulated T cells	
	IL-17 (mCTLA-8)	150, monomer		CD4 memory cells	Induce cytokine production by epithelia, endothelia, and fibroblasts	
	IL-18 (IGIF, interferon-γ inducing factor)	157, monomer	Il-1Rrp (IL-1R related protein)	Activated macrophages and Kupffer cells	Induces IFN-γ production by T cells and NK cells, favors T_H1 induction and later T_H2 responses	Defective NK activity and T_H1 responses
	IL-25	145		T_H2 cells, mast cells	Promotes T_H2 cytokine production	

		Appendix IV. Chemokines and their receptors.		
Chemokine systematic name	**Common names**	**Chromosome**	**Target cell**	**Specific receptor**
CXCL (†ELR⁺)				
1	GROα	4	Neutrophil	CXCR2 >> 1
2	GROβ	4	Neutrophil	CXCR1, 2
3	GROγ	4	Neutrophil	CXCR1, 2
5	ENA-78	4	Neutrophil	CXCR1, 2
6	GCP-2	4	Neutrophil	CXCR1, 2
7	NAP-2 (PBP/CTAP-III/β-TG)	4	Fibroblast, neutrophil	CXCR1, 2
8	IL-8	4	Neutrophil, basophil, T cell	CXCR1, 2
14	BRAK/bolekine	5	T cell, monocyte	Unknown
15	Lungkine/WECHE	5	Neutrophil	Unknown
(†ELR⁻)				
4	PF4	4	Fibroblast	CXCR3 (alternative splice)
9	Mig	4	Activated T cell ($T_H1 > T_H2$)	CXCR3
10	IP-10	4	Activated T cell ($T_H1 > T_H2$)	CXCR3
11	I-TAC	4	Activated T cell ($T_H1 > T_H2$)	CXCR3
12	SDF-1α/β	10	CD34⁺ bone marrow cell, progenitor lymphocytes, T cell, dendritic cell, B cell, plasma cell, activated CD4 T cell	CXCR4
13	BLC/BCA-1	4	Naive B cells, activated CD4 T cells	CXCR5
16	(None)	17	Activated T cell, NK T cell	CXCR6
CCL				
1	I-309	17	Neutrophil (TCA-3 only), T cell	CCR8
2	MCP-1	17	T cell, monocyte, basophil	CCR2
3	MIP-1α	17	Monocyte/macrophage, T cell ($T_H1 > T_H2$), NK cell, basophil, immature dendritic cell, bone marrow cell	CCR1, 5
4	MIP-1β	17	Monocyte/macrophage, T cell ($T_H1 > T_H2$), NK cell, basophil, immature dendritic cell, bone marrow cell	CCR5
5	RANTES	17	Monocyte/macrophage, T cell (memory T cell > T cell; $T_H1 > T_H2$), NK cell, basophil, eosinophil, dendritic cell	CCR1, 3, 5
6	C10	11 (mouse only)	Monocyte	Unknown
7	MCP-3	17	T cell, monocyte, eosinophil, basophil, dendritic cell	CCR1, 2, 3
8	MCP-2	17	T cell, monocyte, eosinophil, basophil	CCR2, 3, 5
9/10	MRP-2/MIP-1γ	11 (mouse only)	T cell, monocyte	Unknown
11	Eotaxin	17	Eosinophil	CCR3
12	MCP-5	11 (mouse only)	Eosinophil, monocyte, T cell	CCR2
13	MCP-4	17	T cell, monocyte, eosinophil, basophil, dendritic cell	CCR2, 3
14	HCC-1	17	Monocyte	CCR1, 5
15	MIP-5/HCC-2	17	T cell, monocyte, neutrophil (?), dendritic cell	CCR1, 3
16	HCC-4	17	Monocyte	CCR1, 2
17	TARC	16	T cell ($T_H1 > T_H2$), immature dendritic cell, IA NK cell, T cell ($T_H1 > T_H2$), thymocyte	CCR4
18	DC-CK1	17	Naive T cell > T cell	Unknown
19	MIP-3β	9	Naive T cell, mature dendritic cell, B cell	CCR7
20	MIP-3α	2	T cell (memory T cell > T cell), peripheral blood mononuclear cell, bone marrow cell-dendritic cell, activated B cells	CCR6
21	6Ckine/SLC	9	Naive T cell, B cell, mesangial cells (?)	CCR7
22	MDC	16	Immature dendritic cell, NK cell, T cell ($T_H1 > T_H2$), thymocyte	CCR4
23	MPIF-1	17	Monocyte, T cell (resting), neutrophil (?)	CCR1
24	**Eotaxin-2/MPIF-2**	7	Eosinophil, basophil, T cell (?)	CCR3
25	TECK	19	Macrophage, thymocytes, dendritic cell, intraepithelial lymphocyte, IgA⁺ plasma cell	CCR9
26	**Eotaxin-3**	7	Eosinophil, basophil	CCR3
27	CTACK	9	T cell	CCR10
28	MEC	5	T cell, eosinophil	CCR10, 3
C and CX3C				
XCL 1	Lymphotactin	1 (1)	T cell, NK cell	XCR1
XCL 2	SCM-1β	1	T cell, NK cell	XCR1
CX3CL 1	Fractalkine	16	T cell, monocyte, neutrophil (?)	CX3CR1

Chromosome locations are for humans. Chemokines for which there is no human homolog are listed with the mouse chromosome.

† ELR refers to the three amino acids that precede the first cysteine residue of the CXC motif. If these amino acids are Glu-Leu-Arg (ie ELR⁺), then the chemokine is chemotactic for neutrophils; if they are not (ELR⁻) then the chemokine is chemotactic for lymphocytes.

Appendix V. Immunological constants.

	Evaluation of the cellular components of the human immune system		
	B cells	**T cells**	**Phagocytes**
Normal numbers ($\times 10^9$ per liter of blood)	Approximately 0.3	Total 1.0–2.5 CD4 0.5–1.6 CD8 0.3–0.9	Monocytes 0.15–0.6 Polymorphonuclear leukocytes Neutrophils 3.00–5.5 Eosinophils 0.05–0.25 Basophils 0.02
Measurement of function *in vivo*	Serum Ig levels Specific antibody levels	Skin test	—
Measurement of function *in vitro*	Induced antibody production in response to pokeweed mitogen	T-cell proliferation in response to phytohemagglutinin or to tetanus toxoid	Phagocytosis Nitro blue tetrazolium uptake Intracellular killing of bacteria
Specific defects	See Fig. 11.8	See Fig. 11.8	See Fig. 11.8

	Evaluation of the humoral components of the human immune system				
	Immunoglobulins				**Complement**
Component	IgG	IgM	IgA	IgE	
Normal levels	600–1400 $mg\,dl^{-1}$	40–345 $mg\,dl^{-1}$	60–380 $mg\,dl^{-1}$	0–200 $IU\,ml^{-1}$	CH_{50} of 125–300 $IU\,ml^{-1}$

BIOGRAPHIES

Emil von Behring (1854–1917) discovered antitoxin antibodies with Shibasaburo Kitasato.

Baruj Benacerraf (1920–) discovered immune response genes and collaborated in the first demonstration of MHC restriction.

Jules Bordet (1870–1961) discovered complement as a heat-labile component in normal serum that would enhance the antimicrobial potency of specific antibodies.

Frank MacFarlane Burnet (1899–1985) proposed the first generally accepted clonal selection hypothesis of adaptive immunity.

Jean Dausset (1916–) was an early pioneer in the study of the human major histocompatibility complex or HLA.

Peter Doherty (1940–) and **Rolf Zinkernagel** (1944–) showed that antigen recognition by T cells is MHC-restricted, thereby establishing the biological role of the proteins encoded by the major histocompatibility complex and leading to an understanding of antigen processing and its importance in the recognition of antigen by T cells.

Gerald Edelman (1929–) made crucial discoveries about the structure of immunoglobulins, including the first complete sequence of an antibody molecule.

Paul Ehrlich (1854–1915) was an early champion of humoral theories of immunity, and proposed a famous side-chain theory of antibody formation that bears a striking resemblance to current thinking about surface receptors.

James Gowans (1924–) discovered that adaptive immunity is mediated by lymphocytes, focusing the attention of immunologists on these small cells.

Michael Heidelberger (1888–1991) developed the quantitative precipitin assay, ushering in the era of quantitative immunochemistry.

Charles A. Janeway, Jr. (1945–2003) recognized the importance of co-stimulation for initiating adaptive immune responses. He predicted the existence of receptors of the innate immune system that would recognize pathogen-associated molecular patterns and would signal activation of the adaptive immune system. His laboratory discovered the first mammalian Toll-like receptor that had this function. He was also the principal original author of this textbook.

Edward Jenner (1749–1823) described the successful protection of humans against smallpox infection by vaccination with cowpox or vaccinia virus. This founded the field of immunology.

Niels Jerne (1911–1994) developed the hemolytic plaque assay and several important immunological theories, including an early version of clonal selection, a prediction that lymphocyte receptors would be inherently biased to MHC recognition, and the idiotype network.

Shibasaburo Kitasato (1852–1931) discovered antibodies in collaboration with Emil von Behring.

Robert Koch (1843–1910) defined the criteria needed to characterize an infectious disease, known as Koch's postulates.

Georges Köhler (1946–1995) pioneered monoclonal antibody production from hybrid antibody-forming cells with César Milstein.

Karl Landsteiner (1868–1943) discovered the ABO blood group antigens. He also carried out detailed studies of the specificity of antibody binding using haptens as model antigens.

Peter Medawar (1915–1987) used skin grafts to show that tolerance is an acquired characteristic of lymphoid cells, a key feature of clonal selection theory.

Elie Metchnikoff (1845–1916) was the first champion of cellular immunology, focusing his studies on the central role of phagocytes in host defense.

César Milstein (1927–2002) pioneered monoclonal antibody production with Georges Köhler.

Louis Pasteur (1822–1895) was a French microbiologist and immunologist who validated the concept of immunization first studied by Jenner. He prepared vaccines against chicken cholera and rabies.

Rodney Porter (1917–1985) worked out the polypeptide structure of the antibody molecule, laying the groundwork for its analysis by protein sequencing.

Ignác Semmelweis (1818–1865) German-Hungarian physician who first determined a connection between hospital hygiene and an infectious disease, puerperal fever, and consquently introduced antisepsis into medical practice.

George Snell (1903–1996) worked out the genetics of the murine major histocompatibility complex and generated the congenic strains needed for its biological analysis, laying the groundwork for our current understanding of the role of the MHC in T-cell biology.

Susumu Tonegawa (1939–) discovered the somatic recombination of immunological receptor genes that underlies the generation of diversity in human and murine antibodies and T-cell receptors.

Don C. Wiley (1944–2001) solved the first crystal structure of an MHC I protein, providing a startling insight into how T cells recognize their antigen in the in the context of MHC molecules.

GLOSSARY

In the context of immunoglobulins, α is the type of heavy chain in IgA.

α:β T cell: see **T cell**.

α:β T-cell receptor: see **T-cell receptor**.

The **ABO blood group system** antigens are expressed on red blood cells. They are used for typing human blood for transfusion. Individuals who do not express A or B antigens on their red blood cells naturally form antibodies that interact with them.

The removal of antibodies specific for one antigen from an antiserum to render it specific for another antigen or antigens is called **absorption**.

Accessory effector cells in adaptive immunity are cells that aid in the response but do not directly mediate specific antigen recognition. They include phagocytes, mast cells, and NK cells.

The **acquired immune deficiency syndrome** (**AIDS**) is a disease caused by infection with the human immunodeficiency virus (HIV-1). AIDS occurs when an infected patient has lost most of his or her CD4 T cells, so that infections with opportunistic pathogens occur.

Acquired immune response: see **adaptive immune response**.

Activation-induced cell death is the normal process by which all immune responses end in the death of most of the responding cells, leaving only a small number of resting memory cells.

The enzyme **activation-induced cytidine deaminase** (**AID**) contributes to somatic hypermutation of immunoglobulin V regions by deaminating DNA directly at cytosine. Depending on how this DNA lesion is repaired, it can lead to a permanent base change at the deaminated site. The enzyme is also involved in isotype switching. An inherited deficiency of the enzyme—**AID deficiency**—blocks both somatic hypermutation and isotype switching, leading to a type of hyper IgM immunodeficiency syndrome.

Immunization with antigen is called **active immunization** to distinguish it from the transfer of antibody to an unimmunized individual, which is called passive immunization.

Acute lymphoblastic leukemia is a highly aggressive, undifferentiated form of lymphoid malignancy derived from a progenitor cell that is thought to be able to give rise to both T and B lineages of lymphoid cells. Most of these leukemias show partial differentiation toward the B-cell lineage (so called B-ALL) whereas a minority show features of T cells (T-ALL).

Acute-phase proteins are found in the blood shortly after the onset of an infection. These proteins participate in early phases of host defense against infection. An example is the mannose-binding lectin.

The **acute-phase response** is a change in the blood that occurs during early phases of an infection. It includes the production of acute-phase proteins and also of cellular elements.

The **adaptive immune response** or **adaptive immunity** is the response of antigen-specific lymphocytes to antigen, including the development of immunological memory. Adaptive immune responses are generated by clonal selection of lymphocytes. Adaptive immune responses are distinct from innate and nonadaptive phases of immunity, which are not mediated by clonal selection of antigen-specific lymphocytes. Adaptive immune responses are also known as **acquired immune responses**.

The **adaptor proteins** are key linkers between receptors and downstream members of signaling pathways. These proteins are functionally heterogeneous, but all use a similar domain, known as an SH2 domain, as the means of interacting with the phosphotyrosine residues generated by the receptor-associated tyrosine kinases. The protein known as Vav is an adaptor protein of this type.

ADCC: see **antibody-dependent cell-mediated cytotoxicity**.

The **adenoids** are mucosal-associated lymphoid tissues located in the nasal cavity.

The enzyme defect **adenosine deaminase deficiency** (**ADA deficiency**) leads to the accumulation of toxic purine nucleosides and nucleotides, resulting in the death of most developing lymphocytes within the thymus. It is a cause of severe combined immunodeficiency.

Adhesion and degranulation promoting protein (**ADAP**) is thought to be involved in cytoskeletal rearrangements and in the increase in integrin affinity that occurs after low-affinity integrin interactions between cells have allowed initial signaling events to take place.

Adhesion molecules mediate the binding of one cell to other cells or to extracellular matrix proteins. Integrins, selectins, members of the immunoglobulin gene superfamily, and CD44 and related proteins are all adhesion molecules important in the operation of the immune system.

An **adjuvant** is any substance that enhances the immune response to an antigen with which it is mixed.

Adoptive immunity is immunity conferred on a naive or irradiated recipient by transfer of lymphoid cells from an actively immunized donor. This is called **adoptive transfer** or **adoptive immunization**.

Afferent lymphatic vessels drain fluid from the tissues and carry macrophages and dendritic cells from sites of infection in most parts of the body to the lymph nodes.

Affinity is the strength of binding of one molecule to another at a single site, such as the binding of a monovalent Fab fragment of antibody to a monovalent antigen. See also **avidity**.

Affinity chromatography is the purification of a substance by means of its affinity for another substance immobilized on a solid support. For example, an antigen can be purified by affinity chromatography on a column of beads to which specific antibody molecules are covalently linked.

Affinity maturation refers to the increase in the affinity for the specific antigen of the antibodies produced during the course of a humoral immune response. It is particularly prominent in secondary and subsequent immunizations.

Agammaglobulinemia: see **X-linked agammaglobulinemia** (**XLA**).

Agglutination is the clumping together of particles, usually by antibody molecules binding to antigens on the surfaces of adjacent particles. Such particles are said to **agglutinate**. When the particles are red blood cells, the phenomenon is called hemagglutination.

Agonist peptides are peptide antigens that activate their specific T cells, inducing them to make cytokines and to proliferate. They are thought to differ from antagonist peptides by their ability to induce T-cell receptor dimerization.

AID: see **activation-induced cytidine deaminase**.

AIDS: see **acquired immune deficiency syndrome**.

Alleles are variants of a single genetic locus.

Allelic exclusion refers to the fact that in a heterozygous individual, only one of the alternative C-region alleles of the heavy or light chain is expressed in a single B cell and in an immunoglobulin molecule. The term has come to be used more generally to describe the expression of a single receptor specificity in cells with the potential to express two or more receptors.

Allergens are antigens that elicit hypersensitivity or allergic reactions.

Allergic asthma is constriction of the bronchial tree due to an allergic reaction to inhaled antigen.

The lining of the eye, called the conjunctiva, manifests **allergic conjunctivitis** in sensitized individuals exposed to allergens.

An **allergic reaction** is a response to innocuous environmental antigens, or allergens, due to preexisting antibody or primed T cells. There are various immune mechanisms of allergic reactions, but the most common is the binding of allergen to IgE antibody on mast cells, which causes asthma, hay fever, and other common allergic reactions.

Allergic rhinitis is an allergic reaction in the nasal mucosa, also known as hay fever, that causes runny nose, sneezing, and tears.

Allergy is a symptomatic reaction to a normally innocuous environmental antigen. It results from the interaction between the antigen and antibody or primed T cells produced by earlier exposure to the same antigen.

Alloantigens are classically defined as polymorphisms at the MHC locus, and are the nonself MHC antigens on an allografted tissue. They stimulate an intense immune reaction.

Two individuals or two mouse strains that differ at the MHC are said to be **allogeneic**. The term can also be used for allelic differences at other loci. Rejection of grafted tissues from unrelated donors usually results from T-cell responses to allogeneic MHC molecules expressed by the grafted tissues. See also **syngeneic**, **xenogeneic**.

An **allograft** is a graft of tissue from an allogeneic or nonself donor of the same species; such grafts are invariably rejected unless the recipient is immunosuppressed.

Alloreactivity describes the stimulation of T cells by MHC molecules other than self; it marks the recognition of allogeneic MHC molecules. Such responses are also called **alloreactions** or **alloreactive** responses.

Allotypes are allelic polymorphisms that can be detected by antibodies specific for the polymorphic gene products. In immunology, **allotypic** differences in immunoglobulin molecules were important in deciphering the genetics of antibodies.

An **altered peptide ligand**, or partial agonist, is a peptide, usually closely related to an agonist peptide in amino acid sequence, that induces only a partial response from T cells specific for the agonist peptide.

The **alternative pathway** of complement activation is not triggered by antibody, as is the classical pathway of complement activation, but by the binding of complement protein C3b to the surface of a pathogen; it is therefore a feature of innate immunity. The alternative pathway also amplifies the classical pathway of complement activation.

Anaphylactic shock or systemic anaphylaxis is an allergic reaction to systemically administered antigen that causes circulatory collapse and suffocation due to tracheal swelling. It results from binding of antigen to IgE antibody on connective tissue mast cells throughout the body, leading to the disseminated release of inflammatory mediators.

Anaphylatoxins are small fragments of complement proteins, released by cleavage during complement activation. These small fragments are recognized by specific receptors, and they recruit fluid and inflammatory cells to sites of their release. The fragments C5a, C3a, and C4a are all anaphylatoxins, listed in order of decreasing potency *in vivo*.

Peptide fragments of antigens are bound to specific MHC class I molecules by **anchor residues**. These are residues of the peptide that have amino acid side chains that bind into pockets lining the peptide-binding groove of the MHC class I molecule. Each MHC class I molecule binds different patterns of anchor residues, called anchor motifs, giving some specificity to peptide binding. Anchor residues exist but are less obvious for peptides that bind to MHC class II molecules.

Anergy is a state of nonresponsiveness to antigen. People are said to be **anergic** when they cannot mount delayed-type hypersensitivity reactions to challenge antigens, whereas T cells and B cells are said to be **anergic** when they cannot respond to their specific antigen under optimal conditions of stimulation.

Antagonist peptides are peptides, usually closely related in sequence to an agonist peptide, that inhibit the response of a cloned T-cell line specific for the agonist peptide.

An **antibody** is a protein that binds specifically to a particular substance—its antigen. Each antibody molecule has a unique structure that enables it to bind specifically to its corresponding antigen, but all antibodies have the same overall structure and are known collectively as immunoglobulins or Igs. Antibodies are produced by plasma cells in response to infection or immunization, and bind to and neutralize pathogens or prepare them for uptake and destruction by phagocytes.

Antibody combining site: see **antigen-binding site**.

Antibody-dependent cell-mediated cytotoxicity (**ADCC**) is the killing of antibody-coated target cells by cells with Fc receptors that recognize the constant region of the bound antibody. Most ADCC is mediated by NK cells that have the Fc receptor FcγRIII or CD16 on their surface.

The **antibody repertoire** or immunoglobulin repertoire describes the total variety of antibodies in the body of an individual.

An **antigen** is any molecule that can bind specifically to an antibody. Their name arises from their ability to **gen**erate **anti**bodies. However, some antigens do not, by themselves, elicit antibody production; those antigens that can induce antibody production are called immunogens.

Antigen:antibody complexes are noncovalently associated groups of antigen and antibody molecules that can vary in size from small soluble complexes to large insoluble complexes that precipitate out of solution; they are also known as immune complexes.

The **antigen-binding site** of an antibody, or **antibody combining site**, is found at the surface of the antibody molecule that makes physical contact with the antigen. Antigen-binding sites are made up of six hypervariable loops, three from the light-chain V region and three from the heavy-chain V region.

In an **antigen-capture assay**, the antigen binds to a specific antibody, and its presence is detected by a second antibody that must be labeled and directed at a different epitope.

Both libraries of cDNA clones in expression vectors and bacteriophage libraries encoding random peptide sequences have been used to identify the targets of specific antibodies and, in some cases, of T cells. Such libraries are termed **antigen display libraries**.

An **antigenic determinant** is the portion of an antigenic molecule that is bound by a given antibody or antigen receptor; it is also known as an epitope.

Influenza virus varies from year to year by a process of **antigenic drift** in which point mutations of viral genes cause small differences in the structure of viral surface antigens. Periodically, influenza viruses undergo an **antigenic shift** through reassortment of their segmented genome with another influenza virus, changing their surface antigens radically. Such antigenic shift variants are not recognized by individuals immune to influenza, so when antigenic shift variants arise, there is widespread and serious disease.

Antigen presentation describes the display of antigen as peptide fragments bound to MHC molecules on the surface of a cell. T cells recognize antigen when it is presented in this way.

Antigen-presenting cells (**APCs**) are highly specialized cells that can process antigens and display their peptide fragments on the cell surface together with molecules required for T-cell activation. The main antigen-presenting cells for T cells are dendritic cells, macrophages, and B cells.

Antigen processing is the degradation of proteins into peptides that can bind to MHC molecules for presentation to T cells. All antigens except peptides must be processed into peptides before they can be presented by MHC molecules.

T and B lymphocytes collectively bear on their surface highly diverse **antigen receptors** capable of recognizing a wide diversity of antigens. Each individual lymphocyte bears receptors of a single antigen specificity.

Antigen spreading: see **epitope spreading**.

Anti-immunoglobulin antibodies are antibodies against immunoglobulin constant domains, useful for detecting bound antibody molecules in immunoassays and other applications. These can be divided into **anti-isotype antibodies** made in a different species, **anti-allotype antibodies** made in the same species against allotypic variants, and **anti-idiotype antibodies**, made against unique determinants to a single antibody.

Anti-lymphocyte globulin is antibody raised in another species against human T cells.

An **antiserum** (plural: **antisera**) is the fluid component of clotted blood from an immune individual that contains antibodies against the molecule used for immunization. Antisera contain heterogeneous collections of antibodies, which bind the antigen used for immunization, but each has its own structure, its own epitope on the antigen, and its own set of cross-reactions. This heterogeneity makes each antiserum unique.

Bites by poisonous snakes can be treated by identification of the snake and injection of an **antivenin** specific for that snake's venom.

APECED: see **autoimmune polyendocrinopathy-candidiasis-ectodermal dystrophy**.

Aplastic anemia is a failure of bone marrow stem cells so that formation of all cellular elements of the blood ceases; it can be treated by bone marrow transplantation.

Apoptosis, or programmed cell death, is a form of cell death in which the cell activates an internal death program. It is characterized by nuclear DNA degradation, nuclear degeneration and condensation, and the phagocytosis of cell remains. Proliferating cells frequently undergo apoptosis, which is a natural process in development, and proliferating lymphocytes undergo high rates of apoptosis in development and during immune responses. Apoptosis contrasts with necrosis, death caused by external factors, which occurs in situations such as poisoning and anoxia.

The **appendix** is a gut-associated lymphoid tissue located at the beginning of the colon.

In this book, we have termed primed effector T cells **armed effector T cells**, because these cells can be triggered to perform their effector functions immediately on contact with cells bearing the peptide:MHC complex for which they are specific. They contrast with memory T cells, which need to be activated by antigen-presenting cells to differentiate into effector T cells before they can mediate effector responses.

The **Arthus reaction** is a skin reaction in which antigen is injected into the dermis and reacts with IgG antibodies in the extracellular spaces, activating complement and phagocytic cells to produce a local inflammatory response.

Ascertainment artifact refers to data that seem to demonstrate some finding, but fail to do so because they are collected from a population that is selected in a biased fashion.

Ataxia telangiectasia is a disease characterized by staggering, multiple disorganized blood vessels, and an immunodeficiency in a protein called ATM, which contains a kinase thought to be important in signaling of double-stranded DNA breaks.

Atopic allergy, or **atopy**, is the increased tendency seen in some people to produce immediate hypersensitivity reactions (usually mediated by IgE antibodies) against innocuous substances.

Atopic dermatitis: see **eczema**.

Pathogens are said to be **attenuated** when they can grow in their host and induce immunity without producing serious clinical disease.

Antibodies specific for self antigens are called **autoantibodies**.

Self antigens to which the immune system makes a response are called **autoantigens**.

A graft of tissue from one site to another on the same individual is called an **autograft**.

Diseases in which the pathology is caused by adaptive immune responses to self antigens are called **autoimmune diseases**.

Autoimmune hemolytic anemia is a pathological condition with low levels of red blood cells (anemia), which is caused by autoantibodies that bind red blood cell surface antigens and target the red blood cell for destruction.

Autoimmune lymphoproliferative syndrome (**ALPS**) is an inherited syndrome in which a defect in the Fas gene leads to a failure in normal apoptosis, causing unregulated immune responses, including autoimmune responses.

In the disease **autoimmune polyendocrinopathy-candidiasis-ectodermal dystrophy** (**APECED**), there is a loss of tolerance to self antigens due to a breakdown of negative selection in the thymus. This is due to defects in the gene *AIRE*, which encodes a transcriptional regulatory protein that enables many self antigens to be expressed by thymic epithelial cells.

An adaptive immune response directed at self antigens is called an **autoimmune response**; likewise, adaptive immunity specific for self antigens is called **autoimmunity**.

In the disease **autoimmune thrombocytopenic purpura**, antibodies against a patient's platelets are made. Antibody binding to platelets causes them to be taken up by cells with Fc receptors and complement receptors, causing a fall in platelet counts that leads to purpura (bleeding).

Autoinflammatory disease characterized by unregulated inflammation occurs as a result of various causes.

Autoreactivity describes immune responses directed at self antigens.

Avidity is the sum total of the strength of binding of two molecules or cells to one another at multiple sites. It is distinct from affinity, which is the strength of binding of one site on a molecule to its ligand.

The **avidity hypothesis** of T-cell selection in the thymus states that T cells must have a measurable affinity for self MHC molecules in order to mature, but not so great an affinity as to cause activation of the cell when it matures, as this would require that the cell be deleted to maintain self tolerance.

Azathioprine is a potent immunosuppressive drug that is converted to its active form *in vivo* and then kills rapidly proliferating cells, including lymphocytes responding to grafted tissues.

4-1BB is a member of the TNF receptor family that specifically binds to 4-1BB ligand.

4-1BB ligand (**41BBL**) is a member of the TNF family that binds to 4-1BB.

The major T-cell co-stimulatory molecules are the **B7 molecules**, B7.1 (CD80) and **B7.2** (CD86). They are closely related members of the immunoglobulin gene superfamily and both bind to the CD28 molecule on T cells. They are expressed differentially on various antigen-presenting cell types. We use the term **B7 molecules** to refer to both B7.1 and B7.2.

B7-RP is a ligand for B7 molecules.

β barrel: see **β sheet**.

A **β sheet** is one of the fundamental structural building blocks of proteins, consisting of adjacent, extended strands of amino acids (**β strands**) that are bonded together by interactions between backbone amide and carbonyl groups. β sheets can be parallel, in which case the adjacent strands run in the same direction, or antiparallel, where adjacent strands run in opposite directions. All immunoglobulin domains are made up of antiparallel β-sheet structures. A **β barrel** or a **β sandwich** is another way of describing the structure of the immunoglobulin domain.

The light chain of the MHC class I proteins is called β_2**-microglobulin**. It binds noncovalently to the heavy or α chain.

A **B cell**, or **B lymphocyte**, is one of the two major types of lymphocyte. The antigen receptor on B lymphocytes, usually called the B-cell receptor, is a cell-surface immunoglobulin. On activation by antigen, B cells differentiate into cells producing antibody molecules of the same antigen specificity as this receptor. B cells are divided into two classes. **B-1 cells**, also known as CD5 B cells, are a class of atypical, self-renewing B cells found mainly in the peritoneal and pleural cavities in adults. They have a far less diverse repertoire of receptors than do **B-2 cells** (also known as conventional B cells), which are generated in the bone marrow throughout life, emerging to populate the blood and lymphoid tissues.

The **B-cell antigen receptor**, or **B-cell receptor** (**BCR**), is the cell-surface receptor of B cells for specific antigen. It is composed of a transmembrane immunoglobulin molecule associated with the invariant Igα and Igβ chains in a noncovalent complex.

A complex of CD19, CD81, and CR2 makes up the **B-cell co-receptor**; co-ligation of this complex with the B-cell antigen receptor increases responsiveness to antigen by about a hundred-fold.

The **B-cell corona** in the spleen is the zone of the white pulp primarily made up of B cells.

B-cell mitogens are substances that cause B cells to proliferate.

B lymphocyte: see **B cell**.

B-lymphocyte chemokine (**BLC**) is a CXC chemokine that attracts B cells and activated T cells into the follicles of peripheral lymphoid tissues by binding to the CXCR5 receptor.

Many infectious diseases are caused by **bacteria**, which are prokaryotic microorganisms that exist as many different species and strains. Bacteria can live on body surfaces, in extracellular spaces, in cellular vesicles, or in the cytosol, and different bacterial species cause distinctive infectious diseases.

BALT: see **bronchial-associated lymphoid tissues**.

Bare lymphocyte syndrome: see **MHC class I deficiency**; **MHC class II deficiency**.

Basophils are white blood cells containing granules that stain with basic dyes, and which are thought to have a function similar to mast cells.

Bb is the large active fragment of complement component factor B. It is produced when factor B is captured by bound C3b and cleaved by factor D. Bb remains associated with C3b and is the serine protease component of the alternative pathway C3 convertase.

The protein known as **Bcl-2** protects cells from apoptosis by binding to the mitochondrial membrane. It is encoded by the *bcl-2* gene, which was discovered at the breakpoint of an oncogenic chromosomal translocation in B-cell leukemia.

Treatments for autoimmune disease or cancer that comprise proteins such as antibodies and cytokines or fragments of proteins or synthetic peptides are called **biologic therapy**. The term also encompasses the use of cells such as bone marrow-derived cells for treatment.

Blk: see **tyrosine kinase**.

The adaptor protein **BLNK** (B-cell linker protein) operates in B cells in the same way as LAT does in T cells; it has multiple tyrosine residues that are targets for phosphorylation, and recruits signaling molecules to membrane lipid rafts.

Blood group antigens are surface molecules on red blood cells that are detectable with antibodies from other individuals. The major blood group antigens are called ABO and Rh (Rhesus), and are used in routine blood banking to type blood. There are many other blood group antigens that can be detected in cross-matching.

In transfusion medicine, **blood typing** is used to determine whether donor and recipient have the same ABO and Rh blood group antigens. A cross-match, in which serum from the donor is tested on the cells of the recipient, and vice versa, is used to rule out other incompatibilities. Transfusion of incompatible blood causes a transfusion reaction, in which red blood cells are destroyed and the released hemoglobin causes toxicity.

Bloom's syndrome is a disease characterized by low T-cell numbers, reduced antibody levels, and an increased susceptibility to respiratory infections, cancer, and radiation damage. It is caused by mutations in a DNA helicase.

The **bone marrow** is the site of hematopoiesis, the generation of the cellular elements of blood, including red blood cells, monocytes, polymorphonuclear leukocytes, and platelets. The bone marrow is also the site of B-cell development in mammals and the source of stem cells that give rise to T cells upon migration to the thymus. Thus, bone-marrow transplantation can restore all the cellular elements of the blood, including the cells required for adaptive immunity.

A **bone marrow chimera** is formed by transferring bone marrow from one mouse to an irradiated recipient mouse, so that all of the lymphocytes and blood cells are of donor genetic origin. Bone marrow chimeras have been crucial in elucidating the development of lymphocytes and other blood cells.

A **booster immunization** is commonly given after a primary immunization, to increase the amount, or titer, of antibodies.

Bradykinin is a vasoactive peptide that is produced as a result of tissue damage and acts as an inflammatory mediator.

The lymphoid cells and organized lymphoid tissues in the respiratory tract are termed the **bronchial-associated lymphoid tissues** (**BALT**). These tissues are very important in the induction of immune responses to inhaled antigens and to respiratory infection.

Bruton's X-linked agammaglobulinemia: see **X-linked agammaglobulinemia**.

Burkitt's lymphoma is caused by Epstein–Barr virus (EBV) and occurs mainly in sub-Saharan Africa.

The constant regions of the polypeptide chains of immunoglobulin molecules are made up of one or more constant domains or **C domains** of similar structure; each immunoglobulin chain also has a single variable or V domain.

The **C1 complex** of complement components comprises one molecule of **C1q** bound to two molecules each of the zymogens **C1r** and **C1s**. C1q initiates the classical pathway of complement activation by binding to a pathogen surface or to bound antibody. This binding activates the associated C1r, which in turn cleaves and activates C1s. The active form of C1s then cleaves the next two components in the pathway, **C4** and **C2**.

C1 inhibitor (**C1INH**) is a protein that inhibits the activity of activated complement component C1 by binding to and inactivating its C1r:C1s enzymatic activity. It also inhibits other serine proteases including kallikrein. Deficiency in C1INH is the cause of the disease hereditary angioneurotic edema, in which the production of vasoactive peptides, kinins, leads to subcutaneous and laryngeal swelling.

The complement fragment **C3b** is the major product of the C3 convertase, and the principal effector molecule of the complement system. It has a highly reactive thioester bond which allows it to bind covalently to the surface on which it is generated. Once bound, it acts as an opsonin to promote the destruction of pathogens by phagocytes and removal of immune complexes; C3b is bound by the complement receptor CR1, while its proteolytic derivative, iC3b, is bound by the complement receptors CR1, CR2, and CR3.

The generation of the enzyme **C3 convertase** on the surface of a pathogen or cell is a crucial step in complement activation. The classical pathway C3 convertase is formed from membrane-bound C4b complexed with the protease C2b. The alternative pathway of complement activation uses a different but homologous C3 convertase, formed from membrane-bound C3b complexed with the protease Bb. These C3 convertases have the same activity, catalyzing the deposition of large numbers of C3b molecules that bind covalently to the pathogen surface, leading to opsonization and the activation of the effector cascade that causes membrane lesions.

C3dg is a breakdown product of C3b that remains attached to the microbial surface, where it can bind to CD21, the complement receptor CR2.

C4b-binding protein (**C4BP**) can inactivate the classical pathway C3 convertase if it forms on host cells, by displacing C2b from the C4bC2b complex. It binds to C4b attached to host cells, but cannot bind C4b attached to pathogens. This is because it has a second binding site specific for sialic acid, a terminal sugar on vertebrate cell surfaces, but not on pathogens.

C5 is an inactive complement component that is cleaved by the **C5 convertase** to release the potent inflammatory peptide **C5a** and a larger fragment, **C5b**, that initiates the formation of a membrane-attack complex from the terminal components of complement.

The receptor for the C5a fragment of complement, the **C5a receptor**, is a seven-transmembrane spanning receptor that couples to a heterotrimeric G protein. Similar receptors bind to **C3a** and **C4a**.

The complement components **C6**, **C7**, and **C8** form a complex with the active complement fragment **C5b** in the late events of complement activation. This complex inserts into the membrane and induces polymerization of **C9** to form a pore known as the membrane-attack complex.

C domain: see **constant domain**.

C region: see **constant region**.

The cytosolic serine/threonine phosphatase **calcineurin** has a crucial role in signaling via the T-cell receptor. The immunosuppressive drugs cyclosporin A and tacrolimus (also known as FK506) form complexes with cellular proteins called immunophilins that bind and inactivate calcineurin, suppressing T-cell responses.

The protein **calnexin** is an 88 kDa protein found in the endoplasmic reticulum. It binds to partly folded members of the immunoglobulin superfamily of proteins and retains them in the endoplasmic reticulum until folding is completed.

Calreticulin is the molecular chaperone that binds initially to MHC class I, MHC class II, and other proteins that contain immunoglobulin-like domains, such as the T-cell and B-cell antigen receptors.

Antibodies or antigens can be measured in various **capture** assays. In these assays, antigens are captured by antibodies bound to plastic (or vice versa). Antibody binding to a plate-bound antigen can be measured using labeled antigen or anti-immunoglobulin. Antigen binding to plate-bound antibody can be measured by using an antibody that binds to a different epitope on the antigen.

Carriers are foreign proteins to which small non-immunogenic antigens, or haptens, can be coupled to render the hapten immunogenic. *In vivo*, self proteins can also serve as carriers if they are correctly modified by the hapten; this is important in allergy to drugs.

Caseation necrosis is a form of necrosis seen in the center of large granulomas, such as the granulomas in tuberculosis. The term comes from the white cheesy appearance of the central necrotic area.

Caspases are a family of closely related cysteine proteases that cleave proteins at aspartic acid residues. They have important roles in apoptosis.

The chemokine **CCL21** (formerly known as SLC) is produced by lymphatic vessels and attracts dendritic cells.

CD: see **clusters of differentiation** and Appendix II.

The **CD3 complex** is the complex of $\alpha{:}\beta$ or $\gamma{:}\delta$ T-cell receptor chains with the invariant subunits CD3γ, δ, and ε, and the dimeric ζ chains.

The cell-surface protein **CD4** is important for recognition by the T-cell receptor of antigenic peptides bound to MHC class II molecules. It acts as a co-receptor by binding to the lateral face of the MHC class II molecules.

CD4 T cells are T cells that carry the co-receptor protein CD4. They recognize peptides derived from intravesicular sources, which are bound to MHC class II molecules, and differentiate into CD4 T_H1 and CD4 T_H2 effector cells that activate macrophages and B-cell responses to antigen.

CD5 B cells are a class of atypical, self-renewing B cells found mainly in the peritoneal and pleural cavities in adults. They have a far less diverse receptor repertoire than conventional B cells, and since they are the first B cells to be produced they are also known as B-1 cells.

The cell-surface protein **CD8** is important for recognition by the T-cell receptor of antigenic peptides bound to MHC class I molecules. It acts as a co-receptor by binding to the lateral face of MHC class I molecules.

CD8 T cells are T cells that carry the co-receptor CD8. They recognize antigens, for example viral antigens, that are synthesized in the cytoplasm of a cell. Peptides derived from these antigens are transported by TAP, assembled with MHC class I molecules in the endoplasmic reticulum, and displayed as peptide:MHC class I complexes on the cell surface. CD8 T cells differentiate into cytotoxic CD8 T cells.

CD11b:CD18: see **CR3**.

CD11c:CD18: see **CR4**.

CD19:CR2:TAPA-1 complex: see **B-cell co-receptor**.

CD21: see **CR2**.

CD31: see **PECAM**.

CD35: see **CR1**.

B-cell growth is triggered in part by the binding of **CD40 ligand**, also known as **CD154**, expressed on activated helper T cells, to **CD40** on the B-cell surface.

CD45, or the leukocyte common antigen, is a transmembrane tyrosine phosphatase found on all leukocytes. It is expressed in different isoforms on different cell types, including the different subtypes of T cells. These isoforms are commonly denoted by the designation of CD45R followed by the exon whose presence gives rise to distinctive antibody-binding patterns.

CD46: see **membrane cofactor of proteolysis** (**MCP**).

CD55: see **decay-accelerating factor** (**DAF**).

CD59: see **protectin**.

CD80 and **CD86**: see **B7.1** and **B7.2**.

CDRs: see **complementarity-determining regions**.

Cell-adhesion molecules (**CAMs**) are cell-surface proteins that are involved in binding cells together in tissues and also in less permanent cell–cell interactions.

Cell-mediated immunity, or a **cell-mediated immune response**, describes any adaptive immune response in which antigen-specific T cells have the main role. It is defined operationally as all adaptive immunity that cannot be transferred to a naive recipient with serum antibody. *Cf.* **humoral immunity**.

Cell-surface immunoglobulin is the B-cell receptor for antigen. See also **B-cell antigen receptor**.

Cellular immunology is the study of the cellular basis of immunity.

Central lymphoid organs are sites of lymphocyte development. In humans, B lymphocytes develop in bone marrow, whereas T lymphocytes develop within the thymus from bone marrow-derived progenitors. They are also sometimes known as the primary lymphoid organs.

Central memory cells are memory cells that are thought to reside in the T-cell areas of secondary lymphoid tissues.

Central tolerance is tolerance that is established in lymphocytes developing in central lymphoid organs. *Cf.* **peripheral tolerance**.

Centroblasts are large, rapidly dividing cells found in germinal centers, and are the cells in which somatic hypermutation is believed to occur. Antibody-secreting and memory B cells derive from these cells.

Centrocytes are the small B cells in germinal centers that derive from centroblasts. They may mature into antibody-secreting plasma cells or memory B cells, or may undergo apoptosis, depending on their receptor's interaction with antigen.

Chediak–Higashi syndrome is caused by a defect in a protein involved in intracellular vesicle fusion. Phagocytic cell function is affected as lysosomes fail to fuse properly with phagosomes and there is impaired killing of ingested bacteria.

Chemokines are small chemoattractant proteins that stimulate the migration and activation of cells, especially phagocytic cells and lymphocytes. They have a central role in inflammatory responses. Chemokines and their receptors are listed in Appendix IV.

Most lymphoid tumors, and many other tumors, bear **chromosomal translocations** that mark points of breakage and rejoining of different chromosomes. These chromosomal breaks are particularly frequent in lymphomas and leukemias.

Chronic granulomatous disease is an immunodeficiency disease in which multiple granulomas form as a result of defective elimination of bacteria by phagocytic cells. It is caused by defects in the NADPH oxidase system of enzymes that generate the superoxide radical involved in bacterial killing.

Chronic lymphocytic leukemias (**CLLs**) are B-cell tumors that are found in the blood. The great majority express CD5 and unmutated V genes and are therefore thought to arise from B-1 cells.

The **class II-associated invariant chain peptide** (**CLIP**) is a peptide of variable length cleaved from the class II invariant chain by proteases. It remains associated with the MHC class II molecule in an unstable form until it is removed by the HLA-DM protein.

Class II transactivator (**CIITA**): see **MHC class II transactivator**.

Class switching: see **isotype switching**.

Classes: see **isotypes**.

The **classical pathway** of complement activation is the pathway activated by C1 binding either directly to bacterial surfaces or to antibody, that serves as a means of flagging the bacteria as foreign. See also **alternative pathway**; **mannose-binding lectin pathway**.

Clonal deletion is the elimination of immature lymphocytes when they bind to self antigens, which produces tolerance to self as required by the clonal selection theory. Clonal deletion is the main mechanism of central tolerance and can also occur in peripheral tolerance.

Clonal expansion is the proliferation of antigen-specific lymphocytes in response to antigenic stimulation and precedes their differentiation into effector cells. It is an essential step in adaptive immunity, allowing rare antigen-specific cells to increase in number so that they can effectively combat the pathogen that elicited the response.

The **clonal selection theory** is a central paradigm of adaptive immunity. It states that adaptive immune responses derive from individual antigen-specific lymphocytes that are self-tolerant. These specific lymphocytes proliferate in response to antigen and differentiate into antigen-specific effector cells that eliminate the eliciting pathogen, and memory cells to sustain immunity. The theory was formulated by Sir Macfarlane Burnet and in earlier forms by Niels Jerne and David Talmage.

A **clone** is a population of cells all derived from a single progenitor cell.

A **cloned T-cell line** is a continuously growing line of T cells derived from a single progenitor cell. Cloned T-cell lines must be stimulated with antigen periodically to maintain growth. They are useful for studying T-cell specificity, growth, and effector functions.

A feature unique to individual cells or members of a clone is said to be **clonotypic**. Thus, a monoclonal antibody that reacts with the receptor on a cloned T-cell line is said to be a clonotypic antibody and to recognize its clonotype, or the clonotypic receptor of that cell.

Clusters of differentiation (**CD**) are groups of monoclonal antibodies that identify the same cell-surface molecule. The cell-surface molecule is designated CD followed by a number (eg, CD1, CD2, etc.). For a current listing of CDs see Appendix II.

The **coagulation system** is a proteolytic cascade of plasma enzymes that triggers blood clotting when blood vessels are damaged.

The expression of a gene is said to be **codominant** when both alleles at one locus are expressed in roughly equal amounts in heterozygotes. Most genes show this property, including the highly polymorphic MHC genes.

A **coding joint** is formed by the imprecise joining of a V gene segment to a (D)J gene segment in immunoglobulin or T-cell receptor genes.

Co-immunoprecipitation: see **immunoprecipitation analysis**.

Collectins are a structurally related family of calcium-dependent sugar-binding proteins or lectins containing collagen-like sequences. An example is mannose-binding lectin.

Antigen receptors manifest two distinct types of **combinatorial diversity** generated by the combination of separate units of genetic information. Receptor gene segments are joined in many different combinations to generate diverse receptor chains, and then two different receptor chains (heavy and light in immunoglobulins; α and β, or γ and δ, in T-cell receptors) are combined to make the antigen-recognition site.

The **common γ chain** (γ_c) is a transmembrane polypeptide chain (CD132) that is common to a subgroup of class I cytokine receptors. It plays a key role in the intracellular signaling mediated by these receptors as shown by gene knockout.

Common lymphoid progenitors are stem cells that give rise to all lymphocytes. They are derived from pluripotent hematopoietic stem cells.

Common variable immunodeficiency is a relatively common deficiency in antibody production whose pathogenesis is not yet understood. There is a strong association with genes mapping within the MHC.

Competitive binding assays are serological assays in which unknowns are detected and quantitated by their ability to inhibit the binding of a labeled known ligand to its specific antibody. When known sources of antibody or antigen are used as competitive inhibitors of antigen–antibody interactions, this assay is referred to as a **competitive inhibition assay**.

Complement receptors (**CRs**) are cell-surface proteins on various cells that recognize and bind complement proteins that have bound an antigen such as a pathogen. Complement receptors on phagocytes allow them to identify pathogens coated with complement proteins and take them up and destroy them. Complement receptors include CR1, CR2, CR3, CR4, and the receptor for C1q.

The **complementarity-determining regions** (**CDRs**) of immunoglobulins and T-cell receptors are the parts of these molecules that determine their specificity and make contact with specific ligand. The CDRs are the most variable part of the molecule, and contribute to the diversity of these molecules. There are three such regions (**CDR1**, **CDR2**, and **CDR3**) in each V domain.

The **complement system** is a set of plasma proteins that act together to attack extracellular forms of pathogens. **Complement activation** can occur spontaneously on certain pathogens or by antibody binding to the pathogen. The pathogen becomes coated with complement proteins that facilitate pathogen removal by phagocytes and can also kill certain pathogens directly.

In **confocal fluorescent microscopy**, it is possible to use optics to produce images at very high resolution by having two origins of fluorescent light that come together only at one plane of a thicker section.

When a protein binds a ligand, the protein often undergoes a change in its tertiary structure, or a **conformational change**, that has an effect on its function, either activating it or inhibiting it.

Conformational epitopes, or discontinuous epitopes, on a protein antigen are formed from several separate regions in the primary sequence of a protein brought together by protein folding. Antibodies that bind conformational epitopes bind only native folded proteins.

Conjugate vaccines are vaccines made from capsular polysaccharides bound to proteins of known immunogenicity, such as tetanus toxoid.

The **constant region** (**C region**) of an immunoglobulin or T-cell receptor is that part of the molecule that is relatively constant in amino acid sequence between different molecules. In an antibody molecule the constant regions of each chain are composed of one or more **constant domains** (**C domains**). The constant region of an antibody determines its particular effector function. *Cf.* **variable region.**

A **contact hypersensitivity reaction** is a form of delayed-type hypersensitivity in which T cells respond to antigens that are introduced by contact with the skin. Poison ivy hypersensitivity is a contact hypersensitivity reaction due to T-cell responses to the chemical antigen pentadecacatechol in poison ivy leaves.

Continuous epitopes, or linear epitopes, are antigenic determinants on proteins that are contiguous in the amino acid sequence and therefore do not require the protein to be folded into its native conformation for antibody to bind. The epitopes detected by T cells are continuous.

A **convertase** is an enzymatic activity that converts a complement protein into its reactive form by cleaving it. Generation of the C3 convertase is the pivotal event in complement activation.

The **Coombs test** is a test for antibody binding to red blood cells. Red blood cells that are coated with antibody are agglutinated if they are exposed to an anti-immunoglobulin antibody. The Coombs test is important in detecting the nonagglutinating antibodies against red blood cells produced by Rh incompatibility in pregnancy.

Two binding sites are said to demonstrate **cooperativity** in binding to their ligand when the binding of ligand to one site enhances the binding of ligand to the second site.

A **co-receptor** is a cell-surface protein that increases the sensitivity of the antigen receptor to antigen by binding to associated ligands and participating in signaling for activation. CD4 and CD8 are MHC-binding co-receptors on T cells, whereas CD19 is part of a complex that makes up a co-receptor on B cells.

Corona: see **B-cell corona.**

Corticosteroids are a family of drugs related to steroids that are naturally produced in the adrenal cortex, such as cortisone. Corticosteroids can kill lymphocytes, especially developing thymocytes, inducing apoptotic cell death. They are useful anti-inflammatory, anti-lymphoid tumor, and immunosuppressive agents.

The proliferation of lymphocytes requires both antigen binding and the receipt of a **co-stimulatory signal**. Co-stimulatory signals are delivered to T cells by the **co-stimulatory molecules** B7.1 and B7.2, related molecules that are expressed on the surface of the cell presenting antigen, and which bind the T-cell surface molecule CD28. B cells may receive co-stimulatory signals from common pathogen components such as LPS, from complement fragments, or from CD40 ligand expressed on the surface of an activated antigen-specific helper T cell.

Cowpox is the common name of the disease produced by vaccinia virus, used by Edward Jenner in the successful vaccination against smallpox, which is caused by the related variola virus.

CR1 (**CD35**) is one of several receptors on cells for various components of complement. It is used to remove immune complexes from the plasma.

CR2 (**CD21**) is part of the B-cell co-receptor complex along with CD19 and CD81. It binds to antigens that have various breakdown products of C3, especially C3dg, bound to them and, by cross-linking to the B-cell receptor, enhances sensitivity to antigen by at least a hundredfold. It is also used by the Epstein–Barr virus to invade B cells and produce the symptoms of infectious mononucleosis.

CR3 (**CD11b:CD18**) is a β_2 integrin that functions both as an adhesion molecule and as a complement receptor. It binds iC3b, and stimulates phagocytosis.

CR4 (**CD11c:CD18**) is a β_2 integrin that binds iC3b and stimulates phagocytosis.

C-reactive protein is an acute-phase protein that binds to phosphorylcholine, which is a constituent of the C-polysaccharide of the bacterium *Streptococcus pneumoniae*, hence its name. Many other bacteria also have surface phosphorylcholine that is accessible to C-reactive protein, so the protein can bind many different bacteria and opsonize them for uptake by phagocytes. C-reactive protein does not bind to mammalian tissues.

Cross-matching is used in blood typing and histocompatibility testing to determine whether donor and recipient have antibodies against each other's cells that might interfere with successful transfusion or grafting.

Extracellular proteins taken up by dendritic cells can give rise to peptides presented by MHC class I molecules, leading to **cross-priming**, by which antigens from extracellular sources can be presented by MHC class I molecules to activate CD8 T cells.

A **cross-reaction** is the binding of antibody to an antigen not used to elicit that antibody. Thus, if antibody raised against antigen A also binds antigen B, it is said to cross-react with antigen B. The term is used generically to describe the reactivity of antibodies or T cells with antigens other than the eliciting antigen.

CRs: see **complement receptors.**

The protein known as **Csk** or **C-terminal Src kinase** is constitutively active in lymphocytes and has the function of phosphorylating the C-terminal tyrosine of Src-family tyrosine kinases, thus inactivating them.

CTLA-4 is the high-affinity receptor for B7 molecules on T cells.

Cutaneous lymphocyte antigen (**CLA**) is a cell-surface molecule that is involved in lymphocyte homing to the skin in humans.

Cutaneous T-cell lymphoma is a malignant growth of T cells that home to the skin.

Cyclic neutropenia is a dominantly inherited disease in which neutrophil numbers fluctuate from near normal to very low or none, with an approximate cycle time of 21 days.

Cyclophosphamide is a DNA alkylating agent that is used as an immunosuppressive drug. It acts by killing rapidly dividing cells, including lymphocytes proliferating in response to antigen.

Cyclosporin A is a powerful immunosuppressive drug that inhibits signaling from the T-cell receptor, preventing T-cell activation and effector function. It binds to cyclophilin, and this complex binds to and inactivates the serine/threonine phosphatase calcineurin.

Cystic fibrosis is an inherited disease in which a defect in a membrane transport protein results in, among other symptoms, the secretion of thick sticky mucus in the airways, which clogs up the lungs and increases the risk of respiratory failure and lung infections.

Cytokine capture: see **antigen-capture assay.**

Cytokine receptors are cellular receptors for cytokines. Binding of the cytokine to the cytokine receptor induces new activities in the cell, such as growth, differentiation, or death. Cytokine receptors are listed in Appendix III.

Cytokines are proteins made by cells that affect the behavior of other cells. Cytokines made by lymphocytes are often called lymphokines or interleukins (abbreviated IL), but the generic term cytokine is used in this book and in most of the literature. Cytokines act via specific cytokine receptors on the cells that they affect. Cytokines and their receptors are listed in Appendix III. See also **chemokines**.

T cells that can kill other cells are called **cytotoxic T cells**. Most cytotoxic T cells are MHC class I-restricted CD8 T cells, but CD4 T cells can also kill in some cases. Cytotoxic T cells are important in host defense against cytosolic pathogens.

Cytotoxins are proteins made by cytotoxic T cells that participate in the destruction of target cells. Perforins, granzymes, and granulysins are the major defined cytotoxins.

In the context of immunoglobulins, δ is the type of heavy chain in IgD.

D gene segments, or **diversity gene segments**, are short DNA sequences that join the V and J gene segments in rearranged immunoglobulin heavy-chain genes and in T-cell receptor β- and δ-chain genes. See **gene segments**.

Dark zone: see **germinal centers**.

ICAM-3 binds with high affinity to a lectin called **DC-SIGN**, which is found only on dendritic cells.

Death domains were originally defined in proteins encoded by genes involved in programmed cell death or apoptosis, and are now known to be involved in protein–protein interactions.

The **decay-accelerating factor** (**DAF** or **CD55**) is a cell-surface molecule that protects cells from lysis by complement. Its absence causes the disease paroxysmal nocturnal hemoglobinuria.

Delayed-type hypersensitivity, or type IV hypersensitivity, is a form of cell-mediated immunity elicited by antigen in the skin and is mediated by CD4 T$_H$1 cells. It is called delayed-type hypersensitivity because the reaction appears hours to days after antigen is injected. *Cf.* **immediate hypersensitivity**.

Dendritic cells, also known as interdigitating dendritic cells, are found in T-cell areas of lymphoid tissues. They have a branched or dendritic morphology and are the most potent stimulators of T-cell responses. Nonlymphoid tissues also contain dendritic cells, but these are not able to stimulate T-cell responses until they are activated and migrate to lymphoid tissues. The dendritic cell derives from bone marrow precursors. It is distinct from the follicular dendritic cell that presents antigen to B cells.

Dendritic epidermal T cells (**dETCs**) are a specialized class of γ:δ T cells found in the skin of mice and some other species, but not humans. All dETCs have the same γ:δ T-cell receptor; their function is unknown.

Immunosuppressive monoclonal antibodies that trigger the destruction of lymphocytes *in vivo* are known as **depleting antibodies**. They are used for treating episodes of acute graft rejection.

Desensitization is a procedure in which an allergic individual is exposed to increasing doses of allergen in hope of inhibiting their allergic reactions. It probably involves shifting the balance between CD4 T$_H$1 and T$_H$2 cells and thus changing the antibody produced from IgE to IgG.

Determinant spreading: see **epitope spreading**.

Diacylglycerol (**DAG**) is most commonly released from inositol phospholipids by the action of phospholipase C-γ. Diacylglycerol production is stimulated by the ligation of many receptors and it acts as an intracellular signaling molecule, activating cytosolic protein kinase C, which further propagates the signal.

Diapedesis is the movement of blood cells, particularly leukocytes, from the blood across blood vessel walls into tissues.

DiGeorge's syndrome is a recessive genetic immunodeficiency disease in which there is a failure to develop thymic epithelium, and is associated with absent parathyroid glands and large vessel anomalies. It seems to be due to a developmental defect in neural crest cells.

Direct allorecognition of a grafted tissue involves donor antigen-presenting cells leaving the graft, migrating via the lymph to regional lymph nodes and activating host T cells bearing the corresponding T-cell receptors.

The **direct Coombs test** uses anti-immunoglobulin to agglutinate red blood cells as a way of detecting whether they are coated with antibody *in vivo* due to autoimmunity or maternal anti-fetal immune responses (see **Coombs test**; **indirect Coombs test**).

Discontinuous epitopes: see **conformational epitopes**.

DNA microarrays are created by placing a different DNA on a small part of a microchip, and using them to assess RNA expression in normal or malignant cells.

DNA vaccination is a novel means of raising an adaptive immune response. For unknown reasons, when DNA is injected into muscle, it is expressed and elicits antibody and T-cell responses to the protein encoded by the DNA.

Dominant immune suppression: see **regulatory tolerance**.

In tissue grafting experiments, the grafted tissues come from a **donor** and are placed in a recipient or host.

Double-negative thymocytes are immature T cells within the thymus that lack expression of the two co-receptors, CD4 and CD8. In a normal thymus, these represent about 5% of thymocytes.

Double-positive thymocytes are an intermediate stage in T-cell development in the thymus and are characterized by expression of both the CD4 and the CD8 co-receptor proteins. They represent the majority (~80%) of thymocytes.

The term **draining lymph node** is used for any lymph node that is downstream of a site of infection and thus receives antigens and microbes from the site via the lymphatic system. Draining lymph nodes often enlarge enormously during an immune response and can be palpated; they were originally called swollen glands.

In the context of immunoglobulins, ε (epsilon) is the heavy chain of IgE.

E-selectin: see **selectins**.

The **early induced responses** or early nonadaptive responses are a series of host defense responses that are triggered by infectious agents early in infection. They are distinct from innate immunity because there is an inductive phase, and from adaptive immunity in that they do not operate by clonal selection of rare antigen-specific lymphocytes.

Early pro-B cell: see **pro-B cells**.

The common skin disease **eczema** or **atopic dermatitis** is seen mainly in children; its etiology is poorly understood.

In immunology, **edema** is the swelling caused by the entry of fluid and cells from the blood into the tissues, which is one of the cardinal features of the process of inflammation.

Effector cells, or **effector lymphocytes**, can mediate the removal of pathogens from the body without the need for further differentiation, as distinct from naive lymphocytes, which must proliferate and differentiate before they can mediate effector functions, and memory cells, which must differentiate and often proliferate before they become effector cells. They are also called armed effector cells in this book, to indicate that they can be triggered to effector function by antigen binding alone.

Effector mechanisms are those processes by which pathogens are destroyed and cleared from the body. Innate and adaptive immune responses use most of the same effector mechanisms to eliminate pathogens.

Effector memory cells are memory cells that are thought to be specialized for quickly entering inflamed tissues after restimulation.

Lymphocytes leave a lymph node through the **efferent lymphatic vessel**.

Electrophoresis is the movement of molecules in a charged field. In immunology, many forms of electrophoresis are used to separate molecules, especially protein molecules, to determine their charge, size, and subunit composition.

ELISA: see **enzyme-linked immunosorbent assay**.

ELISPOT assay is an adaptation of ELISA in which cells are placed over antibodies or antigens attached to a plastic surface. The antigen or antibody traps the cells' secreted products, which can then be detected using an enzyme-coupled antibody that cleaves a colorless substrate to make a localized colored spot.

Embryonic stem (ES) cells are mouse embryonic cells that will grow continuously in culture and that retain the ability to contribute to all cell lineages. ES cells can be genetically manipulated in tissue culture and then inserted into mouse blastocysts to generate mutant lines of mice; most often, genes are deleted in ES cells by homologous recombination and the mutant ES cells are then used to generate gene knockout mice. They have also been used to clone sheep, and could soon be used to replace body parts in humans.

Encapsulated bacteria have thick carbohydrate coats that protect them from phagocytosis. Encapsulated bacteria can cause extracellular infections and are effectively engulfed and destroyed by phagocytes only if they are first coated with antibody and complement produced in an adaptive immune response.

Cytokines that can induce a rise in body temperature are called **endogenous pyrogens,** as distinct from exogenous substances such as endotoxin from Gram-negative bacteria that induce fever by triggering endogenous pyrogen synthesis and release.

The **endoplasmic reticulum-associated aminopeptidase associated with antigen processing (ERAAP)** is an enzyme in the endoplasmic reticulum that trims longer polypeptides to a size at which they can bind to MHC class I molecules.

Antigen taken up by phagocytosis generally enters the **endosomes,** the acidified vesicles present in cells. Protein antigens entering by this route are presented by MHC class II molecules.

Endotoxins are bacterial toxins that are released only when the bacterial cell is damaged, as opposed to exotoxins, which are secreted bacterial toxins. The most important endotoxin is the lipopolysaccharide of Gram-negative bacteria, which is a potent inducer of cytokine synthesis and the proximal cause of endotoxic shock.

Within genomic DNA, there are specific regulatory sequences that act as cell-specific **enhancers** of transcription.

The **enzyme-linked immunosorbent assay (ELISA)** is a serological assay in which bound antigen or antibody is detected by a linked enzyme that converts a colorless substrate into a colored product. The ELISA assay is widely used in biology and medicine as well as in immunology.

Eosinophils are white blood cells thought to be important chiefly in defense against parasitic infections; they are activated by the lymphocytes of the adaptive immune response. The level of eosinophils in the blood is normally quite low. It can increase markedly in several situations, such as atopy, resulting in **eosinophilia,** an abnormally large number of eosinophils in the blood.

Eotaxin-1 (CCL11), eotaxin-2 (CCL24), and **eotaxin-3 (CCL26)** are CC chemokines that act predominantly on eosinophils.

An **epitope** is a site on an antigen recognized by an antibody or an antigen receptor; epitopes are also called antigenic determinants. A T-cell epitope is a short peptide derived from a protein antigen. It binds to an MHC molecule and is recognized by a particular T cell. B-cell epitopes are antigenic determinants recognized by B cells and are typically discontinuous in the primary structure.

Epitope spreading describes the fact that responses to autoantigens tend to become more diverse as the response persists. This is also called determinant spreading or antigen spreading.

The **Epstein–Barr virus (EBV)** is a herpesvirus that selectively infects human B cells by binding to complement receptor 2 (CR2, also known as CD21). It causes infectious mononucleosis and establishes a lifelong latent infection in B cells that is controlled by T cells. Some B cells latently infected with EBV will proliferate *in vitro* to form lymphoblastoid cell lines.

The affinity of an antibody for its antigen can be determined by **equilibrium dialysis,** a technique in which antibody in a dialysis bag is exposed to varying amounts of a small antigen able to diffuse across the dialysis membrane. The amount of antigen inside and outside the bag at the equilibrium diffusion state is determined by the amount and affinity of the antibody in the bag.

Erp57 is a chaperone molecule involved in loading peptide onto MHC class I molecules in the endoplasmic reticulum.

Erythroblastosis fetalis is a severe form of Rh hemolytic disease in which maternal anti-Rh antibody enters the fetus and produces a hemolytic anemia so severe that the fetus has mainly immature erythroblasts in the peripheral blood.

Experimental allergic encephalomyelitis (EAE) is an inflammatory disease of the central nervous system that develops after mice are immunized with neural antigens in a strong adjuvant.

The movement of cells or fluid from within blood vessels to the surrounding tissues is called **extravasation.**

IgG antibody molecules can be cleaved into three fragments by the enzyme papain. Two of these are identical **Fab fragments,** so called because they are the **F**ragment with specific **a**ntigen **b**inding. The Fab fragment consists of the light chain and the amino-terminal half of the heavy chain held together by an interchain disulfide bond. Another protease, pepsin, cuts in the same general region of the antibody molecule as papain but on the carboxy-terminal side of the disulfide bonds. This produces the **F(ab′)$_2$ fragment,** in which the two arms of the antibody molecule remain linked. See also **Fc fragment.**

FACS®: see **fluorescence-activated cell sorter.**

Factor B, factor D, factor H, factor I, and **factor P** are all components of the alternative pathway of complement activation. **Factor B** plays a role very similar to that of C2b in the classical pathway. **Factor D** is a serine protease that cleaves factor B. **Factor H** is an inhibitory protein with a role similar to decay-accelerating factor. **Factor I** is a protease that breaks down various components of the alternative pathway. **Factor P,** or **properdin,** is a positive regulatory component of the alternative pathway. It stabilizes the C3 convertase of the alternative pathway on the surface of bacterial cells.

Familial hemophagocytic lymphohistiocytosis (FHL) is a progressive and potentially lethal inflammatory disease caused by an inherited deficiency of perforin. Polyclonal CD8-positive T cells accumulate in lymphoid and other organs, associated with hemophagocytic activated macrophages.

Farmer's lung is a hypersensitivity disease caused by the interaction of IgG antibodies with large amounts of an inhaled allergen in the alveolar wall of the lung, causing alveolar wall inflammation and compromising gas exchange.

Fas is a member of the TNF receptor family; it is expressed on certain cells and makes them susceptible to killing by cells expressing **Fas ligand,** a cell-surface member of the TNF family of proteins. Binding of Fas ligand to Fas triggers apoptosis in the Fas-bearing cell.

IgG antibody molecules can be cleaved into three fragments by the enzyme papain. One of these is the **Fc fragment,** so-called for Fragment **c**rystallizable. The Fc fragment consists of the carboxy-terminal halves of the two heavy chains disulfide-bonded to each other by the residual hinge region. See also **Fab fragments.**

Fc receptors bind the Fc portions of immunoglobulin isotypes. They include the Fcγ and Fcε receptors.

The high-affinity **Fcε receptor (FcεRI)** on the surface of mast cells and basophils binds the Fc region of free IgE. When antigen binds this IgE and cross-links FcεRI, it causes mast-cell activation.

Fcγ receptors, including **FcγRI, RII,** and **RIII,** are cell-surface receptors that bind the Fc portion of IgG molecules. Most Fcγ receptors bind only aggregated IgG, allowing them to discriminate bound antibody from free IgG. They are expressed on phagocytes, B lymphocytes, NK cells, and follicular dendritic cells. They have a key role in humoral immunity, linking antibody binding to effector cell functions.

FDC: see **follicular dendritic cell**.

The **ficolin pathway** is a primitive complement-activation pathway based on the collectin ficolin, which is present in the urochordate *Ciona*.

When tissue or organ grafts are placed in an unmatched recipient, they are rejected by a **first-set rejection**, which is an immune response by the host against foreign antigens in the graft. *Cf.* **second-set rejection**.

FK506: see **tacrolimus**.

Individual cells can be characterized and separated in a machine called a **fluorescence-activated cell sorter** (**FACS®**) that measures cell size, granularity, and fluorescence due to bound fluorescent antibodies as single cells pass in a stream past photodetectors. The analysis of single cells in this way is called flow cytometry and the instruments that carry out the measurements and/or sort cells are called flow cytometers or cell sorters.

Peripheral lymphoid tissues, such as lymph nodes and Peyer's patches, contain large areas of B cells called **follicles**, which are organized around follicular dendritic cells.

A **follicular center cell lymphoma** is a type of B-cell lymphoma that tends to grow in the follicles of lymphoid tissues.

The **follicular dendritic cells (FDCs)** of lymphoid follicles are cells of uncertain origin. They are characterized by long branching processes that make intimate contact with many different B cells. They have Fc receptors that are not internalized by receptor-mediated endocytosis and thus hold antigen:antibody complexes on the surface for long periods. These cells are crucial in selecting antigen-binding B cells during antibody responses.

The V domains of immunoglobulins and T-cell receptors contain relatively invariant **framework regions** that provide a protein scaffold for the hypervariable regions that make contact with antigen.

Fungi are single-celled and multicellular eukaryotic organisms, including the yeasts and molds, that can cause a variety of diseases. Immunity to fungi is complex and involves both humoral and cell-mediated responses.

Fv: see **single-chain Fv**.

Fyn: see **tyrosine kinase**.

In the context of immunoglobulins, γ is the heavy chain of IgG.

Most T lymphocytes have α:β heterodimeric T-cell receptors, but some bear a distinct γ:δ **T-cell receptor** composed of different antigen-recognition chains, γ and δ, assembled in a γ:δ heterodimer. Cells bearing these receptors are called γ:δ **T cells** and their specificity and function are not yet clear.

G proteins are intracellular proteins that bind GTP and convert it to GDP in the process of cell signal transduction. There are two kinds of G protein, the heterotrimeric (α, β, γ) receptor-associated G proteins, and the small G proteins, such as Ras and Raf, that act downstream of many transmembrane signaling events.

GALT: see **gut-associated lymphoid tissues**.

Plasma proteins can be separated on the basis of electrophoretic mobility into albumin and the α, β, and γ globulins. Most antibodies migrate in electrophoresis as γ **globulins** (or **gamma globulins**), and patients who lack antibodies are said to have agammaglobulinemia.

GEFs: see **guanine-nucleotide exchange factors**.

In birds and rabbits, immunoglobulin receptor diversity is generated mainly by **gene conversion**, in which homologous inactive V gene segments exchange short sequences with an active, rearranged V-region gene.

Gene knockout is jargon for gene disruption by homologous recombination.

Gene rearrangement is the term often used for the recombination of gene segments in the immunoglobulin and T-cell receptor loci to produce a functional variable region sequence.

The V domains of the polypeptide chains of antigen receptors are encoded in sets of **gene segments** that must first undergo somatic recombination to form a complete V-domain exon. There are three types of gene segment: V gene segments that encode the first 95 amino acids, D gene segments that encode about 5 amino acids, and J gene segments that form the last 10–15 amino acids of the V region. There are multiple copies of each type of gene segment in the germline DNA, but only one is expressed for each type of receptor chain in a receptor-bearing lymphocyte.

A gene can be specifically disrupted by a technique known as **gene targeting** or gene knockout. Usually this involves homologous recombination in embryonic stem cells followed by the preparation of chimeric mice by injection of these cells into the blastocyst.

Gene therapy is the correction of a genetic defect by the introduction of a normal gene into bone marrow or other cell types. It is also known as somatic gene therapy because it does not affect the germline genes of the individual.

Mice that are raised in the complete absence of intestinal and other flora are called **germ-free** or **gnotobiotic** mice. Such mice have very depleted immune systems, but they can respond virtually normally to any specific antigen, provided it is mixed with a strong adjuvant.

Germinal centers in secondary lymphoid tissues are sites of intense B-cell proliferation, selection, maturation, and death during antibody responses. Germinal centers form around follicular dendritic cell networks when activated B cells migrate into lymphoid follicles. They can be divided by morphology into the dark zone, which is rich in proliferating B lymphocytes, and a light zone, which contains FDCs and centrocytes.

Immunoglobulin and T-cell receptor genes are said to be in the **germline configuration** in the DNA of germ cells and in all somatic cells in which somatic recombination has not occurred.

The **germline diversity** of antigen receptors is due to the inheritance of multiple gene segments that encode V domains; such diversity is distinguished from the diversity that is generated during gene rearrangement or after receptor gene expression, which is somatically generated.

One theory of antibody diversity, the **germline theory**, proposed that each antibody was encoded in a separate germline gene. This is now known not to be true for people, mice, and most other vertebrates, but appears to occur in elasmobranchs, which have rearranged genes in the germline.

GlyCAM-1 is a mucinlike molecule found on the high endothelial venules of lymphoid tissues. It is an important ligand for the L-selectin molecule expressed on naive lymphocytes, directing these cells to leave the blood and enter the lymphoid tissues.

Gnotobiotic: see **germ-free**.

Goodpasture's syndrome is an autoimmune disease in which autoantibodies against basement membrane or type IV collagen are produced and cause extensive vasculitis. It is rapidly fatal.

Tissue and organ grafts between genetically distinct individuals almost always elicit an adaptive immune response that causes **graft rejection**, the destruction of the grafted tissue by attacking lymphocytes.

When mature T lymphocytes are injected into a nonidentical immunoincompetent recipient, they can attack the recipient, causing a **graft-versus-host** (GVH) reaction. In human patients, mature T cells in allogeneic bone marrow grafts can cause **graft-versus-host disease** (GVHD).

Some of the therapeutic effect of bone marrow transplantation for leukemia can be due to a **graft-versus-leukemia effect**, in which the allogeneic bone marrow recognizes minor histocompatibility antigens or tumor-specific antigens expressed by the recipient's leukemic cells, leading the donor cells to kill the leukemic cells.

Granulocyte: see **polymorphonuclear leukocytes**.

Granulocyte-macrophage colony-stimulating factor (GM-CSF) is a cytokine involved in the growth and differentiation of myeloid and monocytic lineage cells, including dendritic cells, monocytes and tissue macrophages, and cells of the granulocyte lineage.

A **granuloma** is a site of chronic inflammation usually triggered by persistent infectious agents such as mycobacteria or by a nondegradable foreign body. Granulomas have a central area of macrophages, often fused into multinucleate giant cells, surrounded by T lymphocytes.

Granulysin is a cytotoxic protein present in the lytic granules of cytotoxic T cells.

Granzymes are serine proteases produced by cytotoxic T cells and are involved in inducing apoptosis in the target cell.

Graves' disease is an autoimmune disease in which antibodies against the thyroid-stimulating hormone receptor cause overproduction of thyroid hormone and thus hyperthyroidism.

The inherited disease **Griscelli syndrome** (type 2) affects the pathway for secretion of secretory lysosomes. It is caused by mutations in a small GTPase Rab27a, which controls the movement of vesicles within cells.

The **guanine-nucleotide exchange factors** (GEFs) are proteins that can remove the bound GDP from small G proteins; this allows GTP to bind and activate the G protein.

The **gut-associated lymphoid tissues** (GALT) are lymphoid tissues closely associated with the gastrointestinal tract, including the palatine tonsils, Peyer's patches, and intraepithelial lymphocytes. GALT have a distinctive biology related to their exposure to antigens from food and normal intestinal microbial flora.

GVHD: see **graft-versus-host disease**.

H antigens or **histocompatibility antigens**, are known as major histocompatibility antigens when they encode molecules that present foreign peptides to T cells and as minor H antigens when they present polymorphic self peptides to T cells. See also **histocompatibility**.

The major histocompatibility complex of the mouse is called **H-2** (for **histocompatibility-2**). Haplotypes are designated by a lower-case superscript, as in H-2^b.

A **haplotype** is a linked set of genes associated with one haploid genome. The term is used mainly in connection with the linked genes of the major histocompatibility complex, which are usually inherited as one haplotype from each parent. Some MHC haplotypes are overrepresented in the population, a phenomenon known as linkage disequilibrium.

Haptens are molecules that can bind antibody but cannot by themselves elicit an adaptive immune response. Haptens must be chemically linked to protein carriers to elicit antibody and T-cell responses.

Hashimoto's thyroiditis is an autoimmune disease characterized by persistent high levels of antibody against thyroid-specific antigens. These antibodies recruit NK cells to the tissue, leading to damage and inflammation.

All immunoglobulin molecules have two types of chain, a **heavy chain** (**H chain**) of 50–70 kDa and a light chain of 25 kDa. The basic immunoglobulin unit consists of two identical heavy chains and two identical light chains. Heavy chains come in a variety of **heavy-chain classes** or isotypes, each of which confers a distinctive functional activity on the antibody molecule.

Helper CD4 T cells are CD4 T cells that can help B cells make antibody in response to antigenic challenge. The most efficient helper T cells are also known as T$_H$2 cells, which make the cytokines IL-4 and IL-5. Some experts refer to all CD4 T cells, regardless of function, as helper T cells; we do not accept this usage because function can be determined only in cellular assays, and some CD4 T cells kill the cells they interact with.

A **hemagglutinin** is any substance that causes red blood cells to agglutinate, a process known as **hemagglutination**. The hemagglutinins in human blood are antibodies that recognize the ABO blood group antigens. Influenza and some other viruses have hemagglutinin molecules that bind to glycoproteins on host cells to initiate the infectious process.

Hematopoiesis is the generation of the cellular elements of blood, including the red blood cells, leukocytes, and platelets. These cells all originate from pluripotent **hematopoietic stem cells** whose differenti-

ated progeny divide under the influence of **hematopoietic growth factors**.

A **hematopoietic lineage** is any developmental series of cells that derives from hematopoietic stem cells and results in the production of mature blood cells.

Hemolytic disease of the newborn: see **erythroblastosis fetalis**.

In **hemophagocytic syndrome** there is a dysregulated expansion of CD8-positive lymphocytes which is associated with macrophage activation. The activated macrophages phagocytose blood cells, including erythrocytes and leukocytes.

Recombination signal sequences (RSS) flanking gene segments consist of a seven-nucleotide **heptamer** and a nine-nucleotide nonamer of conserved sequence, separated by 12 or 23 nucleotides. RSSs form the target for the site-specific RAG-1:RAG-2 recombinase that joins the gene segments.

Hereditary angioneurotic edema is the clinical name for a genetic deficiency of the C1 inhibitor of the complement system. In the absence of C1 inhibitor, spontaneous activation of the complement system can cause diffuse fluid leakage from blood vessels, the most serious consequence of which is epiglottal swelling leading to suffocation.

Individuals **heterozygous** for a particular gene have two different alleles of that gene.

High endothelial venules (HEVs) are specialized venules found in lymphoid tissues. Lymphocytes migrate from blood into lymphoid tissues by attaching to and migrating across the **high endothelial cells** that make up the walls of these blood vessels.

Tolerance to injected protein antigens occurs at low or high doses of antigen. Tolerance induced by the injection of high doses of antigen is called **high-zone tolerance**, whereas tolerance produced with low doses of antigen is called low-zone tolerance.

The **hinge region** of antibody molecules is a flexible domain that joins the Fab arms to the Fc piece. The flexibility of the hinge region in IgG and IgA molecules allows the Fab arms to adopt a wide range of angles, permitting binding to epitopes spaced variable distances apart.

Histamine is a vasoactive amine stored in mast cell granules. Histamine released by antigen binding to IgE molecules on mast cells causes dilation of local blood vessels and smooth muscle contraction, producing some of the symptoms of immediate hypersensitivity reactions. Antihistamines are drugs that counter histamine action.

Histocompatibility is literally the ability of tissues (Greek: histos) to get along with each other. It is used in immunology to describe the genetic systems that determine the rejection of tissue and organ grafts resulting from immunological recognition of histocompatibility (H) antigens.

Histocompatibility-2: see **H-2**.

HIV: see **human immunodeficiency virus**.

HLA, the acronym for **H**uman **L**eukocyte **A**ntigen, is the genetic designation for the human MHC. Individual loci are designated by uppercase letters, as in HLA-A, and alleles are designated by numbers, as in HLA-A*0201.

The invariant **HLA-DM** molecule in humans is involved in loading peptides onto MHC class II molecules. It is encoded in the MHC within a set of genes resembling MHC class II genes. A homologous protein in mice is called H-2M.

The atypical MHC class II molecule **HLA-DO** acts as a negative regulator of HLA-DM, binding to it and inhibiting the release of CLIP from MHC class II molecules in intracellular vesicles.

Hodgkin's disease is an immune system tumor characterized by large cells called Reed-Sternberg cells, which derive from mutated B-lineage cells. It exists in at least two polar forms, Hodgkin's lymphoma and nodular sclerosis.

Homeostasis is a generic term describing the status of physiological normality. In the case of lymphocytes, homeostasis refers to an uninfected individual who has normal numbers of lymphocytes.

Cellular genes can be disrupted by **homologous recombination** with copies of the gene into which erroneous sequences have been inserted. When these exogenous DNA fragments are introduced into cells, they recombine selectively with the cellular gene through remaining regions of sequence homology, replacing the functional gene with a nonfunctional copy.

Host-versus-graft disease (**HVGD**) is another name for the allograft rejection reaction. The term is used mainly in relation to bone marrow transplantation.

The **human immunodeficiency virus** (**HIV**) is the causative agent of the acquired immune deficiency syndrome (AIDS). HIV is a retrovirus of the lentivirus family that selectively infects macrophages and CD4 T cells, leading to their slow depletion, which eventually results in immunodeficiency. There are two major strains of the virus, HIV-1 and HIV-2, of which HIV-1 causes most disease worldwide. HIV-2 is endemic to West Africa but is spreading.

Humanization is a term used to describe the genetic engineering of mouse hypervariable loops of a desired specificity into otherwise human antibodies. The DNA encoding hypervariable loops of mouse monoclonal antibodies or V regions selected in phage display libraries is inserted into the framework regions of human immunoglobulin genes. This allows the production of antibodies of a desired specificity that do not cause an immune response in humans treated with them.

Human leukocyte antigen: see **HLA**.

Humoral immunity is the antibody-mediated specific immunity made in a **humoral immune response**. Humoral immunity can be transferred to unimmunized recipients by using immune serum containing specific antibody.

Monoclonal antibodies are most commonly produced from **hybridomas**. These are hybrid cell lines formed by fusing a specific antibody-producing B lymphocyte with a myeloma cell that is selected for its ability to grow in tissue culture and for an absence of immunoglobulin chain synthesis.

Hyperacute graft rejection of an allogeneic tissue graft is an immediate reaction caused by natural preformed antibodies that react against antigens on the graft. The antibodies bind to endothelium and trigger the blood clotting cascade, leading to an engorged, ischemic graft and rapid loss of the organ.

Hypereosinophilia is an abnormal state in which there are extremely large numbers of eosinophils in the blood.

Hyper IgM immunodeficiency: see **X-linked hyper IgM syndrome**.

Hyper IgM type 2 syndrome is an inherited immunodeficiency characterized by an abundance of relatively low-affinity IgM antibodies and a lack of antibodies of any other isotype. It is due to defects in the gene for AID (activation-induced cytidine deaminase), an enzyme required for both somatic hypermutation and isotype switching in immunoglobulin genes. *Cf.* X-linked hyper IgM syndrome.

Repeated immunization to achieve a heightened state of immunity is called **hyperimmunization**.

Immune responses to innocuous antigens that lead to symptomatic reactions upon reexposure are called **hypersensitivity reactions**. These can cause **hypersensitivity diseases** if they occur repetitively. This state of heightened reactivity to antigen is called **hypersensitivity**. Hypersensitivity reactions are classified by mechanism: type I hypersensitivity reactions involve IgE antibody triggering of mast cells; type II hypersensitivity reactions involve IgG antibodies against cell-surface or matrix antigens; type III hypersensitivity reactions involve antigen:antibody complexes; and type IV hypersensitivity reactions are T cell-mediated.

The **hypervariable** (**HV**) **regions** of immunoglobulin and T-cell receptor V domains are small regions that make contact with the antigen and differ extensively from one receptor to the next. They are more often known as the complementarity-determining regions. *Cf.* **framework regions**.

Hypohydrotic ectodermal dysplasia with immunodeficiency, also known as **NEMO deficiency**, is an inherited syndrome with some features resembling hyper IgM syndrome. It is caused by defects in the protein NEMO, a component of the NFκB signaling pathway.

The inactive complement fragment **iC3b** is produced by cleavage of C3b and is the first step in C3b inactivation.

The **ICAMs** (intercellular adhesion molecules) are cell-surface ligands for the leukocyte integrins and are crucial in the binding of lymphocytes and other leukocytes to certain cells, including antigen-presenting cells and endothelial cells. They are members of the immunoglobulin superfamily. **ICAM-1** is the most prominent ligand for the integrin CD11a:CD18 or LFA-1. It is rapidly inducible on endothelial cells by infection, and plays a major role in local inflammatory responses. **ICAM-2** is constitutively expressed at relatively low levels by endothelium. **ICAM-3** is expressed only on leukocytes and is thought to play an important part in adhesion between T cells and antigen-presenting cells, particularly dendritic cells.

Iccosomes are small fragments of membrane coated with immune complexes that fragment off the processes of follicular dendritic cells in lymphoid follicles early in a secondary or subsequent antibody response.

ICOS is a CD28-related protein that is induced on activated T cells and can enhance T-cell responses. It binds a ligand known as **LICOS**, which is distinct from the B7 molecules.

Each immunoglobulin molecule has the potential to bind a variety of antibodies directed at its unique features or **idiotype**. An idiotype is made up of a series of **idiotopes** or idiotype epitopes.

IFN: see **interferons**.

Ig: standard abbreviation for **immunoglobulin**. Different immunoglobulin isotypes are called IgM, IgD, IgG, IgA, and IgE.

Igα, Igβ: see **B-cell antigen receptor**.

IgA is the class of immunoglobulin characterized by α heavy chains. IgA antibodies are secreted mainly by mucosal lymphoid tissues.

IgD is the class of immunoglobulin characterized by δ heavy chains. It appears as surface immunoglobulin on mature naive B cells but its function is unknown.

IgE is the class of immunoglobulin characterized by ε heavy chains. It is involved in allergic reactions.

IgG is the class of immunoglobulin characterized by γ heavy chains. It is the most abundant class of immunoglobulin found in the plasma.

IgM is the class of immunoglobulin characterized by μ heavy chains. It is the first immunoglobulin to appear on the surface of B cells and the first to be secreted.

IL: see **interleukin**.

ILLs: see **innate-like lymphocytes**.

Immature B cells are B cells that have rearranged a heavy- and a light-chain V-region gene and express surface IgM, but have not yet matured sufficiently to express surface IgD as well.

Tissues throughout the body contain **immature dendritic cells**, which only leave the tissues in response to an inflammatory mediator or an infection. See also **dendritic cells**.

During allergic reactions, there are normally two phases: the first happens almost immediately and is called the **immediate reaction**. Hypersensitivity reactions that occur within minutes of exposure to antigen are called **immediate hypersensitivity reactions**; such reactions are antibody mediated. *Cf.* **delayed-type hypersensitivity**.

When large amounts of antigen are injected into the blood, they are initially removed slowly by normal catabolic processes that also degrade plasma proteins. However, if the antigen elicits an antibody response, then antigen is removed at an accelerated rate as antigen:antibody complexes, a process known as **immune clearance**.

The binding of antibody to a soluble antigen forms an **immune complex**. Large immune complexes form when sufficient antibody is available to cross-link the antigen; these are readily cleared by the reticuloendothelial system of cells bearing Fc and complement receptors. Small, soluble immune complexes that form when antigen is in excess can be deposited in and damage small blood vessels.

Immune deviation is the deliberate polarization of an immune response from one dominated by T_H1 to one dominated by T_H2, or vice versa.

Any changes that are induced in the course of an immune response are known as **immune modulation**.

The **immune response** is the response made by the host to defend itself against a pathogen.

Immune response (Ir) genes are genetic polymorphisms that control the intensity of the immune response to a particular antigen. Virtually all Ir phenotypes are due to the differential binding of peptide fragments of antigen to MHC molecules, especially MHC class II molecules. The term is little used now. An **immune response (Ir) gene defect** is usually, but not always, due to failure to bind an immunogenic peptide, so that no T-cell response is observed.

It has been proposed that most tumors that arise are detected and eliminated by **immune surveillance** mediated by lymphocytes specific for tumor antigens. There is little evidence for the efficacy of this proposed process, but it remains an important concept in tumor immunology.

The **immune system** is the name used to describe the tissues, cells, and molecules involved in adaptive immunity, or sometimes the totality of host defense mechanisms.

Immunity is the ability to resist infection.

Immunization is the deliberate provocation of an adaptive immune response by introducing antigen into the body. See also **active immunization**; **passive immunization**.

Immunobiology is the study of the biological basis for host defense against infection.

Immunoblotting is a common technique in which proteins separated by gel electrophoresis are blotted onto a nitrocellulose membrane and revealed by the binding of specific labeled antibodies.

Immunodeficiency diseases are a group of inherited or acquired disorders in which some aspect or aspects of host defense are absent or functionally defective.

Immunodiffusion is the detection of antigen or antibody by the formation of an antigen:antibody precipitate in a clear agar gel.

Immunoelectrophoresis is a technique in which antigens are first separated by their electrophoretic mobility and are then detected and identified by immunodiffusion.

Immunofluorescence is a technique for detecting molecules using antibodies labeled with fluorescent dyes. The bound fluorescent antibody can be detected by microscopy, or by flow cytometry depending on the application being used. **Indirect immunofluorescence** uses anti-immunoglobulin antibodies labeled with fluorescent dyes to detect the binding of a specific unlabeled antibody.

There are three ways of detecting molecules in tissues: **immunofluorescent microscopy** that reveals the presence of any molecule against which you have a specific antibody; **immunohistochemistry**, in which one links an enzyme that produces a change in a molecule that is visible under the microscope; and **immunoelectron microscopy**, in which different sized gold particles are linked to antibodies and detected as bound gold particles.

Any molecule that can elicit an adaptive immune response on injection into a person or animal is called an **immunogen**. In practice, only proteins are fully **immunogenic** because only proteins can be recognized by T lymphocytes.

All antibody molecules belong to a family of plasma proteins called **immunoglobulins (Ig)**. Membrane-bound immunoglobulin serves as the specific antigen receptor on B lymphocytes.

Immunoglobulin A: see **IgA**.

Immunoglobulin D: see **IgD**.

Many proteins are partly or entirely composed of protein domains known as **immunoglobulin domains** or **Ig domains** because they were first described in antibody molecules. Immunoglobulin domains are characteristic of proteins of the immunoglobulin superfamily, which includes antibodies, T-cell receptors, MHC molecules, and many other proteins described in this book. The immunoglobulin domain consists of a sandwich of two β sheets held together by a disulfide bond and called the **immunoglobulin fold**. There are two main types of immunoglobulin domain: C domains and V domains. Domains less closely related to the canonical Ig domains are sometimes also called **immunoglobulin-like domains**.

Immunoglobulin E: see **IgE**.

Immunoglobulin G: see **IgG**.

Immunoglobulin M: see **IgM**.

The **immunoglobulin repertoire**, also known as the antibody repertoire, is the total variety of immunoglobulin molecules in the body of an individual.

Many proteins involved in antigen recognition and cell–cell interaction in the immune system and other biological systems are members of a protein family called the **immunoglobulin superfamily**, or **Ig superfamily**, because their shared structural features were first defined in immunoglobulin molecules. All members of the immunoglobulin superfamily have at least one immunoglobulin domain or immunoglobulin-like domain.

The detection of antigens in tissues by means of visible products produced by the degradation of a colorless substrate by antibody-linked enzymes is called **immunohistochemistry**. This technique has the advantage that it can be combined with other stains to be viewed in the light microscope, whereas immunofluorescence microscopy requires a special dark-field or UV microscope.

Immunological ignorance describes a form of self tolerance in which reactive lymphocytes and their target antigen are both detectable within an individual, yet no autoimmune attack occurs. Most autoimmune diseases probably reflect the loss of other lymphocytes known as regulatory or suppressor T cells.

Allogeneic tissue placed in certain sites in the body, such as the brain, does not elicit graft rejection. Such sites are called **immunologically privileged sites**. Immunological privilege results from the effects of both physical barriers to cell and antigen migration, and soluble immunosuppressive mediators such as certain cytokines.

When an antigen is encountered more than once, the adaptive immune response to each subsequent encounter is speedier and more effective, a crucial feature of protective immunity known as **immunological memory**. Immunological memory is specific for a particular antigen and is long-lived.

The contact between T cell and antigen-presenting cell is a highly organized interface known as the **immunological synapse**, in which the spatial organization of the signaling molecules and their temporal organization contribute to the overall signal that is generated on antigen recognition.

Immunology is the study of all aspects of host defense against infection and of adverse consequences of immune responses.

Immunophilins are proteins with peptidyl-prolyl *cis–trans* isomerase activity that bind the immunosuppressive drugs cyclosporin A, tacrolimus, and rapamycin.

Soluble proteins, or membrane proteins solubilized in detergents, can be labeled and then detected by **immunoprecipitation analysis** using specific antibodies. The immunoprecipitated labeled protein is usually detected by SDS-PAGE followed by autoradiography. When proteins that do not react directly with the antibody used are nevertheless precipitated, they are said to co-immunoprecipitate.

The **immunoproteasome** is a form of proteasome found in cells exposed to interferons and contains three different subunits compared with the normal proteasome.

The T- and B-cell antigen receptors are associated with transmembrane molecules that have **immunoreceptor tyrosine-based activation motifs (ITAMs)** in their cytoplasmic domains. These tyrosine-containing motifs are sites of tyrosine phosphorylation and of association with tyrosine kinases and other phosphotyrosine-binding moieties involved in receptor signaling. Related motifs with opposing effects are **immunoreceptor tyrosine-based inhibitory motifs (ITIMs)**, which recruit phosphatases to the receptor site that remove the phosphate groups added by tyrosine kinases.

The ability of the immune system to sense and regulate its own responses is called **immunoregulation**.

Compounds that inhibit adaptive immune responses are called **immunosuppressive drugs**. They are used mainly in the treatment of graft rejection and severe autoimmune disease.

Immunotoxins are antibodies that are chemically coupled to toxic proteins usually derived from plants or microbes. The antibody targets the toxin moiety to the required cells. Immunotoxins are being tested as anticancer agents and as immunosuppressive drugs.

Indirect allorecognition of a grafted tissue involves uptake of allogeneic proteins by the recipient's antigen-presenting cells and their presentation to T cells by self-MHC molecules.

The **indirect Coombs test** is a variation of the direct Coombs test in which an unknown serum is tested for antibodies against normal red blood cells by first mixing the two and then washing out the serum from the red blood cells and reacting them with anti-immunoglobulin antibody. If antibody in the unknown serum binds to the red blood cells, agglutination by anti-immunoglobulin occurs.

Indirect immunofluorescence: see **immunofluorescence**.

Macrophages and many other cells have an **inducible NO synthase**, or **iNOS**, that is induced by many different stimuli to activate NO synthesis. This is a major mechanism of host resistance to intracellular infection in mice, and probably in humans as well.

Infectious mononucleosis, or glandular fever, is the common form of infection with the Epstein–Barr virus. It consists of fever, malaise, and swollen lymph nodes.

Infectious tolerance: see **regulatory tolerance**.

Inflammation is a general term for the local accumulation of fluid, plasma proteins, and white blood cells that is initiated by physical injury, infection, or a local immune response. This is also known as an **inflammatory response**. Acute inflammation is the term used to describe early and often transient episodes, whereas chronic inflammation occurs when the infection persists or during autoimmune diseases. Many different forms of inflammation are seen in different diseases. The cells that invade tissues undergoing inflammatory responses are often called **inflammatory cells** or an **inflammatory infiltrate**.

Influenza hemagglutinin: see **hemagglutinin**.

The early phases of the host response to infection depend on **innate immunity** in which a variety of innate resistance mechanisms recognize and respond to the presence of a pathogen. Innate immunity is present in all individuals at all times, does not increase with repeated exposure to a given pathogen, and discriminates between groups of similar pathogens.

Innate-like lymphocytes (ILLs) are a type of lymphocyte that contribute to rapid responses to infection by acting early but which use a limited set of antigen-receptor gene segments to make immunoglobulins and T-cell receptors.

When inositol phospholipid is cleaved by phospholipase C-γ, it yields **inositol trisphosphate (IP$_3$)** and diacylglycerol. Inositol trisphosphate releases calcium ions from intracellular stores in the endoplasmic reticulum.

In **insulin-dependent diabetes mellitus (IDDM)**, the β cells of the pancreatic islets of Langerhans are destroyed so that no insulin is produced. The disease is believed to result from an autoimmune attack on the β cells.

Integrins are heterodimeric cell-surface proteins involved in cell–cell and cell–matrix interactions. They are important in adhesive interactions between lymphocytes and antigen-presenting cells and in lymphocyte and leukocyte migration into tissues. The **β$_1$-integrins**, or very late antigens (VLA), are a family of integrins with shared β$_1$ chains and different α chains that mediate adhesion to other cells and to extracellular matrix proteins.

Intercellular adhesion molecules: see **ICAMs**.

Interdigitating dendritic cells: see **dendritic cells**.

Interferons-α and -β bind to a common **interferon receptor** that signals through a Janus-family tyrosine kinase.

Interferons are cytokines that can induce cells to resist viral replication. **Interferon-α (IFN-α)** and **interferon-β (IFN-β)** are produced by leukocytes and fibroblasts, respectively, as well as by other cells, whereas **interferon-γ (IFN-γ)** is a product of CD4 T$_H$1 cells, CD8 T cells, and NK cells. IFN-γ has as its primary action the activation of macrophages.

Interleukin, abbreviated **IL**, is a generic term for cytokines produced by leukocytes. We use the more general term cytokine in this book, but the term interleukin is used in the naming of specific cytokines such as IL-2. The interleukins are listed in Appendix III.

Interleukin-2 (IL-2) is the cytokine that is most central to the development of an adaptive immune response.

Staining for cytokines in cells that produce them can be achieved by permeabilizing the cell and reacting it with a labeled fluorescent anticytokine antibody. This procedure is called **intracellular cytokine staining**.

Injections can be administered by a number of routes: **intradermal (i.d.)**—entering the skin or dermis; **subcutaneous (s.c.)**—entering below the skin or dermis; **intramuscular (i.m.)**—entering the muscle; **intranasal (i.n.)**—by way of the nose; and **intravenous (i.v.)**—entering a vein.

Intrathymic dendritic cells: see **dendritic cells**.

The major histocompatibility complex (MHC) class II proteins are assembled in the endoplasmic reticulum with the **invariant chain (Ii)**, which is involved in shielding the MHC class II molecules from binding peptides and in delivering them to cellular vesicles. There Ii is degraded, leaving the MHC class II molecules able to bind peptide fragments of antigen.

IPEX is a very rare inherited condition in which regulatory CD4 CD25 T cells are lacking, leading to the development of autoimmunity.

ISCOMs are **immune stimulatory complexes** of antigen held within a lipid matrix that acts as an adjuvant and enables the antigen to be taken up into the cytoplasm after fusion of the lipid with the plasma membrane.

Isoelectric focusing is an electrophoretic technique in which proteins migrate in a pH gradient until they reach the place in the gradient at which their net charge is neutral—their isoelectric point. Uncharged proteins no longer migrate; thus each protein is focused at its isoelectric point.

Immunoglobulins are made in several distinct **isotypes** or classes—IgM, IgG, IgD, IgA, and IgE—each of which has a distinct heavy-chain C region encoded by a distinct C-region gene. The isotype of an antibody determines the effector mechanisms that it can engage on binding antigen. The different heavy-chain C regions are encoded in exons 3′ to the V(D)J rearrangement site. This allows the same antibody heavy-chain V region to link up with different heavy-chain C-region isotypes as a result of somatic recombination.

The first antibodies produced in a humoral immune response are IgM, but activated B cells subsequently undergo **isotype switching** or class switching to secrete antibodies of different isotypes: IgG, IgA, and IgE.

Isotype switching does not affect antibody specificity significantly, but alters the effector functions that an antibody can engage. Isotype switching occurs by recombination involving the deletion of DNA between the rearranged V region and the selected C-region exon at so-called S regions.

Isotypic exclusion describes the use of one or other of the light-chain isotypes, κ or λ, by a given B cell or antibody.

The **J gene segments**, or **joining gene segments**, are found some distance 5′ to the C genes in immunoglobulin and T-cell receptor loci. In the light-chain locus, the TCRα locus, and the TCRγ locus, a V gene segment joins directly with a J gene segment to form a complete V-region exon. In the case of the heavy-chain locus, the TCRβ locus, and the TCRδ locus, a D gene segment first combines with a J gene segment and the DJ segment then recombines with a V gene segment.

Cytokine receptors signal via **Janus-family tyrosine kinases** (**JAKs**)—tyrosine kinases that are activated by the aggregation of cytokine receptors. These kinases phosphorylate proteins known as STATs, for Signal Transducers and Activators of Transcription. STATs are normally found in the cytosol, but move to the nucleus on phosphorylation and activate a variety of genes.

Junctional diversity is the diversity present in antigen-specific receptors that is created during the process of joining V, D, and J gene segments.

In the context of immunoglobulins, **κ** is one of the two classes of light chain.

Killer T cell is a commonly used term for cytotoxic T cell.

The **kinin system** is an enzymatic cascade of plasma proteins that is triggered by tissue damage to produce several inflammatory mediators, including the vasoactive peptide bradykinin.

Kupffer cells are phagocytes lining the hepatic sinusoids; they remove debris and dying cells from the blood, but are not known to elicit immune responses.

In the context of immunoglobulins, **λ** is one of the two classes of light chain.

λ5: see **surrogate light chain**.

L chain: see **light chain**.

L-selectin is an adhesion molecule of the selectin family found on lymphocytes. L-selectin binds to CD34 and GlyCAM-1 on high endothelial venules to initiate the migration of naive lymphocytes into lymphoid tissue. Also called CD62L.

Langerhans' cells are phagocytic dendritic cells found in the epidermis. They can migrate from the epidermis to regional lymph nodes via the afferent lymphatics. In the lymph node they differentiate into dendritic cells.

The **large pre-B cells** have a cell-surface **pre-B-cell receptor**, which is lost on the transition to small pre-B cells, in which light-chain gene rearrangement occurs.

LAT: see **linker of activation in T cells**.

Some viruses can enter a cell but not replicate, a state known as **latency**. Latency can be established in various ways; when the virus is reactivated and replicates, it can produce disease.

In type I immediate hypersensitivity reactions, the **late-phase reaction** persists and is resistant to treatment with antihistamine.

The **late pro-B cell** is the stage in B-cell development in which V_H to DJ_H joining occurs.

The tyrosine kinase **Lck** associates most strongly with the cytoplasmic tails of CD4 and CD8. It plays a central role in signal transduction and activation of the T-cell receptor.

Lentiviruses are a group of retroviruses that include the human immunodeficiency virus, HIV-1. They cause disease after a long incubation period and can take years to become apparent.

Leprosy is caused by *Mycobacterium leprae* and occurs in a variety of forms. There are two polar forms: **lepromatous leprosy**, which is characterized by abundant replication of leprosy bacilli and abundant antibody production without cell-mediated immunity; and **tuberculoid leprosy**, in which few organisms are seen in the tissues, there is little or no antibody, but cell-mediated immunity is very active. The other forms of leprosy are intermediate between the polar forms.

Leukemia is the unrestrained proliferation of a malignant white blood cell characterized by very high numbers of the malignant cells in the blood. Leukemias can be lymphocytic, myelocytic, or monocytic.

Leukocyte is a general term for a white blood cell. Leukocytes include lymphocytes, polymorphonuclear leukocytes, and monocytes.

Leukocyte adhesion deficiency is an immunodeficiency disease in which the common β chain of the leukocyte integrins is not produced. This mainly affects the ability of leukocytes to enter sites of infection with extracellular pathogens, so that infections cannot be effectively eradicated.

The **leukocyte functional antigens** or **LFAs**, are cell adhesion molecules initially defined with monoclonal antibodies: **LFA-1** is a β_2 integrin; **LFA-2** is a member of the immunoglobulin superfamily, as is **LFA-3**, now called **CD58**. LFA-1 is particularly important in T-cell adhesion to endothelial cells and antigen-presenting cells.

Leukocyte integrins: see **leukocyte functional antigens**.

Leukocytosis is the presence of increased numbers of leukocytes in the blood. It is commonly seen in acute infection.

Leukotrienes are lipid mediators of inflammation that are derived from arachidonic acid. They are produced by macrophages and other cells.

LFA-1, LFA-2, LFA-3: see **leukocyte functional antigens**.

LICOS is the ligand for ICOS, a CD28-related protein that is induced on activated T cells and can enhance T-cell responses. LICOS is produced on activated dendritic cells, monocytes, and B cells.

The immunoglobulin **light chain** (**L chain**) is the smaller of the two types of polypeptide chain that make up all immunoglobulins. It consists of one V and one C domain, and is disulfide-bonded to the heavy chain. There are two classes of light chain, known as κ and λ.

Light zone: see **germinal centers**.

Linear epitopes: see **continuous epitopes**.

Alleles at linked loci within the major histocompatibility complex are said to be in **linkage disequilibrium** if they are inherited together more frequently than predicted from their individual frequencies.

Epitopes recognized by B cells and helper T cells must be physically linked for the helper T cell to activate the B cell. This is called **linked recognition**.

The adaptor protein known as **linker of activation in T cells** (**LAT**) is a cytoplasmic protein with several tyrosines that become phosphorylated by the tyrosine kinase ZAP-70. It becomes associated with membrane lipid rafts and coordinates downstream signaling events in T-cell activation.

Lipid rafts are small, cholesterol-rich areas in the cell membrane that are relatively resistant to solubilization by mild detergents.

Low-zone tolerance: see **high-zone tolerance**.

A molecule of bacterial lipopolysaccharide (LPS) has first to be bound by the **LPS-binding protein** (**LBP**) before it can interact with CD14, an LPS:LBP-binding protein on cells such as macrophages.

Lyme disease is a chronic infection with *Borrelia burgdorferi*, a spirochete that can evade the immune response.

Lymph is the extracellular fluid that accumulates in tissues and is carried by lymphatic vessels back through the lymphatic system to the thoracic duct and into the blood.

The **lymphatic system** is the system of lymphoid channels and tissues that drains extracellular fluid from tissues via the thoracic duct to the blood. It includes the lymph nodes, Peyer's patches, and other organized lymphoid elements apart from the spleen, which communicates directly with the blood.

Lymphatic vessels, or **lymphatics**, are thin-walled vessels that carry lymph through the lymphatic system.

Lymph nodes are a type of peripheral or secondary lymphoid organ. They are found in many locations thoughout the body where lymphatic vessels converge, and are sites where adaptive immune responses are initiated. Antigen-presenting cells and antigen delivered by the lymphatic vessels from a site of infection are displayed to the many recirculating lymphocytes that migrate through the lymph nodes. Some of these lymphocytes will recognize the antigen and respond to it, triggering an adaptive immune response.

A **lymphoblast** is a lymphocyte that has enlarged and increased its rate of RNA and protein synthesis.

Lymphocyte function-associated antigens: see **leukocyte functional antigens.**

The **lymphocyte receptor repertoire** is the totality of the highly variable antigen receptors carried by B and T lymphocytes.

All adaptive immune responses are mediated by **lymphocytes**. Lymphocytes are a class of white blood cells that bear variable cell-surface receptors for antigen. These receptors are encoded in rearranging gene segments. There are two main classes of lymphocyte— B lymphocytes (B cells) and T lymphocytes (T cells)—which mediate humoral and cell-mediated immunity, respectively. Small lymphocytes have little cytoplasm and condensed nuclear chromatin; on antigen recognition, the cell enlarges to form a lymphoblast and then proliferates and differentiates into an antigen-specific effector cell.

Dendritic cells can arise from myeloid cells, in which case they are called myeloid dendritic cells, or from lymphoid tissues, in which case they are called **lymphoid dendritic cells**. Functional differences exist between these two lineages.

Lymphoid tissues contain **lymphoid follicles** made up of follicular dendritic cells and B lymphocytes. The **primary lymphoid follicles** contain resting B lymphocytes. When a primary follicle is entered by activated B cells, a germinal center forms at this site, and the follicle is called a **secondary lymphoid follicle**.

Lymphoid organs are organized tissues characterized by very large numbers of lymphocytes interacting with a nonlymphoid stroma. The central or primary lymphoid organs, where lymphocytes are generated, are the thymus and bone marrow. The main peripheral or secondary lymphoid organs, in which adaptive immune responses are initiated, are the lymph nodes, spleen, and mucosal-associated lymphoid tissues such as tonsils and Peyer's patches.

Lymphokines are cytokines produced by lymphocytes.

Lymphomas are tumors of lymphocytes that grow in lymphoid and other tissues but do not enter the blood in large numbers. There are many types of lymphoma, which represent the transformation of various developmental stages of B or T lymphocytes.

Lymphopoiesis is the differentiation of lymphoid cells from a common lymphoid progenitor.

Lymphotoxin (LT) is also known as tumor necrosis factor-β (TNF-β), a cytokine secreted by inflammatory CD4 T cells that is directly cytotoxic for some cells.

Lyn: see **tyrosine kinase.**

Lysosomes are acidified organelles that contain many degradative hydrolytic enzymes. Material taken up into endosomes is eventually delivered to lysosomes.

Lytic granules containing perforin, granzymes, and granulysin are a defining characteristic of armed effector cytotoxic cells.

In the context of immunoglobulins, μ is the heavy chain of IgM.

Antigens and pathogens enter the body from the intestines through cells called **M cells** (**multi-fenestrated** or **microfold cells**), which are specialized for this function. They are found over the gut-associated lymphoid tissue, or GALT. They may provide a route of infection for HIV.

Macroglobulin describes plasma proteins that are globulins of high molecular weight, including immunoglobulin M (IgM) and α_2-macroglobulin.

Resting macrophages will not destroy certain intracellular bacteria unless the macrophage is activated by a T cell. **Macrophage activation** is important in controlling infection and also causes damage to neighboring tissues.

The **macrophage mannose receptor** is highly specific for certain carbohydrates that occur on the surface of some pathogens but not on host cells.

Macrophages are large mononuclear phagocytic cells important in innate immunity, in early nonadaptive phases of host defense, as antigen-presenting cells, and as effector cells in humoral and cell-mediated immunity. They are migratory cells deriving from bone marrow precursors and are found in most tissues of the body. They have a crucial role in host defense.

Dendritic cells are unique in being able to carry out **macropinocytosis**, a process in which large amounts of extracellular fluid are taken up in single vesicles. This is one means of antigen uptake.

MAdCAM-1 is the mucosal cell adhesion molecule-1 or mucosal addressin that is recognized by the lymphocyte surface proteins L-selectin and VLA-4, allowing specific homing of lymphocytes to mucosal tissues.

Eosinophils can be triggered to release their **major basic protein**, which can then act on mast cells to cause their degranulation.

The **major histocompatibility complex (MHC)** is a cluster of genes on human chromosome 6 or mouse chromosome 17. It encodes a set of membrane glycoproteins called the MHC molecules. The **MHC class I molecules** present peptides generated in the cytosol to CD8 T cells, and the **MHC class II molecules** present peptides degraded in intracellular vesicles to CD4 T cells. The MHC also encodes proteins involved in antigen processing and other aspects of host defense. The MHC is the most polymorphic gene cluster in the human genome, having large numbers of alleles at several different loci. Because this polymorphism is usually detected by using antibodies or specific T cells, the MHC molecules are often called major histocompatibility antigens.

MALT: see **mucosal-associated lymphoid tissue.**

The **mannose-binding lectin (MBL)** is an acute-phase protein that binds to mannose residues. It can opsonize pathogens bearing mannose on their surfaces and can activate the complement system via the **mannose-binding lectin pathway (MB-lectin pathway)** an important part of innate immunity.

The follicular **mantle zone** is a rim of B lymphocytes that surrounds lymphoid follicles. The precise nature and role of mantle zone lymphocytes have not yet been determined.

MAP kinases: see **mitogen-activated protein kinases.**

The **marginal zone** of the lymphoid tissue of the spleen lies at the border of the white pulp. It contains a unique population of B cells, the **marginal zone B cells**, which do not circulate and are distinguished by a distinct set of surface proteins.

The components of the MB-lectin pathway of complement activation include two serine proteases, **MASP-1** and **MASP-2**, that bind to mannose-binding lectin and play the same role in cleaving C4 as do C1r and C1s in the classical pathway.

Mast cells are large cells found in connective tissues throughout the body, most abundantly in the submucosal tissues and the dermis. They contain large granules that store a variety of mediator molecules including the vasoactive amine histamine. Mast cells have high-affinity Fcϵ receptors (FcϵRI) that allow them to bind IgE monomers. Antigen-binding to this IgE triggers mast-cell degranulation and mast-cell activation, producing a local or systemic immediate hypersensitivity reaction. Mast cells have a crucial role in allergic reactions.

Mastocytosis indicates an overproduction of mast cells.

Mature B cells are B cells that have acquired surface IgM and IgD and have become able to respond to antigen.

MBL; **MB-lectin pathway**: see **mannose-binding lectin**.

The **medulla** is generally the central or collecting point of an organ. The thymic medulla is the central area of each thymic lobe, rich in bone marrow-derived antigen-presenting cells and the cells of a distinctive medullary epithelium. The medulla of the lymph node is a site of macrophage and plasma cell concentration through which the lymph flows on its way to the efferent lymphatics.

The **membrane-attack complex** is made up of the terminal complement components, which assemble to generate a membrane-spanning hydrophilic pore, damaging the membrane.

Membrane cofactor of proteolysis (**MCP** or **CD46**) is a host-cell membrane protein that acts in conjunction with factor I to cleave C3b to its inactive derivative iC3b and thus prevent convertase formation.

B cells carry on their surfaces many molecules of **membrane immunoglobulin** (**mIg**) of a single specificity, which acts as the receptor for antigen.

Memory cells are the lymphocytes that mediate immunological memory. They are more sensitive to antigen than are naive lymphocytes and respond rapidly on reexposure to the antigen that originally induced them. Both **memory B cells** and **memory T cells** have been defined.

MHC; **MHC class I**; **MHC class II**: see **major histocompatibility complex**.

The **MHC class IB** molecules encoded within the MHC are not highly polymorphic like the MHC class I and MHC class II molecules, and present a restricted set of antigens.

In **MHC class I deficiency**, MHC class I molecules are not present on the cell surface, usually due to inherited deficiency of either TAP-1 or TAP-2.

The **MHC class II compartment** (**MIIC**) is a site in the cell where MHC class II molecules accumulate, encounter HLA-DM, and bind antigenic peptides, before migrating to the surface of the cell.

In **MHC class II deficiency**, MHC class II molecules are not expressed on cells as a result of one of various inherited defects in regulatory genes. Patients are severely immunodeficient and have few CD4 T cells.

The protein that activates the transcription of MHC class II genes, the **MHC class II transactivator** (**CIITA**), is one of several defective genes in the disease bare lymphocyte syndrome, in which MHC class II molecules are lacking on all cells.

MHC genes are inherited in most cases as an **MHC haplotype**, the set of genes in a haploid genome inherited from one parent. Thus, if the parents are designated as ab and cd, then the offspring are most likely to be ac, ad, bc, or bd.

MHC molecules is the general name given to the highly polymorphic glycoproteins encoded by MHC class I and MHC class II genes, which are involved in the presentation of peptide antigens to T cells. They are also known as histocompatibility antigens.

The development of **MHC:peptide tetramers** held together by fluorescent streptavidin, which has four binding sites for the biotin attached to the tail of the MHC molecule, has made it possible to stain specific T cells in any species.

MHC-restricted antigen recognition, or **MHC restriction**, refers to the fact that a given T cell will recognize a peptide antigen only when it is bound to a particular MHC molecule. Normally, as T cells are stimulated only in the presence of self-MHC molecules, antigen is recognized only as peptides bound to self-MHC molecules.

MIC molecules are MHC class I-like molecules that are expressed in the gut under conditions of stress and are encoded within the class I region of the human MHC. They are not found in mice.

Microfold cells: see **M cells**.

Microorganisms are microscopic organisms, unicellular except for some fungi, that include bacteria, yeasts and other fungi, and protozoa. All these groups contain some microorganisms that cause human disease.

mIg: see **membrane immunoglobulin**.

MIIC: see **MHC class II compartment**.

Minor histocompatibility antigens (**minor H antigens**) are peptides of polymorphic cellular proteins bound to MHC molecules that can lead to graft rejection when they are recognized by T cells.

Mitogen-activated protein kinases (**MAP kinases**) are kinases that become phosphorylated and activated on cellular stimulation by a variety of ligands, and lead to new gene expression by phosphorylating key transcription factors.

When lymphocytes from two unrelated individuals are cultured together, the T cells proliferate in response to the allogeneic MHC molecules on the cells of the other donor. This **mixed lymphocyte reaction** is used in testing for histocompatibility.

It has been proposed that infectious agents could provoke autoimmunity by **molecular mimicry**, the induction of antibodies and T cells that react against the pathogen but also cross-react with self antigens.

Monoclonal antibodies are produced by a single clone of B lymphocytes. Monoclonal antibodies are usually produced by making hybrid antibody-forming cells from a fusion of nonsecreting myeloma cells with immune spleen cells.

Monocytes are white blood cells with a bean-shaped nucleus; they are precursors of macrophages.

Some antibodies recognize all allelic forms of a polymorphic molecule such as an MHC class I protein; these antibodies are thus said to recognize a **monomorphic** epitope.

An individual lymphocyte carries antigen receptors of a single antigen specificity and thus has the property of **monospecificity** in response to antigen.

Mucins are highly glycosylated cell-surface proteins. Mucinlike molecules are bound by L-selectin in lymphocyte homing.

All of the body's internal epithelial organs are lined with epithelium that is coated with mucus, and are therefore called **mucosal epithelia**. This system is the site of entry for virtually all antigens, and is protected by a unique set of lymphoid organs.

The **mucosal-associated lymphoid tissue** (**MALT**) comprises all lymphoid cells in epithelia and in the lamina propria lying below the body's mucosal surfaces. The main sites of mucosal-associated lymphoid tissues are the gut-associated lymphoid tissues (GALT), and the bronchial-associated lymphoid tissues (BALT).

Multi-fenestrated cells: see **M cells**.

Multiple myeloma is a tumor of plasma cells, almost always first detected as multiple foci in bone marrow. Myeloma cells produce a monoclonal immunoglobulin, called a myeloma protein, that is detectable in the patient's plasma.

Multiple sclerosis is a neurological disease characterized by focal demyelination in the central nervous system, lymphocytic infiltration in the brain, and a chronic progressive course. It is caused by an autoimmune response to various antigens found in the myelin sheath.

Mx is an interferon-inducible protein required for cellular resistance to influenza virus replication.

Myasthenia gravis is an autoimmune disease in which autoantibodies against the acetylcholine receptor on skeletal muscle cells cause a block in neuromuscular junctions, leading to progressive weakness and eventually death.

Mycophenolate is an inhibitor of the synthesis of guanosine monophosphate and acts as a cytotoxic immunosuppressive drug. It acts by killing rapidly dividing cells, including lymphocytes proliferating in response to antigen.

Dendritic cells can arise from myeloid cells, in which case they are called **myeloid dendritic cells**, or from lymphoid tissues, in which case they are called lymphoid dendritic cells. Functional differences exist between these two lineages.

Myeloid progenitors are cells in bone marrow that give rise to the granulocytes and macrophages of the immune system.

Myeloma proteins are immunoglobulins secreted by myeloma tumors and are found in the patient's plasma.

Myelopoiesis is the production of monocytes and polymorphonuclear leukocytes in bone marrow.

N-nucleotides are inserted into the junctions between gene segments of T-cell receptor and immunoglobulin heavy-chain V-region genes during gene segment joining. These N-regions are not encoded in either gene segment, but are inserted by the enzyme terminal deoxynucleotidyl transferase (TdT). They markedly increase the diversity of these receptors.

N-regions: see **N-nucleotides**.

Naive lymphocytes are lymphocytes that have never encountered their specific antigen and thus have never responded to it, as distinct from memory or effector lymphocytes. All lymphocytes leaving the central lymphoid organs are naive lymphocytes, those from the thymus being **naive T cells** and those from bone marrow being **naive B cells**.

Natural killer cells (NK cells) are large granular, non-T, non-B lymphocytes, which kill certain tumor cells. NK cells are important in innate immunity to viruses and other intracellular pathogens, as well as in antibody-dependent cell-mediated cytotoxicity (ADCC).

Necrosis is the death of cells or tissues due to chemical or physical injury, as opposed to apoptosis, which is a biologically programmed form of cell death. Necrosis leaves extensive cellular debris that needs to be removed by phagocytes, whereas apoptosis does not.

During intrathymic development, thymocytes that recognize self are deleted from the repertoire, a process known as **negative selection**. Autoreactive B cells undergo a similar process in bone marrow.

NEMO deficiency: see **hypohydrotic ectodermal dysplasia with immunodeficiency**.

Antibodies that can inhibit the infectivity of a virus or the toxicity of a toxin molecule are said to **neutralize** them. Such antibodies are known as **neutralizing antibodies** and the process of inactivation as **neutralization**.

Neutropenia describes the situation in which there are fewer neutrophils in the blood than normal.

Neutrophils, also known as **polymorphonuclear neutrophilic leukocytes**, are the major class of white blood cell in human peripheral blood. They have a multilobed nucleus and neutrophilic granules. Neutrophils are phagocytes and have an important role in engulfing and killing extracellular pathogens.

NFAT: see **nuclear factor of activated T cells**.

The transcription factor called **NFκB** is made up of two chains of 50 kDa and 65 kDa. It is found under normal circumstances in the cytosol, where it is bound to a third chain called IκB, which is an inhibitor of NFκB transcription.

NK cells: see **natural killer cells**.

NK T cells are a class of T cells that express the cell-surface marker NK1.1 normally associated with NK cells, but also have an α:β T-cell receptor, which is, however virtually invariant.

Nodular sclerosis: see **Hodgkin's disease**.

Recombination signal sequences (RSS) flanking gene segments consist of a seven-nucleotide heptamer and a nine-nucleotide **nonamer** of conserved sequence, separated by 12 or 23 nucleotides. RSSs form the target for the site-specific recombinase that joins the gene segments in antigen receptor gene rearrangement.

Noncombinatorial immunoglobulin systems are found in rays and carcharine sharks, which have multiple 'rearranged' V_L regions (and sometimes rearranged V_H regions) in the germline genome.

Nondepleting antibodies being developed for immunosuppression block the function of target proteins on cells without causing the cells to be destroyed.

When T- and B-cell receptor gene segments rearrange, they often form **nonproductive rearrangements** that cannot encode a protein because the coding sequences are in the wrong translational reading frame.

Nonreceptor tyrosine kinase: see **receptor-associated tyrosine kinases**.

The transcription factor called **nuclear factor of activated T cells** (**NFAT**) is a complex of a protein called NFATc, as it is held in the cytosol by serine/threonine phosphorylation, and the Fos/Jun dimer known as AP-1. It moves from the cytosol to the nucleus on cleavage of the phosphate residues by calcineurin, a serine/threonine protein phosphatase.

The *nude* mutation of mice produces hairlessness and defective formation of the thymic stroma, so that nude mice, which are homozygous for this mutation, have no mature T cells.

When a person's work induces allergy, this is called **occupational allergy**.

Patients with the inherited disease **Omenn's syndrome** have defects in either of the *RAG* genes but make small amounts of functional RAG protein, allowing a small amount of V(D)J recombination. They suffer from a severe immunodeficiency with increased susceptibility to multiple opportunistic infections.

Oncogenes are genes involved in regulating cell growth. When these genes are defective in structure or expression, they can cause cells to grow continuously to form a tumor.

An **opportunistic pathogen** is a microorganism that causes disease only in individuals with compromised host defense mechanisms, as occurs in AIDS.

Opsonization is the alteration of the surface of a pathogen or other particle so that it can be ingested by phagocytes. Antibody and complement opsonize extracellular bacteria for destruction by neutrophils and macrophages.

The feeding of foreign antigens leads typically to a state of specific and active unresponsiveness, a phenomenon known as **oral tolerance**.

An autoimmune disease that targets a specific organ is said to be **organ-specific**.

Original antigenic sin describes the tendency of humans to make antibody responses to those epitopes shared between the original strain of a virus and subsequent related viruses, while ignoring other highly immunogenic epitopes on the second and subsequent viruses.

P-nucleotides are nucleotides found in junctions between gene segments of the rearranged V-region genes of antigen receptors. They are an inverse repeat of the sequence at the end of the adjacent gene segment, being generated from a hairpin intermediate during recombination, and hence are called palindromic or P-nucleotides.

P-selectin: see **selectins**.

Lymphocyte subpopulations can be isolated by **panning** on petri dishes coated with monoclonal antibodies against cell-surface markers, to which the lymphocytes bind.

The **paracortical area**, or **paracortex**, is the T-cell area of lymph nodes, lying just below the follicular cortex, which is primarily composed of B cells.

Parasites are organisms that obtain sustenance from a live host. In medical practice, the term is restricted to worms and protozoa, the subject matter of parasitology.

Paroxysmal nocturnal hemoglobinuria (PNH) is a disease in which complement regulatory proteins are defective, so that complement activation leads to episodes of spontaneous hemolysis.

Partial agonist peptide: see **altered peptide ligand**.

Passenger leukocytes are antigen-presenting cells of donor origin carried in as part of an organ graft.

Passive hemagglutination is a technique for detecting antibody in which red blood cells are coated with antigen and the antibody is detected by agglutination of the coated red blood cells.

The injection of antibody or immune serum into a naive recipient is called **passive immunization**. *Cf.* **active immunization**.

Pathogenic microorganisms, or **pathogens**, are microorganisms that can cause disease when they infect a host.

Pathology is the scientific study of disease. The term pathology is also used to describe detectable damage to tissues.

Pattern-recognition receptors are receptors of the innate immune system that recognize common molecular patterns on pathogen surfaces.

The cell-adhesion molecule **PECAM** (**CD31**) is found both on lymphocytes and at endothelial cell junctions. It is believed that CD31–CD31 interactions enable leukocytes to leave blood vessels and enter tissues.

Pentraxins are a family of acute-phase proteins formed of five identical subunits, to which C-reactive protein and serum amyloid protein belong.

Perforin is a protein that can polymerize to form the membrane pores that are an important part of the killing mechanism in cell-mediated cytotoxicity. Perforin is produced by cytotoxic T cells and NK cells and is stored in granules that are released by the cell when it contacts a specific target cell.

The **periarteriolar lymphoid sheath** (**PALS**) is part of the inner region of the white pulp of the spleen, and contains mainly T cells.

Peripheral or **secondary lymphoid organs** are the lymph nodes, spleen, and mucosal-associated lymphoid tissues, in which immune responses are induced, as opposed to the central lymphoid organs, in which lymphocytes develop.

Peripheral blood mononuclear cells are lymphocytes and monocytes isolated from peripheral blood, usually by Ficoll-Hypaque™ density centrifugation.

Peripheral tolerance is tolerance acquired by mature lymphocytes in the peripheral tissues, as opposed to central tolerance, which is acquired by immature lymphocytes during their development.

Peyer's patches are aggregates of lymphocytes along the small intestine, especially the ileum.

Antibody-like phage can be produced by cloning immunoglobulin V-region genes in filamentous phage, which thus express antigen-binding domains on their surfaces, forming a **phage display library**. Antigen-binding phage can be replicated in bacteria and used like antibodies. This technique can be used to develop novel antibodies of any specificity.

Phagocytosis is the internalization of particulate matter by cells. Usually, the **phagocytic cells** or **phagocytes** are macrophages or neutrophils, and the particles are bacteria that are taken up and destroyed. The ingested material is contained in a vesicle called a **phagosome**, which then fuses with one or more lysosomes to form a **phagolysosome**. The lysosomal enzymes are important in pathogen destruction and degradation to small molecules.

Phosphatidylinositol bisphosphate (**PIP$_2$**) is a membrane-associated phospholipid that is cleaved by phospholipase C-γ to give the signaling molecules diacylglycerol and inositol trisphosphate.

Phospholipase C-γ is a key enzyme in signal transduction. It is activated by protein tyrosine kinases that are themselves activated by receptor ligation, and activated phospholipase C-γ cleaves inositol phospholipid into inositol trisphosphate and diacylglycerol.

IFN-α and IFN-β activate a serine/threonine kinase called **PKR kinase**, which phosphorylates the eukaryotic protein synthesis initiation factor eIF-2, inhibiting translation and thus contributing to the inhibition of viral replication.

Plasma is the fluid component of blood containing water, electrolytes, and the plasma proteins.

A **plasmablast** is a B cell in a lymph node that already shows some features of a plasma cell.

Plasma cells are terminally differentiated B lymphocytes and are the main antibody-secreting cells of the body. They are found in the medulla of the lymph nodes, in splenic red pulp, and in bone marrow.

Platelet-activating factor (**PAF**) is a lipid mediator that activates the blood clotting cascade and several other components of the innate immune system.

Platelets are small cell fragments found in the blood that are crucial for blood clotting. They are formed from megakaryocytes.

Antigen activates specific lymphocytes, whereas all mitogens, by definition, activate most or all lymphocytes, a process known as **polyclonal activation** because it involves multiple clones of diverse specificity. Such mitogens are known as **polyclonal mitogens**.

The major histocompatibility complex is both **polygenic**, containing several loci encoding proteins of identical function, and polymorphic, having multiple alleles at each locus.

The **poly-Ig receptor** binds polymeric immunoglobulins, especially IgA, at the basolateral membrane of epithelia and transports them across the cell, where they are released from the apical surface. This transcytosis transfers IgA from its site of synthesis to its site of action at epithelial surfaces.

The **polymerase chain reaction** or **PCR** uses high temperature and unique thermostable enzymes to replicate DNA. It has revolutionized molecular biology.

Polymorphism literally means existing in a variety of different shapes. Genetic polymorphism is variability at a gene locus in which the variants occur at a frequency of greater than 1%. The major histocompatibility complex is the most **polymorphic** gene cluster known in humans.

Polymorphonuclear leukocytes are white blood cells with multilobed nuclei and cytoplasmic granules. There are three types of polymorphonuclear leukocyte: the neutrophils with granules that stain with neutral dyes, the eosinophils with granules that stain with eosin, and the basophils with granules that stain with basic dyes.

Some antibodies show **polyspecificity**, the ability to bind to many different antigens. This is also known as **polyreactivity**.

Only those developing T cells whose receptors can recognize antigens presented by self MHC molecules can mature in the thymus, a process known as **positive selection**. All other developing T cells die before reaching maturity.

Post-streptococcal glomerulonephritis is an autoimmune inflammation of kidney tissue that can follow some streptococcal infections.

Expression of the **pre-B-cell receptor**, or **pre-B-cell receptor complex**, is a critical event in B-cell development. Expression of this receptor, which is a complex of at least five proteins, causes the pre-B cell to enter the cell cycle, to turn off the *RAG* genes, to degrade the RAG proteins, and to expand by several cell divisions. Then the signal ceases, and the pre-B cell is ready to rearrange its light chains.

During B-cell development, **pre-B cells** are cells that have rearranged their heavy-chain genes but not their light-chain genes.

The **precipitin reaction** was the first quantitative technique for measuring antibody production. The amount of antibody is determined from the amount of precipitate obtained with a fixed amount of antigen. The precipitin reaction also can be used to define antigen valence and zones of antibody or antigen excess in mixtures of antigen and antibody.

Prednisone is a synthetic steroid with potent anti-inflammatory and immunosuppressive activity used in treating acute graft rejection, autoimmune disease, and lymphoid tumors.

In T-cell development, TCRβ chains expressed by CD44^{low}CD25$^+$ thymocytes pair with a surrogate α chain called pTα (pre-T-cell α) to form a **pre-T-cell receptor** that exits the endoplasmic reticulum via the Golgi as a complex with the CD3 molecules.

During T-cell dependent antibody responses, a **primary focus** of B-cell activation forms in the vicinity of the margin between T and B cell areas of lymphoid tissue. Here, the T and B cells interact and B cells can differentiate directly into antibody-forming cells or migrate to lymphoid follicles for further proliferation and differentiation.

The **primary immune response** is the adaptive immune response to an initial exposure to antigen. **Primary immunization**, also known as priming, generates both the primary immune response and immunological memory.

The binding of antibody molecules to antigen is called a **primary interaction**, as distinct from secondary interactions in which binding is detected by some associated change such as the precipitation of soluble antigen or agglutination of particulate antigen.

Primary lymphoid organs: see **central lymphoid organs**.

Priming of antigen-specific naive lymphocytes occurs when antigen is presented to them in an immunogenic form; the primed cells will differentiate either into armed effector cells or into memory cells that can respond in second and subsequent immune responses.

During B-cell development, **pro-B cells** are cells that have displayed B-cell surface marker proteins but have not yet completed heavy-chain gene rearrangement. They are divided into early pro-B cells and late pro-B cells.

Any lymphocyte receptor-chain gene can be rearranged in either of two ways, productive and nonproductive. **Productive rearrangements** are in the correct reading frame for the receptor chain in question.

Pro-enzymes are inactive forms of enzymes, often proteases, that must be modified in some way, for example by selective cleavage of the protein chain, before they can become active.

Programmed cell death: see **apoptosis**.

Properdin: see **factor P**.

Prostaglandins, like leukotrienes, are lipid products of the metabolism of arachidonic acid that have a variety of effects on a variety of tissues, including activities as inflammatory mediators.

Cytosolic proteins are degraded by a large catalytic multisubunit protease called a **proteasome**. It is thought that peptides that are presented by MHC class I molecules are generated by the action of proteasomes, and two interferon-inducible subunits of some proteasomes are encoded in the MHC.

Protectin (CD59) is a cell-surface protein that protects host cells from being damaged by complement. It inhibits the formation of the membrane-attack complex by preventing the binding of C8 and C9 to the C5b67 complex.

Protective immunity is the resistance to specific infection that follows infection or vaccination.

Protein A is a membrane component of *Staphylococcus aureus* that binds to the Fc region of IgG and is thought to protect the bacteria from IgG antibodies by inhibiting their interactions with complement and Fc receptors. It is useful for purifying IgG antibodies.

Protein kinase C (PKC) is a family of serine/threonine kinases that are activated by diacylglycerol and calcium as a result of signaling via many different receptors.

Protein kinases add phosphate groups to proteins, and **protein phosphatases** remove these phosphate groups. Enzymes that add phosphate groups to tyrosine residues are called **protein tyrosine kinases**. These enzymes have crucial roles in signal transduction and regulation of cell growth. Their activity is regulated by a second set of molecules called **protein tyrosine phosphatases** that remove the phosphate from the tyrosine residues.

Proto-oncogenes are cellular genes that regulate growth control. When mutated or aberrantly expressed, they can contribute to the malignant transformation of cells, leading to cancer. *Cf.* **oncogenes**.

A **provirus** is the DNA form of a retrovirus when it is integrated into the host cell genome, where it can remain transcriptionally inactive for long periods of time.

pTα: see **pre-T-cell receptor**.

The **pulmonary surfactant A** and **D** proteins are members of the pentraxin family that play various roles in the acute-phase response.

Purine nucleotide phosphorylase (PNP) deficiency is an enzyme defect that results in severe combined immunodeficiency. This enzyme is important in purine metabolism, and its deficiency causes the accumulation of purine nucleosides, which are toxic for developing T cells, causing the immune deficiency.

Pus is the mixture of cell debris and dead neutrophils that is present in wounds and abscesses infected with extracellular encapsulated bacteria.

Bacteria with large capsules are difficult for phagocytes to ingest. Such encapsulated bacteria often produce pus at the site of infection, and are thus called **pyogenic bacteria** or **pus-forming bacteria**. Pyogenic organisms used to kill many young people. Now, pyogenic infections are largely limited to the elderly.

The **qualitative signaling hypothesis** proposes that qualitatively different antigens might mediate the positive and negative selection of T cells in the thymus. *Cf.* **avidity hypothesis**.

The **12/23 rule** states that gene segments of immunoglobulin or T-cell receptors can be joined only if one has a recognition signal sequence with a 12 base pair spacer, and the other has a 23 base pair spacer.

Rac: see **small G proteins**.

Radiation bone marrow chimeras are mice that have been heavily irradiated and then reconstituted with bone marrow cells of a different strain of mouse, so that the lymphocytes differ genetically from the environment in which they develop. Such chimeric mice have been important in studying lymphocyte development.

Antigen–antibody interaction can be studied by **radioimmunoassay (RIA)** in which antigen or antibody is labeled with radioactivity. An unlabeled antigen or antibody is attached to a solid support such as a plastic surface, and the fraction of the labeled antibody or antigen retained on the surface is determined in order to measure binding.

Raf: see **small G proteins**.

The recombination-activating genes *RAG-1* and *RAG-2* encode the proteins **RAG-1** and **RAG-2,** which are essential for receptor gene rearrangement. Mice lacking either of these genes cannot form receptors and thus have no lymphocytes.

Rapamycin, or sirolimus, is an immunosuppressive drug that blocks cytokine action.

Ras: see **small G proteins**.

The antigen receptors of lymphocytes are associated with **receptor-associated tyrosine kinases**, mainly of the Src family, which bind to receptor tails via their SH2 domains.

Receptor-mediated endocytosis is the internalization into endosomes of molecules bound to cell-surface receptors. Antigens bound to B-cell receptors are internalized by this process.

The replacement of a light chain of a self-reactive antigen receptor on immature B cells with a light chain that does not confer autoreactivity is known as **receptor editing**. This has also been shown with heavy chains.

A **recessive lethal gene** encodes a protein that is needed for the human or animal to develop to adulthood; when both copies are defective, the human or animal dies *in utero* or early after birth.

In any situation in which cells or tissues are transplanted, they come from a donor and are placed in a **recipient** or host.

Recombination-activating genes: see *RAG-1* and *RAG-2*.

Recombination signal sequences (RSSs) are short stretches of DNA that flank the gene segments that are rearranged to generate a V-region exon. They always consist of a conserved heptamer and non-amer separated by 12 or 23 base pairs. Gene segments are only joined if one is flanked by an RSS containing a 12 base pair spacer and the other is flanked by an RSS containing a 23 base pair spacer—the 12/23 rule of gene segment joining.

The nonlymphoid area of the spleen in which red blood cells are broken down is called the **red pulp**.

Reed-Sternberg cells are large malignant B cells that are found in Hodgkin's disease.

Regulatory or **suppressor T cells** can inhibit T-cell responses.

Tolerance due to the actions of regulatory T cells is called **regulatory tolerance**.

When neutrophils and macrophages take up opsonized particles this triggers an oxygen-requiring metabolic change in the cell called the **respiratory burst**. It leads to the production of a number of mediators that are involved in killing engulfed microorganisms.

The virus known as **respiratory syncytial virus (RSV)** is a human pathogen that is a common cause of severe chest infection in young children, often associated with wheezing, as well as in immunocompromised patients and patients with AIDS.

The **Rev** protein is the product of the rev gene of the human immunodeficiency virus (HIV). The Rev protein promotes the passage of viral RNA from nucleus to cytoplasm during HIV replication.

The enzyme **reverse transcriptase** is an essential component of retroviruses, as it translates the RNA genome into DNA before integration into host cell DNA. Reverse transcriptase also enables RNA sequences to be converted into complementary DNA (cDNA), and so to be cloned, and thus is an essential reagent in molecular biology.

The **reverse transcriptase–polymerase chain reaction (RT-PCR)** is used to amplify RNA sequences. The enzyme reverse transcriptase is used to convert an RNA sequence into a cDNA sequence, which is then amplified by PCR.

The **Rhesus (Rh) blood group antigen** is a red cell membrane antigen that is also detectable on the red blood cells of rhesus monkeys. Anti-Rh antibodies do not agglutinate human red blood cells, so antibody to Rh antigen must be detected by using a Coombs test.

Rheumatic fever is caused by antibodies elicited by infection with some Streptococcus species. These antibodies cross-react with kidney, joint, and heart antigens.

Rheumatoid arthritis is a common inflammatory joint disease that is probably due to an autoimmune response. The disease is accompanied by the production of **rheumatoid factor**, an IgM anti-IgG antibody that can also be produced in normal immune responses.

RSSs: see **recombination signal sequences**.

The technique of **sandwich ELISA** uses antibody bound to a surface to trap a protein by binding to one of its epitopes. The trapped protein is then detected by an enzyme-linked antibody specific for a different epitope on the protein's surface. This gives the assay a high degree of specificity.

Scatchard analysis is a mathematical analysis of equilibrium binding that allows the affinity and valence of a receptor–ligand interaction to be determined.

Scavenger receptors on macrophages and other cells bind to numerous ligands and remove them from the blood. The Kupffer cells in the liver are particularly rich in scavenger receptors.

SCID, *scid*: see **severe combined immunodeficiency**.

SDS-PAGE is the common abbreviation for polyacrylamide gel electrophoresis (PAGE) of proteins dissolved in the detergent sodium dodecyl sulfate (SDS). This technique is widely used to characterize proteins, especially after labeling and immunoprecipitation.

SEs: see **staphylococcal enterotoxins**.

A **secondary antibody response** is the antibody response induced by a second or booster injection of antigen—a **secondary immunization**. The secondary response starts sooner after antigen injection, reaches higher levels, is of higher affinity than the primary response, and is dominated by IgG antibodies. Therefore, the response to each immunization is increasingly intense, so the secondary, tertiary, and subsequent responses are of increasing magnitude.

Secondary interactions: see **primary interaction**.

Secondary lymphoid organ: see **peripheral lymphoid organ**.

When the recipient of a first tissue or organ graft has rejected that graft, a second graft from the same donor is rejected more rapidly and vigorously in what is called a **second-set rejection**.

The co-stimulatory signal required for lymphocyte activation is often called a **second signal**, with the first signal coming from the binding of antigen by the antigen receptor. Both signals are required for the activation of most lymphocytes.

The **secretory component** attached to IgA antibodies in body secretions is a fragment of the poly-Ig receptor left attached to the IgA after transport across epithelial cells.

A cell is said to be **selected** by antigen when its receptors bind that antigen. If the cell starts to proliferate as a result, this is called clonal selection, and the cell founds a clone; if the cell is killed as a result of binding antigen, this is called negative selection or clonal deletion.

Selectins are a family of cell-surface adhesion molecules of leukocytes and endothelial cells that bind to sugar moieties on specific glycoproteins with mucinlike features.

Selective IgA deficiency is the most common inherited form of immunoglobulin deficiency in populations of European origin. No obvious disease susceptibility is associated with the defect.

Antigens in the body of an individual are by convention called **self antigens**. Lymphocytes are screened during their immature stages for reactivity with self antigens, and those that do respond undergo apoptosis.

Tolerance is the failure to respond to an antigen; when that antigen is **tolerance**.

Allergic reactions require prior immunization, called **sensitization**, by the allergen that elicits the acute response. Allergic reactions occur only in **sensitized** individuals.

Sepsis is infection of the bloodstream. This is a very serious and frequently fatal condition. Infection of the blood with Gram-negative bacteria triggers **septic shock** through the release of the cytokine TNF-α.

A **sequence motif** is a pattern of nucleotides or amino acids shared by different genes or proteins that often have related functions. Sequence motifs observed in peptides that bind a particular MHC glycoprotein are based on the requirements for particular amino acids to achieve binding to that MHC molecule.

Seroconversion is the phase of an infection when antibodies against the infecting agent are first detectable in the blood.

Serology is the use of antibodies to detect and measure antigens using **serological assays**, so called because these assays were originally carried out with serum, the fluid component of clotted blood, from immunized individuals.

Mast cells in mice store the small soluble mediator **serotonin** in their granules.

Different strains of bacteria and other pathogens can sometimes be distinguished by their **serotype**, the ability of an immune serum to agglutinate or lyse some strains of bacteria and not others.

Serpins are a large family of protease inhibitors.

Serum is the fluid component of clotted blood.

Serum sickness occurs when foreign serum or serum proteins are injected into a person. It is caused by the formation of immune complexes between the injected protein and the antibodies formed against it. It is characterized by fever, arthralgias, and nephritis.

Severe combined immunodeficiency (SCID) is an immune deficiency disease, fatal if untreated, in which neither antibody nor T-cell responses are made. It is usually the result of T-cell deficiencies. The *scid* mutation causes severe combined immune deficiency in mice.

In **severe congenital neutropenia**, which can be inherited as a dominant or recessive trait, the neutrophil count is persistently extremely low.

SH2 domain: see **Src-family tyrosine kinases**.

Shock is the name given to the potentially fatal circulatory collapse caused by the systemic actions of cytokines such as TNF-α.

A **signal joint** is formed by the precise joining of recognition signal sequences in the process of somatic recombination that generates T-cell receptor and immunoglobulin genes. The piece of chromosome containing the signal joint is excised from the chromosome as a small circle of DNA.

Signal transducers and activators of transcription (STATs): see **Janus-family tyrosine kinases**.

Signal transduction describes the general process by which cells perceive changes in their environment. More specifically, it refers to the processes by which a cell transforms one type of signal, for example, antigen binding to a lymphocyte antigen receptor, into the intracellular events that signal the cell to make a particular type of response.

A **single-chain Fv** fragment, comprising a V region of a heavy chain linked by a stretch of synthetic peptide to a V region of a light chain, can be made by genetic engineering.

During T-cell maturation in the thymus, mature T cells are detected by the expression of either the CD4 or the CD8 co-receptor and are therefore called **single-positive thymocytes**.

Sirolimus is the drug name that has been adopted for the chemical rapamycin; the two terms are used interchangeably in the literature.

Small G proteins are monomeric G proteins such as Ras, that act as intracellular signaling molecules downstream of many transmembrane signaling events. In their active form they bind GTP, which they hydrolyze to GDP, becoming inactive.

Small pre-B cells: see **large pre-B cells**.

When immunologists discovered that antibodies were variable, they entertained various theories, including the **somatic diversification theory** that postulated that the genes for immunoglobulin were constant, and that they diversified in somatic cells. This turned out to be partly true, as somatic hypermutation is now well established. However, other theories were needed to explain other features of antibody diversity, including somatic gene rearrangement and isotype switching.

Somatic gene therapy: see **gene therapy**.

During B-cell responses to antigen, the V-region DNA sequence undergoes **somatic hypermutation,** resulting in the generation of variant immunoglobulins, some of which bind antigen with a higher affinity. This allows the affinity of the antibody response to increase. These mutations affect only somatic cells, and are not inherited through germline transmission.

During lymphocyte development, receptor gene segments undergo **somatic recombination** to generate intact V-region exons that encode the V region of each immunoglobulin and T-cell receptor chain. These events occur only in somatic cells; the changes are not inherited.

Spacer: see **12/23 rule**.

The **specificity** of an antibody determines its ability to distinguish the immunogen from other antigens.

One uses **spectratyping** to define certain types of DNA gene segments that give a repetitive spacing of three nucleotides, or one codon.

The **spleen** is an organ in the upper left side of the peritoneal cavity containing a red pulp, involved in removing senescent blood cells, and a white pulp of lymphoid cells that respond to antigens delivered to the spleen by the blood.

The **Src-family tyrosine kinases** are receptor-associated protein tyrosine kinases. They have several domains, called Src-homology 1, 2, and 3. The SH1 domain contains the active site of the kinase, the SH2 domain can bind to phosphotyrosine residues, and the SH3 domain is involved in interactions with proline-rich regions in other proteins.

Staphylococcal enterotoxins (SEs) cause food poisoning and also stimulate many T cells by binding to MHC class II molecules and the $V_β$ domain of certain T-cell receptors; the staphylococcal enterotoxins are thus superantigens.

STATs: see **Janus-family tyrosine kinases**.

Stem-cell factor (SCF) is a transmembrane protein on bone marrow stromal cells that binds to c-Kit, a signaling receptor carried on developing B cells and other developing white blood cells.

The development of B lymphocytes and T lymphocytes occurs in association with **stromal cells**, which provide various soluble and cell-bound signals to the developing lymphocyte.

Antigens can be injected into the **subcutaneous** layer (ie, below the skin or dermis) to induce an adaptive immune response. See also **intradermal**.

Superantigens are molecules that stimulate a subset of T cells by binding to MHC class II molecules and $V_β$ domains of T-cell receptors, stimulating the activation of T cells expressing particular $V_β$ gene segments. The staphylococcal enterotoxins are one of the sources of superantigens.

Suppressor T cells: see **regulatory T cells**.

Clustering of T-cell or B-cell receptors after binding their ligands leads to the formation of an organized structure, called the **supramolecular adhesion complex (SMAC)**, in which the antigen receptors are co-localized with other cell-surface signaling and adhesion molecules.

The membrane-bound immunoglobulin that acts as the antigen receptor on B cells is often known as **surface immunoglobulin (sIg)**.

The **surrogate light chain** is made up of two molecules called VpreB and λ5. Together, this chain can pair with an in-frame heavy chain, move to the cell surface, and signal for pre-B-cell growth.

When isotype switching occurs, the active heavy-chain V-region exon undergoes somatic recombination with a 3′ constant-region gene at a **switch region** of DNA. These DNA joints do not need to occur at precise sites, because they occur in intronic DNA. Thus, all **switch recombinations** are productive.

Syk: see **tyrosine kinase**.

When one eye is damaged, there is often an autoimmune response that damages the other eye, a syndrome known as **sympathetic ophthalmia**.

A **syngeneic graft** is a graft between two genetically identical individuals. It is accepted as self.

Syphilis is a chronic disease caused by the spirochete *Treponema pallidum*, a spirochete that can evade the immune response.

Systemic anaphylaxis is the most dangerous form of immediate hypersensitivity reaction. It involves antigen in the bloodstream triggering mast cells all over the body. The activation of these mast cells causes widespread vasodilation, tissue fluid accumulation, epiglottal swelling, and often death.

Systemic lupus erythematosus (SLE) is an autoimmune disease in which autoantibodies against DNA, RNA, and proteins associated with nucleic acids form immune complexes that damage small blood vessels, especially of the kidney.

T-cell antigen receptor: see **T-cell receptor**.

A **T-cell clone** is derived from a single progenitor T cell. See also **cloned T-cell line**.

T-cell hybrids are formed by fusing an antigen-specific, activated T cell with a T-cell lymphoma. The hybrid cells bear the receptor of the specific T-cell parent and grow in culture like the lymphoma.

T-cell lines are cultures of T cells grown by repeated cycles of stimulation, usually with antigen and antigen-presenting cells. When single T cells from these lines are propagated, they can give rise to T-cell clones or cloned T-cell lines.

The **T-cell receptor** (TCR) consists of a disulfide-linked heterodimer of the highly variable α and β chains expressed at the cell membrane as a complex with the invariant CD3 chains. T cells carrying this type of receptor are often called $\alpha{:}\beta$ T cells. An alternative receptor made up of variable γ and δ chains is expressed with CD3 on a subset of T cells. Both of these receptors are expressed with a disulfide-linked homodimer of ζ chains, which carries out the intracellular signaling function of the receptor.

T cells, or **T lymphocytes**, are a subset of lymphocytes defined by their development in the thymus and by heterodimeric receptors associated with the proteins of the CD3 complex. Most T cells have $\alpha{:}\beta$ heterodimeric receptors but $\gamma{:}\delta$ T cells have a $\gamma{:}\delta$ heterodimeric receptor.

The **T-cell zones** in lymphoid tissues are enriched in T cells and are distinct from the B-cell zones and the stromal elements.

T lymphocytes: see **T cells**.

T regulatory 1 cells, T_{reg}, T_R1: see **regulatory T cells**.

Tacrolimus, or FK506, is an immunosuppressive polypeptide drug that inactivates T cells by inhibiting signal transduction from the T-cell receptor. Tacrolimus and cyclosporin A are the most commonly used immunosuppressive drugs in organ transplantation.

TAP-1 and **TAP-2** (transporters associated with antigen processing) are ATP-binding cassette proteins involved in transporting short peptides from the cytosol into the lumen of the endoplasmic reticulum, where they associate with MHC class I molecules.

Tapasin, or the **TAP-associated protein**, is a key molecule in the assembly of MHC class I molecules; a cell deficient in this protein has only unstable MHC class I molecules on the cell surface.

The functions of effector T cells are always assayed by the changes that they produce in antigen-bearing **target cells**. These cells can be B cells, which are activated to produce antibody; macrophages, which are activated to kill bacteria or tumor cells; or labeled cells that are killed by cytotoxic T cells.

The **Tat** protein is a product of the *tat* gene of HIV. It is produced when latently infected cells are activated, and it binds to a transcriptional enhancer in the long terminal repeat of the provirus, increasing the transcription of the proviral genome.

TCRα and **TCRβ** are the two chains of the $\alpha{:}\beta$ **T-cell receptor**.

Activation of the lymphocyte antigen receptors is linked to activation of PLC-γ through members of the **Tec kinase** family of Src-like tyrosine kinases. Other Tec kinases are Btk in B cells, which is mutated in the human immunodeficiency disease X-linked agammaglobulinemia (XLA), and Itk in T lymphocytes.

The complement system can be activated directly or by antibody, but both pathways converge with the activation of the **terminal complement components,** which may assemble to form the membrane-attack complex.

The enzyme **terminal deoxynucleotidyl transferase** (TdT) inserts nontemplated or N-nucleotides into the junctions between gene segments in T-cell receptor and immunoglobulin V-region genes. The N-nucleotides contribute greatly to junctional diversity in V regions.

When the same antigen is injected a third time, the response elicited is called a **tertiary response** and the injection a **tertiary immunization**.

T_H1 cells are a subset of CD4 T cells that are characterized by the cytokines they produce. They are mainly involved in activating macrophages, and are sometimes called inflammatory CD4 T cells.

T_H2 cells are a subset of CD4 T cells that are characterized by the cytokines they produce. They are mainly involved in stimulating B cells to produce antibody, and are often called helper CD4 T cells.

The term **T_H3 cell** has been used to describe unique cells that produce mainly transforming growth factor-β in response to antigen; they develop predominantly in the mucosal immune response to antigens that are presented orally.

The lymph from most of the body, except the head, neck, and right arm, is gathered in a large lymphatic vessel, the **thoracic duct**, which runs parallel to the aorta through the thorax and drains into the left subclavian vein. The thoracic duct thus returns the lymphatic fluid and lymphocytes back into the peripheral blood circulation.

Surgical removal of the thymus is called **thymectomy**.

The **thymic anlage** is the tissue from which the thymic stroma develops during embryogenesis.

The **thymic cortex** is the outer region of each thymic lobule in which thymic progenitor cells proliferate, rearrange their T-cell receptor genes, and undergo thymic selection, especially positive selection on **thymic cortical epithelial cells**.

The **thymic stroma** consists of epithelial cells and connective tissue that form the essential microenvironment for T-cell development.

Thymocytes are lymphoid cells found in the thymus. They consist mainly of developing T cells, although a few thymocytes have achieved functional maturity.

Thymoma is a tumor of thymic stroma.

The **thymus**, the site of T-cell development, is a lymphoepithelial organ in the upper part of the middle of the chest, just behind the breastbone.

Some antigens elicit responses only in individuals that have T cells; they are called **thymus-dependent antigens** or **TD antigens**. Other antigens can elicit antibody production in the absence of T cells and are called **thymus-independent antigens** or **TI antigens**. There are two types of TI antigen: the **TI-1 antigens,** which have intrinsic B-cell activating activity, and the **TI-2 antigens,** which seem to activate B cells by having multiple identical epitopes that cross-link the B-cell receptor.

T cell and T lymphocyte are short designations for **thymus-dependent lymphocyte**, the lymphocyte population that fails to develop in the absence of a functioning thymus.

One uses **time-lapse video microscopy** to examine processes in biology, that are anywhere from cell migration (fast) to a flower blossoming (slow).

During the process of germinal center formation, cells called **tingible body macrophages** appear. These are phagocytic cells engulfing apoptotic B cells, which are produced in large numbers during the height of the germinal center response.

All dendritic cells arise from hematopoietic progenitors that migrate to various locations all over the body. Here, they are referred to as **tissue dendritic cells**.

Transplantation of organs or **tissue grafts** such as skin grafts is used medically to repair organ or tissue deficits.

Some autoimmune diseases attack particular tissues, such as the β cell in the islets of Langerhans in autoimmune diabetes mellitus; such diseases are called **tissue-specific autoimmune disease**.

The **titer** of an antiserum is a measure of its concentration of specific antibodies based on serial dilution to an end point, such as a certain level of color change in an ELISA assay.

TLR-3 is a mammalian Toll-like receptor that recognizes double-stranded RNA.

TLR-4 is a mammalian Toll-like receptor that, in conjunction with the macrophage LPS receptor, recognizes bacterial lipopolysaccharide (LPS).

TNF: see **tumor necrosis factor-α; lymphotoxin**.

There are several members of the **TNF receptor** (**TNFR**) family. Some lead to apoptosis of the cell on which they are expressed (TNFR-I, II, Fas), while others lead to activation (CD40, 4-1BB). All of them signal as trimeric proteins.

Tolerance is the failure to respond to an antigen; the immune system is said to be **tolerant** to self antigens. Tolerance to self antigens is an essential feature of the immune system; when tolerance is lost, the immune system can destroy self tissues, as happens in autoimmune disease. The immune system mainly becomes tolerant to self antigens—is **tolerized**—during lymphocyte development.

All members of the Toll family of receptors so far discovered have been homologous to the original Toll in *Drosophila*. They have been named **Toll-like receptors** (**TLR**) followed by a number, as in **Toll-like receptor 4** or **TLR-4**.

The **Toll pathway** is an ancient signaling pathway that activates the transcription factor NFκB by degrading its inhibitor IκB.

The palatine **tonsils** that lie on either side of the pharynx are large aggregates of lymphoid cells organized as part of the mucosal- or gut-associated immune system.

Toxic shock syndrome is a systemic toxic reaction caused by the massive production of cytokines by CD4 T cells activated by the bacterial superantigen **toxic shock syndrome toxin-1** (**TSST-1**), which is secreted by *Staphylococcus aureus*.

Inactivated toxins called **toxoids** are no longer toxic but retain their immunogenicity so that they can be used for immunization.

T$_R$1: see **regulatory T cells**.

The family of proteins known as TNF receptor-associated factors, or **TRAFs**, consists of at least six members that bind to various TNF family receptors or TNFRs. They share a domain known as a TRAF domain, and have a crucial role as signal transducers between upstream members of the TNFR family and downstream transcription factors.

The active transport of molecules across epithelial cells is called **transcytosis**. Transcytosis of IgA molecules involves transport across intestinal epithelial cells in vesicles that originate on the basolateral surface and fuse with the apical surface in contact with the intestinal lumen.

The insertion of small pieces of DNA into cells is called **transfection**. If the DNA is expressed without integrating into host cell DNA, this is called a transient transfection; if the DNA integrates into host cell DNA, then it replicates whenever host cell DNA is replicated, producing a stable transfection.

Foreign genes can be placed in the mouse genome by **transgenesis**. This generates **transgenic mice** that are used to study the function of the inserted gene, or transgene, and the regulation of its expression.

Some cancers have chromosomal **translocations**, in which a piece of one chromosome is abnormally linked to another chromosome.

The grafting of organs or tissues from one individual to another is called **transplantation**. The **transplanted organs** or grafts can be rejected by the immune system unless the host is tolerant to the graft antigens or immunosuppressive drugs are used to prevent rejection.

Transporters associated with antigen processing: see **TAP-1** and **TAP-2**.

The **tuberculin test** is a clinical test in which a purified protein derivative (PPD) of *Mycobacterium tuberculosis*, the causative agent of tuberculosis, is injected subcutaneously. PPD elicits a delayed-type hypersensitivity reaction in individuals who have had tuberculosis or have been immunized against it.

Tuberculoid leprosy: see **leprosy**.

Tumor immunology is the study of host defenses against tumors, usually studied by tumor transplantation.

Tumor necrosis factor-α (**TNF-α**) is a cytokine produced by macrophages and T cells that has multiple functions in the immune response. It is the defining member of the TNF family of cytokines. These cytokines function as cell-associated or secreted proteins that interact with receptors of the **tumor necrosis factor receptor** (**TNFR**) family, which in turn communicates with the interior of the cell via components known as TRAFs (tumor necrosis factor receptor-associated factors).

Tumor necrosis factor-β (**TNF-β**): see **lymphotoxin**.

Tumors transplanted into syngeneic recipients can grow progressively or can be rejected through T-cell recognition of **tumor-specific transplantation antigens** (**TSTA**) or **tumor rejection antigens**. TSTA are peptides of mutant or overexpressed cellular proteins bound to MHC class I molecules on the tumor cell surface.

The **TUNEL assay** (**T**dT-dependent d**U**TP–biotin **n**ick **e**nd **l**abeling) identifies apoptotic cells *in situ* by the characteristic fragmentation of their DNA. Biotin-tagged dUTP added to the free 3′ ends of the DNA fragments by the enzyme TdT can be detected by immunohistochemical staining with enzyme-linked streptavidin.

In **two-dimensional gel electrophoresis,** proteins are separated by isoelectric focusing in one dimension, followed by SDS-PAGE on a slab gel at right-angles to the first dimension. This can separate and identify large numbers of distinct proteins.

Hypersensitivity reactions are classified by mechanism: **type I hypersensitivity reactions** involve IgE antibody triggering of mast cells; **type II hypersensitivity reactions** involve IgG antibodies against cell surface or matrix antigens; **type III hypersensitivity reactions** involve antigen:antibody complexes; and **type IV hypersensitivity reactions** are T-cell mediated.

A **tyrosine kinase** is an enzyme that specifically phosphorylates tyrosine residues in proteins. They are critical in T- and B-cell activation. The kinases that are critical for B-cell activation are Blk, Fyn, Lyn, and Syk. The tyrosine kinases that are critical for T-cell activation are called Lck, Fyn, and ZAP-70.

Urticaria is the technical term for hives, which are red, itchy skin welts usually brought on by an allergic reaction.

The variable region of the polypeptide chains of an immunoglobulin or T-cell receptor is composed of a single amino-terminal **V domain**. Paired V domains form the antigen-binding sites of immunoglobulins and T-cell receptors.

The first 95 amino acids or so of immunoglobulin or T-cell receptor V domains are encoded in inherited **V gene segments**. There are multiple different V gene segments in the germline genome. To produce a complete exon encoding a V domain, one V gene segment must be rearranged to join up with a J or a rearranged DJ gene segment.

Vaccination is the deliberate induction of adaptive immunity to a pathogen by injecting a **vaccine**, a dead or attenuated (nonpathogenic) form of the pathogen.

The **valence** of an antibody or antigen is the number of different molecules that it can combine with at one time.

The **variability** of a protein is a measure of the difference between the amino acid sequences of different variants of that protein. The most variable proteins known are antibodies and T-cell receptors.

Variable gene segments: see **V gene segments**.

The **variable region** (**V region**) of an immunoglobulin or T-cell receptor is formed of the amino-terminal domains of its component polypeptide chains. These are called the **variable domains** (**V domains**) and are the most variable parts of the molecule. They contain the antigen-binding sites.

Vascular addressins are molecules on endothelial cells to which leukocyte adhesion molecules bind. They have a key role in selective homing of leukocytes to particular sites in the body.

Vav: see **adaptor proteins**.

The adhesion molecule **VCAM-1** is expressed by vascular endothelium at sites of inflammation; it binds the integrin VLA-4, which allows armed effector T cells to enter sites of infection.

The enzyme that joins the gene segments of B-cell and T-cell receptor genes is called the **V(D)J recombinase**. It is made up of several enzymes, but most important are the products the recombination-activating genes *RAG-1* and *RAG-2* whose protein products RAG-1 and RAG-2 are expressed in developing lymphocytes and make up the only known lymphoid-specific components of the V(D)J recombinase.

The process of **V(D)J recombination** is found exclusively in lymphocytes in vertebrates, and allows the recombination of different gene segments into sequences encoding complete protein chains of immunoglobulins and T-cell receptors.

The **very late activation antigens** (**VLA**) are members of the β_1 family of integrins involved in cell–cell and cell–matrix interactions. Some VLAs are important in leukocyte and lymphocyte migration.

Vesicles are small membrane-bounded compartments within the cytosol.

Many viruses that are produced by mammalian cells are enclosed in a **viral envelope** of host cell membrane lipid and proteins bound to the viral core by viral envelope proteins.

Virions are complete virus particles, the form in which viruses spread from cell to cell or from one individual to another.

Viruses are pathogens composed of a nucleic acid genome enclosed in a protein coat. They can replicate only in a living cell, as they do not possess the metabolic machinery for independent life.

VpreB: see **surrogate light chain**.

Weibel–Palade bodies are granules within endothelial cells that contain P-selectin. Activation of the endothelial cell by mediators such as histamine and C5a leads to rapid translocation of P-selectin to the cell surface.

In **Western blotting**, a mixture of proteins is separated, usually by gel electrophoresis and transferred by blotting to a nitrocellulose membrane; labeled antibodies are then used as probes to detect specific proteins.

When small amounts of allergen are injected into the dermis of an allergic individual, a **wheal-and-flare reaction** is observed. This consists of a raised area of skin containing fluid and a spreading, red, itchy circular reaction.

The discrete areas of lymphoid tissue in the spleen are known as the **white pulp**.

The **Wiskott–Aldrich syndrome** (**WAS**) is characterized by defects in the cytoskeleton of cells due to a mutation in the protein **WASP**. Patients with this disease are highly susceptible to pyogenic bacteria.

Animals of different species are **xenogeneic**.

The use of **xenografts**, organs from a different species, is being explored as a solution to the severe shortage of human organs for transplantation. The main problem with xenografting is the presence of natural antibodies against xenograft antigens; attempts are being made to modify these reactions by creating transgenic animals.

Mice with mutations in the *btk* gene have a deficiency in making antibodies, especially in primary responses. These mice are called **xid**, for X-linked immunodeficiency, the mouse equivalent of X-linked agammaglobulinemia, the human form of this disease.

X-linked agammaglobulinemia (**XLA**) is a genetic disorder in which B-cell development is arrested at the pre-B-cell stage and no mature B cells or antibodies are formed. The disease is due to a defect in the gene encoding the protein tyrosine kinase Btk.

X-linked hyper IgM syndrome is a disease in which little or no IgG, IgE, or IgA antibody is produced and even IgM responses are deficient, but serum IgM levels are normal to high. It is due to a defect in the gene encoding the CD40 ligand or CD154.

X-linked lymphoproliferative syndrome is a rare immunodeficiency that results from mutations in a gene named SH2-domain containing gene 1A (*SH2D1A*). Boys with this deficiency typically develop overwhelming EBV infection during childhood, and sometimes lymphomas.

X-linked severe combined immunodeficiency (**X-linked SCID**) is a disease in which T-cell development fails at an early intrathymic stage and no production of mature T cells or T-cell dependent antibody occurs. It is due to a defect in a gene that encodes the γ_c chain that is a component of the receptors for several different cytokines.

The protein called **ZAP-70** is found in T cells and is a relative of Syk in B cells. It contains two SH2 domains that, when bound to the phosphorylated ζ chain, leads to activation of kinase activity. The main cellular substrate of ZAP-70 is a large adaptor protein called LAT.

Zymogen: see **pro-enzymes**.

INDEX

Figures in the Appendix are labeled in the form **Fig. A.1** and those in Chapters 1 to 15 are labeled in the form **Fig. 1.1, Fig. 2.1** etc.

To save space in the index the following abbreviations have been used:

APC – antigen-presenting cells
Btk – Bruton's tyrosine kinase
CDRs – complementarity determining regions
ICAM – intracellular adhesion molecule
IDDM – insulin dependent diabetes mellitus (type I)
ITAMs – immunoreceptor tyrosine-based activating motifs
ITIMs – immunoreceptor tyrosine-based inhibitory motifs
LFA – lymphocyte function-associated antigen
TCR – T cell receptor
TNF – tumor necrosis factor
vs. indicates a differential diagnosis or comparison.

No